19th Edition

HARRISON'S™ PRINCIPLES OF INTERNAL MEDICINE

EDITORS OF PREVIOUS EDITIONS

T. R. Harrison
Editor-in-Chief, Editions 1, 2, 3, 4, 5

W. R. Resnick
Editor, Editions 1, 2, 3, 4, 5

M. M. Wintrobe
Editor, Editions 1, 2, 3, 4, 5
Editor-in-Chief, Editions 6, 7

G. W. Thorn
Editor, Editions 1, 2, 3, 4, 5, 6, 7
Editor-in-Chief, Edition 8

R. D. Adams
Editor, Editions 2, 3, 4, 5, 6, 7, 8, 9, 10

P. B. Beeson
Editor, Editions 1, 2

I. L. Bennett, Jr.
Editor, Editions 3, 4, 5, 6

E. Braunwald
Editor, Editions 6, 7, 8, 9, 10, 12, 13, 14, 16, 17
Editor-in-Chief, Editions 11, 15

K. J. Isselbacher
Editor, Editions 6, 7, 8, 10, 11, 12, 14
Editor-in-Chief, Editions 9, 13

R. G. Petersdorf
Editor, Editions 6, 7, 8, 9, 11, 12
Editor-in-Chief, Edition 10

J. D. Wilson
Editor, Editions 9, 10, 11, 13, 14
Editor-in-Chief, Edition 12

J. B. Martin
Editor, Editions 10, 11, 12, 13, 14

A. S. Fauci
Editor, Editions 11, 12, 13, 15, 16, 18
Editor-in-Chief, Editions 14, 17

R. Root
Editor, Edition 12

D. L. Kasper
Editor, Editions 13, 14, 15, 17, 18
Editor-in-Chief, Editions 16, 19

S. L. Hauser
Editor, Editions 14, 15, 16, 17, 18

D. L. Longo
Editor, Editions 14, 15, 16, 17
Editor-in-Chief, Edition 18

J. L. Jameson
Editor, Editions 15, 16, 17, 18

J. Loscalzo
Editor, Editions 17, 18

ENDOCRINOLOGY AND METABOLISM

GASTROENTEROLOGY AND HEPATOLOGY

HEMATOLOGY AND ONCOLOGY

INFECTIOUS DISEASES

NEPHROLOGY

NEUROLOGY AND PSYCHIATRY

PULMONOLOGY

SYSTEMIC CONDITIONS

19th Edition

HARRISON'S™ PRINCIPLES OF INTERNAL MEDICINE

EDITORS

Dennis L. Kasper, MD
William Ellery Channing Professor of Medicine, Professor of Microbiology and Immunobiology, Department of Microbiology and Immunobiology, Harvard Medical School; Division of Infectious Diseases, Brigham and Women's Hospital
Boston, Massachusetts

Stephen L. Hauser, MD
Robert A. Fishman Distinguished Professor and Chairman, Department of Neurology, University of California, San Francisco
San Francisco, California

J. Larry Jameson, MD, PhD
Robert G. Dunlop Professor of Medicine; Dean, Perelman School of Medicine at the University of Pennsylvania; Executive Vice President, University of Pennsylvania for the Health System
Philadelphia, Pennsylvania

Anthony S. Fauci, MD
Chief, Laboratory of Immunoregulation;
Director, National Institute of Allergy and Infectious Diseases,
National Institutes of Health
Bethesda, Maryland

Dan L. Longo, MD
Professor of Medicine, Harvard Medical School; Senior Physician, Brigham and Women's Hospital; Deputy Editor, *New England Journal of Medicine,* Boston, Massachusetts

Joseph Loscalzo, MD, PhD
Hersey Professor of the Theory and Practice of Medicine, Harvard Medical School; Chairman, Department of Medicine, and Physician-in-Chief, Brigham and Women's Hospital
Boston, Massachusetts

VOLUME I

Mc Graw Hill Education

New York Chicago San Francisco Athens London Madrid Mexico City
Milan New Delhi Singapore Sydney Toronto

Note: Dr. Fauci's work as editor and author was performed outside the scope of his employment as a U.S. government employee. This work represents his personal and professional views and not necessarily those of the U.S. government.

Harrison's™
PRINCIPLES OF INTERNAL MEDICINE
Nineteenth Edition

1 2 3 4 5 6 7 8 9 10 DOW/DOW 19 18 17 16 15

Two Volume Set ISBN 978-0-07-180215-4; MHID 0-07-180215-0
Volume 1 ISBN 978-0-07-180213-0; MHID 0-07-180213-4
Volume 2 ISBN 978-0-07-180214-7; MHID 0-07-180214-2
DVD ISBN 978-0-07-184876-3; MHID 0-07-184876-2
eBook ISBN 978-0-07-1802161; MHID 0-07-180216-9

FOREIGN LANGUAGE EDITIONS

Arabic (13e): McGraw-Hill Libri Italia srl (1996)
Albanian (17e): Tabernakul Publishing, Skopje, Macedonia
Chinese Long Form (15e): McGraw-Hill International, Enterprises, Inc., Taiwan
Chinese Short Form (15e): McGraw-Hill Education (Asia), Singapore
Croatian (16e): Placebo, Split, Croatia
French (16e, 18e): Medecine-Sciences Flammarion, Paris, France
German (17e, 18e): ABW Wissenschaftsverlagsgesellschaft GmbH, Berlin, Germany
Greek (17e): Parissianos, S.A., Athens, Greece
Italian (17e, 18e): The McGraw-Hill Companies, Srl, Milan, Italy
Japanese (17e, 18e): MEDSI-Medical Sciences International Ltd, Tokyo, Japan
Korean (17e, 18e): McGraw-Hill Korea, Inc., Seoul, Korea
Macedonian (17e): Tabernakul Publishing, Skopje, Macedonia
Polish (17e): Czelej Publishing Company, Lubin, Poland
Portuguese (17e, 18e): McGraw-Hill Interamericana Editores, SA de C.V., Mexico City, Mexico
Romanian (17e): Editura All, Bucharest, Romania
Serbian (15e): Publishing House Romanov, Bosnia & Herzegovina, Republic of Serbska
Spanish (17e, 18e): McGraw-Hill Interamericana Editores, SA de C.V., Mexico City, Mexico
Turkish (17e): Nobel Tip Kitabevleri, Ltd., Istanbul, Turkey
Vietnamese (15e): McGraw-Hill Education (Asia), Singapore

This book was set in Minion Pro by Cenveo® Publisher Services. The editors were James F. Shanahan and Kim J. Davis. The production manager was Jeffrey Herzich. Project management was provided by Tania Andrabi, Cenveo Publisher Services. The index was prepared by Susan Hunter. The text designer was Alan Barnett of alan barnett design; the cover design was by Anthony Landi.

R.R. Donnelley and Sons, Inc., was printer and binder.

Library of Congress Cataloging-in-Publication Data

Harrison's principles of internal medicine. — 19th edition / editors, Dennis L. Kasper, Anthony S. Fauci, Stephen L. Hauser, Dan L. Longo, J. Larry Jameson, Joseph Loscalzo.
p. ; cm.
Principles of internal medicine
Includes index.
ISBN 978-0-07-180213-0 (hardback : alk. paper)—ISBN 0-07-180213-4 (hardback : alk. paper)
I. Kasper, Dennis L., editor. II. Title: Principles of internal medicine.
[DNLM: 1. Internal Medicine. WB 115]
RC46
616—dc23

NOTICE

COVER ILLUSTRATION

Budding HIV particle, computer artwork *(Credit: Animate4.com Ltd. / Science Source)*

CONTENTS

CONTENTS

PART 4 Regenerative Medicine

PART 5 Aging

PART 6 Nutrition and Weight Loss

PART 7 Oncology and Hematology

SECTION 1 NEOPLASTIC DISORDERS

SECTION 2 HEMATOPOIETIC DISORDERS

CONTENTS

PART 12 Critical Care Medicine

SECTION 1 RESPIRATORY CRITICAL CARE

SECTION 2 SHOCK AND CARDIAC ARREST

SECTION 3 NEUROLOGIC CRITICAL CARE

SECTION 4 ONCOLOGIC EMERGENCIES

PART 13 Disorders of the Kidney and Urinary Tract

PART 14 Disorders of the Gastrointestinal System

SECTION 1 DISORDERS OF THE ALIMENTARY TRACT

SECTION 2 LIVER AND BILIARY TRACT DISEASE

CONTENTS

CONTENTS

CONTENTS

CONTRIBUTORS

James L. Abbruzzese, MD
Chief, Division of Medical Oncology, Department of Medicine; Associate Director, Clinical Research, Duke Cancer Institute, Durham, North Carolina [120e]

Manal F. Abdelmalek, MD, MPH
Associate Professor of Medicine, Division of Gastroenterology and Hepatology, Duke University, Durham, North Carolina [364]

Jamil Aboulhosn, MD
Assistant Professor of Medicine; Director Ahmanson/UCLA Adult Congenital Heart Disease Center, David Geffen School of Medicine, University of California, Los Angeles, Los Angeles, California [282]

John C. Achermann, MD, PhD, MB
Wellcome Trust Senior Research Fellow in Clinical Science, University College London; Professor of Paediatric Endocrinology, UCL Institute of Child Health, University College London, London, United Kingdom [410]

John W. Adamson, MD
Clinical Professor, Division of Hematology/Oncology, Department of Medicine, University of California at San Diego, San Diego, California [77, 126]

Rizwan Ahmed, MD
General Surgery Resident, Department of General Surgery, Johns Hopkins Hospital, Baltimore, Maryland [353, 354]

Praveen Akuthota, MD
Assistant Professor of Medicine, Harvard Medical School; Beth Israel Deaconess Medical Center, Boston, Massachusetts [310]

Anthony A. Amato, MD
Professor of Neurology, Harvard Medical School; Vice-Chairman, Department of Neurology, Brigham and Women's Hospital, Boston, Massachusetts [459-462e]

Michael J. Aminoff, MD, DSc, FRCP
Professor of Neurology, School of Medicine, University of California, San Francisco, San Francisco, California [30, 31, 442e]

Neil M. Ampel, MD
Professor of Medicine, University of Arizona; Staff Physician, Southern Arizona Veterans Affairs Health Care System, Tucson, Arizona [237]

Kenneth C. Anderson, MD
Kraft Family Professor of Medicine, Harvard Medical School; Chief, Jerome Lipper Multiple Myeloma Center, Dana-Farber Cancer Institute, Boston, Massachusetts [136, 138e]

Rosa M. Andrade, MD
Department of Medicine, Division of Infectious Diseases, University of California, San Diego, San Diego, California [247]

Elliott M. Antman, MD
Professor of Medicine, Cardiovascular Division, Department of Medicine, Brigham and Women's Hospital; Associate Dean for Clinical/Translational Research, Harvard Medical School, Boston, Massachusetts [293, 295]

Frederick R. Appelbaum, MD
Director, Division of Clinical Research, Fred Hutchinson Cancer Research Center, Seattle, Washington [139e]

Cesar A. Arias, MD, PhD, MSc
Associate Professor of Medicine, Microbiology and Molecular Genetics; Director, Laboratory for Antimicrobial Research, University of Texas Medical School at Houston, Houston, Texas; Director, Molecular Genetics and Antimicrobial Unit; Co-Director, International Center for Microbial Genomics, Universidad, El Bosque, Bogota, Colombia [174]

Wiebke Arlt, MD, DSc, FRCP, FMedSci
Professor of Medicine, Centre for Endocrinology, Diabetes and Metabolism, School of Clinical and Experimental Medicine, University of Birmingham; Consultant Endocrinologist, University Hospital Birmingham, Birmingham, United Kingdom [406]

Katrina Armstrong, MD, MS
Jackson Professor of Clinical Medicine, Physician in Chief, Massachusetts General Hospital, Boston Massachusetts [4]

Valder R. Arruda, MD, PhD
Associate Professor, Division of Hematology, Department of Pediatrics, Perelman School of Medicine, University of Pennsylvania, Philadelphia, Pennsylvania [141]

Andrew W. Artenstein, MD
Professor of Medicine, Tufts University School of Medicine, Boston, Massachusetts; Adjunct Professor of Medicine and Health Services, Policy and Practice, Alpert Medical School, Brown University, Providence, Rhode Island; Chair, Department of Medicine, Baystate Health, Springfield, Massachusetts [152e]

Anthony Atala, MD
Professor and Director, Wake Forest Institute for Regenerative Medicine, Wake Forest School of Medicine, Winston-Salem, North Carolina [92e]

John C. Atherton, MD, FRCP
Professor of Gastroenterology and Dean of the School of Medicine, University of Nottingham, Nottingham, United Kingdom [188]

Paul S. Auerbach, MD, MS, FACEP, FAWM
Redich Family Professor of Surgery, Division of Emergency Medicine, Stanford University School of Medicine, Stanford, California [474]

K. Frank Austen, MD
AstraZeneca Professor of Respiratory and Inflammatory Diseases, Director, Inflammation and Allergic Diseases Research Section, Harvard Medical School; Brigham and Women's Hospital, Boston, Massachusetts [376]

Eric H. Awtry, MD
Cardiology Division, Boston Medical Center, Boston, Massachusetts [289e, 290e]

Jamil Azzi, MD
Instructor in Medicine, Harvard Medical School; Associate Physician, Brigham and Women's Hospital, Boston, Massachusetts [337]

Bruce R. Bacon, MD
James F. King, MD Endowed Chair in Gastroenterology; Professor of Internal Medicine, Saint Louis University Liver Center, Saint Louis University School of Medicine, St. Louis, Missouri [365, 367e]

Lindsey R. Baden, MD
Associate Professor of Medicine, Harvard Medical School; Dana-Farber Cancer Institute, Brigham and Women's Hospital, Boston, Massachusetts [215e]

Natalie J. Badowski, MD
Division of Emergency Medicine, Stanford University School of Medicine, Stanford, California [474]

John R. Balmes, MD
Professor of Medicine, University of California, San Francisco; Professor, School of Public Health, University of California, Berkeley; Chief, Division of Occupational and Environmental Medicine, San Francisco General Hospital, San Francisco, California [311]

Manisha Balwani, MD, MS
Assistant Professor, Department of Genetics and Genomic Sciences, Mount Sinai School of Medicine of New York University, New York, New York [430]

Peter A. Banks, MD
Professor of Medicine, Harvard Medical School; Senior Physician, Division of Gastroenterology, Brigham and Women's Hospital, Boston, Massachusetts [370, 371]

Robert L. Barbieri, MD
Kate Macy Ladd Professor of Obstetrics, Gynecology and Reproductive Biology, Harvard Medical School; Chair, Department of Obstetrics and Gynecology, Brigham and Women's Hospital, Boston, Massachusetts [8]

Alan G. Barbour, MD
Professor of Medicine and Microbiology and Molecular Genetics, University of California Irvine, Irvine, California [209]

Joanne M. Bargman, MD, FRCPC
Professor of Medicine, University of Toronto; Staff Nephrologist, University Health Network, Toronto, Canada [335]

Tamar F. Barlam, MD, MSc
Associate Professor of Medicine, Infectious Disease Section, Boston University School of Medicine, Boston, Massachusetts [147, 183e]

Peter J. Barnes, DM, DSc, FMedSci, FRS
Head of Respiratory Medicine, Imperial College, London, United Kingdom [309]

Richard J. Barohn, MD
Chairman, Department of Neurology; Gertrude and Dewey Ziegler Professor of Neurology, University of Kansas Medical Center, Kansas City, Kansas [459]

Rebecca M. Baron, MD
Assistant Professor of Medicine, Harvard Medical School; Associate Physician, Brigham and Women's Hospital, Division of Pulmonary and Critical Care Medicine, Department of Medicine, Boston, Massachusetts [154, 312]

Miriam Baron Barshak, MD
Assistant Professor, Harvard Medical School; Associate Physician, Massachusetts General Hospital, Boston, Massachusetts [154, 159, 312]

Shehzad Basaria, MD
Men's Health: Aging and Metabolism, Brigham and Women's Hospital, Boston, Massachusetts [7e]

Robert C. Basner, MD
Professor of Clinical Medicine, Division of Pulmonary, Allergy, and Critical Care Medicine, Columbia University College of Physicians and Surgeons, New York, New York [Appendix]

Buddha Basnyat, MD, MSc, FACP, FRCP (Edinburgh)
Director, Oxford University Clinical Research Unit, Patan Academy of Health Sciences; Medical Director, Nepal International Clinic, Kathmandu, Nepal [476e]

Shari S. Bassuk, ScD
Epidemiologist, Division of Preventive Medicine, Brigham and Women's Hospital, Boston, Massachusetts [413]

John F. Bateman, PhD
Director, Cell Biology, Murdoch Children's Research Institute, Melbourne, Victoria, Australia; Murdoch Children's Research Institute, Parkville, Victoria, Australia [427]

David W. Bates, MD, MSc
Professor of Medicine, Harvard Medical School; Chief, General Internal Medicine and Primary Care Division, Brigham and Women's Hospital; Medical Director, Clinical and Quality Analysis, Partners HealthCare System, Inc., Boston, Massachusetts [12e]

Robert P. Baughman, MD
Department of Internal Medicine, University of Cincinnati Medical Center, Cincinnati, Ohio [390]

M. Flint Beal, MD
University Professor of Neurology and Neuroscience; Neurologist, New York Presbyterian Hospital; Weill Cornell Medical College, New York, New York [444e, 455]

Laurence H. Beck, MD, PhD
Assistant Professor of Medicine, Boston University School of Medicine, Boston, Massachusetts [340]

Christian D. Becker, MD, PhD, FCCP
Assistant Professor, Department of Internal Medicine, Division of Pulmonary, Critical Care and Sleep Medicine, Icahn School of Medicine at Mount Sinai New York, New York [485e]

Nicholas J. Beeching, MA, BM BCh, FRCP, FRACP, FFTM RCPS(Glasg), DCH, DTM&H
Senior Lecturer (Clinical) in Infectious Diseases, Liverpool School of Tropical Medicine; Clinical Director, Tropical and Infectious Disease Unit, Royal Liverpool University Hospital; NIHR Health Protection Research Unit in Emerging and Zoonotic Infections, Liverpool; Honorary Consultant, Public Health England and Honorary Civilian Consultant in Infectious Diseases, Army Medical Directorate, United Kingdom [194e]

Doron Behar, MD, PhD
Institute of Genetics, Rambam Health Care Campus, Haifa, Israel [85e]

Robert S. Benjamin, MD
P. H. and Faye E. Robinson Distinguished Professor of Medicine, Department of Sarcoma Medical Oncology, The University of Texas M.D. Anderson Cancer Center, Houston, Texas [119e]

Michael H. Bennett, MD, MBBS, MM (Clin Epi)
Conjoint Associate Professor in Anesthesia and Hyperbaric Medicine; Faculty of Medicine, University of New South Wales; Academic Head of Department, Wales Anaesthesia, Prince of Wales Hospital, Sydney, Australia [477e]

Edward J. Benz, Jr., MD
Richard and Susan Smith Professor of Medicine; Professor of Genetics, Harvard Medical School; President and CEO, Dana-Farber Cancer Institute; Director and Principal Investigator, Dana-Farber/Harvard Cancer Center; Boston, Massachusetts [127]

Jean Bergounioux, MD, PhD, PhC
Pediatric Intensive Care Unit, Hôpital Raymond-Poincaré, Université de Versailles-Saint Quentin, Garches, France [191]

John L. Berk, MD
Associate Professor of Medicine, Boston University School of Medicine; Clinical Director, Amyloidosis Center, Boston Medical Center, Boston, Massachusetts [137]

Aaron S. Bernstein, MD, MPH
Instructor, Harvard Medical School; Associate Director, Center for Health and the Global Environment, Harvard School of Public Health; Pediatric Hospitalist, Boston Children's Hospital, Boston, Massachusetts [151e]

Joseph R. Betancourt, MD, MPH
Associate Professor of Medicine, Harvard Medical School; Director, The Disparities Solutions Center, Massachusetts General Hospital, Boston, Massachusetts [16e]

Atul K. Bhan, MD, MBBS
Professor of Pathology, Harvard Medical School, Department of Pathology, Massachusetts General Hospital, Boston, Massachusetts [366e]

Shalender Bhasin, MBBS
Professor of Medicine, Harvard Medical School; Director, Research Program in Men's Health: Aging and Metabolism; Director, Boston Claude D. Pepper Older Americans Independence Center; Site Director, Harvard Catalyst Clinical Research Center at BWH, Brigham and Women's Hospital, Boston, Massachusetts [7e, 411]

Deepak L. Bhatt, MD, MPH
Professor of Medicine, Harvard Medical School; Chief of Cardiology, VA Boston Healthcare System; Senior Physician, Brigham and Women's Hospital; Senior Investigator, TIMI Study Group, Boston, Massachusetts [296e, 297e]

Roby P. Bhattacharyya, MD, PhD
Instructor in Medicine, Harvard Medical School; Assistant in Medicine, Division of Infectious Disease, Massachusetts General Hospital, Boston, Massachusetts [146]

David R. Bickers, MD
Carl Truman Nelson Professor and Chair, Department of Dermatology, Columbia University Medical Center, New York, New York [75]

Henry J. Binder, MD
Professor Emeritus of Medicine, Senior Research Scientist, Yale University, New Haven, Connecticut [349, 350e]

William R. Bishai, MD, PhD
Professor and Co-Director, Center for Tuberculosis Research, Department of Medicine, Division of Infectious Diseases, Johns Hopkins University School of Medicine, Baltimore, Maryland [175]

Bruce R. Bistrian, MD, PhD, MPH
Professor of Medicine, Harvard Medical School; Chief, Clinical Nutrition, Beth Israel Deaconess Medical Center, Boston, Massachusetts [98e]

Martin J. Blaser, MD
Muriel and George Singer Professor of Medicine; Professor of Microbiology; Director, Human Microbiome Program, New York University Langone Medical Center, New York, New York [188, 192]

Chantal P. Bleeker-Rovers, MD, PhD
Department of Internal Medicine, Radboud University Nijmegen Medical Center, Nijmegen, The Netherlands [26]

Gijs Bleijenberg, PhD
Professor Emeritus, Expert Centre for Chronic Fatigue, Radboud University Medical Centre, Nijmegen, The Netherlands [464e]

Clara D. Bloomfield, MD
Distinguished University Professor; William G. Pace, III Professor of Cancer Research; Cancer Scholar and Senior Advisor, The Ohio State University Comprehensive Cancer Center; Arthur G. James Cancer Hospital and Richard J. Solove Research Institute, Columbus, Ohio [132]

Richard S. Blumberg, MD
Chief, Division of Gastroenterology, Hepatology and Endoscopy, Brigham and Women's Hospital, Harvard Medical School, Boston, Massachusetts [351]

Jean L. Bolognia, MD
Professor, Department of Dermatology, Yale University School of Medicine, New Haven, Connecticut [72]

Joseph V. Bonventre, MD, PhD
Samuel A. Levine Professor of Medicine, Harvard Medical School; Chief, Renal Division; Chief, Division of Biomedical Engineering, Brigham and Women's Hospital, Boston, Massachusetts [333e, 334]

George J. Bosl, MD
Professor of Medicine, Weill Cornell Medical College; Chair, Department of Medicine; Patrick M. Byrne Chair in Clinical Oncology, Memorial Sloan-Kettering Cancer Center, New York, New York [116]

Joshua A. Boyce, MD
Professor of Medicine and Pediatrics; Albert L. Sheffer Professor of Medicine, Harvard Medical School; Director, Inflammation and Allergic Disease Research Section, Brigham and Women's Hospital, Boston, Massachusetts [376]

Eugene Braunwald, MD, MA (Hon), ScD (Hon), FRCP
Distinguished Hersey Professor of Medicine, Harvard Medical School; Founding Chairman, TIMI Study Group, Brigham and Women's Hospital, Boston, Massachusetts [50, 288, 294]

Irwin M. Braverman, MD
Professor Emeritus; Senior Research Scientist, Department of Dermatology, Yale University School of Medicine, New Haven, Connecticut [72]

Otis W. Brawley, MD, FACP
Professor of Hematology, Medical Oncology, Medicine and Epidemiology, Emory University; Chief Medical and Scientific Officer, American Cancer Society, Atlanta, Georgia [100]

Joel G. Breman, MD, DTPH
Senior Scientific Advisor, Fogarty International Center, National Institutes of Health, Bethesda, Maryland [248, 250e]

George J. Brewer, MD
Morton S. and Henrietta K. Sellner Emeritus, Professor of Human Genetics, Emeritus Professor of Internal Medicine, University of Michigan Medical School; Senior Vice President for Research and Development, Adeona Pharmaceuticals, Inc., Ann Arbor, Michigan [429]

Josephine P. Briggs, MD
Director, National Center for Complementary and Alternative Medicine (NCCAM) at the National Institutes of Health (NIH), Bethesda, Maryland [14e]

F. Richard Bringhurst, MD
Associate Professor of Medicine, Harvard Medical School; Physician, Massachusetts General Hospital, Boston, Massachusetts [423]

Steven M. Bromley, MD
Director, Outpatient Services, Virtua Neuroscience, Voorhees, New Jersey; Director, Bromley Neurology, PC, Audubon, New Jersey [42]

Darron R. Brown, MD
Professor of Medicine, Microbiology and Immunology, Division of Infectious Diseases, Simon Cancer Center, Indiana University School of Medicine, Indianapolis, Indiana [222]

Kevin E. Brown, MD, MRCp, FRCPath
Virus Reference Department, Public Health England, London, United Kingdom [221]

Robert H. Brown, Jr., MD, PhD
Chairman, Department of Neurology, University of Massachusetts Medical School, Worchester, Massachusetts [452, 462e]

Amy E. Bryant, PhD
Affiliate Assistant Professor, University of Washington School of Medicine, Seattle, Washington; Research Scientist, Veterans Affairs Medical Center, Boise, Idaho [179]

Christopher M. Burns, MD
Associate Professor, Department of Medicine, Section of Rheumatology, Geisel School of Medicine at Dartmouth, Dartmouth Hitchcock Medical Center, Lebanon, New Hampshire [431e]

David M. Burns, MD
Professor Emeritus, Department of Family and Preventive Medicine, University of California, San Diego School of Medicine, San Diego, California [470]

Stephen B. Calderwood, MD
Morton N. Swartz, MD Academy Professor of Medicine (Microbiology and Immunobiology), Harvard Medical School; Chief, Division of Infectious Diseases, Massachusetts General Hospital, Boston, Massachusetts [160]

Michael Camilleri, MD
Atherton and Winifred W. Bean Professor; Professor of Medicine, Pharmacology, and Physiology, Mayo Clinic College of Medicine, Rochester, Minnesota [55]

Christopher P. Cannon, MD
Professor of Medicine, Harvard Medical School; Senior Physician, Cardiovascular Division, Brigham and Women's Hospital, Boston, Massachusetts [294]

Jonathan R. Carapetis, MBBS, PhD, FRACP, FAFPHM
Director, Telethon Kids Institute, The University of Western Australia, Crawley, Western Australia [381]

Kathryn M. Carbone, MD
Deputy Scientific Director, Division of Intramural Research, National Institute of Dental and Craniofacial Research, Bethesda, Maryland [231e]

Brian I. Carr, MD, PhD, FRCP
IRCCS de Bellis National Center for GI Diseases, Castellana Grotte, BA, Italy [111]

John D. Carter, MD
Professor of Medicine, Division of Rheumatology; Director, University of South Florida Morsani College of Medicine, Tampa, Florida [384]

Arturo Casadevall, MD, PhD
Chair, Department of Microbiology and Immunology, Albert Einstein College of Medicine, Bronx, New York [239]

Agustin Castellanos, MD, FACC, FAHA
Professor of Medicine; Director, Clinical Electrophysiology, University of Miami Miller School of Medicine, Cardiovascular Division, Miami, Florida [327]

Bartolome R. Celli, MD
Professor of Medicine, Harvard Medical School; Staff Physician, Division of Pulmonary and Critical Care Medicine, Brigham and Women's Hospital, Boston, Massachusetts [323]

Murali Chakinala, MD
Associate Professor of Medicine, Division of Pulmonary and Critical Care Medicine, Washington University School of Medicine, St. Louis, Missouri [279]

Anil Chandraker, MBChB, FRCP
Associate Professor of Medicine, Harvard Medical School; Medical Director of Kidney and Pancreas Transplantation; Interim Director, Schuster Family Transplantation Research Center, Brigham and Women's Hospital, Boston, Massachusetts [337]

Lan X. Chen, MD, PhD
Penn Presbyterian Medical Center, Philadelphia, Pennsylvania [395]

Yuan-Tsong Chen, MD, PhD
Duke University Medical Center, Division of Medical Genetics, Department of Pediatrics, Durham, North Carolina [433e]

Glenn M. Chertow, MD, MPH
Norman S. Coplon/Satellite Healthcare Professor of Medicine; Chief, Division of Nephrology, Stanford University School of Medicine, Palo Alto, California [336]

John S. Child, MD, FACC, FAHA, FASE
Streisand Professor of Medicine and Cardiology; Director, Ahmanson-UCLA Adult Congenital Heart Disease Center; Director, UCLA Adult Noninvasive Cardiodiagnostics Laboratory Ronald Reagan-UCLA Medical Center, Geffen School of Medicine, University of California, Los Angeles (UCLA), Los Angeles, California [282]

Augustine M. K. Choi, MD
Chairman, Department of Medicine, Weill Cornell Medical College, Physician-in-Chief, New York-Presbyterian Hospital-Weill Cornell Medical Center, New York, New York [305, 307, 322]

Raymond T. Chung, MD
Associate Professor of Medicine, Harvard Medical School; Director of Hepatology and Liver Center; Vice Chief, Gastroenterology, Massachusetts General Hospital, Boston, Massachusetts [368]

Jeffrey W. Clark, MD
Associate Professor of Medicine, Harvard Medical School; Medical Director, Clinical Trials Core, Dana-Farber Harvard Cancer Center; Massachusetts General Hospital, Boston, Massachusetts [102e]

Jeffrey I. Cohen, MD
Chief, Laboratory of Clinical Infectious Diseases, National Institute of Allergy and Infectious Diseases, National Institutes of Health, Bethesda, Maryland [218, 228]

Yehuda Z. Cohen, MD
Clinical Fellow, Department of Medicine, Division of Infectious Diseases and Center for Virology and Vaccine Research, Beth Israel Deaconess Medical Center; Harvard Medical School, Boston, Massachusetts [224]

Ronit Cohen-Poradosu, MD
Senior Physician, Infectious Diseases Unit, Tel Aviv Sourasky Medical Center, Tel Aviv, Israel [201]

Francis S. Collins, MD, PhD
Director, National Institutes of Health, Bethesda, Maryland [101e]

Wilson S. Colucci, MD, FAHA, FACC
Thomas J. Ryan Professor of Medicine, Boston University School of Medicine; Chief of Cardiovascular Medicine, Boston Medical Center, Boston, Massachusetts [289e, 290e]

Laura K. Conlin, PhD
Scientific Director, CytoGenomics Lab, The Children's Hospital of Philadelphia, Assistant Professor of Pathology and Laboratory Medicine, University of Pennsylvania, Philadelphia, Pennsylvania [83e]

Darwin L. Conwell, MD, MS
Professor of Medicine, The Ohio State University College of Medicine; Director, Division of Gastroenterology, Hepatology and Nutrition; The Ohio State University Wexner Medical Center, Columbus, Ohio [370, 371]

Michael J. Corbel, PhD, DSc, FRCPath
Retired (previously Head, Division of Bacteriology, National Institute for Biological Standards and Control, Hertfordshire, United Kingdom) [194e]

William E. Corcoran, V, MD
Staff Anesthesiologist, Allcare Clinical Associates; Medical Director of Analgesia and Sedation, Mission Health; Patient Safety Officer, Mission Health, Asheville, North Carolina [481e]

Kathleen E. Corey, MD, MPH
Clinical and Research Fellow, Harvard Medical School; Fellow, Gastrointestinal Unit, Massachusetts General Hospital, Boston, Massachusetts [59]

Lawrence Corey, MD
Professor, Medicine and Laboratory Medicine, University of Washington; President Emeritus, Fred Hutchinson Cancer Research Center; Member, Vaccine and Infectious Disease Division; Principal Investigator, HIV Vaccine Trials Network, Fred Hutchinson Cancer Research Center, Seattle, Washington [216]

Jorge Cortes, MD
D. B. Lane Cancer Research Distinguished Professor for Leukemia Research; Deputy Chairman; Section Chief of AML and CML, The University of Texas M.D. Anderson Cancer Center, Houston, Texas [133]

Felicia Cosman, MD
Professor of Medicine, Columbia University College of Physicians and Surgeons, New York, New York [425]

Mark A. Creager, MD
Professor of Medicine, Harvard Medical School; Simon C. Fireman Scholar in Cardiovascular Medicine; Director, Vascular Center, Brigham and Women's Hospital, Boston, Massachusetts [301-303]

Leslie J. Crofford, MD
Professor, Division of Rheumatology and Immunology, Vanderbilt University, Nashville, Tennessee; Chief, Division of Rheumatology, University of Kentucky, Lexington, Kentucky [396]

Jennifer M. Croswell, MD, MPH
Medical Officer, Center for Oncology Prevention Trials Research Group, Division of Cancer Prevention, National Cancer Institute, Bethesda, Maryland [100]

Philip E. Cryer, MD
Professor of Medicine Emeritus, Washington University in St. Louis; Physician, Barnes-Jewish Hospital, St. Louis, Missouri [420]

David Cunningham, MD, MB, ChB, FRCP
Professor, Head of Gastrointestinal/Lymphoma Unit; Director of Clinical Research, Royal Marsden NHS Trust, London, United Kingdom [112]

Gary C. Curhan, MD
Professor of Medicine, Harvard Medical School, Professor of Epidemiology, Harvard School of Public Health, Channing Division of Network Medicine/ Renal Division, Brigham and Women's Hospital, Boston, Massachusetts [342]

Brendan D. Curti, MD
Director, Biotherapy Program, Robert W. Franz Cancer Research Center, Providence Portland Medical Center, Portland, Oregon [105]

John J. Cush, MD
Professor of Medicine and Rheumatology, Baylor University Medical Center; Director of Clinical Rheumatology, Baylor Research Institute, Dallas, Texas [393]

Charles A. Czeisler, MD, PhD
Frank Baldino, Jr., PhD Professor of Sleep Medicine, Professor of Medicine and Director, Division of Sleep Medicine, Harvard Medical School; Chief, Division of Sleep and Circadian Disorders, Departments of Medicine and Neurology, Brigham and Women's Hospital, Boston, Massachusetts [38]

Marinos C. Dalakas, MD
Professor of Neurology, University of Athens Medical School, Athens, Greece; Thomas Jefferson University, Philadelphia, Pennsylvania [388]

Josep Dalmau, MD, PhD
ICREA Professor, Institut d'Investigació Biomèdica August Pi i Sunyer, University of Barcelona, Barcelona, Spain; Adjunct Professor, University of Pennsylvania, Philadelphia, Pennsylvania [122]

Daniel F. Danzl, MD
University of Louisville, Department of Emergency Medicine, Louisville, Kentucky [478e, 479e]

Robert B. Daroff, MD
Professor and Chair Emeritus, Department of Neurology, Case Western Reserve University School of Medicine; University Hospitals–Case Medical Center, Cleveland, Ohio [28]

Charles E. Davis, MD
Professor of Pathology and Medicine, Emeritus, University of California, San Diego School of Medicine; Director Emeritus, Microbiology, University of California, San Diego Medical Center, San Diego, California [245e]

Stephen N. Davis, MBBS, FRCP
Theodore E. Woodward Professor and Chairman of the Department of Medicine, University of Maryland School of Medicine; Physician-in-Chief, University of Maryland Medical Center, Baltimore, Maryland [420]

Rafael de Cabo, PhD
Senior Investigator, Experimental Gerontology Section, TGB, National Institute on Aging, National Institutes of Health, Baltimore, Maryland [94e]

Lisa M. DeAngelis, MD
Professor of Neurology, Weill Cornell Medical College; Chair, Department of Neurology, Memorial Sloan Kettering Cancer Center, New York, New York [118]

John Del Valle, MD
Professor and Senior Associate Chair of Medicine, Department of Internal Medicine, University of Michigan School of Medicine, Ann Arbor, Michigan [348]

Marie B. Demay, MD
Professor of Medicine, Harvard Medical School; Physician, Massachusetts General Hospital, Boston, Massachusetts [423]

Bradley M. Denker, MD
Associate Professor of Medicine, Harvard Medical School; Renal Division, Beth Israel Deaconess Medical Center; Chief of Nephrology and Associate Chief of Medical Specialties, Harvard Vanguard Medical Associates, Boston, Massachusetts [61]

David W. Denning, MBBS, FRCP, FRCPath, FMedSci
Professor of Medicine and Medical Mycology; Director, National Aspergillosis Centre, The University of Manchester and Wythenshawe Hospital, Manchester, United Kingdom [241]

Robert J. Desnick, MD, PhD
Dean for Genetics and Genomics, Professor and Chairman Emeritus, Department of Human Genetics and Genomic Sciences, Icahn School of Medicine at Mount Sinai, New York, New York [430]

Richard A. Deyo, MD, MPH
Kaiser Permanente Professor of Evidence-Based Family Medicine, Department of Family Medicine, Department of Medicine, Department of Public Health and Preventive Medicine, Oregon Institute of Occupational Health Sciences; Oregon Health and Science University; Clinical Investigator, Kaiser Permanente Center for Health Research, Portland, Oregon [22]

Betty Diamond, MD
The Feinstein Institute for Medical Research, North Shore LIJ Health System; Center for Autoimmunity and Musculoskeletal Diseases, Manhasset, New York [377e]

Marcelo F. Di Carli, MD
Professor, Department of Radiology, Harvard Medical School; Chief, Division of Nuclear Medicine and Molecular Imaging; Executive Director, Noninvasive Cardiovascular Imaging Program, Brigham and Women's Hospital, Boston, Massachusetts [270e, 271e]

Anna Mae Diehl, MD
Florence McAlister Professor of Medicine; Chief, Division of Gastroenterology, Duke University, Durham, North Carolina [364]

Jules L. Dienstag, MD
Carl W. Walter Professor of Medicine and Dean for Medical Education, Harvard Medical School; Physician, Gastrointestinal Unit, Department of Medicine, Massachusetts General Hospital, Boston, Massachusetts [360-362, 366e, 368]

William P. Dillon, MD
Professor and Executive Vice-Chair; Chief, Section of Neuroradiology, Department of Radiology and Biomedical Imaging, University of California, San Francisco, San Francisco, California [440e, 441e]

Charles A. Dinarello, MD
Professor of Medicine and Immunology, University of Colorado Denver, Aurora, Colorado; Professor of Experimental Medicine, Radboud University Medical Center, Nijmegen, The Netherlands [23]

Raphael Dolin, MD
Maxwell Finland Professor of Medicine (Microbiology and Molecular Genetics), Harvard Medical School; Beth Israel Deaconess Medical Center; Brigham and Women's Hospital, Boston, Massachusetts [215e, 223, 224]

Susan M. Domchek, MD
Basser Professor of Oncology, Abramson Cancer Center, University of Pennsylvania, Philadelphia, Pennsylvania [84]

Richard L. Doty, PhD, MA
Director, Smell and Taste Center; Professor, Department of Otorhinolaryngology: Head and Neck Surgery, Perelman School of Medicine, University of Pennsylvania, Philadelphia, Pennsylvania [42]

Vanja C. Douglas, MD
Assistant Professor of Clinical Neurology and Sara and Evan Williams Foundation Endowed Neurohospitalist Chair, University of California, San Francisco, San Francisco, California [29]

Daniel B. Drachman, MD
Professor of Neurology and Neuroscience, W. W. Smith Charitable Trust Professor of Neuroimmunology, Department of Neurology, Johns Hopkins School of Medicine, Baltimore, Maryland [461]

David F. Driscoll, PhD
Associate Professor of Medicine, University of Massachusetts Medical School, Worchester, Massachusetts [98e]

Thomas D. DuBose, Jr., MD, MACP
Emeritus Professor of Internal Medicine and Nephrology, Wake Forest University School of Medicine, Winston-Salem, North Carolina [64e, 66]

J. Stephen Dumler, MD
Professor, Division of Medical Microbiology, Department of Pathology, Johns Hopkins University School of Medicine, Baltimore, Maryland [211]

Andrea Dunaif, MD
Charles F. Kettering Professor of Endocrinology and Metabolism and Vice-Chair for Research, Department of Medicine, Feinberg School of Medicine, Northwestern University, Chicago, Illinois [6e]

Samuel C. Durso, MD, MBA
Mason F. Lord Professor of Medicine; Director, Division of Geriatric Medicine and Gerontology, Johns Hopkins University School of Medicine, Baltimore, Maryland [45, 46e]

Janice P. Dutcher, MD
Associate Director, Cancer Research Foundation of New York, Chappaqua, New York; Former Professor, New York Medical College, Valhalla, New York [331]

Johanna Dwyer, DSc, RD
Jean Mayer USDA Human Nutrition Research Center on Aging; Professor, Tufts Medical Center and Director, Frances Stern Nutrition Center, Tufts Medical Center, Boston, Massachusetts [95e]

Jeffrey S. Dzieczkowski, MD
Physician, St. Alphonsus Regional Medical Center; Medical Director, Coagulation Clinic, Saint Alphonsus Medical Group, International Medicine and Travel Medicine, Boise, Idaho [138e]

Kim A. Eagle, MD
Albion Walter Hewlett Professor of Internal Medicine; Chief of Clinical Cardiology; Director, Frankel Cardiovascular Center, University of Michigan Health System, Ann Arbor, Michigan [9]

James A. Eastham, MD
Chief, Urology Service, Florence and Theodore Baumritter/Enid Ancell Chair of Urologic Oncology, Department of Surgery, Sidney Kimmel Center for Prostate and Urologic Cancers, Memorial Sloan Kettering Cancer Center, New York, New York [115]

Robert H. Eckel, MD
Professor of Medicine, Division of Endocrinology, Metabolism and Diabetes, Division of Cardiology; Professor of Physiology and Biophysics, Charles A. Boettcher, II Chair in Atherosclerosis, University of Colorado School of Medicine, Anschutz Medical Campus, Director Lipid Clinic, University of Colorado Hospital, Aurora, Colorado [422]

John E. Edwards, Jr., MD
Professor of Medicine, David Geffen School of Medicine, University of California, Los Angeles (UCLA), Los Angeles, California; Chief, Division of Infectious Diseases, Harbor/UCLA Medical Center, Torrance, California [235, 240]

David A. Ehrmann, MD
Professor, Department of Medicine, Section of Endocrinology, Diabetes, and Metabolism, The University of Chicago Pritzker School of Medicine, Chicago, Illinois [68]

Andrew J. Einstein, MD, PhD
Victoria and Esther Aboodi Assistant Professor of Medicine; Director, Cardiac CT Research; Co-Director, Cardiac CT and MRI, Department of Medicine, Cardiology Division, Department of Radiology, Columbia University College of Physicians and Surgeons, New York-Presbyterian Hospital, New York, New York [Appendix]

Ezekiel J. Emanuel, MD, PhD
Chair, Department of Medical Ethics and Health Policy, Levy University Professor, Perelman School of Medicine and Wharton School, University of Pennsylvania, Philadelphia, Pennsylvania [10]

John W. Engstrom, MD
Betty Anker Fife Distinguished Professor and Vice-Chairman; Neurology Residency Program Director, University of California, San Francisco, San Francisco, California [22, 454]

Moshe Ephros, MD
Clinical Associate Professor, Faculty of Medicine, Technion-Israel Institute of Technology; Pediatric Infectious Disease Unit, Carmel Medical Center; Haifa, Israel [197]

Jonathan A. Epstein, MD
William Wikoff Smith Professor; Chair, Department of Cell and Developmental Biology; Scientific Director, Penn Cardiovascular Institute, Perelman School of Medicine, University of Pennsylvania, Philadelphia, Pennsylvania [265e]

Aaron C. Ermel, MD
Assistant Research Professor; Assistant Professor of Clinical Medicine, Department of Internal Medicine, Division of Infectious Disease, Indiana University School of Medicine, Indianapolis, Indiana [222]

Tim Evans, MD, PhD
Senior Director, Health, Nutrition and Population, The World Bank Group, Washington, DC [13e]

Christopher H. Fanta, MD
Professor of Medicine, Harvard Medical School; Pulmonary and Critical Care Division, Brigham and Women's Hospital; Director, Partners Asthma Center, Boston, Massachusetts [48]

Paul Farmer, MD, PhD
Kolokotrones University Professor, Harvard University; Chair, Department of Global Health and Social Medicine, Harvard Medical School; Chief, Division of Global Health Equity, Brigham and Women's Hospital; Co-Founder, Partners In Health, Boston, Massachusetts [2]

Anthony S. Fauci, MD
Chief, Laboratory of Immunoregulation; Director, National Institute of Allergy and Infectious Diseases, National Institutes of Health, Bethesda, Maryland [1, 225e, 226, 261e, 372e, 385, 386e]

Murray J. Favus, MD
Professor of Medicine, Department of Medicine, Section of Endocrinology, Diabetes and Metabolism, Director Bone Program, University of Chicago Pritzker School of Medicine, Chicago, Illinois [426e]

David P. Faxon, MD
Vice Chair of Medicine for Strategic Planning, Department of Medicine, Brigham and Women's Hospital; Senior Lecturer, Harvard Medical School, Boston, Massachusetts [272, 296e, 297]

Darren R. Feldman, MD
Associate Professor in Medicine, Weill Cornell Medical Center; Assistant Attending, Genitourinary Oncology Service, Memorial Sloan-Kettering Cancer Center, New York, New York [116]

David T. Felson, MD, MPH
Professor of Medicine and Epidemiology; Chair, Clinical Epidemiology Unit, Boston University School of Medicine, Boston, Massachusetts [394]

Luigi Ferrucci, MD, PhD
Scientific Director, National Institute of Aging, National Institutes of Health, Baltimore, Maryland [11]

Howard L. Fields, MD, PhD
Professor, Department of Neurology, University of California, San Francisco, San Francisco, California [18]

Gregory A. Filice, MD
Professor of Medicine, Medical School, and Adjunct Professor of Epidemiology and Community Health, School of Public Health, University of Minnesota; Chief, Infectious Disease Section, Veterans Affairs Healthcare System, Minneapolis, Minnesota [199]

Robert W. Finberg, MD
Chair, Department of Medicine, University of Massachusetts Medical School, Worcester, Massachusetts [104, 169]

Joyce Fingeroth, MD
Professor of Medicine and MAPS, Division of Infectious Disease, University of Massachusetts Medical School, Worcester, Massachusetts [169]

Kurt Fink, MD
Palo Alto Medical Foundation, Palo Alto, California [481e]

Alain Fischer, MD, PhD
Director of INSERM U768; Director of Imagine Institute; Professor of Immunology and Pediatric Hematology; Université Paris Descartes, Paris, France [374, 375e]

Jeffrey S. Flier, MD
Caroline Shields Walker Professor of Medicine and Dean, Harvard Medical School, Boston, Massachusetts [415e]

Agnes B. Fogo, MD
John L. Shapiro Professor of Pathology; Professor of Medicine and Pediatrics, Vanderbilt University Medical Center, Nashville, Tennessee [62e]

Larry C. Ford, MD
Clinical Infectious Diseases, Intermountain Healthcare, Provo, Utah [44]

Jane E. Freedman, MD
Professor of Medicine, University of Massachusetts Medical School, Worcester, Massachusetts [142]

Roy Freeman, MD
Professor of Neurology, Harvard Medical School; Director, Center for Autonomic and Peripheral Nerve Disorders, Beth Israel Deaconess Medical Center, Boston, Massachusetts [27]

Gyorgy Frendl, MD, PhD, FCCM
Assistant Professor; Director of Surgical Critical Care Research Center, Department of Anesthesiology, Perioperative Critical Care and Pain Medicine, Harvard Medical School; Brigham and Women's Hospital, Boston, Massachusetts [481e]

Carl E. Freter, MD, PhD, FACP
Professor of Medicine; Director, Division of Hematology and Oncology; Associate Director, Cancer Center, Saint Louis University, St. Louis, Missouri [125]

Lawrence S. Friedman, MD
Professor of Medicine, Harvard Medical School; Professor of Medicine, Tufts University School of Medicine; Assistant Chief of Medicine, Massachusetts General Hospital, Boston, Massachusetts; Anton R. Fried, MD Chair, Department of Medicine, Newton-Wellesley Hospital, Newton, Massachusetts [59]

Sonia Friedman, MD
Associate Professor of Medicine, Harvard Medical School; Associate Physician, Brigham and Women's Hospital, Boston, Massachusetts [351]

Anne L. Fuhlbrigge, MD, MS
Assistant Professor of Medicine, Harvard Medical School, Pulmonary and Critical Care Division; Brigham and Women's Hospital, Boston, Massachusetts [307]

Andre D. Furtado, MD
Assistant Professor, Department of Radiology, School of Medicine, University of Pittsburgh, Pittsburgh, Pennsylvania [441e]

Nicholas B. Galifianakis, MD, MPH
Assistant Clinical Professor, Surgical Movement Disorders Center, Department of Neurology, University of California, San Francisco, San Francisco, California [33e]

John I. Gallin, MD
Director, Clinical Center, National Institutes of Health, Bethesda, Maryland [80]

Charlotte A. Gaydos, DrPh
Professor of Medicine, Johns Hopkins University, Division of Infectious Diseases, Baltimore, Maryland [213]

J. Michael Gaziano, MD, MPH
Professor of Medicine, Harvard Medical School; Chief, Division of Aging, Brigham and Women's Hospital; Director, Massachusetts Veterans Epidemiology Center, Boston VA Healthcare System, Boston, Massachusetts [266e]

Thomas A. Gaziano, MD, MSc
Assistant Professor of Medicine, Harvard Medical School; Assistant Professor, Health Policy and Management, Center for Health Decision Sciences, Harvard School of Public Health; Faculty Co-Leader, Chronic and Cardiovascular Diseases Working Group, Harvard Institute for Global Health, Harvard University; Associate Physician in Cardiovascular Medicine, Department of Cardiology, Brigham and Women's Hospital, Boston, Massachusetts [266e]

Susan L. Gearhart, MD
Associate Professor, Surgery, Johns Hopkins Medical Institutions, Baltimore, Maryland [353]

Robert H. Gelber, MD
Clinical Professor of Medicine and Dermatology, University of California, San Francisco, San Francisco, California [203]

Jeffrey M. Gelfand, MD, MAS
Assistant Professor of Clinical Neurology, Department of Neurology, University of California, San Francisco, San Francisco, California [29]

Alfred L. George, Jr., MD
Magerstadt Professor and Chair, Department of Pharmacology, Feinberg School of Medicine, Northwestern University, Chicago, Illinois [332e]

Dale N. Gerding, MD
Professor of Medicine, Department of Medicine, Loyola University Chicago Stritch School of Medicine, Maywood, Illinois; Research Physician, Edward Hines Jr. Veterans Affairs Hospital, Hines, Illinois [161]

Michael D. Geschwind, MD, PhD
Associate Professor of Neurology, Memory and Aging Center, University of California, San Francisco, San Francisco, California [33e]

Marc G. Ghany, MD, MHSc
Staff Physician, Liver Diseases Branch, National Institute of Diabetes and Digestive and Kidney Diseases, National Institutes of Health, Bethesda, Maryland [357]

Michael Giladi, MD, MSc
Associate Professor of Medicine, Sackler Faculty of Medicine, Tel Aviv University; The Infectious Disease Unit and the Bernard Pridan Laboratory for Molecular Biology of Infectious Diseases, Tel Aviv Medical Center, Tel Aviv, Israel [197]

Roger I. Glass, MD, PhD
Director, Fogarty International Center, Bethesda, Maryland [227]

Eli Glatstein, MD
Professor and Vice Chairman, Department of Radiation Oncology, Hospital of the University of Pennsylvania, Philadelphia, Pennsylvania [263e]

Peter J. Goadsby, MD, PhD, DSc, FRACp, FRCP
Professor, NIHR-Wellcome Trust Clinical Research Facility, King's College, London, United Kingdom; Professor, Department of Neurology, University of California, San Francisco, San Francisco, California [21, 447]

Morton F. Goldberg, MD, FACS, FAOS
Director Emeritus and Joseph Green Professor of Ophthalmology, Wilmer Eye Institute, Johns Hopkins University School of Medicine and Johns Hopkins Hospital, Baltimore, Maryland [40e]

Ary L. Goldberger, MD
Professor of Medicine, Harvard Medical School; Wyss Institute for Biologically Inspired Engineering, Harvard University; Beth Israel Deaconess Medical Center, Boston, Massachusetts [268, 269e, 278e]

David Goldblatt, MB, ChB, PhD
Professor of Vaccinology and Immunology; Consultant in Paediatric Immunology; Director of Clinical Research and Development; Director, NIHR Biomedical Research Centre, Institute of Child Health; University College London; Great Ormond Street Hospital for Children NHS Trust, London, United Kingdom [171]

Samuel Z. Goldhaber, MD
Professor of Medicine, Harvard Medical School; Director, Thrombosis Research Group, Brigham and Women's Hospital, Boston, Massachusetts [300]

Ralph Gonzales, MD, MSPH
Professor of Medicine, University of California, San Francisco, San Francisco, California [44]

Douglas S. Goodin, MD
Professor, Department of Neurology, School of Medicine, University of California, San Francisco, San Francisco, California [458]

Jeffrey I. Gordon, MD
Dr. Robert J. Glaser Distinguished University Professor and Director, Center for Genome Sciences and Systems Biology, Washington University School of Medicine, St. Louis, Missouri [86e]

Maria Luisa Gorno-Tempini, MD, PhD
Professor, Department of Neurology; Language Neurobiology Lab, Memory and Aging Center; Dyslexia Center, University of California, San Francisco, San Francisco, California [37e]

Peter A. Gottlieb, MD
Professor of Pediatrics and Medicine, Barbara Davis Center, University of Colorado School of Medicine, Aurora, Colorado [409]

Gregory A. Grabowski, MD
Adjunct Professor of Pediatrics and Molecular Genetics, Biochemistry, and Microbiology, University of Cincinnati College of Medicine; Division of Human Genetics Cincinnati Children's Hospital Medical Center, Cincinnati, Ohio; Chief Scientific Officer, Synageva BioPharma Corp., Lexington, Massachusetts [432e]

Yonatan H. Grad, MD, PhD
Assistant Professor of Immunology and Infectious Diseases, Harvard School of Public Health; Associate Physician, Division of Infectious Diseases, Brigham and Women's Hospital, Boston, Massachusetts [146]

Christine Grady, RN, PhD
Chief, Department of Bioethics, National Institutes of Health Clinical Center, Bethesda, Maryland [17e]

Alexander R. Green, MD, MPH
Assistant Professor of Medicine, Harvard Medical School; Associate Director, The Disparities Solutions Center, Massachusetts General Hospital, Boston, Massachusetts [16e]

Norton J. Greenberger, MD
Clinical Professor of Medicine, Harvard Medical School; Senior Physician, Division of Gastroenterology, Brigham and Women's Hospital, Boston, Massachusetts [369-371]

Michael F. Greene, MD
Professor of Obstetrics, Gynecology and Reproductive Biology, Harvard Medical School; Vincent Department of Obstetrics and Gynecology, Massachusetts General Hospital, Boston, Massachusetts [124e]

Daryl R. Gress, MD, FAAN, FCCM, FNCS
Associate Professor of Neurology, University of Virginia, Charlottesville, Virginia [330]

Rasim Gucalp, MD
Professor of Clinical Medicine, Albert Einstein College of Medicine; Associate Chairman for Educational Programs, Department of Oncology; Director, Hematology/Oncology Fellowship, Montefiore Medical Center, Bronx, New York [331]

Kalpana Gupta, MD, MPH
Associate Professor, Department of Medicine, Boston University School of Medicine; Chief, Section of Infectious Diseases, VA Boston Healthcare System, Boston, Massachusetts [162]

John G. Haaga, PhD
Deputy Associate Director, Behavioral and Social Research Program, National Institute on Aging, National Institutes of Health, Bethesda, Maryland [93e]

Chadi A. Hage, MD
Assistant Professor of Medicine, Thoracic Transplant Program, Indiana University Health, Indianapolis, Indiana [236]

Bevra Hannahs Hahn, MD
Professor Emerita Division of Rheumatology, University of California, Los Angeles, Los Angeles, California [378]

Colin N. Haile, MD, PhD
Assistant Professor, Menninger Department of Psychiatry and Behavioral Sciences, Baylor College of Medicine; Michael E. DeBakey VA Medical Center, Houston, Texas [468e]

Janet E. Hall, MD, MSc
Professor of Medicine, Harvard Medical School and Associate Chief, Reproductive Endocrine Unit, Massachusetts General Hospital, Boston, Massachusetts [69, 412, 414]

Jesse B. Hall, MD, FCCP
Professor of Medicine, Anesthesia and Critical Care; Chief, Section of Pulmonary and Critical Care Medicine, University of Chicago, Chicago, Illinois [321]

Scott A. Halperin, MD
Professor of Pediatrics and Microbiology and Immunology Head, Pediatric Infectious Diseases, Director, Canadian Center for Vaccinology, Dalhousie University, Halifax, Nova Scotia, Canada [185]

R. Doug Hardy, MD
Infectious Diseases Specialists, PA; Medical City Dallas Hospital and Medical City Children's Hospital, Dallas; Baylor Regional Medical Center, Plano, Texas [212]

Rudy A. Hartskeerl, PhD
Director WHO/FAO/OIE and National Leptospirosis Reference Centre, KIT Biomedical Research, KIT (Royal Tropical Institute), Amsterdam, The Netherlands [208]

William L. Hasler, MD
Professor, Division of Gastroenterology, University of Michigan Health System, Ann Arbor, Michigan [54, 344]

Stephen L. Hauser, MD
Robert A. Fishman Distinguished Professor and Chairman, Department of Neurology, University of California, San Francisco, San Francisco, California [1, 437, 443e, 444e, 455, 456, 458, 460]

Barton F. Haynes, MD
Frederic M. Hanes Professor of Medicine and Immunology, Departments of Medicine and Immunology; Director, Duke Human Vaccine Institute, Duke University School of Medicine, Durham, North Carolina [372e]

Douglas C. Heimburger, MD, MS
Professor of Medicine, Associate Director for Education and Training, Vanderbilt Institute for Global Health, Vanderbilt University School of Medicine, Nashville, Tennessee [97]

J. Claude Hemphill, III, MD, MAS
Professor of Neurology and Neurological Surgery, University of California, San Francisco; Chief of Neurology, San Francisco General Hospital, San Francisco, California [330, 446]

Patrick H. Henry, MD
Clinical Adjunct Professor of Medicine, University of Iowa, Iowa City, Iowa [79]

Katherine A. High, MD
William H. Bennett Professor of Pediatrics, Perelman School of Medicine, University of Pennsylvania; Investigator, Howard Hughes Medical Institute, The Children's Hospital of Philadelphia, Philadelphia, Pennsylvania [91e, 141]

Christine E. Hill-Kayser, MD
Assistant Professor of Radiation Oncology, Perelman School of Medicine, University of Pennsylvania, Philadelphia, Pennsylvania [263e]

Ikuo Hirano, MD
Professor of Medicine, Division of Gastroenterology, Northwestern University Feinberg School of Medicine, Chicago, Illinois [53, 347]

Martin S. Hirsch, MD
Professor of Medicine, Harvard Medical School; Professor of Immunology and Infectious Diseases, Harvard School of Public Health; Physician, Massachusetts General Hospital, Boston, Massachusetts [219]

Helen H. Hobbs, MD
Professor, Internal Medicine and Molecular Genetics, University of Texas Southwestern Medical Center; Investigator, Howard Hughes Medical Institute, Dallas, Texas [421]

Judith S. Hochman, MD
Harold Snyder Family Professor of Cardiology, Clinical Chief, Leon Charney Division of Cardiology, Co-Director, NYU-HHC Clinical and Translational Science Institute; Director, Cardiovascular Clinical Research Center, New York University School of Medicine, New York, New York [326]

A. Victor Hoffbrand, DM
Emeritus Professor of Haematology, University College, London; Honorary Consultant Haematologist, Royal Free Hospital, London, United Kingdom [128]

L. John Hoffer, MD, PhD
Professor, Faculty of Medicine, McGill University; Senior Physician, Divisions of Internal Medicine and Endocrinology, Lady Davis Institute for Medical Research, Jewish General Hospital, Montreal, Quebec, Canada [98e]

Charles W. Hoge, MD
Senior Scientist, Center for Psychiatry and Neuroscience, Walter Reed Army Institute of Research, Silver Spring, Maryland [471e]

Elizabeth L. Hohmann, MD
Associate Professor of Medicine and Infectious Diseases, Harvard Medical School; Massachusetts General Hospital, Boston, Massachusetts [176]

Steven M. Holland, MD
Chief, Laboratory of Clinical Infectious Diseases, National Institute of Allergy and Infectious Diseases, National Institutes of Health, Bethesda, Maryland [80, 204]

King K. Holmes, MD, PhD
Chair, Global Health; Professor of Medicine and Global Health; Adjunct Professor, Epidemiology; Director, Center for AIDS and STD; University of Washington School of Medicine; Head, Infectious Diseases Section, Harborview Medical Center, Seattle, Washington [163]

Jay H. Hoofnagle, MD
Director, Liver Diseases Research Branch, National Institute of Diabetes and Digestive and Kidney Diseases, National Institutes of Health, Bethesda, Maryland [357]

David C. Hooper, MD
Professor, Harvard Medical School; Chief, Infection Control Unit; Associate Chief, Division of Infectious Diseases, Massachusetts General Hospital, Boston, Massachusetts [170]

Robert J. Hopkin, MD
Associate Professor, Cincinnati Children's Hospital Medical Center, Cincinnati, Ohio [432e]

Leora Horn, MD, MSc
Assistant Professor, Division of Hematology and Medical Oncology, Vanderbilt University School of Medicine, Nashville, Tennessee [107]

Jonathan C. Horton, MD, PhD
William F. Hoyt Professor of Neuro-ophthalmology, Professor of Ophthalmology, Neurology and Physiology, University of California, San Francisco School of Medicine, San Francisco, California [39]

Howard Hu, MD, MPH, ScD
Dean; Professor of Environmental Health, Epidemiology and Global Health, Dalla Lana School of Public Health; Professor of Medicine, University of Toronto, Toronto, Ontario, Canada [472e]

Deborah T. Hung, MD, PhD
Associate Professor of Microbiology and Molecular Genetics, Assistant Professor of Medicine, Harvard Medical School; Brigham and Women's Hospital; Massachusetts General Hospital, Boston, Massachusetts; Co-director, Infectious Disease Initiative, Broad Institute of Harvard University and Massachusetts Institute of Technology, Cambridge, Massachusetts [146]

Sharon A. Hunt, MD, FACC
Professor of Medicine, Cardiovascular Medicine, Stanford University, Palo Alto, California [281]

Charles G. Hurst, MD
Chief, Chemical Casualty Care Division, United States Medical Research Institute of Chemical Defense, APG-Edgewood Area, Maryland [262e]

Ashraf S. Ibrahim, PhD
Professor, Department of Medicine, Geffen School of Medicine, University of California, Los Angeles (UCLA); Division of Infectious Diseases, Los Angeles Biomedical Research Institute at Harbor–UCLA Medical Center, Torrance, California [242]

David H. Ingbar, MD
Professor of Medicine, Pediatrics, and Physiology; Director, Pulmonary Allergy, Critical Care and Sleep Division, University of Minnesota School of Medicine, Minneapolis, Minnesota [326]

Alan C. Jackson, MD, FRCPC
Professor of Medicine (Neurology) and of Medical Microbiology, University of Manitoba; Section Head of Neurology, Winnipeg Regional Health Authority, Winnipeg, Manitoba, Canada [232]

Lisa A. Jackson, MD, MPH
Senior Investigator, Group Health Research Institute, Seattle, Washington [148]

Danny O. Jacobs, MD, MPH, FACS
Executive Vice President, Provost, and Dean of the School of Medicine; Thomas N. and Gleaves T. James Distinguished Chair, The University of Texas Medical Branch at Galveston, Galveston, Texas [20, 355, 356]

Richard F. Jacobs, MD
Robert H. Fiser, Jr., MD Endowed Chair in Pediatrics; Professor and Chairman, Department of Pediatrics, University of Arkansas for Medical Sciences; President, Arkansas Children's Hospital Research Institute, Little Rock, Arkansas [195]

J. Larry Jameson, MD, PhD
Robert G. Dunlop Professor of Medicine; Dean, Perelman School of Medicine at the University of Pennsylvania; Executive Vice President, University of Pennsylvania for the Health System, Philadelphia, Pennsylvania [1, 56, 82, 84, 121, 399-403, 405, 410, 411, 436e]

Robert T. Jensen, MD
Chief, Cell Biology Section, National Institutes of Diabetes, Digestive and Kidney Diseases, National Institutes of Health, Bethesda, Maryland [113]

Roy M. John, MBBS, PhD, FRCP
Assistant Professor of Medicine, Harvard Medical School; Department of Medicine, Brigham and Women's Hospital, Boston, Massachusetts [277]

Savio John, MD
Assistant Professor of Medicine, Division of Gastroenterology and Hepatology, State University of New York Upstate Medical University, Syracuse, New York [58]

David H. Johnson, MD
Donald W. Seldin Distinguished Chair in Internal Medicine; Professor and Chairman, Department of Internal Medicine, University of Texas Southwestern School of Medicine, Dallas, Texas [107]

James R. Johnson, MD
Professor of Medicine, University of Minnesota, Minneapolis, Minnesota [186]

Stuart Johnson, MD
Associate Professor of Medicine, Loyola University Chicago Stritch School of Medicine; Staff Physician, Edward Hines Jr. VA Hospital, Hines, Illinois [161]

S. Clairborne Johnston, MD, PhD
Dean, Dell Medical School; Frank Denius Distinguished Dean's Chair in Medical Leadership; Vice President for Medical Affairs, University of Texas, Austin, Austin, Texas [446]

S. Andrew Josephson, MD
Associate Professor; Vice Chairman, Department of Neurology, University of California, San Francisco, San Francisco, California [34, 329e, 463e]

Harald Jüppner, MD
Professor of Pediatrics, Endocrine Unit and Pediatric Nephrology Unit, Massachusetts General Hospital, Boston, Massachusetts [424]

Peter J. Kahrilas, MD
Gilbert H. Marquardt Professor of Medicine, Feinberg School of Medicine, Northwestern University, Chicago, Illinois [53, 347]

Gail Kang, MD
San Francisco, California [33e]

Hagop Kantarjian, MD
Chairman, Leukemia Department; Professor of Leukemia, The University of Texas M.D. Anderson Cancer Center, Houston, Texas [133]

Adolf W. Karchmer, MD
Professor of Medicine, Harvard Medical School, Division of Infectious Diseases, Beth Israel Deaconess Medical Center, Boston, Massachusetts [155]

Dennis L. Kasper, MD, MA
William Ellery Channing Professor of Medicine, Professor of Microbiology and Immunobiology, Department of Microbiology and Immunobiology, Harvard Medical School; Division of Infectious Diseases, Brigham and Women's Hospital, Boston, Massachusetts [1, 144, 147, 159, 183e, 201]

Lloyd H. Kasper, MD
Professor of Microbiology/Immunology and Medicine, Geisel School of Medicine, Dartmouth College, Hanover, New Hampshire [253]

Daniel L. Kastner, MD, PhD
Scientific Director, National Human Genome Research Institute, National Institutes of Health, Bethesda, Maryland [392]

Carol A. Kauffman, MD
Professor of Internal Medicine, University of Michigan Medical School; Chief, Infectious Diseases Section, Veterans Affairs Ann Arbor Healthcare System, Ann Arbor, Michigan [243]

Elaine T. Kaye, MD
Assistant Clinical Professor of Dermatology, Harvard Medical School; Boston Children's Hospital, Boston, Massachusetts [24, 25e]

Kenneth M. Kaye, MD
Associate Professor of Medicine, Harvard Medical School; Division of Infectious Diseases, Brigham and Women's Hospital, Boston, Massachusetts [24, 25e]

John A. Kessler, MD
Davee Professor of Stem Cell Biology, Department of Neurology, Feinberg School of Medicine, Northwestern University, Chicago, Illinois [90e]

Jay S. Keystone, MD, FRCPC, MSc(CTM)
Professor of Medicine, University of Toronto, Toronto, Ontario, Canada [149]

Sundeep Khosla, MD
Professor of Medicine and Physiology, College of Medicine, Mayo Clinic, Rochester, Minnesota [65]

Elliott Kieff, MD, PhD
Harriet Ryan Albee Professor of Medicine, Harvard Medical School; Brigham and Women's Hospital, Boston, Massachusetts [214e]

Anthony A. Killeen, MD, PhD
Professor, Department of Laboratory Medicine and Pathology, University of Minnesota, Minneapolis, Minnesota [480e]

Kami Kim, MD
Professor, Departments of Medicine, Pathology, and Microbiology and Immunology, Albert Einstein College of Medicine, Bronx, New York [253]

Charles H. King, MD, MS
Professor, Center for Global Health and Diseases, School of Medicine, Case Western Reserve University, Cleveland, Ohio [259]

Lindsay King, MD, MPH
Advanced Transplant/Hepatology Fellow, Department of Medicine, Gastrointestinal Unit, Massachusetts General Hospital, Boston, Massachusetts [483e]

Talmadge E. King, Jr., MD
Professor and Chair, Department of Medicine, University of California, San Francisco, San Francisco, California [315]

Louis V. Kirchhoff, MD, MPH
Professor, Departments of Internal Medicine (Infectious Diseases) and Epidemiology, University of Iowa; Staff Physician, Department of Veterans Affairs Medical Center, Iowa City, Iowa [252]

Priya S. Kishnani, MD
Professor of Pediatrics, Division Chief, Medical Genetics, Duke University Medical Center, Durham, North Carolina [433e]

Rob Knight, PhD
Professor, Howard Hughes Medical Institute; Departments of Chemistry and Biochemistry and Computer Science, Biofrontiers Institute, University of Colorado, Boulder, Colorado [86e]

Minoru S. H. Ko, MD, PhD
Mitsunada Sakaguchi Professor and Chair, Department of Systems Medicine, Keio University School of Medicine, Tokyo, Japan [88]

Barbara A. Konkle, MD
Professor of Medicine, Hematology, University of Washington; Director, Translational Research, Puget Sound Blood Center, Seattle, Washington [78, 140]

Peter Kopp, MD
Associate Professor, Division of Endocrinology, Metabolism and Molecular Science and Center for Genetic Medicine, Northwestern University Feinberg School of Medicine, Chicago, Illinois [82]

Walter J. Koroshetz, MD
National Institute of Neurological Disorders and Stroke, National Institutes of Health, Bethesda, Maryland [165]

Thomas R. Kosten, MD
J. H. Waggoner Professor of Psychiatry, Pharmacology, Immunology, Neuroscience, Baylor College of Medicine, Houston, Texas [468e]

Theodore A. Kotchen, MD
Professor Emeritus, Department of Medicine; Associate Dean for Clinical Research, Medical College of Wisconsin, Milwaukee, Wisconsin [298]

Camille Nelson Kotton, MD, FIDSA
Clinical Director, Transplant and Immunocompromised Host Infectious Diseases, Infectious Diseases Division, Massachusetts General Hospital; Harvard Medical School, Boston, Massachusetts [219]

Phyllis E. Kozarsky, MD
Professor of Medicine and Infectious Diseases, Emory University School of Medicine, Atlanta, Georgia [149]

Barnett S. Kramer, MD, MPH, FACP
Director, Division of Cancer Prevention, National Cancer Institute, Bethesda, Maryland [100]

Joel Kramer, PsyD
Professor of Neuropsychology in Neurology; Director of Neuropsychology, Memory and Aging Center, University of California, San Francisco, San Francisco, California [37e]

Stephen M. Krane, MD
Persis, Cyrus and Marlow B. Harrison Distinguished Professor of Medicine, Harvard Medical School; Massachusetts General Hospital, Boston, Massachusetts [423]

Alexander Kratz, MD, MPH, PhD
Associate Professor of Clinical Pathology and Cell Biology, Columbia University College of Physicians and Surgeons; Director, Core Laboratory, Columbia University Medical Center and the New York Presbyterian Hospital; Director, the Allen Hospital Laboratory, New York, New York [Appendix]

Peter J. Krause, MD
Senior Research Scientist, Yale School of Public Health; Yale School of Medicine, New Haven, Connecticut [249]

John P. Kress, MD
Professor of Medicine, Director, Medical Intensive Care Unit, University of Chicago, Chicago, Illinois [321]

Stephen Krieger, MD
Assistant Professor, Department of Neurology; Director, Neurology Residency Program, Icahn School of Medicine at Mount Sinai; Attending Physician, The Corinne Goldsmith Dickinson Center for MS, New York, New York [486e]

Patricia A. Kritek, MD, EdM
Associate Professor, Division of Pulmonary and Critical Care Medicine, University of Washington, Seattle, Washington [48, 305, 308e]

Henry M. Kronenberg, MD
Professor of Medicine, Harvard Medical School; Chief, Endocrine Unit, Massachusetts General Hospital, Boston, Massachusetts [423]

Jens H. Kuhn, MD, PhD, MS
Principal, Tunnell Government Services (TGS), Inc.; Lead Virologist, Integrated Research Facility at Fort Detrick (IRF-Frederick); TGS IRF-Frederick Team Leader, NIH/NIAID/DCR, Fort Detrick, Frederick, Maryland [233, 234]

Robert F. Kushner, MD, MS
Professor of Medicine, Northwestern University Feinberg School of Medicine, Chicago, Illinois [416]

Raymond Y. Kwong, MD, MPH
Associate Professor of Medicine, Harvard Medical School; Director of Cardiac Magnetic Resonance Imaging, Cardiovascular Division, Department of Medicine, Brigham and Women's Hospital, Boston, Massachusetts [270e, 271e]

Loren Laine, MD
Professor of Medicine, Yale University School of Medicine, New Haven, Connecticut; VA Connecticut Healthcare System, West Haven, Connecticut [57]

Neil K. Lakdawala, MD
Instructor in Medicine, Harvard Medical School; Associate Physician, Cardiovascular Medicine, Brigham and Women's Hospital; Boston VA Healthcare; Boston, Massachusetts [287]

Anil K. Lalwani, MD
Professor and Vice Chair for Research; Director, Division of Otology, Neurotology and Skull Base Surgery; Director, Columbia Cochlear Implant Center, Columbia University College of Physicians and Surgeons, New York, New York [43]

H. Clifford Lane, MD
Clinical Director, National Institute of Allergy and Infectious Diseases, National Institutes of Health, Bethesda, Maryland [226, 261e]

Carol A. Langford, MD, MHS
Harold C. Schott Endowed Chair; Director, Center for Vasculitis Care and Research, Department of Rheumatic and Immunologic Diseases, Cleveland Clinic, Cleveland, Ohio [385, 386e, 389, 397, 398]

Regina C. LaRocque, MD, MPH
Assistant Professor of Medicine, Harvard Medical School; Assistant Physician, Massachusetts General Hospital, Boston, Massachusetts [160]

Wei C. Lau, MD, FAHA
Emeritus Associate Professor, Department of Anesthesiology, Section Cardiovascular Anesthesiology, University of Michigan Health System Cardiovascular Center, Ann Arbor, Michigan [9]

Leslie P. Lawley, MD
Assistant Professor, Department of Dermatology, School of Medicine, Emory University, Atlanta, Georgia [71]

Thomas J. Lawley, MD
William P. Timmie Professor of Dermatology, Dean, Emory University School of Medicine, Atlanta, Georgia [70, 71, 73, 76e]

David G. Le Couteur, MD, PhD, FRACP
Professor of Geriatric Medicine, Director of the Centre for Education and Research on Ageing, University of Sydney and Sydney Research, Sydney, Australia [94e]

William M. Lee, MD
Professor of Internal Medicine; Meredith Mosle Chair in Liver Diseases, University of Texas Southwestern Medical Center at Dallas, Dallas, Texas [361]

Charles Lei, MD
Assistant Professor, Department of Emergency Medicine, Vanderbilt University Medical Center, Nashville, Tennessee [474]

Jane A. Leopold, MD
Associate Professor of Medicine, Harvard Medical School; Brigham and Women's Hospital, Boston, Massachusetts [272, 297e]

Nelson Leung, MD
Associate Professor of Medicine, Division of Nephrology and Hypertension, Division of Hematology, Mayo Clinic Rochester, Rochester, Minnesota [341]

Bruce D. Levy, MD
Associate Professor of Medicine, Harvard Medical School; Pulmonary and Critical Care Medicine, Brigham and Women's Hospital, Boston, Massachusetts [322]

Julia B. Lewis, MD
Professor, Department of Medicine, Division of Nephrology, Vanderbilt University Medical Center, Nashville, Tennessee [338]

Peter Libby, MD
Mallinckrodt Professor of Medicine, Harvard Medical School; Chief, Cardiovascular Medicine, Brigham and Women's Hospital, Boston, Massachusetts [265e, 291e, 292e]

Richard W. Light, MD
Professor of Medicine, Division of Allergy, Pulmonary, and Critical Care Medicine, Vanderbilt University, Nashville, Tennessee [316, 317]

Julie Lin, MD, MPH
Lecturer on Medicine, Harvard Medical School; Associate Physician, Renal Division, Brigham and Women's Hospital, Boston, Massachusetts, Boston, Massachusetts [61]

Yusen E. Lin, PhD, MBA
Professor and Director, Center for Environmental Laboratory Services; National Kaohsiung Normal University, Kaohsiung, Taiwan [184]

Robert Lindsay, MD, PhD
Chief, Internal Medicine; Professor of Clinical Medicine, Helen Hayes Hospital, West Haverstraw, New York [425]

Marc E. Lippman, MD, MACP, FRCP
Kathleen and Stanley Glaser Professor, Department of Medicine, Deputy Director, Sylvester Comprehensive Cancer Center, University of Miami Miller School of Medicine, Miami, Florida [108]

Peter E. Lipsky, MD
Charlottesville, Virginia [377e]

Kathleen D. Liu, MD, PhD, MAS
Associate Professor, Division of Nephrology, Department of Medicine, Division of Critical Care Medicine, Department of Anesthesiology, University of California, San Francisco, San Francisco, California [336]

Bernard Lo, MD
President, The Greenwall Foundation, New York; Professor of Medicine Emeritus and Director Emeritus of the Program in Medical Ethics, University of California, San Francisco, San Francisco, California [17e]

Dan L. Longo, MD
Professor of Medicine, Harvard Medical School; Senior Physician, Brigham and Women's Hospital; Deputy Editor, *New England Journal of Medicine*, Boston, Massachusetts [1, 77, 79, 81e, 89e, 99, 102e, 103e, 121, 123e, 124e, 125, 134, 135e, 136, 225e]

Nicola Longo, MD, PhD
Professor and Chief, Division of Medical Genetics, Departments of Pediatrics and Pathology; Medical Co-Director, Biochemical Genetics Laboratory, ARUP Laboratories, University of Utah, Salt Lake City, Utah [434e, 435e]

Joseph Loscalzo, MD, PhD
Hersey Professor of the Theory and Practice of Medicine, Harvard Medical School; Chairman, Department of Medicine; Physician-in-Chief, Brigham and Women's Hospital, Boston, Massachusetts [1, 49-52, 87e, 142, 264, 265e, 267, 283-287, 293, 295, 301-304]

Christine M. Lovly, MD, PhD
Academic, Vanderbilt Ingram Cancer Center, Vanderbilt University School of Medicine, Nashville, Tennessee [107]

Phillip A. Low, MD, FRACP, FRCP(Hon)
Robert D. and Patricia E. Kern Professor of Neurology, Mayo Clinic, College of Medicine, Rochester, Minnesota [454]

Daniel H. Lowenstein, MD
Dr. Robert B. and Mrs. Ellinor Aird Professor of Neurology; Director, Epilepsy Center, University of California, San Francisco, San Francisco, California [437, 438e, 445]

Elyse E. Lower, MD
Medical Oncology and Hematology, University of Cincinnati, Oncology Hematology Care, Inc., Cincinnati, Ohio [390]

Franklin D. Lowy, MD
Professor of Medicine and Pathology, Columbia University College of Physicians and Surgeons, New York, New York [172]

Sheila A. Lukehart, PhD
Professor, Departments of Medicine and Global Health, University of Washington, Seattle, Washington [206, 207e]

Lucio Luzzatto, MD, FRCP, FRCPath
Professor of Hematology, University of Genova, Genova; Scientific Director, Istituto Toscano Tumori, Florence, Italy [129]

Lawrence C. Madoff, MD
Professor of Medicine, University of Massachusetts Medical School, Worcester, Massachusetts; Director, Division of Epidemiology and Immunization, Massachusetts Department of Public Health, Jamaica Plain, Massachusetts [157, 166e, 167e]

Adel A. F. Mahmoud, MD, PhD
Professor in Molecular Biology and Public Policy, Princeton University, Princeton, New Jersey [259]

Ronald V. Maier, MD
Jane and Donald D. Trunkey Professor and Vice-Chair, Surgery, University of Washington; Surgeon-in-Chief, Harborview Medical Center, Seattle, Washington [324]

Mark E. Mailliard, MD
Frederick F. Paustian Professor; Chief, Division of Gastroenterology and Hepatology, Department of Internal Medicine, University of Nebraska College of Medicine, Omaha, Nebraska [363]

Mahmoud Malas, MD, MHS, FACS
Associate Professor of Surgery, Johns Hopkins University; Director of Endovascular Surgery; Director of The Vascular and Endovascular Clinical Research Center, Johns Hopkins Bayview Medical Center, Baltimore, Maryland [354]

Hari R. Mallidi, MD
Associate Professor of Surgery and Chief, Division of Transplant and Assist Devices; Lester and Sue Smith Endowed Chair in Surgery, Baylor College of Medicine, Houston, Texas [281]

Susan J. Mandel, MD, MPH
Professor of Medicine; Associate Chief, Division of Endocrinology, Diabetes and Metabolism, Perelman School of Medicine, University of Pennsylvania, Philadelphia, Pennsylvania [405]

Brian F. Mandell, MD, PhD
Professor and Chairman of Medicine, Cleveland Clinic Lerner College of Medicine, Department of Rheumatic and Immunologic Disease, Cleveland Clinic, Cleveland, Ohio [397]

Lionel A. Mandell, MD, FRCPC
Professor of Medicine, McMaster University, Hamilton, Ontario, Canada [153]

Douglas L. Mann, MD
Lewin Chair and Chief, Cardiovascular Division; Professor of Medicine, Cell Biology and Physiology, Washington University School of Medicine, Cardiologist-in-Chief, Barnes Jewish Hospital, St. Louis, Missouri [279]

JoAnn E. Manson, MD, DrPH
Professor of Medicine and the Elizabeth Fay Brigham Professor of Women's Health, Harvard Medical School; Chief, Division of Preventive Medicine, Brigham and Women's Hospital, Boston, Massachusetts [413]

Eleftheria Maratos-Flier, MD
Professor of Medicine, Harvard Medical School; Division of Endocrinology, Beth Israel Deaconess Medical Center, Boston, Massachusetts [415e]

Guido Marcucci, MD
Professor of Medicine; John B. and Jane T. McCoy Chair in Cancer Research; Associate Director of Translational Research, Comprehensive Cancer Center, The Ohio State University College of Medicine, Columbus, Ohio [132]

Daniel B. Mark, MD, MPH
Professor of Medicine, Duke University Medical Center; Director, Outcomes Research, Duke Clinical Research Institute, Durham, North Carolina [3]

Alexander G. Marneros, MD, PhD
Assistant Professor, Department of Dermatology, Harvard Medical School; Cutaneous Biology Research Center, Massachusetts General Hospital, Boston, Massachusetts [75]

Jeanne M. Marrazzo, MD, MPH
Professor of Medicine, Division of Allergy and Infectious Diseases, University of Washington, Seattle, Washington [163]

Thomas Marrie, MD
Dean, Faculty of Medicine; Professor, Department of Medicine, Dalhousie University, Halifax, Nova Scotia, Canada [211]

Gary J. Martin, MD
Raymond J. Langenbach, MD Professor of Medicine; Vice Chairman for Faculty Affairs, Department of Medicine, Northwestern University Feinberg School of Medicine, Chicago, Illinois [4]

Joseph B. Martin, MD, PhD
Edward R. and Anne G. Lefler Professor, Department of Neurobiology, Harvard Medical School, Boston, Massachusetts [437]

Susan Maslanka, PhD
Enteric Diseases Laboratory Branch, Centers for Disease Control and Prevention, Atlanta, Georgia [178]

Henry Masur, MD
Chief, Critical Care Medicine Department, Clinical Center, National Institutes of Health, Bethesda, Maryland [244]

Jeremy Matloff, MD
Fellow, Department of Gastroenterology, Icahn School of Medicine at Mount Sinai, New York, New York [485e, 486e]

Robert J. Mayer, MD
Faculty Vice President for Academic Affairs, Dana-Farber Cancer Institute; Stephen B. Kay Family Professor of Medicine, Harvard Medical School, Boston, Massachusetts [109, 110]

Alexander J. McAdam, MD, PhD
Associate Professor of Pathology, Harvard Medical School; Medical Director, Infectious Diseases Diagnostic Laboratory, Children's Hospital of Boston, Boston, Massachusetts [150e]

Calvin O. McCall, MD
Associate Professor, Department of Dermatology, Virginia Commonwealth University Medical Center, Richmond, Virginia; Chief, Dermatology Section, Hunter Holmes McGuire Veterans Affairs Medical Center, Richmond, Virginia [71, 76e]

John F. McConville, MD
Associate Professor of Medicine and Director, Internal Medicine Residency Program, University of Chicago, Chicago, Illinois [318]

Corey A. McGraw, MD
Assistant Professor, The Saul R. Korey Department of Neurology, Albert Einstein College of Medicine, Yeshiva University, New York, New York [486e]

Kevin T. McVary, MD, FACS
Professor and Chairman, Division of Urology, Southern Illinois University School of Medicine, Springfield, Illinois [67]

Mandeep R. Mehra, MD, FACC, FACP
Professor of Medicine, Harvard Medical School; Executive Director, Center for Advanced Heart Disease, Brigham and Women's Hospital; Co-Director, Brigham and Women's Hospital Heart and Vascular Center, Boston, Massachusetts [280]

Nancy K. Mello,† PhD
Professor of Psychology (Neuroscience), Harvard Medical School, Boston, Massachusetts; Director, Alcohol and Drug Abuse Research Center, McLean Hospital, Belmont, Massachusetts [469e]

Shlomo Melmed, MD
Senior Vice President and Dean of the Medical Faculty, Cedars-Sinai Medical Center, Los Angeles, California [401e-403]

Jack H. Mendelson,† MD
Professor of Psychiatry (Neuroscience), Harvard Medical School, Belmont, Massachusetts [469e]

Robert O. Messing, MD
Professor, Division of Pharmacology and Toxicology, College of Pharmacy; Associate Director, Waggoner Center for Alcohol and Addiction Research, University of Texas at Austin, Austin, Texas [465e]

M.-Marsel Mesulam, MD
Professor of Neurology, Psychiatry and Psychology, Cognitive Neurology and Alzheimer's Disease Center, Northwestern University Feinberg School of Medicine, Chicago, Illinois [36]

Gregory F. Michaud, MD
Assistant Professor of Medicine, Harvard Medical School; Brigham and Women's Hospital, Boston, Massachusetts [276]

Susan Miesfeldt, MD
Medical Oncology, Medical Director, Cancer Risk and Prevention Clinic, Maine Medical Center, Scarborough, Maine [84]

Edgar L. Milford, MD
Associate Professor of Medicine, Harvard Medical School; Director, Tissue Typing Laboratory, Brigham and Women's Hospital, Boston, Massachusetts [337]

Bruce L. Miller, MD
A. W. and Mary Margaret Clausen Distinguished Professor of Neurology, University of California, San Francisco School of Medicine, San Francisco, California [34, 35, 37e, 448, 453e]

Samuel I. Miller, MD
Professor, Departments of Microbiology, Medicine and Genome Sciences, University of Washington, Seattle, Washington [190]

Simon J. Mitchell, MB ChB, PhD, FUHM, FANZCA
Associate Professor, Department of Anaesthesiology, University of Auckland and Auckland City Hospital, Auckland, New Zealand [477e]

Babak Mokhlesi, MD, MSc
Professor of Medicine, Department of Medicine, Section of Pulmonary and Critical Care; Director, Sleep Disorders Center and Sleep Fellowship Program, University of Chicago, Chicago, Illinois [318]

Thomas A. Moore, MD, FACP, FIDSA
Chairman, Department of Infectious Diseases, Ochsner Health System, New Orleans, Louisiana [246e]

Pat J. Morin, PhD
Senior Director, Scientific Review and Grants Administration, American Association for Cancer Research, Philadelphia, Pennsylvania [101e]

Alison Morris, MD, MS
Associate Professor, Departments of Medicine and Immunology; Director, University of Pittsburgh HIV Lung Research Center, Division of Pulmonary, Allergy, and Critical Care Medicine, University of Pittsburgh School of Medicine, Pittsburgh, Pennsylvania [244]

Charles A. Morris, MD, MPH
Instructor in Medicine, Harvard Medical School; Staff Physician, Brigham and Women's Hospital, Boston, Massachusetts [482e, 484e]

David A. Morrow, MD, MPH
Associate Professor of Medicine, Harvard Medical School; Director, Levine Cardiac Intensive Care Unit; Senior Investigator, TIMI Study Group, Brigham and Women's Hospital, Boston, Massachusetts [19]

William J. Moss, MD, MPH
Professor, Departments of Epidemiology, International Health, and Molecular Microbiology and Immunology, Johns Hopkins Bloomberg School of Public Health, Baltimore, Maryland [229]

Robert J. Motzer, MD
Professor of Medicine, Joan and Sanford Weill College of Medicine of Cornell University D. Attending Physician, Genitourinary Oncology Service, Memorial Sloan-Kettering Cancer Center, New York, New York [114, 116]

David B. Mount, MD
Assistant Professor of Medicine, Harvard Medical School; Renal Division, Brigham and Women's Hospital, Renal Division, Boston VA Healthcare System, Boston, Massachusetts [63, 64e]

Haralampos M. Moutsopoulos, MD, FACP, FRCP(hc), Master ACR
Professor and Director, Department of Pathophysiology, Medical School, National University of Athens, Athens, Greece [379, 383, 387]

Robert S. Munford, MD
Senior Clinician, Laboratory of Clinical Infectious Diseases, National Institute of Allergy and Infectious Diseases, National Institutes of Health, Bethesda, Maryland [325]

Nikhil C. Munshi, MD
Professor of Medicine, Harvard Medical School; Boston VA Healthcare System; Director of Basic and Correlative Sciences; Associate Director, Jerome Lipper Myeloma Center, Dana-Farber Cancer Institute, Boston, Massachusetts [136]

John R. Murphy, PhD
Professor of Medicine and Microbiology; Director ad interim, National Emerging Infectious Diseases Laboratories Institute, Boston University School of Medicine, Boston, Massachusetts [175]

Timothy F. Murphy, MD
SUNY Distinguished Professor; Director, Clinical and Translational Research Center, University at Buffalo, the State University of New York, Buffalo, New York [182]

Barbara E. Murray, MD
J. Ralph Meadows Professor and Director, Division of Infectious Diseases, University of Texas Medical School, Houston, Texas [174]

Joseph A. Murray, MD
Professor of Medicine, Departments of Internal Medicine and Immunology, Mayo Clinic, Rochester, Minnesota [55]

Mark B. Mycyk, MD
Associate Professor, Department of Emergency Medicine, Northwestern University Feinberg School of Medicine; Associate Professor, Department of Emergency Medicine, Rush University School of Medicine; Research Director, Toxikon Consortium; Attending Physician, Department of Emergency Medicine, Cook County Hospital, Chicago, Illinois [473e]

Robert J. Myerburg, MD
Professor, Departments of Medicine and Physiology, Division of Cardiology; AHA Chair in Cardiovascular Research, University of Miami Miller School of Medicine, Miami, Florida [327]

Avindra Nath, MD
Chief, Section of Infections of the Nervous System; Clinical Director, National Institute of Neurological Disorders and Stroke (NINDS), National Institutes of Health, Bethesda, Maryland [165]

Edward T. Naureckas, MD
Professor of Medicine, and Director, Pulmonary Function Laboratory, and Adult Cystic Fibrosis Laboratory, Section of Pulmonary and Critical Care Medicine, University of Chicago, Chicago, Illinois [306e]

Eric G. Neilson, MD
Lewis Landsberg Dean, and Vice President, Medical Affairs, Feinberg School of Medicine, Northwestern University, Chicago, Illinois [62e, 332e, 338]

Emily Page Nelson, MD
Clinical Instructor, Department of Anesthesiology, Perioperative, and Pain Medicine, Brigham and Women's Hospital, Boston, Massachusetts [484e]

Gerald T. Nepom, MD, PhD
Professor (Affiliate), University of Washington School of Medicine; Director, Benaroya Research Institute at Virginia Mason; Director, Immune Tolerance Network, Seattle, Washington [373e]

†Deceased

Eric J. Nestler, MD, PhD
Nash Family Professor and Chair, Department of Neuroscience; Director, Friedman Brain Institute, Ichan School of Medicine at Mount Sinai, New York, New York [465e]

Hartmut P. H. Neumann, MD
Universitaet Freiburg, Medizinische Universitaetsklinik, Freiburg im Breisgau, Germany [407]

Joseph P. Newhouse, PhD
John D. MacArthur Professor of Health Policy and Management, Department of Health Care Policy, Harvard Medical School; Faculty, John F. Kennedy School of Government, Harvard School of Public Health, Faculty of Arts and Sciences, Harvard University, Boston, Massachusetts [15e]

Jonathan Newmark, MD
Colonel, Medical Corps, U.S. Army; Deputy Joint Program Executive Officer, Medical Systems, Joint Program Executive Office for Chemical/Biological Defense, U.S. Department of Defense, Falls Church, Virginia; Adjunct Professor of Neurology, F. Edward Hebert School of Medicine, Uniformed Services University of the Health Sciences, Bethesda, Maryland [262e]

Rathel L. Nolan, III, MD
Professor, Department of Medicine, Division of Infectious Diseases, University of Mississippi Medical Center, Jackson, Mississippi [238]

Robert L. Norris, MD
Professor, Department of Surgery; Chief, Division of Emergency Medicine, Stanford University School of Medicine, Stanford, California [474]

Scott A. Norton, MD, MPH, MSc
Chief of Dermatology, Children's National Health Systems, Washington, DC [475]

Thomas B. Nutman, MD
Head, Helminth Immunology Section, Head, Clinical Parasitology Unit, Laboratory of Parasitic Diseases, National Institute of Allergy and Infectious Diseases, National Institutes of Health, Bethesda, Maryland [257, 258]

Jose A. Obeso, MD
Professor of Neurology and Director, CIINAC, Hospital de Madrid; Medical School, CEU-San Pablo, Madrid, Spain [449]

Katherine L. O'Brien, MD, MPH
Professor, Department of International Health, Bloomberg School of Public Health, Johns Hopkins University, Baltimore, Maryland [171]

Max R. O'Donnell, MD, MPH
Assistant Professor of Medicine and Epidemiology, Division of Pulmonary, Allergy, and Critical Care Medicine, Columbia University Medical Center, New York, New York [205e]

Nigel O'Farrell, MD, MSc, FRCP
Ealing Hospital, London, United Kingdom [198e]

Jennifer Ogar, MS CCC-SLP
Speech-Language Pathologist, Memory and Aging Center, University of California, San Francisco, San Francisco, California [37e]

Patrick T. O'Gara, MD
Professor of Medicine, Harvard Medical School; Director, Clinical Cardiology, Brigham and Women's Hospital, Boston, Massachusetts [51e, 267, 283-286]

C. Warren Olanow, MD, FRCPC, FRCP(hon)
Henry P. and Georgette Goldschmidt Professor and Chairman Emeritus, Department of Neurology; Professor, Department of Neuroscience, Mount Sinai School of Medicine, New York, New York [449]

Andrew B. Onderdonk, PhD
Professor of Pathology, Harvard Medical School; Brigham and Women's Hospital, Boston, Massachusetts [150e]

Chung Owyang, MD
H. Marvin Pollard Professor of Internal Medicine; Chief, Division of Gastroenterology, University of Michigan Health System, Ann Arbor, Michigan [344, 352]

Umesh D. Parashar, MBBS, MPH
Lead, Viral Gastroenteritis Epidemiology Team, Division of Viral Diseases, National Center for Immunization and Respiratory Diseases, Centers for Disease Control and Prevention, Atlanta, Georgia [227]

Shreyaskumar R. Patel, MD
Robert R. Herring Distinguished Professor of Medicine; Center Medical Director, Sarcoma Center, The University of Texas M.D. Anderson Cancer Center, Houston, Texas [119e]

David L. Paterson, MD, PhD
Professor of Medicine, University of Queensland Centre for Clinical Research; Royal Brisbane and Women's Hospital, Brisbane, Australia [187]

Gustav Paumgartner, MD
Professor Emeritus of Medicine, University of Munich, Munich, Germany [369]

M. Luisa Pedro-Botet, MD, PhD
Professor of Medicine, Autonomous University of Barcelona; Infectious Diseases Section (Senior Consultant), Germans Trias i Pujol University Hospital, Badalona, Barcelona, Spain [184]

David A. Pegues, MD
Professor of Medicine, Division of Infectious Diseases, Perelman School of Medicine, University of Pennsylvania, Philadelphia, Pennsylvania [190]

Anton Y. Peleg, MBBS, PhD, MPH, FRACP
Associate Professor, Department of Infectious Diseases and Microbiology, The Alfred Hospital and Monash University, Melbourne, Victoria, Australia [187]

Florencia Pereyra, MD
Instructor in Medicine, Harvard Medical School; Associate Physician, Infectious Disease Division, Brigham and Women's Hospital, Boston, Massachusetts [166e, 167e]

Michael A. Pesce, PhD
Professor Emeritus of Pathology and Cell Biology, Columbia University College of Physicians and Surgeons; Director, Biochemical Genetics Laboratory, Columbia University Medical Center, New York Presbyterian Hospital, New York, New York [Appendix]

Clarence J. Peters, MD
John Sealy Distinguished University Chair in Tropical and Emerging Virology; Professor, Department of Microbiology and Immunology; Department of Pathology; Director for Biodefense, Center for Biodefense and Emerging Infectious Diseases, University of Texas Medical Branch, Galveston, Texas [233]

Gerald B. Pier, PhD
Professor of Medicine (Microbiology and Immunobiology), Harvard Medical School; Brigham and Women's Hospital, Division of Infectious Diseases, Boston, Massachusetts [145e]

Richard J. Pollack, PhD
Instructor, Department of Immunology and Infectious Disease, Harvard School of Public Health, Boston, Massachusetts; Senior Environmental Public Health Officer, Department of Environmental Health and Safety, Harvard University, Cambridge, Massachusetts; President and Chief Scientific Officer, IdentifyUS LLC, Newton, Massachusetts [475]

Martin R. Pollak, MD
Professor of Medicine, Harvard Medical School; Beth Israel Deaconess Medical Center, Boston, Massachusetts [339]

Andrew J. Pollard, PhD, FRCPCH
Professor of Paediatric Infection and Immunity, Department of Paediatrics, University of Oxford, Oxford, United Kingdom [180]

Reuven Porat, MD
Professor of Medicine, Department of Internal Medicine, Tel Aviv Souarsky Medical Center; Sackler Faculty of Medicine, Tel Aviv University, Tel Aviv, Israel [23]

Daniel A. Portnoy, PhD
Professor, Department of Molecular and Cell Biology and the School of Public Health, University of California, Berkeley, Berkeley, California [176]

John T. Potts, Jr., MD
Jackson Distinguished Professor of Clinical Medicine, Harvard Medical School; Physician-in-Chief and Director of Research Emeritus, Massachusetts General Hospital, Boston, Massachusetts [424]

Lawrie W. Powell, MD, PhD
Professor of Medicine, The University of Queensland; Director, Centre for the Advancement of Clinical Research, Royal Brisbane and Women's Hospital, Brisbane, Australia [428]

Alvin C. Powers, MD
Joe C. Davis Chair in Biomedical Science; Professor of Medicine, Molecular Physiology and Biophysics; Director, Vanderbilt Diabetes Center; Chief, Division of Diabetes, Endocrinology, and Metabolism, Vanderbilt University School of Medicine, Nashville, Tennessee [417-419]

Daniel S. Pratt, MD
Assistant Professor of Medicine, Harvard Medical Center; Massachusetts General Hospital, Boston, Massachusetts [58, 358]

Michael B. Prentice, MB ChB, PhD, MRCP(UK), FRCPath, FFPRCPI
Professor of Medical Microbiology, Departments of Microbiology and Pathology, University College Cork, Cork, Ireland [196]

Darwin J. Prockop, MD, PhD
Director and Professor, Institute for Regenerative Medicine, Texas A&M Health Science Center College of Medicine at Scott & White, Temple, Texas [427]

Stanley B. Prusiner, MD
Director, Institute for Neurodegenerative Diseases; Professor, Department of Neurology, University of California, San Francisco, San Francisco, California [444e, 453e]

Thomas C. Quinn, MD
Professor of Medicine, Johns Hopkins University, Baltimore, Maryland; Senior Investigator, National Institute of Allergy and Infectious Diseases, National Institutes of Health, Bethesda, Maryland [213]

Gil Rabinovici, MD
Associate Professor in Neurology, Memory and Aging Center, University of California, San Francisco, San Francisco, California [37e]

Daniel J. Rader, MD
Seymour Gray Professor of Molecular Medicine; Chair, Department of Genetics; Chief, Division of Translational Medicine and Human Genetics, Department of Medicine, Perelman School of Medicine at the University of Pennsylvania, Philadelphia, Pennsylvania [421]

Kaitlin Rainwater-Lovett, PhD, MPH
Research Fellow, Division of Infectious Diseases, Department of Pediatrics, Johns Hopkins University School of Medicine, Baltimore, Maryland [229]

Sanjay Ram, MBBS
Associate Professor of Medicine, Division of Infectious Diseases and Immunology, University of Massachusetts Medical School, Worcester, Massachusetts [181]

Reuben Ramphal, MD
Adjunct Professor of Medicine, Division of Infectious Diseases and Global Medicine, University of Florida College of Medicine, Gainesville, Florida [189]

Agam K. Rao, MD
Medical Officer, Division of Foodborne, Waterborne, and Environmental Diseases, Centers for Disease Control and Prevention, Atlanta, Georgia [178]

Beth Rapaport, MD
Attending Physician, Elmhurst Hospital Center, Mount Sinai Medical Affiliate, Elmhurst, New York [486e]

Kumanan Rasanathan, MBChB, MPH, FAFPHM
Technical Officer, Department of Ethics, Equity, Trade, and Human Rights, World Health Organization, Geneva, Switzerland [13e]

Neil H. Raskin, MD
Department of Neurology, University of California, San Francisco, San Francisco, California [21, 447]

Anis Rassi, Jr., MD, PhD, FACC, FACP, FAHA
Scientific Director, Anis Rassi Hospital, Goiânia, Brazil [252]

James P. Rathmell, MD
Henry Knowles Beecher Professor of Anesthesiology, Harvard Medical School; Executive Vice Chair and Chief, Division of Pain Medicine, Department of Anesthesia, Critical Care and Pain Medicine, Massachusetts General Hospital, Boston, Massachusetts [18]

Mario C. Raviglione, MD
Director, Global TB Programme, World Health Organization, Geneva, Switzerland [202]

Divya Reddy, MBBS, MPH
Faculty, Department of Medicine, Pulmonary Division, Albert Einstein College of Medicine; Montefiore Medical Center, Bronx, New York [205e]

Susan Redline, MD, MPH
Peter C. Farrell Professor of Sleep Medicine, Harvard Medical School; Brigham and Women's Hospital; Beth Israel Deaconess Medical Center, Boston, Massachusetts [319]

Sharon L. Reed, MD, MSCTM, D(ABMM)
Professor of Pathology and Medicine; Director, Microbiology Laboratory, University of California, San Diego School of Medicine, La Jolla, California [245e, 247]

Susan E. Reef, MD
Medical Epidemiologist, Centers for Disease Control and Prevention, Atlanta, Georgia [230e]

John J. Reilly, Jr., MD
Jack D. Myers Professor of Medicine and Chair, Department of Medicine; Vice Chair for Clinical Affairs, University of Pittsburgh, Pittsburgh, Pennsylvania [308e, 314]

John T. Repke, MD, FACOG
University Professor and Chairman, Department of Obstetrics and Gynecology, Pennsylvania State University College of Medicine; Obstetrician-Gynecologist In-Chief, The Milton S. Hershey Medical Center, Hershey, Pennsylvania [8]

Victor I. Reus, MD
Department of Psychiatry, University of California, San Francisco School of Medicine; Langley Porter Neuropsychiatric Institute, San Francisco, California [466]

Joseph J. Rhatigan, MD
Assistant Professor, Harvard Medical School, Harvard School of Public Health; Associate Chief, Division of Global Health Equity, Brigham and Women's Hospital, Boston, Massachusetts [2]

Peter A. Rice, MD
Professor of Medicine, Division of Infectious Diseases and Immunology, University of Massachusetts Medical School, Worcester, Massachusetts [181]

Elizabeth Robbins, MD
Clinical Professor of Pediatrics, University of California, San Francisco, San Francisco, California [443e]

Gary L. Robertson, MD
Emeritus Professor of Medicine, Northwestern University School of Medicine, Chicago, Illinois [404]

Russell G. Robertson, MD
Professor of Family Medicine, Chicago Medical School, Rosalind Franklin University of Medicine and Science, Chicago, Illinois [56]

Dan M. Roden, MD
William Stokes Professor of Experimental Therapeutics; Professor of Medicine and Pharmacology, Assistant Vice-Chancellor for Personalized Medicine, Director, Oates Institute for Experimental Therapeutics, Vanderbilt University School of Medicine, Nashville, Tennessee [5]

James A. Romano, Jr., PhD, DABT
Principal Senior Life Scientist Advisor, Tunnell Government Services, Inc., Rockville, Maryland [262e]

Karen L. Roos, MD
John and Nancy Nelson Professor of Neurology; Professor of Neurological Surgery, Indiana University School of Medicine, Indianapolis, Indiana [164]

Allan H. Ropper, MD, FRCP, FACP
Professor of Neurology, Harvard Medical School; Raymond D. Adams Master Clinician; Executive Vice Chair, Department of Neurology, Brigham and Women's Hospital, Boston, Massachusetts [328, 456, 457e]

Jonathan E. Rosenberg, MD
Associate Attending; Section Chief, Non-Prostate Program, Division of Solid Tumor Oncology, Department of Medicine, Memorial Sloan-Kettering Cancer Center, New York, New York [114]

Roger N. Rosenberg, MD
Zale Distinguished Chair and Professor of Neurology, Department of Neurology, University of Texas Southwestern Medical Center, Dallas, Texas [450, 451e]

Myrna R. Rosenfeld, MD, PhD
Department of Neurology, Hospital Clínic/IDIBAPS, Barcelona, Spain [122]

Michael A. Rubin, MD, PhD
Assistant Professor of Medicine, University of Utah School of Medicine, Salt Lake City, Utah [44]

Steven A. Rubin, PhD
Acting Principal Investigator, Center for Biologics Evaluation and Research, Food and Drug Administration, Bethesda, Maryland [231e]

Robert M. Russell, MD
Professor Emeritus of Medicine and Nutrition, Tufts University, Boston, Massachusetts; Office of Dietary Supplements, National Institutes of Health, Bethesda, Maryland [96e]

Thomas A. Russo, MD, CM
Staff Physician, Western New York VA Healthcare System; Professor of Medicine and Microbiology and Immunology; Vice Chair of Medicine; Head, Division of Infectious Disease, University at Buffalo, State University of New York, Buffalo, New York [186, 200]

Anna E. Rutherford, MD, MPH
Assistant Professor, Harvard Medical School; Associate Physician, Brigham and Women's Hospital, Boston, Massachusetts [483e]

Edward T. Ryan, MD, FACP, FIDSA, FASTMH
Professor of Medicine, Harvard Medical School; Professor of Immunology and Infectious Diseases, Harvard School of Public Health; Director, Global Infectious Diseases, Division of Infectious Diseases, Massachusetts General Hospital, Boston, Massachusetts [160, 193]

Sean Sadikot, MD
Department of Internal Medicine, Critical Care and Pulmonary Disease, Hackensack University Medical Center, Hackensack, New Jersey [485e, 486e]

David J. Salant, MD
Professor of Medicine, Boston University School of Medicine; Chief, Section of Nephrology, Boston Medical Center, Boston, Massachusetts [340]

Martin A. Samuels, MD
Professor of Neurology, Harvard Medical School; Chair, Department of Neurology, Brigham and Women's Hospital, Boston, Massachusetts [439e, 463e]

Philippe J. Sansonetti, MD
Professor, Collège de France; Institut Pasteur, Paris, France [191]

Clifford B. Saper, MD, PhD
James Jackson Putnam Professor of Neurology and Neuroscience, Harvard Medical School; Chairman, Department of Neurology, Beth Israel Deaconess Medical Center, Boston, Massachusetts [38]

Jussi J. Saukkonen, MD
Associate Professor of Medicine, Section of Pulmonary, Allergy, and Critical Care Medicine, Boston University School of Medicine, Boston, Massachusetts [205e]

Edward A. Sausville, MD, PhD
Professor of Medicine, University of Maryland School of Medicine; Associate Director for Clinical Research, Marlene and Stewart Greenbaum Cancer Center, Baltimore, Maryland [103e]

Mohamed H. Sayegh, MD
Raja N. Khuri Dean, Faculty of Medicine; Professor of Medicine and Immunology; Vice President of Medical Affairs, American University of Beirut, Beirut, Lebanon; Senior Lecturer, Harvard Medical School; Schuster Family Transplantation Center, Brigham and Women's Hospital, Boston, Massachusetts [337]

David T. Scadden, MD
Gerald and Darlene Professor of Medicine; Co-Chair, Harvard Stem Cell Institute; Co-chair, Department of Stem Cell and Regenerative Biology, Harvard Medical School; Director, Center for Regenerative Medicine; Chief, Hematologic Malignancies, Cancer Center, Massachusetts General Hospital, Boston, Massachusetts [89e]

Thomas E. Scammell, MD
Professor, Harvard Medical School; Beth Israel Deaconess Medical Center; Boston Children's Hospital, Boston, Massachusetts [38]

Anthony H. V. Schapira, MD, DSc, FRCP, FMedSci
Chair and Professor of Clinical Neurosciences, UCL Institute of Neurology, London, United Kingdom [449]

Howard I. Scher, MD
Professor of Medicine, Joan and Sanford Weill College of Medicine of Cornell University; D. Wayne Calloway Chair in Urologic Oncology; Attending Physician and Chief, Genitourinary Oncology Service, Department of Medicine, Memorial Sloan-Kettering Cancer Center, New York, New York [114, 115]

Anne Schuchat, MD
RADM, U.S. Public Health Service; Assistant Surgeon General, National Center for Immunization and Respiratory Diseases, Centers for Disease Control and Prevention, Atlanta, Georgia [148]

Marc A. Schuckit, MD
Distinguished Professor of Psychiatry, University of California, San Diego School of Medicine, La Jolla, California [467]

H. Ralph Schumacher, Jr., MD
Professor of Medicine, Division of Rheumatology, University of Pennsylvania, School of Medicine, Philadelphia, Pennsylvania [395]

Gordon E. Schutze, MD, FAAP
Professor of Pediatrics; Vice-Chairman for Educational Affairs; Martin I. Lorin, MD Chair in Medical Education, Department of Pediatrics, Section of Retrovirology, Vice President, Baylor International Pediatric AIDS Initiative at Texas Children's Hospital, Baylor College of Medicine, Texas Children's Hospital, Houston, Texas [195]

Richard M. Schwartzstein, MD
Ellen and Melvin Gordon Professor of Medicine and Medical Education, Harvard Medical School; Associate Division Chief, Division of Pulmonary, Critical Care, and Sleep Medicine, Beth Israel Deaconess Medical Center, Boston, Massachusetts [47e]

William W. Seeley, MD
Associate Professor of Neurology and Pathology, Memory and Aging Center, University of California, San Francisco, San Francisco, California [35, 448]

Michael V. Seiden, MD, PhD
Chief Medical Officer, McKesson Specialty Health, The Woodlands, Texas [117]

Julian L. Seifter, MD
Associate Professor of Medicine, Harvard Medical School; Brigham and Women's Hospital, Boston, Massachusetts [343]

David C. Seldin, MD, PhD
Professor, Departments of Medicine and Microbiology; Chief, Section of Hematology-Oncology; Director, Amyloidosis Center, Boston University School of Medicine; Boston Medical Center, Boston, Massachusetts [137]

Ankoor Shah, MD
Assistant Professor, Department of Medicine, Division of Rheumatology and Immunology, Duke University Medical Center, Durham, North Carolina [380]

Steven D. Shapiro, MD
Jack D. Myers Professor and Chair, Department of Medicine, University of Pittsburgh, Pittsburgh, Pennsylvania [314]

Erica S. Shenoy, MD, PhD
Instructor in Medicine, Harvard Medical School; Assistant Chief, Infection Control Unit, Massachusetts General Hospital, Boston, Massachusetts [170]

Kanade Shinkai, MD, PhD
Assistant Professor, Department of Dermatology, University of California, San Francisco, San Francisco, California [74]

William Silen, MD
Johnson and Johnson Professor Emeritus of Surgery, Harvard Medical School, Auburndale, Massachusetts [20]

Edwin K. Silverman, MD, PhD
Professor of Medicine, Harvard Medical School; Chief, Channing Division of Network Medicine, Department of Medicine, Brigham and Women's Hospital, Boston, Massachusetts [314]

Karl Skorecki, MD, FRCP(C), FASN
Annie Chutick Professor in Medicine (Nephrology); Director, Rappaport Research Institute, Technion-Israel Institute of Technology; Director of Medical and Research Development, Rambam Health Care Campus, Haifa, Israel [85e, 335]

Wade S. Smith, MD, PhD
Professor of Neurology, Daryl R. Gress Endowed Chair of Neurocritical Care and Stroke; Director, University of California, San Francisco Neurovascular Service, San Francisco, California [330, 446]

Elizabeth Smyth, MB BAO, MSc
Department of Gastrointestinal Oncology, Royal Marsden NHS Foundation Trust, London and Sutton, United Kingdom [112]

Kelly A. Soderberg, PhD, MPH
Associate Director, Duke Center for HIV/AIDS Vaccine Immunology-Immunogen Discovery, Duke Human Vaccine Institute, Duke University, Durham, North Carolina [372e]

Scott D. Solomon, MD
Professor, Harvard Medical School; Director, Noninvasive Cardiology, Brigham and Women's Hospital, Boston, Massachusetts [270e, 271e]

Julian Solway, MD
Walter L. Palmer Distinguished Service Professor of Medicine and Pediatrics; Associate Dean for Translational Medicine, Biological Sciences Division; Vice Chair for Research, Department of Medicine; Chair, Committee on Molecular Medicine, University of Chicago, Chicago, Illinois [306e, 318]

Michael F. Sorrell, MD
Robert L. Grissom Professor of Medicine, Department of Internal Medicine, University of Nebraska Medical Center, Omaha, Nebraska [363]

Eric J. Sorscher, MD
Professor, Departments of Medicine and Genetics, Gwaltney Chair for Medical Research; Director, Gregory Fleming James Cystic Fibrosis Research Center, University of Alabama at Birmingham, Birmingham, Alabama [313]

Frank E. Speizer, MD
E. H. Kass Distinguished Professor of Medicine, Harvard Medical School; Channing Division of Network Medicine, Department of Medicine, Brigham and Women's Hospital; Professor of Environmental Science, Department of Environmental Health, Harvard School of Public Health, Boston, Massachusetts [311]

Brad Spellberg, MD
Professor of Medicine; Associate Medical Director for Inpatient Services, Harbor–UCLA Medical Center and Los Angeles Biomedical Research Institute, Torrance, California [242]

Nancy B. Spinner, PhD, FACMG
Professor of Pathology and Laboratory Medicine, Perelman School of Medicine, University of Pennsylvania; Chief, Division of Genomic Diagnostics, Children's Hospital of Philadelphia, Philadelphia, Pennsylvania [83e]

Jerry L. Spivak, MD
Professor of Medicine and Oncology, Hematology Division, Johns Hopkins University School of Medicine, Baltimore, Maryland [131]

David D. Spragg, MD
Associate Professor, Department of Medicine, Johns Hopkins University; Director, Electrophysiology Laboratory, Johns Hopkins Bayview Medical Center, Baltimore, Maryland [273e-275]

E. William St. Clair, MD
Professor of Medicine and Immunology, Department of Medicine, Duke University Medical Center, Durham, North Carolina [380]

Allen C. Steere, MD
Professor of Medicine, Harvard Medical School; Massachusetts General Hospital, Boston, Massachusetts [210]

Robert S. Stern, MD
Carl J. Herzog Professor of Dermatology, Harvard Medical School; Chair, Department of Dermatology, Beth Israel Deaconess Medical Center, Boston, Massachusetts [74]

Dennis L. Stevens, MD, PhD
Professor of Medicine, University of Washington School of Medicine, Seattle, Washington [156, 179]

Lynne Warner Stevenson, MD
Professor of Medicine, Harvard Medical School; Director, Heart Failure Program, Brigham and Women's Hospital, Boston, Massachusetts [287]

William G. Stevenson, MD
Brigham and Women's Hospital; Cardiovascular Division, Department of Medicine, Harvard Medical School, Boston, Massachusetts [276, 277]

John H. Stone, MD, MPH
Professor of Medicine, Harvard Medical School; Director, Clinical Rheumatology, Massachusetts General Hospital, Boston, Massachusetts [391e]

Stephanie Studenski, MD, MPH
Director, Longitudinal Studies Section, Intramural Research Program, National Institute on Aging, National Institutes of Health, Baltimore, Maryland [11]

Lewis Sudarsky, MD
Associate Professor of Neurology, Harvard Medical School; Director of Movement Disorders, Brigham and Women's Hospital, Boston, Massachusetts [32]

Donna C. Sullivan, PhD
Professor, Department of Medicine, Division of Infectious Diseases, University of Mississippi Medical School, Jackson, Mississippi [238]

Shyam Sundar, MD, FRCP, FNA
Professor of Medicine, Institute of Medical Sciences, Banaras Hindu University, Varanasi, India [251]

Neeraj K. Surana, MD, PhD
Instructor in Pediatrics, Harvard Medical School; Assistant in Medicine, Boston Children's Hospital, Boston, Massachusetts [144]

Paolo M. Suter, MD, MS
Professor, Clinic and Policlinic of Internal Medicine, University Hospital, Zurich, Switzerland [96e]

Richard M. Suzman, PhD
Director, Behavioral and Social Research Program, National Institute on Aging, National Institutes of Health, Bethesda, Maryland [93e]

Robert A. Swerlick, MD
Alicia Leizman Stonecipher Professor and Chair of Dermatology, Emory University School of Medicine, Atlanta, Georgia [76e]

Homayoun Tabandeh, MD
Retina-Vitreous Associates Medical Group, Los Angeles, California [40e]

Geoffrey Tabin, MD
John and Marva Warnock Presidential Professor, University of Utah School of Medicine; Director, International Ophthalmology Division, John A. Moran Eye Center; Director, Himalayan Cataract Project, Salt Lake City, Utah [476e]

Maria Carmela Tartaglia, MD
Assistant Professor, Tanz Centre for Research in Neurodegenerative Diseases, University of Toronto, Toronto, Ontario, Canada [37e]

Joel D. Taurog, MD
Professor of Internal Medicine, Rheumatic Diseases Division, University of Texas Southwestern Medical Center at Dallas, Dallas, Texas [384]

Ayalew Tefferi, MD
Professor of Medicine and Hematology, Mayo Clinic, Rochester, Minnesota [135e]

Stephen C. Textor, MD
Professor of Medicine, Division of Nephrology and Hypertension, Mayo Clinic, Rochester, Minnesota [299, 341]

Rajesh V. Thakker, MD, FMedSci, FR
May Professor of Medicine, Academic Endocrine Unit, University of Oxford; O.C.D.E.M., Churchill Hospital, Headington, Oxford, United Kingdom [408]

C. Louise Thwaites, MD, MBBS
Oxford University Clinical Research Unit, Hospital for Tropical Diseases, Ho Chi Minh City, Vietnam [177]

Zelig A. Tochner, MD
Professor of Radiation Oncology, University of Pennsylvania School of Medicine; Medical Director, Proton Therapy Center, Philadelphia, Pennsylvania [263e]

Gordon F. Tomaselli, MD
Michel Mirowski, MD Professor of Cardiology; Professor of Medicine and Cellular and Molecular Medicine; Chief, Division of Cardiology, Johns Hopkins University, Baltimore, Maryland [273e-275]

Karina A. Top, MD, MS
Assistant Professor of Pediatrics, Dalhousie University, Halifax, Nova Scotia, Canada [185]

Mark Topazian, MD
Professor of Medicine, Mayo Clinic, Rochester, Minnesota [345, 346e]

Barbara W. Trautner, MD, PhD
Assistant Professor, Section of Infectious Diseases, Department of Medicine, Baylor College of Medicine; Houston VA Health Services Research and Development Center of Excellence, Houston, Texas [162]

Jeffrey M. Trent, PhD, FACMG
President and Research Director, Translational Genomics Research Institute, Phoenix, Arizona; Van Andel Research Institute, Grand Rapids, Michigan [101e]

Elbert P. Trulock, III, MD
Rosemary and I. Jerome Flance Professor in Pulmonary Medicine, Washington University School of Medicine, St. Louis, Missouri [320e]

Kenneth L. Tyler, MD
Reuler-Lewin Family Professor and Chair of Neurology; Professor of Medicine, Immunology, and Microbiology, University of Colorado School of Medicine, Aurora, Colorado; Neurologist, Denver Veterans Affairs Medical Center, Denver, Colorado [164]

Athanasios G. Tzioufas, MD
Professor, Department of Pathophysiology, School of Medicine, National University of Athens, Athens, Greece [383]

Walter J. Urba, MD, PhD
Director of Research, Earle A. Chiles Research Institute, Providence Cancer Center, Portland, Oregon [105]

Jos W. M. van der Meer, MD, PhD
Professor of Medicine; Head, Department of General Internal Medicine, Radboud University Nijmegen Medical Centre, Nijmegen, The Netherlands [26, 464e]

Edouard G. Vannier, PharmD, PhD
Assistant Professor, Division of Geographic Medicine and Infectious Diseases, Department of Medicine, Tufts Medical Center and Tufts University School of Medicine, Boston, Massachusetts [249]

Gauri R. Varadhachary, MD
Professor, Department of Gastrointestinal Medical Oncology, The University of Texas M.D. Anderson Cancer Center, Houston, Texas [120e]

John Varga, MD
John Hughes Professor of Medicine, Northwestern University Feinberg School of Medicine, Chicago, Illinois [382]

Christy A. Varughese, PharmD
Infectious Disease Specialist, Department of Pharmacy, Massachusetts General Hospital, Boston, Massachusetts [170]

Panayiotis G. Vlachoyiannopoulos, MD
Professor of Medicine-Immunology, Department of Pathophysiology, Medical School, National University of Athens, Athens, Greece [379]

Bert Vogelstein, MD
Investigator, Howard Hughes Medical Institute; Director, Ludwig Center at the Sidney Kimmel Comprehensive Cancer Center; Clayton Professor of Oncology and Pathology; Johns Hopkins Medical Institutions, Baltimore, Maryland [101e]

Everett E. Vokes, MD
John E. Ultmann Professor; Chairman, Department of Medicine; Physician-in-Chief, University of Chicago Medical Center, Chicago, Illinois [106]

Tamara J. Vokes, MD
Professor, Department of Medicine, Section of Endocrinology, University of Chicago, Chicago, Illinois [426e]

Jiři F. P. Wagenaar, MD, PhD
Senior Scientist, WHO/FAO/OIE and National Leptospirosis Reference Centre, KIT Biomedical Research, KIT (Royal Tropical Institute), Amsterdam, The Netherlands [208]

Sushrut S. Waikar, MD, MPH
Associate Professor, Harvard Medical School; Director, Renal Ambulatory Services, Brigham and Women's Hospital, Boston, Massachusetts [334]

Matthew K. Waldor, MD, PhD
Edward H. Kass Professor of Medicine, Channing Laboratory, Brigham and Women's Hospital; Harvard Medical School and Howard Hughes Medical Institute, Boston, Massachusetts [193]

David H. Walker, MD
The Carmage and Martha Walls Distinguished University Chair in Tropical Diseases; Professor and Chairman, Department of Pathology; Executive Director, Center for Biodefense and Emerging Infectious Diseases, University of Texas Medical Branch, Galveston, Texas [211]

Mark F. Walker, MD
Associate Professor, Neurology, Case Western Reserve University; Cleveland VA Medical Center, Cleveland, Ohio [28]

Fred Wang, MD
Professor of Medicine, Harvard Medical School and Brigham and Women's Hospital, Boston, Massachusetts [214e, 220e]

John W. Warren, MD
Professor of Medicine, University of Maryland School of Medicine, Baltimore, Maryland [60e]

Aaron B. Waxman, MD, PhD, FACP, FCCP
Associate Professor of Medicine, Harvard Medical School; Executive Director, Center for Pulmonary-Heart Diseases, Brigham and Women's Hospital Heart and Vascular Center, Boston, Massachusetts [304]

Michael E. Wechsler, MD, MMSc
Professor of Medicine; Director, Asthma Program, National Jewish Health, Denver, Colorado [310]

Anthony P. Weetman, MD, DSc
University of Sheffield, School of Medicine Sheffield, United Kingdom [405]

Robert A. Weinstein, MD
The C. Anderson Hedberg, MD Professor of Internal Medicine, Rush Medical College; Chief Academic Officer, Cook County Health and Hospitals System, Chicago, Illinois [168]

Jeffrey I. Weitz, MD, FRCP(C), FACP
Professor of Medicine and Biochemistry, McMaster University; Executive Director, Thrombosis and Atherosclerosis Research Institute, Hamilton, Ontario, Canada [143]

Peter F. Weller, MD
Chief, Infectious Disease Division; Chief, Allergy and Inflammation Division; Beth Israel Deaconess Medical Center, Boston, Massachusetts [254-258, 260]

Andrew Wellman, MD, PhD
Assistant Professor of Medicine, Division of Sleep Medicine, Harvard Medical School; Brigham and Women's Hospital, Boston, Massachusetts [319]

Patrick Y. Wen, MD
Professor of Neurology, Harvard Medical School; Director, Center for Neuro-Oncology, Dana-Farber Cancer Institute; Director, Division of Neuro-Oncology, Department of Neurology, Brigham and Women's Hospital; Dana-Farber Cancer Institute, Boston, Massachusetts [118]

Michael R. Wessels, MD
John F. Enders Professor of Pediatrics; Professor of Medicine, Harvard Medical School; Chief, Division of Infectious Diseases, Boston Children's Hospital, Boston, Massachusetts [173]

L. Joseph Wheat, MD
President and Medical Director, MiraVista Diagnostics, LLC, Indianapolis, Indiana [236]

A. Clinton White, Jr., MD
Paul R. Stalnaker Distinguished Professor; Director, Infectious Disease Division, Department of Internal Medicine, University of Texas Medical Branch, Galveston, Texas [260]

Nicholas J. White, DSc, MD, FRCP, F Med Sci, FRS
Professor of Tropical Medicine, Faculty of Tropical Medicine, Mahidol University, Mahidol-Oxford Research Unit, Bangkok, Thailand [248, 250e]

Richard J. Whitley, MD
Distinguished Professor of Pediatrics; Loeb Eminent Scholar Chair in Pediatrics; Professor of Microbiology, Medicine and Neurosurgery, The University of Alabama at Birmingham, Birmingham, Alabama [217]

Bruce U. Wintroub, MD
Professor and Chair, Department of Dermatology, University of California, San Francisco, San Francisco, California [74]

Andrea S. Wolf, MD, MPH
Assistant Professor, and Director, Women's Lung Cancer Program, Mt. Sinai Medical Center, New York, New York [482e]

Allan W. Wolkoff, MD
The Herman Lopata Chair in Liver Disease Research; Professor of Medicine and Anatomy and Structural Biology; Associate Chair of Medicine for Research; Chief, Division of Gastroenterology and Liver Diseases; Director, Marion Bessin Liver Research Center, Albert Einstein College of Medicine and Montefiore Medical Center, Bronx, New York [359]

John B. Wong, MD
Professor of Medicine, Tufts University School of Medicine; Chief, Division of Clinical Decision Making, Department of Medicine, Tufts Medical Center, Boston, Massachusetts [3]

Louis Michel Wong Kee Song, MD
Associate Professor, Division of Gastroenterology and Hepatology, Mayo Clinic College of Medicine, Rochester, Minnesota [345, 346e]

Robert L. Wortmann, MD, FACP, MACR
Professor Emeritus, Department of Medicine, Geisel School of Medicine at Dartmouth, Lebanon, New Hampshire [431e]

Shirley H. Wray, MD, PhD, FRCP
Professor of Neurology, Harvard Medical School; Master Clinician, Department of Neurology, Massachusetts General Hospital, Boston, Massachusetts [41e]

Richard G. Wunderink, MD
Professor, Pulmonary and Critical Care, Northwestern University Feinberg School of Medicine, Chicago, Illinois [153]

Kim B. Yancey, MD
Professor and Chair, Department of Dermatology, University of Texas Southwestern Medical Center in Dallas, Dallas, Texas [70, 73]

Janet A. Yellowitz, DMD, MPH
Associate Professor; Director, Geriatric Dentistry, University of Maryland Dental School, Baltimore, Maryland [46e]

Lam Minh Yen, MD
Director, Tetanus Intensive Care Unit, Hospital for Tropical Diseases, Ho Chi Minh City, Vietnam [177]

Maria A. Yialamas, MD
Assistant Professor of Medicine, Harvard Medical School; Associate Program Director, Internal Medicine Residency, Brigham and Women's Hospital, Boston, Massachusetts [481e, 483e]

Neal S. Young, MD
Chief, Hematology Branch, National Heart, Lung and Blood Institute; Director, NIH Center for Human Immunology, Autoimmunity and Inflammation, National Institutes of Health, Bethesda, Maryland [130]

Victor L. Yu, MD
Professor of Medicine, Department of Medicine, University of Pittsburgh Medical Center, Pittsburgh, Pennsylvania [184]

Jing Zhou, MD, PhD, FASN
Director, Laboratory of Molecular Genetics and Developmental Biology of Disease, Renal Division; Director, Center for Polycystic Kidney Disease Research, Brigham and Women's Hospital; Harvard Medical School, Boston, Massachusetts [339]

Werner Zimmerli, MD
Professor of Medicine, Basel University; Interdisciplinary Unit of Orthopaedic Infection, Kantonspital Baselland, Liestal, Switzerland [158]

Laura A. Zimmerman, MPH
Epidemiologist, Centers for Disease Control and Prevention, Atlanta, Georgia [230e]

PREFACE

The Editors are pleased to present the 19th edition of *Harrison's Principles of Internal Medicine.* Since the first edition was published 65 years ago, virtually every area of medicine and medical education has evolved remarkably, and many new fields have emerged.

While retaining the founding goals of *Harrison's*, this edition has been modified extensively in light of the varied needs of the book's readers and the diverse methods and formats by which information is now acquired and applied. The focus of medical education worldwide is shifting from the classic structure/function/disease approach to an integrated, often case-based approach in which basic and population sciences are specifically linked to the practical diagnosis and management of disease. Many of the updates and changes described here have been undertaken with the modern educational and clinical environments in mind.

This new edition offers a thoroughly updated presentation of the classic pathophysiologic basis of clinical medicine and details the cutting-edge methods and tools that are now available for the assessment of symptoms and the effective management of diseases in the modern patient-care environment. The text is supplemented by germane new photographs, radiographs, illustrations, atlases, patient-care algorithms, tables, and practical demonstrative videos.

In the interest of producing the most practical format possible for the 19th edition, a new system of referencing has been used. Detailed bibliographic listings, with summaries of articles' relevance to practice, appear in the online edition, replacing the general and limited collection of Suggested Readings that appeared in the prior print editions.

The 19th edition of *Harrison's* is designed for accessibility and flexibility. The print textbook is available in two volumes. Volume 1 focuses on the foundations of medicine and the understanding and assessment of cardinal disease manifestations; Volume 2 focuses on specific diseases, by system. This functional division will be helpful to students who are mastering the basis of clinical medicine and to clinicians who are more focused on gaining an advanced understanding of mechanisms and patient care in specific diseases. In terms of digital media, *Harrison's* is now available as an eBook on multiple platforms, as an enhanced "app" developed especially for tablet and smartphone devices that offer high-definition resolution of multimedia content and interactive features, and as an updated online edition. All of these options provide access to our numerous e-chapters as well as to videos and atlases. Additional resources include the *Harrison's Self-Assessment and Board Review*, a useful study guide based on information in the 19th edition, and the *Harrison's Manual of Medicine*, a pocket version of *Harrison's Principles of Internal Medicine.* A new *Harrison's* collection of case vignettes emphasizing differential diagnostic considerations in the assessment of cardinal manifestations will also be available.

Advances in medical science have been spectacular since *Harrison's* was first published in 1949. At that time, peptic ulcer disease was thought to be caused by stress, nearly every tumor that was not resected resulted in death, rheumatic heart disease was widely prevalent, and hepatitis B and HIV infection were unknown. In the intervening years, both the infectious cause of and the cure for peptic ulcer disease were identified; advances in diagnosis and treatment made it possible to cure two-thirds of cancers; rheumatic heart disease virtually disappeared; atherosclerotic coronary artery disease waxed and then—at least in part through management of modifiable risk factors—began to wane; hepatitis B and its consequences, cirrhosis and hepatocellular carcinoma, became preventable by a vaccine; and HIV, first viewed as a uniformly fatal worldwide scourge, became a treatable chronic disease. Notably, emerging and reemerging diseases have presented significant challenges to medical research and practice, while a new understanding of systems-wide concepts such as the microbiome offers exciting new possibilities for understanding and managing health and disease in ways never before possible.

Of particular note in this 19th edition are critical updates in the classic chapter on HIV/AIDS, which offers both a clinically pragmatic focus and a comprehensive and analytical approach to pathogenesis. The updates cover the latest treatment protocols and address the issue of combination prevention modalities, making the chapter the most up-to-date and comprehensive treatise on HIV disease available.

Several other chapters likewise reflect the rapid pace of advancement in the field of immune-related diseases and their treatment. In this regard, Chapter 372e, "Introduction to the Immune System," serves as a mini-textbook of immunology for use in immunology courses. In addition, a new chapter on IgG4-mediated disease summarizes an important and newly recognized constellation of entities.

Readers will find expanded coverage of the neurodegenerative diseases, highlighting advances in their classification and management and delineating the new understanding of mechanisms responsible for the deposition and spread of pathogenic protein aggregates in these disorders. The chapter on chronic hepatitis discusses in detail the dramatic new discoveries in the use of direct-acting antiviral agents for the treatment of hepatitis C virus disease; these agents are responsible for some of the most exciting therapeutic advances in medicine today.

The rapidly expanding application of genetic knowledge to medicine is covered in many chapters, including a new chapter on microbial genomics and infectious diseases and substantially updated chapters on the human microbiome and chromosomal genetic disorders. Other new chapters address timely topics such as the impact of climate change on disease, infections in U.S. veterans returning from foreign wars, and advances in contraception and the treatment of infertility. Another topic of increasing interest, the impact of aging on health and disease, is addressed by several chapters, including a newly authored chapter on the biology of aging. A new chapter on men's health complements the updated chapter on women's health. New chapters also address diverse topics including the emerging field of tissue engineering, the examination of the comatose patient, the management of heart failure, the major characteristics of helminths and helminthic infections, specific cardiac valvular disorders, venous and lymphatic diseases of the extremities, renovascular disease, late complications of diabetes, chronic myeloid leukemia, heat-related illnesses, fatigue, polyglandular failure syndromes, and nonalcoholic fatty liver disease and nonalcoholic steatohepatitis.

Supplementing new content and updates on diseases and patient care, new videos in this edition cover sleep disorders, tissue engineering, noninvasive cardiac imaging, examination of the comatose patient, and myasthenia gravis and other diseases of the neuromuscular junction. New atlases for this edition address noninvasive imaging, percutaneous revascularization, and gastrointestinal endoscopy.

We have many people to thank for their efforts in producing this book. First, the authors have done a superb job of producing authoritative chapters that synthesize vast amounts of scientific and clinical data to create state-of-the-art descriptions of medical disorders encompassed by internal medicine. In today's information-rich, rapidly evolving environment, they have ensured that this information is current. Helpful suggestions and critical input have been provided by a number of colleagues; particularly notable was the advice of Chung Owyang on the Gastroenterology Section. We are most grateful to our colleagues in each of our editorial offices who have kept track of the work in its various phases and facilitated communication with the authors, with the McGraw-Hill Education staff, and among the editors: Patricia Conrad, Patricia L. Duffey, Gregory K. Folkers, Julie B. McCoy, Elizabeth Robbins, Anita Rodriguez, and Stephanie Tribuna.

The staff at McGraw-Hill Education has been a constant source of support and expertise. James Shanahan, Associate Publisher for McGraw-Hill Education's Professional Publishing Division, has been a superb and insightful partner to the editors, guiding the development of the book and its related products in new formats. Kim Davis, as Associate Managing Editor, has adeptly ensured that the complex production of this multi-authored textbook proceeded smoothly and efficiently. Dominik Pucek oversaw the production of the new procedural videos. Jeffrey Herzich ably served as production manager for this new edition.

We are privileged to have compiled this 19th edition and are enthusiastic about all that it offers our readers. We learned much in the process of editing *Harrison's* and hope that you will find this edition a uniquely valuable educational resource.

THE EDITORS

1 The Practice of Medicine

The Editors

THE PHYSICIAN IN THE TWENTY-FIRST CENTURY

No greater opportunity, responsibility, or obligation can fall to the lot of a human being than to become a physician. In the care of the suffering, [the physician] needs technical skill, scientific knowledge, and human understanding.... Tact, sympathy, and understanding are expected of the physician, for the patient is no mere collection of symptoms, signs, disordered functions, damaged organs, and disturbed emotions. [The patient] is human, fearful, and hopeful, seeking relief, help, and reassurance.

—*Harrison's Principles of Internal Medicine*, 1950

The practice of medicine has changed in significant ways since the first edition of this book appeared more than 60 years ago. The advent of molecular genetics, molecular and systems biology, and molecular pathophysiology; sophisticated new imaging techniques; and advances in bioinformatics and information technology have contributed to an explosion of scientific information that has fundamentally changed the way physicians define, diagnose, treat, and attempt to prevent disease. This growth of scientific knowledge is ongoing and accelerating.

The widespread use of electronic medical records and the Internet have altered the way doctors practice medicine and access and exchange information (Fig. 1-1). As today's physicians strive to integrate copious amounts of scientific knowledge into everyday practice, it is critically important that they remember two things: first, that the ultimate goal of medicine is to prevent disease and treat patients; and second, that despite more than 60 years of scientific advances since the first edition of this text, cultivation of the intimate relationship between physician and patient still lies at the heart of successful patient care.

THE SCIENCE AND ART OF MEDICINE

Deductive reasoning and applied technology form the foundation for the solution to many clinical problems. Spectacular advances in biochemistry, cell biology, and genomics, coupled with newly developed imaging techniques, allow access to the innermost parts of the cell and provide a window into the most remote recesses of the body. Revelations about the nature of genes and single cells have opened a portal for formulating a new molecular basis for the physiology of systems. Increasingly, physicians are learning how subtle changes in many different genes can affect the function of cells and organisms. Researchers are deciphering the complex mechanisms by which genes are regulated. Clinicians have developed a new appreciation of the role of stem cells in normal tissue function; in the development of cancer, degenerative diseases, and other disorders; and in the treatment of certain diseases. Entirely new areas of research, including studies of the human microbiome, have become important in understanding both health and disease. The knowledge gleaned from the ***science of medicine*** continues to enhance physicians' understanding of complex disease processes and provide new approaches to treatment and prevention. Yet skill in the most sophisticated applications of laboratory technology and in the use of the latest therapeutic modality alone does not make a good physician.

When a patient poses challenging clinical problems, an effective physician must be able to identify the crucial elements in a complex history and physical examination; order the appropriate laboratory, imaging, and diagnostic tests; and extract the key results from densely populated computer screens to determine whether to treat or to "watch." As the number of tests increases, so does the likelihood that some incidental finding, completely unrelated to the clinical problem at hand, will be uncovered. Deciding whether a clinical clue is worth pursuing or should be dismissed as a "red herring" and weighing whether a proposed test, preventive measure, or treatment entails a greater risk than the disease itself are essential judgments that a skilled clinician must make many times each day. This combination of medical knowledge, intuition, experience, and judgment defines the ***art of medicine***, which is as necessary to the practice of medicine as is a sound scientific base.

CLINICAL SKILLS

History-Taking The written history of an illness should include all the facts of medical significance in the life of the patient. Recent events should be given the most attention. Patients should, at some early point, have the opportunity to tell their own story of the illness without frequent interruption and, when appropriate, should receive expressions of interest, encouragement, and empathy from the physician. Any event related by a patient, however trivial or seemingly irrelevant, may provide the key to solving the medical problem. In general, only patients who feel comfortable with the physician will offer complete information; thus putting the patient at ease to the greatest extent possible contributes substantially to obtaining an adequate history.

An informative history is more than an orderly listing of symptoms. By listening to patients and noting the way in which they describe their symptoms, physicians can gain valuable insight. Inflections of voice, facial expression, gestures, and attitude (i.e., "body language") may offer important clues to patients' perception of their symptoms. Because patients vary in their medical sophistication and ability to recall facts, the reported medical history should be corroborated whenever possible. The social history also can provide important insights into the types of diseases that should be considered. The family history not only identifies rare Mendelian disorders within a family but often reveals risk factors for common disorders, such as coronary heart disease, hypertension, and asthma. A thorough family history may require input from multiple relatives to ensure completeness and accuracy; once recorded, it can be updated readily. The process of history-taking provides an opportunity to observe the patient's behavior and to watch for features to be pursued more thoroughly during the physical examination.

The very act of eliciting the history provides the physician with an opportunity to establish or enhance the unique bond that forms the basis for the ideal patient-physician relationship. This process helps the physician develop an appreciation of the patient's view of the illness, the patient's expectations of the physician and the health care system, and the financial and social implications of the illness for the patient. Although current health care settings may impose time constraints on patient visits, it is important not to rush the history-taking. A hurried approach may lead patients to believe that what they are relating is not of importance to the physician, and thus they may withhold relevant information. The confidentiality of the patient-physician relationship cannot be overemphasized.

Physical Examination The purpose of the physical examination is to identify physical signs of disease. The significance of these objective indications of disease is enhanced when they confirm a functional or structural change already suggested by the patient's history. At times, however, physical signs may be the only evidence of disease.

The physical examination should be methodical and thorough, with consideration given to the patient's comfort and modesty. Although attention is often directed by the history to the diseased organ or part of the body, the examination of a new patient must extend from head to toe in an objective search for abnormalities. Unless the physical examination is systematic and is performed consistently from patient to patient, important segments may be omitted inadvertently. The results of the examination, like the details of the history, should be recorded at the time they are elicited—not hours later, when they are subject to the distortions of memory. Skill in physical diagnosis is acquired with experience, but it is not merely technique that determines success in eliciting signs of disease. The detection of a few

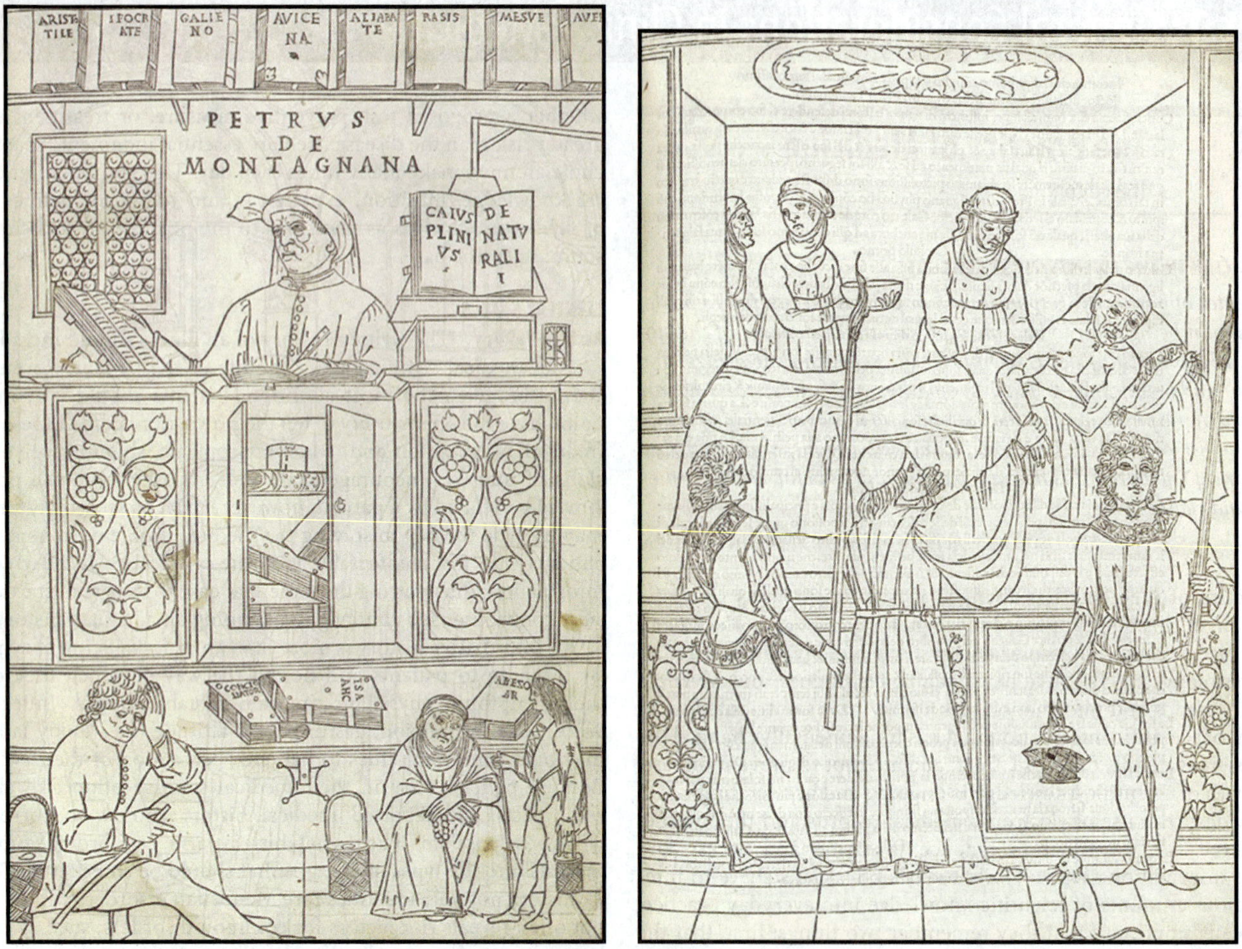

FIGURE 1-1 Woodcuts from Johannes de Ketham's *Fasciculus Medicinae,* the first illustrated medical text ever printed, show methods of information access and exchange in medical practice during the early Renaissance. Initially published in 1491 for use by medical students and practitioners, *Fasciculus Medicinae* appeared in six editions over the next 25 years. *Left:* Petrus de Montagnana, a well-known physician and teacher at the University of Padua and author of an anthology of instructive case studies, consults medical texts dating from antiquity up to the early Renaissance. *Right:* A patient with plague is attended by a physician and his attendants. *(Courtesy, U.S. National Library of Medicine.)*

scattered petechiae, a faint diastolic murmur, or a small mass in the abdomen is not a question of keener eyes and ears or more sensitive fingers but of a mind alert to those findings. Because physical findings can change with time, the physical examination should be repeated as frequently as the clinical situation warrants.

Given the many highly sensitive diagnostic tests now available (particularly imaging techniques), it may be tempting to place less emphasis on the physical examination. Indeed, many patients are seen by consultants after a series of diagnostic tests have been performed and the results are known. This fact should not deter the physician from performing a thorough physical examination since important clinical findings may have escaped detection by the barrage of prior diagnostic tests. The act of examining (touching) the patient also offers an opportunity for communication and may have reassuring effects that foster the patient-physician relationship.

Diagnostic Studies Physicians rely increasingly on a wide array of laboratory tests to solve clinical problems. However, accumulated laboratory data do not relieve the physician from the responsibility of carefully observing, examining, and studying the patient. It is also essential to appreciate the limitations of diagnostic tests. By virtue of their impersonal quality, complexity, and apparent precision, they often gain an aura of certainty regardless of the fallibility of the tests themselves, the instruments used in the tests, and the individuals performing or interpreting the tests. Physicians must weigh the expense involved in laboratory procedures against the value of the information these procedures are likely to provide.

Single laboratory tests are rarely ordered. Instead, physicians generally request "batteries" of multiple tests, which often prove useful. For example, abnormalities of hepatic function may provide the clue to nonspecific symptoms such as generalized weakness and increased fatigability, suggesting a diagnosis of chronic liver disease. Sometimes a single abnormality, such as an elevated serum calcium level, points to a particular disease, such as hyperparathyroidism or an underlying malignancy.

The thoughtful use of screening tests (e.g., measurement of low-density lipoprotein cholesterol) may be of great value. A group of laboratory values can conveniently be obtained with a single specimen at relatively low cost. Screening tests are most informative when they are directed toward common diseases or disorders and when their results indicate whether other useful—but often costly—tests or interventions are needed. On the one hand, biochemical measurements, together with simple laboratory determinations such as blood count, urinalysis, and erythrocyte sedimentation rate, often provide a major clue to the presence of a pathologic process. On the other hand, the physician must learn to evaluate occasional screening-test abnormalities that do not necessarily connote significant disease. An in-depth workup after the report of an isolated laboratory abnormality in a person who is otherwise well is almost invariably wasteful and unproductive. Because so many tests are performed routinely for screening purposes, it is not unusual for one or two values to be slightly abnormal. Nevertheless, even if there is no reason to suspect an underlying illness, tests yielding abnormal results ordinarily are repeated to rule out laboratory error. If an abnormality is confirmed, it is important to consider its potential significance in the context of the patient's condition and other test results.

The development of technically improved imaging studies with greater sensitivity and specificity proceeds apace. These tests provide remarkably detailed anatomic information that can be a pivotal factor in medical decision-making. Ultrasonography, a variety of isotopic scans, CT, MRI, and positron emission tomography have supplanted older, more invasive approaches and opened new diagnostic vistas. In light of their capabilities and the rapidity with which they can lead to a diagnosis, it is tempting to order a battery of imaging studies. All physicians have had experiences in which imaging studies revealed findings that led to an unexpected diagnosis. Nonetheless, patients must endure each of these tests, and the added cost of unnecessary testing is substantial. Furthermore, investigation of an unexpected abnormal finding may be associated with risk and/or expense and may lead to the diagnosis of an irrelevant or incidental problem. A skilled physician must learn to use these powerful diagnostic tools judiciously, always considering whether the results will alter management and benefit the patient.

PRINCIPLES OF PATIENT CARE

Evidence-Based Medicine *Evidence-based medicine* refers to the making of clinical decisions that are formally supported by data, preferably data derived from prospectively designed, randomized, controlled clinical trials. This approach is in sharp contrast to anecdotal experience, which is often biased. Unless they are attuned to the importance of using larger, more objective studies for making decisions, even the most experienced physicians can be influenced to an undue extent by recent encounters with selected patients. Evidence-based medicine has become an increasingly important part of routine medical practice and has led to the publication of many practice guidelines.

Practice Guidelines Many professional organizations and government agencies have developed formal clinical-practice guidelines to aid physicians and other caregivers in making diagnostic and therapeutic decisions that are evidence-based, cost-effective, and most appropriate to a particular patient and clinical situation. As the evidence base of medicine increases, guidelines can provide a useful framework for managing patients with particular diagnoses or symptoms. Clinical guidelines can protect patients—particularly those with inadequate health care benefits—from receiving substandard care. These guidelines also can protect conscientious caregivers from inappropriate charges of malpractice and society from the excessive costs associated with the overuse of medical resources. There are, however, caveats associated with clinical-practice guidelines since they tend to oversimplify the complexities of medicine. Furthermore, groups with different perspectives may develop divergent recommendations regarding issues as basic as the need for screening of women in their forties by mammography or of men over age 50 by serum prostate-specific antigen (PSA) assay. Finally, guidelines, as the term implies, do not—and cannot be expected to—account for the uniqueness of each individual and his or her illness. The physician's challenge is to integrate into clinical practice the useful recommendations offered by experts without accepting them blindly or being inappropriately constrained by them.

Medical Decision-Making Medical decision-making is an important responsibility of the physician and occurs at each stage of the diagnostic and therapeutic process. The decision-making process involves the ordering of additional tests, requests for consultations, and decisions about treatment and predictions concerning prognosis. This process requires an in-depth understanding of the pathophysiology and natural history of disease. As discussed above, medical decision-making should be evidence-based so that patients derive full benefit from the available scientific knowledge. Formulating a differential diagnosis requires not only a broad knowledge base but also the ability to assess the relative probabilities of various diseases. Application of the scientific method, including hypothesis formulation and data collection, is essential to the process of accepting or rejecting a particular diagnosis. Analysis of the differential diagnosis is an iterative process. As new information or test results are acquired, the group of disease processes being considered can be contracted or expanded appropriately.

Despite the importance of evidence-based medicine, much medical decision-making relies on good clinical judgment, an attribute that is difficult to quantify or even to assess qualitatively. Physicians must use their knowledge and experience as a basis for weighing known factors, along with the inevitable uncertainties, and then making a sound judgment; this synthesis of information is particularly important when a relevant evidence base is not available. Several quantitative tools may be invaluable in synthesizing the available information, including diagnostic tests, Bayes' theorem, and multivariate statistical models. *Diagnostic tests* serve to reduce uncertainty about an individual's diagnosis or prognosis and help the physician decide how best to manage that individual's condition. The battery of diagnostic tests complements the history and the physical examination. The accuracy of a particular test is ascertained by determining its sensitivity (true-positive rate) and specificity (true-negative rate) as well as the predictive value of a positive and a negative result. *Bayes' theorem* uses information on a test's sensitivity and specificity, in conjunction with the pretest probability of a diagnosis, to determine mathematically the posttest probability of the diagnosis. More complex clinical problems can be approached with *multivariate statistical models*, which generate highly accurate information even when multiple factors are acting individually or together to affect disease risk, progression, or response to treatment. Studies comparing the performance of statistical models with that of expert clinicians have documented equivalent accuracy, although the models tend to be more consistent. Thus, multivariate statistical models may be particularly helpful to less experienced clinicians. See Chap. 3 for a more thorough discussion of decision-making in clinical medicine.

Electronic Medical Records Both the growing reliance on computers and the strength of information technology now play central roles in medicine. Laboratory data are accessed almost universally through computers. Many medical centers now have electronic medical records, computerized order entry, and bar-coded tracking of medications. Some of these systems are interactive, sending reminders or warning of potential medical errors.

Electronic medical records offer rapid access to information that is invaluable in enhancing health care quality and patient safety, including relevant data, historical and clinical information, imaging studies, laboratory results, and medication records. These data can be used to monitor and reduce unnecessary variations in care and to provide real-time information about processes of care and clinical outcomes. Ideally, patient records are easily transferred across the health care system. However, technologic limitations and concerns about privacy and cost continue to limit broad-based use of electronic health records in many clinical settings.

As valuable as it is, information technology is merely a tool and can never replace the clinical decisions that are best made by the physician. Clinical knowledge and an understanding of a patient's needs, supplemented by quantitative tools, still represent the best approach to decision-making in the practice of medicine.

Evaluation of Outcomes Clinicians generally use *objective* and readily measurable parameters to judge the outcome of a therapeutic intervention. These measures may oversimplify the complexity of a clinical condition as patients often present with a major clinical problem in the context of multiple complicating background illnesses. For example, a patient may present with chest pain and cardiac ischemia, but with a background of chronic obstructive pulmonary disease and renal insufficiency. For this reason, outcome measures such as mortality, length of hospital stay, or readmission rates are typically risk-adjusted. An important point is that patients usually seek medical attention for *subjective* reasons; they wish to obtain relief from pain, to preserve or regain function, and to enjoy life. The components of a patient's health status or quality of life can include bodily comfort, capacity for physical activity, personal and professional function, sexual function, cognitive function, and overall perception of health. Each of these important areas can be assessed through structured interviews or specially designed questionnaires. Such assessments provide useful parameters by which a physician can judge patients' subjective views of their disabilities and responses to treatment, particularly in chronic illness. The practice of medicine requires consideration and integration of both objective and subjective outcomes.

Women's Health and Disease Although past epidemiologic studies and clinical trials have often focused predominantly on men, more recent studies have included more women, and some, like the Women's Health Initiative, have exclusively addressed women's health issues. Significant sex-based differences exist in diseases that afflict both men and women. Much is still to be learned in this arena, and ongoing studies should enhance physicians' understanding of the mechanisms underlying these differences in the course and outcome of certain diseases. For a more complete discussion of women's health, see Chap. 6e.

Care of the Elderly The relative proportion of elderly individuals in the populations of developed nations has grown considerably over the past few decades and will continue to grow. The practice of medicine is greatly influenced by the health care needs of this growing demographic group. The physician must understand and appreciate the decline in physiologic reserve associated with aging; the differences in appropriate doses, clearance, and responses to medications; the diminished responses of the elderly to vaccinations such as those against influenza; the different manifestations of common diseases among the elderly; and the disorders that occur commonly with aging, such as depression, dementia, frailty, urinary incontinence, and fractures. For a more complete discussion of medical care for the elderly, see Chap. 11 and Part 5, Chaps. 93e and 94e.

Errors in the Delivery of Health Care A 1999 report from the Institute of Medicine called for an ambitious agenda to reduce medical error rates and improve patient safety by designing and implementing fundamental changes in health care systems. Adverse drug reactions occur in at least 5% of hospitalized patients, and the incidence increases with the use of a large number of drugs. Whatever the clinical situation, it is the physician's responsibility to use powerful therapeutic measures wisely, with due regard for their beneficial actions, potential dangers, and cost. It is the responsibility of hospitals and health care organizations to develop systems to reduce risk and ensure patient safety. Medication errors can be reduced through the use of ordering systems that rely on electronic processes or, when electronic options are not available, that eliminate misreading of handwriting. Implementation of infection control systems, enforcement of hand-washing protocols, and careful oversight of antibiotic use can minimize the complications of nosocomial infections. Central-line infection rates have been dramatically reduced at many centers by careful adherence of trained personnel to standardized protocols for introducing and maintaining central lines. Rates of surgical infection and wrong-site surgery can likewise be reduced by the use of standardized protocols and checklists. Falls by patients can be minimized by judicious use of sedatives and appropriate assistance with bed-to-chair and bed-to-bathroom transitions. Taken together, these and other measures are saving thousands of lives each year.

The Physician's Role in Informed Consent The fundamental principles of medical ethics require physicians to act in the patient's best interest and to respect the patient's autonomy. These requirements are particularly relevant to the issue of informed consent. Patients are required to sign a consent form for essentially any diagnostic or therapeutic procedure. Most patients possess only limited medical knowledge and must rely on their physicians for advice. Communicating in a clear and understandable manner, physicians must fully discuss the alternatives for care and explain the risks, benefits, and likely consequences of each alternative. In every case, the physician is responsible for ensuring that the patient thoroughly understands these risks and benefits; encouraging questions is an important part of this process. This is the very definition of *informed consent*. Full, clear explanation and discussion of the proposed procedures and treatment can greatly mitigate the fear of the unknown that commonly accompanies hospitalization. Excellent communication can also help alleviate misunderstandings in situations where complications of intervention occur. Often the patient's understanding is enhanced by repeatedly discussing the issues in an unthreatening and supportive way, answering new questions that occur to the patient as they arise.

Special care should be taken to ensure that a physician seeking a patient's informed consent has no real or apparent conflict of interest involving personal gain.

The Approach to Grave Prognoses and Death No circumstance is more distressing than the diagnosis of an incurable disease, particularly when premature death is inevitable. What should the patient and family be told? What measures should be taken to maintain life? What can be done to maintain the quality of life?

Honesty is absolutely essential in the face of a terminal illness. The patient must be given an opportunity to talk with the physician and ask questions. A wise and insightful physician uses such open communication as the basis for assessing what the patient wants to know and when he or she wants to know it. On the basis of the patient's responses, the physician can assess the right tempo for sharing information. Ultimately, the patient must understand the expected course of the disease so that appropriate plans and preparations can be made. The patient should participate in decision-making with an understanding of the goal of treatment (palliation) and its likely effects. The patient's religious beliefs must be taken into consideration. Some patients may find it easier to share their feelings about death with their physician, who is likely to be more objective and less emotional, than with family members.

The physician should provide or arrange for emotional, physical, and spiritual support and must be compassionate, unhurried, and open. In many instances, there is much to be gained by the laying on of hands. Pain should be controlled adequately, human dignity maintained, and isolation from family and close friends avoided. These aspects of care tend to be overlooked in hospitals, where the intrusion of life-sustaining equipment can detract from attention to the whole person and encourage concentration instead on the life-threatening disease, against which the battle ultimately will be lost in any case. In the face of terminal illness, the goal of medicine must shift from *cure* to *care* in the broadest sense of the term. *Primum succurrere*, first hasten to help, is a guiding principle. In offering care to a dying patient, a physician must be prepared to provide information to family members and deal with their grief and sometimes their feelings of guilt or even anger. It is important for the doctor to assure the family that everything reasonable has been done. A substantial problem in these discussions is that the physician often does not know how to gauge the prognosis. In addition, various members of the health care team may offer different opinions. Good communication among providers is essential so that consistent information is provided to patients. This is especially important when the best path forward is uncertain. Advice from experts in palliative and terminal care should be sought whenever necessary to ensure that clinicians are not providing patients with unrealistic expectations. For a more complete discussion of end-of-life care, see Chap. 10.

THE PATIENT-PHYSICIAN RELATIONSHIP

> *The significance of the intimate personal relationship between physician and patient cannot be too strongly emphasized, for in an extraordinarily large number of cases both the diagnosis and treatment are directly dependent on it. One of the essential qualities of the clinician is interest in humanity,* ***for the secret of the care of the patient is in caring for the patient.***
>
> —Francis W. Peabody, October 21, 1925,
> Lecture at Harvard Medical School

Physicians must never forget that patients are individual human beings with problems that all too often transcend their physical complaints. They are not "cases" or "admissions" or "diseases." Patients do not fail treatments; treatments fail to benefit patients. This point is particularly important in this era of high technology in clinical medicine. Most patients are anxious and fearful. Physicians should instill confidence and offer reassurance but must never come across as arrogant or patronizing. A professional attitude, coupled with warmth and openness, can do much to alleviate anxiety and to encourage patients to share all aspects of their medical history. Empathy and compassion are the essential features of a caring physician. The physician needs to consider the setting in which an illness occurs—in terms not only of patients themselves but also of their familial, social, and cultural backgrounds. The ideal patient-physician relationship is based on thorough knowledge of the patient, mutual trust, and the ability to communicate.

The Dichotomy of Inpatient and Outpatient Internal Medicine The hospital environment has changed dramatically over the last few decades. Emergency departments and critical care units have evolved to identify and manage critically ill patients, allowing them to survive formerly fatal diseases. At the same time, there is increasing pressure to reduce the length of stay in the hospital and to manage complex disorders in the outpatient setting. This transition has been driven not only by efforts to reduce costs but also by the availability of new outpatient technologies, such as imaging and percutaneous infusion catheters for long-term antibiotics or nutrition, minimally invasive surgical procedures, and evidence that outcomes often are improved by minimizing inpatient hospitalization.

In these circumstances, two important issues arise as physicians cope with the complexities of providing care for hospitalized patients. On the one hand, highly specialized health professionals are essential to the provision of optimal acute care in the hospital; on the other, these professionals—with their diverse training, skills, responsibilities, experiences, languages, and "cultures"—need to work as a team.

In addition to traditional medical beds, hospitals now encompass multiple distinct levels of care, such as the emergency department, procedure rooms, overnight observation units, critical care units, and palliative care units. A consequence of this differentiation has been the emergence of new trends, including specialties (e.g., emergency medicine and end-of-life care) and the provision of in-hospital care by hospitalists and intensivists. Most *hospitalists* are board-certified internists who bear primary responsibility for the care of hospitalized patients and whose work is limited entirely to the hospital setting. The shortened length of hospital stay that is now standard means that most patients receive only acute care while hospitalized; the increased complexities of inpatient medicine make the presence of a generalist with specific training, skills, and experience in the hospital environment extremely beneficial. *Intensivists* are board-certified physicians who are further certified in critical care medicine and who direct and provide care for very ill patients in critical care units. Clearly, then, an important challenge in internal medicine today is to ensure the continuity of communication and information flow between a patient's primary care doctor and these physicians who are in charge of the patient's hospital care. Maintaining these channels of communication is frequently complicated by patient "handoffs"—i.e., from the outpatient to the inpatient environment, from the critical care unit to a general medicine floor, and from the hospital to the outpatient environment. The involvement of many care providers in conjunction with these transitions can threaten the traditional one-to-one relationship between patient and primary care physician. Of course, patients can benefit greatly from effective collaboration among a number of health care professionals; however, *it is the duty of the patient's principal or primary physician to provide cohesive guidance through an illness*. To meet this challenge, primary care physicians must be familiar with the techniques, skills, and objectives of specialist physicians and allied health professionals who care for their patients in the hospital. In addition, primary care doctors must ensure that their patients will benefit from scientific advances and from the expertise of specialists when they are needed both in and out of the hospital. Primary care physicians can also explain the role of these specialists to reassure patients that they are in the hands of the physicians best trained to manage an acute illness. However, the primary care physician should retain ultimate responsibility for making major decisions about diagnosis and treatment and should assure patients and their families that decisions are being made in consultation with these specialists by a physician who has an overall and complete perspective on the case.

A key factor in mitigating the problems associated with multiple care providers is a commitment to interprofessional teamwork. Despite the diversity in training, skills, and responsibilities among health care professionals, common values need to be reinforced if patient care is not to be adversely affected. This component of effective medical care is widely recognized, and several medical schools have integrated interprofessional teamwork into their curricula. The evolving concept of the "medical home" incorporates team-based primary care with linked subspecialty care in a cohesive environment that ensures smooth transitions of care cost-effectively.

Appreciation of the Patient's Hospital Experience The hospital is an intimidating environment for most individuals. Hospitalized patients find themselves surrounded by air jets, buttons, and glaring lights; invaded by tubes and wires; and beset by the numerous members of the health care team—hospitalists, specialists, nurses, nurses' aides, physicians' assistants, social workers, technologists, physical therapists, medical students, house officers, attending and consulting physicians, and many others. They may be transported to special laboratories and imaging facilities replete with blinking lights, strange sounds, and unfamiliar personnel; they may be left unattended at times; and they may be obligated to share a room with other patients who have their own health problems. It is little wonder that a patient's sense of reality may be compromised. Physicians who appreciate the hospital experience from the patient's perspective and who make an effort to develop a strong relationship within which they can guide the patient through this experience may make a stressful situation more tolerable.

Trends in the Delivery of Health Care: A Challenge to the Humane Physician Many trends in the delivery of health care tend to make medical care impersonal. These trends, some of which have been mentioned already, include (1) vigorous efforts to reduce the escalating costs of health care; (2) the growing number of managed-care programs, which are intended to reduce costs but in which the patient may have little choice in selecting a physician or in seeing that physician consistently; (3) increasing reliance on technological advances and computerization for many aspects of diagnosis and treatment; and (4) the need for numerous physicians to be involved in the care of most patients who are seriously ill.

In light of these changes in the medical care system, it is a major challenge for physicians to maintain the *humane* aspects of medical care. The American Board of Internal Medicine, working together with the American College of Physicians–American Society of Internal Medicine and the European Federation of Internal Medicine, has published a *Charter on Medical Professionalism* that underscores three main principles in physicians' contract with society: (1) the primacy of patient welfare, (2) patient autonomy, and (3) social justice. While medical schools appropriately place substantial emphasis on professionalism, a physician's personal attributes, including integrity, respect, and compassion, also are extremely important. Availability to the patient, expression of sincere concern, willingness to take the time to explain all aspects of the illness, and a nonjudgmental attitude when dealing with patients whose cultures, lifestyles, attitudes, and values differ from those of the physician are just a few of the characteristics of a humane physician. Every physician will, at times, be challenged by patients who evoke strongly negative or positive emotional responses. Physicians should be alert to their own reactions to such patients and situations and should consciously monitor and control their behavior so that the patient's best interest remains the principal motivation for their actions at all times.

An important aspect of patient care involves an appreciation of the patient's "quality of life," a subjective assessment of what each patient values most. This assessment requires detailed, sometimes intimate knowledge of the patient, which usually can be obtained only through deliberate, unhurried, and often repeated conversations. Time pressures will always threaten these interactions, but they should not diminish the importance of understanding and seeking to fulfill the priorities of the patient.

EXPANDING FRONTIERS IN MEDICAL PRACTICE

The Era of "Omics": Genomics, Epigenomics, Proteomics, Microbiomics, Metagenomics, Metabolomics, Exposomics . . . In the spring of 2003, announcement of the complete sequencing of the human genome officially ushered in the genomic era. However, even before that landmark accomplishment, the practice of medicine had been evolving as a result of the insights into both the human genome and the genomes of a wide variety of microbes. The clinical implications of these insights are illustrated by the complete genome sequencing of H1N1 influenza virus in 2009 and the rapid identification of H1N1 influenza as a potentially fatal pandemic illness, with swift development and dissemination of an effective protective vaccine. Today, gene expression profiles are being used to guide therapy and inform prognosis for a number of diseases, the use of genotyping is providing a new means to assess the risk of certain diseases as well as variations in response to a number of drugs, and physicians are better understanding the role of certain genes in the causality of common conditions such as obesity and allergies. Despite these advances, the use of complex genomics in the diagnosis, prevention, and treatment of disease is still in its early stages. The task of physicians is complicated by the fact that phenotypes generally are determined not by genes alone but by the interplay of genetic and environmental factors. Indeed, researchers have just begun to scratch the surface of the potential applications of genomics in the practice of medicine.

Rapid progress also is being made in other areas of molecular medicine. *Epigenomics* is the study of alterations in chromatin and histone proteins and methylation of DNA sequences that influence gene expression. Every cell of the body has identical DNA sequences; the diverse phenotypes a person's cells manifest are the result of epigenetic regulation of gene expression. Epigenetic alterations are associated with a number of cancers and other diseases. *Proteomics*, the study of the entire library of proteins made in a cell or organ and its complex relationship to disease, is enhancing the repertoire of the 23,000 genes in the human genome through alternate splicing, posttranslational processing, and posttranslational modifications that often have unique functional consequences. The presence or absence of particular proteins in the circulation or in cells is being explored for diagnostic and disease-screening applications. *Microbiomics* is the study of the resident microbes in humans and other mammals. The human haploid genome has ~20,000 genes, while the microbes residing on and in the human body comprise over 3–4 million genes; the contributions of these resident microbes are likely to be of great significance with regard to health status. In fact, research is demonstrating that the microbes inhabiting human mucosal and skin surfaces play a critical role in maturation of the immune system, in metabolic balance, and in disease susceptibility. A variety of environmental factors, including the use and overuse of antibiotics, have been tied experimentally to substantial increases in disorders such as obesity, metabolic syndrome, atherosclerosis, and immune-mediated diseases in both adults and children. *Metagenomics*, of which microbiomics is a part, is the genomic study of environmental species that have the potential to influence human biology directly or indirectly. An example is the study of exposures to microorganisms in farm environments that may be responsible for the lower incidence of asthma among children raised on farms. *Metabolomics* is the study of the range of metabolites in cells or organs and the ways they are altered in disease states. The aging process itself may leave telltale metabolic footprints that allow the prediction (and possibly the prevention) of organ dysfunction and disease. It seems likely that disease-associated patterns will be sought in lipids, carbohydrates, membranes, mitochondria, and other vital components of cells and tissues. Finally, *exposomics* refers to efforts to catalogue and capture environmental exposures such as smoking, sunlight, diet, exercise, education, and violence, which together have an enormous impact on health. All of this new information represents a challenge to the traditional reductionist approach to medical thinking. The variability of results in different patients, together with the large number of variables that can be assessed, creates difficulties in identifying preclinical disease and defining disease states unequivocally. Accordingly, the tools of *systems biology* and *network medicine* are being applied to the enormous body of information now obtainable for every patient and may eventually provide new approaches to classifying disease. **For a more complete discussion of a complex systems approach to human disease, see Chap. 87e.**

The rapidity of these advances may seem overwhelming to practicing physicians. However, physicians have an important role to play in ensuring that these powerful technologies and sources of new information are applied with sensitivity and intelligence to the patient. Since "omics" are evolving so rapidly, physicians and other health care professionals must continue to educate themselves so that they can apply this new knowledge to the benefit of their patients' health and well-being. Genetic testing requires wise counsel based on an understanding of the value and limitations of the tests as well as the implications of their results for specific individuals. **For a more complete discussion of genetic testing, see Chap. 84.**

The Globalization of Medicine Physicians should be cognizant of diseases and health care services beyond local boundaries. Global travel has implications for disease spread, and it is not uncommon for diseases endemic to certain regions to be seen in other regions after a patient has traveled to and returned from those regions. In addition, factors such as wars, the migration of refugees, and climate change are contributing to changing disease profiles worldwide. Patients have broader access to unique expertise or clinical trials at distant medical centers, and the cost of travel may be offset by the quality of care at those distant locations. As much as any other factor influencing global aspects of medicine, the Internet has transformed the transfer of medical information throughout the world. This change has been accompanied by the transfer of technological skills through telemedicine and international consultation—for example, regarding radiologic images and pathologic specimens. **For a complete discussion of global issues, see Chap. 2.**

Medicine on the Internet On the whole, the Internet has had a very positive effect on the practice of medicine; through personal computers, a wide range of information is available to physicians and patients almost instantaneously at any time and from anywhere in the world. This medium holds enormous potential for the delivery of current information, practice guidelines, state-of-the-art conferences, journal content, textbooks (including this text), and direct communications with other physicians and specialists, expanding the depth and breadth of information available to the physician regarding the diagnosis and care of patients. Medical journals are now accessible online, providing rapid sources of new information. By bringing them into direct and timely contact with the latest developments in medical care, this medium also serves to lessen the information gap that has hampered physicians and health care providers in remote areas.

Patients, too, are turning to the Internet in increasing numbers to acquire information about their illnesses and therapies and to join Internet-based support groups. Patients often arrive at a clinic visit with sophisticated information about their illnesses. In this regard, physicians are challenged in a positive way to keep abreast of the latest relevant information while serving as an "editor" as patients navigate this seemingly endless source of information, the accuracy and validity of which are not uniform.

A critically important caveat is that virtually anything can be published on the Internet, with easy circumvention of the peer-review process that is an essential feature of academic publications. Both physicians and patients who search the Internet for medical information must be aware of this danger. Notwithstanding this limitation, appropriate use of the Internet is revolutionizing information access for physicians and patients and in this regard represents a remarkable resource that was not available to practitioners a generation ago.

Public Expectations and Accountability The general public's level of knowledge and sophistication regarding health issues has grown rapidly over the last few decades. As a result, expectations of the health care system in general and of physicians in particular have risen. Physicians are expected to master rapidly advancing fields (the *science* of medicine) while considering their patients' unique needs (the *art* of medicine). Thus, physicians are held accountable not only for the technical aspects of the care they provide but also for their patients' satisfaction with the delivery and costs of care.

In many parts of the world, physicians increasingly are expected to account for the way in which they practice medicine by meeting certain standards prescribed by federal and local governments. The hospitalization of patients whose health care costs are reimbursed by the government and other third parties is subjected to utilization review. Thus, a physician must defend the cause for and duration of a patient's hospitalization if it falls outside certain "average" standards. Authorization for reimbursement increasingly is based on documentation of the nature and complexity of an illness, as reflected by recorded elements of the history and physical examination. A growing "pay-for-performance" movement seeks to link reimbursement to quality of care. The goal of this movement is to improve standards of health care and contain spiraling health care costs. In many parts of the United States, managed (capitated) care contracts with insurers have replaced traditional fee-for-service care, placing the onus of managing the cost of all care directly on the providers and increasing the emphasis on preventive strategies. In addition, physicians are expected to give evidence of their current competence through mandatory continuing education, patient record audits, maintenance of certification, and relicensing.

Medical Ethics and New Technologies The rapid pace of technological advance has profound implications for medical applications that go far beyond the traditional goals of disease prevention, treatment, and cure. Cloning, genetic engineering, gene therapy, human–computer interfaces, nanotechnology, and use of designer drugs have the potential to modify inherited predispositions to disease, select desired characteristics in embryos, augment "normal" human performance, replace failing tissues, and substantially prolong life span. Given their unique training, physicians have a responsibility to help shape the debate on the appropriate uses of and limits placed on these new techniques and to consider carefully the ethical issues associated with the implementation of such interventions.

The Physician as Perpetual Student From the time doctors graduate from medical school, it becomes all too apparent that their lot is that of the "perpetual student" and that the mosaic of their knowledge and experiences is eternally unfinished. This realization is at the same time exhilarating and anxiety-provoking. It is exhilarating because doctors can apply constantly expanding knowledge to the treatment of their patients; it is anxiety-provoking because doctors realize that they will never know as much as they want or need to know. Ideally, doctors will translate the latter feeling into energy through which they can continue to improve themselves and reach their potential as physicians. It is the physician's responsibility to pursue new knowledge continually by reading, attending conferences and courses, and consulting colleagues and the Internet. This is often a difficult task for a busy practitioner; however, a commitment to continued learning is an integral part of being a physician and must be given the highest priority.

The Physician as Citizen Being a physician is a privilege. The capacity to apply one's skills for the benefit of one's fellow human beings is a noble calling. The doctor–patient relationship is inherently unbalanced in the distribution of power. In light of their influence, physicians must always be aware of the potential impact of what they do and say and must always strive to strip away individual biases and preferences to find what is best for the patient. To the extent possible, physicians should also act within their communities to promote health and alleviate suffering. Meeting these goals begins by setting a healthy example and continues in taking action to deliver needed care even when personal financial compensation may not be available.

A goal for medicine and its practitioners is to strive to provide the means by which the poor can cease to be unwell.

Learning Medicine It has been a century since the publication of the Flexner Report, a seminal study that transformed medical education and emphasized the scientific foundations of medicine as well as the acquisition of clinical skills. In an era of burgeoning information and access to medical simulation and informatics, many schools are implementing new curricula that emphasize lifelong learning and the acquisition of competencies in teamwork, communication skills, system-based practice, and professionalism. These and other features of the medical school curriculum provide the foundation for many of the themes highlighted in this chapter and are expected to allow physicians to progress, with experience and learning over time, from competency to proficiency to mastery.

At a time when the amount of information that must be mastered to practice medicine continues to expand, increasing pressures both within and outside of medicine have led to the implementation of restrictions on the amount of time a physician-in-training can spend in the hospital. Because the benefits associated with continuity of medical care and observation of a patient's progress over time were thought to be outstripped by the stresses imposed on trainees by long hours and by the fatigue-related errors they made in caring for patients, strict limits were set on the number of patients that trainees could be responsible for at one time, the number of new patients they could evaluate in a day on call, and the number of hours they could spend in the hospital. In 1980, residents in medicine worked in the hospital more than 90 hours per week on average. In 1989, their hours were restricted to no more than 80 per week. Resident physicians' hours further decreased by ~10% between 1996 and 2008, and in 2010 the Accreditation Council for Graduate Medical Education further restricted (i.e., to 16 hours per shift) consecutive in-hospital duty hours for first-year residents. The impact of these changes is still being assessed, but the evidence that medical errors have decreased as a consequence is sparse. An unavoidable by-product of fewer hours at work is an increase in the number of "handoffs" of patient responsibility from one physician to another. These transfers often involve a transition from a physician who knows the patient well, having evaluated that individual on admission, to a physician who knows the patient less well. It is imperative that these transitions of responsibility be handled with care and thoroughness, with all relevant information exchanged and acknowledged.

Research, Teaching, and the Practice of Medicine The word *doctor* is derived from the Latin *docere*, "to teach." As teachers, physicians should share information and medical knowledge with colleagues, students of medicine and related professions, and their patients. The practice of medicine is dependent on the sum total of medical knowledge, which in turn is based on an unending chain of scientific discovery, clinical observation, analysis, and interpretation. Advances in medicine depend on the acquisition of new information through research, and improved medical care requires the transmission of that information. As part of their broader societal responsibilities, physicians should encourage patients to participate in ethical and properly approved clinical investigations if these studies do not impose undue hazard, discomfort, or inconvenience. However, physicians engaged in clinical research must be alert to potential conflicts of interest between their research goals and their obligations to individual patients. The best interests of the patient must always take priority.

To wrest from nature the secrets which have perplexed philosophers in all ages, to track to their sources the causes of disease, to correlate the vast stores of knowledge, that they may be quickly available for the prevention and cure of disease—these are our ambitions.

—William Osler, 1849–1919

2 Global Issues in Medicine

Paul Farmer, Joseph Rhatigan

WHY GLOBAL HEALTH?

Global health is not a discipline; it is, rather, a collection of problems. Some scholars have defined global health as the field of study and practice concerned with improving the health of all people and achieving health equity worldwide, with an emphasis on addressing transnational problems. No single review can do much more than identify the leading problems in applying evidence-based medicine in settings of great poverty or across national boundaries. However, this is a moment of opportunity: only recently, persistent epidemics, improved metrics, and growing interest have been matched by an unprecedented investment in addressing the health problems of poor people in the developing world. To ensure that this opportunity is not wasted, the facts need to be laid out for specialists and laypeople alike. This chapter introduces the major international bodies that address health problems; identifies the more significant barriers to improving the health of people who to date have not, by and large, had access to modern medicine; and summarizes population-based data on the most common health problems faced by people living in poverty. Examining specific problems—notably HIV/AIDS (Chap. 226) but also tuberculosis (TB, Chap. 202), malaria (Chap. 248), and key "noncommunicable" chronic diseases (NCDs)—helps sharpen the discussion of barriers to prevention, diagnosis, and care as well as the means of overcoming them. This chapter closes by discussing global health equity, drawing on notions of social justice that once were central to international public health but had fallen out of favor during the last decades of the twentieth century.

A BRIEF HISTORY OF GLOBAL HEALTH INSTITUTIONS

Concern about health across national boundaries dates back many centuries, predating the Black Plague and other pandemics. One of the first organizations founded explicitly to tackle cross-border health issues was the Pan American Sanitary Bureau, which was formed in 1902 by 11 countries in the Americas. The primary goal of what later became the Pan American Health Organization was the control of infectious diseases across the Americas. Of special concern was yellow fever, which had been running a deadly course through much of South and Central America and halted the construction of the Panama Canal. In 1948, the United Nations formed the first truly global health institution: the World Health Organization (WHO). In 1958, under the aegis of the WHO and in line with a long-standing focus on communicable diseases that cross borders, leaders in global health initiated the effort that led to what some see as the greatest success in international health: the eradication of smallpox. Naysayers were surprised when the smallpox eradication campaign, which engaged public health officials throughout the world, proved successful in 1979 despite the ongoing Cold War.

At the International Conference on Primary Health Care in Alma-Ata (in what is now Kazakhstan) in 1978, public health officials from around the world agreed on a commitment to "Health for All by the Year 2000," a goal to be achieved by providing universal access to primary health care worldwide. Critics argued that the attainment of this goal by the proposed date was impossible. In the ensuing years, a strategy for the provision of selective primary health care emerged that included four inexpensive interventions collectively known as GOBI: *g*rowth monitoring, *o*ral rehydration, *b*reast-feeding, and *i*mmunizations for diphtheria, whooping cough, tetanus, polio, TB, and measles. GOBI later was expanded to GOBI-FFF, which also included *f*emale education, *f*ood, and *f*amily planning. Some public health figures saw GOBI-FFF as an interim strategy to achieve "health for all," but others criticized it as a retreat from the bolder commitments of Alma-Ata.

The influence of the WHO waned during the 1980s. In the early 1990s, many observers argued that, with its vastly superior financial resources and its close—if unequal—relationships with the governments of poor countries, the World Bank had eclipsed the WHO as the most important multilateral institution working in the area of health. One of the stated goals of the World Bank was to help poor countries identify "cost-effective" interventions worthy of public funding and international support. At the same time, the World Bank encouraged many of those nations to reduce public expenditures in health and education in order to stimulate economic growth as part of (later discredited) structural adjustment programs whose restrictions were imposed as a condition for access to credit and assistance through international financial institutions such as the World Bank and the International Monetary Fund. There was a resurgence of many diseases, including malaria, trypanosomiasis, and schistosomiasis, in Africa. TB, an eminently curable disease, remained the world's leading infectious killer of adults. Half a million women per year died in childbirth during the last decade of the twentieth century, and few of the world's largest philanthropic or funding institutions focused on global health equity.

HIV/AIDS, first described in 1981, precipitated a change. In the United States, the advent of this newly described infectious killer marked the culmination of a series of events that discredited talk of "closing the book" on infectious diseases. In Africa, which would emerge as the global epicenter of the pandemic, HIV disease strained TB control programs, and malaria continued to take as many lives as ever. At the dawn of the twenty-first century, these three diseases alone killed nearly 6 million people each year. New research, new policies, and new funding mechanisms were called for. The past decade has seen the rise of important multilateral global health financing institutions such as the Global Fund to Fight AIDS, Tuberculosis, and Malaria; bilateral efforts such as the U.S. President's Emergency Plan for AIDS Relief (PEPFAR); and private philanthropic organizations such as the Bill & Melinda Gates Foundation. With its 193 member states and 147 country offices, the WHO remains important in matters relating to the cross-border spread of infectious diseases and other health threats. In the aftermath of the epidemic of severe acute respiratory syndrome in 2003, the WHO's International Health Regulations—which provide a legal foundation for that organization's direct investigation into a wide range of global health problems, including pandemic influenza, in any member state—were strengthened and brought into force in May 2007.

Even as attention to and resources for health problems in poor countries grow, the lack of coherence in and among global health institutions may undermine efforts to forge a more comprehensive and effective response. The WHO remains underfunded despite the ever-growing need to engage a wider and more complex range of health issues. In another instance of the paradoxical impact of success, the rapid growth of the Gates Foundation, which is one of the most important developments in the history of global health, has led some foundations to question the wisdom of continuing to invest their more modest resources in this field. This indeed may be what some have called "the golden age of global health," but leaders of major organizations such as the WHO, the Global Fund, the United Nations Children's Fund (UNICEF), the Joint United Nations Programme on HIV/AIDS (UNAIDS), PEPFAR, and the Gates Foundation must work together to design an effective architecture that will make the most of opportunities to link new resources for and commitments to global health equity with the emerging understanding of disease burden and unmet need. To this end, new and old players in global health must invest heavily in *discovery* (relevant basic science), *development* of new tools (preventive, diagnostic, and therapeutic), and modes of *delivery* that will ensure the equitable provision of health products and services to all who need them.

THE ECONOMICS OF GLOBAL HEALTH

Political and economic concerns have often guided global health interventions. As mentioned, early efforts to control yellow fever were tied to the completion of the Panama Canal. However, the precise nature of the link between economics and health remains a matter for debate. Some economists and demographers argue that improving the health status of populations must begin with economic development; others maintain that addressing ill health is the starting point for development in poor countries. In either case, investment in health care, especially the control of communicable diseases, should lead to increased productivity. The question is where to find the necessary resources to start the predicted "virtuous cycle."

During the past two decades, spending on health in poor countries has increased dramatically. According to a study from the Institute for Health Metrics and Evaluation (IHME) at the University of Washington, total development assistance for health worldwide grew to $28.2 billion in 2010—up from $5.6 billion in 1990. In 2010, the leading contributors included U.S. bilateral agencies such as PEPFAR, the Global Fund, nongovernmental organizations (NGOs), the WHO, the World Bank, and the Gates Foundation. It appears, however, that total development assistance for health plateaued in 2010, and it is unclear whether growth will continue in the upcoming decade.

To reach the United Nations Millennium Development Goals, which include targets for poverty reduction, universal primary education, and gender equality, spending in the health sector must be increased above the 2010 levels. To determine by how much and for how long, it is imperative to improve the ability to assess the global burden of disease and to plan interventions that more precisely match need.

MORTALITY AND THE GLOBAL BURDEN OF DISEASE

Refining metrics is an important task for global health: only recently have there been solid assessments of the global burden of disease. The first study to look seriously at this issue, conducted in 1990, laid the foundation for the first report on *Disease Control Priorities in Developing Countries* and for the World Bank's 1993 World Development Report *Investing in Health*. Those efforts represented a major advance in the understanding of health status in developing countries. *Investing in Health* has been especially influential: it familiarized a broad audience with cost-effectiveness analysis for specific health interventions and with the notion of disability-adjusted life years (DALYs). The DALY, which has become a standard measure of the impact of a specific health condition on a population, combines absolute years of life lost and years lost due to disability for incident cases of a condition. (See Fig. 2-1 and Table 2-1 for an analysis of the global disease burden by DALYs.)

In 2012, the IHME and partner institutions began publishing results from the Global Burden of Diseases, Injuries, and Risk Factors Study 2010 (GBD 2010). GBD 2010 is the most comprehensive effort to date to produce longitudinal, globally complete, and comparable estimates of the burden of diseases, injuries, and risk factors. This report reflects the expansion of the available data on health in the poorest countries and of the capacity to quantify the impact of specific conditions on a population. It measures current levels and recent trends in all major diseases, injuries, and risk factors among 21 regions and for 20 age groups and both sexes. The GBD 2010 team revised and improved the health-state severity weight system, collated published data, and used household surveys to enhance the breadth and accuracy of disease burden data. As analytic methods and data quality improve, important trends can be identified in a comparison of global disease burden estimates from 1990 to 2010.

GLOBAL MORTALITY

Of the 52.8 million deaths worldwide in 2010, 24.6% (13 million) were due to communicable diseases, maternal and perinatal conditions, and nutritional deficiencies—a marked decrease compared with figures for 1990, when these conditions accounted for 34% of global mortality. Among the fraction of all deaths related to communicable diseases, maternal and perinatal conditions, and nutritional deficiencies, 76% occurred in sub-Saharan Africa and southern Asia. While the proportion of deaths due to these conditions has decreased significantly in the past decade, there has been a dramatic rise in the number of deaths from NCDs, which constituted the top five causes of death in 2010. The leading cause of death among adults in 2010 was ischemic heart disease, accounting for 7.3 million deaths (13.8% of total deaths) worldwide. In high-income countries ischemic heart disease accounted for 17.9% of total deaths, and in developing (low- and middle-income) countries it accounted for 10.1%. It is noteworthy that ischemic heart disease was responsible for just 2.6% of total deaths in sub-Saharan Africa (Table 2-2). In second place—causing 11.1% of global mortality—was cerebrovascular disease, which accounted for 9.9% of deaths in high-income countries, 10.5% in developing countries, and 4.0% in sub-Saharan Africa. Although the third leading cause of death in high-income countries was lung cancer (accounting for 5.6% of all deaths), this condition did not figure among the top 10 causes in low- and middle-income countries. Among the 10 leading causes of death in sub-Saharan Africa, 6 were infectious diseases, with malaria and HIV/AIDS ranking as the dominant contributors to disease burden. In high-income countries, however, only one infectious disease—lower respiratory infection—ranked among the top 10 causes of death.

The GBD 2010 found that the worldwide mortality figure among children <5 years of age dropped from 16.39 million in 1970 to 11.9 million in 1990 and to 6.8 million in 2010—a decrease that surpassed predictions. Of childhood deaths in 2010, 3.1 million (40%) occurred in the neonatal period. About one-third of deaths among children <5 years old occurred in southern Asia and almost one-half in sub-Saharan Africa; <1% occurred in high-income countries.

The global burden of death due to HIV/AIDS and malaria was on an upward slope until 2004; significant improvements have since been documented. Global deaths from HIV infection fell from 1.7 million in 2006 to 1.5 million in 2010, while malaria deaths dropped from 1.2 million to 0.98 million over the same period. Despite these improvements, malaria and HIV/AIDS continue to be major burdens in particular regions, with global implications. Although it has a minor impact on mortality outside sub-Saharan Africa and Southeast Asia, malaria is the eleventh leading cause of death worldwide. HIV infection ranked thirty-third in global DALYs in 1990 but was the fifth leading cause of disease burden in 2010, with sub-Saharan Africa bearing the vast majority of this burden (Fig. 2-1).

The world's population is living longer: global life expectancy has increased significantly over the past 40 years from 58.8 years in 1970 to 70.4 years in 2010. This demographic change, accompanied by the fact that the prevalence of NCDs increases with age, is dramatically shifting the burden of disease toward NCDs, which have surpassed communicable, maternal, nutritional, and neonatal causes. By 2010, 65.5% of total deaths at all ages and 54% of all DALYs were due to NCDs. Increasingly, the global burden of disease comprises conditions and injuries that cause disability rather than death.

Worldwide, although both life expectancy and years of life lived in good health have risen, years of life lived with disability have also increased. Despite the higher prevalence of diseases common in older populations (e.g., dementia and musculoskeletal disease) in developed and high-income countries, best estimates from 2010 reveal that disability resulting from cardiovascular diseases, chronic respiratory diseases, and the long-term impact of communicable diseases was greater in low- and middle-income countries. In most developing countries, people lived shorter lives and experienced disability and poor health for a greater proportion of their lives. Indeed, 50% of the global burden of disease occurred in southern Asia and sub-Saharan Africa, which together account for only 35% of the world's population.

HEALTH AND WEALTH

Clear disparities in burden of disease (both communicable and noncommunicable) across country income levels are strong indicators that poverty and health are inherently linked. Poverty remains one of the most important root causes of poor health worldwide, and the global burden of poverty continues to be high. Among the 6.7 billion people alive in 2008, 19% (1.29 billion) lived on less than $1.25 a day—one standard measurement of extreme poverty—and another 1.18 billion lived on $1.25 to $2 a day. Approximately 600 million children—more than 30% of those in low-income countries—lived in extreme poverty in 2005. Comparison of national health indicators with gross domestic product per capita among nations shows a clear relationship between higher gross domestic product and better health, with only a few outliers. Numerous studies have also documented the link between poverty and health within nations as well as across them.

RISK FACTORS FOR DISEASE BURDEN

The GBD 2010 study found that the three leading risk factors for global disease burden in 2010 were (in order of frequency) high blood pressure, tobacco smoking (including secondhand smoke), and alcohol use—a substantial change from 1990, when childhood undernutrition was ranked first. Though ranking eighth in 2010, childhood undernutrition remains the leading risk factor for death worldwide among children <5 years of age. In an era that has seen obesity become a major health concern in many developed countries—and the sixth leading risk factor worldwide—the persistence of undernutrition is surely cause for great consternation. Low body weight is still the dominant risk factor for disease burden in sub-Saharan Africa. Inability to feed the hungry reflects many years of failed development projects and must be addressed as a problem of the highest priority. Indeed, no health care initiative, however generously funded, will be effective without adequate nutrition.

In a 2006 publication that examined how specific diseases and injuries are affected by environmental risk, the WHO estimated that roughly one-quarter of the total global burden of disease, one-third of the global disease burden among children, and 23% of all deaths were due to modifiable environmental factors. Many of these factors lead to deaths from infectious diseases; others lead to deaths

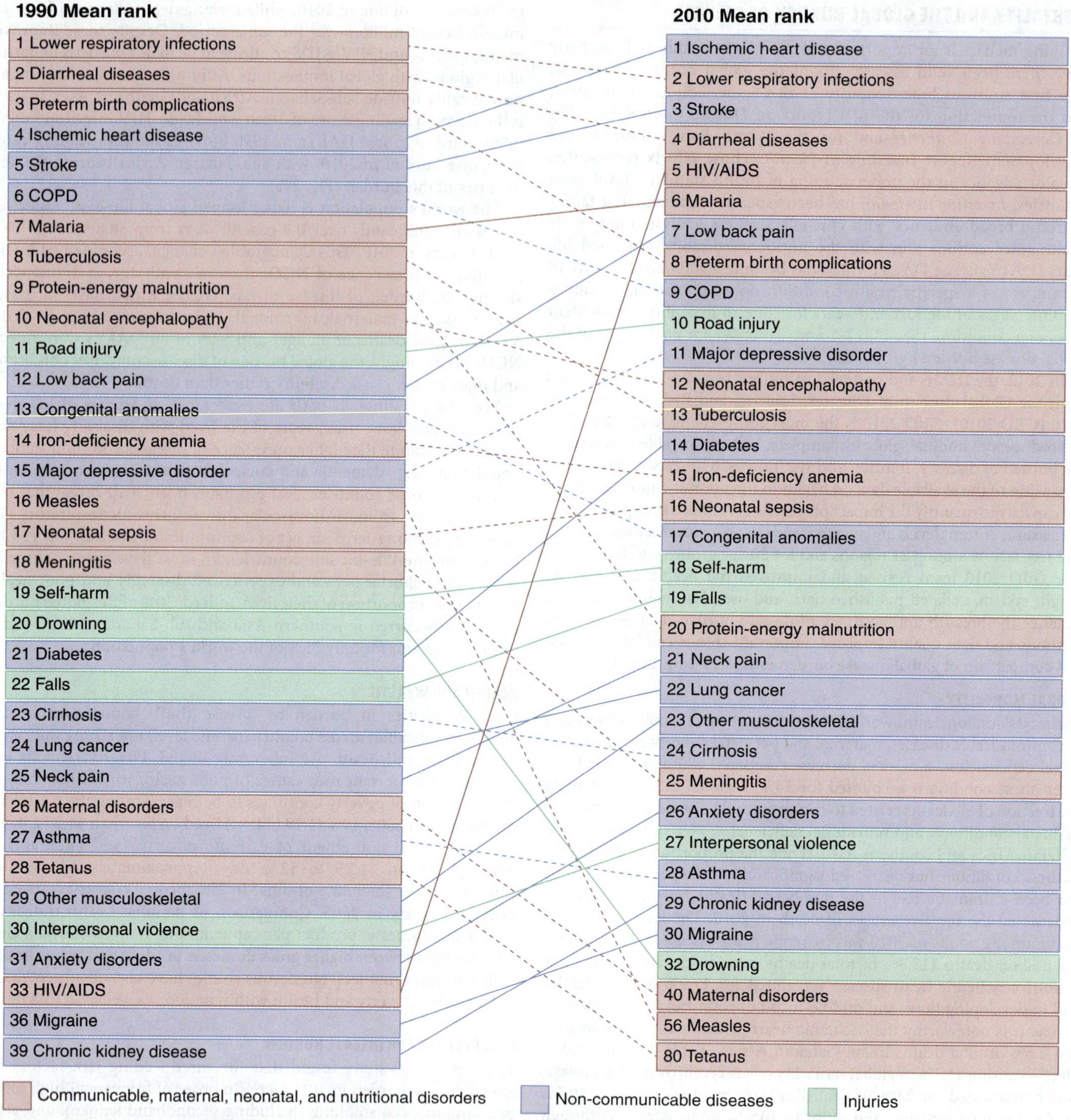

FIGURE 2-1 Global DALY (disability-adjusted life year) ranks for the top causes of disease burden in 1990 and 2010. COPD, chronic obstructive pulmonary disease. *(Reproduced with permission from C Murray et al: Disability-adjusted life years [DALYs] for 291 diseases and injuries in 21 regions, 1990–2010: A systematic analysis for the Global Burden of Disease Study 2010. Lancet 380:2197–2223, 2012.)*

from malignancies. Etiology and nosology are increasingly difficult to parse. As much as 94% of diarrheal disease, which is linked to unsafe drinking water and poor sanitation, can be attributed to environmental factors. Risk factors such as indoor air pollution due to use of solid fuels, exposure to secondhand tobacco smoke, and outdoor air pollution account for 20% of lower respiratory infections in developed countries and for as many as 42% of such infections in developing countries. Various forms of unintentional injury and malaria top the list of health problems to which environmental factors contribute. Some 4 million children die every year from causes related to unhealthy environments, and the number of infant deaths due to environmental factors in developing countries is 12 times that in developed countries.

The second edition of *Disease Control Priorities in Developing Countries*, published in 2006, is a document of great breadth and ambition, providing cost-effectiveness analyses for more than 100 interventions and including 21 chapters focused on strategies for strengthening health systems. Cost-effectiveness analyses that compare relatively equivalent interventions and facilitate the best choices under constraint are necessary; however, these analyses are often based on an incomplete knowledge of cost and evolving evidence of effectiveness. As both resources and objectives for global health grow, cost-effectiveness analyses (particularly those based on older evidence) must not hobble the increased worldwide commitment to providing resources and accessible health care services to all who need them. This is why we use the term *global health equity*. To illustrate these points, it

TABLE 2-1 LEADING CAUSES OF DISEASE BURDEN, 2010

Disease or Injury	DALYs (Millions)	Percent of Total DALYs	Disease or Injury	DALYs (Millions)	Percent of Total DALYs
World			**High-income countries**[b]		
1 Ischemic heart disease	129.8	5.2	1 Ischemic heart disease	21.8	8.2
2 Lower respiratory infections	115.2	4.7	2 Low back pain	17.0	6.4
3 Cerebrovascular disease	102.2	4.1	3 Cerebrovascular disease	11.3	4.2
4 Diarrheal disease	89.5	3.6	4 Major depressive disorder	9.7	3.7
5 HIV/AIDS	81.5	3.3	5 Lung cancer	9.2	3.5
6 Malaria	82.7	3.3	6 COPD	8.6	3.2
7 Low back pain	80.7	3.2	7 Other musculoskeletal disorders	8.2	3.1
8 Preterm birth complications	77.0	3.1	8 Diabetes mellitus	7.3	2.8
9 COPD	76.8	3.1	9 Neck pain	7.2	2.7
10 Road injury	75.5	3.1	10 Falls	6.8	2.5
Developing countries[a]			**Sub-Saharan Africa**		
1 Lower respiratory infections	109.0	5.2	1 Malaria	76.6	13.3
2 Diarrheal disease	88.0	4.2	2 HIV/AIDS	57.8	10.1
3 Ischemic heart disease	85.5	4.1	3 Lower respiratory infections	43.5	7.6
4 Malaria	82.7	3.9	4 Diarrheal diseases	39.2	6.8
5 Cerebrovascular disease	79.4	3.8	5 Protein-energy malnutrition	22.3	3.9
6 HIV/AIDS	77.0	3.7	6 Preterm birth complications	20.0	3.5
7 Preterm birth complications	74.4	3.5	7 Neonatal sepsis	18.9	3.3
8 Road injury	66.2	3.2	8 Meningitis	16.3	2.8
9 COPD	65.6	3.1	9 Neonatal encephalopathy	14.9	2.6
10 Low back pain	58.4	2.8	10 Road injury	13.9	2.5

[a]The term *developing countries* refers to low- and middle-income economies. See *data.worldbank.org/about/country-classifications.* [b]The World Bank classifies high-income countries as those whose gross national income per capita is $12,476 or more. See *data.worldbank.org/about/country-classifications.*

Abbreviations: COPD, chronic obstructive pulmonary disease; DALYs, disability-adjusted life years.

Source: Institute for Health Metrics and Evaluation, University of Washington (2013). Data are available through *www.healthmetricsandevaluation.org/gbd/visualizations/country.*

TABLE 2-2 LEADING CAUSES OF DEATH WORLDWIDE, 2010

Disease or Injury	Deaths (Millions)	Percent of Total Deaths	Disease or Injury	Deaths (Millions)	Percent of Total Deaths
World			**High-income countries**[b]		
1 Ischemic heart disease	7.3	13.3	1 Ischemic heart disease	1.6	17.9
2 Cerebrovascular disease	5.9	11.1	2 Cerebrovascular disease	0.9	9.9
3 COPD	2.9	5.5	3 Lung cancer	0.5	5.6
4 Lower respiratory infections	2.8	5.3	4 Lower respiratory infections	0.4	4.7
5 Lung cancer	1.5	2.9	5 COPD	0.4	4.5
6 HIV/AIDS	1.5	2.8	6 Alzheimer's and other dementias	0.4	4.0
7 Diarrheal diseases	1.4	2.7	7 Colon and rectum cancers	0.3	3.3
8 Road injury	1.3	2.5	8 Diabetes	0.2	2.6
9 Diabetes	1.3	2.4	9 Other cardiovascular and circulatory diseases	0.2	2.5
10 Tuberculosis	1.2	2.3	10 Chronic kidney disease	0.2	2.0
Developing countries[a]			**Sub-Saharan Africa**		
1 Cerebrovascular disease	4.2	10.5	1 Malaria	1.1	12.7
2 Ischemic heart disease	4.0	10.1	2 HIV/AIDS	1.0	12.0
3 COPD	2.4	6.1	3 Lower respiratory infections	0.8	9.3
4 Lower respiratory infections	2.3	5.9	4 Diarrheal diseases	0.5	6.6
5 Diarrheal diseases	1.4	3.6	5 Cerebrovascular disease	0.3	4.0
6 HIV/AIDS	1.4	3.4	6 Protein-energy malnutrition	0.3	4.0
7 Malaria	1.2	2.9	7 Tuberculosis	0.3	3.6
8 Road injury	1.2	2.9	8 Road injury	0.2	2.8
9 Tuberculosis	1.1	2.9	9 Preterm birth complications	0.2	2.8
10 Diabetes	1.0	2.6	10 Meningitis	0.2	2.6

[a]The term *developing countries* refers to low- and middle-income economies. See *data.worldbank.org/about/country-classifications.* [b]The World Bank classifies high-income countries as those whose gross national income per capita is $12,476 or more. See *data.worldbank.org/about/country-classifications.*

Abbreviation: COPD, chronic obstructive pulmonary disease.

Source: Institute for Health Metrics and Evaluation, University of Washington (2013). Data available through *www.healthmetricsandevaluation.org/gbd/visualizations/country.*

is instructive to look to HIV/AIDS, which in the course of the last three decades has become the world's leading infectious cause of adult death.

HIV INFECTION/AIDS

Chapter 226 provides an overview of the HIV epidemic in the world today. Here the discussion will be limited to HIV/AIDS in the developing world. Lessons learned from tackling HIV/AIDS in resource-constrained settings are highly relevant to discussions of other chronic diseases, including NCDs, for which effective therapies have been developed.

Approximately 34 million people in all countries worldwide were living with HIV infection in 2011; more than 8 million of those in low- and middle-income countries were receiving antiretroviral therapy (ART)—a number representing a 20-fold increase over the corresponding figure for 2003. By the end of 2011, 54% of people eligible for treatment were receiving ART. (It remains to be seen how many of these people are receiving ART regularly and with the requisite social support.)

In the United States, the availability of ART has transformed HIV/AIDS from an inescapably fatal destruction of cell-mediated immunity into a manageable chronic illness. In high-income countries, improved ART has prolonged life by an estimated average of 35 years per patient—up from 6.8 years in 1993 and 24 years in 2006. This success rate exceeds that obtained with almost any treatment for adulthood cancer or for complications of coronary artery disease. In developing countries, treatment has been offered broadly only since 2003, and only in 2009 did the number of patients receiving treatment exceed 40% of the number who needed it. Before 2003, many arguments were raised to justify not moving forward rapidly with ART programs for people living with HIV/AIDS in resource-limited settings. The standard litany included the price of therapy compared with the poverty of the patient, the complexity of the intervention, the lack of infrastructure for laboratory monitoring, and the lack of trained health care providers. Narrow cost-effectiveness arguments that created false dichotomies—prevention *or* treatment rather than both—too often went unchallenged. As a cumulative result of these delays in the face of health disparities, old and new, there were millions of premature deaths.

Disparities in access to HIV treatment gave rise to widespread moral indignation and a new type of health activism. In several middle-income countries, including Brazil, public programs have helped bridge the access gap. Other innovative projects pioneered by international NGOs in diverse settings such as Haiti and Rwanda have established that a simple approach to ART that is based on intensive community engagement and support can achieve remarkable results (Fig. 2-2).

During the past decade, the availability of ART has increased sharply in the low- and middle-income countries that have borne the greatest burden of the HIV/AIDS pandemic. In 2000, very few people living with HIV/AIDS in these nations had access to ART, whereas by 2011, as stated above, 8 million people, a majority of those deemed eligible, in these countries were receiving ART. This scale-up was made possible by a number of developments: a staggering drop in the cost of ART, the development of a standardized approach to treatment, substantial investments by funders, and the political commitment of governments to make ART available. Civil-society AIDS activists spurred many of these efforts.

Starting in the early 2000s, a combination of factors, including work by the Clinton Foundation HIV/AIDS Initiative and Médecins Sans Frontières, led to the availability of generic ART medications. While first-line ART cost more than $10,000 per patient per year in 2000, first-line regimens in low- and middle-income countries are now available for less than $100 per year. At the same time, fixed-dose combination drugs that are easier to administer have become more widely available.

Also around this time, the WHO began advocating a public health approach to the treatment of people with AIDS in resource-limited settings. This approach, derived from models of care pioneered by the NGO Partners In Health and other groups, proposed standard first-line treatment regimens based on a simple five-drug formulary, with a more complex (and more expensive) set of second-line options in reserve. Clinical protocols were standardized, and intensive training packages for health professionals and community health workers were developed and implemented in many countries. These efforts were supported by new funding from the World Bank, the Global Fund, and PEPFAR. In 2003, lack of access to ART was declared a global public health emergency by the WHO and UNAIDS, and those two agencies launched the "3 by 5 initiative," setting an ambitious target: to have 3 million people in developing countries on treatment by the end of 2005. Worldwide funding for HIV/AIDS treatment increased dramatically during this period, rising from $300 million in 1996 to over $15 billion in 2010.

Many countries set corresponding national targets and have worked to integrate ART into their national AIDS programs and health systems and to harness the synergies between HIV/AIDS treatment and prevention activities. Further lessons with implications for policy and action have come from efforts now under way among lower-income countries. Rwanda provides an example: Over the past decade, mortality from HIV disease has fallen by >78% as the country—despite its relatively low gross national income (Fig. 2-3)—has provided almost universal access to ART. The reasons for this success include strong national leadership, evidence-based policy, cross-sector collaboration, community-based care, and a deliberate focus on a health system approach that embeds HIV/AIDS treatment and prevention in the primary health care service delivery platform. As we will discuss later in this chapter, these principles can be applied to other conditions, including NCDs.

TUBERCULOSIS

Chapter 202 provides a concise overview of the pathophysiology and treatment of TB. In 2011, an estimated 12 million people were living with active TB, and 1.4 million died from it. The disease is closely linked to HIV infection in much of the world: of the 8.7 million estimated new cases of TB in 2011, 1.2 million occurred among people living with HIV. Indeed, a substantial proportion of the TB resurgence

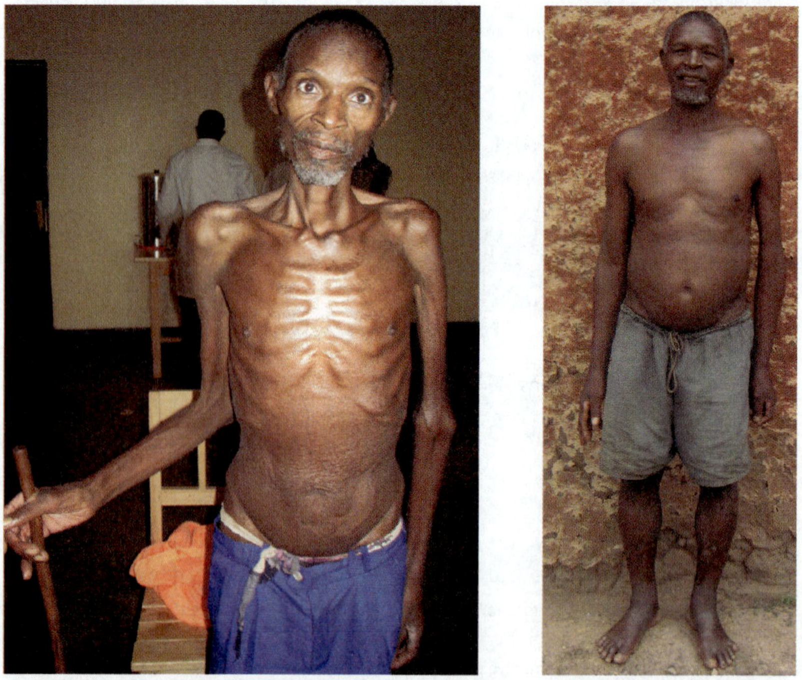

FIGURE 2-2 An HIV/TB-co-infected patient in Rwanda before (***left***) and after (***right***) 6 months of treatment.

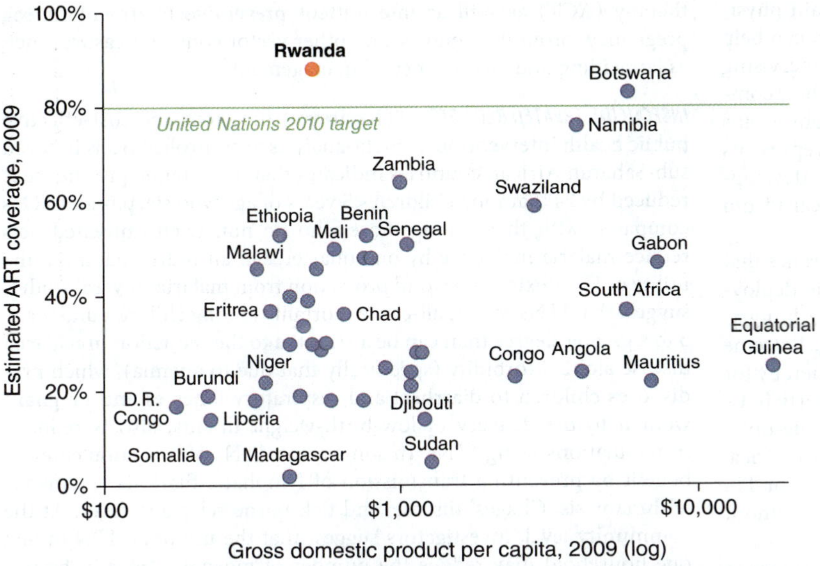

FIGURE 2-3 Antiretroviral therapy (ART) coverage in sub-Saharan Africa, 2009.

registered in southern Africa is attributed to HIV co-infection. Even before the advent of HIV, however, it was estimated that fewer than one-half of all cases of TB in developing countries were ever diagnosed, much less treated. Primarily because of the common failure to diagnose and treat TB, international authorities devised a single strategy to reduce the burden of disease. In the early 1990s, the World Bank, the WHO, and other international bodies promoted the DOTS strategy (*d*irectly *o*bserved *t*herapy using *s*hort-course isoniazid- and rifampin-based regimens) as highly cost-effective. Passive case-finding of smear-positive patients was central to the strategy, and an uninterrupted drug supply was, of course, deemed necessary for cure.

DOTS was clearly effective for most uncomplicated cases of drug-susceptible TB, but a number of shortcomings were soon identified. First, the diagnosis of TB based solely on sputum smear microscopy—a method dating from the late nineteenth century—is not sensitive. Many cases of pulmonary TB and all cases of exclusively extrapulmonary TB are missed by smear microscopy, as are most cases of active disease in children. Second, passive case-finding relies on the availability of health care services, which is uneven in the settings where TB is most prevalent. Third, patients with multidrug-resistant TB (MDR-TB) are by definition infected with strains of *Mycobacterium tuberculosis* resistant to isoniazid and rifampin; thus exclusive reliance on these drugs is unwarranted in settings in which drug resistance is an established problem.

The crisis of antibiotic resistance registered in U.S. hospitals is not confined to the industrialized world or to common bacterial infections. The great majority of patients sick with and dying from TB are afflicted with strains susceptible to all first-line drugs. In some settings, however, a substantial minority of patients with TB are infected with *M. tuberculosis* strains resistant to at least one first-line anti-TB drug. A 2012 article in a leading journal reported that, in China, 10% of all patients with TB and 26% of all previously treated patients were sick with MDR strains of *M. tuberculosis*. Most of these cases were the result of primary transmission. To improve DOTS-based responses to MDR-TB, global health authorities adopted DOTS-Plus, which adds the diagnostics and drugs necessary to manage drug-resistant disease. Even as DOTS-Plus was being piloted in resource-constrained settings, however, new strains of extensively drug-resistant (XDR) *M. tuberculosis* (resistant to isoniazid and rifampin, any fluoroquinolone, and at least one injectable second-line drug) had already threatened the success of TB control programs in beleaguered South Africa, for example, where high rates of HIV infection have led to a doubling of TB incidence over the last decade. Despite the poor capacity for detection of MDR- and XDR-TB in most resource-limited settings, an estimated 630,000 cases of MDR-TB were thought to occur in 2011. Approximately 9% of these drug-resistant cases were caused by XDR strains. It is clear that poor infection control in hospitals and clinics is associated with explosive and lethal epidemics due to these strains and that patients may be infected with multiple strains.

TUBERCULOSIS AND AIDS AS CHRONIC DISEASES: LESSONS LEARNED

Strategies effective against MDR-TB have implications for the management of drug-resistant HIV infection and even drug-resistant malaria, which, through repeated infections and a lack of effective therapy, has become a chronic disease in parts of Africa (see "Malaria," below). As new therapies, whether for TB or for hepatitis C infection, become available, many of the problems encountered in the past will recur. Indeed, examining AIDS and TB as chronic diseases—instead of simply communicable diseases—makes it possible to draw a number of conclusions, many of them pertinent to global health in general.

First, the chronic infections discussed here are best treated with multidrug regimens to which the infecting strains are susceptible. This is true of chronic infections due to many bacteria, fungi, parasites, or viruses; even acute infections such as those caused by *Plasmodium* species are not reliably treated with a single drug.

Second, charging fees for AIDS prevention and care poses insurmountable problems for people living in poverty, many of whom are unable to pay even modest amounts for services or medications. Like efforts to battle airborne TB, such services might best be seen as a *public good* promoting public health. Initially, a subsidy approach will require sustained donor contributions, but many African countries have set targets for increased national investments in health—a pledge that could render ambitious programs sustainable in the long run, as the Rwanda experience suggests. Meanwhile, as local investments increase, the price of AIDS care is decreasing. The development of generic medications means that ART can now cost <$0.25 per day; costs continue to decrease.

Third, the effective scale-up of pilot projects requires strengthening and sometimes rebuilding of health care systems, including those charged with delivering primary care. In the past, the lack of health care infrastructure has been cited as a barrier to providing ART in the world's poorest regions; however, AIDS resources, which are at last considerable, may be marshaled to rebuild public health systems in sub-Saharan Africa and other HIV-burdened regions—precisely the settings in which TB is resurgent.

Fourth, the lack of trained health care personnel, most notably doctors and nurses, in resource-poor settings must be addressed. This personnel deficiency is invoked as a reason for the failure to treat AIDS in poor countries. In what is termed the *brain drain*, many physicians and nurses emigrate from their home countries to pursue opportunities abroad, leaving behind health systems that are understaffed and ill equipped to deal with the epidemic diseases that ravage local populations. The WHO recommends a minimum of 20 physicians and 100 nurses per 100,000 persons, but recent reports from that organization and others confirm that many countries, especially in sub-Saharan Africa, fall far short of those target numbers. Specifically, more than one-half of those countries register fewer than 10 physicians per 100,000 population. In contrast, the United States and Cuba register 279 and 596 doctors per 100,000 population, respectively. Similarly, the majority of sub-Saharan African countries do not have even half of the WHO-recommended minimum number of nurses. Further inequalities in health care staffing exist *within* countries. Rural–urban disparities in health care personnel mirror disparities of both wealth and health. For instance, nearly 90% of Malawi's population lives in rural areas, but more than 95% of clinical officers work at urban facilities, and 47% of nurses work at tertiary care facilities. Even community health workers trained to provide first-line services to rural populations often transfer to urban districts.

One reason doctors and nurses leave sub-Saharan Africa and other resource-poor areas is that they lack the tools to practice their trade there. Funding for "vertical" (disease-specific) programs can be used not only to strengthen health systems but to recruit and train physicians and nurses to underserved regions where they, in turn, can help to train and then work with community health workers in supervising care for patients with AIDS and many other diseases within their communities. Such training should be undertaken even where physicians are abundant, since close community-based supervision represents the highest standard of care for chronic disease, whether in developing or developed countries. The United States has much to learn from Rwanda.

Fifth, the barriers to adequate health care and patient adherence that are raised by extreme poverty can be removed only with the deployment of "wrap-around services": food supplements for the hungry, help with transportation to clinics, child care, and housing. Extreme poverty makes it difficult for many patients to comply with therapy for chronic diseases, whether communicable or not. Indeed, poverty in its many dimensions is far and away the greatest barrier to the scale-up of treatment and prevention programs. In many rural regions of Africa, hunger is the major coexisting condition in patients with AIDS or TB, and those consumptive diseases cannot be treated effectively without adequate caloric intake.

Finally, there is a need for a renewed basic-science commitment to the discovery and development of vaccines; more reliable, less expensive diagnostic tools; and new classes of therapeutic agents. This need applies not only to the three leading infectious killers—against none of which is there an effective vaccine—but also to most other neglected diseases of poverty.

MALARIA

Chapter 248 reviews the etiology, pathogenesis, and clinical treatment of malaria, the world's third-ranking infectious killer. Malaria's human cost is enormous, with the highest toll among children—especially African children—living in poverty. In 2010, there were ~219 million cases of malaria, and the disease is thought to have killed 660,000 people; 86% of these deaths (~568,000) occurred among children <5 years old. The poor disproportionately experience the burden of malaria: more than 80% of estimated malaria deaths occur in just 14 countries, and mortality rates are highest in sub-Saharan Africa. The Democratic Republic of the Congo and Nigeria account for more than 40% of total estimated malaria deaths globally.

Microeconomic analyses focusing on direct and indirect costs estimate that malaria may consume >10% of a household's annual income. A study in rural Kenya shows that mean direct-cost burdens vary between the wet and dry seasons (7.1% and 5.9% of total household expenditure, respectively) and that this proportion is >10% in the poorest households in both seasons. A Ghanaian study that categorized the population by income group highlighted the regressive nature of this cost: responding to malaria consumed only 1% of a wealthy family's income but 34% of a poor household's income.

Macroeconomic analyses estimate that malaria may reduce the per capita gross national product of a disease-endemic country by 50% relative to that of a non-malaria-endemic country. The causes of this drag include impaired cognitive development of children, decreased schooling, decreased savings, decreased foreign investment, and restriction of worker mobility. In light of this enormous cost, it is little wonder that an important review by the economists Sachs and Malaney concludes that "where malaria prospers most, human societies have prospered least."

Rolling Back Malaria In part because of differences in vector distribution and climate, resource-rich countries offer few blueprints for malaria control and treatment that are applicable in tropical (and resource-poor) settings. In 2001, African heads of state endorsed the WHO Roll Back Malaria (RBM) campaign, which prescribes strategies appropriate for sub-Saharan African countries. In 2008, the RBM partnership launched the Global Malaria Action Plan (GMAP). This strategy *integrates prevention and care* and calls for an avoidance of single-dose regimens and an awareness of existing drug resistance. The GMAP recommends a number of key tools to reduce malaria-related morbidity and mortality rates: the use of insecticide-treated bed nets (ITNs), indoor residual spraying, and artemisinin-based combination therapy (ACT) as well as intermittent preventive treatment during pregnancy, prompt diagnosis, and other vector control measures such as larviciding and environmental management.

INSECTICIDE-TREATED BED NETS ITNs are an efficacious and cost-effective public health intervention. A meta-analysis of controlled trials in seven sub-Saharan African countries indicates that parasitemia prevalence is reduced by 24% among children <5 years of age who sleep under ITNs compared with that among those who do not. Even untreated nets reduce malaria incidence by one-quarter. On an individual level, the utility of ITNs extends beyond protection from malaria. Several studies suggest that ITNs reduce all-cause mortality among children under age 5 to a greater degree than can be attributed to the reduction in malarial disease alone. Morbidity (specifically that due to anemia), which predisposes children to diarrheal and respiratory illnesses and pregnant women to the delivery of low-birth-weight infants, also is reduced in populations using ITNs. In some areas, ITNs offer a supplemental benefit by preventing transmission of lymphatic filariasis, cutaneous leishmaniasis, Chagas' disease, and tick-borne relapsing fever. At the community level, investigators suggest that the use of an ITN in just one household may reduce the number of mosquito bites in households up to a hundred meters away by reducing mosquito density. The cost of ITNs per DALY saved—estimated at $29—makes ITNs a good-value public health investment.

The WHO recommends that all individuals living in malaria-endemic areas sleep under protective ITNs. About 140 million long-lasting ITNs were distributed in high-burden African countries in 2006–2008, and rates of household ownership of ITNs in high-burden countries increased to 31%. Although the RBM partnership has seen modest success, the WHO's 2009 World Malaria Report states that the percentage of children <5 years of age using an ITN (24%) remains well below the World Health Assembly's target of 80%. Limited success in scaling up ITN coverage reflects the inadequately acknowledged economic barriers that prevent the destitute sick from gaining access to critical preventive technologies and the challenges faced in designing and implementing effective delivery platforms for these products. In other words, this is a *delivery* failure rather than a lack of knowledge of how best to reduce malaria deaths.

INDOOR RESIDUAL SPRAYING Indoor residual spraying is one of the most common interventions for preventing the transmission of malaria in endemic areas. Vector control using insecticides approved by the WHO, including DDT, can effectively reduce or even interrupt malaria transmission. However, studies have indicated that spraying is effective in controlling malaria transmission only if most (~80%) of the structures in the targeted community are treated. Moreover, since a successful program depends on well-trained spraying teams as well as on effective monitoring and planning, indoor residual spraying is difficult to employ and is often reliant on health systems with a strong infrastructure. Regardless of the limitations of indoor residual spraying, the WHO recommends its use in combination with ITNs. Neither intervention alone is sufficient to prevent transmission of malaria entirely.

ARTEMISININ-BASED COMBINATION THERAPY The emergence and spread of chloroquine resistance have increased the need for antimalarial combination therapy. To limit the spread of resistance, the WHO now recommends that only ACT (as opposed to artemisinin monotherapy) be used for uncomplicated falciparum malaria. Like that of other antimalarial interventions, the use of ACT has increased in the last few years, but coverage rates remain very low in several countries in sub-Saharan Africa. The RBM partnership has invested significantly in measures to enhance access to ACT by facilitating its delivery through the public health sector and developing innovative funding mechanisms (e.g., the Affordable Medicines Facility—malaria) that reduce its cost significantly so that ineffective monotherapies can be eliminated from the market.

In the last several years, resistance to antimalarial medicines and insecticides has become an even larger problem than in the past. In 2009, confirmation of artemisinin resistance was reported. Although the WHO has called for an end to the use of artemisinin monotherapy, the marketing of such therapies continues in many countries. Ongoing use of artemisinin monotherapy increases the likelihood of drug resistance, a deadly prospect that will make malaria far more difficult to treat.

Between 2001 and 2011, global malaria deaths were reduced by an estimated 38%, with reductions of ≥50% in 10 African countries as well as in most endemic countries in other regions. Again the experience in Rwanda is instructive: from 2005 to 2011, malaria deaths dropped by >85% for the same reasons mentioned earlier in recounting that nation's successes in battling HIV.

Meeting the challenge of malaria control will continue to require careful study of appropriate preventive and therapeutic strategies in the context of an increasingly sophisticated molecular understanding of pathogen, vector, and host. However, an appreciation of the economic and social devastation wrought by malaria—like that inflicted by diarrhea, AIDS, and TB—on the most vulnerable populations should heighten the level of commitment to critical analysis of ways to implement proven strategies for prevention and treatment.

Funding from the Global Fund, the Gates Foundation, the World Bank's International Development Association, and the U.S. President's Malaria Initiative, along with leadership from public health authorities, is critical to sustain the benefits of prevention and treatment. Building on the growing momentum of the last decade with adequate financial support, innovative strategies, and effective tools for prevention, diagnosis, and treatment, we may one day achieve the goal of a world free of malaria.

"NONCOMMUNICABLE" CHRONIC DISEASES

Although the burden of communicable diseases—especially HIV infection, TB, and malaria—still accounts for the majority of deaths in resource-poor regions such as sub-Saharan Africa, 63% of all deaths worldwide in 2008 were held to be due to NCDs. Although we will use this term to describe cardiovascular diseases, cancers, diabetes, and chronic lung diseases, this usage masks important distinctions. For instance, two significant NCDs in low-income countries, rheumatic heart disease (RHD) and cervical cancer, represent the chronic sequelae of infections with group A *Streptococcus* and human papillomavirus, respectively. It is in these countries that the burden of disease due to NCDs is rising most rapidly. Close to 80% of deaths attributable to NCDs occur in low- and middle-income countries, where 86% of the global population lives. The WHO reports that ~25% of global NCD-related deaths take place before the age of 60—a figure representing ~5.7 million people and exceeding the total number of deaths due to AIDS, TB, and malaria combined. In almost all high-income countries, the WHO reported that NCD deaths accounted for ~70% of total deaths in 2008. By 2020, NCDs will account for 80% of the global burden of disease and for 7 of every 10 deaths in developing countries. The recent increase in resources for and attention to communicable diseases is both welcome and long overdue, but developing countries are already carrying a "double burden" of communicable and noncommunicable diseases.

Diabetes, Cardiovascular Disease, and Cancer: A Global Perspective In contrast to TB, HIV infection, and malaria—diseases caused by single pathogens that damage multiple organs—cardiovascular diseases reflect injury to a single organ system downstream of a variety of insults, both infectious and noninfectious. Some of these insults result from rapid changes in diet and labor conditions.

Other insults are of a less recent vintage. The burden of cardiovascular disease in low-income countries represents one consequence of decades of neglect of health systems. Furthermore, cardiovascular research and investment have long focused on the ischemic conditions that are increasingly common in high- and middle-income countries. Meanwhile, despite awareness of its health impact in the early twentieth century, cardiovascular damage in response to infection and malnutrition has fallen out of view until recently.

The misperception of cardiovascular diseases as a problem primarily of elderly populations in middle- and high-income countries has contributed to the neglect of these diseases by global health institutions. Even in Eastern Europe and Central Asia, where the collapse of the Soviet Union was followed by a catastrophic surge in cardiovascular disease deaths (mortality rates from ischemic heart disease nearly doubled between 1991 and 1994 in Russia, for example), the modest flow of overseas development assistance to the health sector focused on the communicable causes that accounted for <1 in 20 excess deaths during that period.

DIABETES The International Diabetes Federation reports that the number of diabetic patients in the world is expected to increase from 366 million in 2011 to 552 million by 2030. Already, a significant proportion of diabetic patients live in developing countries where, because those affected are far more frequently between ages 40 and 59, the complications of micro- and macrovascular disease take a far greater toll. Globally, these complications are a major cause of disability and reduced quality of life. A high fasting plasma glucose level alone ranks seventh among risks for disability and is the sixth leading risk factor for global mortality. The GBD 2010 estimates that diabetes accounted for 1.28 million deaths in 2010, with almost 80% of those deaths occurring in low- and middle-income countries.

Predictions of an imminent rise in the share of deaths and disabilities due to NCDs in developing countries have led to calls for preventive policies to improve diet, increase exercise, and restrict tobacco use, along with the prescription of multidrug regimens for persons at high-level vascular risk. Although this agenda could do much to prevent pandemic NCD, it will do little to help persons with established heart disease stemming from nonatherogenic pathologies.

CARDIOVASCULAR DISEASE Because systemic investigation of the causes of stroke and heart failure in sub-Saharan Africa has begun only recently, little is known about the impact of elevated blood pressure in this portion of the continent. Modestly elevated blood pressure in the absence of tobacco use in populations with low rates of obesity may confer little risk of adverse events in the short run. In contrast, persistently elevated blood pressure above 180/110 goes largely undetected, untreated, and uncontrolled in this part of the world. In the cohort of men assessed in the Framingham Heart Study, the prevalence of blood pressures above 210/120—severe hypertension—declined from 1.8% in the 1950s to 0.1% by the 1960s with the introduction of effective antihypertensive agents. Although debate continues about appropriate screening strategies and treatment thresholds, rural health centers staffed largely by nurses must quickly gain access to essential antihypertensive medications.

The epidemiology of heart failure reflects inequalities in risk factor prevalence and in treatment. The reported burden of this condition has remained unchanged since the 1950s, but the causes of heart failure and the age of the people affected vary across the globe. Heart failure as a consequence of pericardial, myocardial, endocardial, or valvular injury accounts for as many as 5% of all medical admissions to hospitals around the world. In high-income countries, coronary artery disease and hypertension among the elderly account for most cases of heart failure. For example, in the United States, coronary artery disease is present in 60% of patients with heart failure and hypertension in 70%. Among the world's poorest 1 billion people, however, heart failure reflects poverty-driven exposure of children and young adults to rheumatogenic strains of streptococci and cardiotropic microorganisms (e.g., HIV, *Trypanosoma cruzi*, enteroviruses, *M. tuberculosis*), untreated high blood pressure, and nutrient deficiencies. The mechanisms underlying other causes of heart failure common in these populations—such as idiopathic dilated cardiomyopathy, peripartum cardiomyopathy, and endomyocardial fibrosis—remain unclear.

In stark contrast to the extraordinary lengths to which clinicians in wealthy countries will go to treat ischemic cardiomyopathy, little attention has been paid to young patients with nonischemic cardiomyopathies in resource-poor settings. Nonischemic cardiomyopathies, such as those due to hypertension, RHD, and chronic lung disease, account for >90% of cases of cardiac failure in sub-Saharan Africa and include poorly understood entities such as peripartum cardiomyopathy (which has an incidence in rural Haiti of 1 per 300 live births) and HIV-associated cardiomyopathy. Multidrug regimens that include beta blockers, angiotensin-converting enzyme inhibitors, and other agents can dramatically reduce mortality risk and improve quality of life for these patients. Lessons learned in the scale-up of chronic care for HIV infection and TB may be illustrative as progress is made in establishing the means to deliver heart-failure therapies.

Some of the lessons learned from the chronic infections discussed above are, of course, relevant to cardiovascular disease, especially those classified as NCDs but caused by infectious pathogens. Integration of prevention and care remains as important today as in 1960 when Paul Dudley White and his colleagues found little evidence of myocardial infarction in the region near the Albert Schweitzer Hospital in Lambaréné, Gabon, but reported that "the high prevalence of mitral stenosis is astonishing…. We believe strongly that it is a duty to help bring to these sufferers the benefits of better penicillin prophylaxis and of cardiac surgery when indicated. The same responsibility exists for those with correctable congenital cardiovascular defects."

RHD affects more than 15 million people worldwide, with more than 470,000 new cases each year. Among the 2.4 million annual cases of pediatric RHD, an estimated 42% occur in sub-Saharan Africa. This disease, which may cause endocarditis or stroke, leads to more than 345,000 deaths per year—almost all occurring in developing countries. Researchers in Ethiopia have reported annual death rates as high as 12.5% in rural areas. In part because the prevention of RHD has not advanced since the disease's disappearance in wealthy countries, no part of sub-Saharan Africa has eradicated RHD despite examples of success in Costa Rica, Cuba, and some Caribbean nations. A survey of acute heart failure among adults in sub-Saharan Africa showed that ~14.3% of these cases were due to RHD.

Strategies to eliminate rheumatic heart disease may depend on active case-finding, with confirmation by echocardiography, among high-risk groups as well as on efforts to expand access to surgical interventions among children with advanced valvular damage. Partnerships between established surgical programs and areas with limited or nonexistent facilities may help expand the capacity to provide life-saving interventions to patients who otherwise would die early and painfully. A long-term goal is the establishment of regional centers of excellence equipped to provide consistent, accessible, high-quality services.

Clinicians from tertiary care centers in sub-Saharan Africa and elsewhere have continued to call for prevention and treatment of the cardiovascular conditions of the poor. The reconstruction of health services in response to pandemic infectious disease offers an opportunity to identify and treat patients with organ damage and to undertake the prevention of cardiovascular and other chronic conditions of poverty.

CANCER Cancers account for ~5% of the global burden of disease. Low- and middle-income countries accounted for more than two-thirds of the 12.6 million cases and 7.6 million deaths due to cancer in 2008. By 2030, annual mortality from cancer will increase by 4 million—with developing countries experiencing a sharper increase than developed nations. "Western" lifestyle changes will be responsible for the increased incidence of cancers of the breast, colon, and prostate among populations in low- and middle-income countries, but historic realities, sociocultural and behavioral factors, genetics, and poverty itself also will have a profound impact on cancer-related mortality and morbidity rates. At least 2 million cancer cases per year—18% of the global cancer burden—are attributable to infectious causes, which are responsible for <10% of cancers in developed countries but account for up to 20% of all malignancies in low- and middle-income countries. Infectious causes of cancer such as human papillomavirus, hepatitis B virus, and *Helicobacter pylori* will continue to have a much larger impact in developing countries. Environmental and dietary factors, such as indoor air pollution and high-salt diets, also contribute to increased rates of certain cancers (e.g., lung and gastric cancers). Tobacco use (both smoking and chewing) is the most important source of increased mortality rates from lung and oral cancers. In contrast to decreasing tobacco use in many developed countries, the number of smokers is growing in developing countries, especially among women and young persons.

For many reasons, outcomes of malignancies are far worse in developing countries than in developed nations. As currently funded, overstretched health systems in poor countries are not capable of early detection; the majority of patients already have incurable malignancies at diagnosis. Treatment of cancers is available for only a very small number of mostly wealthy citizens in the majority of poor countries, and, even when treatment is available, the range and quality of services are often substandard. Yet this need not be the future. Only a decade ago, MDR-TB and HIV infection were considered untreatable in settings of great poverty. The feasibility of creating innovative programs that reduce technical and financial barriers to the provision of care for treatable malignancies among the world's poorest populations is now clear (Fig. 2-4). Several middle-income countries, including Mexico, have expanded publicly funded cancer care to reach poorer populations. This commitment of resources has dramatically improved outcomes for cancers, from childhood leukemia to cervical cancer.

Prevention of Noncommunicable Diseases False debates, including those pitting prevention against care, continue in global health and reflect, in part, outmoded paradigms or a partial understanding of disease burden and etiology as well as the dramatic variations in risk within a single nation. Moreover, debates are sometimes politicized as a

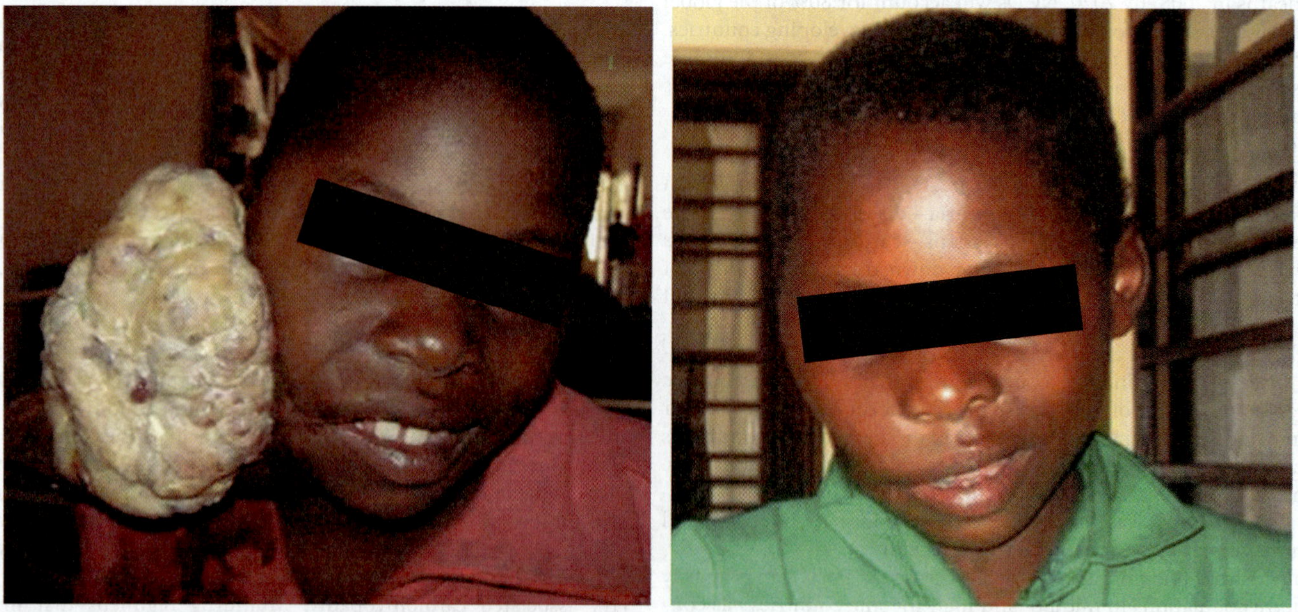

A B

FIGURE 2-4 An 11-year-old Rwandan patient with embryonal rhabdomyosarcoma before (***left***) and after (***right***) 48 weeks of chemotherapy plus surgery. Five years later, she is healthy with no evidence of disease.

result of vested interests. For example, in 2004, the WHO released its Global Strategy on Diet, Physical Activity, and Health, which focused on the population-wide promotion of healthy diet and regular physical activity in an effort to reduce the growing global problem of obesity. Passing this strategy at the World Health Assembly proved difficult because of strong opposition from the food industry and from a number of WHO member states, including the United States. Although globalization has had many positive effects, one negative effect has been the growth in both developed and developing countries of well-financed lobbies that have aggressively promoted unhealthy dietary changes and increased consumption of alcohol and tobacco. Foreign direct investment in tobacco, beverage, and food products in developing countries reached $90.3 billion in 2010—a figure nearly 490 times greater than the $185 million spent during that year to address NCDs by bilateral funding agencies, the WHO, the World Bank, and all other sources of development assistance for health combined. Investment in curbing NCDs remains disproportionately low despite the WHO's 2008–2013 Action Plan for the Global Strategy for the Prevention and Control of Noncommunicable Diseases.

The WHO estimates that 80% of all cases of cardiovascular disease and type 2 diabetes as well as 40% of all cancers can be prevented through healthier diets, increased physical activity, and avoidance of tobacco. These estimates mask large local variations. Although some evidence indicates that population-based measures can have some impact on these behaviors, it is sobering to note that increasing obesity levels have not been reversed in any population. Tobacco avoidance may be the most important and most difficult behavioral modification of all. In the twentieth century, 100 million people worldwide died of tobacco-related diseases; it is projected that more than 1 billion people will die of these diseases in the twenty-first century, with the vast majority of those deaths in developing countries. The WHO's 2003 Framework Convention on Tobacco Control represented a major advance, committing all of its signatories to a set of policy measures shown to reduce tobacco consumption. Today, ~80% of the world's 1 billion smokers live in low- and middle-income countries. If trends continue, tobacco-related deaths will increase to 8 million per year by 2030, with 80% of those deaths in low- and middle-income countries.

MENTAL HEALTH

The WHO reports that some 450 million people worldwide are affected by mental, neurologic, or behavioral problems at any given time and that ~877,000 people die by suicide every year. Major depression is the leading cause of years lost to disability in the world today. One in four patients visiting a health service has at least one mental, neurologic, or behavioral disorder, but most of these disorders are neither diagnosed nor treated. Most low- and middle-income countries devote <1% of their health expenditures to mental health.

Increasingly effective therapies exist for many of the major causes of mental disorders. Effective treatments for many neurologic diseases, including seizure disorders, have long been available. One of the greatest barriers to delivery of such therapies is the paucity of skilled personnel. Most sub-Saharan African countries have only a handful of psychiatrists, for example; most of them practice in cities and are unavailable within the public sector or to patients living in poverty.

Among the few patients who are fortunate enough to see a psychiatrist or neurologist, fewer still are able to adhere to treatment regimens: several surveys of already diagnosed patients ostensibly receiving daily therapy have revealed that, among the poor, multiple barriers prevent patients from taking their medications as prescribed. In one study from Kenya, no patients being seen in an epilepsy clinic had therapeutic blood levels of anti-seizure medications, even though all had had these drugs prescribed. Moreover, many patients had no detectable blood levels of these agents. The same barriers that prevent the poor from having reliable access to insulin or ART prevent them from benefiting from antidepressant, antipsychotic, and antiepileptic agents. To alleviate this problem, some authorities are proposing the training of health workers to provide community-based adherence support, counseling services, and referrals for patients in need of mental health services. One such program instituted in Goa, India, used "lay" counselors and resulted in a significant reduction in symptoms of common mental disorders among the target population.

World Mental Health: Problems and Priorities in Low-Income Countries still offers a comprehensive analysis of the burden of mental, behavioral, and social problems in low-income countries and relates the mental health consequences of social forces such as violence, dislocation, poverty, and disenfranchisement of women to current economic, political, and environmental concerns. In the years since this report was published, however, a number of pilot projects designed to deliver community-based care to patients with chronic mental illness have been launched in settings as diverse as Goa, India; Banda Aceh, Indonesia; rural China; post-earthquake Haiti; and Fiji. Some of these programs have been school-based and have sought to link prevention to care.

CONCLUSION: TOWARD A SCIENCE OF IMPLEMENTATION

Public health strategies draw largely on quantitative methods—epidemiology, biostatistics, and economics. Clinical practice, including the practice of internal medicine, draws on a rapidly expanding knowledge base but remains focused on individual patient care; clinical interventions are rarely population-based. But global health equity depends on avoiding the false debates of the past: neither public health nor clinical approaches alone are adequate to address the problems of global health. There is a long way to go before evidence-based internal medicine is applied effectively among the world's poor. Complex infectious diseases such as HIV/AIDS and TB have proved difficult but not impossible to manage; drug resistance and lack of effective health systems have complicated such work. Beyond what is usually termed "communicable diseases"—i.e., in the arena of chronic diseases such as cardiovascular disease and mental illness—global health is a nascent endeavor. Efforts to address any one of these problems in settings of great scarcity need to be integrated into broader efforts to strengthen failing health systems and alleviate the growing personnel crisis within these systems.

Such efforts must include the building of "platforms" for care delivery that are robust enough to incorporate new preventive, diagnostic, and therapeutic technologies rapidly in response to changes both in the burden of disease and in the needs not met by dominant paradigms and systems of health delivery. Academic medical centers have tried to address this "know–do" gap as new technologies are introduced and assessed through clinical trials, but the reach of these institutions into settings of poverty is limited in rich and poor countries alike. When such centers link their capacities effectively to the public institutions charged with the delivery of health care to the poor, great progress can be made.

For these reasons, scholarly work and practice in the field once known as "international health" and now often designated "global health equity" are changing rapidly. That work is still informed by the tension between clinical practice and population-based interventions, between analysis and action, and between prevention and care. Once metrics are refined, how might they inform efforts to lessen premature morbidity and mortality rates among the world's poor? As in the nineteenth century, human rights perspectives have proved helpful in turning attention to the problems of the destitute sick; such perspectives may also inform strategies for delivering care equitably.

A number of university hospitals are developing training programs for physicians with an interest in global health. In medical schools across the United States and in other wealthy countries, interest in global health has exploded. One study has shown that more than 25% of medical students take part in at least one global health experience prior to graduation. Half a century or even a decade ago, such high levels of interest would have been unimaginable.

An estimated 12 million people die each year simply because they live in poverty. An absolute majority of these premature deaths occur in Africa, with the poorer regions of Asia not far behind. Most of these deaths occur because the world's poorest do not have access to the fruits of science. They include deaths from vaccine-preventable illness, deaths during childbirth, deaths from infectious diseases that might be cured with access to antibiotics and other essential medicines, deaths from malaria that would have been prevented by bed nets and access to therapy, and deaths from waterborne illnesses. Other excess mortality is attributable to the inadequacy of efforts to develop new preventive, diagnostic, and therapeutic tools. Those funding the discovery and development of new tools typically neglect the concurrent need for strategies to make them available to the poor. Indeed, some would argue that the biggest challenge facing those who seek to address this outcome gap is the lack of practical means of distribution in the most heavily affected regions.

The development of tools must be followed quickly by their equitable distribution. When new preventive and therapeutic tools are developed without concurrent attention to delivery or implementation, one encounters what are sometimes termed *perverse effects:* even as new tools are developed, inequalities of outcome—lower morbidity and mortality rates among those who can afford access, with sustained high morbidity and mortality among those who cannot—will grow in the absence of an equity plan to deliver the tools to those most at risk. Preventing such a future is the most important goal of global health.

3 Decision-Making in Clinical Medicine

Daniel B. Mark, John B. Wong

INTRODUCTION

To a medical student who requires hours to collect a patient's history, perform a physical examination, and organize that information into a coherent presentation, an experienced clinician's ability to decide on a diagnosis and management plan in minutes may seem extraordinary. What separates the master clinician from the novice is an elusive quality called "expertise." The first part of this chapter provides an overview of our current understanding of expertise in clinical reasoning, what it is, and how it can be developed.

The proper use of diagnostic tests and the integration of the results into the patient's clinical assessment may also be equally bewildering to students. Hoping to hit the unknown diagnostic target, novice medical practitioners typically apply a "shotgun" approach to testing. The expert, in contrast, usually focuses her testing strategy to specific diagnostic hypotheses. The second part of the chapter reviews basic statistical concepts useful for interpreting diagnostic tests and quantitative tools useful for clinical decision-making.

Evidence-based medicine (EBM) constitutes the integration of the best available research evidence with clinical judgment as applied to the care of individual patients. The third part of the chapter provides an overview of the tools of EBM.

BRIEF INTRODUCTION TO CLINICAL REASONING

Clinical Expertise Defining "clinical expertise" remains surprisingly difficult. Chess has an objective ranking system based on skill and performance criteria. Athletics, similarly, have ranking systems to distinguish novices from Olympians. But in medicine, after physicians complete training and pass the boards, no further tests or benchmarks identify those who have attained the highest levels of clinical performance. Of course, physicians often consult a few "elite" clinicians for their "special problem-solving prowess" when particularly difficult or obscure cases have baffled everyone else. Yet despite their skill, even master clinicians typically cannot explain their exact processes and methods, thereby limiting the acquisition and dissemination of the expertise used to achieve their impressive results. Furthermore, clinical virtuosity appears not to be generalizable, e.g., an expert on hypertrophic cardiomyopathy may be no better (and possibly worse) than a first-year medical resident at diagnosing and managing a patient with neutropenia, fever, and hypotension.

Broadly construed, clinical expertise includes not only cognitive dimensions and the integration of verbal and visual cues or information but also complex fine-motor skills necessary for invasive and noninvasive procedures and tests. In addition, "the complete package" of expertise in medicine includes the ability to communicate effectively with patients and work well with members of the medical team. Research on medical expertise remains relatively sparse overall, with most of the work focused on diagnostic reasoning, and much less work focused on treatment decisions or the technical skills involved in the performance of procedures. Thus, in this chapter, we focus primarily on the cognitive elements of clinical reasoning.

Because clinical reasoning takes place in the heads of doctors, it is therefore not readily observable, making it obviously difficult to study. One method of research on reasoning asks doctors to "think out loud" as they receive increments of clinical information in a manner meant to simulate a clinical encounter. Another research approach has focused on how doctors *should* reason diagnostically rather than on how they actually *do* reason. Much of what is known about clinical reasoning comes from empirical studies of nonmedical problem-solving behavior. Because of the diverse perspectives contributing to this area, with important contributions from cognitive psychology, sociology, medical education, economics, informatics, and decision sciences, no single integrated model of clinical reasoning exists, and not infrequently, different terms and models describe similar phenomena.

Intuitive versus Analytic Reasoning A contemporary model of reasoning, *dual-process theory* distinguishes two general systems of cognitive processes. *Intuition* (System 1) provides rapid effortless judgments from memorized associations using pattern recognition and other simplifying "rules of thumb" (i.e., heuristics). For example, a very simple pattern that could be useful in certain situations is "African-American women plus hilar adenopathy equals sarcoid." Because no effort is involved in recalling the pattern, typically, the clinician is unable to say how those judgments were formulated. In contrast, *analysis* (System 2), the other form of reasoning in the dual-process model, is slow, methodical, deliberative, and effortful. These are, of course, idealized extremes of the cognitive continuum. How these systems interact in different decision problems, how experts use them differently from novices, and when their use can lead to errors in judgment remain the subject of considerable study and debate.

Pattern recognition is a complex cognitive process that appears largely effortless. One can recognize people's faces, the breed of a dog, or an automobile model without necessarily being able to say what specific features prompted the recognition. Analogously, experienced clinicians often recognize familiar diagnosis patterns quickly. In the absence of an extensive stored repertoire of diagnostic patterns, students (as well as more experienced clinicians operating outside their area of expertise) often use the more laborious System 2 analytic approach along with more intensive and comprehensive data collection to reach the diagnosis.

The following three brief scenarios of a patient with hemoptysis demonstrate three distinct patterns:

- A 46-year-old man presents to his internist with a chief complaint of hemoptysis. An otherwise healthy nonsmoker, he is recovering from an apparent viral bronchitis. This presentation pattern suggests that the small amount of blood-streaked sputum is due to acute bronchitis, so that a chest x-ray provides sufficient reassurance that a more serious disorder is absent.
- In the second scenario, a 46-year-old patient who has the same chief complaint but with a 100-pack-year smoking history, a productive morning cough, and episodes of blood-streaked sputum fits the pattern of carcinoma of the lung. Consequently, along with the chest x-ray, the physician obtains a sputum cytology examination and refers this patient for a chest computed tomography (CT) scan.
- In the third scenario, a 46-year-old patient with hemoptysis who immigrated from a developing country has an echocardiogram as well, because the physician hears a soft diastolic rumbling murmur at the apex on cardiac auscultation, suggesting rheumatic mitral stenosis and possibly pulmonary hypertension.

Although rapid, pattern recognition used without sufficient reflection can result in *premature closure*: mistakenly concluding that one already knows the correct diagnosis and therefore failing to complete the data collection that would demonstrate the lack of fit of the initial pattern selected. For example, a 45-year-old man presents with a 3-week history of a "flulike" upper respiratory infection (URI) including symptoms of dyspnea and a productive cough. On the basis of the presenting complaints, the clinician uses a "URI assessment form" to improve the quality and efficiency of care by standardizing the information gathered. After quickly acquiring the requisite structured examination components and noting in particular the absence of fever and a clear chest examination, the physician prescribes medication for acute bronchitis and sends the patient home with the reassurance that his illness was not serious. Following a sleepless night with significant dyspnea, the patient develops nausea and vomiting and collapses. He presents to the emergency department in cardiac arrest and is unable to be resuscitated. His autopsy shows a posterior wall myocardial infarction and a fresh thrombus in an atherosclerotic right coronary artery. What went wrong? The clinician had decided, based on the patient's appearance, even before starting the history, that the patient's complaints were not serious. Therefore, he felt confident that he could perform an abbreviated and focused examination by using the URI assessment protocol rather than considering the broader range of possibilities and performing appropriate tests to confirm or refute his initial hypotheses. In particular, by concentrating on the URI, the clinician failed to elicit the full dyspnea history, which would have suggested a far more serious disorder, and he neglected to search for other symptoms that could have directed him to the correct diagnosis.

Heuristics, also referred to as cognitive shortcuts or rules of thumb, are simplifying decision strategies that ignore part of the data available so as to provide an efficient path to the desired judgment. They are generally part of the intuitive system tools. Two major research programs have come to different conclusions about the value of heuristics in clinical judgment. The "heuristics and biases" program focused on understanding how heuristics in problem solving could be biased by testing the numerical intuition of psychology undergraduates against the rules of statistics. In contrast, the "fast and frugal heuristics" research program explored how and when decision makers' reliance on simple heuristics can produce good decisions. Although many heuristics have relevance to clinical reasoning, only four will be mentioned here.

When assessing a particular patient, clinicians often weigh the similarity of that patient's symptoms, signs, and risk factors against those of their mental representations of the diagnostic hypotheses being considered. In other words, among the diagnostic possibilities, clinicians identify the diagnosis for which the patient appears to be a representative example. Analogous to pattern recognition, this cognitive shortcut is called the *representativeness heuristic*. However, physicians using the representativeness heuristic can reach erroneous conclusions if they fail to consider the underlying prevalence (i.e., the prior, or pretest, probabilities) of the two competing diagnoses that could explain the patient's symptoms. Consider a patient with hypertension and headache, palpitations, and diaphoresis. Inexperienced clinicians might judge pheochromocytoma to be quite likely based on the representativeness heuristic with this classic symptom triad suggesting pheochromocytoma. Doing so would be incorrect given that other causes of hypertension are much more common than pheochromocytoma, and this triad of symptoms can occur in patients who do not have pheochromocytoma. Less experience with a particular diagnosis and with the breadth of presentations (e.g., diseases that affect multiple organ systems such as sarcoid) may also lead to errors.

A second commonly used cognitive shortcut, the *availability heuristic*, involves judgments based of how easily prior similar cases or outcomes can be brought to mind. For example, an experienced clinician may recall 20 elderly patients seen over the last few years who presented with painless dyspnea of acute onset and were found to have acute myocardial infarction (MI). A novice clinician may spend valuable time seeking a pulmonary cause for the symptoms before considering and then confirming the cardiac diagnosis. In this situation, the patient's clinical pattern does not fit the most common pattern of acute MI, but experience with this atypical presentation, along with the ability to recall it, directs the physician to the diagnosis.

Errors with the availability heuristic arise from several sources of recall bias. Rare catastrophes are likely to be remembered with a clarity and force disproportionate to their likelihood for future diagnosis—for example, a patient with a sore throat eventually found to have leukemia or a young athlete with leg pain eventually found to have a sarcoma—and those publicized in the media or that are recent experiences are, of course, easier to recall and therefore more influential on clinical judgments.

The third commonly used cognitive shortcut, the *anchoring heuristic* (also called conservatism or stickiness), involves estimating a probability of disease (the anchor) and then insufficiently adjusting that probability up or down (compared with Bayes' rule) when interpreting new data about the patient, i.e., sticking to their initial diagnosis. For example, a clinician may still judge the probability of coronary artery disease (CAD) to be high after a negative exercise thallium test and proceed to cardiac catheterization (see "Measures of Disease Probability and Bayes' Rule," below).

The fourth heuristic states that clinicians should use the simplest explanation possible that will account adequately for the patient's symptoms or findings (Occam's razor or, alternatively, the *simplicity heuristic*). Although this is an attractive and often used principle, it is important to remember that no biologic basis for it exists. Errors from the simplicity heuristic include premature closure leading to the neglect of unexplained significant symptoms or findings.

Even experienced physicians use analytic reasoning processes (System 2) when the problem they face is recognized to be complex or to involve important unfamiliar elements or features. In such situations, clinicians proceed much more methodically in what has been referred to as the hypothetico-deductive model of reasoning. From the outset, expert clinicians working analytically generate, refine, and discard diagnostic hypotheses. The hypotheses drive questions asked during history taking and may change based on the working hypotheses of the moment. Even the physical examination is focused by the working hypotheses. Is the spleen enlarged? How big is the liver? Is it tender? Are there any palpable masses or nodules? Each question must be answered (with the exclusion of all other inputs) before the examiner can move on to the next specific question. Each diagnostic hypothesis provides testable predictions and sets a context for the next question or step to follow. For example, if the enlarged and quite tender liver felt on physical examination is due to acute hepatitis (the hypothesis), certain specific liver function tests should be markedly elevated (the prediction). If the tests come back normal, the hypothesis may have to be discarded or substantially modified.

Negative findings often are neglected but are as important as positive ones because they often reduce the likelihood of the diagnostic hypotheses under consideration. Chest discomfort that is not provoked or worsened by exertion in an active patient reduces the likelihood that chronic ischemic heart disease is the underlying cause. The absence of a resting tachycardia and thyroid gland enlargement reduces the likelihood of hyperthyroidism in a patient with paroxysmal atrial fibrillation.

The acuity of a patient's illness may override considerations of prevalence and the other issues described above. "Diagnostic imperatives" recognize the significance of relatively rare but potentially catastrophic diagnoses if undiagnosed and untreated. For example, clinicians are taught to consider aortic dissection routinely as a possible cause of acute severe chest discomfort. Even though the typical history of dissection differs from that of MI, dissection is far less prevalent, so diagnosing dissection remains challenging unless it is explicitly and routinely considered as a diagnostic imperative (Chap. 301). If the clinician fails to elicit any of the characteristic features of dissection by history and finds equivalent blood pressures in both arms and no pulse deficits, he may feel comfortable discarding the aortic dissection hypothesis. If, however, the chest x-ray shows a possible widened mediastinum, the hypothesis may be reinstated and an appropriate imaging test ordered (e.g., thoracic CT scan, transesophageal echocardiogram) to evaluate more fully. In nonacute situations, the prevalence of potential alternative diagnoses should play a much more prominent role in diagnostic hypothesis generation.

Cognitive scientists studying the thought processes of expert clinicians have observed that clinicians group data into packets, or "chunks," that are stored in short-term or "working memory" and manipulated to generate diagnostic hypotheses. Because short-term memory can typically retain only 5–9 items at a time, the number of packets that can be actively integrated into hypothesis-generating activities is similarly limited. For this reason, the cognitive shortcuts discussed above play a key role in the generation of diagnostic hypotheses, many of which are discarded as rapidly as they are formed (thereby demonstrating that the distinction between analytic and intuitive reasoning is an arbitrary and simplistic, but nonetheless useful, representation of cognition).

Research into the hypothetico-deductive model of reasoning has had surprising difficulty identifying the elements of the reasoning process that distinguish experts from novices. This has led to a shift from examining the problem-solving process of experts to analyzing the organization of their knowledge. For example, diagnosis may be based on the resemblance of a new case to prior individual instances (exemplars). Experts have a much larger store of memorized cases, for example, visual long-term memory in radiology. However, clinicians do not simply rely on literal recall of specific cases but have constructed elaborate conceptual networks of memorized information or models of disease to aid in arriving at their conclusions. That is, expertise involves an increased ability to connect symptoms, signs, and risk factors to one another in meaningful ways; relate those findings to possible diagnoses; and identify the additional information necessary to confirm the diagnosis.

No single theory accounts for all the key features of expertise in medical diagnosis. Experts have more knowledge about more things and a larger repertoire of cognitive tools to employ in problem solving than do novices. One definition of expertise highlights the ability to make powerful distinctions. In this sense, expertise involves a working knowledge of the diagnostic possibilities and what features distinguish one disease from another. Memorization alone is insufficient. Memorizing a medical textbook would not make one an expert. But having access to detailed and specific relevant information is critically important. Clinicians of the past primarily accessed their own remembered experience. Clinicians of the future will be able to access the experience of large numbers of clinicians using electronic tools, but, as with the memorized textbook, the data alone will not create an instant expert. The expert adds these data to an extensive internalized database of knowledge and experience not available to the novice (and nonexpert).

Despite all the work that has been done to understand expertise, in medicine and other disciplines, it remains uncertain whether there is any didactic program that can accelerate the progression from novice to expert or from experienced clinician to master clinician. Deliberate effortful practice (over an extended period of time, sometimes said to be 10 years or 10,000 practice hours) and personal coaching are two strategies that are often used outside medicine (e.g., music, athletics, chess) to promote expertise. Their use in developing medical expertise and maintaining or enhancing it has not yet been adequately explored.

DIAGNOSTIC VERSUS THERAPEUTIC DECISION MAKING

The modern ideal of medical therapeutic decision making is to "personalize" the recommendation. In the abstract, personalizing treatment involves combining the best available evidence about what works with an individual patient's unique features (e.g., risk factors) and his or her preferences and health goals to craft an optimal treatment recommendation with the patient. Operationally, there are two different and complementary levels of personalization possible: individualizing the evidence for the specific patient based on relevant clinical and other characteristics, and personalizing the patient interaction by incorporating their values, often referred to as shared decision-making, which is critically important, but falls outside the scope of this chapter.

Individualizing the evidence about therapy **does not** mean relying on physician impressions of what works based on personal experience. Because of small sample sizes and rare events, the chance of drawing erroneous causal inferences from one's own clinical experience is very high. For most chronic diseases, therapeutic effectiveness is only demonstrable statistically in patient populations. It would be incorrect to infer with any certainty, for example, that treating a hypertensive patient with angiotensin-converting enzyme (ACE) inhibitors necessarily prevented a stroke from occurring during treatment, or that an untreated patient would definitely have avoided a stroke had he or she been treated. For many chronic diseases, a majority of patients will remain event free regardless of treatment choices; some will have events regardless of which treatment is selected; and those who avoided having an event through treatment cannot be individually identified. Blood pressure lowering, a readily observable surrogate endpoint, does not have a tightly coupled relationship with strokes prevented. Consequently, demonstrating therapeutic effectiveness cannot rely simply on observing the outcome of an individual patient but should instead be based on large groups of patients carefully studied and properly analyzed.

Therapeutic decision making, therefore, should be based on the best available evidence from clinical trials and well-done outcome studies. Authoritative, well-done clinical practice guidelines that synthesize such evidence offer readily available, reliable, and trustworthy information relevant to many treatment decisions clinicians face. However, all guidelines recognize that their "one size fits all" recommendations may not apply to individual patients. Increased attention is now being paid to understand how best to adjust group-level clinical evidence of treatment harms and benefits to account for the absolute level of risks faced by subgroups and even individual patients, using, for example, validated clinical risk scores.

NONCLINICAL INFLUENCES ON CLINICAL DECISION-MAKING

More than a decade of research on variations in clinician practice patterns has shed much light on the forces that shape clinical decisions. These factors can be grouped conceptually into three overlapping categories: (1) factors related to physicians' personal characteristics and practice style, (2) factors related to the practice setting, and (3) factors related to economic incentives.

Factors Related to Practice Style To ensure that necessary care is provided at a high level of quality, physicians fulfill a key role in medical care by serving as the patient's agent. Factors that influence performance in this role include the physician's knowledge, training, and experience. Clearly, physicians cannot practice EBM (described later in the chapter) if they are unfamiliar with the evidence. As would be expected, specialists generally know the evidence in their field better than do generalists. Beyond published evidence and practice guidelines, a major set of influences on physician practice can be subsumed under the general concept of "practice style." The practice style serves to define norms of clinical behavior. Beliefs about effectiveness of different therapies and preferred patterns of diagnostic test use are examples of different facets of a practice style. The physician beliefs that drive these different practice styles may be based on personal experience, recollection, and interpretation of the available medical evidence. For example, heart failure specialists are much more likely than generalists to achieve target doses of ACE inhibitor therapy in their heart failure patients because they are more familiar with what the targets are (as defined by large clinical trials), have more familiarity with the specific drugs (including adverse effects), and are less likely to overreact to foreseeable problems in therapy such as a rise in creatinine levels or asymptomatic hypotension.

Beyond the patient's welfare, physician perceptions about the risk of a malpractice suit resulting from either an erroneous decision or a bad outcome may drive clinical decisions and create a practice referred to as *defensive medicine*. This practice involves using tests and therapies with very small marginal benefit, ostensibly to preclude future criticism should an adverse outcome occur. Without any conscious awareness of a connection to the risk of litigation, however, over time such patterns of care may become accepted as part of the practice norm, thereby perpetuating their overuse, e.g., annual cardiac exercise testing in asymptomatic patients.

Practice Setting Factors Factors in this category relate to the physical resources available to the physician's practice and the practice environment. *Physician-induced demand* is a term that refers to the repeated observation that once medical facilities and technologies are made available to physicians, they will use them. Other environmental factors that can influence decision-making include the local availability of specialists for consultations and procedures; "high-tech" advanced imaging or procedure facilities such as MRI machines and proton beam therapy centers; and fragmentation of care.

Economic Incentives Economic incentives are closely related to the other two categories of practice-modifying factors. Financial issues can exert both stimulatory and inhibitory influences on clinical practice. In general, physicians are paid on a fee-for-service, capitation, or salary basis. In fee-for-service, physicians who do more get paid more, thereby encouraging overuse, consciously or unconsciously. When fees are reduced (discounted reimbursement), doctors tend to increase the number of services provided to maintain revenue. Capitation, in contrast, provides a fixed payment per patient per year to encourage physicians to consider a global population budget in managing individual patients and ideally reducing the use of interventions with small marginal benefit. In contrast to inexpensive preventive services, however, this type of incentive is more likely to affect expensive interventions. To discourage volume-based excessive utilization, fixed salary compensation plans pay physicians the same regardless of the clinical effort expended, but may provide an incentive to see fewer patients.

INTERPRETATION OF DIAGNOSTIC TESTS IN THE CONTEXT OF DECISION-MAKING

Despite the great technological advances in medicine over the last century, uncertainty remains a key challenge in all aspects of medical decision-making. Compounding this challenge is the massive information overload that characterizes modern medicine. Today's clinician needs access to close to 2 million pieces of information to practice medicine. According to one estimate, doctors subscribe to an average of seven journals, representing over 2500 new articles each year. Of course, to be useful, this information must be sifted for applicability to and then integrated with patient-specific data. Although computers appear to offer an obvious solution both for information management and for quantification of medical care uncertainties, many practical problems must be solved before computerized decision support can be routinely incorporated into the clinical reasoning process in a way that demonstrably improves the quality of care. For the present, understanding the nature of diagnostic test information can help clinicians become more efficient users of such data. The next section reviews important concepts related to diagnostic testing.

DIAGNOSTIC TESTING: MEASURES OF TEST ACCURACY

The purpose of performing a test on a patient is to reduce uncertainty about the patient's diagnosis or prognosis in order to facilitate optimal management. Although diagnostic tests commonly are thought of as laboratory tests (e.g., blood count) or procedures (e.g., colonoscopy or bronchoscopy), any technology that changes a physician's understanding of the patient's problem qualifies as a diagnostic test. Thus, even the history and physical examination can be considered a form of diagnostic test. In clinical medicine, it is common to reduce the results of a test to a dichotomous outcome, such as positive or negative, normal or abnormal. Although this simplification ignores useful information (such as the degree of abnormality), such simplification does make it easier to demonstrate the fundamental principles of test interpretation discussed below.

The accuracy of diagnostic tests is defined in relation to an accepted "gold standard," which defines the presumably true state of the patient (Table 3-1). Characterizing the diagnostic performance of a new test requires identifying an appropriate population (ideally, patients in whom the new test would be used) and applying both the new and the gold standard tests to all subjects. Biased estimates of test performance

TABLE 3-1 MEASURES OF DIAGNOSTIC TEST ACCURACY

	Disease Status	
Test Result	**Present**	**Absent**
Positive	True positive (TP)	False positive (FP)
Negative	False negative (FN)	True negative (TN)
Test Characteristics in Patients with Disease		
True-positive rate (sensitivity) = TP/(TP + FN)		
False-negative rate = FN/(TP + FN)		
True-positive rate = 1 – false-negative rate		
Test Characteristics in Patients without Disease		
True-negative rate (specificity) = TN/(TN + FP)		
False-positive rate = FP/(TN + FP)		
True-negative rate = 1 – false-positive rate		

may occur from using an inappropriate population or from incompletely applying the gold standard test. By comparing the two tests, the characteristics of the new test are determined. The *sensitivity* or *true-positive rate* of the new test is the proportion of patients with disease (defined by the gold standard) who have a positive (new) test. This measure reflects how well the new test identifies patients with disease. The proportion of patients with disease who have a negative test is the *false-negative rate* and is calculated as 1 – sensitivity. Among patients without disease, the proportion who have a negative test is the *specificity*, or *true-negative rate*. This measure reflects how well the new test correctly identifies patients without disease. Among patients without disease, the proportion who have a positive test is the *false-positive rate*, calculated as 1 – specificity. A perfect test would have a sensitivity of 100% and a specificity of 100% and would completely distinguish patients with disease from those without it.

Calculating sensitivity and specificity requires selection of a threshold value or cut point above which the test is considered "positive." Making the cut point "stricter" (e.g., raising it) lowers sensitivity but improves specificity, whereas making it "laxer" (e.g., lowering it) raises sensitivity but lowers specificity. This dynamic trade-off between more accurate identification of subjects with disease versus those without disease is often displayed graphically as a receiver operating characteristic (ROC) curve (Fig. 3-1) by plotting sensitivity (*y* axis) versus 1 – specificity (*x* axis). Each point on the curve represents a potential cut point with an associated sensitivity and specificity value. The area under the ROC curve often is used as a quantitative measure of the information content of a test. Values range from 0.5 (no diagnostic information from testing at all; the test is equivalent to flipping a coin) to 1.0 (perfect test). The choice of cut point should depend on the relative harms and benefits of treatment for those without versus those with disease. For example, if treatment was safe with substantial benefit, then choosing a high-sensitivity cut point (upper right of the ROC curve) for a low-risk test may be appropriate (e.g., phenylketonuria in newborns), but if treatment had substantial risk for harm, then choosing a high-specificity cut point (lower left of the ROC curve) may be appropriate (e.g., amniocentesis that may lead to therapeutic abortion of a normal fetus). The choice of cut point may also depend on the likelihood of disease, with low likelihoods placing a greater emphasis on the harms of treating false-positive tests and higher likelihoods placing a greater emphasis on missed benefit by not treating false-negative tests.

MEASURES OF DISEASE PROBABILITY AND BAYES' RULE

Unfortunately, there are no perfect tests. After every test is completed, the true disease state of the patient remains uncertain. Quantifying this residual uncertainty can be done with Bayes' rule, which provides a simple way to calculate the likelihood of disease after a test result or posttest probability from three parameters: the pretest probability of disease, the test sensitivity, and the test specificity. The pretest probability is a quantitative estimate of the likelihood of the diagnosis before the test is performed and is usually the prevalence of the disease in the underlying population although occasionally it can be the disease

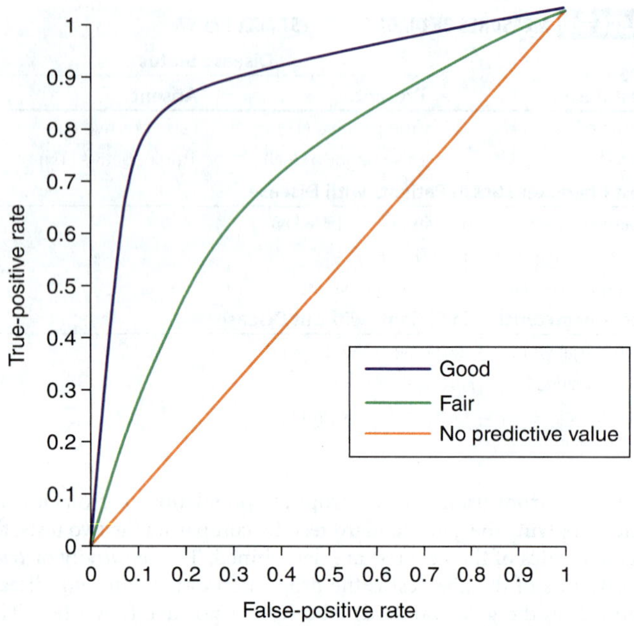

FIGURE 3-1 Each receiver operating characteristic (ROC) curve illustrates a trade-off that occurs between improved test sensitivity (accurate detection of patients with disease) and improved test specificity (accurate detection of patients without disease), because the test value defining when the test turns from "negative" to "positive" is varied. A 45° line would indicate a test with no predictive value (sensitivity = specificity at every test value). The area under each ROC curve is a measure of the information content of the test. Thus, a larger ROC area signifies increased diagnostic accuracy.

incidence. For some common conditions, such as CAD, nomograms and statistical models generate estimates of pretest probability that account for history, physical examination, and test findings. The posttest probability (also called the predictive value of the test) is a revised statement of the likelihood of the diagnosis, accounting for both pretest probability and test results. For the likelihood of disease following a positive test (i.e., positive predictive value), Bayes' rule is calculated as:

$$\text{Posttest probability} = \frac{\text{Pretest probability} \times \text{Sensitivity}}{\text{Pretest probability} \times \text{Sensitivity} + (1 - \text{Pretest probability}) \times \text{False-positive Rate}}$$

For example, with a pretest probability of 0.50 and a "positive" diagnostic test result (test sensitivity = 0.90 and specificity = 0.90):

$$\text{Posttest probability} = \frac{0.50 \times 0.90}{0.50 \times 0.90 + (1 - 0.50) \times 0.10} = 0.90$$

The term *predictive value* often is used as a synonym for the posttest probability. Unfortunately, clinicians commonly misinterpret reported predictive values as intrinsic measures of test accuracy. Studies of diagnostic tests compound the confusion by calculating predictive values on the same sample used to measure sensitivity and specificity. Since all posttest probabilities are a function of the prevalence of disease in the tested population, such calculations may be misleading unless the test is applied subsequently to populations with the same disease prevalence. For these reasons, the term *predictive value* is best avoided in favor of the more informative *posttest probability* following a positive or a negative test result.

The nomogram version of Bayes' rule (Fig. 3-2) helps us to conceptually understand how it estimates the posttest probability of disease. In this nomogram, the impact of the diagnostic test result is summarized by the *likelihood ratio*, which is defined as the ratio of the probability of a given test result (e.g., "positive" or "negative") in a patient with disease to the probability of that result in a patient without disease, thereby providing a measure of how well the test distinguishes those with from those without disease.

For a positive test, the likelihood ratio positive is calculated as the ratio of the true-positive rate to the false-positive rate (or sensitivity/[1 – specificity]). For example, a test with a sensitivity of 0.90 and a specificity of 0.90 has a likelihood ratio of 0.90/(1 – 0.90), or 9. Thus, for this hypothetical test, a "positive" result is nine times more likely in a patient with the disease than in a patient without it. Most tests in medicine have likelihood ratios for a positive result between 1.5 and 20. Higher values are associated with tests that more substantially increase the posttest likelihood of disease. A very high likelihood ratio positive (exceeding 10) usually implies high specificity, so a positive high-specificity test helps "rule in" disease. If sensitivity is excellent but specificity is less so, the likelihood ratio will be reduced substantially (e.g., with a 90% sensitivity but a 55% specificity, the likelihood ratio is 2.0).

For a negative test, the corresponding likelihood ratio negative is the ratio of the false-negative rate to the true-negative rate (or [1 – sensitivity]/specificity). Lower likelihood ratio values more substantially lower the posttest likelihood of disease. A very low likelihood ratio negative (falling below 0.10) usually implies high sensitivity, so a negative high-sensitivity test helps "rule out" disease. The hypothetical test considered above with a sensitivity of 0.9 and a specificity of 0.9 would have a likelihood ratio for a negative test result of (1 – 0.9)/0.9, or 0.11, meaning that a negative result is about one-tenth as likely in patients with disease than in those without disease (or 10 times more likely in those without disease than in those with disease).

APPLICATIONS TO DIAGNOSTIC TESTING IN CAD

Consider two tests commonly used in the diagnosis of CAD: an exercise treadmill test and an exercise single-photon emission CT (SPECT) myocardial perfusion imaging test (Chap. 270e). Meta-analysis has shown that a positive treadmill ST-segment response has an average sensitivity of 66% and an average specificity of 84%, yielding a likelihood ratio of 4.1 (0.66/[1 – 0.84]) (consistent with small discriminatory ability because it falls between 2 and 5). For a patient with a 10% pretest probability of CAD, the posttest probability of disease after a positive result rises to only about 30%. If a patient with a pretest probability of CAD of 80% has a positive test result, the posttest probability of disease is about 95%.

In contrast, exercise SPECT myocardial perfusion test is more accurate for CAD. For simplicity, assume that the finding of a reversible exercise-induced perfusion defect has both a sensitivity and a specificity of 90%, yielding a likelihood ratio for a positive test of 9.0 (0.90/[1 – 0.90]) (consistent with moderate discriminatory ability because it falls between 5 and 10). For the same 10% pretest probability patient, a positive test raises the probability of CAD to 50% (Fig. 3-2). However, despite the differences in posttest probabilities between these two tests (30% versus 50%), the more accurate test may not improve diagnostic likelihood enough to change patient management (e.g., decision to refer to cardiac catheterization) because the more accurate test has only moved the physician from being fairly certain that the patient did not have CAD to a 50:50 chance of disease. In a patient with a pretest probability of 80%, exercise SPECT test raises the posttest probability to 97% (compared with 95% for the exercise treadmill). Again, the more accurate test does not provide enough improvement in posttest confidence to alter management, and neither test has improved much on what was known from clinical data alone.

In general, positive results with an accurate test (e.g., likelihood ratio positive 10) when the pretest probability is low (e.g., 20%) do not move the posttest probability to a range high enough to rule in disease (e.g., 80%). In screening situations, pretest probabilities are often particularly low because patients are asymptomatic. In such cases, specificity becomes particularly important. For example, in screening first-time female blood donors without risk factors for HIV, a positive test raised the likelihood of HIV to only 67% despite a specificity of 99.995% because the prevalence was 0.01%. Conversely, with a high pretest

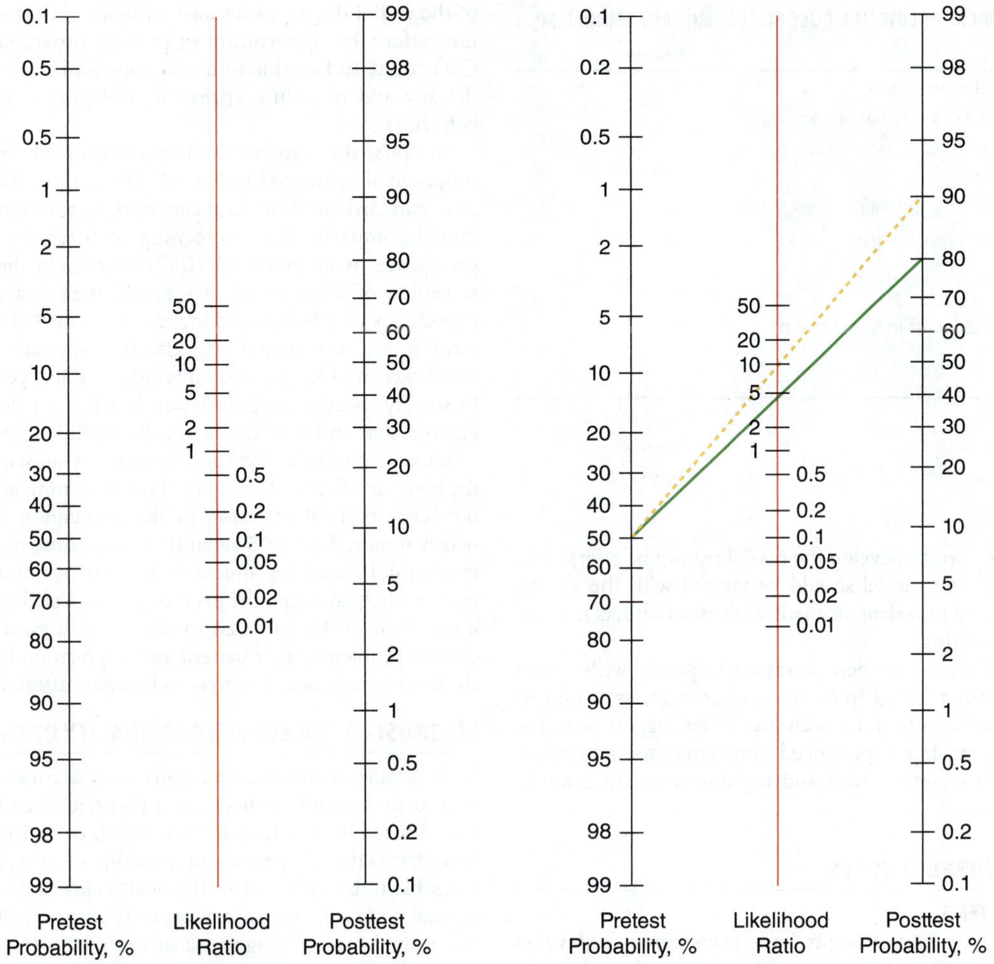

FIGURE 3-2 **Nomogram version of Bayes' rule** used to predict the posttest probability of disease (right-hand scale) using the pretest probability of disease (left-hand scale) and the likelihood ratio for a positive test (middle scale). See text for information on calculation of likelihood ratios. To use, place a straight edge connecting the pretest probability and the likelihood ratio and read off the posttest probability. The right-hand part of the figure illustrates the value of a positive exercise treadmill test (likelihood ratio 4, green line) and a positive exercise thallium single-photon emission computed tomography perfusion study (likelihood ratio 9, broken yellow line) in a patient with a pretest probability of coronary artery disease of 50%. *(Adapted from Centre for Evidence-Based Medicine: Likelihood ratios. Available at http://www.cebm.net/index.aspx?o=1043.)*

probability, a negative test may not rule out disease adequately if it is not sufficiently sensitive. Thus, the largest change in diagnostic likelihood following a test result occurs when the clinician is most uncertain (i.e., pretest probability between 30% and 70%). For example, if a patient has a pretest probability for CAD of 50%, a positive exercise treadmill test will move the posttest probability to 80% and a positive exercise SPECT perfusion test will move it to 90% (Fig. 3-2).

As presented above, Bayes' rule employs a number of important simplifications that should be considered. First, few tests have only positive or negative results, and many tests provide multiple outcomes (e.g., ST-segment depression and exercise duration with exercise testing). Although Bayes' rule can be adapted to this more detailed test result format, it is computationally more complex to do so. Similarly, when multiple tests are performed, the posttest probability may be used as the pretest probability to interpret the second test. However, this simplification assumes conditional independence—that is, that the results of the first test do not affect the likelihood of the second test result—and this is often not true.

Finally, it has long been asserted that sensitivity and specificity are prevalence-independent parameters of test accuracy, and many texts still make this statement. This statistically useful assumption, however, is clinically simplistic. A treadmill exercise test, for example, has a sensitivity in a population of patients with one-vessel CAD of around 30%, whereas its sensitivity in patients with severe three-vessel CAD approaches 80%. Thus, the best estimate of sensitivity to use in a particular decision may vary, depending on the severity of disease in the local population. A hospitalized, symptomatic, or referral population typically has a higher prevalence of disease and, in particular, a higher prevalence of more advanced disease than does an outpatient population. Consequently, test sensitivity will likely be higher in hospitalized patients, and test specificity higher in outpatients.

STATISTICAL PREDICTION MODELS

Bayes' rule, while illustrative as presented above, provides an unrealistically simple solution to most problems a clinician faces. Predictions based on multivariable statistical models, however, can more accurately address these more complex problems by accounting for specific patient characteristics. In particular, these models explicitly account for multiple possibly overlapping pieces of patient-specific information and assign a relative weight to each on the basis of its unique contribution to the prediction in question. For example, a logistic regression model to predict the probability of CAD considers all the relevant independent factors from the clinical examination and diagnostic testing and their significance instead of the limited data that clinicians can manage in their heads or with Bayes' rule. However, despite this strength, prediction models are usually too complex computationally to use without a calculator or computer (although this limitation may be overcome once medicine is practiced from a fully computerized platform).

To date, only a handful of prediction models have been validated properly (for example, Wells criteria for pulmonary embolism) (Table 3-2). The importance of independent validation in a population

TABLE 3-2 WELLS CLINICAL PREDICTION RULE FOR PULMONARY EMBOLISM

Clinical Feature	Points
Clinical signs of deep vein thrombosis	3
Alternative diagnosis is less likely than pulmonary embolism	3
Heart rate >100 beats/min	1.5
Immobilization ≥3 days or surgery in previous 4 weeks	1.5
History of deep vein thrombosis or pulmonary embolism	1.5
Hemoptysis	1
Malignancy (with treatment within 6 months) or palliative	1
Interpretation	
Score >6.0	High
Score 2.0–6.0	Intermediate
Score <2.0	Low

separate from the one used to develop the model cannot be overstated. An unvalidated prediction model should be viewed with the skepticism appropriate for any new drug or medical device that has not had rigorous clinical trial testing.

When statistical models have been compared directly with expert clinicians, they have been found to be more consistent, as would be expected, but not significantly more accurate. Their biggest promise, then, may be in helping less-experienced clinicians identify critical discriminating patient characteristics and become more accurate in their predictions.

FORMAL DECISION SUPPORT TOOLS

DECISION SUPPORT SYSTEMS

Over the last 40 years, many attempts have been made to develop computer systems to aid clinical decision-making and patient management. Conceptually attractive because computers offer ready access to the vast information available to today's physicians, they may also support management decisions by making accurate predictions of outcome, simulating the whole decision process, or providing algorithmic guidance. Computer-based predictions using Bayesian or statistical regression models inform a clinical decision but do not actually reach a "conclusion" or "recommendation." Artificial intelligence systems attempt to simulate or replace human reasoning with a computer-based analogue. To date, such approaches have achieved only limited success. Reminder or protocol-directed systems do not make predictions but use existing algorithms, such as guidelines, to guide clinical practice. In general, however, decision support systems have had little impact on practice. Reminder systems, although not yet in widespread use, have shown the most promise, particularly in correcting drug dosing and promoting adherence to guidelines. Checklists, as used by pilots for example, have garnered recent support as an approach to avoid or reduce errors.

DECISION ANALYSIS

Compared with the decision support methods discussed above, decision analysis represents a prescriptive approach to decision making in the face of uncertainty. Its principal application is in complex decisions that involve substantial risk, abundant uncertainty, trade-offs in the outcomes emphasizing a role for preferences, or absence of evidence due to an idiosyncratic feature. For a public health example, Fig. 3-3 displays a decision tree to evaluate strategies for screening for HIV infection. Infected individuals who are unaware of their illness cause up to 20,000 new cases of HIV infection annually in the United States, and about 40% of HIV-positive patients progress to AIDS within a year of the initial diagnosis because of delayed diagnosis. Early identification offers the opportunity to prevent progression to AIDS through CD4 count and viral load monitoring and combination antiretroviral therapy and to reduce spread by reducing risky injection or sexual behaviors.

In 2003, the Centers for Disease Control and Prevention (CDC) proposed that routine universal HIV testing should be incorporated into standard adult medical care and, in part, cited a decision analysis model comparing HIV screening with usual care. Assuming a 1% prevalence of unidentified HIV infection in the population, routine screening of a cohort of 43-year-old men and women increased life expectancy by 5.5 days and lifetime costs by $194 per person screened, yielding an incremental cost-effectiveness ratio for screening versus usual care of $15,078 per quality-adjusted life-year (the additional cost to society to increase population health by 1 year of perfect health). Factors that influenced the results included assumptions about the effectiveness of behavior modification on subsequent sexual behavior, the benefits of early therapy for HIV infection, and the prevalence and incidence of HIV infection in the population targeted. This model, which required over 75 separate data points, provided novel insights into a public health problem in the absence of a randomized clinical trial and helped weigh the pros and cons of such a health policy recommendation. Although such models have been developed for selected clinical problems, their benefit and application to individual real-time clinical management have yet to be demonstrated.

DIAGNOSIS AS AN ELEMENT OF QUALITY OF CARE

High-quality medical care begins with accurate diagnosis. Recently, diagnostic errors have been re-envisioned: the old view was that they were caused by a lack of sufficient skill of an individual clinician; the new view is that they represent a quality of care patient-safety problem traceable to breakdowns in the health care system. Whether this conceptual shift will lead to new ways to improve diagnosis is uncertain. An annual rate of diagnostic errors of 10–15%, possibly leading to 40,000 deaths in the United States, is commonly cited, but these figures are imprecise.

Solutions to the "diagnostic errors as a system of care problem" have focused on system-level approaches, such as decision support and other tools integrated into electronic medical records. The use of checklists has been proposed as a means of reducing some of the cognitive errors discussed earlier in the chapter, such as premature closure. Although checklists have been shown to be useful in certain medical contexts, such as operating rooms and intensive care units, their value in preventing diagnostic errors that lead to patient adverse events remains to be shown.

EVIDENCE-BASED MEDICINE

Clinical medicine is defined traditionally as a practice combining medical knowledge (including scientific evidence), intuition, and judgment in the care of patients (Chap. 1). EBM updates this construct by placing much greater emphasis on the processes by which clinicians gain knowledge of the most up-to-date and relevant clinical research

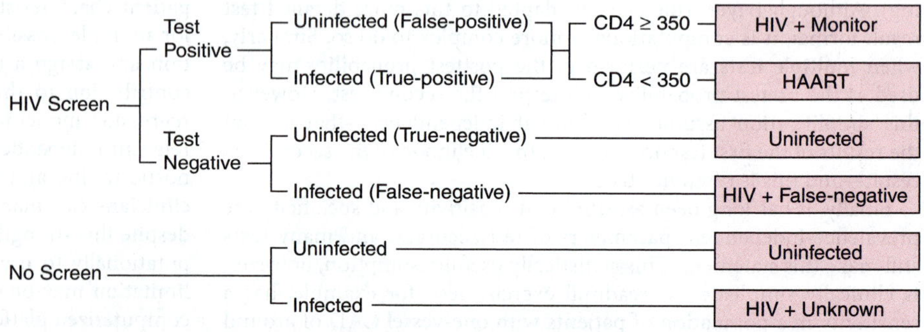

FIGURE 3-3 Basic structure of decision model used to evaluate strategies for screening for HIV in the general population. HAART, highly active antiretroviral therapy. *(Provided courtesy of G. Sanders, with permission.)*

to determine for themselves whether medical interventions alter the disease course and improve the length or quality of life. The meaning of practicing EBM becomes clearer through an examination of its four key steps:

1. Formulating the management question to be answered
2. Searching the literature and online databases for applicable research data
3. Appraising the evidence gathered with regard to its validity and relevance
4. Integrating this appraisal with knowledge about the unique aspects of the patient (including the patient's preferences about the possible outcomes)

The process of searching the world's research literature and appraising the quality and relevance of studies thus identified can be quite time-consuming and requires skills and training that most clinicians do not possess. Thus, identifying recent systematic overviews of the problem in question (Table 3-3) may offer the best starting point for most EBM searches.

Generally, the EBM tools listed in Table 3-3 provide access to research information in one of two forms. The first, primary research reports, is the original peer-reviewed research work that is published in medical journals and accessible through MEDLINE in abstract form. However, without training in using MEDLINE, quickly and efficiently locating reports that are on point in a huge sea of irrelevant or unhelpful citations may be difficult, and important studies could also be missed. The second form, systematic reviews, is the highest level of evidence in the hierarchy because it comprehensively summarizes the available evidence on a particular topic up to a certain date. To avoid the potential biases in review articles, predefined explicit search strategies and inclusion and exclusion criteria are used to find all of the relevant scientific research and grade its quality. The prototype for this kind of resource is the Cochrane Database of Systematic Reviews. When appropriate, a meta-analysis quantitatively summarizes the systematic review findings. The next two sections explicate the major types of clinical research reports available in the literature and the process of aggregating those data into meta-analyses.

SOURCES OF EVIDENCE: CLINICAL TRIALS AND REGISTRIES

The notion of learning from observation of patients is as old as medicine itself. Over the last 50 years, physicians' understanding of how best to turn raw observation into useful evidence has evolved considerably. Case reports, personal anecdotal experience, and small single-center case series are now recognized as having severe limitations in validity and generalizability, and although they may generate hypotheses or be the first reports of adverse events, they have no role in formulating modern standards of practice. The major tools used to develop reliable evidence consist of the randomized clinical trial and the large observational registry. A registry or database typically is focused on a disease or syndrome (e.g., cancer, CAD, heart failure), a clinical procedure (e.g., bone marrow transplantation, coronary revascularization), or an administrative process (e.g., claims data used for billing and reimbursement).

By definition, in observational data, the investigator does not control patient care. Carefully collected *prospective* observational data, however, can achieve a level of evidence quality approaching that of major clinical trial data. At the other end of the spectrum, data collected retrospectively (e.g., chart review) are limited in form and content to what previous observers recorded, which may not include the specific research data being sought, e.g., claims data. Advantages of observational data include the inclusion of a broader population as encountered in practice than is typically represented in clinical trials because of their restrictive inclusion and exclusion criteria. In addition, observational data provide primary evidence for research questions when a randomized trial cannot be performed. For example, it would be difficult to randomize patients to test diagnostic or therapeutic strategies that are unproven but widely accepted in practice, and it would be unethical to randomize based on sex, racial/ethnic group, socioeconomic status, or country of residence or to randomize patients to a potentially harmful intervention, such as smoking or deliberately overeating to develop obesity.

A well-done prospective observational study of a particular management strategy differs from a well-done randomized clinical trial most importantly by its lack of protection from treatment selection bias. The use of observational data to compare diagnostic or therapeutic strategies assumes that sufficient uncertainty exists in clinical practice to ensure that similar patients will be managed differently by different physicians. In short, the analysis assumes that a sufficient element of randomness (in the sense of disorder rather than in the formal statistical sense) exists in clinical management. In such cases, statistical models attempt to adjust for important imbalances to "level the playing field" so that a fair comparison among treatment options can be made. When management is clearly not random (e.g., all eligible left main CAD patients are referred for coronary bypass surgery), the problem may be too confounded (biased) for statistical correction, and observational data may not provide reliable evidence.

In general, the use of concurrent controls is vastly preferable to that of historical controls. For example, comparison of current surgical management of left main CAD with left main CAD patients treated medically during the 1970s (the last time these patients were routinely treated with medicine alone) would be extremely misleading because "medical therapy" has substantially improved in the interim.

TABLE 3-3 SELECTED TOOLS FOR FINDING THE EVIDENCE IN EVIDENCE-BASED MEDICINE (EBM)

Name	Description	Web Address	Availability
Evidence-Based Medicine Reviews	Comprehensive electronic database that combines and integrates: 1. The Cochrane Database of Systematic Reviews 2. ACP Journal Club 3. The Database of Abstracts of Reviews of Effectiveness	*www.ovid.com*	Subscription required. Available through medical center libraries and other institutions.
Cochrane Library	Collection of EBM databases, including The Cochrane Database of Systematic Reviews—full text articles reviewing specific health care topics.	*www.cochrane.org*	Subscription required. Abstracts of systematic reviews available free online. Some countries have funding to provide free access to all residents.
ACP Journal Club	Collection of summaries of original studies and systematic reviews. Published bimonthly. All data since 1991 available on website, updated yearly.	*www.acpjc.org*	Subscription required.
Clinical Evidence	Monthly updated directory of concise overviews of common clinical interventions.	*www.clinicalevidence.com*	Subscription required. Free access for United Kingdom and developing countries.
MEDLINE	National Library of Medicine database with citations back to 1966.	*www.nlm.nih.gov*	Free via Internet.

Randomized controlled clinical trials include the careful prospective design features of the best observational data studies but also include the use of random allocation of treatment. This design provides the best protection against measured and unmeasured confounding due to treatment selection bias (a major aspect of internal validity). However, the randomized trial may not have good external validity (generalizability) if the process of recruitment into the trial resulted in the exclusion of many patients seen in clinical practice.

Consumers of medical evidence need to be aware that randomized trials vary widely in their quality and applicability to practice. The process of designing such a trial often involves many compromises. For example, trials designed to gain U.S. Food and Drug Administration (FDA) approval for an investigational drug or device must fulfill regulatory requirements that may result in a trial population and design that differs substantially from what practicing clinicians would find most useful.

META-ANALYSIS

The Greek prefix *meta* signifies something at a later or higher stage of development. Meta-analysis is research that combines and summarizes the available evidence quantitatively. Although occasionally used to examine nonrandomized studies, meta-analysis is used most typically to summarize all randomized trials examining a particular therapy. Ideally, unpublished trials should be identified and included to avoid publication bias (i.e., missing "negative" trials that may not be published). Furthermore, the best meta-analyses obtain and analyze individual patient-level data from all trials rather than working only the summary data in published reports of each trial. Nonetheless, not all published meta-analyses yield reliable evidence for a particular problem, so their methodology should be scrutinized carefully to ensure proper study design and analysis. The results of a well-done meta-analysis are likely to be most persuasive if they include at least several large-scale, properly performed randomized trials. Meta-analysis can especially help detect benefits when individual trials are inadequately powered (e.g., the benefits of streptokinase thrombolytic therapy in acute MI demonstrated by ISIS-2 in 1988 were evident by the early 1970s through meta-analysis). However, in cases in which the available trials are small or poorly done, meta-analysis should not be viewed as a remedy for the deficiency in primary trial data.

Meta-analyses typically focus on summary measures of relative treatment benefit, such as odds ratios or relative risks. Clinicians also should examine what absolute risk reduction (ARR) can be expected from the therapy. A useful summary metric of absolute treatment benefit is the number needed to treat (NNT) to prevent one adverse outcome event (e.g., death, stroke). NNT is simply 1/ARR. For example, if a hypothetical therapy reduced mortality rates over a 5-year follow-up by 33% (the relative treatment benefit) from 12% (control arm) to 8% (treatment arm), the ARR would be 12% – 8% = 4%, and the NNT would be 1/0.04, or 25. Thus, it would be necessary to treat 25 patients for 5 years to prevent 1 death. If the hypothetical treatment was applied to a lower-risk population, say, with a 6% 5-year mortality, the 33% relative treatment benefit would reduce absolute mortality by 2% (from 6% to 4%), and the NNT for the same therapy in this lower-risk group of patients would be 50. Although not always made explicit, comparisons of NNT estimates from different studies should account for the duration of follow-up used to create each estimate.

CLINICAL PRACTICE GUIDELINES

According to the 1990 Institute of Medicine definition, clinical practice guidelines are "systematically developed statements to assist practitioner and patient decisions about appropriate health care for specific clinical circumstances." This definition emphasizes several crucial features of modern guideline development. First, guidelines are created by using the tools of EBM. In particular, the core of the development process is a systematic literature search followed by a review of the relevant peer-reviewed literature. Second, guidelines usually are focused on a clinical disorder (e.g., adult diabetes, stable angina pectoris) or a health care intervention (e.g., cancer screening). Third, the primary objective of guidelines is to improve the quality of medical care by identifying care practices that should be routinely implemented, based on high-quality evidence and high benefit-to-harm ratios for the interventions. Guidelines are intended to "assist" decision-making, not to define explicitly what decisions should be made in a particular situation, in part because evidence alone is never sufficient for clinical decision-making (e.g., deciding whether to intubate and administer antibiotics for pneumonia in a terminally ill individual, in an individual with dementia, or in an otherwise healthy 30-year-old mother).

Guidelines are narrative documents constructed by expert panels whose composition often is determined by interested professional organizations. These panels vary in the degree to which they represent all relevant stakeholders. The guideline documents consist of a series of specific management recommendations, a summary indication of the quantity and quality of evidence supporting each recommendation, an assessment of the benefit-to-harm ratio for the recommendation, and a narrative discussion of the recommendations. Many recommendations simply reflect the expert consensus of the guideline panel because literature-based evidence is absent. The final step in guideline construction is peer review, followed by a final revision in response to the critiques provided. To improve the reliability and trustworthiness of guidelines, the Institute of Medicine has made methodologic recommendations for guideline development.

Guidelines are closely tied to the process of quality improvement in medicine through their identification of evidence-based best practices. Such practices can be used as quality indicators. Examples include the proportion of acute MI patients who receive aspirin upon admission to a hospital and the proportion of heart failure patients with a depressed ejection fraction treated with an ACE inhibitor.

CONCLUSIONS

In this era of EBM, it is tempting to think that all the difficult decisions practitioners face have been or soon will be solved and digested into practice guidelines and computerized reminders. However, EBM provides practitioners with an ideal rather than a finished set of tools with which to manage patients. Moreover, even with such evidence, it is always worth remembering that the response to therapy of the "average" patient represented by the summary clinical trial outcomes may not be what can be expected for the specific patient sitting in front of a physician in the clinic or hospital. In addition, meta-analyses cannot generate evidence when there are no adequate randomized trials, and most of what clinicians confront in practice will never be thoroughly tested in a randomized trial. For the foreseeable future, excellent clinical reasoning skills, experience supplemented by well-designed quantitative tools, and a keen appreciation for the role of individual patient preferences in their health care will continue to be of paramount importance in the practice of clinical medicine.

4 Screening and Prevention of Disease

Katrina Armstrong, Gary J. Martin

A primary goal of health care is to prevent disease or detect it early enough that intervention will be more effective. Tremendous progress has been made toward this goal over the last 50 years. Screening tests are available for many common diseases and encompass biochemical (e.g., cholesterol, glucose), physiologic (e.g., blood pressure, growth curves), radiologic (e.g., mammogram, bone densitometry), and cytologic (e.g., Pap smear) approaches. Effective preventive interventions have resulted in dramatic declines in mortality from many diseases, particularly infections. Preventive interventions include counseling about risk behaviors, vaccinations, medications, and, in some relatively uncommon settings, surgery. Preventive services (including screening tests, preventive interventions, and counseling) are different than other medical interventions because they are proactively administered to healthy individuals instead of in response to a symptom, sign, or diagnosis. Thus, the decision to recommend a screening test or preventive intervention requires a particularly high bar of evidence that testing and intervention are both practical and effective.

Because population-based screening and prevention strategies must be extremely low risk to have an acceptable benefit-to-harm ratio, the ability to target individuals who are more likely to develop disease could enable the application of a wider set of potential approaches and increase efficiency. Currently, there are many types of data that can predict disease incidence in an asymptomatic individual. Genomic data have received the most attention to date, at least in part because mutations in high-penetrance genes have clear implications for preventive care (Chap. 84). Women with mutations in either *BRCA1* or *BRCA2*, the two major breast cancer susceptibility genes identified to date, have a markedly increased risk (5- to 20-fold) of breast and ovarian cancer. Screening and prevention recommendations include prophylactic oophorectomy and breast magnetic resonance imaging (MRI), both of which are considered to incur too much harm for women at average cancer risk. Some women opt for prophylactic mastectomy to dramatically reduce their breast cancer risk. Although the proportion of common disease explained by high-penetrance genes appears to be relatively small (5–10% of most diseases), mutations in rare, moderate-penetrance genes, and variants in low-penetrance genes, also contribute to the prediction of disease risk. The advent of affordable whole exome/whole genome sequencing is likely to speed the dissemination of these tests into clinical practice and may transform the delivery of preventive care.

Other forms of "omic" data also have the potential to provide important predictive information, including proteomics and metabolomics. These fields are earlier in development and have yet to move into clinical practice. Imaging and other clinical data may also be integrated into a risk-stratified paradigm as evidence grows about the predictive ability of these data and the feasibility of their collection. Of course, all of these data may also be helpful in predicting the risk of harms from screening or prevention, such as the risk of a false-positive mammogram. To the degree that this information can be incorporated into personalized screening and prevention strategies, it could also improve delivery and efficiency.

In addition to advances in risk prediction, there are several other factors that are likely to promote the importance of screening and prevention in the near term. New imaging modalities are being developed that promise to detect changes at the cellular and subcellular levels, greatly increasing the probability that early detection improves outcomes. The rapidly growing understanding of the biologic pathways underlying initiation and progression of many common diseases has the potential to transform the development of preventive interventions, including chemoprevention. Furthermore, screening and prevention offer the promise of both improving health and sparing the costs of disease treatment, an issue that has gained national attention with the continued growth in health care costs.

This chapter will review the basic principles of screening and prevention in the primary care setting. Recommendations for specific disorders such as cardiovascular disease, diabetes, and cancer are provided in the chapters dedicated to those topics.

BASIC PRINCIPLES OF SCREENING

The basic principles of screening populations for disease were published by the World Health Organization in 1968 (Table 4-1).

TABLE 4-1 PRINCIPLES OF SCREENING

The condition should be an important health problem.
There should be a treatment for the condition.
Facilities for diagnosis and treatment should be available.
There should be a latent stage of the disease.
There should be a test or examination for the condition.
The test should be acceptable to the population.
The natural history of the disease should be adequately understood.
There should be an agreed policy on whom to treat.
The cost of finding a case should be balanced in relation to overall medical expenditure.

In general, screening is most effective when applied to relatively common disorders that carry a large disease burden (Table 4-2). The five leading causes of mortality in the United States are heart diseases, malignant neoplasms, accidents, cerebrovascular diseases, and chronic obstructive pulmonary disease. Thus, many screening strategies are targeted at these conditions. From a global health perspective, these conditions are priorities, but malaria, malnutrition, AIDS, tuberculosis, and violence also carry a heavy disease burden (Chap. 2).

Having an effective treatment for early disease has proven challenging for some common diseases. For example, although Alzheimer's disease is the sixth leading cause of death in the United States, there are no curative treatments and no evidence that early treatment improves outcomes. Lack of facilities for diagnosis and treatment is a particular challenge for developing countries and may change screening strategies, including the development of "see and treat" approaches such as those currently used for cervical cancer screening in some countries. A long latent or preclinical phase where early treatment increases the chance of cure is a hallmark of many cancers; for example, polypectomy prevents progression to colon cancer. Similarly, early identification of hypertension or hyperlipidemia allows therapeutic interventions that reduce the long-term risk of cardiovascular or cerebrovascular events. In contrast, lung cancer screening has historically proven more challenging because most tumors are not curable by the time they can be detected on a chest x-ray. However, the length of the preclinical phase also depends on the level of resolution of the screening test, and this situation changed with the development of chest computed tomography (CT). Low-dose chest CT scanning can detect tumors earlier and was recently demonstrated to reduce lung cancer mortality by 20% in individuals who had at least a 30-pack-year history of smoking. The short interval between the ability to detect disease on a screening test and the development of incurable disease also contributes to the limited effectiveness of mammography screening in reducing breast cancer mortality among premenopausal women. Similarly, the early detection of prostate cancer may not lead to a difference in the mortality rate because the disease is often indolent and competing morbidities, such as coronary artery disease, may ultimately cause mortality (Chap. 100). This uncertainty about the natural history is also reflected in the controversy about treatment of prostate cancer, further contributing to the challenge of screening in this disease. Finally, screening programs can incur significant economic costs that must be considered in the context of the available resources and alternative strategies for improving health outcomes.

METHODS OF MEASURING HEALTH BENEFITS

Because screening and preventive interventions are recommended to asymptomatic individuals, they are held to a high standard for demonstrating a favorable risk-benefit ratio before implementation. In general, the principles of evidence-based medicine apply to demonstrating the efficacy of screening tests and preventive interventions, where randomized controlled trials (RCTs) with mortality outcomes are the gold standard. However, because RCTs are often not feasible, observational studies, such as case-control designs, have been used to assess the effectiveness of some interventions such as colorectal cancer screening. For some strategies, such as cervical cancer screening, the only data available are ecologic data demonstrating dramatic declines in mortality.

TABLE 4-2 LIFETIME CUMULATIVE RISK

Breast cancer for women	10%
Colon cancer	6%
Cancer of the cervix for women[a]	2%
Domestic violence for women	Up to 15%
Hip fracture for white women	16%

[a]Assuming an unscreened population.

Irrespective of the study design used to assess the effectiveness of screening, it is critical that disease incidence or mortality is the primary endpoint rather than length of disease survival. This is important because lead time bias and length time bias can create the appearance of an improvement in disease survival from a screening test when there is no actual effect. Lead time bias occurs because screening identifies a case before it would have presented clinically, thereby creating the perception that a patient lived longer after diagnosis simply by moving the date of diagnosis earlier rather than the date of death later. Length time bias occurs because screening is more likely to identify slowly progressive disease than rapidly progressive disease. Thus, within a fixed period of time, a screened population will have a greater proportion of these slowly progressive cases and will appear to have better disease survival than an unscreened population.

A variety of endpoints are used to assess the potential gain from screening and preventive interventions.

1. *The absolute and relative impact of screening on disease incidence or mortality.* The absolute difference in disease incidence or mortality between a screened and nonscreened group allows the comparison of size of the benefit across preventive services. A meta-analysis of Swedish mammography trials (ages 40–70) found that ~1.2 fewer women per 1000 would die from breast cancer if they were screened over a 12-year period. By comparison, ~3 lives per 1000 would be saved from colon cancer in a population (ages 50–75) screened with annual fecal occult blood testing (FOBT) over a 13-year period. Based on this analysis, colon cancer screening may actually save more women's lives than does mammography. However, the relative impact of FOBT (30% reduction in colon cancer death) is similar to the relative impact of mammography (14–32% reduction in breast cancer death), emphasizing the importance of both relative and absolute comparisons.
2. *The number of subjects screened to prevent disease or death in one individual.* The inverse of the absolute difference in mortality is the number of subjects who would need to be screened or receive a preventive intervention to prevent one death. For example, 731 women ages 65–69 would need to be screened by dual-energy x-ray absorptiometry (DEXA) (and treated appropriately) to prevent one hip fracture from osteoporosis.
3. *Increase in average life expectancy for a population.* Predicted increases in life expectancy for various screening and preventive interventions are listed in Table 4-3. It should be noted, however, that the increase in life expectancy is an average that applies to a population, not to an individual. In reality, the vast majority of the population does not derive any benefit from a screening test or preventive intervention. A small subset of patients, however, will benefit greatly. For example, Pap smears do not benefit the 98% of women who never develop cancer of the cervix. However, for the 2% who would have developed cervical cancer, Pap smears may add as much as 25 years to their lives. Some studies suggest that a 1-month gain of life expectancy is a reasonable goal for a population-based screening or prevention strategy.

TABLE 4-3 ESTIMATED AVERAGE INCREASE IN LIFE EXPECTANCY FOR A POPULATION

Screening or Preventive Intervention	Average Increase
Mammography:	
Women, 40–50 years	0–5 days
Women, 50–70 years	1 month
Pap smears, age 18–65	2–3 months
Getting a 35-year-old smoker to quit	3–5 years
Beginning regular exercise for a 40-year-old man (30 min, 3 times a week)	9 months–2 years

ASSESSING THE HARMS OF SCREENING AND PREVENTION

Just as with most aspects of medical care, screening and preventive interventions also incur the possibility of adverse outcomes. These adverse outcomes include side effects from preventive medications and vaccinations, false-positive screening tests, overdiagnosis of disease from screening tests, anxiety, radiation exposure from some screening tests, and discomfort from some interventions and screening tests. The risk of side effects from preventive medications is analogous to the use of medications in therapeutic settings and is considered in the Food and Drug Administration (FDA) approval process. Side effects from currently recommended vaccinations are primarily limited to discomfort and minor immune reactions. However, the concern about associations between vaccinations and serious adverse outcomes continues to limit the acceptance of many vaccinations despite the lack of data supporting the causal nature of these associations.

The possibility of a false-positive test occurs with nearly all screening tests, although the definition of what constitutes a false-positive result often varies across settings. For some tests such as screening mammography and screening chest CT, a false-positive result occurs when an abnormality is identified that is not malignant, requiring either a biopsy diagnosis or short-term follow-up. For other tests such as Pap smears, a false-positive result occurs because the test identifies a wide range of potentially premalignant states, only a small percentage of which would ever progress to an invasive cancer. This risk is closely tied to the risk of overdiagnosis in which the screening test identifies disease that would not have presented clinically in the patient's lifetime. Assessing the degree of overdiagnosis from a screening test is very difficult given the need for long-term follow-up of an unscreened population to determine the true incidence of disease over time. Recent estimates suggest that as much as 15–25% of breast cancers identified by mammography screening and 15–37% of prostate cancers identified by prostate-specific antigen testing may never have presented clinically. Screening tests also have the potential to create unwarranted anxiety, particularly in conjunction with false-positive findings. Although multiple studies have documented increased anxiety through the screening process, there are few data suggesting this anxiety has long-term adverse consequences, including subsequent screening behavior. Screening tests that involve radiation (e.g., mammography, chest CT) add to the cumulative radiation exposure for the screened individual. The absolute amount of radiation is very small from any of these tests, but the overall impact of repeated exposure from multiple sources is still being determined. Some preventive interventions (e.g., vaccinations) and screening tests (e.g., mammography) may lead to discomfort at the time of administration, but again, there is little evidence of long-term adverse consequences.

WEIGHING THE BENEFITS AND HARMS

The decision to implement a population-based screening and prevention strategy requires weighing the benefits and harms, including the economic impact of the strategy. The costs include not only the expense of the intervention but also time away from work, downstream costs from false-positive results or adverse events, and other potential harms. Cost-effectiveness is typically assessed by calculating the cost per year of life saved, with adjustment for the quality of life impact of different interventions and disease states (i.e., quality-adjusted life-year). Typically, strategies that cost <$50,000 to $100,000 per quality-adjusted year of life saved are considered "cost-effective" (Chap. 3).

The U.S. Preventive Services Task Force (USPSTF) is an independent panel of experts in preventive care that provides evidence-based recommendations for screening and preventive strategies based on an assessment of the benefit-to-harm ratio (Tables 4-4 and 4-5). Because there are multiple advisory organizations providing recommendations for preventive services, the agreement among the organizations varies across the different services. For example, all advisory groups support screening for hyperlipidemia and colorectal cancer, whereas consensus is lower for breast cancer screening among women in their 40s and almost nonexistent for prostate cancer screening. Because the guidelines are only updated periodically, differences across advisory organizations may also reflect the data that were available when the guideline was issued. For example, multiple organizations have recently issued recommendations supporting lung cancer screening among heavy smokers based on the results of the National Lung Screening Trial (NLST) published in 2011, whereas the USPSTF did not review lung cancer screening until 2014.

TABLE 4-4 SCREENING TESTS RECOMMENDED BY THE U.S. PREVENTIVE SERVICES TASK FORCE FOR AVERAGE-RISK ADULTS

Disease	Test	Population	Frequency	Chapter
Abdominal aortic aneurysm	Ultrasound	Men 65–75 who have ever smoked	Once	
Alcohol misuse	Alcohol Use Disorders Identification Test	>18	Unknown	467
Breast cancer	Mammography with or without clinical breast examination	Women 50–75	Every 2 years	
Cervical cancer	Pap smear	Women 21–65	Every 3 years	100
	Pap smear and HPV testing	Women 30–65	Every 5 years if HPV negative	
Chlamydia/gonorrhea	Nucleic acid amplification test on urine or cervical swab	Sexually active women <25	Unknown	213
Colorectal cancer	Fecal occult blood testing	50–75	Every year	100, 110
	Sigmoidoscopy	50–75	Every 5 years	
	Colonoscopy	50–75	Every 10 years	
Depression	Screening questions	All adults	Periodically	
Diabetes	Fasting blood glucose	Adults with hypertension	Every 3 years	417
Hepatitis C	Anti-HCV antibody followed by confirmatory PCR	Adults born between 1945 and 1965	Once	
HIV	Reactive immunoassay or rapid HIV followed by confirmatory test	15–65	Once	
Hyperlipidemia	Cholesterol	Men >35	Every 5 years	291e
		Women >45	Every 5 years	
Hypertension	Blood pressure	All adults	Periodically	298
Intimate partner violence	Screening questions	Women of childbearing age	Unknown	
Obesity	Body mass index	All adults	Unknown	
Osteoporosis	DEXA	Women >65 or >60 with risk factors	Unknown	425

Abbreviations: DEXA, dual-energy x-ray absorptiometry; HCV, hepatitis C virus; HPV, human papillomavirus; PCR, polymerase chain reaction.

Source: Adapted from the U.S. Preventive Services Task Force 2013. *http://www.uspreventiveservicestaskforce.org/adultrec.htm.*

For many screening tests and preventive interventions, the balance of benefits and harms may be uncertain for the average-risk population but more favorable for individuals at higher risk for disease. Although age is the most commonly used risk factor for determining screening and prevention recommendations, the USPSTF also recommends some screening tests in populations with other risk factors for the disease (e.g., syphilis). In addition, being at increased risk for the disease often supports initiating screening at an earlier age than that recommended for the average-risk population. For example, when there is a significant family history of breast or colon cancer, it is prudent to initiate screening 10 years before the age at which the youngest family member was diagnosed with cancer.

Although informed consent is important for all aspects of medical care, shared decision-making may be a particularly important approach to decisions about preventive services when the benefit-to-harm ratio is uncertain for a specific population. For example, many expert groups, including the USPSTF, recommend an individualized discussion about prostate cancer screening, because the decision-making process is complex and relies heavily on personal issues. Some men may decline screening, whereas others may be more willing to accept the risks of an early detection strategy. Recent analysis suggests that many men may be better off not screening for prostate cancer because watchful waiting was the preferred strategy when quality-adjusted life-years were considered. Another example of

TABLE 4-5 PREVENTIVE INTERVENTIONS RECOMMENDED FOR AVERAGE-RISK ADULTS

Intervention	Disease	Population	Frequency	Chapter
Adult immunization				148, 149
Tetanus-diphtheria		>18	Every 10 years	
Varicella		Susceptibles only, >18	Two doses	
Measles-mumps-rubella		Women, childbearing age	One dose	
Pneumococcal		>65	One dose	
Influenza		>50	Yearly	
Human papillomavirus		Boys >21	If not done prior	
		Girls >26		
Zoster		>60	Once	
Chemoprevention				
Aspirin	Cardiovascular disease	Men 45–79		
		Women 55–79		
Folic acid	Neural tube defects in baby	Women planning or capable of pregnancy		
Tamoxifen/raloxifene	Breast cancer	Women at high risk for breast cancer		
Vitamin D	Fracture/falls	>65 at increased risk for falls		

shared decision-making involves the choice of techniques for colon cancer screening (Chap. 100). In controlled studies, the use of annual FOBT reduces colon cancer deaths by 15–30%. Flexible sigmoidoscopy reduces colon cancer deaths by ~60%. Colonoscopy offers the same benefit as or greater benefit than flexible sigmoidoscopy, but its use incurs additional costs and risks. These screening procedures have not been compared directly in the same population, but the estimated cost to society is similar: $10,000–25,000 per year of life saved. Thus, although one patient may prefer the ease of preparation, less time disruption, and the lower risk of flexible sigmoidoscopy, others may prefer the sedation and thoroughness of colonoscopy.

TABLE 4-6 PREVENTIVE COUNSELING RECOMMENDED BY THE USPSTF

Topic	Chapter Reference
Alcohol and drug use	467, 468e
Genetic counseling for *BRCA1/2* testing among women at increased risk for deleterious mutations	
Nutrition and diet	
Sexually transmitted infections	163, 226
Sun exposure	75
Tobacco use	470

COUNSELING ON HEALTHY BEHAVIORS

In considering the impact of preventive services, it is important to recognize that tobacco and alcohol use, diet, and exercise constitute the vast majority of factors that influence preventable deaths in developed countries. Perhaps the single greatest preventive health care measure is to help patients quit smoking (Chap. 470). However, efforts in these areas frequently involve behavior changes (e.g., weight loss, exercise, seat belts) or the management of addictive conditions (e.g., tobacco and alcohol use) that are often recalcitrant to intervention. Although these are challenging problems, evidence strongly supports the role of counseling by health care providers (Table 4-6) in effecting health behavior change. Educational campaigns, public policy changes, and community-based interventions have also proven to be important parts of a strategy for addressing these factors in some settings. Although the USPSTF found that the evidence was conclusive to recommend a relatively small set of counseling activities, counseling in areas such as physical activity and injury prevention (including seat belts and bicycle and motorcycle helmets) has become a routine part of primary care practice.

IMPLEMENTING DISEASE PREVENTION AND SCREENING

The implementation of disease prevention and screening strategies in practice is challenging. A number of techniques can assist physicians with the delivery of these services. An appropriately configured electronic health record can provide reminder systems that make it easier for physicians to track and meet guidelines. Some systems give patients secure access to their medical records, providing an additional means to enhance adherence to routine screening. Systems that provide nurses and other staff with standing orders are effective for smoking prevention and immunizations. The Agency for Healthcare Research and Quality and the Centers for Disease Control and Prevention have developed flow sheets and electronic tools as part of their "Put Prevention into Practice" program (*http://www.uspreventiveservicestaskforce.org/tools.htm*). Many of these tools use age categories to help guide implementation. Age-specific recommendations for screening and counseling are summarized in Table 4-7.

Many patients see a physician for ongoing care of chronic illnesses, and this visit provides an opportunity to include a "measure of prevention" for other health problems. For example, a patient seen for management of hypertension or diabetes can have breast cancer screening incorporated into one visit and a discussion about colon cancer screening at the next visit. Other patients may respond more favorably to a clearly defined visit that addresses all relevant screening and prevention interventions. Because of age or comorbidities, it may be appropriate with some patients to abandon certain screening and prevention activities, although there are fewer data about when to "sunset" these services. For many screening tests, the benefit of screening does not accrue until 5 to 10 years of follow-up, and there are generally few data to support continuing screening for most diseases past age 75. In addition, for patients with advanced diseases and limited life expectancy, there is considerable benefit from shifting the focus from screening procedures to the conditions and interventions more likely to affect quality and length of life.

TABLE 4-7 AGE-SPECIFIC CAUSES OF MORTALITY AND CORRESPONDING PREVENTIVE OPTIONS

Age Group	Leading Causes of Age-Specific Mortality	Screening Prevention Interventions to Consider for Each Specific Population
15–24	1. Accident	• Counseling on routine seat belt use, bicycle/motorcycle/ATV helmets (1)
	2. Homicide	• Counseling on diet and exercise (5)
	3. Suicide	• Discuss dangers of alcohol use while driving, swimming, boating (1)
	4. Malignancy	• Assess and update vaccination status (tetanus, diphtheria, hepatitis B, MMR, rubella, varicella, meningitis, HPV)
	5. Heart disease	• Ask about gun use and/or gun possession (2,3)
		• Assess for substance abuse history including alcohol (2,3)
		• Screen for domestic violence (2,3)
		• Screen for depression and/or suicidal/homicidal ideation (2,3)
		• Pap smear for cervical cancer screening after age 21 (4)
		• Discuss skin, breast awareness, and testicular self-exams (4)
		• Recommend UV light avoidance and regular sunscreen use (4)
		• Measurement of blood pressure, height, weight, and body mass index (5)
		• Discuss health risks of tobacco use, consider emphasis on cosmetic and economic issues to improve quit rates for younger smokers (4,5)
		• Chlamydia and gonorrhea screening and contraceptive counseling for sexually active females, discuss STD prevention
		• Hepatitis B, and syphilis testing if there is high-risk sexual behavior(s) or any prior history of sexually transmitted disease
		• HIV testing
		• Continue annual influenza vaccination

(Continued)

TABLE 4-7 AGE-SPECIFIC CAUSES OF MORTALITY AND CORRESPONDING PREVENTIVE OPTIONS (*CONTINUED*)

Age Group	Leading Causes of Age-Specific Mortality	Screening Prevention Interventions to Consider for Each Specific Population
25–44	1. Accident	*As above plus consider the following:*
	2. Malignancy	• Readdress smoking status, encourage cessation at every visit (2,3)
	3. Heart disease	• Obtain detailed family history of malignancies and begin early screening/prevention program if patient is at significant increased risk (2)
	4. Suicide	• Assess all cardiac risk factors (including screening for diabetes and hyperlipidemia) and consider primary prevention with aspirin for patients at >3% 5-year risk of a vascular event (3)
	5. Homicide	• Assess for chronic alcohol abuse, risk factors for viral hepatitis, or other risks for development of chronic liver disease
	6. HIV	• Consider individualized breast cancer screening with mammography at age 40 (2)
45–64	1. Malignancy	• Consider prostate cancer screen with annual PSA and digital rectal exam at age 50 (or possibly earlier in African Americans or patients with family history) (1)
	2. Heart disease	• Begin colorectal cancer screening at age 50 with fecal occult blood testing, flexible sigmoidoscopy, or colonoscopy (1)
	3. Accident	• Reassess and update vaccination status at age 50 and vaccinate all smokers against *S. pneumoniae* at age 50 (6)
	4. Diabetes mellitus	• Consider screening for coronary disease in higher-risk patients (2,5)
	5. Cerebrovascular disease	• Consider screening for hepatitis C in adults born between 1945 and 1965 (7)
	6. Chronic lower respiratory disease	• Zoster vaccination at age 60
	7. Chronic liver disease and cirrhosis	• Begin mammography screening by age 50
	8. Suicide	
≥65	1. Heart disease	*As above plus consider the following:*
	2. Malignancy	• Readdress smoking status, encourage cessation at every visit (1,2,3,4)
	3. Cerebrovascular disease	• One-time ultrasound for AAA in men 65–75 who have ever smoked
	4. Chronic lower respiratory disease	• Consider pulmonary function testing for all long-term smokers to assess for development of chronic obstructive pulmonary disease (4,6)
	5. Alzheimer's disease	
	6. Influenza and pneumonia	• Screen all postmenopausal women (and all men with risk factors) for osteoporosis
	7. Diabetes mellitus	• Continue annual influenza vaccination and vaccinate against *S. pneumoniae* at age 65 (4, 6)
	8. Kidney disease	• Screen for dementia and depression (5)
	9. Accidents	• Screen for visual and hearing problems, home safety issues, and elder abuse (9)
	10. Septicemia	

Note: The numbers in parentheses refer to areas of risk in the mortality column affected by the specified intervention.

Abbreviations: AAA, abdominal aortic aneurysm; ATV, all-terrain vehicle; HPV, human papillomavirus; MMR, measles-mumps-rubella; PSA, prostate-specific antigen; STD, sexually transmitted disease; UV, ultraviolet.

5 Principles of Clinical Pharmacology

Dan M. Roden

Drugs are the cornerstone of modern therapeutics. Nevertheless, it is well recognized among physicians and in the lay community that the outcome of drug therapy varies widely among individuals. While this variability has been perceived as an unpredictable, and therefore inevitable, accompaniment of drug therapy, this is not the case. The goal of this chapter is to describe the principles of clinical pharmacology that can be used for the safe and optimal use of available and new drugs.

Drugs interact with specific target molecules to produce their beneficial and adverse effects. The chain of events between administration of a drug and production of these effects in the body can be divided into two components, both of which contribute to variability in drug actions. The first component comprises the processes that determine drug delivery to, and removal from, molecular targets. The resulting description of the relationship between drug concentration and time is termed *pharmacokinetics*. The second component of variability in drug action comprises the processes that determine variability in drug actions despite equivalent drug delivery to effector drug sites. This description of the relationship between drug concentration and effect is termed *pharmacodynamics*. As discussed further below, pharmacodynamic variability can arise as a result of variability in function of the target molecule itself or of variability in the broad biologic context in which the drug-target interaction occurs to achieve drug effects.

Two important goals of the discipline of clinical pharmacology are (1) to provide a description of conditions under which drug actions vary among human subjects; and (2) to determine mechanisms underlying this variability, with the goal of improving therapy with available drugs as well as pointing to new drug mechanisms that may be effective in the treatment of human disease. The first steps in the discipline were empirical descriptions of the influence of disease on drug actions and of individuals or families with unusual sensitivities to adverse drug effects. These important descriptive findings are now being replaced by an understanding of the molecular mechanisms underlying variability in drug actions. Thus, the effects of disease, drug coadministration, or familial factors in modulating drug action can now be reinterpreted as variability in expression or function of specific genes whose products determine pharmacokinetics and pharmacodynamics. Nevertheless, it is often the personal interaction of the patient with the physician or other health care provider that first identifies unusual variability in drug actions; maintained alertness to unusual drug responses continues to be a key component of improving drug safety.

Unusual drug responses, segregating in families, have been recognized for decades and initially defined the field of *pharmacogenetics*. Now, with an increasing appreciation of common and rare polymorphisms across the human genome, comes the opportunity to reinterpret descriptive mechanisms of variability in drug action as a consequence of specific DNA variants, or sets of variants, among individuals. This approach defines the field of *pharmacogenomics*, which may hold the opportunity of allowing practitioners to integrate a molecular understanding of the basis of disease with an individual's genomic makeup to prescribe personalized, highly effective, and safe therapies.

IDENTIFYING DRUG TARGETS

Drug therapy is an ancient feature of human culture. The first treatments were plant extracts discovered empirically to be effective for indications like fever, pain, or breathlessness. This symptom-based empiric approach to drug development was supplanted in the twentieth century by identification of compounds targeting more fundamental biologic processes such as bacterial growth or elevated blood pressure; the term "magic bullet," coined by Paul Ehrlich to describe the search for effective compounds for syphilis, captures the essence of the hope that understanding basic biologic processes will lead to highly effective new therapies. An integral step in modern drug development follows identification of a chemical lead with biologic activity with increasingly sophisticated medicinal chemistry-based structural modifications to develop compounds with specificity for the chosen target, lack of "off-target" effects, and pharmacokinetic properties suitable for human use (e.g., consistent bioavailability, long elimination half-life, no high-risk pharmacokinetic features described further below).

A common starting point for contemporary drug development is basic biologic discovery that implicates potential target molecules: examples of such target molecules include HMG-CoA reductase or the *BRAF* V600E mutation in many malignant melanomas. The development of compounds targeting these molecules has not only revolutionized treatment for diseases such as hypercholesterolemia or malignant melanoma, but has also revealed new biologic features of disease. Thus, for example, initial spectacular successes with vemurafenib (which targets *BRAF* V600E) were followed by near-universal tumor relapse, strongly suggesting that inhibition of this pathway alone would be insufficient for tumor control. This reasoning, in turn, supports a view that many complex diseases will not lend themselves to cure by targeting a single magic bullet, but rather single drugs or combinations will need to attack multiple pathways whose perturbation results in disease. The use of combination therapy in settings such as hypertension, tuberculosis, HIV infection, and many cancers highlights potential for such a "systems biology" view of drug therapy.

GLOBAL CONSIDERATIONS

It is true across all cultures and diseases that factors such as compliance, genetic variants affecting pharmacokinetics or pharmacodynamics, and drug interactions contribute to drug responses. In addition, culture- or ancestry-specific factors play a role. For example, the frequency of specific genetic variants modulating drug responses often varies by ancestry, as discussed later. Cost issues or cultural factors may determine the likelihood that specific drugs, drug combinations, or over-the-counter (OTC) remedies are prescribed. The broad principles of clinical pharmacology enunciated here can be used to analyze the mechanisms underlying successful or unsuccessful therapy with any drug.

INDICATIONS FOR DRUG THERAPY: RISK VERSUS BENEFIT

It is self-evident that the benefits of drug therapy should outweigh the risks. Benefits fall into two broad categories: those designed to alleviate a symptom and those designed to prolong useful life. An increasing emphasis on the principles of evidence-based medicine and techniques such as large clinical trials and meta-analyses have defined benefits of drug therapy in broad patient populations. Establishing the balance between risk and benefit is not always simple. An increasing body of evidence supports the idea, with which practitioners are very familiar, that individual patients may display responses that are not expected from large population studies and often have comorbidities that typically exclude them from large clinical trials. In addition, therapies that provide symptomatic benefits but shorten life may be entertained in patients with serious and highly symptomatic diseases such as heart failure or cancer. These considerations illustrate the continuing, highly personal nature of the relationship between the prescriber and the patient.

Adverse Effects Some adverse effects are so common and so readily associated with drug therapy that they are identified very early during clinical use of a drug. By contrast, serious adverse effects may be sufficiently uncommon that they escape detection for many years after a drug begins to be widely used. The issue of how to identify rare but serious adverse effects (that can profoundly affect the benefit-risk perception in an individual patient) has not been satisfactorily resolved. Potential approaches range from an increased understanding of the molecular and genetic basis of variability in drug actions to expanded postmarketing surveillance mechanisms. None of these have been completely effective, so practitioners must be continuously vigilant to the possibility that unusual symptoms may be related to specific drugs, or combinations of drugs, that their patients receive.

Therapeutic Index Beneficial and adverse reactions to drug therapy can be described by a series of dose-response relations (Fig. 5-1). Well-tolerated drugs demonstrate a wide margin, termed the *therapeutic ratio*, *therapeutic index*, or *therapeutic window*, between the doses required to produce a therapeutic effect and those producing toxicity. In cases where there is a similar relationship between plasma drug concentration and effects, monitoring plasma concentrations can be a highly effective aid in managing drug therapy by enabling concentrations to be maintained above the minimum required to produce an effect and below the concentration range likely to produce toxicity. Such monitoring has been widely used to guide therapy with specific agents, such as certain antiarrhythmics, anticonvulsants, and antibiotics. Many of the principles in clinical pharmacology and examples

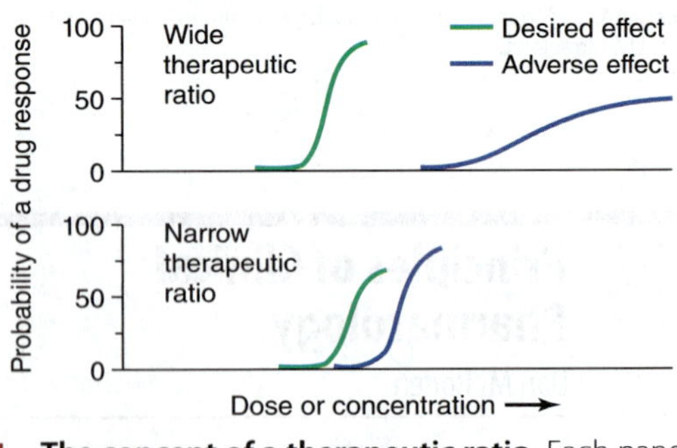

FIGURE 5-1 The concept of a therapeutic ratio. Each panel illustrates the relationship between increasing dose and cumulative probability of a desired or adverse drug effect. ***Top.*** A drug with a wide therapeutic ratio, i.e., a wide separation of the two curves. ***Bottom.*** A drug with a narrow therapeutic ratio; here, the likelihood of adverse effects at therapeutic doses is increased because the curves are not well separated. Further, a steep dose-response curve for adverse effects is especially undesirable, as it implies that even small dosage increments may sharply increase the likelihood of toxicity. When there is a definable relationship between drug concentration (usually measured in plasma) and desirable and adverse effect curves, concentration may be substituted on the abscissa. Note that not all patients necessarily demonstrate a therapeutic response (or adverse effect) at any dose, and that some effects (notably some adverse effects) may occur in a dose-independent fashion.

outlined below, which can be applied broadly to therapeutics, have been developed in these arenas.

PRINCIPLES OF PHARMACOKINETICS

The processes of absorption, distribution, metabolism, and excretion—collectively termed *drug disposition*—determine the concentration of drug delivered to target effector molecules.

ABSORPTION AND BIOAVAILABILITY

When a drug is administered orally, subcutaneously, intramuscularly, rectally, sublingually, or directly into desired sites of action, the amount of drug actually entering the systemic circulation may be less than with the intravenous route (Fig. 5-2*A*). The fraction of drug available to the systemic circulation by other routes is termed *bioavailability*. Bioavailability may be <100% for two main reasons: (1) absorption is reduced, or (2) the drug undergoes metabolism or elimination prior to entering the systemic circulation. Occasionally, the administered drug formulation is inconsistent or has degraded with time; for example, the anticoagulant dabigatran degrades rapidly (over weeks) once exposed to air, so the amount administered may be less than prescribed.

When a drug is administered by a nonintravenous route, the peak concentration occurs later and is lower than after the same dose given by rapid intravenous injection, reflecting absorption from the site of administration (Fig. 5-2). The extent of absorption may be reduced because a drug is incompletely released from its dosage form, undergoes destruction at its site of administration, or has physicochemical properties such as insolubility that prevent complete absorption from its site of administration. Slow absorption rates are deliberately designed into "slow-release" or "sustained-release" drug formulations in order to minimize variation in plasma concentrations during the interval between doses.

"First-Pass" Effect When a drug is administered orally, it must traverse the intestinal epithelium, the portal venous system, and the liver prior

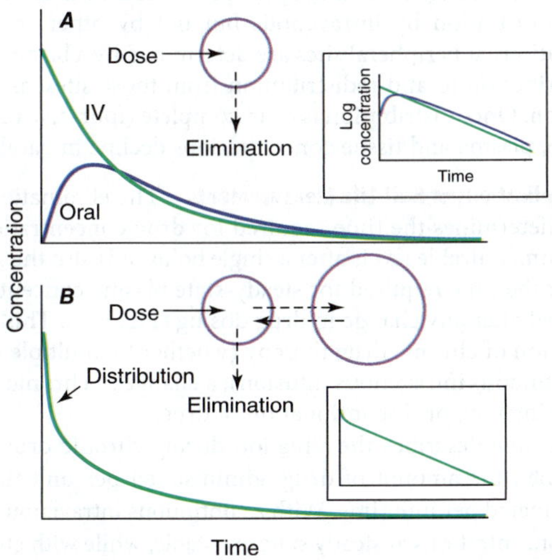

FIGURE 5-2 Idealized time-plasma concentration curves after a single dose of drug. ***A.*** The time course of drug concentration after an instantaneous IV bolus or an oral dose in the one-compartment model shown. The area under the time-concentration curve is clearly less with the oral drug than the IV, indicating incomplete bioavailability. Note that despite this incomplete bioavailability, concentration after the oral dose can be higher than after the IV dose at some time points. The inset shows that the decline of concentrations over time is linear on a log-linear plot, characteristic of first-order elimination, and that oral and IV drugs have the same elimination (parallel) time course. ***B.*** The decline of central compartment concentration when drug is distributed both to and from a peripheral compartment and eliminated from the central compartment. The rapid initial decline of concentration reflects not drug elimination but distribution.

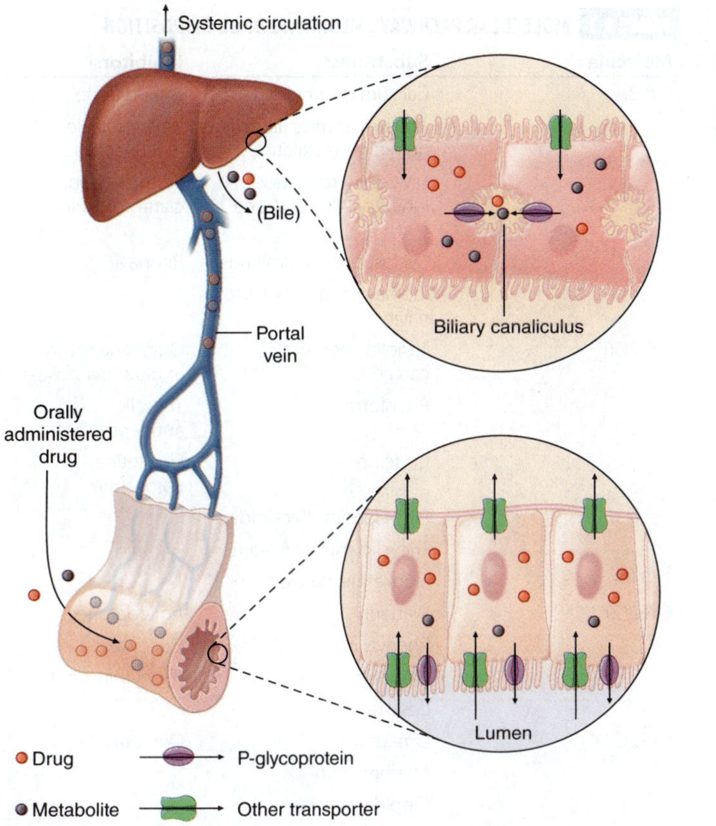

FIGURE 5-3 Mechanism of presystemic clearance. After drug enters the enterocyte, it can undergo metabolism, excretion into the intestinal lumen, or transport into the portal vein. Similarly, the hepatocyte may accomplish metabolism and biliary excretion prior to the entry of drug and metabolites to the systemic circulation. *(Adapted by permission from DM Roden, in DP Zipes, J Jalife [eds]: Cardiac Electrophysiology: From Cell to Bedside, 4th ed. Philadelphia, Saunders, 2003. Copyright 2003 with permission from Elsevier.)*

to entering the systemic circulation (Fig. 5-3). Once a drug enters the enterocyte, it may undergo metabolism, be transported into the portal vein, or be excreted back into the intestinal lumen. Both excretion into the intestinal lumen and metabolism decrease systemic bioavailability. Once a drug passes this enterocyte barrier, it may also be taken up into the hepatocyte, where bioavailability can be further limited by metabolism or excretion into the bile. This elimination in intestine and liver, which reduces the amount of drug delivered to the systemic circulation, is termed *presystemic elimination*, *presystemic extraction*, or *first-pass elimination*.

Drug movement across the membrane of any cell, including enterocytes and hepatocytes, is a combination of passive diffusion and active transport, mediated by specific drug uptake and efflux molecules. One widely studied drug transport molecule is P-glycoprotein, the product of the *MDR1* gene. P-glycoprotein is expressed on the apical aspect of the enterocyte and on the canalicular aspect of the hepatocyte (Fig. 5-3). In both locations, it serves as an efflux pump, limiting availability of drug to the systemic circulation. P-glycoprotein–mediated drug efflux from cerebral capillaries limits drug brain penetration and is an important component of the blood-brain barrier.

Drug metabolism generates compounds that are usually more polar and, hence, more readily excreted than parent drug. Metabolism takes place predominantly in the liver but can occur at other sites such as kidney, intestinal epithelium, lung, and plasma. "Phase I" metabolism involves chemical modification, most often oxidation accomplished by members of the cytochrome P450 (CYP) monooxygenase superfamily. CYPs that are especially important for drug metabolism are presented in Table 5-1, and each drug may be a substrate for one or more of these enzymes. "Phase II" metabolism involves conjugation of specific endogenous compounds to drugs or their metabolites. The enzymes

TABLE 5-1 MOLECULAR PATHWAYS MEDIATING DRUG DISPOSITION

Molecule	Substrates[a]	Inhibitors[a]
CYP3A	Calcium channel blockers	Amiodarone
	Antiarrhythmics (lidocaine, quinidine, mexiletine)	Ketoconazole, itraconazole
	HMG-CoA reductase inhibitors ("statins"; see text)	Erythromycin, clarithromycin
	Cyclosporine, tacrolimus	Ritonavir
	Indinavir, saquinavir, ritonavir	
CYP2D6[b]	Timolol, metoprolol, carvedilol	Quinidine (even at ultra-low doses)
	Phenformin	Tricyclic antidepressants
	Codeine	Fluoxetine, paroxetine
	Propafenone, flecainide	
	Tricyclic antidepressants	
	Fluoxetine, paroxetine	
CYP2C9[b]	Warfarin	Amiodarone
	Phenytoin	Fluconazole
	Glipizide	Phenytoin
	Losartan	
CYP2C19[b]	Omeprazole	Omeprazole
	Mephenytoin	
	Clopidogrel	
CYP2B6[b]	Efavirenz	
Thiopurine S-methyltransferase[b]	6-Mercaptopurine, azathioprine	
N-acetyltransferase[b]	Isoniazid	
	Procainamide	
	Hydralazine	
	Some sulfonamides	
UGT1A1[b]	Irinotecan	
Pseudocholinesterase[b]	Succinylcholine	
P-glycoprotein	Digoxin	Quinidine
	HIV protease inhibitors	Amiodarone
	Many CYP3A substrates	Verapamil
		Cyclosporine
		Itraconazole
		Erythromycin
SLCO1B1[b]	Simvastatins and some other statins	

[a]Inhibitors affect the molecular pathway, and thus may affect substrate. [b]Clinically important genetic variants described; see Table 5-2.

Note: A listing of CYP substrates, inhibitors, and inducers is maintained at *http://medicine.iupui.edu/flockhart/table.htm*.

that accomplish phase II reactions include glucuronyl-, acetyl-, sulfo-, and methyltransferases. Drug metabolites may exert important pharmacologic activity, as discussed further below.

Clinical Implications of Altered Bioavailability Some drugs undergo near-complete presystemic metabolism and, thus, cannot be administered orally. Nitroglycerin cannot be used orally because it is completely extracted prior to reaching the systemic circulation. The drug is, therefore, used by the sublingual or transdermal routes, which bypass presystemic metabolism.

Some drugs with very extensive presystemic metabolism can still be administered by the oral route, using much higher doses than those required intravenously. Thus, a typical intravenous dose of verapamil is 1–5 mg, compared to the usual single oral dose of 40–120 mg. Administration of low-dose aspirin can result in exposure of cyclooxygenase in platelets in the portal vein to the drug, but systemic sparing because of first-pass aspirin deacylation in the liver. This is an example of presystemic metabolism being exploited to therapeutic advantage.

PHARMACOKINETIC CONCEPTS

Most pharmacokinetic processes, such as elimination, are first-order; that is, the rate of the process depends on the amount of drug present. Elimination can occasionally be zero-order (fixed amount eliminated per unit time), and this can be clinically important (see "Principles of Dose Selection"). In the simplest pharmacokinetic model (Fig. 5-2*A*), a drug bolus (D) is administered instantaneously to a central compartment, from which drug elimination occurs as a first-order process. Occasionally, central and other compartments correspond to physiologic spaces (e.g., plasma volume), whereas in others they are simply mathematical functions used to describe drug disposition. The first-order nature of drug elimination leads directly to the relationship describing drug concentration (*C*) at any time (*t*) following the bolus:

$$C = \frac{D}{V_c} \bullet e^{(-0.69t/t_{1/2})}$$

where V_c is the volume of the compartment into which drug is delivered and $t_{1/2}$ is elimination half-life. As a consequence of this relationship, a plot of the logarithm of concentration versus time is a straight line (Fig. 5-2*A*, inset). *Half-life* is the time required for 50% of a first-order process to be complete. Thus, 50% of drug elimination is achieved after one drug-elimination half-life, 75% after two, 87.5% after three, etc. In practice, first-order processes such as elimination are near-complete after four–five half-lives.

In some cases, drug is removed from the central compartment not only by elimination but also by distribution into peripheral compartments. In this case, the plot of plasma concentration versus time after a bolus may demonstrate two (or more) exponential components (Fig. 5-2*B*). In general, the initial rapid drop in drug concentration represents not elimination but drug distribution into and out of peripheral tissues (also first-order processes), while the slower component represents drug elimination; the initial precipitous decline is usually evident with administration by intravenous but not by other routes. Drug concentrations at peripheral sites are determined by a balance between drug distribution to and redistribution from those sites, as well as by elimination. Once distribution is near-complete (four–five distribution half-lives), plasma and tissue concentrations decline in parallel.

Clinical Implications of Half-Life Measurements The elimination half-life not only determines the time required for drug concentrations to fall to near-immeasurable levels after a single bolus, it is also the sole determinant of the time required for steady-state plasma concentrations to be achieved after any change in drug dosing (Fig. 5-4). This applies to the initiation of chronic drug therapy (whether by multiple oral doses or by continuous intravenous infusion), a change in chronic drug dose or dosing interval, or discontinuation of drug.

Steady state describes the situation during chronic drug administration when the amount of drug administered per unit time equals drug eliminated per unit time. With a continuous intravenous infusion, plasma concentrations at steady state are stable, while with chronic oral drug administration, plasma concentrations vary during the dosing interval but the time-concentration profile between dosing intervals is stable (Fig. 5-4).

DRUG DISTRIBUTION

In a typical 70-kg human, plasma volume is ~3 L, blood volume is ~5.5 L, and extracellular water outside the vasculature is ~20 L. The volume of distribution of drugs extensively bound to plasma proteins but not to tissue components approaches plasma volume; warfarin is one such example. By contrast, for drugs highly bound to tissues, the volume of distribution can be far greater than any physiologic space. For example, the volume of distribution of digoxin and tricyclic antidepressants is hundreds of liters, obviously exceeding total-body volume. Such drugs are not readily removed by dialysis, an important consideration in overdose.

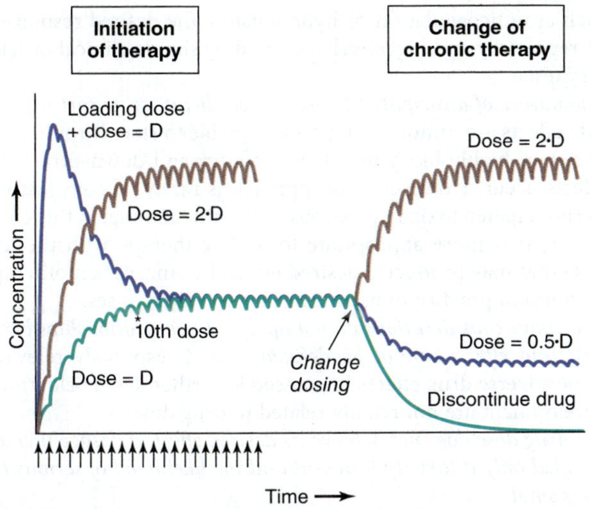

FIGURE 5-4 Drug accumulation to steady state. In this simulation, drug was administered (arrows) at intervals = 50% of the elimination half-life. Steady state is achieved during initiation of therapy after ~5 elimination half-lives, or 10 doses. A loading dose did not alter the eventual steady state achieved. A doubling of the dose resulted in a doubling of the steady state but the same time course of accumulation. Once steady state is achieved, a change in dose (increase, decrease, or drug discontinuation) results in a new steady state in ~5 elimination half-lives. *(Adapted by permission from DM Roden, in DP Zipes, J Jalife [eds]: Cardiac Electrophysiology: From Cell to Bedside, 4th ed. Philadelphia, Saunders, 2003. Copyright 2003 with permission from Elsevier.)*

Clinical Implications of Drug Distribution In some cases, pharmacologic effects require drug distribution to peripheral sites. In this instance, the time course of drug delivery to and removal from these sites determines the time course of drug effects; anesthetic uptake into the central nervous system (CNS) is an example.

LOADING DOSES For some drugs, the indication may be so urgent that administration of "loading" dosages is required to achieve rapid elevations of drug concentration and therapeutic effects earlier than with chronic maintenance therapy (Fig. 5-4). Nevertheless, the time required for true steady state to be achieved is still determined only by the elimination half-life.

RATE OF INTRAVENOUS ADMINISTRATION Although the simulations in Fig. 5-2 use a single intravenous bolus, this is usually inappropriate in practice because side effects related to transiently very high concentrations can result. Rather, drugs are more usually administered orally or as a slower intravenous infusion. Some drugs are so predictably lethal when infused too rapidly that special precautions should be taken to prevent accidental boluses. For example, solutions of potassium for intravenous administration >20 mEq/L should be avoided in all but the most exceptional and carefully monitored circumstances. This minimizes the possibility of cardiac arrest due to accidental increases in infusion rates of more concentrated solutions.

Transiently high drug concentrations after rapid intravenous administration can occasionally be used to advantage. The use of midazolam for intravenous sedation, for example, depends upon its rapid uptake by the brain during the distribution phase to produce sedation quickly, with subsequent egress from the brain during the redistribution of the drug as equilibrium is achieved.

Similarly, adenosine must be administered as a rapid bolus in the treatment of reentrant supraventricular tachycardias (Chap. 276) to prevent elimination by very rapid ($t_{1/2}$ of seconds) uptake into erythrocytes and endothelial cells before the drug can reach its clinical site of action, the atrioventricular node.

Clinical Implications of Altered Protein Binding Many drugs circulate in the plasma partly bound to plasma proteins. Since only unbound (free) drug can distribute to sites of pharmacologic action, drug response is related to the free rather than the total circulating plasma drug concentration. In chronic kidney or liver disease, protein binding may be decreased and thus drug actions increased. In some situations (myocardial infarction, infection, surgery), acute phase reactants transiently increase drug binding and thus decrease efficacy. These changes assume the greatest clinical importance for drugs that are highly protein-bound since even a small change in protein binding can result in large changes in free drug; for example, a decrease in binding from 99% to 98% doubles the free drug concentration from 1% to 2%. For some drugs (e.g., phenytoin), monitoring free rather than total drug concentrations can be useful.

ELIMINATION

Drug elimination reduces the amount of drug in the body over time. An important approach to quantifying this reduction is to consider that drug concentrations at the beginning and end of a time period are unchanged and that a specific volume of the body has been "cleared" of the drug during that time period. This defines clearance as volume/time. Clearance includes both drug metabolism and excretion.

Clinical Implications of Altered Clearance While elimination half-life determines the time required to achieve steady-state plasma concentration (C_{ss}), the *magnitude* of that steady state is determined by clearance (*Cl*) and dose alone. For a drug administered as an intravenous infusion, this relationship is:

$$C_{ss} = \text{dosing rate}/Cl \quad \text{or} \quad \text{dosing rate} = Cl \cdot C_{ss}$$

When drug is administered orally, the average plasma concentration within a dosing interval ($C_{avg,ss}$) replaces C_{ss}, and the dosage (dose per unit time) must be increased if bioavailability (F) is less than 1:

$$\text{Dose/time} = Cl \cdot C_{avg,ss}/F$$

Genetic variants, drug interactions, or diseases that reduce the activity of drug-metabolizing enzymes or excretory mechanisms lead to decreased clearance and, hence, a requirement for downward dose adjustment to avoid toxicity. Conversely, some drug interactions and genetic variants increase the function of drug elimination pathways, and hence, increased drug dosage is necessary to maintain a therapeutic effect.

ACTIVE DRUG METABOLITES

Metabolites may produce effects similar to, overlapping with, or distinct from those of the parent drug. Accumulation of the major metabolite of procainamide, *N*-acetylprocainamide (NAPA), likely accounts for marked QT prolongation and torsades des pointes ventricular tachycardia (Chap. 276) during therapy with procainamide. Neurotoxicity during therapy with the opioid analgesic meperidine is likely due to accumulation of normeperidine, especially in renal disease.

Prodrugs are inactive compounds that require metabolism to generate active metabolites that mediate the drug effects. Examples include many angiotensin-converting enzyme (ACE) inhibitors, the angiotensin receptor blocker losartan, the antineoplastic irinotecan, the antiestrogen tamoxifen, the analgesic codeine (whose active metabolite morphine probably underlies the opioid effect during codeine administration), and the antiplatelet drug clopidogrel. Drug metabolism has also been implicated in bioactivation of procarcinogens and in generation of reactive metabolites that mediate certain adverse drug effects (e.g., acetaminophen hepatotoxicity, discussed below).

THE CONCEPT OF HIGH-RISK PHARMACOKINETICS

When plasma concentrations of active drug depend exclusively on a single metabolic pathway, any condition that inhibits that pathway (be it disease-related, genetic, or due to a drug interaction) can lead to dramatic changes in drug concentrations and marked variability in drug action. This problem of high-risk pharmacokinetics is especially pronounced in two settings. *First*, variability in bioactivation of a prodrug can lead to striking variability in drug action; examples include decreased CYP2D6 activity, which prevents analgesia by codeine, and decreased CYP2C19 activity, which reduces the antiplatelet effects of clopidogrel. The *second* setting is drug elimination that relies on a single pathway. In this case, inhibition of the elimination pathway by genetic variants or by administration of inhibiting drugs leads to marked elevation of drug concentration and, for drugs with a narrow therapeutic window, an increased likelihood of dose-related toxicity. Individuals with loss-of-function alleles in CYP2C9, responsible for metabolism of the active S-enantiomer of warfarin, appear to be at increased risk for bleeding. When drugs undergo elimination by multiple-drug metabolizing or excretory pathways, absence of one pathway (due to a genetic variant or drug interaction) is much less likely to have a large impact on drug concentrations or drug actions.

PRINCIPLES OF PHARMACODYNAMICS

The Onset of Drug Action For drugs used in the urgent treatment of acute symptoms, little or no delay is anticipated (or desired) between the drug-target interaction and the development of a clinical effect. Examples of such acute situations include vascular thrombosis, shock, or status epilepticus.

For many conditions, however, the indication for therapy is less urgent, and a delay between the interaction of a drug with its pharmacologic target(s) and a clinical effect is clinically acceptable. Common pharmacokinetic mechanisms that can contribute to such a delay include slow elimination (resulting in slow accumulation to steady state), uptake into peripheral compartments, or accumulation of active metabolites. Another common explanation for such a delay is that the clinical effect develops as a downstream consequence of the initial molecular effect the drug produces. Thus, administration of a proton pump inhibitor or an H_2-receptor blocker produces an immediate increase in gastric pH but ulcer healing that is delayed. Cancer chemotherapy similarly produces delayed therapeutic effects.

Drug Effects May Be Disease Specific A drug may produce no action or a different spectrum of actions in unaffected individuals compared to patients with underlying disease. Further, concomitant disease can complicate interpretation of response to drug therapy, especially adverse effects. For example, high doses of anticonvulsants such as phenytoin may cause neurologic symptoms, which may be confused with the underlying neurologic disease. Similarly, increasing dyspnea in a patient with chronic lung disease receiving amiodarone therapy could be due to drug, underlying disease, or an intercurrent cardiopulmonary problem. Thus, the presence of chronic lung disease may argue against the use of amiodarone.

While drugs interact with specific molecular receptors, drug effects may vary over time, even if stable drug and metabolite concentrations are maintained. The drug-receptor interaction occurs in a complex biologic milieu that can vary to modulate the drug effect. For example, ion channel blockade by drugs, an important anticonvulsant and antiarrhythmic effect, is often modulated by membrane potential, itself a function of factors such as extracellular potassium or local ischemia. Receptors may be up- or downregulated by disease or by the drug itself. For example, β-adrenergic blockers upregulate β-receptor density during chronic therapy. While this effect does not usually result in resistance to the therapeutic effect of the drugs, it may produce severe agonist-mediated effects (such as hypertension or tachycardia) if the blocking drug is abruptly withdrawn.

PRINCIPLES OF DOSE SELECTION

The desired goal of therapy with any drug is to maximize the likelihood of a beneficial effect while minimizing the risk of adverse effects. Previous experience with the drug, in controlled clinical trials or in postmarketing use, defines the relationships between dose or plasma concentration and these dual effects (Fig. 5-1) and has important implications for initiation of drug therapy:

1. *The target drug effect should be defined when drug treatment is started.* With some drugs, the desired effect may be difficult to measure objectively, or the onset of efficacy can be delayed for weeks or months; drugs used in the treatment of cancer and psychiatric disease are examples. Sometimes a drug is used to treat a symptom, such as pain or palpitations, and here it is the patient who will report whether the selected dose is effective. In yet other settings, such as anticoagulation or hypertension, the desired response can be repeatedly and objectively assessed by simple clinical or laboratory tests.
2. *The nature of anticipated toxicity often dictates the starting dose.* If side effects are minor, it may be acceptable to start chronic therapy at a dose highly likely to achieve efficacy and down-titrate if side effects occur. However, this approach is rarely, if ever, justified if the anticipated toxicity is serious or life-threatening; in this circumstance, it is more appropriate to initiate therapy with the lowest dose that may produce a desired effect. In cancer chemotherapy, it is common practice to use maximum-tolerated doses.
3. *The above considerations do not apply if these relationships between dose and effects cannot be defined.* This is especially relevant to some adverse drug effects (discussed in further detail below) whose development are not readily related to drug dose.
4. *If a drug dose does not achieve its desired effect, a dosage increase is justified only if toxicity is absent and the likelihood of serious toxicity is small.*

Failure of Efficacy Assuming the diagnosis is correct and the correct drug is prescribed, explanations for failure of efficacy include drug interactions, noncompliance, or unexpectedly low drug dosage due to administration of expired or degraded drug. These are situations in which measurement of plasma drug concentrations, if available, can be especially useful. Noncompliance is an especially frequent problem in the long-term treatment of diseases such as hypertension and epilepsy, occurring in ≥25% of patients in therapeutic environments in which no special effort is made to involve patients in the responsibility for their own health. Multidrug regimens with multiple doses per day are especially prone to noncompliance.

Monitoring response to therapy, by physiologic measures or by plasma concentration measurements, requires an understanding of the relationships between plasma concentration and anticipated effects. For example, measurement of QT interval is used during treatment with sotalol or dofetilide to avoid marked QT prolongation that can herald serious arrhythmias. In this setting, evaluating the electrocardiogram at the time of anticipated peak plasma concentration and effect (e.g., 1–2 h postdose at steady state) is most appropriate. Maintained high vancomycin levels carry a risk of nephrotoxicity, so dosages should be adjusted on the basis of plasma concentrations measured at trough (predose). Similarly, for dose adjustment of other drugs (e.g., anticonvulsants), concentration should be measured at its lowest during the dosing interval, just prior to a dose at steady state (Fig. 5-4), to ensure a maintained therapeutic effect.

Concentration of Drugs in Plasma as a Guide to Therapy Factors such as interactions with other drugs, disease-induced alterations in elimination and distribution, and genetic variation in drug disposition combine to yield a wide range of plasma levels in patients given the same dose. Hence, if a predictable relationship can be established between plasma drug concentration and beneficial or adverse drug effect, measurement of plasma levels can provide a valuable tool to guide selection of an optimal dose, especially when there is a narrow range between the plasma levels yielding therapeutic and adverse effects. Monitoring is commonly used with certain types of drugs including many anticonvulsants, antirejection agents, antiarrhythmics, and antibiotics. By contrast, if no such relationship can be established (e.g., if drug access to important sites of action outside plasma is highly variable), monitoring plasma concentration may not provide an accurate guide to therapy (Fig. 5-5*A*).

The common situation of first-order elimination implies that average, maximum, and minimum steady-state concentrations are related linearly to the dosing rate. Accordingly, the maintenance dose may be adjusted on the basis of the ratio between the desired and measured concentrations *at steady state*; for example, if a doubling of the steady-state plasma concentration is desired, the dose should be doubled. This does not apply to drugs eliminated by zero-order kinetics (fixed amount per unit time), where small dosage increases will produce disproportionate increases in plasma concentration; examples include phenytoin and theophylline.

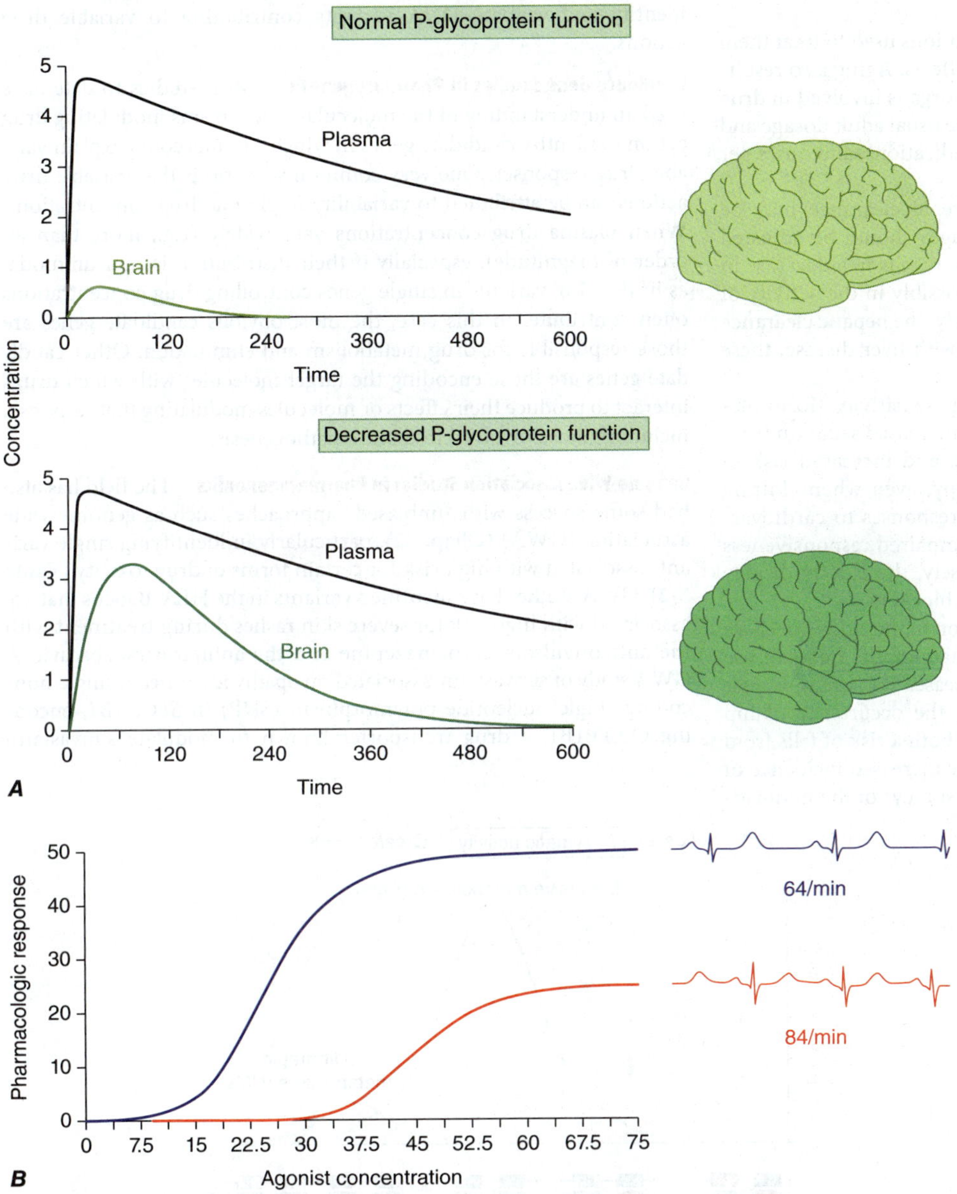

FIGURE 5-5 ***A.*** The efflux pump P-glycoprotein excludes drugs from the endothelium of capillaries in the brain and so constitutes a key element of the blood-brain barrier. Thus, reduced P-glycoprotein function (e.g., due to drug interactions or genetically determined variability in gene transcription) increases penetration of substrate drugs into the brain, even when plasma concentrations are unchanged. ***B.*** The graph shows an effect of a β_1-receptor polymorphism on receptor function in vitro. Patients with the hypofunctional variant (red) may display lesser heart-rate slowing or blood pressure lowering on exposure to a receptor blocking agent.

An increase in dosage is usually best achieved by changing the drug dose but not the dosing interval (e.g., by giving 200 mg every 8 h instead of 100 mg every 8 h). However, this approach is acceptable only if the resulting maximum concentration is not toxic and the trough value does not fall below the minimum effective concentration for an undesirable period of time. Alternatively, the steady state may be changed by altering the frequency of intermittent dosing but not the size of each dose. In this case, the magnitude of the fluctuations around the average steady-state level will change—the shorter the dosing interval, the smaller the difference between peak and trough levels.

EFFECTS OF DISEASE ON DRUG CONCENTRATION AND RESPONSE

RENAL DISEASE

Renal excretion of parent drug and metabolites is generally accomplished by glomerular filtration and by specific drug transporters. If a drug or its metabolites are primarily excreted through the kidneys and increased drug levels are associated with adverse effects, drug dosages must be reduced in patients with renal dysfunction to avoid toxicity. The antiarrhythmics dofetilide and sotalol undergo predominant renal excretion and carry a risk of QT prolongation and arrhythmias if doses are not reduced in renal disease. In end-stage renal disease, sotalol has been given as 40 mg after dialysis (every second day), compared to the usual daily dose, 80–120 mg every 12 h. The narcotic analgesic meperidine undergoes extensive hepatic metabolism, so that renal failure has little effect on its plasma concentration. However, its metabolite, normeperidine, does undergo renal excretion, accumulates in renal failure, and probably accounts for the signs of CNS excitation, such as irritability, twitching, and seizures, that appear when multiple doses of meperidine are administered to patients with renal disease. Protein binding of some drugs (e.g., phenytoin) may be altered in uremia, so measuring free drug concentration may be desirable.

In non-end-stage renal disease, changes in renal drug clearance are generally proportional to those in creatinine clearance, which may be measured directly or estimated from the serum creatinine (Chap. 333e). This estimate, coupled with the knowledge of how much drug is normally excreted renally versus nonrenally, allows an estimate of the dose adjustment required. In practice, most decisions involving dosing adjustment in patients with renal failure use published recommended adjustments in dosage or dosing interval based on the severity of renal dysfunction indicated by creatinine clearance. Any such modification of dose is a first approximation and should be followed by plasma concentration data (if available) and clinical observation to further optimize therapy for the individual patient.

LIVER DISEASE

Standard tests of liver function are not useful in adjusting doses in diseases like hepatitis or cirrhosis. First-pass metabolism may decrease, leading to increased oral bioavailability as a consequence of disrupted hepatocyte function, altered liver architecture, and portacaval shunts. The oral bioavailability for high first-pass drugs such as morphine, meperidine, midazolam, and nifedipine is almost doubled in patients with cirrhosis, compared to those with normal liver function. Therefore, the size of the oral dose of such drugs should be reduced in this setting.

HEART FAILURE AND SHOCK

Under conditions of decreased tissue perfusion, the cardiac output is redistributed to preserve blood flow to the heart and brain at the expense of other tissues (Chap. 279). As a result, drugs may be distributed into a smaller volume of distribution, higher drug concentrations will be present in the plasma, and the tissues that are best perfused (the brain and heart) will be exposed to these higher concentrations, resulting in increased CNS or cardiac effects. As well, decreased perfusion of the kidney and liver may impair drug clearance. Another consequence of severe heart failure is decreased gut perfusion, which may reduce drug absorption and, thus, lead to reduced or absent effects of orally administered therapies.

DRUG USE IN THE ELDERLY

In the elderly, multiple pathologies and medications used to treat them result in more drug interactions and adverse effects. Aging also results in changes in organ function, especially of the organs involved in drug disposition. Initial doses should be less than the usual adult dosage and should be increased slowly. The number of medications, and doses per day, should be kept as low as possible.

Even in the absence of kidney disease, renal clearance may be reduced by 35–50% in elderly patients. Dosages should be adjusted on the basis of creatinine clearance. Aging also results in a decrease in the size of, and blood flow to, the liver and possibly in the activity of hepatic drug-metabolizing enzymes; accordingly, the hepatic clearance of some drugs is impaired in the elderly. As with liver disease, these changes are not readily predicted.

Elderly patients may display altered drug sensitivity. Examples include increased analgesic effects of opioids, increased sedation from benzodiazepines and other CNS depressants, and increased risk of bleeding while receiving anticoagulant therapy, even when clotting parameters are well controlled. Exaggerated responses to cardiovascular drugs are also common because of the impaired responsiveness of normal homeostatic mechanisms. Conversely, the elderly display decreased sensitivity to β-adrenergic receptor blockers.

Adverse drug reactions are especially common in the elderly because of altered pharmacokinetics and pharmacodynamics, the frequent use of multidrug regimens, and concomitant disease. For example, use of long half-life benzodiazepines is linked to the occurrence of hip fractures in elderly patients, perhaps reflecting both a risk of falls from these drugs (due to increased sedation) and the increased incidence of osteoporosis in elderly patients. In population surveys of the noninstitutionalized elderly, as many as 10% had at least one adverse drug reaction in the previous year.

DRUG USE IN CHILDREN

While most drugs used to treat disease in children are the same are those in adults, there are few studies that provide solid data to guide dosing. Drug metabolism pathways mature at different rates after birth, and disease mechanisms may be different in children. In practice, doses are adjusted for size (weight or body surface area) as a first approximation unless age-specific data are available.

GENETIC DETERMINANTS OF THE RESPONSE TO DRUGS

PRINCIPLES OF GENETIC VARIATION AND HUMAN TRAITS (SEE ALSO CHAPS. 82 AND 84)

The concept that genetically determined variations in drug metabolism might be associated with variable drug levels and hence, effect, was advanced at the end of the nineteenth century, and the examples of familial clustering of unusual drug responses were noted in the mid-twentieth century. A goal of traditional Mendelian genetics is to identify DNA variants associated with a distinct phenotype in multiple related family members (Chap. 84). However, it is unusual for a drug response phenotype to be accurately measured in more than one family member, let alone across a kindred. Thus, non-family-based approaches are generally used to identify and validate DNA variants contributing to variable drug actions.

Candidate Gene Studies in Pharmacogenetics Most studies to date have used an understanding of the molecular mechanisms modulating drug action to identify candidate genes in which variants could explain variable drug responses. One very common scenario is that variable drug actions can be attributed to variability in plasma drug concentrations. When plasma drug concentrations vary widely (e.g., more than an order of magnitude), especially if their distribution is non-unimodal as in Fig. 5-6, variants in single genes controlling drug concentrations often contribute. In this case, the most obvious candidate genes are those responsible for drug metabolism and elimination. Other candidate genes are those encoding the target molecules with which drugs interact to produce their effects or molecules modulating that response, including those involved in disease pathogenesis.

Genome-Wide Association Studies in Pharmacogenomics The field has also had some success with "unbiased" approaches such as genome-wide association (GWA) (Chap. 82), particularly in identifying single variants associated with high risk for certain forms of drug toxicity (Table 5-2). GWA studies have identified variants in the HLA-B locus that are associated with high risk for severe skin rashes during treatment with the anticonvulsant carbamazepine and the antiretroviral abacavir. A GWA study of simvastatin-associated myopathy identified a single noncoding single nucleotide polymorphism (SNP) in *SLCO1B1*, encoding OATP1B1, a drug transporter known to modulate simvastatin

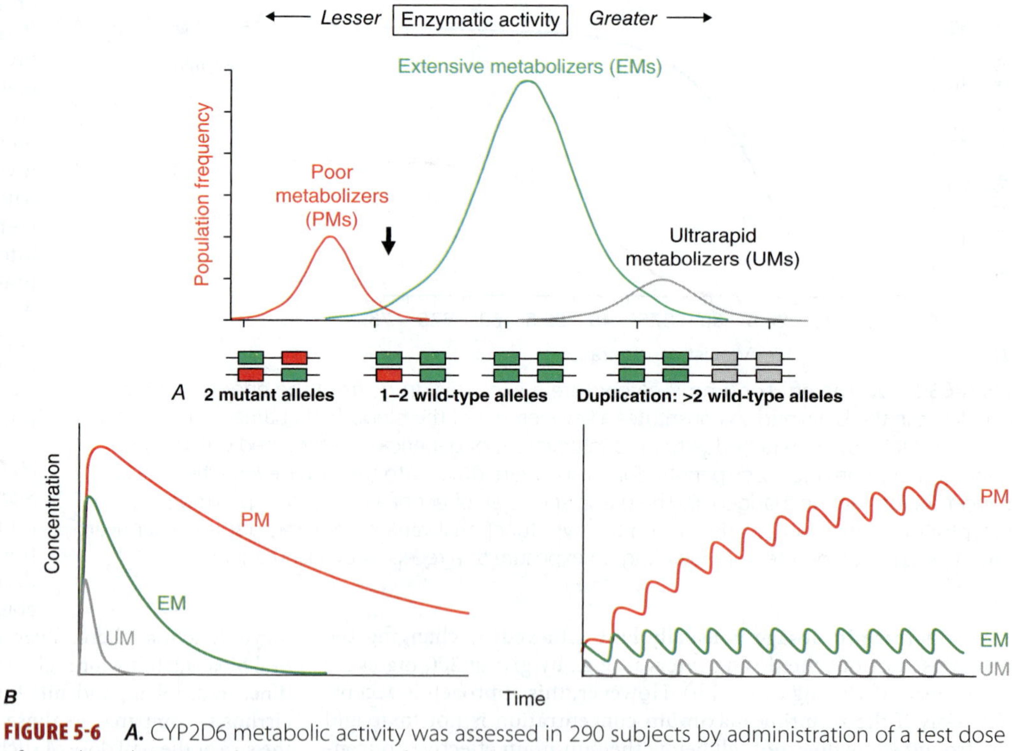

FIGURE 5-6 ***A.*** CYP2D6 metabolic activity was assessed in 290 subjects by administration of a test dose of a probe substrate and measurement of urinary formation of the CYP2D6-generated metabolite. The heavy arrow indicates a clear antimode, separating poor metabolizer subjects (PMs, red), with two loss-of-function CYP2D6 alleles, indicated by the intron-exon structures below the chart. Individuals with one or two functional alleles are grouped together as extensive metabolizers (EMs, green). Also shown are ultra-rapid metabolizers (UMs), with 2–12 functional copies of the gene (gray), displaying the greatest enzyme activity. *(Adapted from M-L Dahl et al: J Pharmacol Exp Ther 274:516, 1995.)* ***B.*** These simulations show the predicted effects of CYP2D6 genotype on disposition of a substrate drug. With a single dose (left), there is an inverse "gene-dose" relationship between the number of active alleles and the areas under the time-concentration curves (smallest in UM subjects; highest in PM subjects); this indicates that clearance is greatest in UM subjects. In addition, elimination half-life is longest in PM subjects. The right panel shows that these single dose differences are exaggerated during chronic therapy: steady-state concentration is much higher in PM subjects (decreased clearance), as is the time required to achieve steady state (longer elimination half-life).

TABLE 5-2 GENETIC VARIANTS AND DRUG RESPONSES

Gene	Drugs	Effect of Genetic Variants[a]
Variants in Drug Metabolism Pathways		
CYP2C9	Losartan	Decreased bioactivation and effects (PMs)
	Warfarin	Decreased dose requirements; possible increased bleeding risk (PMs)
CYP2C19	Omeprazole, voriconazole	Decreased effect in extensive metabolizers (EMs)
	Celecoxib	Exaggerated effect in PMs
	Clopidogrel	Decreased effect in PMs
CYP2D6	Codeine, tamoxifen	Decreased bioactivation and drug effects in PMs
	Codeine	Morphine-like adverse effects in UMs
	Tricyclic antidepressants	Increased adverse effects in PMs; decreased therapeutic effects in UMs
	Metoprolol, carvedilol, timolol, propafenone	Increased beta blockade in PMs
CYP3A5	Tacrolimus, vincristine	Decreased drug concentrations and effect
Dihydropyrimidine dehydrogenase	Capecitabine, fluorouracil	Possible severe toxicity (PMs)
NAT2	Rifampin, isoniazid, pyrazinamide, hydralazine, procainamide	Increased risk of toxicity in PMs
Thiopurine S-methyltransferase (*TPMT*)	Azathioprine, 6-mercaptopurine	*3A/*3A (PMs): increased risk of bone marrow aplasia; wild-type homozygote: possible decreased drug action at usual dosages
Uridine diphosphate glucuronosyltransferase (*UGT1A1*)	Irinotecan	*28/*28 PM homozygotes: increased risk of severe adverse effects (diarrhea, bone marrow aplasia)
Variants in Other Genes		
Glucose 6-phosphate dehydrogenase (G6PD)	Rasburicase, primaquine, chloroquine	Increased risk of hemolytic anemia in G6PD-deficient subjects
HLA-B*1501	Carbamazepine	Carriers (1 or 2 alleles) at increased risk of severe skin toxicity
HLA-B*5701	Abacavir	Carriers (1 or 2 alleles) at increased risk of severe skin toxicity
IL28B	Interferon	Variable response in hepatitis C therapy
IL15	Childhood leukemia therapy	Variability in response
SLCO1B1	Simvastatin	Encodes a drug uptake transporter; variant non-synonymous single nucleotide polymorphism increases myopathy risk
VKORC1	Warfarin	Decreased dose requirements with variant promoter haplotype
ITPA	Ribavirin	Variants modulate risk for hemolytic anemia
Variants in Other Genomes (Infectious Agents, Tumors)		
Chemokine C-C motif receptor (CCR5)	Maraviroc	Drug effective only in HIV strains with CCR5 detectible
C-KIT	Imatinib	In gastrointestinal stromal tumors, drug indicated only with c-kit–positive cases
Epidermal growth factor receptor (EGFR)	Cetuximab	Clinical trials conducted in patients with EGFR-positive tumors
Her2/neu overexpression	Trastuzumab, lapatinib	Drugs indicated only with tumor overexpression
K-ras mutation	Panitumumab, cetuximab	Lack of efficacy with *KRAS* mutation
Philadelphia chromosome	Busulfan, dasatinib, nilotinib, imatinib	Decreased efficacy in Philadelphia chromosome–negative chronic myelogenous leukemia

[a]Drug effect in homozygotes unless otherwise specified.

Note: EM, extensive metabolizer (normal enzymatic activity); PM, poor metabolizer (homozygote for reduced or loss of function allele); UM, ultra-rapid metabolizer (enzymatic activity much greater than normal, e.g., with gene duplication, Fig. 5-6). Further data at U.S. Food and Drug Administration: *http://www.fda.gov/Drugs/ScienceResearch/ResearchAreas/Pharmacogenetics/ucm083378.htm*; or Pharmacogenetics Research Network/Knowledge Base: *http://www.pharmgkb.org*.

uptake into the liver, which accounts for 60% of myopathy risk. GWA approaches have also implicated interferon variants in antileukemic responses and in response to therapy in hepatitis C. Ribavirin, used as therapy in hepatitis C, causes hemolytic anemia, and this has been linked to variants in *ITPA*, encoding inosine triphosphatase.

GENETIC VARIANTS AFFECTING PHARMACOKINETICS

Clinically important genetic variants have been described in multiple molecular pathways of drug disposition (Table 5-2). A distinct multimodal distribution of drug disposition (as shown in Fig. 5-6) argues for a predominant effect of variants in a single gene in the metabolism of that substrate. Individuals with two alleles (variants) encoding for nonfunctional protein make up one group, often termed *poor metabolizers* (PM phenotype); for some genes, many variants can produce such a loss of function, complicating the use of genotyping in clinical practice. Individuals with one functional allele make up a second (*intermediate metabolizers*) and may or may not be distinguishable from those with two functional alleles (*extensive metabolizers*, EMs). *Ultra-rapid metabolizers* with especially high enzymatic activity (occasionally due to gene duplication; Fig. 5-6) have also been described for some traits. Many drugs in widespread use can inhibit specific drug disposition pathways (Table 5-1), and so EM individuals receiving such inhibitors can respond like PM patients (*phenocopying*). Polymorphisms in genes encoding drug uptake or drug efflux transporters may be other contributors to variability in drug delivery to target sites and, hence, in drug effects.

CYP Variants Members of the CYP3A family (CYP3A4, 3A5) metabolize the greatest number of drugs in therapeutic use. CYP3A4 activity is highly variable (up to an order of magnitude) among individuals, but the underlying mechanisms are not well understood. In whites, but not African Americans, there is a common loss-of-function polymorphism in the closely related CYP3A5 gene. Decreased efficacy of the antirejection agent tacrolimus in African-American subjects has been attributed to more rapid elimination due to relatively greater CYP3A5 activity. A lower risk of vincristine-associated neuropathy has been reported in CYP3A5 "expressers."

CYP2D6 is second to CYP3A4 in the number of commonly used drugs that it metabolizes. CYP2D6 activity is polymorphically distributed, with about 7% of European- and African-derived populations (but very few Asians) displaying the PM phenotype (Fig. 5-6). Dozens of loss-of-function variants in the CYP2D6 gene have been described; the PM phenotype arises in individuals with two such alleles. In addition, ultra-rapid metabolizers with multiple functional copies of the CYP2D6 gene have been identified.

Codeine is biotransformed by CYP2D6 to the potent active metabolite morphine, so its effects are blunted in PMs and exaggerated in ultra-rapid metabolizers. In the case of drugs with beta-blocking properties metabolized by CYP2D6, greater signs of beta blockade (e.g., bronchospasm, bradycardia) are seen in PM subjects than in EMs. This can be seen not only with orally administered beta blockers such as metoprolol and carvedilol, but also with ophthalmic timolol and with the sodium channel–blocking antiarrhythmic propafenone, a CYP2D6 substrate with beta-blocking properties. Ultra-rapid metabolizers may require very high dosages of tricyclic antidepressants to achieve a therapeutic effect and, with codeine, may display transient euphoria and nausea due to very rapid generation of morphine. Tamoxifen undergoes CYP2D6-mediated biotransformation to an active metabolite, so its efficacy may be in part related to this polymorphism. In addition, the widespread use of selective serotonin reuptake inhibitors (SSRIs) to treat tamoxifen-related hot flashes may also alter the drug's effects because many SSRIs, notably fluoxetine and paroxetine, are also CYP2D6 inhibitors.

The PM phenotype for CYP2C19 is common (20%) among Asians and rarer (2–3%) in European-derived populations. The impact of polymorphic CYP2C19-mediated metabolism has been demonstrated with the proton pump inhibitor omeprazole, where ulcer cure rates with "standard" dosages were much lower in EM patients (29%) than in PMs (100%). Thus, understanding the importance of this polymorphism would have been important in developing the drug, and knowing a patient's *CYP2C19* genotype should improve therapy. CYP2C19 is responsible for bioactivation of the antiplatelet drug clopidogrel, and several large studies have documented decreased efficacy (e.g., increased myocardial infarction after placement of coronary stents) among Caucasian subjects with reduction of function alleles. In addition, some studies suggest that omeprazole and possibly other proton pump inhibitors phenocopy this effect.

There are common variants of *CYP2C9* that encode proteins with loss of catalytic function. These variant alleles are associated with increased rates of neurologic complications with phenytoin, hypoglycemia with glipizide, and reduced warfarin dose required to maintain stable anticoagulation. The angiotensin-receptor blocker losartan is a prodrug that is bioactivated by CYP2C9; as a result, PMs and those receiving inhibitor drugs may display little response to therapy.

Transferase Variants One of the most extensively studied phase II polymorphisms is the PM trait for thiopurine S-methyltransferase (TPMT). TPMT bioinactivates the antileukemic drug 6-mercaptopurine. Further, 6-mercaptopurine is itself an active metabolite of the immunosuppressive azathioprine. Homozygotes for alleles encoding the inactive TPMT (1 in 300 individuals) predictably exhibit severe and potentially fatal pancytopenia on standard doses of azathioprine or 6-mercaptopurine. On the other hand, homozygotes for fully functional alleles may display less anti-inflammatory or antileukemic effect with the drugs.

N-acetylation is catalyzed by hepatic *N*-acetyl transferase (NAT), which represents the activity of two genes, *NAT-1* and *NAT-2*. Both enzymes transfer an acetyl group from acetyl coenzyme A to the drug; polymorphisms in *NAT-2* are thought to underlie individual differences in the rate at which drugs are acetylated and thus define "rapid acetylators" and "slow acetylators." Slow acetylators make up ~50% of European- and African-derived populations but are less common among Asians. Slow acetylators have an increased incidence of the drug-induced lupus syndrome during procainamide and hydralazine therapy and of hepatitis with isoniazid. Induction of CYPs (e.g., by rifampin) also increases the risk of isoniazid-related hepatitis, likely reflecting generation of reactive metabolites of acetylhydrazine, itself an isoniazid metabolite.

Individuals homozygous for a common promoter polymorphism that reduces transcription of uridine diphosphate glucuronosyltransferase (*UGT1A1*) have benign hyperbilirubinemia (Gilbert's syndrome; Chap. 358). This variant has also been associated with diarrhea and increased bone marrow depression with the antineoplastic prodrug irinotecan, whose active metabolite is normally detoxified by UGT1A1-mediated glucuronidation. The antiretroviral atazanavir is a UGT1A1 inhibitor, and individuals with the Gilbert's variant develop higher bilirubin levels during treatment.

VARIABILITY IN THE MOLECULAR TARGETS WITH WHICH DRUGS INTERACT

Multiple polymorphisms identified in the β_2-adrenergic receptor appear to be linked to specific phenotypes in asthma and congestive heart failure, diseases in which β_2-receptor function might be expected to determine prognosis. Polymorphisms in the β_2-receptor gene have also been associated with response to inhaled β_2-receptor agonists, while those in the β_1-adrenergic receptor gene have been associated with variability in heart rate slowing and blood pressure lowering (Fig. 5-5*B*). In addition, in heart failure, a common polymorphism in the β_1-adrenergic receptor gene has been implicated in variable clinical outcome during therapy with the investigational beta blocker bucindolol. Response to the 5-lipoxygenase inhibitor zileuton in asthma has been linked to polymorphisms that determine the expression level of the 5-lipoxygenase gene.

Drugs may also interact with genetic pathways of disease to elicit or exacerbate symptoms of the underlying conditions. In the porphyrias, CYP inducers are thought to increase the activity of enzymes proximal to the deficient enzyme, exacerbating or triggering attacks (Chap. 430). Deficiency of glucose-6-phosphate dehydrogenase (G6PD), most often in individuals of African, Mediterranean, or South Asian descent, increases the risk of hemolytic anemia in response to the antimalarial primaquine (Chap. 129) and the uric acid–lowering agent rasburicase, which do not cause hemolysis in patients with normal amounts of the enzyme. Patients with mutations in the ryanodine receptor, which controls intracellular calcium in skeletal muscle and other tissues, may be asymptomatic until exposed to certain general anesthetics, which trigger the rare syndrome of malignant hyperthermia. Certain antiarrhythmics and other drugs can produce marked QT prolongation and torsades des pointes (Chap. 276), and in some patients, this adverse effect represents unmasking of previously subclinical congenital long QT syndrome. Up to 50% of the variability in steady-state warfarin dose requirement is attributable to polymorphisms in the promoter of *VKORC1*, which encodes the warfarin target, and in the coding region of *CYP2C9*, which mediates its elimination.

Tumor and Infectious Agent Genomes The actions of drugs used to treat infectious or neoplastic disease may be modulated by variants in these nonhuman germline genomes. Genotyping tumors is a rapidly evolving approach to target therapies to underlying mechanisms and to avoid potentially toxic therapy in patients who would derive no benefit (Chap. 101e). Trastuzumab, which potentiates anthracycline-related cardiotoxicity, is ineffective in breast cancers that do not express the herceptin receptor. Imatinib targets a specific tyrosine kinase, BCR-Abl1, that is generated by the translocation that creates the Philadelphia chromosome typical of chronic myelogenous leukemia (CML). BCR-Abl1 is not only active but may be central to the pathogenesis of CML; its use in BCR-Abl1-positive tumors has resulted in remarkable antitumor efficacy. Similarly, the anti–epidermal growth factor receptor (EGFR) antibodies cetuximab and panitumumab appear especially effective in colon cancers in which K-ras, a G protein in the EGFR pathway, is not mutated. Vemurafenib does not inhibit wild-type *BRAF* but is active against the V600E mutant form of the kinase.

PROSPECTS FOR INCORPORATING PHARMACOGENETIC INFORMATION INTO CLINICAL PRACTICE

The description of genetic variants linked to variable drug responses naturally raises the question of if and how to use this information in practice. Indeed, the U.S. Food and Drug Administration (FDA) now incorporates pharmacogenetic data into information ("package inserts") meant to guide prescribing. A decision to adopt pharmacogenetically guided dosing for a given drug depends on multiple factors. The most important are the magnitude and clinical importance of the genetic effect and the strength of evidence linking genetic variation to variable drug effects (e.g., anecdote versus post-hoc analysis of clinical trial data versus randomized prospective clinical trial). The evidence can be strengthened if statistical arguments from clinical trial data are complemented by an understanding of underlying physiologic mechanisms. Cost versus expected benefit may also be a factor.

When the evidence is compelling, alternate therapies are not available, and there are clear recommendations for dosage adjustment in subjects with variants, there is a strong argument for deploying genetic testing as a guide to prescribing. The association between HLA-B*5701 and severe skin toxicity with abacavir is an example. In other situations, the arguments are less compelling: the magnitude of the genetic effect may be smaller, the consequences may be less serious, alternate therapies may be available, or the drug effect may be amenable to monitoring by other approaches. Ongoing clinical trials are addressing the utility of preprescription genotyping in large populations exposed to drugs with known pharmacogenetic variants (e.g., warfarin). Importantly, technological advances are now raising the possibility of inexpensive whole genome sequencing. Incorporating a patient's whole genome sequence into their electronic medical record would allow the information to be accessed as needed for many genetic and pharmacogenetic applications, and the argument has been put forward that this approach would lower logistic barriers to use of pharmacogenomic variant data in prescribing. There are multiple issues (e.g., economic, technological, and ethical) that need to be addressed if such a paradigm is to be adopted (Chap. 82). While barriers to bringing genomic and pharmacogenomic information to the bedside seem daunting, the field is very young and evolving rapidly. Indeed, one major result of understanding the role of genetics in drug action has been improved screening of drugs during the development process to reduce the likelihood of highly variable metabolism or unanticipated toxicity.

INTERACTIONS BETWEEN DRUGS

Drug interactions can complicate therapy by increasing or decreasing the action of a drug; interactions may be based on changes in drug disposition or in drug response in the absence of changes in drug levels. *Interactions must be considered in the differential diagnosis of any unusual response occurring during drug therapy.* Prescribers should recognize that patients often come to them with a legacy of drugs acquired during previous medical experiences, often with multiple physicians who may not be aware of all the patient's medications. A meticulous drug history should include examination of the patient's medications and, if necessary, calls to the pharmacist to identify prescriptions. It should also address the use of agents not often volunteered during questioning, such as OTC drugs, health food supplements, and topical agents such as eye drops. Lists of interactions are available from a number of electronic sources. While it is unrealistic to expect the practicing physician to memorize these, certain drugs consistently run the risk of generating interactions, often by inhibiting or inducing specific drug elimination pathways. Examples are presented below and in Table 5-3. Accordingly, when these drugs are started or stopped, prescribers must be especially alert to the possibility of interactions.

PHARMACOKINETIC INTERACTIONS CAUSING DECREASED DRUG EFFECTS

Gastrointestinal absorption can be reduced if a drug interaction results in drug binding in the gut, as with aluminum-containing antacids, kaolin-pectin suspensions, or bile acid sequestrants. Drugs such as histamine H_2-receptor antagonists or proton pump inhibitors that alter gastric pH may decrease the solubility and hence absorption of weak bases such as ketoconazole.

Expression of some genes responsible for drug elimination, notably *CYP3A* and *MDR1*, can be markedly increased by inducing drugs, such as rifampin, carbamazepine, phenytoin, St. John's wort, and glutethimide, and by smoking, exposure to chlorinated insecticides such as DDT (CYP1A2), and chronic alcohol ingestion. Administration of inducing agents lowers plasma levels, and thus effects, over 2–3 weeks as gene expression is increased. If a drug dose is stabilized in the presence of an inducer that is subsequently stopped, major toxicity can occur as clearance returns to preinduction levels and drug concentrations rise. Individuals vary in the extent to which drug metabolism can be induced, likely through genetic mechanisms.

Interactions that inhibit the bioactivation of prodrugs will decrease drug effects (Table 5-1).

Interactions that decrease drug delivery to intracellular sites of action can decrease drug effects: tricyclic antidepressants can blunt the antihypertensive effect of clonidine by decreasing its uptake into adrenergic neurons. Reduced CNS penetration of multiple HIV protease inhibitors (with the attendant risk of facilitating viral replication in a sanctuary site) appears attributable to P-glycoprotein-mediated exclusion of the drug from the CNS; indeed, inhibition of P-glycoprotein has been proposed as a therapeutic approach to enhance drug entry to the CNS (Fig. 5-5*A*).

PHARMACOKINETIC INTERACTIONS CAUSING INCREASED DRUG EFFECTS

The most common mechanism here is inhibition of drug elimination. In contrast to induction, new protein synthesis is not involved, and the effect develops as drug and any inhibitor metabolites accumulate (a function of their elimination half-lives). Since shared substrates of a single enzyme can compete for access to the active site of the protein, many CYP substrates can also be considered inhibitors. However, some drugs are especially potent as inhibitors (and occasionally may not even be substrates) of specific drug elimination pathways, and so it is in the use of these agents that clinicians must be most alert to the potential for interactions (Table 5-3). Commonly implicated interacting drugs of this type include amiodarone, cimetidine,

TABLE 5-3 DRUGS WITH A HIGH RISK OF GENERATING PHARMACOKINETIC INTERACTIONS

Drug	Mechanism	Examples
Antacids Bile acid sequestrants	Reduced absorption	Antacids/tetracyclines Cholestyramine/digoxin
Proton pump inhibitors H_2-receptor blockers	Altered gastric pH	Ketoconazole absorption decreased
Rifampin Carbamazepine Barbiturates Phenytoin St. John's wort Glutethimide Nevirapine (CYP3A; CYP2B6)	Induction of CYPs and/or P-glycoprotein	Decreased concentration and effects of warfarin quinidine cyclosporine losartan oral contraceptives methadone, dabigatran
Tricyclic antidepressants Fluoxetine Quinidine	Inhibitors of CYP2D6	Increased effect of many β blockers Decreased codeine effect; possible decreased tamoxifen effect
Cimetidine	Inhibitor of multiple CYPs	Increased concentration and effects of warfarin theophylline phenytoin
Ketoconazole, itraconazole Erythromycin, clarithromycin Calcium channel blockers Ritonavir	Inhibitor of CYP3A	Increased concentration and toxicity of some HMG-CoA reductase inhibitors cyclosporine, cisapride, terfenadine (now withdrawn) Increased concentration and effects of indinavir (with ritonavir) Decreased clearance and dose requirement for cyclosporine (with calcium channel blockers)
Allopurinol	Xanthine oxidase inhibitor	Azathioprine and 6-mercaptopurine toxicity
Amiodarone	Inhibitor of many CYPs and of P-glycoprotein	Decreased clearance (risk of toxicity) for warfarin digoxin quinidine
Gemfibrozil (and other fibrates)	CYP3A inhibition	Rhabdomyolysis when co-prescribed with some HMG-CoA reductase inhibitors
Quinidine Amiodarone Verapamil Cyclosporine Itraconazole Erythromycin	P-glycoprotein inhibition	Risk of toxicity with P-glycoprotein substrates (e.g., digoxin, dabigatran)
Phenylbutazone Probenecid Salicylates	Inhibition of renal tubular transport	Increased risk of methotrexate toxicity with salicylates

erythromycin and some other macrolide antibiotics (clarithromycin but not azithromycin), ketoconazole and other azole antifungals, the antiretroviral agent ritonavir, and high concentrations of grapefruit juice (Table 5-3). The consequences of such interactions will depend on the drug whose elimination is being inhibited (see "The Concept of High-Risk Pharmacokinetics," above). Examples include CYP3A inhibitors increasing the risk of cyclosporine toxicity or of rhabdomyolysis with some HMG-CoA reductase inhibitors (lovastatin, simvastatin, atorvastatin, but not pravastatin), and P-glycoprotein inhibitors increasing the risk of toxicity with digoxin therapy or of bleeding with the thrombin inhibitor dabigatran.

These interactions can occasionally be exploited to therapeutic benefit. The antiviral ritonavir is a very potent CYP3A4 inhibitor that is sometimes added to anti-HIV regimens, not because of its antiviral effects but because it decreases clearance, and hence increases efficacy, of other anti-HIV agents. Similarly, calcium channel blockers have been deliberately coadministered with cyclosporine to reduce its clearance and thus its maintenance dosage and cost.

Phenytoin, an inducer of many systems, including CYP3A, inhibits CYP2C9. CYP2C9 metabolism of losartan to its active metabolite is inhibited by phenytoin, with potential loss of antihypertensive effect.

Grapefruit (but not orange) juice inhibits CYP3A, especially at high doses; patients receiving drugs where even modest CYP3A inhibition may increase the risk of adverse effects (e.g., cyclosporine, some HMG-CoA reductase inhibitors) should therefore avoid grapefruit juice.

CYP2D6 is markedly inhibited by quinidine, a number of neuroleptic drugs (chlorpromazine and haloperidol), and the SSRIs fluoxetine and paroxetine. The clinical consequences of fluoxetine's interaction with CYP2D6 substrates may not be apparent for weeks after the drug is started, because of its very long half-life and slow generation of a CYP2D6-inhibiting metabolite.

6-Mercaptopurine is metabolized not only by TPMT but also by xanthine oxidase. When allopurinol, an inhibitor of xanthine oxidase, is administered with standard doses of azathioprine or 6-mercaptopurine, life-threatening toxicity (bone marrow suppression) can result.

A number of drugs are secreted by the renal tubular transport systems for organic anions. Inhibition of these systems can cause excessive drug accumulation. Salicylate, for example, reduces the renal clearance of methotrexate, an interaction that may lead to methotrexate toxicity. Renal tubular secretion contributes substantially to the elimination of penicillin, which can be inhibited (to increase its therapeutic effect) by probenecid. Similarly, inhibition of the tubular cation transport system by cimetidine decreases the renal clearance of dofetilide.

DRUG INTERACTIONS NOT MEDIATED BY CHANGES IN DRUG DISPOSITION

Drugs may act on separate components of a common process to generate effects greater than either has alone. Antithrombotic therapy with combinations of antiplatelet agents (glycoprotein IIb/IIIa inhibitors, aspirin, clopidogrel) and anticoagulants (warfarin, heparins) is often used in the treatment of vascular disease, although such combinations carry an increased risk of bleeding.

Nonsteroidal anti-inflammatory drugs (NSAIDs) cause gastric ulcers, and in patients treated with warfarin, the risk of upper gastrointestinal bleeding is increased almost threefold by concomitant use of an NSAID.

Indomethacin, piroxicam, and probably other NSAIDs antagonize the antihypertensive effects of β-adrenergic receptor blockers, diuretics, ACE inhibitors, and other drugs. The resulting elevation in blood pressure ranges from trivial to severe. This effect is not seen with aspirin and sulindac but has been found with the cyclooxygenase 2 (COX-2) inhibitor celecoxib.

Torsades des pointes ventricular tachycardia during administration of QT-prolonging antiarrhythmics (quinidine, sotalol, dofetilide) occurs much more frequently in patients receiving diuretics, probably reflecting hypokalemia. In vitro, hypokalemia not only prolongs the QT interval in the absence of drug but also potentiates drug block of ion channels that results in QT prolongation. Also, some diuretics have direct electrophysiologic actions that prolong QT.

The administration of supplemental potassium leads to more frequent and more severe hyperkalemia when potassium elimination is reduced by concurrent treatment with ACE inhibitors, spironolactone, amiloride, or triamterene.

The pharmacologic effects of sildenafil result from inhibition of the phosphodiesterase type 5 isoform that inactivates cyclic guanosine monophosphate (GMP) in the vasculature. Nitroglycerin and related nitrates used to treat angina produce vasodilation by elevating cyclic GMP. Thus, coadministration of these nitrates with sildenafil can cause profound hypotension, which can be catastrophic in patients with coronary disease.

Sometimes, combining drugs can increase overall efficacy and/or reduce drug-specific toxicity. Such therapeutically useful interactions are described in chapters dealing with specific disease entities.

ADVERSE REACTIONS TO DRUGS

The beneficial effects of drugs are coupled with the inescapable risk of untoward effects. The morbidity and mortality from these adverse effects often present diagnostic problems because they can involve every organ and system of the body and may be mistaken for signs of underlying disease. As well, some surveys have suggested that drug therapy for a range of chronic conditions such as psychiatric disease or hypertension does not achieve its desired goal in up to half of treated patients; thus, the most common "adverse" drug effect may be failure of efficacy.

Adverse reactions can be classified in two broad groups. One type results from exaggeration of an intended pharmacologic action of the drug, such as increased bleeding with anticoagulants or bone marrow suppression with antineoplastics. The second type of adverse reaction ensues from toxic effects unrelated to the intended pharmacologic actions. The latter effects are often unanticipated (especially with new drugs) and frequently severe and may result from recognized as well as previously undescribed mechanisms.

Drugs may increase the frequency of an event that is common in a general population, and this may be especially difficult to recognize; an excellent example is the increase in myocardial infarctions with the COX-2 inhibitor rofecoxib. Drugs can also cause rare and serious adverse effects, such as hematologic abnormalities, arrhythmias, severe skin reactions, or hepatic or renal dysfunction. Prior to regulatory approval and marketing, new drugs are tested in relatively few patients who tend to be less sick and to have fewer concomitant diseases than those patients who subsequently receive the drug therapeutically. Because of the relatively small number of patients studied in clinical trials and the selected nature of these patients, rare adverse effects are generally not detected prior to a drug's approval; indeed, if they are detected, the new drugs are generally not approved. Therefore, physicians need to be cautious in the prescription of new drugs and alert for the appearance of previously unrecognized adverse events.

Elucidating mechanisms underlying adverse drug effects can assist development of safer compounds or allow a patient subset at especially high risk to be excluded from drug exposure. National adverse reaction reporting systems, such as those operated by the FDA (suspected adverse reactions can be reported online at *http://www.fda.gov/safety/medwatch/default.htm*) and the Committee on Safety of Medicines in Great Britain, can prove useful. The publication or reporting of a newly recognized adverse reaction can in a short time stimulate many similar such reports of reactions that previously had gone unrecognized.

Occasionally, "adverse" effects may be exploited to develop an entirely new indication for a drug. Unwanted hair growth during minoxidil treatment of severely hypertensive patients led to development of the drug for hair growth. Sildenafil was initially developed as an antianginal, but its effects to alleviate erectile dysfunction not only led to a new drug indication but also to increased understanding of the role of type 5 phosphodiesterase in erectile tissue. These examples further reinforce the concept that prescribers must remain vigilant to the possibility that unusual symptoms may reflect unappreciated drug effects.

Some 25–50% of patients make errors in self-administration of prescribed medicines, and these errors can be responsible for adverse drug effects. Similarly, patients commit errors in taking OTC drugs by not reading or following the directions on the containers. Health care providers must recognize that providing directions with prescriptions does not always guarantee compliance.

In hospitals, drugs are administered in a controlled setting, and patient compliance is, in general, ensured. Errors may occur nevertheless—the wrong drug or dose may be given or the drug may be given to the wrong patient—and improved drug distribution and administration systems are addressing this problem.

SCOPE OF THE PROBLEM

Patients receive, on average, 10 different drugs during each hospitalization. The sicker the patient, the more drugs are given, and there is a corresponding increase in the likelihood of adverse drug reactions. When <6 different drugs are given to hospitalized patients, the probability of an adverse reaction is ~5%, but if >15 drugs are given, the probability is >40%. Retrospective analyses of ambulatory patients have revealed adverse drug effects in 20%. Serious adverse reactions are also well-recognized with "herbal" remedies and OTC compounds; examples include kava-associated hepatotoxicity, L-tryptophan-associated eosinophilia-myalgia, and phenylpropanolamine-associated stroke, each of which has caused fatalities.

A small group of widely used drugs accounts for a disproportionate number of reactions. Aspirin and other NSAIDs, analgesics, digoxin, anticoagulants, diuretics, antimicrobials, glucocorticoids, antineoplastics, and hypoglycemic agents account for 90% of reactions.

TOXICITY UNRELATED TO A DRUG'S PRIMARY PHARMACOLOGIC ACTIVITY

Drugs or more commonly reactive metabolites generated by CYPs can covalently bind to tissue macromolecules (such as proteins or DNA) to cause tissue toxicity. Because of the reactive nature of these metabolites, covalent binding often occurs close to the site of production, typically the liver.

The most common cause of drug-induced hepatotoxicity is acetaminophen overdosage (Chap. 361). Normally, reactive metabolites are detoxified by combining with hepatic glutathione. When glutathione becomes depleted, the metabolites bind instead to hepatic protein, with resultant hepatocyte damage. The hepatic necrosis produced by the ingestion of acetaminophen can be prevented or attenuated by the administration of substances such as *N*-acetylcysteine that reduce the binding of electrophilic metabolites to hepatic proteins. The risk of acetaminophen-related hepatic necrosis is increased in patients receiving drugs such as phenobarbital or phenytoin, which increase the rate of drug metabolism, or ethanol, which exhausts glutathione stores. Such toxicity has even occurred with therapeutic dosages, so patients at risk through these mechanisms should be warned.

Most pharmacologic agents are small molecules with low molecular weights (<2000) and thus are poor immunogens. Generation of an immune response to a drug therefore usually requires in vivo activation and covalent linkage to protein, carbohydrate, or nucleic acid.

Drug stimulation of antibody production may mediate tissue injury by several mechanisms. The antibody may attack the drug when the drug is covalently attached to a cell and thereby destroy the cell. This occurs in penicillin-induced hemolytic anemia. Antibody-drug-antigen complexes may be passively adsorbed by a bystander cell, which is then destroyed by activation of complement; this occurs in quinine- and quinidine-induced thrombocytopenia. Heparin-induced thrombocytopenia arises when antibodies against complexes of platelet factor 4 peptide and heparin generate immune complexes that activate platelets; thus, the thrombocytopenia is accompanied by "paradoxical" thrombosis and is treated with thrombin inhibitors. Drugs or their reactive metabolites may alter a host tissue, rendering it antigenic and eliciting autoantibodies. For example, hydralazine and procainamide (or their reactive metabolites) can chemically alter nuclear material, stimulating the formation of antinuclear antibodies and occasionally causing lupus erythematosus. Drug-induced pure red cell aplasia **(Chap. 130)** is due to an immune-based drug reaction.

Serum sickness **(Chap. 376)** results from the deposition of circulating drug-antibody complexes on endothelial surfaces. Complement activation occurs, chemotactic factors are generated locally, and an inflammatory response develops at the site of complex entrapment. Arthralgias, urticaria, lymphadenopathy, glomerulonephritis, or cerebritis may result. Foreign proteins (vaccines, streptokinase, therapeutic antibodies) and antibiotics are common causes. Many drugs, particularly antimicrobial agents, ACE inhibitors, and aspirin, can elicit anaphylaxis with production of IgE, which binds to mast cell membranes. Contact with a drug antigen initiates a series of biochemical events in the mast cell and results in the release of mediators that can produce the characteristic urticaria, wheezing, flushing, rhinorrhea, and (occasionally) hypotension.

Drugs may also elicit cell-mediated immune responses. Topically administered substances may interact with sulfhydryl or amino groups in the skin and react with sensitized lymphocytes to produce the rash characteristic of contact dermatitis. Other types of rashes may also result from the interaction of serum factors, drugs, and sensitized lymphocytes.

DIAGNOSIS AND TREATMENT OF ADVERSE DRUG REACTIONS

The manifestations of drug-induced diseases frequently resemble those of other diseases, and a given set of manifestations may be produced by different and dissimilar drugs. Recognition of the role of a drug or drugs in an illness depends on appreciation of the possible adverse reactions to drugs in any disease, on identification of the temporal relationship between drug administration and development of the illness, and on familiarity with the common manifestations of the drugs. A suspected adverse drug reaction developing after introduction of a new drug naturally implicates that drug; however, it is also important to remember that a drug interaction may be responsible. Thus, for example, a patient on a chronic stable warfarin dose may develop a bleeding complication after introduction of amiodarone; this does not reflect a direct reaction to amiodarone but rather its effect to inhibit warfarin metabolism. Many associations between particular drugs and specific reactions have been described, but there is always a "first time" for a novel association, and any drug should be suspected of causing an adverse effect if the clinical setting is appropriate.

Illness related to a drug's intended pharmacologic action is often more easily recognized than illness attributable to immune or other mechanisms. For example, side effects such as cardiac arrhythmias in patients receiving digitalis, hypoglycemia in patients given insulin, or bleeding in patients receiving anticoagulants are more readily related to a specific drug than are symptoms such as fever or rash, which may be caused by many drugs or by other factors.

Electronic listings of adverse drug reactions can be useful. However, exhaustive compilations often provide little sense of perspective in terms of frequency and seriousness, which can vary considerably among patients.

Eliciting a drug history from each patient is important for diagnosis. Attention must be directed to OTC drugs and herbal preparations as well as to prescription drugs. Each type can be responsible for adverse drug effects, and adverse interactions may occur between OTC drugs and prescribed drugs. Loss of efficacy of oral contraceptives or cyclosporine with concurrent use of St. John's wort (a P-glycoprotein inducer) is an example. In addition, it is common for patients to be cared for by several physicians, and duplicative, additive, antagonistic, or synergistic drug combinations may therefore be administered if the physicians are not aware of the patients' drug histories. Every physician should determine what drugs a patient has been taking, for the previous month or two ideally, before prescribing any medications. Medications stopped for inefficacy or adverse effects should be documented to avoid pointless and potentially dangerous reexposure. A frequently overlooked source of additional drug exposure is topical therapy; for example, a patient complaining of bronchospasm may not mention that an ophthalmic beta blocker is being used unless specifically asked. A history of previous adverse drug effects in patients is common. Since these patients have shown a predisposition to drug-induced illnesses, such a history should dictate added caution in prescribing new drugs.

Laboratory studies may include demonstration of serum antibody in some persons with drug allergies involving cellular blood elements, as in agranulocytosis, hemolytic anemia, and thrombocytopenia. For example, both quinine and quinidine can produce platelet agglutination in vitro in the presence of complement and the serum from a patient who has developed thrombocytopenia following use of this drug. Biochemical abnormalities such as G6PD deficiency, serum pseudocholinesterase level, or genotyping may also be useful in diagnosis, often after an adverse effect has occurred in the patient or a family member.

Once an adverse reaction is suspected, discontinuation of the suspected drug followed by disappearance of the reaction is presumptive evidence of a drug-induced illness. Confirming evidence may be sought by cautiously reintroducing the drug and seeing if the reaction reappears. However, that should be done only if confirmation would be useful in the future management of the patient and if the attempt would not entail undue risk. With concentration-dependent adverse reactions, lowering the dosage may cause the reaction to disappear, and raising it may cause the reaction to reappear. When the reaction is thought to be allergic, however, readministration of the drug may be hazardous, since anaphylaxis may develop.

If the patient is receiving many drugs when an adverse reaction is suspected, the drugs likeliest to be responsible can usually be identified; this should include both potential culprit agents as well as drugs that alter their elimination. All drugs may be discontinued at once or, if this is not practical, discontinued one at a time, starting with the ones most suspect, and the patient observed for signs of improvement. The time needed for a concentration-dependent adverse effect to disappear depends on the time required for the concentration to fall below the range associated with the adverse effect; that, in turn, depends on the initial blood level and on the rate of elimination or metabolism of the drug. Adverse effects of drugs with long half-lives or those not directly related to serum concentration may take a considerable time to disappear.

SUMMARY

Modern clinical pharmacology aims to replace empiricism in the use of drugs with therapy based on in-depth understanding of factors that determine an individual's response to drug treatment. Molecular pharmacology, pharmacokinetics, genetics, clinical trials, and the educated prescriber all contribute to this process. No drug response should ever be termed *idiosyncratic*; all responses have a mechanism whose understanding will help guide further therapy with that drug or successors. This rapidly expanding understanding of variability in drug actions makes the process of prescribing drugs increasingly daunting for the practitioner. However, fundamental principles should guide this process:

- The benefits of drug therapy, however defined, should always outweigh the risk.
- The smallest dosage necessary to produce the desired effect should be used.
- The number of medications and doses per day should be minimized.
- Although the literature is rapidly expanding, accessing it is becoming easier; electronic tools to search databases of literature and unbiased opinion will become increasingly commonplace.
- Genetics play a role in determining variability in drug response and may become a part of clinical practice.
- Electronic medical record and pharmacy systems will increasingly incorporate prescribing advice, such as indicated medications not used; unindicated medications being prescribed; and potential dosing errors, drug interactions, or genetically determined drug responses.
- Prescribers should be particularly wary when adding or stopping specific drugs that are especially liable to provoke interactions and adverse reactions.
- Prescribers should use only a limited number of drugs, with which they are thoroughly familiar.

6e Women's Health

Andrea Dunaif

This is a digital-only chapter. It is available on the DVD that accompanies this book, as well as on Access Medicine/Harrison's Online, and the eBook and "app" editions of HPIM 19e.

The National Institutes of Health's Office of Research on Women's Health celebrated its twentieth anniversary in 2010 with a new strategic plan recognizing the study of the biologic basis of sex differences as a distinct scientific discipline. It has become clear that both sex chromosomes and sex hormones contribute to these differences. Indeed, it is recommended that the term *sex difference* be used for biologic processes that differ between males and females and the term *gender difference* be used for features related to social influences. The clinical discipline of women's health emphasizes greater attention to patient education and involvement in disease prevention and medical decision-making and has become a model for patient-centered health care.

7e Men's Health

Shalender Bhasin, Shehzad Basaria

This is a digital-only chapter. It is available on the DVD that accompanies this book, as well as on Access Medicine/Harrison's Online, and the eBook and "app" editions of HPIM 19e.

The emergence of men's health as a distinct discipline within internal medicine is founded on the evidence that men and women differ across their life span in their susceptibility to disease, in the clinical manifestations of the disease, and in their response to treatment. Furthermore, men and women weigh the health consequences of illness differently and have different motivations for seeking care. Men and women experience different types of disparities in access to health care services and in the manner in which health care is delivered to them because of a complex array of socioeconomic and cultural factors. Attitudinal and institutional barriers to accessing care, fear and embarrassment due to the perception by some that it is not manly to seek medical help, and reticence on the part of patients and physicians to discuss issues related to sexuality, drug use, and aging have heightened the need for programs tailored to address the specific health needs of men.

8 Medical Disorders During Pregnancy

Robert L. Barbieri, John T. Repke

Each year, approximately 4 million births occur in the United States, and more than 130 million births occur worldwide. A significant proportion of births are complicated by medical disorders. In the past, many medical disorders were contraindications to pregnancy. Advances in obstetrics, neonatology, obstetric anesthesiology, and medicine have increased the expectation that pregnancy will result in a positive outcome for both mother and fetus despite most of these conditions. A successful pregnancy requires important physiologic adaptations, such as a marked increase in cardiac output. Medical problems that interfere with the physiologic adaptations of pregnancy increase the risk for poor pregnancy outcome; conversely, in some instances, pregnancy may adversely impact an underlying medical disorder.

HYPERTENSION

(See also Chap. 298) In pregnancy, cardiac output increases by 40%, with most of the increase due to an increase in stroke volume. Heart rate increases by ~10 beats/min during the third trimester. In the second trimester, systemic vascular resistance decreases, and this decline is associated with a fall in blood pressure. During pregnancy, a blood pressure of 140/90 mmHg is considered to be abnormally elevated and is associated with an increase in perinatal morbidity and mortality. In all pregnant women, the measurement of blood pressure should be performed in the sitting position, because the lateral recumbent position may result in a blood pressure lower than that recorded in the sitting position. The diagnosis of hypertension requires the measurement of two elevated blood pressures at least 6 h apart. Hypertension during pregnancy is usually caused by preeclampsia, chronic hypertension, gestational hypertension, or renal disease.

PREECLAMPSIA

Approximately 5–7% of all pregnant women develop *preeclampsia*, the new onset of hypertension (blood pressure >140/90 mmHg) and proteinuria (either a 24 hour urinary protein >300 mg/24 h, or a protein-creatinine ratio ≥0.3) after 20 weeks of gestation. Although the precise pathophysiology of preeclampsia remains unknown, recent studies show excessive placental production of antagonists to both vascular epithelial growth factor (VEGF) and transforming growth factor β (TGF-β). These antagonists to VEGF and TGF-β disrupt endothelial and renal glomerular function resulting in edema, hypertension, and proteinuria. The renal histological feature of preeclampsia is glomerular endotheliosis. Glomerular endothelial cells are swollen and encroach on the vascular lumen. Preeclampsia is associated with abnormalities of cerebral circulatory autoregulation, which increase the risk of stroke at mildly and moderately elevated blood pressures. Risk factors for the development of preeclampsia include nulliparity, diabetes mellitus, a history of renal disease or chronic hypertension, a prior history of preeclampsia, extremes of maternal age (>35 years or <15 years), obesity, antiphospholipid antibody syndrome, and multiple gestation. Low-dose aspirin (81 mg daily, initiated at the end of the first trimester) may reduce the risk of preeclampsia in pregnant women at high risk of developing the disease.

In December, 2013 The American College of Obstetricians and Gynecologists issued a report summarizing the findings and recommendations of their Task Force on Hypertension in Pregnancy. With respect to preeclampsia several pertinent revisions to the diagnostic criteria were made including: proteinuria is no longer an absolute requirement for making the diagnosis; the terms mild and severe preeclampsia have been replaced, and the disease is now termed preeclampsia either with or without severe features; removal of fetal growth restriction as a defining criterion for severe preeclampsia.

Preeclampsia with severe features is the presence of new-onset hypertension and proteinuria accompanied by end-organ damage. Features may include severe elevation of blood pressure (>160/110 mmHg), evidence of central nervous system (CNS) dysfunction (headaches, blurred vision, seizures, coma), renal dysfunction (oliguria or creatinine >1.5 mg/dL), pulmonary edema, hepatocellular injury (serum alanine aminotransferase level more than twofold the upper limit of normal), hematologic dysfunction (platelet count <100,000/L or disseminated intravascular coagulation [DIC]). The *HELLP syndrome* (*h*emolysis, *e*levated *l*iver enzymes, *l*ow *p*latelets) is a special subtype of severe preeclampsia and is a major cause of morbidity and mortality in this disease. Platelet dysfunction and coagulation disorders further increase the risk of stroke.

TREATMENT PREECLAMPSIA

Preeclampsia resolves within a few weeks after delivery. For pregnant women with preeclampsia prior to 37 weeks of gestation, delivery reduces the mother's morbidity but exposes the fetus to the risk of premature birth. The management of preeclampsia is challenging because it requires the clinician to balance the health of the mother and fetus simultaneously. In general, prior to term, women with *mild* preeclampsia without severe features may be managed conservatively with limited physical activity, although bed rest is not recommended, close monitoring of blood pressure and renal function, and careful fetal surveillance. For women with preeclampsia with severe features, delivery is recommended unless the patient is eligible for expectant management in a tertiary hospital setting. Expectant management of preeclampsia with severe features remote from term affords some benefits for the fetus but significant risks for the mother.

The definitive treatment of preeclampsia is delivery of the fetus and placenta. For women with preeclampsia with severe features, aggressive management of blood pressures >160/110 mmHg reduces the risk of cerebrovascular accidents. IV labetalol or hydralazine is most commonly used to acutely manage severe hypertension in preeclampsia; labetalol is associated with fewer episodes of maternal hypotension. Oral nifedipine and labetalol are commonly used to manage hypertension in pregnancy. Elevated arterial pressure should be reduced slowly to avoid hypotension and a decrease in blood flow to the fetus. Angiotensin-converting enzyme (ACE) inhibitors as well as angiotensin-receptor blockers should be avoided in the second and third trimesters of pregnancy because of their adverse effects on fetal development.

Magnesium sulfate is the preferred agent for the prevention and treatment of eclamptic seizures. Large, randomized clinical trials have demonstrated the superiority of magnesium sulfate over phenytoin and diazepam in reducing the risk of seizure and, possibly, the risk of maternal death. Magnesium may prevent seizures by interacting with *N*-methyl-D-aspartate (NMDA) receptors in the CNS. Given the difficulty of predicting eclamptic seizures on the basis of disease severity, once the decision to proceed with delivery is made, most patients carrying a diagnosis of preeclampsia should be treated with magnesium sulfate. Women who have had preeclampsia appear to be at increased risk of cardiovascular and renal disease later in life.

CHRONIC ESSENTIAL HYPERTENSION

Pregnancy complicated by chronic essential hypertension is associated with intrauterine growth restriction and increased perinatal mortality. Pregnant women with chronic hypertension are at increased risk for superimposed preeclampsia and abruptio placentae. Women with chronic hypertension should have a thorough prepregnancy evaluation, both to identify remediable causes of hypertension and to ensure that the prescribed antihypertensive agents (e.g., ACE inhibitors, angiotensin-receptor blockers) are not associated with an adverse outcome of pregnancy. α-Methyldopa, labetalol, and nifedipine are the most commonly used medications for the treatment of chronic hypertension in pregnancy. The target blood pressure is in the range of 130–150 mmHg systolic and 80–100 mmHg diastolic. Should hypertension worsen during pregnancy, baseline evaluation of renal function (see below) is necessary to help differentiate the effects of chronic hypertension from those of superimposed preeclampsia. There are no convincing data that the treatment of mild chronic hypertension improves perinatal outcome.

GESTATIONAL HYPERTENSION

The development of elevated blood pressure during pregnancy or in the first 24 h post-partum in the absence of preexisting chronic hypertension or proteinuria is referred to as *gestational hypertension*. Mild gestational hypertension that does not progress to preeclampsia has not been associated with adverse pregnancy outcome or adverse long-term prognosis.

RENAL DISEASE

(See also Chaps. 333 and 341) Normal pregnancy is characterized by an increase in glomerular filtration rate and creatinine clearance. This increase occurs secondary to a rise in renal plasma flow and increased glomerular filtration pressures. Patients with underlying renal disease and hypertension may expect a worsening of hypertension during pregnancy. If superimposed preeclampsia develops, the additional endothelial injury results in a capillary leak syndrome that may make management challenging. In general, patients with underlying renal disease and hypertension benefit from aggressive management of blood pressure. Preconception counseling is also essential for these patients so that accurate risk assessment and medication changes can occur prior to pregnancy. In general, a prepregnancy serum creatinine level <133 μmol/L (<1.5 mg/dL) is associated with a favorable prognosis. When renal disease worsens during pregnancy, close collaboration between the internist and the maternal-fetal medicine specialist is essential so that decisions regarding delivery can be weighed to balance the sequelae of prematurity for the neonate versus long-term sequelae for the mother with respect to future renal function.

CARDIAC DISEASE

VALVULAR HEART DISEASE

(See also Chaps. 283–286) Valvular heart disease is the most common cardiac problem complicating pregnancy.

Mitral Stenosis This is the valvular disease most likely to cause death during pregnancy. The pregnancy-induced increase in blood volume, cardiac output, and tachycardia can increase the transmitral pressure gradient and cause pulmonary edema in women with mitral stenosis. Women with moderate to severe mitral stenosis who are planning pregnancy and have either symptomatic disease or pulmonary hypertension should undergo valvuloplasty prior to conception. Pregnancy associated with long-standing mitral stenosis may result in pulmonary hypertension. Sudden death has been reported when hypovolemia occurs. Careful control of heart rate, especially during labor and delivery, minimizes the impact of tachycardia and reduced ventricular filling times on cardiac function. Pregnant women with mitral stenosis are at increased risk for the development of atrial fibrillation and other tachyarrhythmias. Medical management of severe mitral stenosis and atrial fibrillation with digoxin and beta blockers is recommended. Balloon valvulotomy can be carried out during pregnancy. The immediate postpartum period is a time of particular concern secondary to rapid volume shifts. Careful monitoring of cardiac and fluid status should be observed.

Mitral Regurgitation and Aortic Regurgitation and Stenosis The pregnancy-induced decrease in systemic vascular resistance reduces the risk of cardiac failure with these conditions. As a rule, mitral valve prolapse does not present problems for the pregnant patient, and aortic stenosis, unless very severe, is well tolerated. In the most severe cases of aortic stenosis, limitation of activity or balloon valvuloplasty may be indicated.

CONGENITAL HEART DISEASE

(See also Chap. 282) Reparative surgery has markedly increased the number of women with surgically repaired congenital heart disease. Maternal morbidity and mortality are greater among these women than among those without surgical repairs. When pregnant, these patients should be jointly managed by a cardiologist and an obstetrician familiar with these problems. The presence of a congenital cardiac lesion in the mother increases the risk of congenital cardiac disease in the newborn. Prenatal screening of the fetus for congenital cardiac disease with ultrasound is recommended. Atrial or ventricular septal defect is usually well tolerated during pregnancy in the absence of pulmonary hypertension, provided that the woman's prepregnancy cardiac status is favorable. Use of air filters on IV sets during labor and delivery in patients with intracardiac shunts is recommended.

OTHER CARDIAC DISORDERS

Supraventricular tachycardia (Chap. 276) is a common cardiac complication of pregnancy. Treatment is the same as in the nonpregnant patient, and fetal tolerance of medications such as adenosine and calcium channel blockers is acceptable. When necessary, pharmacologic or electric cardioversion may be performed to improve cardiac performance and reduce symptoms. This intervention is generally well tolerated by mother and fetus.

Peripartum cardiomyopathy (Chap. 287) is an uncommon disorder of pregnancy associated with myocarditis, and its etiology remains unknown. Treatment is directed toward symptomatic relief and improvement of cardiac function. Many patients recover completely; others are left with progressive dilated cardiomyopathy. Recurrence in a subsequent pregnancy has been reported, and women who do not have normal baseline left-ventricular function after an episode of peripartum cardiomyopathy should be counseled to avoid pregnancy.

SPECIFIC HIGH-RISK CARDIAC LESIONS

Marfan Syndrome (See also Chap. 427) This autosomal dominant disease is associated with a high risk of maternal morbidity. Approximately 15% of pregnant women with Marfan syndrome develop a major cardiovascular manifestation during pregnancy, with almost all women surviving. An aortic root diameter <40 mm is associated with a favorable outcome of pregnancy. Prophylactic therapy with beta blockers has been advocated, although large-scale clinical trials in pregnancy have not been performed. *Ehlers-Danlos syndrome* (EDS) may be associated with premature labor, and in type IV EDS there is increased risk of organ or vascular rupture that may cause death.

Pulmonary Hypertension (See also Chap. 304) Maternal mortality in the setting of severe pulmonary hypertension is high, and primary pulmonary hypertension is a contraindication to pregnancy. Termination of pregnancy may be advisable in these circumstances to preserve the life of the mother. In the *Eisenmenger syndrome*, i.e., the combination of pulmonary hypertension with right-to-left shunting due to congenital abnormalities (Chap. 282), maternal and fetal deaths occur frequently. Systemic hypotension may occur after blood loss, prolonged Valsalva maneuver, or regional anesthesia; sudden death secondary to hypotension is a dreaded complication. Management of these patients is challenging, and invasive hemodynamic monitoring during labor and delivery is recommended in severe cases.

In patients with pulmonary hypertension, vaginal delivery is less stressful hemodynamically than cesarean section, which should be reserved for accepted obstetric indications.

DEEP VENOUS THROMBOSIS AND PULMONARY EMBOLISM

(See also Chap. 300) A hypercoagulable state is characteristic of pregnancy, and deep venous thrombosis (DVT) occurs in about 1 in 500 pregnancies. In pregnant women, most unilateral DVTs occur in the left leg because the left iliac vein is compressed by the right iliac artery and the uterus compresses the inferior vena cava. Pregnancy is associated with an increase in procoagulants such as factors V and VII and a decrease in anticoagulant activity, including proteins C and S. Pulmonary embolism is one of the most common causes of maternal death in the United States. Activated protein C resistance caused by the factor V Leiden mutation increases the risk for DVT and pulmonary embolism during pregnancy. Approximately 25% of women with DVT during pregnancy carry the factor V Leiden allele. Additional genetic mutations associated with DVT during pregnancy include the prothrombin G20210A mutation (heterozygotes and homozygotes) and the methylenetetrahydrofolate reductase C677T mutation (homozygotes).

TREATMENT DEEP VENOUS THROMBOSIS

Aggressive diagnosis and management of DVT and suspected pulmonary embolism optimize the outcome for mother and fetus. In general, all diagnostic and therapeutic modalities afforded the nonpregnant patient should be utilized in pregnancy except for D-dimer measurement, in which values are elevated in normal pregnancy. Anticoagulant therapy with low-molecular-weight heparin (LMWH) or unfractionated heparin is indicated in pregnant women with DVT. LMWH may be associated with an increased risk of epidural hematoma in women receiving an epidural anesthetic in labor. Four weeks prior to anticipated delivery, LMWH should be switched to unfractionated heparin. Warfarin therapy is contraindicated in the first trimester due to its association with fetal chondrodysplasia punctata. In the second and third trimesters, warfarin may cause fetal optic atrophy and mental retardation. When DVT occurs in the postpartum period, LMWH therapy for 7–10 days may be followed by warfarin therapy for 3–6 months. Warfarin is not contraindicated in breast-feeding women. For women at moderate or high risk of DVT who have a cesarean delivery, mechanical and/or pharmacologic prophylaxis is warranted.

ENDOCRINE DISORDERS

DIABETES MELLITUS

(See also Chaps. 417–419) In pregnancy, the fetoplacental unit induces major metabolic changes, the purpose of which is to shunt glucose and amino acids to the fetus while the mother uses ketones and triglycerides to fuel her metabolic needs. These metabolic changes are accompanied by maternal insulin resistance caused in part by placental production of steroids, a growth hormone variant, and placental lactogen. Although pregnancy has been referred to as a state of "accelerated starvation," it is better characterized as "accelerated ketosis." In pregnancy, after an overnight fast, plasma glucose is lower by 0.8–1.1 mmol/L (15–20 mg/dL) than in the nonpregnant state. This difference is due to the use of glucose by the fetus. In early pregnancy, fasting may result in circulating glucose concentrations in the range of 2.2 mmol/L (40 mg/dL) and may be associated with symptoms of hypoglycemia. In contrast to the decrease in maternal glucose concentration, plasma hydroxybutyrate and acetoacetate levels rise to two to four times normal after a fast.

TREATMENT DIABETES MELLITUS IN PREGNANCY

Pregnancy complicated by diabetes mellitus is associated with higher maternal and perinatal morbidity and mortality rates. Preconception counseling and treatment are important for the diabetic patient contemplating pregnancy and can reduce the risk of congenital malformations and improve pregnancy outcome. Folate supplementation reduces the incidence of fetal neural tube defects, which occur with greater frequency in fetuses of diabetic mothers. In addition, optimizing glucose control during key periods of organogenesis reduces other congenital anomalies, including sacral agenesis, caudal dysplasia, renal agenesis, and ventricular septal defect.

Once pregnancy is established, glucose control should be managed more aggressively than in the nonpregnant state. In addition to dietary changes, this enhanced management requires more frequent blood glucose monitoring and often involves additional injections of insulin or conversion to an insulin pump. Fasting blood glucose levels should be maintained at <5.8 mmol/L (<105 mg/dL), with avoidance of values >7.8 mmol/L (140 mg/dL). Commencing in the third trimester, regular surveillance of maternal glucose control as well as assessment of fetal growth (obstetric sonography) and fetoplacental oxygenation (fetal heart rate monitoring or biophysical profile) optimize pregnancy outcome. Pregnant diabetic patients without vascular disease are at greater risk for delivering a macrosomic fetus, and attention to fetal growth via clinical and ultrasound examination is important. Fetal macrosomia is associated with an increased risk of maternal and fetal birth trauma, including permanent newborn *Erb's palsy*. Pregnant women with diabetes have an increased risk of developing preeclampsia, and those with vascular disease are at greater risk for developing intrauterine growth restriction, which is associated with an increased risk of fetal and neonatal death. Excellent pregnancy outcomes in patients with diabetic nephropathy and proliferative retinopathy have been reported with aggressive glucose control and intensive maternal and fetal surveillance.

As pregnancy progresses, glycemic control may become more difficult to achieve due to an increase in insulin resistance. Because of delayed pulmonary maturation of the fetuses of diabetic mothers, early delivery should be avoided unless there is biochemical evidence of fetal lung maturity. In general, efforts to control glucose and avoid preterm delivery result in the best overall outcome for both mother and newborn. Preterm delivery is generally performed only for the usual obstetric indications (e.g., preeclampsia, fetal growth restriction, non-reassuring fetal testing) or for worsening maternal renal or active proliferative retinopathy.

GESTATIONAL DIABETES

Gestational diabetes occurs in approximately 4% of pregnancies. All pregnant women should be screened for gestational diabetes unless they are in a low-risk group. Women at low risk for gestational diabetes are those <25 years of age; those with a body mass index <25 kg/m^2, no maternal history of macrosomia or gestational diabetes, and no diabetes in a first-degree relative; and those who are not members of a high-risk ethnic group (African American, Hispanic, Native American). A typical two-step strategy for establishing the diagnosis of gestational diabetes involves administration of a 50-g oral glucose challenge with a single serum glucose measurement at 60 min. If the plasma glucose is <7.8 mmol/L (<130 mg/dL), the test is considered normal. Plasma glucose >7.8 mmol/L (>130 mg/dL) warrants administration of a 100-g oral glucose challenge with plasma glucose measurements obtained in the fasting state and at 1, 2, and 3 h. Normal plasma glucose concentrations at these time points are <5.8 mmol/L (<105 mg/dL), 10.5 mmol/L (190 mg/dL), 9.1 mmol/L (165 mg/dL), and 8.0 mmol/L (145 mg/dL), respectively. Some centers have adopted more sensitive criteria, using values of <5.3 mmol/L (<95 mg/dL), <10 mmol/L (<180 mg/dL), <8.6 mmol/L (<155 mg/dL), and <7.8 mmol/L (<140 mg/dL) as the upper norms for a 3-h glucose tolerance test. Two elevated glucose values indicate a positive test. Adverse pregnancy outcomes for mother and fetus appear to increase with glucose as a continuous variable; thus it is challenging to define the optimal threshold for establishing the diagnosis of gestational diabetes.

Pregnant women with gestational diabetes are at increased risk of stillbirth, preeclampsia, and delivery of infants who are large for their gestational age, with resulting birth lacerations, shoulder dystocia, and birth trauma including brachial plexus injury. These fetuses are at risk of hypoglycemia, hyperbilirubinemia, and polycythemia. Tight control of blood sugar during pregnancy and labor can reduce these risks.

TREATMENT GESTATIONAL DIABETES

Treatment of gestational diabetes with a two-step strategy—dietary intervention followed by insulin injections if diet alone does not adequately control blood sugar [fasting glucose <5.6 mmol/L (<100 mg/dL) and 2-h postprandial glucose <7.0 mmol/L (<126 mg/dL)]—is associated with a decreased risk of birth trauma for the fetus. Oral hypoglycemic agents such as glyburide and metformin have become more commonly utilized for managing gestational diabetes refractory to nutritional management, but many experts favor insulin therapy. For women with gestational diabetes, there is a 40% risk of being diagnosed with diabetes within the 10 years after the index pregnancy. In women with a history of gestational diabetes, exercise, weight loss, and treatment with metformin reduce the risk of developing diabetes. All women with a history of gestational diabetes should be counseled about prevention strategies and evaluated regularly for diabetes.

OBESITY

(See also Chap. 416) Pregnant women who are obese have an increased risk of stillbirth, congenital fetal malformations, gestational diabetes, preeclampsia, urinary tract infections, post-date delivery, and cesarean delivery. Women contemplating pregnancy should attempt to attain a healthy weight prior to conception. For morbidly obese women who have not been able to lose weight with lifestyle changes, bariatric surgery may result in weight loss and improve pregnancy outcomes. Following bariatric surgery, women should delay conception for 1 year to avoid pregnancy during an interval of rapid metabolic changes.

THYROID DISEASE

(See also Chap. 405) In pregnancy, the estrogen-induced increase in thyroxine-binding globulin increases circulating levels of total T_3 and total T_4. The normal range of circulating levels of free T_4, free T_3, and thyroid-stimulating hormone (TSH) remain unaltered by pregnancy.

The thyroid gland normally enlarges during pregnancy. Many physiologic adaptations to pregnancy may mimic subtle signs of *hyperthyroidism*. Maternal hyperthyroidism occurs at a rate of ~2 per 1000 pregnancies and is generally well tolerated by pregnant women. Clinical signs and symptoms should alert the physician to the occurrence of this condition. Hyperthyroidism in pregnancy is most commonly caused by Graves' disease, but autonomously functioning nodules and gestational trophoblastic disease should also be considered. Although pregnant women are able to tolerate mild hyperthyroidism without adverse sequelae, more severe hyperthyroidism can cause spontaneous abortion or premature labor, and thyroid storm is associated with a significant risk of maternal death.

Testing for *hypothyroidism* using TSH measurements before or early in pregnancy may be warranted in symptomatic women and in women with a personal or family history of thyroid disease. With use of this case-finding approach, about 30% of pregnant women with mild hypothyroidism remain undiagnosed, leading some to recommend universal screening. Children born to women with an elevated serum TSH (and a normal total thyroxine) during pregnancy may have impaired performance on neuropsychologic tests.

TREATMENT HYPERTHYROIDISM IN PREGNANCY

HYPERTHYROIDISM

Methimazole crosses the placenta to a greater degree than propylthiouracil and has been associated with fetal aplasia cutis. However, propylthiouracil can be associated with liver failure. Some experts recommend propylthiouracil in the first trimester and methimazole thereafter. Radioiodine should not be used during pregnancy, either for scanning or for treatment, because of effects on the fetal thyroid. In emergent circumstances, additional treatment with beta blockers may be necessary. Hyperthyroidism is most difficult to control in the first trimester of pregnancy and easiest to control in the third trimester.

HYPOTHYROIDISM

The goal of therapy for hypothyroidism is to maintain the serum TSH in the normal range, and thyroxine is the drug of choice. During pregnancy, the dose of thyroxine required to keep the TSH in the normal range rises. In one study, the mean replacement dose of thyroxine required to maintain the TSH in the normal range was 0.1 mg daily before pregnancy and increased to 0.15 mg daily during pregnancy. Since the increased thyroxine requirement occurs as early as the fifth week of pregnancy, one approach is to increase the thyroxine dose by 30% (two additional pills weekly) as soon as pregnancy is diagnosed and then adjust the dose by serial measurements of TSH.

HEMATOLOGIC DISORDERS

Pregnancy has been described as a state of physiologic anemia. Part of the reduction in hemoglobin concentration is dilutional, but iron and folate deficiencies are major causes of correctable anemia during pregnancy.

In populations at high risk for hemoglobinopathies (Chap. 127), hemoglobin electrophoresis should be performed as part of the prenatal screen. Hemoglobinopathies can be associated with increased maternal and fetal morbidity and mortality. Management is tailored to the specific hemoglobinopathy and is generally the same for both pregnant and nonpregnant women. Prenatal diagnosis of hemoglobinopathies in the fetus is readily available and should be discussed with prospective parents either prior to or early in pregnancy.

Thrombocytopenia occurs commonly during pregnancy. The majority of cases are benign gestational thrombocytopenias, but the differential diagnosis should include immune thrombocytopenia (Chap. 140), thrombotic thrombocytopenic purpura, and preeclampsia. Maternal thrombocytopenia may also be caused by DIC, which is a consumptive coagulopathy characterized by thrombocytopenia, prolonged prothrombin time (PT) and activated partial thromboplastin time (aPTT), elevated fibrin degradation products, and a low fibrinogen concentration. Several catastrophic obstetric events are associated with the development of DIC, including retention of a dead fetus, sepsis, abruptio placentae, and amniotic fluid embolism.

NEUROLOGIC DISORDERS

Headache appearing during pregnancy is usually due to migraine (Chap. 21), a condition that may worsen, improve, or be unaffected by pregnancy. A new or worsening headache, particularly if associated with visual blurring, may signal eclampsia (above) or pseudotumor cerebri (benign intracranial hypertension); diplopia due to a sixth-nerve palsy suggests pseudotumor cerebri (Chap. 39). The risk of seizures in patients with epilepsy increases in the postpartum period but not consistently during pregnancy; management is discussed in Chap. 445. The risk of stroke is generally thought to increase during pregnancy because of a hypercoagulable state; however, studies suggest that the period of risk occurs primarily in the postpartum period and that both ischemic and hemorrhagic strokes may occur at this time. Guidelines for use of heparin therapy are summarized above (see "Deep Venous Thrombosis and Pulmonary Embolism"); warfarin is teratogenic and should be avoided.

The onset of a new movement disorder during pregnancy suggests *chorea gravidarum*, a variant of Sydenham's chorea associated with rheumatic fever and streptococcal infection (Chap. 381); the chorea may recur with subsequent pregnancies. Patients with preexisting *multiple sclerosis* (Chap. 458) experience a gradual decrease in the risk of relapses as pregnancy progresses and, conversely, an increase in attack risk during the postpartum period. Disease-modifying agents, including interferon β, should *not* be administered to pregnant multiple sclerosis patients, but moderate or severe relapses can be safely treated with pulse glucocorticoid therapy. Finally, certain tumors, particularly pituitary adenoma and meningioma (Chap. 403), may manifest during pregnancy because of accelerated growth, possibly driven by hormonal factors.

Peripheral nerve disorders associated with pregnancy include *Bell's palsy* (idiopathic facial paralysis) (Chap. 459), which is approximately threefold more likely to occur during the third trimester and immediate postpartum period than in the general population. Therapy with glucocorticoids should follow the guidelines established for nonpregnant patients. Entrapment neuropathies are common in the later stages of pregnancy, presumably as a result of fluid retention. *Carpal tunnel syndrome* (median nerve) presents first as pain and paresthesia in the hand (often worse at night) and later with weakness in the thenar muscles. Treatment is generally conservative; wrist splints may be helpful, and glucocorticoid injections or surgical section of the carpal tunnel can usually be postponed. *Meralgia paresthetica* (lateral femoral cutaneous nerve entrapment) consists of pain and numbness in the lateral aspect of the thigh without weakness. Patients are usually reassured to learn that these symptoms are benign and can be expected to remit spontaneously after the pregnancy has been completed. *Restless leg syndrome* is the most common peripheral nerve and movement disorder in pregnancy. Disordered iron metabolism is the suspected etiology. Management is expectant in most cases.

GASTROINTESTINAL AND LIVER DISEASE

Up to 90% of pregnant women experience nausea and vomiting during the first trimester of pregnancy. *Hyperemesis gravidarum* is a severe form that prevents adequate fluid and nutritional intake and may require hospitalization to prevent dehydration and malnutrition.

Crohn's disease may be associated with exacerbations in the second and third trimesters. Ulcerative colitis is associated with disease exacerbations in the first trimester and during the early postpartum period. Medical management of these diseases during pregnancy is similar to management in the nonpregnant state (Chap. 351).

Exacerbation of gallbladder disease is common during pregnancy. In part, this aggravation may be due to pregnancy-induced alteration in the metabolism of bile and fatty acids. Intrahepatic cholestasis of pregnancy is generally a third-trimester event. Profound pruritus may accompany this condition, and it may be associated with increased fetal mortality. Placental bile salt deposition may contribute to progressive uteroplacental insufficiency. Therefore, regular fetal surveillance should be undertaken once the diagnosis of intrahepatic cholestasis is made, and delivery should be planned once the fetus reaches about 37 weeks of gestation. Favorable results with ursodiol have been reported.

Acute fatty liver is a rare complication of pregnancy. Frequently confused with the HELLP syndrome (see "Preeclampsia" above) and severe preeclampsia, the diagnosis of acute fatty liver of pregnancy may be facilitated by imaging studies and laboratory evaluation. Acute fatty liver of pregnancy is generally characterized by markedly increased serum levels of bilirubin and ammonia and by hypoglycemia. Management of acute fatty liver of pregnancy is supportive; recurrence in subsequent pregnancies has been reported.

All pregnant women should be screened for hepatitis B. This information is important for pediatricians after delivery of the infant. All infants receive hepatitis B vaccine. Infants born to mothers who are carriers of hepatitis B surface antigen should also receive hepatitis B immune globulin as soon after birth as possible and preferably within the first 72 h. Screening for hepatitis C is recommended for individuals at high risk for exposure.

INFECTIONS

BACTERIAL INFECTIONS

Other than bacterial vaginosis, the most common bacterial infections during pregnancy involve the urinary tract (Chap. 162). Many pregnant women have asymptomatic bacteriuria, most likely due to stasis caused by progestational effects on ureteral and bladder smooth muscle and later in pregnancy due to compression effects of the enlarging uterus. In itself, this condition is not associated with an adverse outcome of pregnancy. However, if asymptomatic bacteriuria is left untreated, symptomatic pyelonephritis may occur. Indeed, ~75% of pregnancy-associated pyelonephritis cases are the result of untreated asymptomatic bacteriuria. All pregnant women should be screened with a urine culture for asymptomatic bacteriuria at the first prenatal visit. Subsequent screening with nitrite/leukocyte esterase strips is indicated for high-risk women, such as those with sickle cell trait or a history of urinary tract infections. All women with positive screens should be treated. Pregnant women who develop pyelonephritis need careful monitoring, including inpatient IV antibiotic administration due to the elevated risk of urosepsis and acute respiratory distress syndrome in pregnancy.

Abdominal pain and fever during pregnancy create a clinical dilemma. The diagnosis of greatest concern is intrauterine amniotic infection. While amniotic infection most commonly follows rupture of the membranes, this is not always the case. In general, antibiotic therapy is not recommended as a temporizing measure in these circumstances. If intrauterine infection is suspected, induced delivery with concomitant antibiotic therapy is generally indicated. Intrauterine amniotic infection is most often caused by pathogens such as *Escherichia coli* and group B *Streptococcus* (GBS). In high-risk patients at term or in preterm patients, routine intrapartum prophylaxis of GBS disease is recommended. Penicillin G and ampicillin are the drugs of choice. In penicillin-allergic patients with a low risk of anaphylaxis, cefazolin is recommended. If the patient is at high risk of anaphylaxis, vancomycin is recommended. If the organism is known to be sensitive to clindamycin, this antibiotic may be used. For the reduction of neonatal morbidity due to GBS, universal screening of pregnant women for GBS between 35 and 37 weeks of gestation, with intrapartum antibiotic treatment of infected women, is recommended.

Postpartum infection is a significant cause of maternal morbidity and mortality. Postpartum endomyometritis is more common after cesarean delivery than vaginal delivery and develops in 2% of women after elective repeat cesarean section and in up to 10% after emergency cesarean section following prolonged labor. To reduce the risk of endomyometritis, prophylactic antibiotics should be given to all patients undergoing cesarean section, and administration 30–60 min prior to skin incision is preferable to administration at the time of umbilical cord clamping. As most cases of postpartum endomyometritis are polymicrobial, broad-spectrum antibiotic coverage with a penicillin, an aminoglycoside, and metronidazole is recommended (Chap. 201). Most cases resolve within 72 h. Women who do not respond to antibiotic treatment for postpartum endomyometritis should be evaluated for septic pelvic thrombophlebitis. Imaging studies may be helpful in establishing the diagnosis, which is primarily a clinical diagnosis of exclusion. Patients with septic pelvic thrombophlebitis generally have tachycardia out of proportion to their fever and respond rapidly to IV administration of heparin.

All pregnant patients are screened prenatally for gonorrhea and chlamydial infections, and the detection of either should result in prompt treatment. Ceftriaxone and azithromycin are the agents of choice (Chaps. 181 and 213).

VIRAL INFECTIONS

Influenza (See also Chap. 224) Pregnant women with influenza are at increased risk of serious complications and death. All women who are pregnant or plan to become pregnant in the near future should receive inactivated influenza vaccine. The prompt initiation of antiviral treatment is recommended for pregnant women in whom influenza is suspected. Treatment can be reconsidered once the results of high-sensitivity tests are available. Prompt initiation of treatment lowers the risk of admission to an intensive care unit and death.

Cytomegalovirus Infection The most common cause of congenital viral infection in the United States is cytomegalovirus (CMV) (Chap. 219). As many as 50–90% of women of childbearing age have antibodies to CMV, but only rarely does CMV reactivation result in neonatal infection. More commonly, primary CMV infection during pregnancy creates a risk of congenital CMV. No currently accepted treatment of CMV infection during pregnancy has been demonstrated to protect the fetus effectively. Moreover, it is difficult to predict which fetus will sustain a life-threatening CMV infection. Severe CMV disease in the newborn is characterized most often by petechiae, hepatosplenomegaly, and jaundice. Chorioretinitis, microcephaly, intracranial calcifications, hepatitis, hemolytic anemia, and purpura may also develop. CNS involvement, resulting in the development of psychomotor, ocular, auditory, and dental abnormalities over time, has been described.

Rubella (See also Chap. 230e) Rubella virus is a known teratogen; first-trimester rubella carries a high risk of fetal anomalies, though the risk significantly decreases later in pregnancy. Congenital rubella may be diagnosed by percutaneous umbilical-blood sampling with the detection of IgM antibodies in fetal blood. All pregnant women and all women of childbearing age should be tested for their immune status to rubella. All nonpregnant women who are not immune to rubella should be vaccinated. The incidence of congenital rubella in the United States is extremely low.

Herpesvirus Infection (See also Chap. 216) The acquisition of genital herpes during pregnancy is associated with spontaneous abortion, prematurity, and congenital and neonatal herpes. A cohort study of pregnant women without evidence of previous herpesvirus infection demonstrated that ~2% acquired a new herpesvirus infection during the pregnancy. Approximately 60% of the newly infected women had no clinical symptoms. Infection occurred with equal frequency in all three trimesters. If herpesvirus seroconversion occurred early in pregnancy, the risk of transmission to the newborn was very low. In women who acquired genital herpes shortly before delivery, the risk of transmission was high. The risk of active genital herpes lesions at term can be reduced by prescribing acyclovir for the last 4 weeks of pregnancy to women who have had their first episode of genital herpes during the pregnancy.

Herpesvirus infection in the newborn can be devastating. Disseminated neonatal herpes carries with it high mortality and morbidity rates from CNS involvement. It is recommended that pregnant women with active genital herpes lesions at the time of presentation in labor be delivered by cesarean section.

Parvovirus Infection (See also Chap. 221) Parvovirus infection (caused by human parvovirus B19) may occur during pregnancy. It rarely causes sequelae, but susceptible women infected during pregnancy may be at risk for fetal hydrops secondary to erythroid aplasia and profound anemia.

HIV Infection (See also Chap. 226) The predominant cause of HIV infection in children is transmission of the virus from mother to newborn during the perinatal period. All pregnant women should be screened for HIV infection. Factors that increase the risk of mother-to-newborn transmission include high maternal viral load, low maternal CD4+ T cell count, prolonged labor, prolonged duration of membrane rupture, and the presence of other genital tract infections, such as syphilis or herpes. Prior to the widespread use of antiretroviral treatment, the perinatal transmission rate was in the range of 20%. In women with a good response to antiretroviral treatment, the transmission rate is about 1%. Measurement of maternal plasma HIV RNA copy number guides the decision for vaginal versus cesarean delivery. For women with <1000 copies of plasma HIV RNA/ml who are receiving combination antiretroviral therapy, the risk of transmission to the newborn is approximately 1% regardless of mode of delivery or duration of membrane rupture. These women may elect to attempt a vaginal birth following the spontaneous onset of labor. For women with a viral load of ≥1000 copies/ml prior to 38 weeks of gestation, a scheduled prelabor cesarean at 38 weeks is recommended to reduce the risk of HIV transmission to the newborn. To reduce the risk of mother-to-newborn transmission, women with >400 copies of HIV RNA/ml should be treated during the intrapartum interval with zidovudine. All newborns of HIV-infected mothers should be treated with zidovudine for 6 months after birth. Women who are HIV-positive may transmit the virus through their breast milk. In developed countries, HIV-infected mothers are advised not to breast-feed.

VACCINATIONS

(See also Chap. 148) For rubella-nonimmune individuals contemplating pregnancy, measles-mumps-rubella vaccine should be administered, ideally at least 3 months prior to conception but otherwise in the immediate postpartum period. In addition, pregnancy is not a contraindication for vaccination against influenza, tetanus, diphtheria, and pertussis (Tdap), and these vaccines are recommended for appropriate individuals.

MATERNAL MORTALITY

Maternal death is defined as death occurring during pregnancy or within 42 days of completion of pregnancy from a cause related to or aggravated by pregnancy, but not due to accident or incidental causes. From 1935 to 2007, the U.S. maternal death rate decreased from nearly 600/100,000 births to 12.7/100,000 births. There are significant health disparities in the maternal mortality rate, with the highest rates among non-Hispanic black women. In 2007, maternal mortality rates (per 100,000) by race were 10.5 among non-Hispanic white women, 8.9 among Hispanic women, and 28.4 among non-Hispanic black women. The most common causes of maternal death in the United States today are pulmonary embolism, obstetric hemorrhage, hypertension, sepsis, cardiovascular conditions (including peripartum cardiomyopathy), and ectopic pregnancy.

As stated above, the maternal mortality rate in the United States is about 12.7/100,00 births. In some countries in sub-Saharan Africa and southern Asia, the maternal mortality rate is about 500/100,000 live births. The most common cause of maternal death in these countries is maternal hemorrhage. The high maternal death rates are due in part to inadequate contraceptive and family-planning services, an insufficient number of skilled birth attendants, and difficulty in accessing birthing centers and emergency obstetrical care units. Maternal death is a global public-health tragedy that could be mitigated with the application of modest resources.

SUMMARY

With improved diagnostic and therapeutic modalities as well as advances in the treatment of infertility, more patients with medical complications will be seeking and will require complex obstetric care. Improved outcomes of pregnancy in these women will be best attained by a team of internists, maternal-fetal medicine (high-risk obstetrics) specialists, and anesthesiologists assembled to counsel these patients about the risks of pregnancy and to plan their treatment prior to conception. The importance of preconception counseling cannot be overstated. It is the responsibility of all physicians caring for women in the reproductive age group to assess their patients' reproductive plans as part of their overall health evaluation.

9 Medical Evaluation of the Surgical Patient

Wei C. Lau, Kim A. Eagle

Cardiovascular and pulmonary complications continue to account for major morbidity and mortality in patients undergoing noncardiac surgery. Emerging evidence-based practices dictate that the internist should perform an individualized evaluation of the surgical patient to provide an accurate preoperative risk assessment and stratification that will guide optimal perioperative risk-reduction strategies. This chapter reviews cardiovascular and pulmonary preoperative risk assessment, targeting intermediate- and high-risk patients with the goal of improving outcome. It also reviews perioperative management and prophylaxis of diabetes mellitus, endocarditis, and venous thromboembolism.

EVALUATION OF INTERMEDIATE- AND HIGH-RISK PATIENTS

Simple, standardized preoperative screening questionnaires, such as the one shown in Table 9-1, have been developed for the purpose of identifying patients at intermediate or high risk who may benefit from a more detailed clinical evaluation. Evaluation of such patients for surgery should always begin with a thorough history and physical examination and with a 12-lead resting electrocardiogram (ECG), in accordance with the American College of Cardiology/American Heart Association (ACC/AHA) guidelines. The history should focus on symptoms of occult cardiac or pulmonary disease. The urgency of the surgery should be determined, as true emergency procedures are associated with unavoidably higher morbidity and mortality risk. Preoperative laboratory testing should be carried out only for specific clinical conditions, as noted during clinical examination. Thus, healthy patients of any age who are undergoing elective surgical procedures without coexisting medical conditions should not require any testing unless the degree of surgical stress may result in unusual changes from the baseline state.

TABLE 9-1 STANDARDIZED PREOPERATIVE QUESTIONNAIRE[a]

1. Age, weight, height
2. Are you:
   Female and 55 years of age or older or male and 45 years of age of older?
   If yes, are you 70 years of age or older?
3. Do you take anticoagulant medications ("blood thinners")?
4. Do you have or have you had any of the following heart-related conditions?
   Heart disease
   Heart attack within the last 6 months
   Angina (chest pain)
   Irregular heartbeat
   Heart failure
5. Do you have or have you ever had any of the following?
   Rheumatoid arthritis
   Kidney disease
   Liver disease
   Diabetes
6. Do you get short of breath when you lie flat?
7. Are you currently on oxygen treatment?
8. Do you have a chronic cough that produces any discharge or fluid?
9. Do you have lung problems or diseases?
10. Have you or any blood member of your family ever had a problem other than nausea with any anesthesia?
    If yes, describe:
11. If female, is it possible that you are pregnant?
    Pregnancy test:
    Please list date of last menstrual period:

[a]University of Michigan Health System patient information report. Patients who answer yes to any of questions 2–9 should receive a more detailed clinical evaluation.

Source: Adapted from KK Tremper, P Benedict: Anesthesiology 92:1212, 2000; with permission.

PREOPERATIVE CARDIAC RISK ASSESSMENT

A stepwise approach to cardiac risk assessment and stratification in patients undergoing noncardiac surgery is illustrated in Fig. 9-1. Assessment of exercise tolerance in the prediction of in-hospital perioperative risk is most helpful in patients who self-report worsening exercise-induced cardiopulmonary symptoms; those who may benefit from noninvasive or invasive cardiac testing regardless of a scheduled surgical procedure; and those with known coronary artery disease (CAD) or with multiple risk factors who are able to exercise. For predicting perioperative events, poor exercise tolerance has been defined as the inability to walk four blocks or climb two flights of stairs at a normal pace or to meet a metabolic equivalent (MET) level of 4 (e.g., carrying objects of 15–20 lb or playing golf or doubles tennis) because of the development of dyspnea, angina, or excessive fatigue (Table 9-2).

Previous studies have compared several cardiac risk indices. The American College of Surgeons' National Surgical Quality Improvement

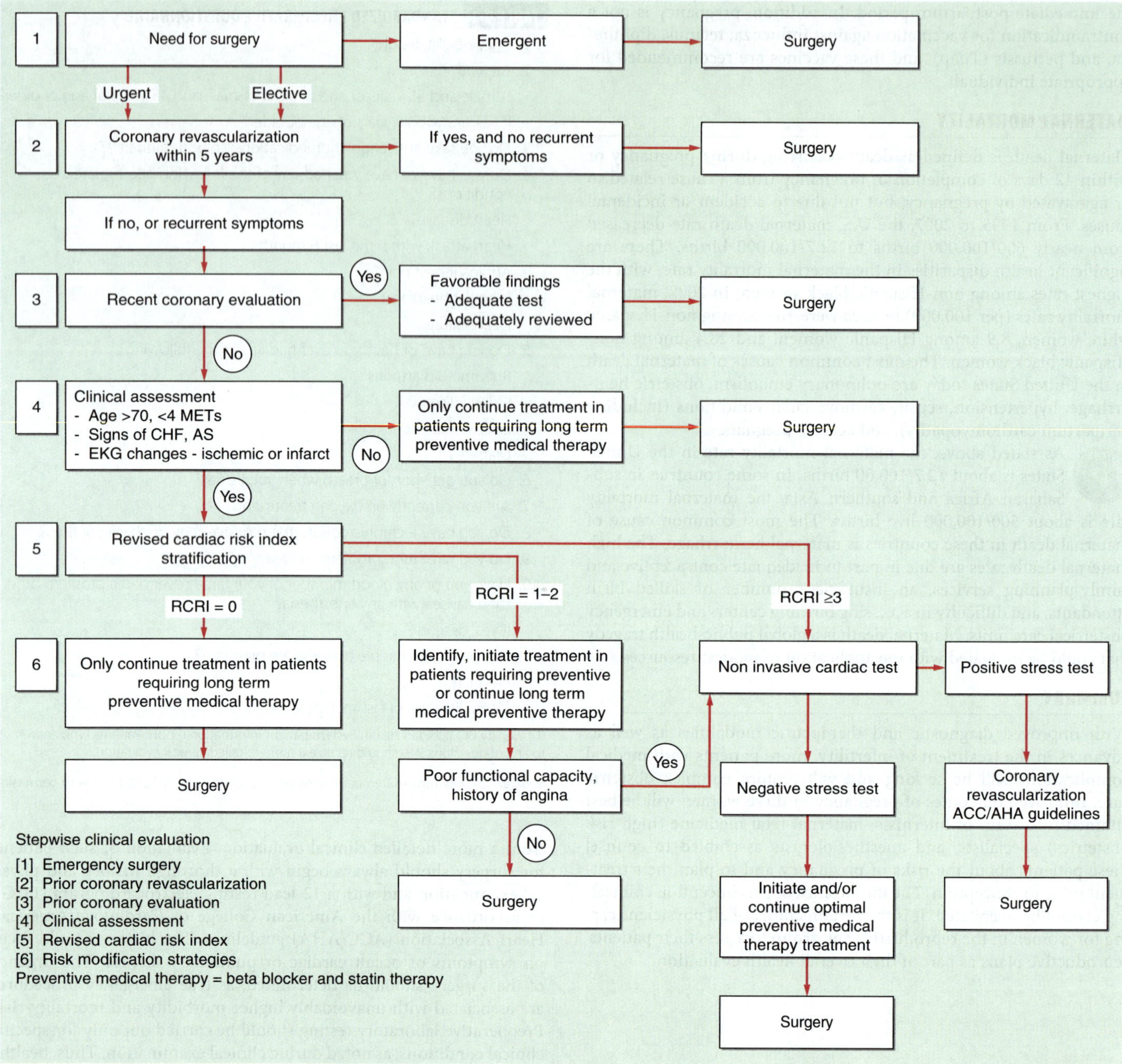

FIGURE 9-1 Composite algorithm for cardiac risk assessment and stratification in patients undergoing noncardiac surgery. Stepwise clinical evaluation: [1] emergency surgery; [2] prior coronary revascularization; [3] prior coronary evaluation; [4] clinical assessment; [5] RCRI; [6] risk modification strategies. Preventive medical therapy = beta blocker and statin therapy. RCRI, revised cardiac risk index. *(Adapted from LA Fleisher et al: Circulation 116:1971, 2007, with permission.)*

Program prospective database has identified five predictors of perioperative myocardial infarction (MI) and cardiac arrest based on increasing age, American Society of Anesthesiologists class, type of surgery, dependent functional status, and abnormal serum creatinine level. However, given its accuracy and simplicity, the revised cardiac risk

TABLE 9-2 ASSESSMENT OF CARDIAC RISK BY FUNCTIONAL STATUS

Risk	Higher	• Has difficulty with adult activities of daily living
		• Cannot walk four blocks or up two flights of stairs or does not meet a MET level of 4
		• Is inactive but has no limitations
		• Is active: easily does vigorous tasks
	Lower	• Performs regular vigorous exercises

Source: From LA Fleisher et al: Circulation 116:1971, 2007.

index (RCRI) (Table 9-3) is favored. The RCRI relies on the presence or absence of six identifiable predictive factors: high-risk surgery, ischemic heart disease, congestive heart failure, cerebrovascular disease, diabetes mellitus, and renal dysfunction. Each of these predictors is assigned one point. The risk of major cardiac events—defined as myocardial infarction, pulmonary edema, ventricular fibrillation or primary cardiac arrest, and complete heart block—can then be predicted. Based on the presence of none, one, two, three, or more of these clinical predictors, the rate of development of one of these four major cardiac events is estimated to be 0.4, 0.9, 7, and 11%, respectively (Fig. 9-2). An RCRI score of 0 signifies a 0.4–0.5% risk of cardiac events; RCRI 1, 0.9–1.3%; RCRI 2, 4–7%; and RCRI ≥3, 9–11%. The clinical utility of the RCRI is to identify patients with three or more predictors who are at very high risk (≥11%) for cardiac complications and who may benefit from further risk stratification with noninvasive cardiac testing or initiation of preoperative preventive medical management.

TABLE 9-3 CLINICAL MARKERS INCLUDED IN THE REVISED CARDIAC RISK INDEX

High-Risk Surgical Procedures
Vascular surgery
Major intraperitoneal or intrathoracic procedures
Ischemic Heart Disease
History of myocardial infarction
Current angina considered to be ischemic
Requirement for sublingual nitroglycerin
Positive exercise test
Pathological Q-waves on ECG
History of PCI and/or CABG with current angina considered to be ischemic
Congestive Heart Failure
Left ventricular failure by physical examination
History of paroxysmal nocturnal dyspnea
History of pulmonary edema
S_3 gallop on cardiac auscultation
Bilateral rales on pulmonary auscultation
Pulmonary edema on chest x-ray
Cerebrovascular Disease
History of transient ischemic attack
History of cerebrovascular accident
Diabetes Mellitus
Treatment with insulin
Chronic Renal Insufficiency
Serum creatinine >2 mg/dL

Abbreviations: CABG, coronary artery bypass grafting; ECG, electrocardiogram; PCI, percutaneous coronary interventions.

Source: Adapted from TH Lee et al: Circulation 100:1043, 1999.

PREOPERATIVE NONINVASIVE CARDIAC TESTING FOR RISK STRATIFICATION

There is little evidence to support widespread application of preoperative noninvasive cardiac testing for all patients undergoing major surgery. Rather, a discriminative approach based on clinical risk categorization appears to be both clinically useful and cost-effective. There is potential benefit in identifying asymptomatic but high-risk patients, such as those with left main or left main–equivalent CAD or those with three-vessel CAD and poor left ventricular function, who may benefit from coronary revascularization (Chap. 293). However, evidence does not support aggressive attempts to identify patients at intermediate risk who have asymptomatic but advanced coronary artery disease, in whom coronary revascularization appears to offer little advantage over medical therapy.

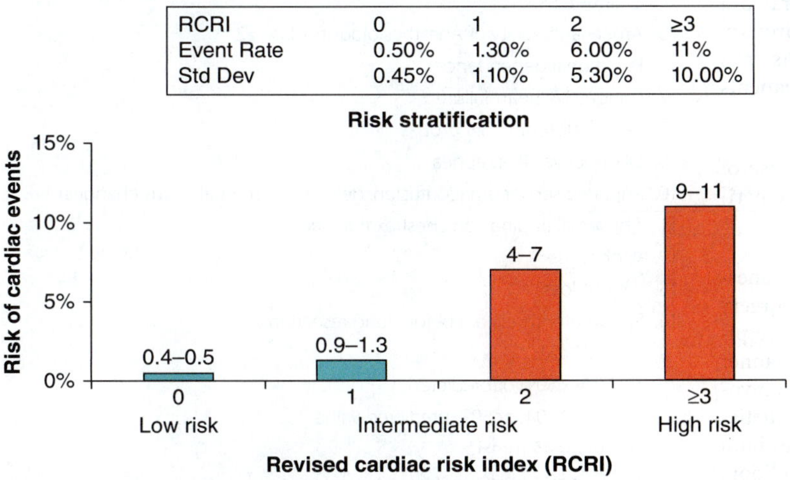

FIGURE 9-2 Risk stratification based on the RCRI: derivation and prospective validation of a simple index for prediction of cardiac risk in patients undergoing major noncardiac surgery. Cardiac events include myocardial infarction, pulmonary edema, ventricular fibrillation, cardiac asystole, and complete heart block. *(Adapted from TH Lee et al: Circulation 100:1043, 1999.)*

An RCRI score ≥3 in patients with severe myocardial ischemia on stress testing should lead to consideration of coronary revascularization prior to noncardiac surgery. Noninvasive cardiac testing is most appropriate if it is anticipated that, in the event of a strongly positive test, a patient will meet guidelines for coronary angiography and coronary revascularization. Pharmacologic stress tests are more useful than exercise testing in patients with functional limitations. Dobutamine echocardiography and persantine, adenosine, or dobutamine nuclear perfusion testing (Chap. 270e) have excellent negative predictive values (near 100%) but poor positive predictive values (<20%) in the identification of patients at risk for perioperative MI or death. Thus, a negative study is reassuring, but a positive study is a relatively weak predictor of a "hard" perioperative cardiac event.

RISK MODIFICATION: PREVENTIVE STRATEGIES TO REDUCE CARDIAC RISK

Perioperative Coronary Revascularization Currently, potential options for reducing perioperative cardiovascular risk include coronary artery revascularization and/or perioperative preventive medical therapies (Chap. 293). *Prophylactic* coronary revascularization with either coronary artery bypass grafting (CABG) or percutaneous coronary intervention (PCI) provides no short- or midterm survival benefit for patients *without* left main CAD or three-vessel CAD in the presence of poor left ventricular systolic function and is *not recommended* for patients with stable CAD before noncardiac surgery. Although PCI is associated with lower procedural risk than is CABG in the perioperative setting, the placement of a coronary artery stent soon before noncardiac surgery may increase the risk of bleeding during surgery if dual antiplatelet therapy (aspirin and thienopyridine) is administered; moreover, stent placement shortly before noncardiac surgery increases the perioperative risk of MI and cardiac death due to stent thrombosis if such therapy is withdrawn prematurely (Chap. 296e). It is recommended that, if possible, noncardiac surgery be delayed 30–45 days after placement of a bare metal coronary stent and for 365 days after a drug-eluting stent. For patients who *must* undergo noncardiac surgery early (>14 days) after PCI, balloon angioplasty without stent placement appears to be a reasonable alternative because dual antiplatelet therapy is not necessary in such patients. One recent clinical trial further suggests that after 6 months, bare metal and drug eluting stents may not pose a threat.

PERIOPERATIVE PREVENTIVE MEDICAL THERAPIES The goal of perioperative preventive medical therapies with β-adrenergic antagonists, HMG-CoA reductase inhibitors (statins), antiplatelet agents, and α_2 agonists is to reduce perioperative adrenergic stimulation, ischemia, and inflammation, which are triggered during the perioperative period.

β-ADRENERGIC ANTAGONISTS The use of perioperative beta blockade should be based on a thorough assessment of a patient's perioperative clinical and surgery-specific cardiac risk (RCRI ≥2). For patients with or without mild to moderate reactive airway disease, the cardioselective beta blocker of choice should be used and titrated to maintain a target heart rate of 60–80 beats/min in the absence of hypotension in the operative and perioperative period. In RCRI ≥2 patients without a long-term indication for beta blockers, the medications can be administered IV as a preoperative medication on the day of surgery, with a targeted heart rate of 60–80 beats/min without hypotension, and continued for >7 days (preferably 30 days) postoperatively. Abrupt perioperative beta blocker withdrawal should be avoided unless necessary because of the associated increase in risk of MI and angina. IV preparations should be substituted for oral medications if patients are unable to swallow or absorb pills in the perioperative period. The results from the Perioperative Ischemic Evaluation (POISE) trial showed that, although cardiac death, nonfatal myocardial infarction, or cardiac arrest was reduced among patients who received metoprolol rather than placebo, there was an increased incidence of death and stroke among metoprolol recipients because of a high and rapidly loading dose of this drug.

The POISE trial highlights the importance of a clear risk-and-benefit assessment, with careful initiation and titration to therapeutic efficacy of preoperative beta blockers in patients undergoing noncardiac surgery. A recent meta-analysis which included the POISE study further supports that excessive beta blocker dosing is, in fact, harmful.

The ACC/AHA guidelines recommend the following: (1) Beta blockers *should be continued* in patients with active cardiac conditions who are undergoing surgery and are receiving beta blockers. (2) Beta blockers titrated to heart rate and blood pressure are *probably recommended* for patients undergoing vascular surgery who are at high cardiac risk defined by CAD or cardiac ischemia on preoperative testing. (3) Beta blockers are *reasonable* for high-risk patients (RCRI ≥2) who undergo vascular surgery. (4) Beta blockers are *reasonable* for patients with known CAD or high risk (RCRI ≥2) who undergo intermediate-risk surgery. (5) Nondiscriminant administration of high-dose beta blockers without dose titration to effectiveness is *contraindicated* for patients who have never been treated with a beta blocker.

HMG-CoA REDUCTASE INHIBITORS (STATINS) A number of prospective and retrospective studies support the perioperative prophylactic use of statins for reduction of cardiac complications in patients with established atherosclerosis. The ACC/AHA Guidelines support the protective efficacy of perioperative statins on cardiac complications in intermediate risk patients undergoing major noncardiac surgery. For patients undergoing noncardiac surgery and currently taking statins, statin therapy *should be continued* to reduce perioperative cardiac risk. Statins are *reasonable* for patients undergoing vascular surgery with or without clinical risk factors (RCRI ≥1).

ANGIOTENSIN-CONVERTING ENZYME (ACE) INHIBITORS Evidence supports the discontinuation of ACE inhibitors and angiotensin receptor blockers for 24 h prior to noncardiac surgery due to adverse circulatory effects after induction of anesthesia.

ORAL ANTIPLATELET AGENTS Evidence-based recommendations regarding perioperative use of aspirin and/or thienopyridine to reduce cardiac risk currently lack clarity. A substantial increase in perioperative bleeding and in the need for transfusion in patients receiving dual antiplatelet therapy has been observed. The discontinuation of thienopyridine and aspirin for 5–7 days prior to major surgery to minimize the risk of perioperative bleeding and transfusion must be balanced with the potential increased risk of an acute coronary syndrome and of subacute stent thrombosis in patients with recent coronary stent implantation. If clinicians elect to withhold antiplatelet agents prior to surgery, these agents should be restarted as soon as possible postoperatively.

α_2 AGONISTS Several prospective and retrospective meta-analyses of perioperative α_2 agonists (clonidine and mivazerol) demonstrated a reduction of cardiac death rates among patients with known coronary artery disease who underwent noncardiac surgery. α_2 agonists thus *may be considered* for perioperative control of hypertension in patients with known coronary artery disease or an RCRI score ≥2.

CALCIUM CHANNEL BLOCKERS Evidence is lacking to support the use of calcium channel blockers as a prophylactic strategy to decrease perioperative risk in major noncardiac surgery.

ANESTHETICS Mortality risk is low with safe delivery of modern anesthesia, especially among low-risk patients undergoing low-risk surgery (Table 9-4). Inhaled anesthetics have predictable circulatory and respiratory effects: all decrease arterial pressure in a dose-dependent manner by reducing sympathetic tone and causing systemic vasodilation, myocardial depression, and decreased cardiac output. Inhaled anesthetics also cause respiratory depression, with diminished responses to both hypercapnia and hypoxemia, in a dose-dependent manner; in addition, these agents have a variable effect on heart rate. Prolonged residual neuromuscular blockade also increases the risk of postoperative pulmonary complications due to reduction in functional residual lung capacity, loss of diaphragmatic and intercostal muscle function, atelectasis, and arterial hypoxemia from ventilation-perfusion mismatch.

TABLE 9-4 GRADATION OF MORTALITY RISK OF COMMON NONCARDIAC SURGICAL PROCEDURES

Higher	• Emergent major operations, especially in the elderly • Aortic and other noncarotid major vascular surgery (endovascular and nonendovascular) • Prolonged surgery associated with large fluid shift and/or blood loss
Intermediate	• Major thoracic surgery • Major abdominal surgery • Carotid endarterectomy surgery • Head/neck surgery • Orthopedic surgery • Prostate surgery
Lower	• Eye, skin, and superficial surgery • Endoscopic procedures

Source: From LA Fleisher et al: Circulation 116:1971, 2007, with permission.

Several meta-analyses have shown that rates of pneumonia and respiratory failure are lower among patients receiving neuroaxial anesthesia (epidural or spinal) rather than general anesthesia (inhaled). However, there were no significant differences in cardiac events between the two approaches. Evidence from a meta-analysis of randomized controlled trials supports postoperative epidural analgesia for >24 h for the purpose of pain relief. However, the risk of epidural hematoma in the setting of systemic anticoagulation for venous thromboembolism prophylaxis (see below) and postoperative epidural catheterization must be considered.

PREOPERATIVE PULMONARY RISK ASSESSMENT

Perioperative pulmonary complications occur frequently and lead to significant morbidity and mortality. The guidelines from the American College of Physicians recommend the following:

1. All patients undergoing noncardiac surgery should be assessed for risk of pulmonary complications (Table 9-5).
2. Patients undergoing emergency or prolonged (3- to 4-h) surgery; aortic aneurysm repair; vascular surgery; major abdominal, thoracic, neurologic, head, or neck surgery; and general anesthesia

TABLE 9-5 PREDISPOSING RISK FACTORS FOR PULMONARY COMPLICATIONS

1. Upper respiratory tract infection: cough, dyspnea
2. Age >60 years
3. Chronic obstructive pulmonary disease
4. Cigarette use
5. American Society of Anesthesiologists Class ≥2
6. Functional dependence
7. Congestive heart failure
8. Serum albumin <3.5 g/dL
9. Obstructive sleep apnea
10. Impaired sensorium (confusion, delirium, or mental status changes)
11. Abnormal findings on chest examination
12. Alcohol use
13. Weight loss
14. Spirometry threshold before lung resection
    a. FEV_1 <2 L
    b. MVV <50% of predicted
    c. PEF <100 L or 50% predicted value
    d. PCO_2 ≥45 mmHg
    e. PO_2 ≤50 mmHg

Abbreviations: FEV_1, forced expiratory volume in 1 s; MVV, maximal voluntary ventilation; PEF, peak expiratory flow rate; PCO_2, partial pressure of carbon dioxide; PO_2, partial pressure of oxygen.

Source: A Qaseem et al: Ann Intern Med 144:575-80. Modified from GW Smetana et al: Ann Intern Med 144:581, 2006, and from DN Mohr et al: Postgrad Med 100:247, 1996.

TABLE 9-6 RISK MODIFICATION TO REDUCE PERIOPERATIVE PULMONARY COMPLICATIONS
Preoperatively
• Cessation of smoking for at least 8 weeks before and until at least 10 days after surgery
• Training in proper lung expansion techniques
• Inhalation bronchodilator and/or steroid therapy, when indicated
• Control of infection and secretion, when indicated
• Weight reduction, when appropriate
Intraoperatively
• Limited duration of anesthesia
• Avoidance of long-acting neuromuscular blocking drugs, when indicated
• Prevention of aspiration and maintenance of optimal bronchodilation
Postoperatively
• Optimization of inspiratory capacity maneuvers, with attention to:
Mobilization of secretions
Early ambulation
Encouragement of coughing
Selective use of a nasogastric tube
Adequate pain control without excessive narcotics

Source: From VA Lawrence et al: Ann Intern Med 144:596, 2006, and WF Dunn, PD Scanlon: Mayo Clin Proc 68:371, 1993.

should be considered to be at elevated risk for postoperative pulmonary complications.

3. Patients at higher risk of pulmonary complications should undergo incentive spirometry, deep-breathing exercises, cough encouragement, postural drainage, percussion and vibration, suctioning and ambulation, intermittent positive-pressure breathing, continuous positive airway pressure, and selective use of a nasogastric tube for postoperative nausea, vomiting, or symptomatic abdominal distention to reduce postoperative risk (Table 9-6).
4. Routine preoperative spirometry and chest radiography should not be used routinely for predicting risk of postoperative pulmonary complications but may be appropriate for patients with chronic obstructive pulmonary disease or asthma.
5. Spirometry is of value before lung resection in determining candidacy for coronary artery bypass; however, it does not provide a spirometric threshold for extrathoracic surgery below which the risks of surgery are unacceptable.
6. Pulmonary artery catheterization, administration of total parenteral nutrition (as opposed to no supplementation), or total enteral nutrition has no benefit in reducing postoperative pulmonary complications.

PERIOPERATIVE MANAGEMENT AND PROPHYLAXIS

DIABETES MELLITUS

(See also Chaps. 417–419) Many patients with diabetes mellitus have significant symptomatic or asymptomatic CAD and may have silent myocardial ischemia due to autonomic dysfunction. Evidence supports intensive perioperative glycemic control to achieve near-normal glucose levels (90–110 mg/dL) rather than moderate glycemic control (120–200 mg/dL), using insulin infusion. This practice must be balanced against the risk of hypoglycemic complications. Oral hypoglycemic agonists should not be given on the morning of surgery. Perioperative hyperglycemia should be treated with IV infusion of short-acting insulin or SC sliding-scale insulin. Patients whose diabetes is diet controlled may proceed to surgery with close postoperative monitoring.

INFECTIVE ENDOCARDITIS

(See also Chap. 155) Perioperative prophylactic antibiotics should be administered to patients with congenital or valvular heart disease, prosthetic valves, mitral valve prolapse, or other cardiac abnormalities, in accordance with ACC/AHA practice guidelines.

VENOUS THROMBOEMBOLISM

(See also Chap. 300) Perioperative prophylaxis of venous thromboembolism should follow established guidelines of the American College of Chest Physicians. Aspirin is not supported as a single agent for thromboprophylaxis. Low-dose unfractionated heparin (≤5000 units SC bid), low-molecular weight heparin (e.g., enoxaparin, 30 mg bid or 40 mg qd), or a pentasaccharide (fondaparinux, 2.5 mg qd) is appropriate for patients at moderate risk; unfractionated heparin (5000 units SC tid) is appropriate for patients at high risk. Graduated compression stockings and pneumatic compression devices are useful supplements to anticoagulant therapy.

10 Palliative and End-of-Life Care

Ezekiel J. Emanuel

EPIDEMIOLOGY

In 2010, according to the Centers for Disease Control and Prevention, 2,468,435 individuals died in the United States (Table 10-1). Approximately 73% of all deaths occur in those >65 years of age. The epidemiology of mortality is similar in most developed countries; cardiovascular diseases and cancer are the predominant causes of death, a marked change since 1900, when heart disease caused ~8% of all deaths and cancer accounted for <4% of all deaths. In 2010, the year with the most recent available data, AIDS did not rank among the top 15 causes of death, causing just 8369 deaths. Even among people age 35–44, heart disease, cancer, chronic liver disease, and accidents all cause more deaths than AIDS.

It is estimated that in developed countries ~70% of all deaths are preceded by a disease or condition, making it reasonable to plan for dying in the foreseeable future. Cancer has served as the paradigm for terminal care, but it is not the only type of illness with a recognizable and predictable terminal phase. Because heart failure, chronic obstructive pulmonary disease (COPD), chronic liver failure, dementia, and many other conditions have recognizable terminal phases, a systematic approach to end-of-life care should be part of all medical specialties. Many patients with illness-related suffering also can benefit from palliative care regardless of prognosis. Ideally, palliative care should be considered part of comprehensive care for all patients. Palliative care can be improved by coordination between caregivers, doctors, and patients for advance care planning, as well as dedicated teams of physicians, nurses, and other providers.

The rapid increases in life expectancy in developed countries over the last century have been accompanied by new difficulties facing individuals, families, and society as a whole in addressing the needs of an aging population. These challenges include both more complicated conditions and technologies to address them at the end of life. The development of technologies that can prolong life without restoring full health has led many Americans to seek out alternative end-of-life care settings and approaches that relieve suffering for those with terminal diseases. Over the last few decades in the United States, a significant change in the site of death has occurred that coincides with patient and family preferences. Nearly 60% of Americans died as inpatients in hospitals in 1980. By 2000, the trend was reversing, with ~31% of Americans dying as hospital inpatients (Fig. 10-1). This shift has been most dramatic for those dying from cancer and COPD and for younger and very old individuals. In the last decade, it has been associated with the increased use of hospice care; in 2008, approximately 39% of all decedents in the United States received such care. Cancer patients currently constitute ~36.9% of hospice users. About 79% of patients receiving hospice care die out of the hospital, and around 42% of those receiving hospice care die in a private residence. In addition, in 2008, for the first time, the American Board of Medical Specialties (ABMS) offered certification in hospice and palliative medicine. With shortening of hospital stays,

TABLE 10-1 TEN LEADING CAUSES OF DEATH IN THE UNITED STATES AND BRITAIN

	United States			Britain	
Cause of Death	Number of Deaths	Percentage of Total	Number of Deaths Among People ≥65 Years of Age	Number of Deaths	Percentage of Total
All deaths	2,468,435	100	1,798,276	499,331	100
Heart disease	597,689	24.2	477,338	141,362	28.3
Malignant neoplasms	574,743	23.3	396,670	142,107	28.5
Chronic lower respiratory diseases	138,080	5.6	118,031	27,132	5.4
Cerebrovascular diseases	129,476	5.2	109,990	35,846	7.2
Accidents	120,859	4.9	41,300	11,256	2.3
Alzheimer's disease	83,494	3.4	82,616	8859	1.8
Diabetes mellitus	69,071	2.8	49,191	4931	1.0
Nephritis, nephritic syndrome, nephrosis	50,476	2.0	41,994	4102	0.8
Influenza and pneumonia	50,097	2.0	42,846	26,138	5.2
Intentional self-harm	38,364	1.6	6008	3671	0.7

Source: National Center for Health Statistics (data for all age groups from 2010), *http://www.cdc.gov/nchs*; National Statistics (England and Wales, 2012), *http://www.statistics.gov.uk*.

many serious conditions are being treated at home or on an outpatient basis. Consequently, providing optimal palliative and end-of-life care requires ensuring that appropriate services are available in a variety of settings, including noninstitutional settings.

HOSPICE AND THE PALLIATIVE CARE FRAMEWORK

Central to this type of care is an interdisciplinary team approach that typically encompasses pain and symptom management, spiritual and psychological care for the patient, and support for family caregivers during the patient's illness and the bereavement period.

Terminally ill patients have a wide variety of advanced diseases, often with multiple symptoms that demand relief, and require noninvasive therapeutic regimens to be delivered in flexible care settings. Fundamental to ensuring quality palliative and end-of-life care is a focus on four broad domains: (1) physical symptoms; (2) psychological symptoms; (3) social needs that include interpersonal relationships, caregiving, and economic concerns; and (4) existential or spiritual needs.

A comprehensive assessment screens for and evaluates needs in each of these four domains. Goals for care are established in discussions with the patient and/or family, based on the assessment in each of the domains. Interventions then are aimed at improving or managing symptoms and needs. Although physicians are responsible

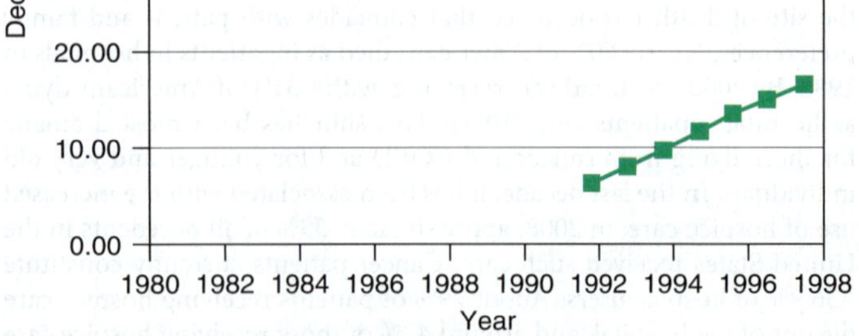

FIGURE 10-1 Graph showing trends in the site of death in the last two decades. ◆, percentage of hospital inpatient deaths; ■, percentage of decedents enrolled in a hospice.

for certain interventions, especially technical ones, and for coordinating the interventions, they cannot be responsible for providing all of them. Because failing to address any one of the domains is likely to preclude a good death, a well-coordinated, effectively communicating interdisciplinary team takes on special importance in end-of-life care. Depending on the setting, critical members of the interdisciplinary team will include physicians, nurses, social workers, chaplains, nurse's aides, physical therapists, bereavement counselors, and volunteers.

ASSESSMENT AND CARE PLANNING

Comprehensive Assessment Standardized methods for conducting a comprehensive assessment focus on evaluating the patient's condition in all four domains affected by illness: physical, psychological, social, and spiritual. The assessment of physical and mental symptoms should follow a modified version of the traditional medical history and physical examination that emphasizes symptoms. Questions should aim at elucidating symptoms and discerning sources of suffering and gauging how much those symptoms interfere with the patient's quality of life. Standardized assessment is critical. Currently, there are 21 symptom assessment instruments for cancer alone. Further research on and validation of these assessment tools, especially taking into account patient perspectives, could improve their effectiveness. Instruments with good psychometric properties that assess a wide range of symptoms include the Memorial Symptom Assessment Scale (MSAS), the Rotterdam Symptom Checklist, the Worthing Chemotherapy Questionnaire, and the Computerized Symptom Assessment Instrument. These instruments are long and may be useful for initial clinical or for research assessments. Shorter instruments are useful for patients whose performance status does not permit comprehensive assessments. Suitable shorter instruments include the Condensed Memorial Symptom Assessment Scale, the Edmonton Symptom Assessment System, the M.D. Anderson Symptom Assessment Inventory, and the Symptom Distress Scale. Using such instruments ensures that the assessment is comprehensive and does not focus only on pain and a few other physical symptoms. Invasive tests are best avoided in end-of-life care, and even minimally invasive tests should be evaluated carefully for their benefit-to-burden ratio for the patient. Aspects of the physical examination that are uncomfortable and unlikely to yield useful information can be omitted.

Regarding social needs, health care providers should assess the status of important relationships, financial burdens, caregiving needs, and access to medical care. Relevant questions will include the following: *How often is there someone to feel close to? How has this illness been for your family? How has it affected your relationships? How much help do you need with things like getting meals and getting around? How much trouble do you have getting the medical care you need?* In the area of existential needs, providers should assess distress and the patient's sense of being emotionally and existentially settled and of finding purpose or meaning. Helpful assessment questions can include the following: *How much are you able to find meaning since your illness began? What things are most important to you at this stage?* In addition, it can be helpful to ask how the patient perceives his or her care: *How much do you feel your doctors and nurses respect you? How clear is the information from us about what to expect regarding your illness? How much do you feel that the medical care you are getting fits with your goals?* If concern is detected in any of these areas, deeper evaluative questions are warranted.

Communication Especially when an illness is life-threatening, there are many emotionally charged and potentially conflict-creating moments, collectively called "bad news" situations, in which empathic and effective communication skills are essential. Those moments include communicating with the patient and/or family about a terminal diagnosis, the patient's prognosis, any treatment failures, deemphasizing efforts to cure and prolong life while focusing more on symptom management and palliation, advance care planning, and the patient's death. Although these conversations can be difficult and lead to tension, research indicates that end-of-life discussions can lead to earlier hospice referrals rather than overly aggressive treatment, benefiting quality of life for patients and improving the bereavement process for families.

Just as surgeons plan and prepare for major operations and investigators rehearse a presentation of research results, physicians and health care providers caring for patients with significant or advanced illness can develop a practiced approach to sharing important information and planning interventions. In addition, families identify as important both how well the physician was prepared to deliver bad news and the setting in which it was delivered. For instance, 27% of families making critical decisions for patients in an intensive care unit (ICU) desired better and more private physical space to communicate with physicians, and 48% found having clergy present reassuring.

An organized and effective seven-step procedure for communicating bad news goes by the acronym P-SPIKES: (1) ***p***repare for the discussion, (2) ***s***et up a suitable environment, (3) begin the discussion by finding out what the ***p***atient and/or family understand, (4) determine how they will comprehend new ***i***nformation best and how much they want to know, (5) provide needed new ***k***nowledge accordingly, (6) allow for ***e***motional responses, and (7) ***s***hare plans for the next steps in care. Table 10-2 provides a summary of these steps along with

TABLE 10-2 ELEMENTS OF COMMUNICATING BAD NEWS—THE P-SPIKES APPROACH

Acronym	Steps	Aim of the Interaction	Preparations, Questions, or Phrases
P	Preparation	Mentally prepare for the interaction with the patient and/or family.	Review what information needs to be communicated. Plan how you will provide emotional support. Rehearse key steps and phrases in the interaction.
S	Setting of the interaction	Ensure the appropriate setting for a serious and potentially emotionally charged discussion.	Ensure that patient, family, and appropriate social supports are present. Devote sufficient time. Ensure privacy and prevent interruptions by people or beeper. Bring a box of tissues.
P	Patient's perception and preparation	Begin the discussion by establishing the baseline and whether the patient and family can grasp the information. Ease tension by having the patient and family contribute.	Start with open-ended questions to encourage participation. Possible phrases to use: *What do you understand about your illness?* *When you first had symptom X, what did you think it might be?* *What did Dr. X tell you when he or she sent you here?* *What do you think is going to happen?*
I	Invitation and information needs	Discover what information needs the patient and/or family have and what limits they want regarding the bad information.	Possible phrases to use: *If this condition turns out to be something serious, do you want to know?* *Would you like me to tell you all the details of your condition? If not, who would you like me to talk to?*
K	Knowledge of the condition	Provide the bad news or other information to the patient and/or family sensitively.	Do not just dump the information on the patient and family. Check for patient and family understanding. Possible phrases to use: *I feel badly to have to tell you this, but . . .* *Unfortunately, the tests showed . . .* *I'm afraid the news is not good . . .*
E	Empathy and exploration	Identify the cause of the emotions—e.g., poor prognosis. Empathize with the patient and/or family's feelings. Explore by asking open-ended questions.	Strong feelings in reaction to bad news are normal. Acknowledge what the patient and family are feeling. Remind them such feelings are normal, even if frightening. Give them time to respond. Remind patient and family you won't abandon them. Possible phrases to use: *I imagine this is very hard for you to hear.* *You look very upset. Tell me how you are feeling.* *I wish the news were different.* *We'll do whatever we can to help you.*
S	Summary and planning	Delineate for the patient and the family the next steps, including additional tests or interventions.	It is the unknown and uncertain that can increase anxiety. Recommend a schedule with goals and landmarks. Provide your rationale for the patient and/or family to accept (or reject). If the patient and/or family are not ready to discuss the next steps, schedule a follow-up visit.

Source: Adapted from R Buckman: *How to Break Bad News: A Guide for Health Care Professionals.* Baltimore, Johns Hopkins University Press, 1992.

suggested phrases and underlying rationales for each one. Additional research that further considers the response of patients to systematic methods of delivering bad news could build the evidence base for even more effective communication procedures.

Continuous Goal Assessment Major barriers to ensuring quality palliative and end-of-life care include difficulty providing an accurate prognosis and emotional resistance of patients and their families to accepting the implications of a poor prognosis. There are two practical solutions to these barriers. One is to integrate palliative care with curative care regardless of prognosis. With this approach, palliative care no longer conveys the message of failure, having no more treatments, or "giving up hope." Fundamental to integrating palliative care with curative therapy is to include continuous goal assessment as part of the routine patient reassessment that occurs at most patient-physician encounters. Alternatively, some practices may find it useful to implement a standard point in the clinical course to address goals of care and advance care planning. For example, some oncology practices ask all patients whose Eastern Cooperative Oncology Group (ECOG) performance status is 3 or less—meaning they spend 50% or more of the day in bed—or those who develop metastatic disease about their goals of care and advance care preferences.

Goals for care are numerous, ranging from cure of a specific disease, to prolonging life, to relief of a symptom, to delaying the course of an incurable disease, to adapting to progressive disability without disrupting the family, to finding peace of mind or personal meaning, to dying in a manner that leaves loved ones with positive memories. Discernment of goals for care can be approached through a seven-step protocol: (1) ensure that medical and other information is as complete as reasonably possible and is understood by all relevant parties (see above); (2) explore what the patient and/or family are hoping for while identifying relevant and realistic goals; (3) share all the options with the patient and family; (4) respond with empathy as they adjust to changing expectations; (5) make a plan, emphasizing what can be done toward achieving the realistic goals; (6) follow through with the plan; and (7) review and revise the plan periodically, considering at every encounter whether the goals of care should be reviewed with the patient and/or family. Each of these steps need not be followed in rote order, but together they provide a helpful framework for interactions with patients and their families about goals for care. It can be especially challenging if a patient or family member has difficulty letting go of an unrealistic goal. One strategy is to help them refocus on more realistic goals and also suggest that while hoping for the best, it is still prudent to plan for other outcomes as well.

Advance Care Planning • ***PRACTICES*** Advance care planning is a process of planning for future medical care in case the patient becomes incapable of making medical decisions. A 2010 study of adults 60 or older who died between 2000 and 2006 found that 42% required decision making about treatment in the final days of life but 70% lacked decision-making capacity. Among those lacking decision-making capacity, around one-third did not have advance planning directives. Ideally, such planning would occur before a health care crisis or the terminal phase of an illness. Diverse barriers prevent this. Polls suggest 80% of Americans endorse advance care planning and completing living wills. However, data suggest between 33 and 42% have actually completed one. Other countries have even lower completion rates. Most patients expect physicians to initiate advance care planning and will wait for physicians to broach the subject. Patients also wish to discuss advance care planning with their families. Yet patients with unrealistic expectations are significantly more likely to prefer aggressive treatments. Fewer than one-third of health care providers have completed advance care planning for themselves. Hence, a good first step is for health care providers to complete their own advance care planning. This makes providers aware of the critical choices in the process and the issues that are especially charged and allows them to tell their patients truthfully that they personally have done advance planning. Lessons from behavioral economics suggest that setting this kind of social norming helps people view completing an advance directive as acceptable and even expected.

Steps in effective advance care planning center on (1) introducing the topic, (2) structuring a discussion, (3) reviewing plans that have been discussed by the patient and family, (4) documenting the plans, (5) updating them periodically, and (6) implementing the advance care directives (Table 10-3). Two of the main barriers to advance care planning are problems in raising the topic and difficulty in structuring a succinct discussion. Raising the topic can be done efficiently as a routine matter, noting that it is recommended for all patients, analogous to purchasing insurance or estate planning. Many of the most difficult cases have involved unexpected, acute episodes of brain damage in young individuals.

Structuring a focused discussion is a central communication skill. Identify the health care proxy and recommend his or her involvement in the process of advance care planning. Select a worksheet, preferably one that has been evaluated and demonstrated to produce reliable and valid expressions of patient preferences, and orient the patient and proxy to it. Such worksheets exist for both general and disease-specific situations. Discuss with the patient and proxy one scenario as an example to demonstrate how to think about the issues. It is often helpful to begin with a scenario in which the patient is likely to have settled preferences for care, such as being in a persistent vegetative state. Once the patient's preferences for interventions in this scenario are determined, suggest that the patient and proxy discuss and complete the worksheet for the others. If appropriate, suggest that they involve other family members in the discussion. On a return visit, go over the patient's preferences, checking and resolving any inconsistencies. After having the patient and proxy sign the document, place it in the medical chart and be sure that copies are provided to relevant family members and care sites. Because patients' preferences can change, these documents have to be reviewed periodically.

TYPES OF DOCUMENTS Advance care planning documents are of three broad types. The first includes living wills or instructional directives; these are advisory documents that describe the types of decisions that should direct care. Some are more specific, delineating different scenarios and interventions for the patient to choose from. Among these, some are for general use and others are designed for use by patients with a specific type of disease, such as cancer or HIV. A second type is a less specific directive that provides general statements of not wanting life-sustaining interventions or forms that describe the values that should guide specific discussions about terminal care. These can be problematic because, when critical decisions about specific treatments are needed, they require assessments by people other than the patient of whether a treatment fulfills a particular wish. The third type of advance directive allows the designation of a health care proxy (sometimes also referred to as a durable attorney for health care), who is an individual selected by the patient to make decisions. The choice is not either/or; a combined directive that includes a living will and designates a proxy is often used, and the directive should indicate clearly whether the specified patient preferences or the proxy's choice takes precedence if they conflict. The Five Wishes and the Medical Directive are such combined forms. Some states have begun to put into practice a "Physician Orders for Life-Sustaining Treatment (POLST)" paradigm, which builds on communication between providers and patients to include guidance for end-of-life care in a color-coordinated form that follows the patient across treatment settings. The procedures for completing advance care planning documents vary according to state law.

A potentially misleading distinction relates to statutory as opposed to advisory documents. Statutory documents are drafted to fulfill relevant state laws. Advisory documents are drafted to reflect the patient's wishes. Both are legal, the first under state law and the latter under common or constitutional law.

LEGAL ASPECTS The U.S. Supreme Court has ruled that patients have a constitutional right to decide about refusing and terminating medical interventions, including life-sustaining interventions, and that mentally incompetent patients can exercise this right by providing "clear and convincing evidence" of their preferences. Because advance care directives permit patients to provide such evidence, commentators agree that

TABLE 10-3 STEPS IN ADVANCE CARE PLANNING

Step	Goals to be Achieved and Measures to Cover	Useful Phrases or Points to Make
Introducing advance care planning	Ask the patient what he or she knows about advance care planning and if he or she has already completed an advance care directive.	*I'd like to talk with you about something I try to discuss with all my patients. It's called advance care planning. In fact, I feel that this is such an important topic that I have done this myself. Are you familiar with advance care planning or living wills?*
	Indicate that you as a physician have completed advance care planning.	*Have you thought about the type of care you would want if you ever became too sick to speak for yourself? That is the purpose of advance care planning.*
	Indicate that you try to perform advance care planning with all patients regardless of prognosis.	*There is no change in health that we have not discussed. I am bringing this up now because it is sensible for everyone, no matter how well or ill, old or young.*
	Explain the goals of the process as empowering the patient and ensuring that you and the proxy understand the patient's preferences.	Have many copies of advance care directives available, including in the waiting room, for patients and families.
	Provide the patient relevant literature, including the advance care directive that you prefer to use.	Know resources for state-specific forms (available at *www.nhpco.org*).
	Recommend the patient identify a proxy decision-maker who should attend the next meeting.	
Structured discussion of scenarios and patient	Affirm that the goal of the process is to follow the patient's wishes if the patient loses decision-making capacity.	Use a structured worksheet with typical scenarios.
	Elicit the patient's overall goals related to health care.	Begin the discussion with persistent vegetative state and consider other scenarios, such as recovery from an acute event with serious disability, asking the patient about his or her preferences regarding specific interventions, such as ventilators, artificial nutrition, and CPR, and then proceeding to less invasive interventions, such as blood transfusions and antibiotics.
	Elicit the patient's preferences for specific interventions in a few salient and common scenarios.	
	Help the patient define the threshold for withdrawing and withholding interventions.	
	Define the patient's preference for the role of the proxy.	
Review the patient's preferences	After the patient has made choices of interventions, review them to ensure they are consistent and the proxy is aware of them.	
Document the patient's preferences	Formally complete the advance care directive and have a witness sign it.	
	Provide a copy for the patient and the proxy.	
	Insert a copy into the patient's medical record and summarize in a progress note.	
Update the directive	Periodically, and with major changes in health status, review the directive with the patient and make any modifications.	
Apply the directive	The directive goes into effect only when the patient becomes unable to make medical decisions for himself or herself.	
	Reread the directive to be sure about its content.	
	Discuss your proposed actions based on the directive with the proxy.	

Abbreviation: CPR, cardiopulmonary resuscitation.

they are constitutionally protected. Most commentators believe that a state is required to honor any clear advance care directive whether or not it is written on an "official" form. Many states have enacted laws explicitly to honor out-of-state directives. If a patient is not using a statutory form, it may be advisable to attach a statutory form to the advance care directive being used. State-specific forms are readily available free of charge for health care providers and patients and families through the National Hospice and Palliative Care Organization's "Caring Connections" website *(http://www.caringinfo.org)*.

In January 2014, Texas judge R. H. Wallace ruled that a brain dead woman who was 23 weeks pregnant should be removed from life support. This was after several months of disagreement between the woman's family and the hospital providing care. The hospital cited Texas law that states that life-sustaining treatment must be administered to a pregnant woman, but the judge sided with the woman's family saying that the law did not apply because the patient was legally dead.

As of 2013, advance directives are legal in all states and the District of Columbia either through state specific legislation, state judicial rulings, or United States Supreme Court rulings. Many states have their own statutory forms. Massachusetts and Michigan do not have living will laws, although both have health care proxy laws. In 27 states, the laws state that the living will is not valid if a woman is pregnant. However, like all other states except Alaska, these states have enacted durable power of attorney for health care laws that permit patients to designate a proxy decision-maker with authority to terminate life-sustaining treatments. Only in Alaska does the law prohibit proxies from terminating life-sustaining treatments. The health reform legislation, the Affordable Care Act of 2010, raised substantial controversy when early versions of the law included Medicare reimbursement for advance care planning consultations. These provisions were withdrawn over accusations that they would lead to the rationing of care for the elderly.

INTERVENTIONS

PHYSICAL SYMPTOMS AND THEIR MANAGEMENT

Great emphasis has been placed on addressing dying patients' pain. Some institutions have made pain assessment a fifth vital sign to emphasize its importance. This also has been advocated by large health care systems such as the Veterans' Administration and accrediting bodies such as the Joint Commission. Although this embrace of pain as the fifth vital sign has been symbolically important, no data document that it has improved pain management practices. Although good palliative care requires good pain management, it also requires more. The frequency of symptoms varies by disease and other factors. The most common physical and psychological symptoms among all terminally ill patients include pain, fatigue, insomnia, anorexia, dyspnea, depression, anxiety, and nausea and vomiting. In the last days of life, terminal delirium is also common. Assessments of patients with advanced cancer have shown that patients experienced an average of 11.5 different physical and psychological symptoms (Table 10-4).

Evaluations to determine the etiology of these symptoms usually can be limited to the history and physical examination. In some cases, radiologic or other diagnostic examinations will provide sufficient

TABLE 10-4 COMMON PHYSICAL AND PSYCHOLOGICAL SYMPTOMS OF TERMINALLY ILL PATIENTS

Physical Symptoms	Psychological Symptoms
Pain	Anxiety
Fatigue and weakness	Depression
Dyspnea	Hopelessness
Insomnia	Meaninglessness
Dry mouth	Irritability
Anorexia	Impaired concentration
Nausea and vomiting	Confusion
Constipation	Delirium
Cough	Loss of libido
Swelling of arms or legs	
Itching	
Diarrhea	
Dysphagia	
Dizziness	
Fecal and urinary incontinence	
Numbness/tingling in hands/feet	

benefit in directing optimal palliative care to warrant the risks, potential discomfort, and inconvenience, especially to a seriously ill patient. Only a few of the common symptoms that present difficult management issues will be addressed in this chapter. **Additional information on the management of other symptoms, such as nausea and vomiting, insomnia, and diarrhea, can be found in Chaps. 54 and 99, Chap. 38, and Chap. 55, respectively.**

Pain • ***FREQUENCY*** The frequency of pain among terminally ill patients varies widely. Substantial pain occurs in 36–90% of patients with advanced cancer. In the SUPPORT study of hospitalized patients with diverse conditions and an estimated survival ≤6 months, 22% reported moderate to severe pain, and caregivers of those patients noted that 50% had similar levels of pain during the last few days of life. A meta-analysis found pain prevalence of 58–69% in studies that included patients characterized as having advanced, metastatic, or terminal cancer; 44–73% in studies that included patients characterized as undergoing cancer treatment; and 21–46% in studies that included posttreatment individuals.

ETIOLOGY *Nociceptive pain* is the result of direct mechanical or chemical stimulation of nociceptors and normal neural signaling to the brain. It tends to be localized, aching, throbbing, and cramping. The classic example is bone metastases. *Visceral pain* is caused by nociceptors in gastrointestinal, respiratory, and other organ systems. It is a deep or colicky type of pain classically associated with pancreatitis, myocardial infarction, or tumor invasion of viscera. *Neuropathic pain* arises from disordered nerve signals. It is described by patients as burning, electrical, or shocklike pain. Classic examples are poststroke pain, tumor invasion of the brachial plexus, and herpetic neuralgia.

ASSESSMENT Pain is a subjective experience. Depending on the patient's circumstances, perspective, and physiologic condition, the same physical lesion or disease state can produce different levels of reported pain and need for pain relief. Systematic assessment includes eliciting the following: (1) type: throbbing, cramping, burning, etc.; (2) periodicity: continuous, with or without exacerbations, or incident; (3) location; (4) intensity; (5) modifying factors; (6) effects of treatments; (7) functional impact; and (8) impact on patient. Several validated pain assessment measures may be used, such as the Visual Analogue Scale, the Brief Pain Inventory, and the pain component of one of the more comprehensive symptom assessment instruments. Frequent reassessments are essential to assess the effects of interventions.

INTERVENTIONS Interventions for pain must be tailored to each individual, with the goal of preempting chronic pain and relieving breakthrough pain. At the end of life, there is rarely reason to doubt a patient's report of pain. Pain medications are the cornerstone of management. If they are failing and nonpharmacologic interventions—including radiotherapy and anesthetic or neurosurgical procedures such as peripheral nerve blocks or epidural medications—are required, a pain consultation is appropriate.

Pharmacologic interventions follow the World Health Organization three-step approach involving nonopioid analgesics, mild opioids, and strong opioids, with or without adjuvants (Chap. 18). Nonopioid analgesics, especially nonsteroidal anti-inflammatory drugs (NSAIDs), are the initial treatments for mild pain. They work primarily by inhibiting peripheral prostaglandins and reducing inflammation but also may have central nervous system (CNS) effects. They have a ceiling effect. Ibuprofen, up to a total dose of 1600 mg/d given in four doses of 400 mg each, has a minimal risk of causing bleeding and renal impairment and is a good initial choice. In patients with a history of severe gastrointestinal (GI) or other bleeding, it should be avoided. In patients with a history of mild gastritis or gastroesophageal reflux disease (GERD), acid-lowering therapy such as a proton pump inhibitor should be used. Acetaminophen is an alternative in patients with a history of GI bleeding and can be used safely at up to 4 g/d given in four doses of 1 g each. In patients with liver dysfunction due to metastases or other causes and in patients with heavy alcohol use, doses should be reduced.

If nonopioid analgesics are insufficient, opioids should be introduced. They work by interacting with μ opioid receptors in the CNS to activate pain-inhibitory neurons; most are receptor antagonists. The mixed agonist/antagonist opioids useful for postacute pain should not be used for the chronic pain in end-of-life care. Weak opioids such as codeine can be used initially. However, if they are escalated and fail to relieve pain, strong opioids such as morphine, 5–10 mg every 4 h, should be used. Nonopioid analgesics should be combined with opioids because they potentiate the effect of opioids.

For continuous pain, opioids should be administered on a regular, around-the-clock basis consistent with their duration of analgesia. They should not be provided only when the patient experiences pain; the goal is to prevent patients from experiencing pain. Patients also should be provided rescue medication, such as liquid morphine, for breakthrough pain, generally at 20% of the baseline dose. Patients should be informed that using the rescue medication does not obviate the need to take the next standard dose of pain medication. If after 24 h the patient's pain remains uncontrolled and recurs before the next dose, requiring the patient to use the rescue medication, the daily opioid dose can be increased by the total dose of rescue medications used by the patient, or by 50% for moderate pain and 100% for severe pain of the standing opioid daily dose.

It is inappropriate to start with extended-release preparations. Instead, an initial focus on using short-acting preparations to determine how much is required in the first 24–48 h will allow clinicians to determine opioid needs. Once pain relief is obtained with short-acting preparations, one should switch to extended-release preparations. Even with a stable extended-release preparation regimen, the patient may have incident pain, such as during movement or dressing changes. Short-acting preparations should be taken before such predictable episodes. Although less common, patients may have "end-of-dose failure" with long-acting opioids, meaning that they develop pain after 8 h in the case of an every-12-h medication. In these cases, a trial of giving an every-12-h medication every 8 h is appropriate.

Because of differences in opioid receptors, cross-tolerance among opioids is incomplete, and patients may experience different side effects with different opioids. Therefore, if a patient is not experiencing pain relief or is experiencing too many side effects, a change to another opioid preparation is appropriate. When switching, one should begin with 50–75% of the published equianalgesic dose of the new opioid.

Unlike NSAIDs, opioids have no ceiling effect; therefore, there is no maximum dose no matter how many milligrams the patient is receiving. The appropriate dose is the dose needed to achieve pain relief. This is an important point for clinicians to explain to patients and families. Addiction or excessive respiratory depression is extremely unlikely in the terminally ill; fear of these side effects should neither prevent escalating opioid medications when the patient is experiencing insufficient pain relief nor justify using opioid antagonists.

Opioid side effects should be anticipated and treated preemptively. Nearly all patients experience constipation that can be debilitating (see below). Failure to prevent constipation often results in noncompliance with opioid therapy. Methylnaltrexone is a drug that targets opioid-induced constipation by blocking peripheral opioid receptors but not central receptors for analgesia. In placebo-controlled trials, it has been shown to cause laxation within 24 h of administration. As with the use of opioids, about a third of patients using methylnaltrexone experience nausea and vomiting, but unlike constipation, tolerance develops, usually within a week. Therefore, when one is beginning opioids, an antiemetic such as metoclopramide or a serotonin antagonist often is prescribed prophylactically and stopped after 1 week. Olanzapine also has antinausea properties and can be effective in countering delirium or anxiety, with the advantage of some weight gain.

Drowsiness, a common side effect of opioids, also usually abates within a week. During this period, drowsiness can be treated with psychostimulants such as dextroamphetamine, methylphenidate, and modafinil. Modafinil has the advantage of everyday dosing. Pilot reports suggest that donepezil may also be helpful for opiate-induced drowsiness as well as relieving fatigue and anxiety. Metabolites of morphine and most opioids are cleared renally; doses may have to be adjusted for patients with renal failure.

Seriously ill patients who require chronic pain relief rarely if ever become addicted. Suspicion of addiction should not be a reason to withhold pain medications from terminally ill patients. Patients and families may withhold prescribed opioids for fear of addiction or dependence. Physicians and health care providers should reassure patients and families that the patient will not become addicted to opioids if they are used as prescribed for pain relief; this fear should not prevent the patient from taking the medications around the clock. However, diversion of drugs for use by other family members or illicit sale may occur. It may be necessary to advise the patient and caregiver about secure storage of opioids. Contract writing with the patient and family can help. If that fails, transfer to a safe facility may be necessary.

Tolerance is the need to increase medication dosage for the same pain relief without a change in disease. In the case of patients with advanced disease, the need for increasing opioid dosage for pain relief usually is caused by disease progression rather than tolerance. Physical dependence is indicated by symptoms from the abrupt withdrawal of opioids and should not be confused with addiction.

Adjuvant analgesic medications are nonopioids that potentiate the analgesic effects of opioids. They are especially important in the management of neuropathic pain. Gabapentin and pregabalin, calcium channel alpha 2-delta ligands, are now the first-line treatments for neuropathic pain from a variety of causes. Gabapentin is begun at 100–300 mg bid or tid, with 50–100% dose increments every 3 days. Usually 900–3600 mg/d in two or three doses is effective. The combination of gabapentin and nortriptyline may be more effective than gabapentin alone. One potential side effect of gabapentin to be aware of is confusion and drowsiness, especially in the elderly. Pregabalin has the same mechanism of action as gabapentin but is absorbed more efficiently from the GI tract. It is started at 75 mg bid and increased to 150 mg bid. The maximum dose is 225 mg bid. Carbamazepine, a first-generation agent, has been proved effective in randomized trials for neuropathic pain. Other potentially effective anticonvulsant adjuvants include topiramate (25–50 mg qd or bid, rising to 100–300 mg/d) and oxcarbazepine (75–300 mg bid, rising to 1200 mg bid). Glucocorticoids, preferably dexamethasone given once a day, can be useful in reducing inflammation that causes pain while elevating mood, energy, and appetite. Its main side effects include confusion, sleep difficulties, and fluid retention. Glucocorticoids are especially effective for bone pain and abdominal pain from distention of the GI tract or liver. Other drugs, including clonidine and baclofen, can be effective in pain relief. These drugs are adjuvants and generally should be used in conjunction with—not instead of—opioids. Methadone, carefully dosed because of its unpredictable half-life in many patients, has activity at the *N*-methyl-D-aspartamate (NMDA) receptor and is useful for complex pain syndromes and neuropathic pain. It generally is reserved for cases in which first-line opioids (morphine, oxycodone, hydromorphone) are either ineffective or unavailable.

Radiation therapy can treat bone pain from single metastatic lesions. Bone pain from multiple metastases can be amenable to radiopharmaceuticals such as strontium-89 and samarium-153. Bisphosphonates (such as pamidronate [90 mg every 4 weeks]) and calcitonin (200 IU intranasally once or twice a day) also provide relief from bone pain but have an onset of action of days.

Constipation • ***FREQUENCY*** Constipation is reported in up to 87% of patients requiring palliative care.

ETIOLOGY Although hypercalcemia and other factors can cause constipation, it is most frequently a predictable consequence of the use of opioids for the relief of pain and dyspnea and of tricyclic antidepressants, from their anticholinergic effects, and of the inactivity and poor diet that are common among seriously ill patients. If untreated, constipation can cause substantial pain and vomiting and also is associated with confusion and delirium. Whenever opioids and other medications known to cause constipation are used, preemptive treatment for constipation should be instituted.

ASSESSMENT The physician should establish the patient's previous bowel habits, including the frequency, consistency, and volume. Abdominal and rectal examinations should be performed to exclude impaction or acute abdomen. A number of constipation assessment scales are available, although guidelines issued in the *Journal of Palliative Medicine* did not recommend them for routine practice. Radiographic assessments beyond a simple flat plate of the abdomen in cases in which obstruction is suspected are rarely necessary.

INTERVENTION Intervention to reestablish comfortable bowel habits and relieve pain and discomfort should be the goals of any measures to address constipation during end-of-life care. Although physical activity, adequate hydration, and dietary treatments with fiber can be helpful, each is limited in its effectiveness for most seriously ill patients, and fiber may exacerbate problems in the setting of dehydration and if impaired motility is the etiology. Fiber is contraindicated in the presence of opioid use. Stimulant and osmotic laxatives, stool softeners, fluids, and enemas are the mainstays of therapy (Table 10-5). In preventing constipation from opioids and other medications, a combination of a laxative and a stool softener (such as senna and docusate) should be used. If after several days of treatment, a bowel movement has not occurred, a rectal examination to remove impacted stool and place a suppository is necessary. For patients with impending bowel obstruction or gastric stasis, octreotide to reduce secretions can be helpful. For patients in whom the suspected mechanism is dysmotility, metoclopramide can be helpful.

Nausea • ***FREQUENCY*** Up to 70% of patients with advanced cancer have nausea, defined as the subjective sensation of wanting to vomit.

ETIOLOGY Nausea and vomiting are both caused by stimulation at one of four sites: the GI tract, the vestibular system, the chemoreceptor trigger zone (CTZ), and the cerebral cortex. Medical treatments for nausea are aimed at receptors at each of these sites: the GI tract contains mechanoreceptors, chemoreceptors, and 5-hydroxytryptamine type 3 (5-HT_3) receptors; the vestibular system probably contains histamine and acetylcholine receptors; and the CTZ contains chemoreceptors, dopamine type 2 receptors, and 5-HT_3 receptors. An example of nausea that most likely is mediated by the cortex is anticipatory nausea before a dose of chemotherapy or other noxious stimuli.

Specific causes of nausea include metabolic changes (liver failure, uremia from renal failure, hypercalcemia), bowel obstruction, constipation, infection, GERD, vestibular disease, brain metastases, medications (including antibiotics, NSAIDs, proton pump inhibitors, opioids, and chemotherapy), and radiation therapy. Anxiety can also contribute to nausea.

INTERVENTION Medical treatment of nausea is directed at the anatomic and receptor-mediated cause that a careful history and physical examination reveals. When a single specific cause is not found, many advocate beginning treatment with a dopamine antagonist such as haloperidol or prochlorperazine. Prochlorperazine is usually more

TABLE 10-5 MEDICATIONS FOR THE MANAGEMENT OF CONSTIPATION

Intervention	Dose	Comment
Stimulant laxatives		These agents directly stimulate peristalsis and may reduce colonic absorption of water.
Prune juice	120–240 mL/d	Work in 6–12 h.
Senna (Senokot)	2–8 tablets PO bid	
Bisacodyl	5–15 mg/d PO, PR	
Osmotic laxatives		These agents are not absorbed. They attract and retain water in the gastrointestinal tract.
Lactulose	15–30 mL PO q4–8h	Lactulose may cause flatulence and bloating.
Magnesium hydroxide (Milk of Magnesia)	15–30 mL/d PO	Lactulose works in 1 day, magnesium products in 6 h.
Magnesium citrate	125–250 mL/d PO	
Stool softeners		These agents work by increasing water secretion and as detergents, increasing water penetration into the stool.
Sodium docusate (Colace)	300–600 mg/d PO	Work in 1–3 days.
Calcium docusate	300–600 mg/d PO	
Suppositories and enemas		
Bisacodyl	10–15 PR qd	
Sodium phosphate enema	PR qd	Fixed dose, 4.5 oz, Fleet's.

sedating than haloperidol. When decreased motility is suspected, metoclopramide can be an effective treatment. When inflammation of the GI tract is suspected, glucocorticoids such as dexamethasone are an appropriate treatment. For nausea that follows chemotherapy and radiation therapy, one of the 5-HT$_3$ receptor antagonists (ondansetron, granisetron, dolasetron, palonosetron) is recommended. Studies suggest palonosetron has higher receptor binding affinity and clinical superiority to the other 5-HT$_3$ receptor antagonists. Clinicians should attempt prevention of postchemotherapy nausea rather than provide treatment after the fact. Current clinical guidelines recommend tailoring the strength of treatments to the specific emetic risk posed by a specific chemotherapy drug. When a vestibular cause (such as "motion sickness" or labyrinthitis) is suspected, antihistamines such as meclizine (whose primary side effect is drowsiness) or anticholinergics such as scopolamine can be effective. In anticipatory nausea, a benzodiazepine such as lorazepam is indicated. As with antihistamines, drowsiness and confusion are the main side effects.

Dyspnea • ***FREQUENCY*** Dyspnea is a subjective experience of being short of breath. Frequencies vary among causes of death, but it can affect 80–90% of dying patients with lung cancer, COPD, and heart disease. Dyspnea is among the most distressing physical symptoms and can be even more distressing than pain.

ASSESSMENT As with pain, dyspnea is a subjective experience that may not correlate with objective measures of P_{O_2}, P_{CO_2}, or respiratory rate. Consequently, measurements of oxygen saturation through pulse oximetry or blood gases are rarely helpful in guiding therapy. Despite the limitations of existing assessment methods, physicians should regularly assess and document patients' experience of dyspnea and its intensity. Guidelines recommend visual or analogue dyspnea scales to assess the severity of symptoms and the effects of treatment. Potentially reversible or treatable causes of dyspnea include infection, pleural effusions, pulmonary emboli, pulmonary edema, asthma, and tumor encroachment on the airway. However, the risk-versus-benefit ratio of the diagnostic and therapeutic interventions for patients with little time left to live must be considered carefully before one undertakes diagnostic steps. Frequently, the specific etiology cannot be identified, and dyspnea is the consequence of progression of the underlying disease that cannot be treated. The anxiety caused by dyspnea and the choking sensation can significantly exacerbate the underlying dyspnea in a negatively reinforcing cycle.

TABLE 10-6 MEDICATIONS FOR THE MANAGEMENT OF DYSPNEA

Intervention	Dose	Comments
Weak opioids		For patients with mild dyspnea
Codeine (or codeine with 325 mg acetaminophen)	30 mg PO q4h	For opioid-naïve patients
Hydrocodone	5 mg PO q4h	
Strong opioids		For opioid-naïve patients with moderate to severe dyspnea
Morphine	5–10 mg PO q4h 30–50% of baseline opioid dose q4h	For patients already taking opioids for pain or other symptoms
Oxycodone	5–10 mg PO q4h	
Hydromorphone	1–2 mg PO q4h	
Anxiolytics		Give a dose every hour until the patient is relaxed, then provide a dose for maintenance
Lorazepam	0.5–2.0 mg PO/SL/IV qh then q4–6h	
Clonazepam	0.25–2.0 mg PO q12h	
Midazolam	0.5 mg IV q15min	

INTERVENTIONS When reversible or treatable etiologies are diagnosed, they should be treated as long as the side effects of treatment, such as repeated drainage of effusions or anticoagulants, are less burdensome than the dyspnea itself. More aggressive treatments such as stenting a bronchial lesion may be warranted if it is clear that the dyspnea is due to tumor invasion at that site and if the patient and family understand the risks of such a procedure. Usually, treatment will be symptomatic (Table 10-6). A dyspnea scale and careful monitoring should guide dose adjustment. Low-dose opioids reduce the sensitivity of the central respiratory center and the sensation of dyspnea. If patients are not receiving opioids, weak opioids can be initiated; if patients are already receiving opioids, morphine or other strong opioids should be used. Controlled trials do not support the use of nebulized opioids for dyspnea at the end of life. Phenothiazines and chlorpromazine may be helpful when combined with opioids. Benzodiazepines can be helpful if anxiety is present but should be neither used as first-line therapy nor used alone in the treatment of dyspnea. If the patient has a history of COPD or asthma, inhaled bronchodilators and glucocorticoids may be helpful. If the patient has pulmonary edema due to heart failure, diuresis with a medication such as furosemide is indicated. Excess secretions can be dried with scopolamine, transdermally or intravenously. Use of oxygen is controversial. There are conflicting data on its effectiveness for patients with proven hypoxemia. But there is no clear benefit of oxygen compared to room air for nonhypoxemic patients. Noninvasive positive-pressure ventilation using a facemask or nasal plugs may be used for some patients for symptom relief. For some families and patients, oxygen is distressing; for others, it is reassuring. More general interventions that medical staff can do include sitting the patient upright, removing smoke or other irritants such as perfume, ensuring a supply of fresh air with sufficient humidity, and minimizing other factors that can increase anxiety.

Fatigue • ***FREQUENCY*** More than 90% of terminally ill patients experience fatigue and/or weakness. Fatigue is one of the most commonly reported symptoms of cancer treatment as well as in the palliative care of multiple sclerosis, COPD, heart failure, and HIV. Fatigue frequently is cited as among the most distressing symptoms.

ETIOLOGY The multiple causes of fatigue in the terminally ill can be categorized as resulting from the underlying disease; from disease-induced factors such as tumor necrosis factor and other cytokines; and from secondary factors such as dehydration, anemia, infection, hypothyroidism, and drug side effects. Apart from low caloric intake, loss of muscle mass and changes in muscle enzymes may play an important role in fatigue of terminal illness. The importance of changes in the CNS, especially the reticular activating system, have been hypothesized based on reports of fatigue in patients receiving cranial radiation, experiencing depression, or having chronic pain in the absence of cachexia or other physiologic changes. Finally, depression and other causes of psychological distress can contribute to fatigue.

ASSESSMENT Like pain and dyspnea, fatigue is subjective. Objective changes, even in body mass, may be absent. Consequently, assessment must rely on patient self-reporting. Scales used to measure fatigue, such as the Edmonton Functional Assessment Tool, the Fatigue Self-Report Scales, and the Rhoten Fatigue Scale, are usually appropriate for research rather than clinical purposes. In clinical practice, a simple performance assessment such as the Karnofsky Performance Status or the ECOG's question "How much of the day does the patient spend in bed?" may be the best measure. In this 0–4 performance status assessment, 0 = normal activity; 1 = symptomatic without being bedridden; 2 = requiring some, but <50%, bed time; 3 = bedbound more than half the day; and 4 = bedbound all the time. Such a scale allows for assessment over time and correlates with overall disease severity and prognosis. A 2008 review by the European Association of Palliative Care also described several longer assessment tools with 9–20 items, including the Piper Fatigue Inventory, the Multidimensional Fatigue Inventory, and the Brief Fatigue Inventory (BFI).

INTERVENTIONS For some patients, there are reversible causes such as anemia, but for most patients at the end of life, fatigue will not be "cured." The goal is to ameliorate it and help patients and families adjust expectations. Behavioral interventions should be used to avoid blaming the patient for inactivity and to educate both the family and the patient that the underlying disease causes physiologic changes that produce low energy levels. Understanding that the problem is physiologic and not psychological can help alter expectations regarding the patient's level of physical activity. Practically, this may mean reducing routine activities such as housework and cooking or social events outside the house and making it acceptable to receive guests lying on a couch. At the same time, institution of exercise regimens and physical therapy can raise endorphins, reduce muscle wasting, and reduce the risk of depression. In addition, ensuring good hydration without worsening edema may help reduce fatigue. Discontinuing medications that worsen fatigue may help, including cardiac medications, benzodiazepines, certain antidepressants, or opioids if pain is well-controlled. As end-of-life care proceeds into its final stages, fatigue may protect patients from further suffering, and continued treatment could be detrimental.

There are woefully few pharmacologic interventions that target fatigue and weakness. Glucocorticoids can increase energy and enhance mood. Dexamethasone is preferred for its once-a-day dosing and minimal mineralocorticoid activity. Benefit, if any, usually is seen within the first month. Psychostimulants such as dextroamphetamine (5–10 mg PO) and methylphenidate (2.5–5 mg PO) may also enhance energy levels, although a randomized trial did not show methylphenidate beneficial compared with placebo in cancer fatigue. Doses should be given in the morning and at noon to minimize the risk of counterproductive insomnia. Modafinil, developed for narcolepsy, has shown some promise in the treatment of severe fatigue and has the advantage of once-daily dosing. Its precise role in fatigue at the end of life has not been determined. Anecdotal evidence suggests that L-carnitine may improve fatigue, depression, and sleep disruption. Similarly, some studies suggest ginseng can reduce fatigue.

PSYCHOLOGICAL SYMPTOMS AND THEIR MANAGEMENT

Depression • ***FREQUENCY*** Depression at the end of life presents an apparently paradoxical situation. Many people believe that depression is normal among seriously ill patients because they are dying. People frequently say, "Wouldn't you be depressed?" However, depression is not a necessary part of terminal illness and can contribute to needless suffering. Although sadness, anxiety, anger, and irritability are normal responses to a serious condition, they are typically of modest intensity and transient. Persistent sadness and anxiety and the physically disabling symptoms that they can lead to are abnormal and suggestive of major depression. Although as many as 75% of terminally ill patients experience emotional distress and depressive symptoms, <30% of terminally ill patients have major depression. Depression is not limited to cancer patients but found in patients with end-stage renal disease, Parkinson's disease, multiple sclerosis, and other terminal conditions.

ETIOLOGY Previous history of depression, family history of depression or bipolar disorder, and prior suicide attempts are associated with increased risk for depression among terminally ill patients. Other symptoms, such as pain and fatigue, are associated with higher rates of depression; uncontrolled pain can exacerbate depression, and depression can cause patients to be more distressed by pain. Many medications used in the terminal stages, including glucocorticoids, and some anticancer agents, such as tamoxifen, interleukin 2, interferon α, and vincristine, also are associated with depression. Some terminal conditions, such as pancreatic cancer, certain strokes, and heart failure, have been reported to be associated with higher rates of depression, although this is controversial. Finally, depression may be attributable to grief over the loss of a role or function, social isolation, or loneliness.

ASSESSMENT Diagnosing depression among seriously ill patients is complicated because many of the vegetative symptoms in the DSM-V (*Diagnostic and Statistical Manual of Mental Disorders*) criteria for clinical depression—insomnia, anorexia and weight loss, fatigue, decreased libido, and difficulty concentrating—are associated with the dying process itself. The assessment of depression in seriously ill patients therefore should focus on the dysphoric mood, helplessness, hopelessness, and lack of interest and enjoyment and concentration in normal activities. The single questions "How often do you feel downhearted and blue?" (more than a good bit of the time or similar responses) and "Do you feel depressed most of the time?" are appropriate for screening. Visual Analog Scales can also be useful in screening.

INTERVENTIONS Physicians must treat any physical symptom, such as pain, that may be causing or exacerbating depression. Fostering adaptation to the many losses that the patient is experiencing can also be helpful. Nonpharmacologic interventions, including group or individual psychological counseling, and behavioral therapies such as relaxation and imagery can be helpful, especially in combination with drug therapy.

Pharmacologic interventions remain the core of therapy. The same medications are used to treat depression in terminally ill as in non-terminally ill patients. Psychostimulants may be preferred for patients with a poor prognosis or for those with fatigue or opioid-induced somnolence. Psychostimulants are comparatively fast acting, working within a few days instead of the weeks required for selective serotonin reuptake inhibitors (SSRIs). Dextroamphetamine or methylphenidate should be started at 2.5–5.0 mg in the morning and at noon, the same starting doses used for treating fatigue. The dose can be escalated up to 15 mg bid. Modafinil is started at 100 mg qd and can be increased to 200 mg if there is no effect at the lower dose. Pemoline is a nonamphetamine psychostimulant with minimal abuse potential. It is also effective as an antidepressant beginning at 18.75 mg in the morning and at noon. Because it can be absorbed through the buccal mucosa, it is preferred for patients with intestinal obstruction or dysphagia. If it is used for prolonged periods, liver function must be monitored. The psychostimulants can also be combined with more traditional antidepressants while waiting for the antidepressants to become effective and then tapered after a few weeks if necessary. Psychostimulants have side effects, particularly initial anxiety, insomnia, and rarely paranoia, which may necessitate lowering the dose or discontinuing treatment.

Mirtazapine, an antagonist at the postsynaptic serotonin receptors, is a promising psychostimulant. It should be started at 7.5 mg before bed. It has sedating, antiemetic, and anxiolytic properties with few drug interactions. Its side effect of weight gain may be beneficial for seriously ill patients; it is available in orally disintegrating tablets.

For patients with a prognosis of several months or longer, SSRIs, including fluoxetine, sertraline, paroxetine, citalopram, escitalopram, and fluvoxamine, and serotonin-noradrenaline reuptake inhibitors such as venlafaxine, are the preferred treatment because of their efficacy and comparatively few side effects. Because low doses of these medications may be effective for seriously ill patients, one should use half the usual starting dose for healthy adults. The starting dose for fluoxetine is 10 mg once a day. In most cases, once-a-day dosing is possible. The choice of which SSRI to use should be driven by (1) the patient's past success or failure with the specific medication, (2) the most favorable side effect profile for that specific agent, and (3) the time it takes to reach steady-state drug levels. For instance, for a patient in whom fatigue is a major symptom, a more activating SSRI (fluoxetine) would be appropriate. For a patient in whom anxiety and sleeplessness are major symptoms, a more sedating SSRI (paroxetine) would be appropriate.

Atypical antidepressants are recommended only in selected circumstances, usually with the assistance of a specialty consultation. Trazodone can be an effective antidepressant but is sedating and can cause orthostatic hypotension and, rarely, priapism. Therefore, it should be used only when a sedating effect is desired and is often used for patients with insomnia, at a dose starting at 25 mg. In addition to its antidepressant effects, bupropion is energizing, making it useful for depressed patients who experience fatigue. However, it can cause seizures, preventing its use for patients with a risk of CNS neoplasms or terminal delirium. Finally, alprazolam, a benzodiazepine, starting at 0.25–1.0 mg tid, can be effective in seriously ill patients who have a combination of anxiety and depression. Although it is potent and works quickly, it has many drug interactions and may cause delirium, especially among very ill patients, because of its strong binding to the benzodiazepine–γ-aminobutyric acid (GABA) receptor complex.

Unless used as adjuvants for the treatment of pain, tricyclic antidepressants are not recommended. Similarly, monoamine oxidase (MAO) inhibitors are not recommended because of their side effects and dangerous drug interactions.

Delirium (See Chap. 34) • ***FREQUENCY*** In the weeks or months before death, delirium is uncommon, although it may be significantly underdiagnosed. However, delirium becomes relatively common in the hours and days immediately before death. Up to 85% of patients dying from cancer may experience terminal delirium.

ETIOLOGY Delirium is a global cerebral dysfunction characterized by alterations in cognition and consciousness. It frequently is preceded by anxiety, changes in sleep patterns (especially reversal of day and night), and decreased attention. In contrast to dementia, delirium has an acute onset, is characterized by fluctuating consciousness and inattention, and is reversible, although reversibility may be more theoretical than real for patients near death. Delirium may occur in a patient with dementia; indeed, patients with dementia are more vulnerable to delirium.

Causes of delirium include metabolic encephalopathy arising from liver or renal failure, hypoxemia, or infection; electrolyte imbalances such as hypercalcemia; paraneoplastic syndromes; dehydration; and primary brain tumors, brain metastases, or leptomeningeal spread of tumor. Commonly, among dying patients, delirium can be caused by side effects of treatments, including radiation for brain metastases, and medications, including opioids, glucocorticoids, anticholinergic drugs, antihistamines, antiemetics, benzodiazepines, and chemotherapeutic agents. The etiology may be multifactorial; e.g., dehydration may exacerbate opioid-induced delirium.

ASSESSMENT Delirium should be recognized in any terminally ill patient with new onset of disorientation, impaired cognition, somnolence, fluctuating levels of consciousness, or delusions with or without agitation. Delirium must be distinguished from acute anxiety and depression as well as dementia. The central distinguishing feature is altered consciousness, which usually is not noted in anxiety, depression, and dementia. Although "hyperactive" delirium characterized by overt confusion and agitation is probably more common, patients also should be assessed for "hypoactive" delirium characterized by sleep-wake reversal and decreased alertness.

In some cases, use of formal assessment tools such as the Mini-Mental Status Examination (which does not distinguish delirium from dementia) and the Delirium Rating Scale (which does distinguish delirium from dementia) may be helpful in distinguishing delirium from other processes. The patient's list of medications must be evaluated carefully. Nonetheless, a reversible etiologic factor for delirium is found in fewer than half of terminally ill patients. Because most terminally ill patients experiencing delirium will be very close to death and may be at home, extensive diagnostic evaluations such as lumbar punctures and neuroradiologic examinations are usually inappropriate.

INTERVENTIONS One of the most important objectives of terminal care is to provide terminally ill patients the lucidity to say goodbye to the people they love. Delirium, especially with agitation during the final days, is distressing to family and caregivers. A strong determinant of bereavement difficulties is witnessing a difficult death. Thus, terminal delirium should be treated aggressively.

At the first sign of delirium, such as day-night reversal with slight changes in mentation, the physician should let the family members know that it is time to be sure that everything they want to say has been said. The family should be informed that delirium is common just before death.

If medications are suspected of being a cause of the delirium, unnecessary agents should be discontinued. Other potentially reversible causes, such as constipation, urinary retention, and metabolic abnormalities, should be treated. Supportive measures aimed at providing a familiar environment should be instituted, including restricting visits only to individuals with whom the patient is familiar and eliminating new experiences; orienting the patient, if possible, by providing a clock and calendar; and gently correcting the patient's hallucinations or cognitive mistakes.

Pharmacologic management focuses on the use of neuroleptics and, in the extreme, anesthetics (Table 10-7). Haloperidol remains first-line therapy. Usually, patients can be controlled with a low dose (1–3 mg/d), usually given every 6 h, although some may require as much as 20 mg/d. It can be administered PO, SC, or IV. IM injections should not be used, except when this is the only way to get a patient under control. Newer atypical neuroleptics, such as olanzapine, risperidone, and quetiapine, have shown significant effectiveness in completely resolving delirium in cancer patients. These drugs also have fewer side effects than haloperidol, along with other beneficial effects for terminally ill patients, including antinausea, antianxiety, and weight gain. They are useful for patients with longer anticipated life expectancy because they are less likely to cause dysphoria and have a lower risk of dystonic reactions. Also, because they are metabolized through multiple pathways, they can be used in patients with hepatic and renal

TABLE 10-7 MEDICATIONS FOR THE MANAGEMENT OF DELIRIUM

Interventions	Dose
Neuroleptics	
Haloperidol	0.5–5 mg q2–12h, PO/IV/SC/IM
Thioridazine	10–75 mg q4–8h, PO
Chlorpromazine	12.5–50 mg q4–12h, PO/IV/IM
Atypical neuroleptics	
Olanzapine	2.5–5 mg qd or bid, PO
Risperidone	1–3 mg q12h, PO
Quetiapine	50 mg qd, PO
Anxiolytics	
Lorazepam	0.5–2 mg q1–4h, PO/IV/IM
Midazolam	1–5 mg/h continuous infusion, IV/SC
Anesthetics	
Propofol	0.3–2.0 mg/h continuous infusion, IV

dysfunction. Olanzapine has the disadvantage that it is available only orally and that it takes a week to reach steady state. The usual dose is 2.5–5 mg PO bid. Chlorpromazine (10–25 mg every 4–6 h) can be useful if sedation is desired and can be administered IV or PR in addition to PO. Dystonic reactions resulting from dopamine blockade are a side effect of neuroleptics, although they are reported to be rare when these drugs are used to treat terminal delirium. If patients develop dystonic reactions, benztropine should be administered. Neuroleptics may be combined with lorazepam to reduce agitation when the delirium is the result of alcohol or sedative withdrawal.

If no response to first-line therapy is seen, a specialty consultation should be obtained with a change to a different medication. If patients fail to improve after a second neuroleptic, sedation with an anesthetic such as propofol or continuous-infusion midazolam may be necessary. By some estimates, at the very end of life, as many as 25% of patients experiencing delirium, especially restless delirium with myoclonus or convulsions, may require sedation.

Physical restraints should be used with great reluctance and only when the patient's violence is threatening to self or others. If they are used, their appropriateness should be reevaluated frequently.

Insomnia • *FREQUENCY* Sleep disorders, defined as difficulty initiating sleep or maintaining sleep, sleep difficulty at least 3 nights a week, or sleep difficulty that causes impairment of daytime functioning, occur in 19–63% of patients with advanced cancer. Some 30–74% of patients with other end-stage conditions, including AIDS, heart disease, COPD, and renal disease, experience insomnia.

ETIOLOGY Patients with cancer may have changes in sleep efficiency such as an increase in stage I sleep. Other etiologies of insomnia are coexisting physical illness such as thyroid disease and coexisting psychological illnesses such as depression and anxiety. Medications, including antidepressants, psychostimulants, steroids, and β agonists, are significant contributors to sleep disorders, as are caffeine and alcohol. Multiple over-the-counter medications contain caffeine and antihistamines, which can contribute to sleep disorders.

ASSESSMENT Assessment should include specific questions concerning sleep onset, sleep maintenance, and early-morning wakening as these will provide clues to the causative agents and to management. Patients should be asked about previous sleep problems, screened for depression and anxiety, and asked about symptoms of thyroid disease. Caffeine and alcohol are prominent causes of sleep problems, and a careful history of the use of these substances should be obtained. Both excessive use and withdrawal from alcohol can be causes of sleep problems.

INTERVENTIONS The mainstays of intervention include improvement of sleep hygiene (encouragement of regular time for sleep, decreased nighttime distractions, elimination of caffeine and other stimulants and alcohol), intervention to treat anxiety and depression, and treatment for the insomnia itself. For patients with depression who have insomnia and anxiety, a sedating antidepressant such as mirtazapine can be helpful. In the elderly, trazodone, beginning at 25 mg at nighttime, is an effective sleep aid at doses lower than those which cause its antidepressant effect. Zolpidem may have a decreased incidence of delirium in patients compared with traditional benzodiazepines, but this has not been clearly established. When benzodiazepines are prescribed, short-acting ones (such as lorazepam) are favored over longer-acting ones (such as diazepam). Patients who receive these medications should be observed for signs of increased confusion and delirium.

SOCIAL NEEDS AND THEIR MANAGEMENT

Financial Burdens • *FREQUENCY* Dying can impose substantial economic strains on patients and families, causing distress. In the United States, with one of the least comprehensive health insurance systems among the developed countries, ~20% of terminally ill patients and their families spend >10% of family income on health care costs over and above health insurance premiums. Between 10 and 30% of families sell assets, use savings, or take out a mortgage to pay for the patient's health care costs. Nearly 40% of terminally ill patients in the United States report that the cost of their illness is a moderate or great economic hardship for their family.

The patient is likely to reduce and eventually stop working. In 20% of cases, a family member of the terminally ill patient also stops working to provide care. The major underlying causes of economic burden are related to poor physical functioning and care needs, such as the need for housekeeping, nursing, and personal care. More debilitated patients and poor patients experience greater economic burdens.

INTERVENTION This economic burden should not be ignored as a private matter. It has been associated with a number of adverse health outcomes, including preferring comfort care over life-prolonging care as well as consideration of euthanasia or physician-assisted suicide. Economic burdens increase the psychological distress of families and caregivers of terminally ill patients, and poverty is associated with many adverse health outcomes. Importantly, recent studies found that "patients with advanced cancer who reported having end-of-life conversations with physicians had significantly lower health care costs in their final week of life. Higher costs were associated with worse quality of death." Assistance from a social worker, early on if possible, to ensure access to all available benefits may be helpful. Many patients, families, and health care providers are unaware of options for long-term care insurance, respite care, the Family Medical Leave Act (FMLA), and other sources of assistance. Some of these options (such as respite care) may be part of a formal hospice program, but others (such as the FMLA) do not require enrollment in a hospice program.

Relationships • *FREQUENCY* Settling personal issues and closing the narrative of lived relationships are universal needs. When asked if sudden death or death after an illness is preferable, respondents often initially select the former but soon change to the latter as they reflect on the importance of saying goodbye. Bereaved family members who have not had the chance to say goodbye often have a more difficult grief process.

INTERVENTIONS Care of seriously ill patients requires efforts to facilitate the types of encounters and time spent with family and friends that are necessary to meet those needs. Family and close friends may need to be accommodated with unrestricted visiting hours, which may include sleeping near the patient even in otherwise regimented institutional settings. Physicians and other health care providers may be able to facilitate and resolve strained interactions between the patient and other family members. Assistance for patients and family members who are unsure about how to create or help preserve memories, whether by providing materials such as a scrapbook or memory box or by offering them suggestions and informational resources, can be deeply appreciated. Taking photographs and creating videos can be especially helpful to terminally ill patients who have younger children or grandchildren.

Family Caregivers • *FREQUENCY* Caring for seriously ill patients places a heavy burden on families. Families frequently are required to provide transportation and homemaking as well as other services. Typically, paid professionals such as home health nurses and hospice workers supplement family care; only about a quarter of all caregiving consists of exclusively paid professional assistance. The trend toward more out-of-hospital deaths will increase reliance on families for end-of-life care. Increasingly, family members are being called upon to provide physical care (such as moving and bathing patients) and medical care (such as assessing symptoms and giving medications) in addition to emotional care and support.

Three-quarters of family caregivers of terminally ill patients are women—wives, daughters, sisters, and even daughters-in-law. Because many are widowed, women tend to be able to rely less on family for caregiving assistance and may need more paid assistance. About 20% of terminally ill patients report substantial unmet needs for nursing and personal care. The impact of caregiving on family caregivers is substantial: both bereaved and current caregivers have a higher mortality rate than that of non-caregiving controls.

INTERVENTIONS It is imperative to inquire about unmet needs and to try to ensure that those needs are met either through the family or by paid professional services when possible. Community assistance through houses of worship or other community groups often can be mobilized by telephone calls from the medical team to someone the patient or family identifies. Sources of support specifically for family caregivers should be identified through local sources or nationally through groups such as the National Family Caregivers Association (*www.nfcacares.org*), the American Cancer Society (*www.cancer.org*), and the Alzheimer's Association (*www.alz.org*).

EXISTENTIAL NEEDS AND THEIR MANAGEMENT

Frequency Religion and spirituality are often important to dying patients. Nearly 70% of patients report becoming more religious or spiritual when they became terminally ill, and many find comfort in religious or spiritual practices such as prayer. However, ~20% of terminally ill patients become less religious, frequently feeling cheated or betrayed by becoming terminally ill. For other patients, the need is for existential meaning and purpose that is distinct from and may even be antithetical to religion or spirituality. When asked, patients and family caregivers frequently report wanting their professional caregivers to be more attentive to religion and spirituality.

ASSESSMENT Health care providers are often hesitant about involving themselves in the religious, spiritual, and existential experiences of their patients because it may seem private or not relevant to the current illness. But physicians and other members of the care team should be able at least to detect spiritual and existential needs. Screening questions have been developed for a physician's spiritual history taking. Spiritual distress can amplify other types of suffering and even masquerade as intractable physical pain, anxiety, or depression. The screening questions in the comprehensive assessment are usually sufficient. Deeper evaluation and intervention are rarely appropriate for the physician unless no other member of a care team is available or suitable. Pastoral care providers may be helpful, whether from the medical institution or from the patient's own community.

INTERVENTIONS Precisely how religious practices, spirituality, and existential explorations can be facilitated and improve end-of-life care is not well established. What is clear is that for physicians, one main intervention is to inquire about the role and importance of spirituality and religion in a patient's life. This will help a patient feel heard and help physicians identify specific needs. In one study, only 36% of respondents indicated that a clergy member would be comforting. Nevertheless, the increase in religious and spiritual interest among a substantial fraction of dying patients suggests inquiring of individual patients how this need can be addressed. Some evidence supports specific methods of addressing existential needs in patients, ranging from establishing a supportive group environment for terminal patients to individual treatments emphasizing a patient's dignity and sources of meaning.

MANAGING THE LAST STAGES

WITHDRAWING AND WITHHOLDING LIFE-SUSTAINING TREATMENT

LEGAL ASPECTS For centuries, it has been deemed ethical to withhold or withdraw life-sustaining interventions. The current legal consensus in the United States and most developed countries is that patients have a moral as well as constitutional or common law right to refuse medical interventions. American courts also have held that incompetent patients have a right to refuse medical interventions. For patients who are incompetent and terminally ill and who have not completed an advance care directive, next of kin can exercise that right, although this may be restricted in some states, depending how clear and convincing the evidence is of the patient's preferences. Courts have limited families' ability to terminate life-sustaining treatments in patients who are conscious, incompetent, but not terminally ill. In theory, patients' right to refuse medical therapy can be limited by four countervailing interests: (1) preservation of life, (2) prevention of suicide, (3) protection of third parties such as children, and (4) preservation of the integrity of the medical profession. In practice, these interests almost never override the right of competent patients and incompetent patients who have left explicit and advance care directives.

For incompetent patients who either appointed a proxy without specific indications of their wishes or never completed an advance care directive, three criteria have been suggested to guide the decision to terminate medical interventions. First, some commentators suggest that ordinary care should be administered but extraordinary care could be terminated. Because the ordinary/extraordinary distinction is too vague, courts and commentators widely agree that it should not be used to justify decisions about stopping treatment. Second, many courts have advocated the use of the substituted-judgment criterion, which holds that the proxy decision-makers should try to imagine what the incompetent patient would do if he or she were competent. However, multiple studies indicate that many proxies, even close family members, cannot accurately predict what the patient would have wanted. Therefore, substituted judgment becomes more of a guessing game than a way of fulfilling the patient's wishes. Finally, the best-interests criterion holds that proxies should evaluate treatments by balancing their benefits and risks and select those treatments in which the benefits maximally outweigh the burdens of treatment. Clinicians have a clear and crucial role in this by carefully and dispassionately explaining the known benefits and burdens of specific treatments. Yet even when that information is as clear as possible, different individuals can have very different views of what is in the patient's best interests, and families may have disagreements or even overt conflicts. This criterion has been criticized because there is no single way to determine the balance between benefits and burdens; it depends on a patient's personal values. For instance, for some people, being alive even if mentally incapacitated is a benefit, whereas for others, it may be the worst possible existence. As a matter of practice, physicians rely on family members to make decisions that they feel are best and object only if those decisions seem to demand treatments that the physicians consider not beneficial.

PRACTICES Withholding and withdrawing acutely life-sustaining medical interventions from terminally ill patients are now standard practice. More than 90% of American patients die without cardiopulmonary resuscitation (CPR), and just as many forgo other potentially life-sustaining interventions. For instance, in ICUs in the period 1987–1988, CPR was performed 49% of the time, but it was performed only 10% of the time in 1992–1993. On average, 3.8 interventions, such as vasopressors and transfusions, were stopped for each dying ICU patient. However, up to 19% of decedents in hospitals received interventions such as extubation, ventilation, and surgery in the 48 h preceding death. However, practices vary widely among hospitals and ICUs, suggesting an important element of physician preferences rather than objective data.

Mechanical ventilation may be the most challenging intervention to withdraw. The two approaches are *terminal extubation*, which is the removal of the endotracheal tube, and *terminal weaning*, which is the gradual reduction of the or ventilator rate. One-third of ICU physicians prefer to use the terminal weaning technique, and 13% extubate; the majority of physicians use both techniques. The American Thoracic Society's 2008 clinical policy guidelines note that there is no single correct process of ventilator withdrawal and that physicians use and should be proficient in both methods but that the chosen approach should carefully balance benefits and burdens as well as patient and caregiver preferences. Physicians' assessment of patients' likelihood of survival, their prediction of possible cognitive damage, and patients' preferences about the use of life support are primary factors in determining the likelihood of withdrawal of mechanical ventilation. Some recommend terminal weaning because patients do not develop upper airway obstruction and the distress caused by secretions or stridor; however, terminal weaning can prolong the dying process and not allow a patient's family to be with him or her unencumbered by an endotracheal tube. To ensure comfort for conscious or semiconscious patients before withdrawal of the ventilator, neuromuscular blocking agents should be terminated and sedatives and analgesics administered. Removing the neuromuscular blocking agents permits patients to show discomfort, facilitating the titration of sedatives and analgesics; it also permits interactions between patients and their families. A common practice is to inject a bolus of midazolam (2–4 mg) or lorazepam (2–4 mg) before withdrawal, followed by 5–10 mg of morphine and continuous infusion of morphine (50% of the bolus dose per hour) during weaning. In patients who have significant upper airway secretions, IV scopolamine at a rate of 100 μg/h can be administered. Additional boluses of morphine or increases in the infusion rate should be administered for respiratory distress or signs of pain. Higher doses will be needed for patients already receiving sedatives and opioids. Families need to be reassured about treatments for common symptoms after withdrawal of ventilatory support, such as dyspnea and agitation, and warned about the uncertainty of length of survival after withdrawal of ventilatory support: up to 10% of patients unexpectedly survive for 1 day or more after mechanical ventilation is stopped.

FUTILE CARE

Beginning in the late 1980s, some commentators argued that physicians could terminate futile treatments demanded by the families of terminally ill patients. Although no objective definition or standard of futility exists, several categories have been proposed. Physiologic futility means that an intervention will have no physiologic effect. Some have defined qualitative futility as applying to procedures that "fail to end a patient's total dependence on intensive medical care." Quantitative futility occurs "when physicians conclude (through personal experience, experiences shared with colleagues, or consideration of reported empiric data) that in the last 100 cases, a medical treatment has been useless." The term conceals subjective value judgments about when a treatment is "not beneficial." Deciding whether a treatment that obtains an additional 6 weeks of life or a 1% survival advantage confers benefit depends on patients' preferences and goals. Furthermore, physicians' predictions of when treatments were futile deviated markedly from the quantitative definition. When residents thought CPR was quantitatively futile, more than one in five patients had a >10% chance of survival to hospital discharge. Most studies that purport to guide determinations of futility are based on insufficient data to provide statistical confidence for clinical decision making. Quantitative futility rarely applies in ICU settings. Many commentators reject using futility as a criterion for withdrawing care, preferring instead to consider futility situations as ones that represent conflict that calls for careful negotiation between families and health care providers.

In the wake of a lack of consensus over quantitative measures of futility, many hospitals adopted process-based approaches to resolve disputes over futility and enhance communication with patients and surrogates, including focusing on interests and alternatives rather than opposing positions and generating a wide range of options. Some hospitals have enacted "unilateral do not resuscitate (DNR)" policies to allow clinicians to provide a DNR order in cases in which consensus cannot be reached with families and medical opinion is that resuscitation would be futile if attempted. This type of a policy is not a replacement for careful and patient communication and negotiation but recognizes that agreement cannot always be reached. Over the last 15 years, many states, such as Texas, Virginia, Maryland, and California, have enacted so-called medical futility laws that provide physicians a "safe harbor" from liability if they refuse a patient or family's request for life-sustaining interventions. For instance, in Texas when a disagreement about terminating interventions between the medical team and the family has not been resolved by an ethics consultation, the hospital is supposed to try to facilitate transfer of the patient to an institution willing to provide treatment. If this fails after 10 days, the hospital and physician may unilaterally withdraw treatments determined to be futile. The family may appeal to a state court. Early data suggest that the law increases futility consultations for the ethics committee and that although most families concur with withdrawal, about 10–15% of families refuse to withdraw treatment. Approximately 12 cases have gone to court in Texas in the 7 years since the adoption of the law. As of 2007, there had been 974 ethics committee consultations on medical futility cases and 65 in which committees ruled against families and gave notice that treatment would be terminated. Treatment was withdrawn for 27 of those patients, and the remainder were transferred to other facilities or died while awaiting transfer.

EUTHANASIA AND PHYSICIAN-ASSISTED SUICIDE

Euthanasia and physician-assisted suicide are defined in Table 10-8. Terminating life-sustaining care and providing opioid medications to manage symptoms have long been considered ethical by the medical profession and legal by courts and should not be confused with euthanasia or physician-assisted suicide.

LEGAL ASPECTS Euthanasia is legal in the Netherlands, Belgium, and Luxembourg. It was legalized in the Northern Territory of Australia in 1995, but that legislation was repealed in 1997. Euthanasia is not legal in any state in the United States. With certain conditions, in Switzerland, a layperson can legally assist suicide. In the United States, physician-assisted suicide is legal in four states: Oregon, Vermont, and Washington State by legislation and Montana by court ruling. In jurisdictions where physician-assisted suicide is legal, physicians wishing to prescribe the necessary medication must fulfill multiple criteria and complete processes that include a waiting period. In other countries and all other states in the United States, physician-assisted suicide and euthanasia are illegal explicitly or by common law.

PRACTICES Fewer than 10–20% of terminally ill patients actually consider euthanasia and/or physician-assisted suicide for themselves. In the Netherlands and Oregon, >70% of patients using these interventions are dying of cancer; in Oregon, in 2013, just 1.2% of physician-assisted suicide cases involved patients with HIV/AIDS and 7.2% involved patients with amyotrophic lateral sclerosis. In the Netherlands, the share of deaths attributable to euthanasia or physician-assisted suicide declined from around 2.8% of all deaths in 2001 to around 1.8% in 2005. In 2013, the last year with complete data, around 71 patients in Oregon (just 0.2% of all deaths) died by physician-assisted suicide, although this may be an underestimate. In Washington State, between March 2009 (when the law allowing physician-assisted suicide went into force) and December 2009, 36 individuals died from prescribed lethal doses.

Pain is not a primary motivator for patients' requests for or interest in euthanasia and/or physician-assisted suicide. Fewer than 25% of all patients in Oregon cite inadequate pain control as the reason for desiring physician-assisted suicide. Depression, hopelessness, and, more profoundly, concerns about loss of dignity or autonomy or being a burden on family members appear to be primary factors motivating a desire for euthanasia or physician-assisted suicide. Over 75% cite loss of autonomy or dignity and inability to engage in enjoyable activities as the reason for wanting physician-assisted suicide. About 40% cite being a burden on family. A study from the Netherlands showed that depressed terminally ill cancer patients were four times more likely

TABLE 10-8 DEFINITIONS OF ASSISTED SUICIDE AND EUTHANASIA

Term	Definition	Legal Status
Voluntary active euthanasia	Intentionally administering medications or other interventions to cause the patient's death with the patient's informed consent	Netherlands, Belgium
Involuntary active euthanasia	Intentionally administering medications or other interventions to cause the patient's death when the patient was competent to consent but did not—e.g., the patient may not have been asked	Nowhere
Passive euthanasia	Withholding or withdrawing life-sustaining medical treatments from a patient to let him or her die (terminating life-sustaining treatments)	Everywhere
Physician-assisted suicide	A physician provides medications or other interventions to a patient with the understanding that the patient can use them to commit suicide	Oregon, Netherlands, Belgium, Switzerland

to request euthanasia and confirmed that uncontrolled pain was not associated with greater interest in euthanasia. Interestingly, despite the importance of emotional distress in motivating requests for euthanasia and physician-assisted suicide, few patients receive psychiatric care. For instance, in Oregon, only 5.9% of patients have been referred for psychiatric evaluation.

Euthanasia and physician-assisted suicide are no guarantee of a painless, quick death. Data from the Netherlands indicate that in as many as 20% of cases technical and other problems arose, including patients waking from coma, not becoming comatose, regurgitating medications, and experiencing a prolonged time to death. Data from Oregon indicate that between 1997 and 2013, 22 patients (~5%) regurgitated after taking prescribed medication, 1 patient awaked, and none experienced seizures. Problems were significantly more common in physician-assisted suicide, sometimes requiring the physician to intervene and provide euthanasia.

Whether practicing in a setting where euthanasia is legal or not, over a career, 12–54% of physicians receive a request for euthanasia or physician-assisted suicide from a patient. Competency in dealing with such a request is crucial. Although challenging, the request can also provide a chance to address intense suffering. After receiving a request for euthanasia and/or physician-assisted suicide, health care providers should carefully clarify the request with empathic, open-ended questions to help elucidate the underlying cause for the request, such as "What makes you want to consider this option?" Endorsing either moral opposition or moral support for the act tends to be counterproductive, giving an impression of being judgmental or of endorsing the idea that the patient's life is worthless. Health care providers must reassure the patient of continued care and commitment. The patient should be educated about alternative, less controversial options, such as symptom management and withdrawing any unwanted treatments and the reality of euthanasia and/or physician-assisted suicide, because the patient may have misconceptions about their effectiveness as well as the legal implications of the choice. Depression, hopelessness, and other symptoms of psychological distress as well as physical suffering and economic burdens are likely factors motivating the request, and such factors should be assessed and treated aggressively. After these interventions and clarification of options, most patients proceed with another approach, declining life-sustaining interventions, possibly including refusal of nutrition and hydration.

CARE DURING THE LAST HOURS

Most laypersons have limited experiences with the actual dying process and death. They frequently do not know what to expect of the final hours and afterward. The family and other caregivers must be prepared, especially if the plan is for the patient to die at home.

Patients in the last days of life typically experience extreme weakness and fatigue and become bedbound; this can lead to pressure sores. The issue of turning patients who are near the end of life, however, must be balanced against the potential discomfort that movement may cause. Patients stop eating and drinking with drying of mucosal membranes and dysphagia. Careful attention to oral swabbing, lubricants for lips, and use of artificial tears can provide a form of care to substitute for attempts at feeding the patient. With loss of the gag reflex and dysphagia, patients may also experience accumulation of oral secretions, producing noises during respiration sometimes called "the death rattle." Scopolamine can reduce the secretions. Patients also experience changes in respiration with periods of apnea or Cheyne-Stokes breathing. Decreased intravascular volume and cardiac output cause tachycardia, hypotension, peripheral coolness, and livedo reticularis (skin mottling). Patients can have urinary and, less frequently, fecal incontinence. Changes in consciousness and neurologic function generally lead to two different paths to death (Fig. 10-2).

Each of these terminal changes can cause patients and families distress, requiring reassurance and targeted interventions (Table 10-9). Informing families that these changes might occur and providing them with an information sheet can help preempt problems and minimize distress. Understanding that patients stop eating because they are dying, not dying because they have stopped eating, can reduce family and caregiver anxiety. Similarly, informing the family and caregivers that the "death rattle" may occur and that it is not indicative of suffocation, choking, or pain can reduce their worry from the breathing sounds.

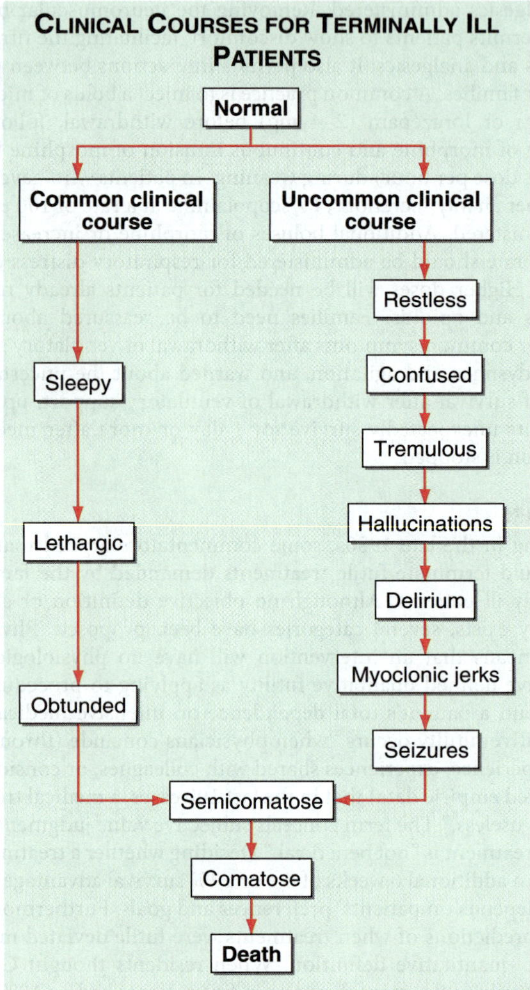

FIGURE 10-2 Common and uncommon clinical courses in the last days of terminally ill patients. *(Adapted from FD Ferris et al: Module 4: Palliative care, in Comprehensive Guide for the Care of Persons with HIV Disease. Toronto: Mt. Sinai Hospital and Casey Hospice, 1995, http://www.cpsonline.info/content/resources/hivmodule/module4complete.pdf.)*

Families and caregivers may also feel guilty about stopping treatments, fearing that they are "killing" the patient. This may lead to demands for interventions, such as feeding tubes, that may be ineffective. In such cases, the physician should remind the family and caregivers about the inevitability of events and the palliative goals. Interventions may prolong the dying process and cause discomfort. Physicians also should emphasize that withholding treatments is both legal and ethical and that the family members are not the cause of the patient's death. This reassurance may have to be provided multiple times.

Hearing and touch are said to be the last senses to stop functioning. Whether this is the case or not, families and caregivers can be encouraged to communicate with the dying patient. Encouraging them to talk directly to the patient, even if he or she is unconscious, and hold the patient's hand or demonstrate affection in other ways can be an effective way to channel their urge "to do something" for the patient.

When the plan is for the patient to die at home, the physician must inform the family and caregivers how to determine that the patient has died. The cardinal signs are cessation of cardiac function and respiration; the pupils become fixed; the body becomes cool; muscles relax; and incontinence may occur. Remind the family and caregivers that the eyes may remain open even after the patient has died because

TABLE 10-9 MANAGING CHANGES IN THE PATIENT'S CONDITION DURING THE FINAL DAYS AND HOURS

Changes in the Patient's Condition	Potential Complication	Family's Possible Reaction and Concern	Advice and Intervention
Profound fatigue	Bedbound with development of pressure ulcers that are prone to infection, malodor, and pain, and joint pain	Patient is lazy and giving up.	Reassure family and caregivers that terminal fatigue will not respond to interventions and should not be resisted. Use an air mattress if necessary.
Anorexia	None	Patient is giving up; patient will suffer from hunger and will starve to death.	Reassure family and caregivers that the patient is not eating because he or she is dying; not eating at the end of life does not cause suffering or death. Forced feeding, whether oral, parenteral, or enteral, does not reduce symptoms or prolong life.
Dehydration	Dry mucosal membranes (see below)	Patient will suffer from thirst and die of dehydration.	Reassure family and caregivers that dehydration at the end of life does not cause suffering because patients lose consciousness before any symptom distress. Intravenous hydration can worsen symptoms of dyspnea by pulmonary edema and peripheral edema as well as prolong dying process.
Dysphagia	Inability to swallow oral medications needed for palliative care		Do not force oral intake. Discontinue unnecessary medications that may have been continued, including antibiotics, diuretics, antidepressants, and laxatives. If swallowing pills is difficult, convert essential medications (analgesics, antiemetics, anxiolytics, and psychotropics) to oral solutions, buccal, sublingual, or rectal administration.
"Death rattle"—noisy breathing		Patient is choking and suffocating.	Reassure the family and caregivers that this is caused by secretions in the oropharynx and the patient is not choking. Reduce secretions with scopolamine (0.2–0.4 mg SC q4h or 1–3 patches q3d). Reposition patient to permit drainage of secretions. Do not suction. Suction can cause patient and family discomfort and is usually ineffective.
Apnea, Cheyne-Stokes respirations, dyspnea		Patient is suffocating.	Reassure family and caregivers that unconscious patients do not experience suffocation or air hunger. Apneic episodes are frequently a premorbid change. Opioids or anxiolytics may be used for dyspnea. Oxygen is unlikely to relieve dyspneic symptoms and may prolong the dying process.
Urinary or fecal incontinence	Skin breakdown if days until death Potential transmission of infectious agents to caregivers	Patient is dirty, malodorous, and physically repellent.	Remind family and caregivers to use universal precautions. Frequent changes of bedclothes and bedding. Use diapers, urinary catheter, or rectal tube if diarrhea or high urine output.
Agitation or delirium	Day/night reversal Hurt self or caregivers	Patient is in horrible pain and going to have a horrible death.	Reassure family and caregivers that agitation and delirium do not necessarily connote physical pain. Depending on the prognosis and goals of treatment, consider evaluating for causes of delirium and modify medications. Manage symptoms with haloperidol, chlorpromazine, diazepam, or midazolam.
Dry mucosal membranes	Cracked lips, mouth sores, and candidiasis can also cause pain. Odor	Patient may be malodorous or physically repellent.	Use baking soda mouthwash or saliva preparation q15–30min. Use topical nystatin for candidiasis. Coat lips and nasal mucosa with petroleum jelly q60–90min. Use ophthalmic lubricants q4h or artificial tears q30min.

the retroorbital fat pad may be depleted, permitting the orbit to fall posteriorly, which makes it difficult for the eyelids to cover the eyeball.

The physician should establish a plan for who the family or caregivers will contact when the patient is dying or has died. Without a plan, they may panic and call 911, unleashing a cascade of unwanted events, from arrival of emergency personnel and resuscitation to hospital admission. The family and caregivers should be instructed to contact the hospice (if one is involved), the covering physician, or the on-call member of the palliative care team. They should also be told that the medical examiner need not be called unless the state requires it for all deaths. Unless foul play is suspected, the health care team need not contact the medical examiner either.

Just after the patient dies, even the best-prepared family may experience shock and loss and be emotionally distraught. They need time to assimilate the event and be comforted. Health care providers are likely to find it meaningful to write a bereavement card or letter to the family. The purpose is to communicate about the patient, perhaps emphasizing the patient's virtues and the honor it was to care for the patient, and to express concern for the family's hardship. Some physicians attend the funerals of their patients. Although this is beyond any medical obligation, the presence of the physician can be a source of support to the grieving family and provides an opportunity for closure for the physician.

Death of a spouse is a strong predictor of poor health, and even mortality, for the surviving spouse. It may be important to alert the spouse's physician about the death so that he or she is aware of symptoms that might require professional attention.

PALLIATIVE CARE SERVICES: HOW AND WHERE

Determining the best approach to providing palliative care to patients will depend on patient preferences, the availability of caregivers and specialized services in close proximity, institutional resources, and reimbursement. Hospice is a leading, but not the only, model of palliative care services. In the United States, a plurality—41.5%—of hospice care is provided in residential homes. In 2012, just over 17% of hospice care was provided in nursing homes. In the United States, Medicare pays for hospice services under Part A, the hospital insurance part of reimbursement. Two physicians must certify that the patient has a prognosis of ≤6 months if the disease runs its usual course. Prognoses are probabilistic by their nature; patients are not required to die within 6 months but rather to have a condition from which half the individuals with it would not be alive within 6 months. Patients sign a hospice enrollment form that states their intent to forgo curative services related to their terminal illness, but they can still receive medical services for other comorbid conditions. Patients also can withdraw enrollment and reenroll later; the hospice Medicare benefit can be revoked later to secure traditional Medicare benefits. Payments to the hospice are per diem (or capitated), not fee-for-service. Payments are intended to cover physician services for the medical direction of the care team; regular home care visits by registered nurses and licensed practical nurses; home health aid and homemaker services; chaplain services; social work services; bereavement counseling; and medical equipment, supplies, and medications. No specific therapy is excluded, and the goal is for each therapy to be considered for its symptomatic (as opposed to disease-modifying) effect. Additional clinical care, including services of the primary physician, is covered by Medicare Part B even while the hospice Medicare benefit is in place. The health reform legislation signed into law in March 2010—the Affordable Care Act—directs the Secretary of Health and Human Services to gather data on Medicare hospice reimbursement with the goal of reforming payment rates to account for resource use over an entire episode of care. The legislation also requires additional evaluations and reviews of eligibility for hospice care by hospice physicians or nurses. Finally, the legislation establishes a demonstration project for concurrent hospice care in Medicare, which would test and evaluate allowing patients to remain eligible for regular Medicare during hospice care.

By 2012, the mean length of enrollment in a hospice was around 71.8 days, with the median being 18.7 days. Such short stays create barriers to establishing high-quality palliative services in patients' homes and also place financial strains on hospice providers because the initial assessments are resource intensive. Physicians should initiate early referrals to the hospice to allow more time for patients to receive palliative care.

Hospice care has been the main method in the United States for securing palliative services for terminally ill patients. However, efforts are being made to ensure continuity of palliative care across settings and through time. Palliative care services are becoming available as consultative services and more rarely as palliative care units in hospitals, in day care and other outpatient settings, and in nursing homes. Palliative care consultations for nonhospice patients can be billed as for other consultations under Medicare Part B, the physician reimbursement part. Many believe palliative care should be offered to patients regardless of their prognosis. A patient, his or her family, and physicians should not have to make a "curative versus palliative care" decision because it is rarely possible to make such a decisive switch to embracing mortality.

FUTURE DIRECTIONS

OUTCOME MEASURES

Care near the end of life cannot be measured by most of the available validated outcome measures because palliative care does not consider death a bad outcome. Similarly, the family and patients receiving end-of-life care may not desire the elements elicited in current quality-of-life measurements. Symptom control, enhanced family relationships, and quality of bereavement are difficult to measure and are rarely the primary focus of carefully developed or widely used outcome measures. Nevertheless, outcomes are as important in end-of-life care as in any other field of medical care. Specific end-of-life care instruments are being developed both for assessment, such as The Brief Hospice Inventory and NEST (*n*eeds near the *e*nd of life *s*creening *t*ool), and for outcome measures, such as the Palliative Care Outcomes Scale, as well as for prognosis, such as the Palliative Prognostic Index. The field of end-of-life care is entering an era of evidence-based practice and continuous improvement through clinical trials.

11 Clinical Problems of Aging

Luigi Ferrucci, Stephanie Studenski

While an in-depth understanding of internal medicine serves as a foundation, proper care of older adults should be complemented by insight into the multidimensional effects of aging on disease manifestations, consequences, and response to treatment. In younger adults, individual diseases tend to have a more distinct pathophysiology with well-defined risk factors; the same diseases in older persons may have a less distinct pathophysiology and are often the result of failed homeostatic mechanisms. Causes and clinical manifestations are less specific and can vary widely between individuals. Therefore, the care of older patients demands an understanding of the effects of aging on human physiology and a broader perspective that incorporates geriatric syndromes, disability, social contexts, and goals of care. For example, care planning for the older patient should account for the substantial portion of the wide variability in life expectancy across individuals of the same age that can be predicted by simple and inexpensive measures such as walking speed. Estimation of the expected remaining years of life can guide recommendations about appropriate preventive and other long-term interventions and can shape discussions about treatment alternatives.

DEMOGRAPHY

(See also Chap. 93e) Population aging emerged as a worldwide phenomenon for the first time in history within the past century. Since aging influences many facets of life, governments and societies—as well as families and communities—now face new social and economic challenges that affect health care. Fig. 11-1 highlights recent and predicted changes in U.S. population structure.

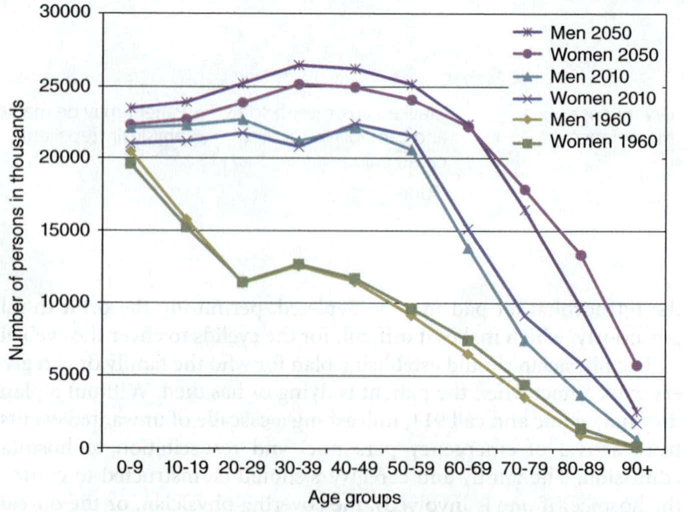

FIGURE 11-1 Change in the structure of the U.S. population between 1960 and 2050. *(From United Nations World Population Prospects: The 2008 Revision, http://www.un.org/esa/population/publications/wpp2008/wpp2008_highlights.pdf.)*

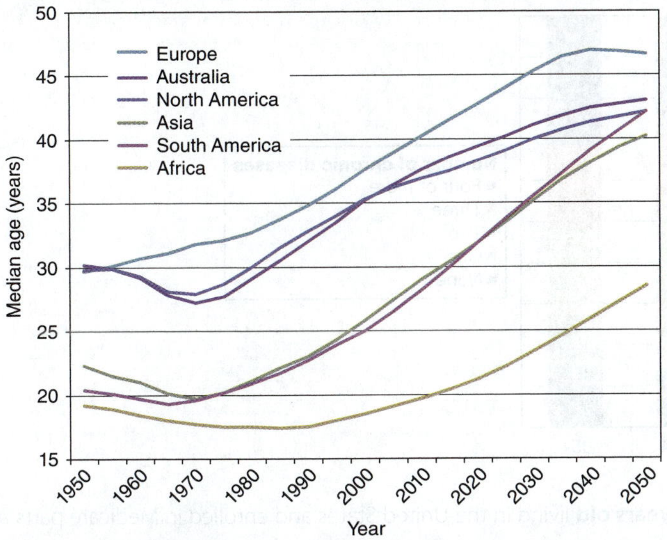

FIGURE 11-2 Population aging in different geographic regions. *(From United Nations World Population Prospects: The 2008 Revision, http://www.un.org/esa/population/publications/wpp2008/wpp2008_highlights.pdf.)*

The overall number of children has remained relatively stable, but explosive growth has occurred among older populations. The percentage of growth is particularly dramatic among the oldest of the old. For example, the number of persons aged 80–89 years more than tripled between 1960 and 2010 and will increase over tenfold between 1960 and 2050. Women already outlive men by many years, and the sex discrepancy in longevity is projected to increase further in the future.

Population aging occurs at different rates in varying geographic regions of the world. Over the past century, Europe, Australia, and North America have had the populations with the greatest proportions of older persons, but the populations of Asia and South America are aging rapidly, and the population structure on these continents will resemble that of "older" countries by around 2050 (Fig. 11-2). Among older persons, the oldest old (those >80 years of age) are the fastest-growing segment of the population (Fig. 11-3), and the pace of population aging is projected to accelerate in most countries over the next 50 years. There is no evidence that the rate of population aging is decreasing.

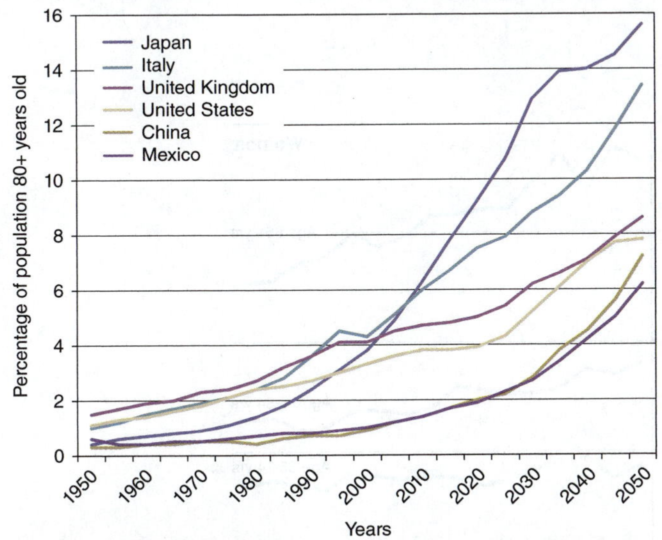

FIGURE 11-3 Percentage of the population age >80 years from 1950 to 2050 in representative nations. The pace of population aging will accelerate. *(From United Nations World Population Prospects: The 2008 Revision, http://www.un.org/esa/population/publications/wpp2008/wpp2008_highlights.pdf.)*

POPULATION AGING AND HEALTH

Many chronic diseases increase in prevalence with age. It is not unusual for older persons to have multiple chronic diseases (Fig. 11-4), although some seem more susceptible than others to co-occurring problems. Functional problems that pose difficulties or require help in performing basic activities of daily living (ADLs) (Table 11-1) increase with age and are more common among women than among men. In recent decades, the age-specific prevalence of disability has declined, especially in the oldest old. Estimated rates are shown in Fig. 11-5 as the percentage of persons who reported severe difficulty or needed help in bathing, and data on other basic ADLs show similar trends. Although the age-specific prevalence of disability is decreasing, the magnitude of this decline is small compared to the overwhelming effect of population aging. Thus, the number of people with disability in the United States and other countries is rapidly expanding. Rates of cognitive impairments, such as memory problems, also increase with aging (Fig. 11-6). Chronic disease and disability lead to increased use of health care resources. Health care expenditures increase with age, increase more with disability, and are highest in the last year of life. However, new medical technologies and expensive medications are greater influences on health care costs than population aging itself. General practitioners and internists with little specific training in geriatric medicine provide the bulk of care for older persons.

SYSTEMIC EFFECTS OF AGING

Systemic consequences of aging are widespread but can be clustered into four main domains or processes (Fig. 11-7): (1) body composition; (2) balance between energy availability and energy demand; (3) signaling networks that maintain homeostasis; and (4) neurodegeneration. Each domain can be assessed with routine clinical tests, although more detailed research techniques are also available (Table 11-2).

Body Composition Profound changes in body composition may be the most evident and inescapable effect of aging (Fig. 11-8). Over the life span, body weight tends to increase through childhood, puberty, and adulthood until late middle age. Weight tends to decline in men between ages 65 and 70 years and in women somewhat later. Lean body mass, composed predominantly of muscle and visceral organs, decreases steadily after the third decade. In muscle, this atrophy is greater in fast-twitch than in slow-twitch fibers. The origin of this change is unknown, but several lines of evidence suggest that progressive loss of motor neurons probably plays an important role. Fat mass tends to increase in middle age and then declines in late life, reflecting the trajectory of weight change. Waist circumference continues to increase across the life span, a pattern suggesting that visceral fat, which is responsible for most of the pathologic consequences of obesity, continues to accumulate. In some individuals, fat also accumulates inside muscle, affecting muscle quality and function. With age, fibroconnective tissue tends to increase in many organ systems. In muscle, fibroconnective tissue buildup also affects muscle quality and function. In combination, the loss of muscle mass and quality result in reduced muscle strength, which ultimately affects functional capacity and mobility. Muscle strength declines with aging; this decrease not only affects functional status but also is a strong independent predictor of mortality (Fig. 11-9). Progressive demineralization and architectural modification occur in bone, resulting in a decline of bone strength. Loss of bone strength increases the risk of fracture. Sex differences in the effects of aging on bone mass are due to differences in peak bone mass and the effects of gonadal hormones on bone. Overall, compared with men, women tend to lose bone mass at a younger age and more quickly reach the threshold of low bone strength that increases fracture risk.

All of these changes in body composition can be attributed to disruptions in the links between synthesis, degradation, and repair that normally serve to remodel tissues. Such changes in body composition are influenced not only by aging and illness but also by lifestyle factors such as physical activity and diet. Body composition can be approximated in clinical practice on the basis of weight, height, body mass index (BMI; weight in kilograms divided by height in meters squared), and waist circumference or, more precisely, with dual-energy x-ray

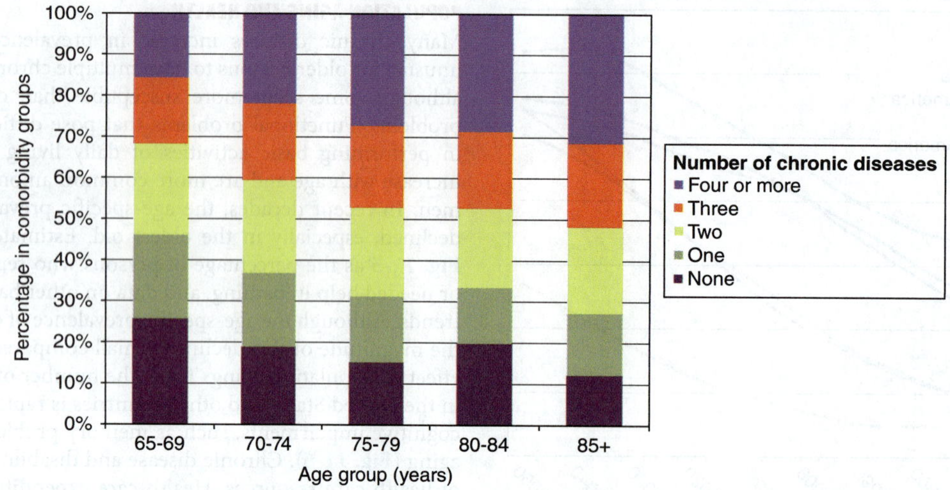

FIGURE 11-4 Prevalence of comorbidity by age group in persons ≥65 years old living in the United States and enrolled in Medicare parts A and B in 1999. *(From JL Wolff et al: Arch Intern Med 162:2269, 2002.)*

TABLE 11-1 BASIC AND INSTRUMENTAL ACTIVITIES OF DAILY LIVING

***Basic* Activities of Daily Living: Self-Care Tasks**
• Personal hygiene
• Dressing and undressing
• Eating
• Transferring from bed to chair and back
• Voluntarily controlling urinary and fecal discharge
• Using the toilet
• Moving around (as opposed to being bedridden)
***Instrumental* Activities of Daily Living: Not Necessary for Fundamental Functioning, but Permit an Individual to Live Independently in a Community**
• Doing light housework
• Preparing meals
• Taking medications
• Shopping for groceries or clothes
• Using the telephone
• Managing money
• Using technology[a]

[a]With the recognition that older persons may not be that technologically savvy since they were not as extensively exposed to technology during their lifetime.

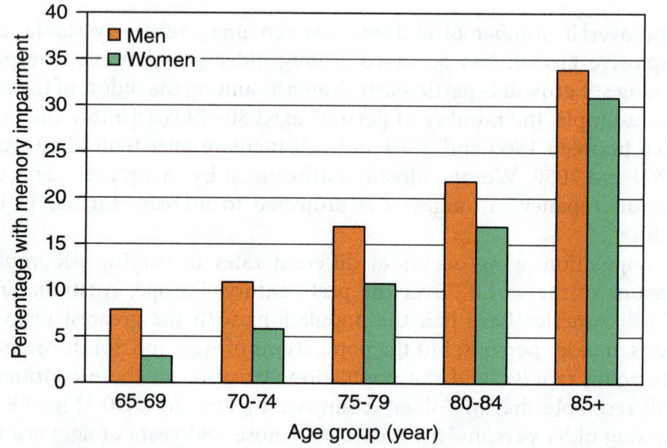

FIGURE 11-6 Rates of memory impairment in different age groups. The definition of "moderate or severe memory impairment" is 4 or fewer words recalled out of 20. *(Source: Health and Retirement Survey. Accessed November 15, 2013, at aoa.gov/agingstatsdotnet/Main_Site/Data/2000_Documents/healthstatus.aspx.)*

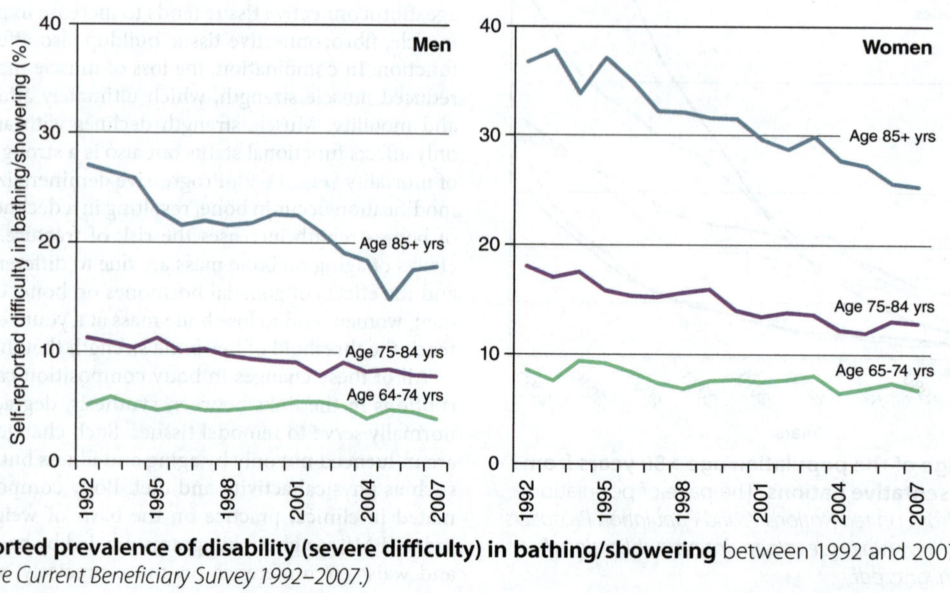

FIGURE 11-5 Self-reported prevalence of disability (severe difficulty) in bathing/showering between 1992 and 2007, according to age and sex.) *(From Medicare Current Beneficiary Survey 1992–2007.)*

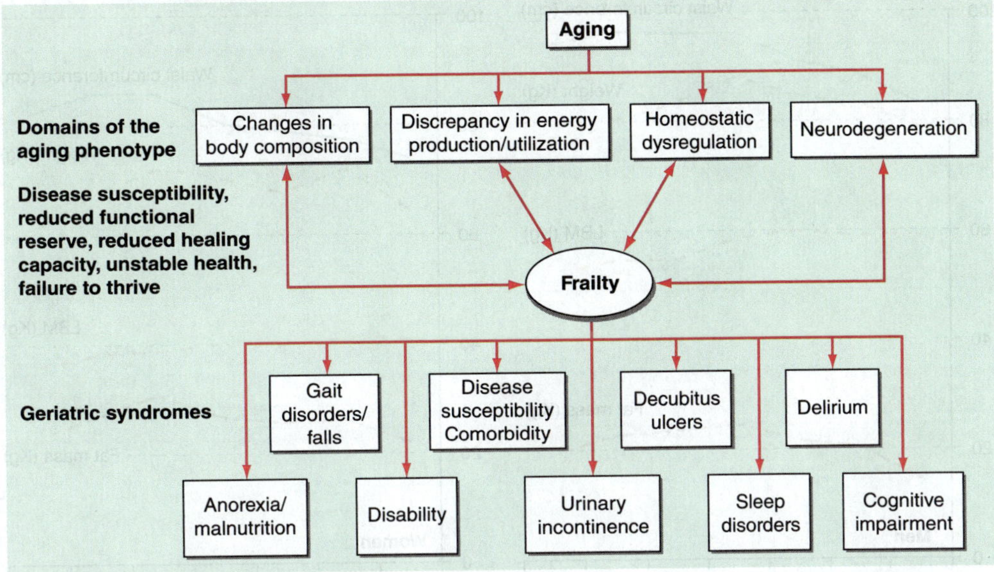

FIGURE 11-7 **A unifying model of aging, frailty, and the geriatric syndromes.**

absorptiometry, CT, or MRI. In healthy men and women in their twenties, lean body mass is, on average, 85% of body weight, with roughly 50% of lean mass represented by skeletal muscle. With aging, both the percentage of lean mass and the percentage represented by muscle decline rapidly, and these changes have important health and functional consequences.

Balance Between Energy Availability and Energy Demand Release of phosphate from ATP provides every living cell with the energy required for life. However, the storage of ATP is only enough for 6 sec; therefore, ATP is constantly resynthesized. Although ATP can be resynthesized by anaerobic glycolysis, most of the energy used in the body is generated through aerobic metabolism. Therefore, energy consumption is usually estimated indirectly by oxygen consumption (indirect calorimetry). There is currently no method to measure true "fitness," which is the maximal energy that can be produced by an organism over extended periods. Thus, fitness is estimated indirectly from peak oxygen consumption ($MVo_{2\ peak}$), often during a maximal treadmill test. Longitudinal studies have demonstrated that $MVo_{2\ peak}$ declines progressively with aging (Fig. 11-10), and the rate of decline is accelerated in persons who are sedentary and in those affected by chronic diseases.

A large portion of energy is consumed as the "resting metabolic rate" (RMR)—i.e., the amount of energy expended at rest in a neutral temperature environment and in a postabsorptive state. In healthy men and women, RMR declines with aging, and such decline is only partially explained by the parallel decline in the highly metabolically active tissues that make up lean body mass (Fig. 11-11). However, persons with unstable homeostasis due to illness require additional

TABLE 11-2 **EXAMPLES OF ASSESSMENT OF THE FOUR DOMAINS OF THE AGING PHENOTYPE**

Approach to Assessment	Body Composition	Energetics	Homeostatic Regulation	Neurodegeneration
Self-report		Self-reported questionnaires investigating physical activity, sense of fatigue/exhaustion, exercise tolerance		
Physical examination	Muscle strength testing (isometric and isokinetic) Anthropometrics (weight, height, BMI, waist circumference, arm and leg circumference, skin folds)	Performance-based tests of physical function		Objective assessment of gait, balance, reaction time, coordination Standard neurologic exam, including assessment of global cognition[a]
Laboratory values	Biomarkers (24-h creatinuria or 3-methyl-histidine)		Nutritional biomarkers (e.g., vitamins, antioxidants) Baseline levels of biomarkers and hormone levels Inflammatory markers (e.g., ESR, CRP, IL-6, TNF-α)	
Imaging	CT and MRI, DEXA	Magnetic resonance spectroscopy		MRI, fMRI, PET, and other dynamic imaging techniques
Other	Hydrostatic weighing	Resting metabolic rate Treadmill testing of oxygen consumption during walking Objective measures of physical activity (accelerometers, double-labeled water)	Stress response Response to provocative tests, such as oral glucose tolerance test, dexamethasone test, and others	Evoked potentials Electroneurography and electromyography

[a]Mini Mental State; Montreal Cognitive Assessment.

Abbreviations: BMI, body mass index; CRP, C-reactive protein; DEXA, dual-energy x-ray absorptiometry; ESR, erythrocyte sedimentation rate; fMRI, functional MRI; IL-6, interleukin 6; PET, positron emission tomography; TNFα, tumor necrosis factor α.

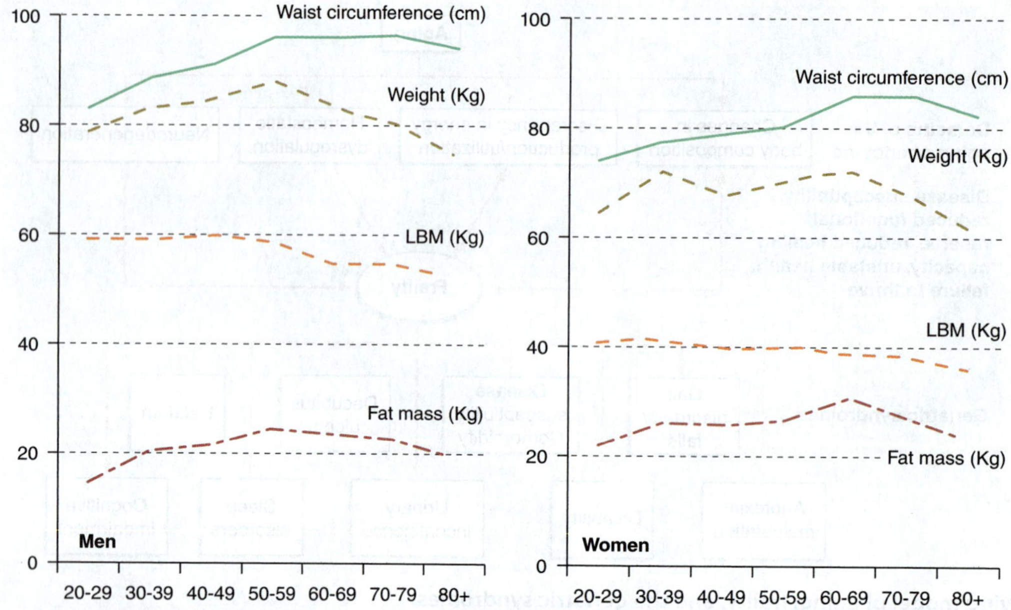

FIGURE 11-8 Longitudinal changes of weight, body composition, and waist circumference over the life span, estimated in 1167 participants in the Baltimore Longitudinal Study of Aging. Lean body mass (LBM) and fat mass were estimated with dual-energy x-ray absorptiometry. *(Source: The Baltimore Longitudinal study of Aging 2010; unpublished data.)*

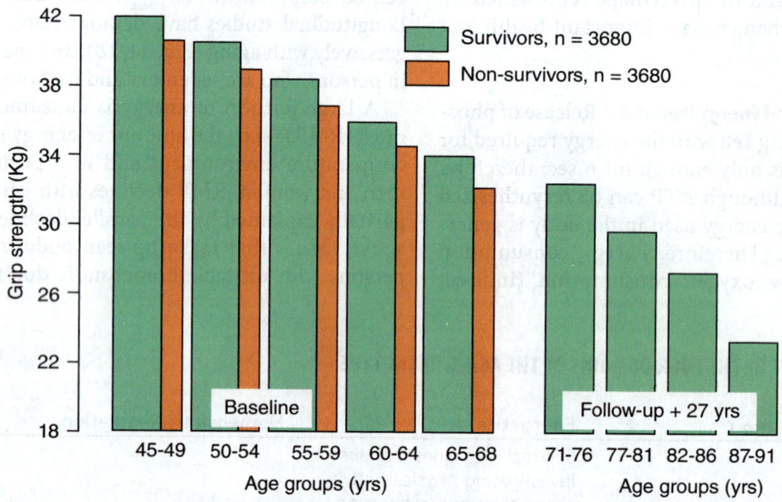

FIGURE 11-9 Cross-sectional differences and longitudinal changes in muscle strength over a 27-year follow-up. Note that persons who died during the follow-up had lower baseline muscle strength. *(From T Rantanen et al: J Appl Physiol 85:2047, 1998.)*

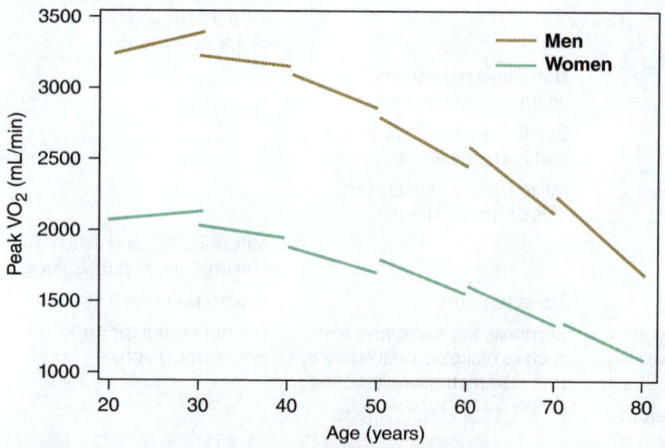

FIGURE 11-10 Longitudinal changes in aerobic capacity in participants in the Baltimore Longitudinal Study of Aging. *(From JL Fleg: Circulation 112:674, 2005.)*

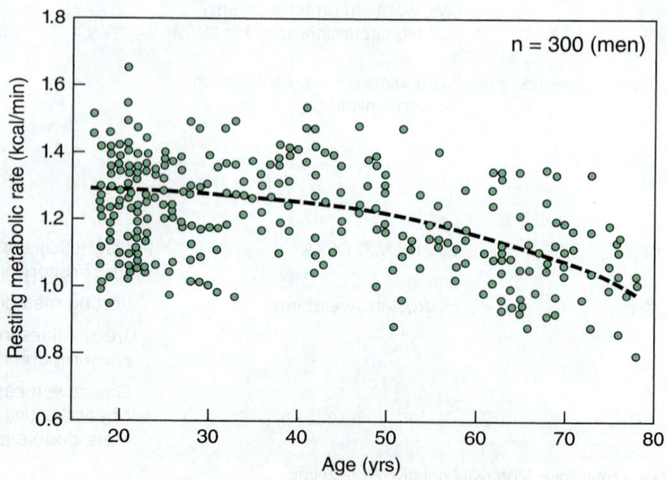

FIGURE 11-11 Changes in resting metabolic rate with aging. *(Unpublished data from the Baltimore Longitudinal Study of Aging.)*

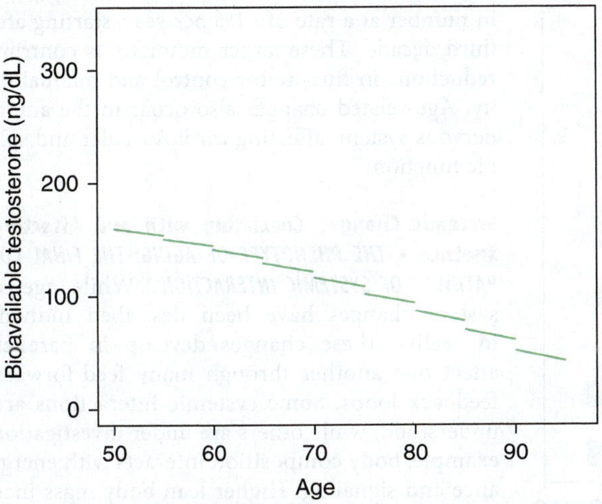

FIGURE 11-12 Longitudinal trajectory of bioavailable testosterone plasma concentration in the Baltimore Longitudinal Study of Aging (BLSA). The plot is based on 584 men who were 50 years or older with a total of 1455 data points. The average follow up for each subject was 3.2 years. *(Figure created using unpublished data from the BLSA.)*

energy for compensatory mechanisms. Indeed, observational studies have demonstrated (1) that older persons with poor health status and substantial morbidity have a higher RMR than healthier individuals of the same age and sex and (2) that a high RMR is an independent risk factor for mortality and may contribute to the weight loss that often accompanies severe illness. Finally, for reasons that are not yet completely clear but certainly involve changes in the biomechanical characteristics of movement, older age, pathology, and physical impairment increase the energy cost of motor activities such as walking. Overall, older individuals with multiple chronic conditions have low available energy levels and require more energy both at rest and during physical activity. Thus, sick older people may consume all their available energy performing the most basic ADLs, and consequent fatigue and restriction may lead to a sedentary existence. Energy status can be assessed clinically by simply asking patients about their perceived level of fatigue during daily activities such as walking or dressing. Energy capacity can be assessed more precisely by exercise tolerance during a walking test or a treadmill test coupled with spirometry.

The main signaling pathways that control homeostasis involve hormones, inflammatory mediators, and antioxidants; all are profoundly affected by aging. Sex hormone levels, such as testosterone in men (Fig. 11-12) and estrogen in women, decrease with age, while other hormone systems may change more subtly (Table 11-3). Most aging individuals, even those who remain healthy and fully functional, tend to develop a mild proinflammatory state characterized by high levels of proinflammatory markers, including interleukin 6 (IL-6) and C-reactive protein (CRP) (Fig. 11-13). Aging is also thought to be associated with increased oxidative stress damage, either because the production of reactive oxygen species increases or because antioxidant buffers are less effective. Since hormones, inflammatory markers, and antioxidants are integrated into complex signaling networks, levels of individual biomarkers may well reflect adaptation within homeostatic feedback loops rather than true causative factors. Thus, the therapeutic strategy of single-molecule replacement may be ineffective or even counterproductive. The presence of such signaling networks and feedback loops may help explain why single-hormone "replacement therapy" for problems of aging has demonstrated little benefit. The focus of research in this area is now on multiple-hormone

TABLE 11-3 HORMONES THAT DECREASE, REMAIN STABLE, AND INCREASE WITH AGING

Decrease	No Change	Increase
Growth hormone	Prolactin	Cholecystokinin
Luteinizing hormone (men)	Thyrotropin	Luteinizing hormone (women)
Insulin growth factor 1	Thyroid hormones	Follicle-stimulating hormone
Testosterone	Epinephrine	Cortisol
Estradiol	Glucagon-like peptide 1	Prolactin
Dehydroepiandrosterone	Gastric inhibitory polypeptide	Norepinephrine
Pregnenolone		Insulin
25-Hydroxyvitamin D		Parathormone
Aldosterone		
Vasoactive intestinal peptide		
Melatonin		

dysregulation. For example, taken one at a time, levels of testosterone, dehydroepiandrosterone (DHEA), and insulin-like growth factor 1 (IGF-1) do not predict mortality, but in combination they are highly predictive of longevity. This combination effect is especially strong in the setting of congestive heart failure. Similarly, several micronutrients, such as vitamins (especially vitamin D), minerals (selenium and magnesium), and antioxidants (vitamins D and E), also regulate aspects of metabolism. Low levels of these micronutrients have been associated with accelerated aging and a high risk of adverse outcomes. However, except for vitamin D, no clear evidence suggests that supplementation has positive effects on health. Unfortunately, no standard criteria exist that allow the detection and quantification of homeostatic dysregulation as a general phenomenon.

Neurodegeneration It was long generally believed that neurons stop reproducing shortly after birth and that their number declines throughout life. However, results from animal models and even some studies in humans suggest that neurogenesis in the hippocampus continues at low levels throughout life. Brain atrophy occurs with aging after the age of 60 years. Atrophy proceeds at varying rates in different parts of the brain (Fig. 11-14) and is often accompanied by an inflammatory response and microglial activation. Age-associated brain atrophy may contribute to age-related declines in cognitive and motor function. Atrophy may also be a factor in some brain diseases that can occur with aging, such as mild cognitive impairment, in which persons have mild but detectable impairments on tests of cognition but no severe disability in daily activities. In mild cognitive impairment, atrophy has been found mostly in the prefrontal cortex and hippocampus,

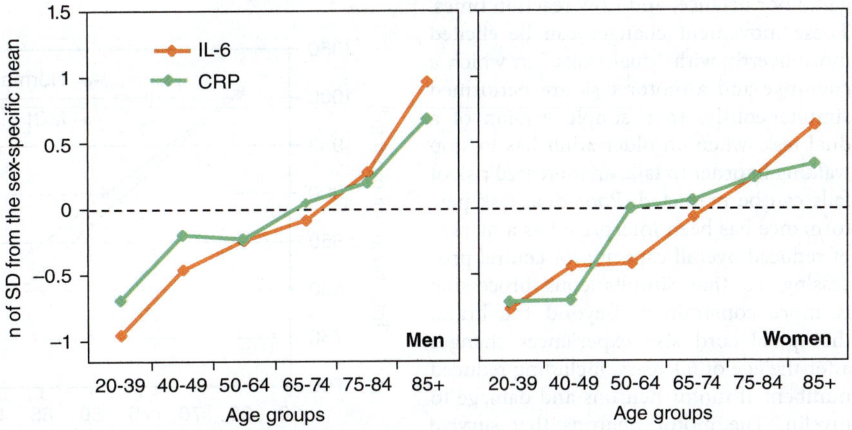

FIGURE 11-13 Change in interleukin 6 (IL-6) and C-reactive protein (CRP) with aging. Values are expressed as Z-scores to make them comparable. *(From L Ferrucci et al: Blood 105:2294, 2005.)*

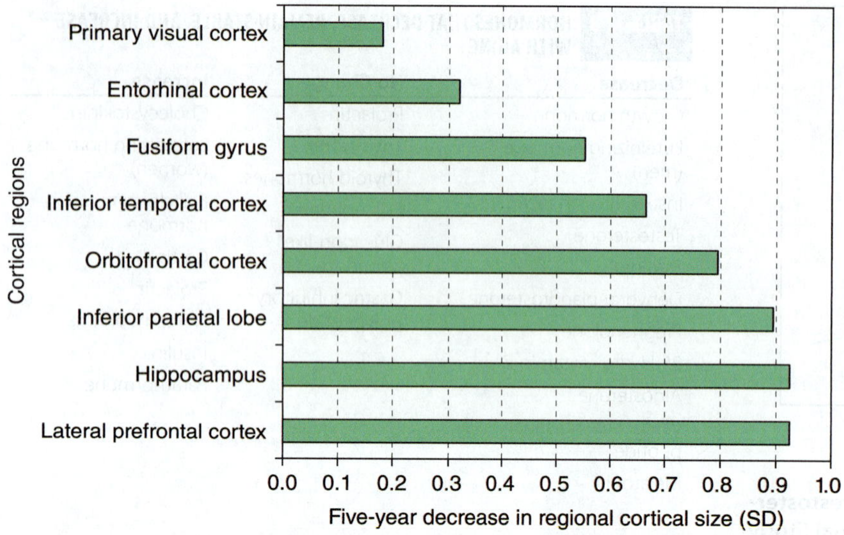

FIGURE 11-14 Five-year decline in mean volumes of different brain regions, measured in standard deviation (SD) units (Cohen's *d*). The primary visual cortex shows the least average shrinkage, and the prefrontal and inferior parietal cortex and hippocampus show the most average shrinkage. *(From N Raz et al: Ann N Y Acad Sci 1097:84, 2007.)*

but these findings are not specific and their diagnostic utility is unclear (Fig. 11-15). Other neurophysiologic changes in the brain frequently occur with aging and may contribute to cognitive decline. Functional imaging studies have shown that some older people have diminished coordination between the brain regions responsible for higher-order cognitive functions and that such diminished coordination is correlated with poor cognitive performance. In young healthy individuals, the brain activity associated with executive cognitive functions (e.g., problem-solving, decision-making) is very well localized; in contrast, in healthy older individuals, the pattern of cortical activation is more diffuse. Brain pathology has typically been associated with specific diseases; amyloid plaques and neurofibrillary tangles are considered the pathologic hallmarks of Alzheimer's disease. However, these pathologic markers have been found at autopsy in many older individuals who had normal cognition, as assessed by extensive testing in the year before death.

Taken together, trends in brain changes with aging suggest that some neurophysiologic manifestations are compensatory adaptations rather than primary contributors to age-related declines. Because the brain is capable of reorganization and compensation, extensive neurodegeneration may not be clinically evident. Therefore, early detection requires careful testing. Clinically, cortical and subcortical changes are reflected in the high prevalence of "soft," nonspecific neurologic signs, often reflected in slow and unstable gait, poor balance, and slow reaction times. These movement changes can be elicited more overtly with "dual tasks," in which a cognitive and a motor task are performed simultaneously. In a simple version of a dual task, when an older adult has to stop walking in order to talk, an increased risk of falls can be predicted. Poor dual-task performance has been interpreted as a marker of reduced overall capacity for central processing, so that simultaneous processing is more constrained. Beyond the brain, the spinal cord also experiences changes after the age of 60 years, including reduced numbers of motor neurons and damage to myelin. The motor neurons that survive compensate by increased branching complexity and by service to larger motor units. As motor units become larger, they decline in number at a rate of ~1% per year, starting after the third decade. These larger motor units contribute to reductions in fine-motor control and manual dexterity. Age-related changes also occur in the autonomic nervous system, affecting cardiovascular and splanchnic function.

Systemic Changes Coexisting with and Affecting One Another • ***THE PHENOTYPE OF AGING: THE FINAL COMMON PATHWAY OF SYSTEMIC INTERACTION*** While age-related system changes have been described individually, in reality, these changes develop in parallel and affect one another through many feed-forward and feedback loops. Some systemic interactions are well understood, while others are under investigation. For example, body composition interacts with energy balance and signaling. Higher lean body mass increases energy consumption and improves insulin sensitivity and carbohydrate metabolism. Higher fat mass, especially visceral fat mass, is the culprit in the metabolic syndrome and is associated with low testosterone levels, high sex hormone–binding globulin levels, and increased levels of proinflammatory markers such as CRP and IL-6. Altered signaling can affect neurodegeneration; insulin resistance and adipokines such as leptin and adiponectin are associated with declines in cognitive function. Combined with loss of motor neurons and dysfunction of the motor unit, a state of inflammation and reduced levels of testosterone and IGF-1 have been linked to accelerated decline of muscle mass and strength. Normal intersystem coordination is also affected by aging. The hypothalamus normally functions as a central regulator of metabolism and energy use and coordinates physiologic responses of the entire organism through hormonal signaling; aging-related changes in the hypothalamus alter this control. The central nervous system (CNS) also controls adaptive sympathetic/parasympathetic activity, so that age-related CNS degeneration may have implications for autonomic function.

The phenotype that results from the aging process is characterized by increased susceptibility to diseases, high risk of multiple coexisting diseases, impaired response to stress (including limited ability to heal or recover after an acute disease), emergence of "geriatric syndromes" (characterized by stereotyped clinical manifestations but multifactorial causes), altered response to treatment, high risk of disability, and loss of personal autonomy with all its psychological and social consequences. In addition, these key aging processes may interfere with the typical pathophysiology of specific diseases, thereby altering expected clinical manifestations and confounding diagnosis. Clinically, patients may present with obvious problems within only one of these domains, but, since systems interact, all four main domains should be evaluated

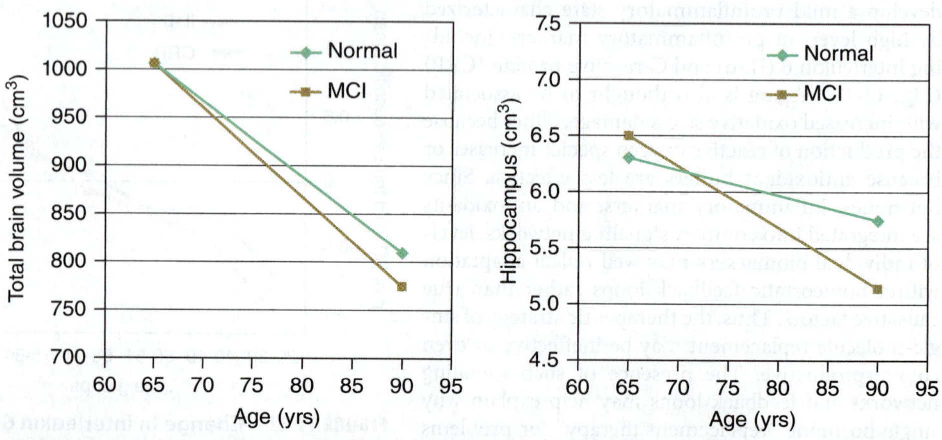

FIGURE 11-15 Longitudinal changes of regional brain volumes in normal aging and mild cognitive impairment (MCI). *(From I Driscoll et al: Neurology 72:1906, 2009.)*

and considered potential therapeutic targets. When patients present with obvious problems in multiple main systems affected by aging, they tend toward extreme degrees of susceptibility and loss of resilience, a condition that is globally referred to as *frailty*.

BIOLOGIC UNDERPINNINGS OF THE DOMAINS OF THE AGING PHENOTYPE The changes that occur with aging encompass multiple physiologic systems. Although they are often described in isolation, they are likely attributable to the progressive dysfunction of a unique mechanism that affects some fundamental housekeeping mechanism of cellular physiology. An important goal of future research is to connect the aging phenotype in humans to theories of aging that have largely been developed from studies in cell or animal models. If the main theories of aging could be operationalized into assessments that are feasible in humans, it would be possible to test the hypothesis that some of these processes are correlated with all the domains of the aging phenotype, above and beyond chronologic age. Review of the biologic theories (hallmarks) of aging provides an excellent template for a working hypothesis that, at least theoretically, could be tested in longitudinal studies. Candidate mechanisms of mammalian aging include genomic instability, telomere attrition, epigenetic alterations, loss of proteostasis, deregulated nutrient sensing, mitochondrial dysfunction, cellular senescence, stem cell exhaustion, and altered intercellular communication.

Frailty Frailty has been described as a physiologic syndrome that is characterized by decreased reserve and diminished resistance to stressors, that results from cumulative decline across multiple physiologic systems, and that causes vulnerability to adverse outcomes and a high risk of death. A proposed "phenotype" definition characterized by weight loss, fatigue, impaired grip strength, diminished physical activity, and slow gait has shown good internal consistency and strong predictive validity and has been used in many clinical and epidemiologic studies. An alternative approach, the Frailty Index, assesses cumulative physiologic and functional burden. When combined with a structured clinical assessment (the Comprehensive Geriatric Assessment), the Frailty Index can be applied in clinical settings and has low rates of missing data; it predicts survival in community-dwelling older people as well as survival, length of stay and discharge location in acute-care settings. Regardless of the definition, an extensive body of literature shows that older persons who are considered frail by any definition have overt changes in the same four main processes: body composition, homeostatic dysregulation, energetic failure, and neurodegeneration—the characteristics of the aging phenotype. A classic clinical case would be an older woman with sarcopenic obesity characterized by increased body fat and decreased muscle (body composition changes); extremely low exercise tolerance and extreme fatigue (energetic failure); high insulin levels, low IGF-1 levels, inadequate intake of calories, and low levels of vitamins D and E and carotenoids (signal dysregulation); and memory problems, slow gait, and unstable balance (neurodegeneration). This woman is likely to exhibit all the manifestations of frailty, including a high risk of multiple diseases, disability, urinary incontinence, falls, delirium, depression, and other geriatric syndromes. It is expected that the biologic process underlying a particular "aging theory" would be more advanced in this woman than would be expected on the basis of chronologic age.

A goal of future research in geriatric medicine that has strong potential for clinical translation is to demonstrate that the hypothetical patient described above is biologically older, according to some robust biomarkers of biologic aging, than would be estimated from chronologic age alone. Conceptualizing frailty through the four main underlying processes is a step in this direction that stems from accumulated evidence and recognizes the heterogeneity and dynamic nature of the aging phenotype. Aging is universal but proceeds at highly variable rates, with wide heterogeneity in the emergence of the aging phenotype. Thus, the question is not whether an older patient is frail, but rather whether the severity of frailty is beyond the threshold of clinical and behavioral relevance. Understanding frailty through the lens of four interacting underlying processes also provides an interface with diseases that, like aging itself, affect the aging phenotype. For example, congestive heart failure is associated with low energy availability, multiple hormonal derangements, and a proinflammatory state, thereby contributing to frailty severity. Parkinson's disease provides an example of neurodegeneration that, in an advanced state, affects body composition, energy metabolism, and homeostatic signaling, resulting in a syndrome that closely resembles frailty. Diabetes is especially important to aging and frailty because it harms body composition, energy metabolism, homeostatic dysregulation, and neuronal integrity. Accordingly, a number of studies have found that type 2 diabetes is a strong risk factor for frailty and for many of its consequences. Since disease and aging interact, careful and appropriate treatment of disease is critical to prevent or reduce frailty.

CONSEQUENCES OF AGING PROCESSES, THE AGING PHENOTYPE, AND FRAILTY

While the pathophysiology of frailty is still being elucidated, its consequences have been well characterized in prospective studies. Four main consequences are important for clinical practice: (1) ineffective or incomplete homeostatic response to stress, (2) multiple coexisting diseases (multi- or comorbidity) and polypharmacy, (3) physical disability, and (4) the so-called geriatric syndromes. We will briefly address each one of these consequences.

Low Resistance to Stress Frailty can be considered a progressive loss of reserve in multiple physiologic functions. At an early stage and in the absence of stress, mildly frail older individuals may appear to be normal. However, they have reduced ability to cope with challenges, such as acute diseases, traumas, surgical procedures, or chemotherapy. Acute illness involving a hospital stay is associated with undernutrition and inactivity, which sometimes may be of such magnitude that the residual muscle mass fails to meet the minimal requirement for walking. Even when nutrition is reinstated, energy reserves may be insufficient to adequately rebuild muscle mass. Older persons have a reduced ability to tolerate infections, in part because they are less able than younger people to build a dynamic inflammatory response to vaccination or infectious exposure; thus, infections are more likely to become severe and systemic and to resolve more slowly. In the context of tolerance to stress, assessing aspects of frailty can help estimate the individual's ability to withstand the rigors of aggressive treatments and to respond to interventions aimed at infection as well as the caregiver's ability to anticipate and prevent complications of hospitalization and generally to estimate prognosis. Accordingly, treatment plans may be adjusted to improve tolerance and safety; bed rest and hospitalization should be used sparingly; and infections should be prevented, anticipated, and managed assertively.

Comorbidity and Polypharmacy Older age is associated with high rates of many chronic diseases (Fig. 11-4). Thus, not unexpectedly, the percentage of individuals affected by multiple medical conditions (co- or multimorbidity) also increases with age. In frail older individuals, comorbidity occurs at higher rates than would be expected from the combined probability of the component conditions. It is likely that frailty and comorbidity affect each other, so that multiple diseases contribute to frailty and frailty increases susceptibility to diseases.

Clinically, patients with multiple conditions present unique diagnostic and treatment challenges. Standard diagnostic criteria may not be informative because there are additional confusing signs and symptoms. A classic example is the coexistence of deficiencies in iron and vitamin B_{12}, creating an apparently normocytic anemia. The risk/benefit ratio for many medical and surgical treatment options may be reduced in the face of other diseases. Drug treatment planning is made more complex because comorbid diseases may affect the absorption, volume of distribution, protein binding, and, especially, elimination of many drugs, leading to fluctuation in therapeutic levels and increased risk of under- or overdosing. Drug excretion is affected by renal and hepatic changes with aging that may not be detectable with the usual clinical tests. Formulas for estimating glomerular filtration rate in older patients are available, whereas the estimation of changes in hepatic excretion remains a challenge.

Patients with many diseases are usually prescribed multiple drugs, especially when they are cared for by multiple specialists who do not communicate. The risk of adverse drug reactions, drug–drug interactions, and poor compliance increases geometrically with the number of drugs prescribed and with the severity of frailty. Some general rules to minimize the chances of adverse drug events are as follows: (1) Always ask patients to bring in all medications, including prescription drugs, over-the-counter products, vitamin supplements, and herbal preparations (the "brown bag test"). (2) Screen for unnecessary drugs; those without a clear indication should be discontinued. (3) Simplify the regimen in terms of number of agents and schedules, try to avoid frequent changes, and use single-daily-dose regimens whenever possible. (4) Avoid drugs that are expensive or not covered by insurance whenever possible. (5) Minimize the number of drugs to those that are absolutely essential, and always check for possible interactions. (6) Make sure that the patient or an available caregiver understands the administered regimen, and provide legible written instructions. (7) Schedule periodic medication reviews.

Disability and Impaired Recovery from Acute-Onset Disability The prevalence of disability in self-care and home management increases steeply with aging and tends to be higher among women than among men (Fig. 11-5). Physical and cognitive function in older persons reflects overall health status and predicts health care utilization, institutionalization, and mortality more accurately than any other known biomedical measure. Thus, assessment of function and disability and prediction of the risk of disability are cornerstones of geriatric medicine. Frailty, regardless of the criteria used for its definition, is a robust and powerful risk factor for disability. Because of this strong relationship, measures of physical function and mobility have been proposed as standard criteria for frailty. However, disability occurs late in the frailty process, after reserve and compensation are exhausted. Early in the development of frailty, body composition changes, reductions in fitness, homeostatic deregulation, and neurodegeneration can begin without affecting daily function. As opposed to disability in younger persons, in which the rule is to look for a clear dominant cause, disability in frail older persons is almost always multifactorial. Multiple disrupted aging processes are usually involved, even when the precipitating cause seems unique. Excess fat mass, poor muscle strength, reduced lean body mass, poor fitness, reduced energy efficiency, poor nutritional intake, low circulating levels of antioxidant micronutrients, high levels of proinflammatory markers, objective signs of neurologic dysfunction, and cognitive impairment all contribute to disability. The multifactorial nature of disability in frail older persons reduces the capacity for compensation and interferes with functional recovery. For example, a small lacunar stroke that causes problems with balance in a young hypertensive individual can be overcome by standing and walking with the feet further apart, a strategy that requires brain adaptation, strong muscles, and a high energy capacity. The same small lacunar stroke may cause catastrophic disability in an older person already affected by neurodegeneration and weakness, who is less able to compensate. As a consequence, interventions aimed at preventing and reducing disability in older persons should have a dual focus on both the precipitating cause and the systems needed for compensation. In the case of the lacunar stroke, interventions to promote mobility function might include stroke prevention, balance rehabilitation, and strength training.

As a rule of thumb, the assessment of contributing causes and the design of intervention strategies for disability in older persons should always consider the four main aging processes that contribute to frailty. One of the most popular approaches to disability measurement is a modification of the International Classification of Impairments, Disabilities and Handicaps (World Health Organization, 1980) proposed by the Institute of Medicine (1992). This classification infers a causal pathway in four steps: pathology (diseases), impairment (the physical manifestation of diseases), functional limitation (global functions such as walking, grasping, climbing stairs), and disability (ability to fulfill social roles in the environment). In practice, the assessment of functional limitation and disability is performed either by (1) self-reported questionnaire concerning the degree of ability to perform basic self-care or more complex ADLs or by (2) performance-based measures of physical function that assess specific domains, such as balance, gait, manual dexterity, coordination, flexibility, and endurance. A concise list of standard tools that can be used to assess physical function in older persons is provided in Table 11-4. In 2001, the WHO officially endorsed a new classification system, the International Classification of Functioning, Disability and Health, known more commonly as the ICF. In the ICF, health measures are classified from bodily, individual, and societal perspectives by means of two lists: a list of body functions and

TABLE 11-4 TOOLS FOR FUNCTIONAL ASSESSMENT IN OLDER PATIENTS

Measurement Instrument	Evaluation	Activities/Reference	Notes
Index of independence in ADLs	Self-reported	Difficulty/need for help in bathing, dressing, using toilet, transferring, continence, feeding *(S Katz et al: JAMA 185:914, 1963)*	Short and simple, but subjective
Instrumental ADLs	Self-reported	Difficulty using the telephone, using a car/public transportation, shopping, preparing meals, housework, managing medications, financial management *(MP Lawton et al: Psychopharmacol Bull 24:609, 1988)*	Short and simple; sex-biased and culturally biased items
Functional Independence Measure	Consensus multidisciplinary team	Motor (eating, grooming, bathing, dressing, toileting, managing bladder/bowels, transferring, walking, climbing stairs); cognitive (auditory comprehension, verbal expression, social interaction, problem solving, memory) *(RA Keith et al: Adv Clin Rehabil 1:6, 1987)*	Administered by trained health professionals
Barthel Index	Professionally evaluated	Independence and need for help in feeding, transferring from bed to chair and back, grooming, transferring to and from toilet, bathing, walking, climbing stairs, dressing, continence *(FI Mahoney et al: Md State Med J 14:61, 1965)*	Administered by trained health professionals
Mobility Questionnaire	Self-reported	Severe difficulty walking ¼ mile and/or climbing stairs	Short and simple
Short Physical Performance Battery	Objective performance based	Time required to walk 4 m, rise from a chair 5 times, maintain balance for 10 sec in the side-by-side, semi-tandem, and tandem positions *(JM Guralnik et al: J Gerontol 49:M85, 1994)*	Some training required
Berg Balance Scale	Objective and professionally evaluated	Performance in 14 tasks related to balance *(KO Berg et al: Arch Phys Med Rehabil 73:1073, 1992)*	Typically used by physical therapists
Walking speed	Objective performance	Measure walking speed over a 4 m course *(S Studenski: J Nutr Health Aging 13:878, 2009)*	Simple and powerful, but limited to patients who can walk
6-Minute walk	Objective performance based	Distance covered in 6 min *(GH Guyatt: Can Med Assoc J 132:919, 1985)*	Good measure of fitness, walking capacity/endurance
Long-Distance Corridor Walk (400 m)	Objective performance based	Time to fast-walk 400 m *(AB Newman et al: JAMA 295:2018, 2006)*	More challenging than the 6-min walk

Abbreviation: ADLs, activities of daily living.

structure and a list of domains of activity and participation. Since an individual's functioning and disability occur in a context, the ICF also includes a list of environmental factors. A detailed list of codes that allow the classification of body functions, activities, and participation is being developed. The ICF system is widely implemented in Europe and is gaining popularity in the United States. Whatever classification system is used, the health care provider should try to identify factors that can be modified to minimize disability. Many of these factors are discussed in this chapter. Important issues related to aging that are not addressed in this chapter but are covered elsewhere include dementia (Chap. 35) and other cognitive disorders including aphasia, memory loss, and other focal cerebral disorders (Chap. 36).

Geriatric Syndromes The term *geriatric syndrome* encompasses clinical conditions that are frequently encountered in older persons; have a deleterious effect on function and quality of life; have a multifactorial pathophysiology, often involving systems unrelated to the apparent chief symptom; and are manifested by stereotypical clinical presentations. The list of geriatric syndromes includes incontinence, delirium, falls, pressure ulcers, sleep disorders, problems with eating or feeding, pain, and depressed mood. In addition, dementia and physical disability are sometimes considered to be geriatric syndromes. The term *syndrome* is somewhat misleading in this context since it is most commonly used to describe a pattern of symptoms and signs that have a single underlying cause. The term *geriatric syndromes*, by contrast, refers to "multifactorial health conditions that occur when the accumulated effects of impairments in multiple systems render an older person vulnerable to situational challenges." According to this definition, geriatric syndromes reflect the complex interactions between an individual's vulnerabilities and exposure to stressors or challenges. This definition aligns well with the concept that geriatric syndromes should be considered as phenotypic consequences of frailty and that a limited number of shared risk factors contribute to their etiology. Indeed, in various combinations and frequencies, virtually all geriatric syndromes are characterized by body composition changes, energy gaps, signaling disequilibria, and neurodegeneration. For example, detrusor (bladder) underactivity is a multifactorial geriatric condition that contributes to urinary retention in the frail elderly. It is characterized by detrusor muscle loss, fibrosis, and axonal degeneration. A proinflammatory state and a lack of estrogen signaling cause bladder muscle loss and detrusor underactivity, while a chronic urinary tract infection may cause detrusor hyperactivity; all of these factors may contribute to urinary incontinence.

Because of limited space, only delirium, falls, chronic pain, incontinence, and anorexia are addressed here. Interested readers are referred to textbooks on geriatric medicine for a discussion of other geriatric syndromes.

Delirium (See also Chap. 34) Delirium is an acute disorder of disturbed attention that fluctuates with time. It affects 15–55% of hospitalized older patients. Delirium has previously been considered to be transient and reversible and a normal consequence of surgery, chronic disease, or infections in older people. Delirium may be associated with a substantially increased risk for dementia and is an independent risk factor for morbidity, prolonged hospitalization, and death. These associations are particularly strong in the oldest old. Fig. 11-16 shows an algorithm for assessment and management of delirium in hospitalized older patients. The clinical presentation of delirium is heterogeneous, but frequent features are (1) a rapid decline in the level of consciousness, with difficulty focusing, shifting, or sustaining attention; (2) cognitive change (rumbling incoherent speech, memory gaps, disorientation, hallucinations) not explained by dementia; and (3) a medical history suggestive of preexisting cognitive impairment, frailty, and comorbidity. The strongest predisposing factors for delirium are dementia, any other condition associated with chronic or transient neurologic dysfunction (neurologic diseases, dehydration, alcohol consumption, psychoactive drugs), and sensory (visual and hearing) deprivation; these associations suggest that delirium is a condition of brain function susceptibility (neurodegeneration or transient neuronal impairment) that precludes the avoidance of decompensation in the face of a stressful event. Many stressful conditions have been implicated as precipitating factors, including surgery;

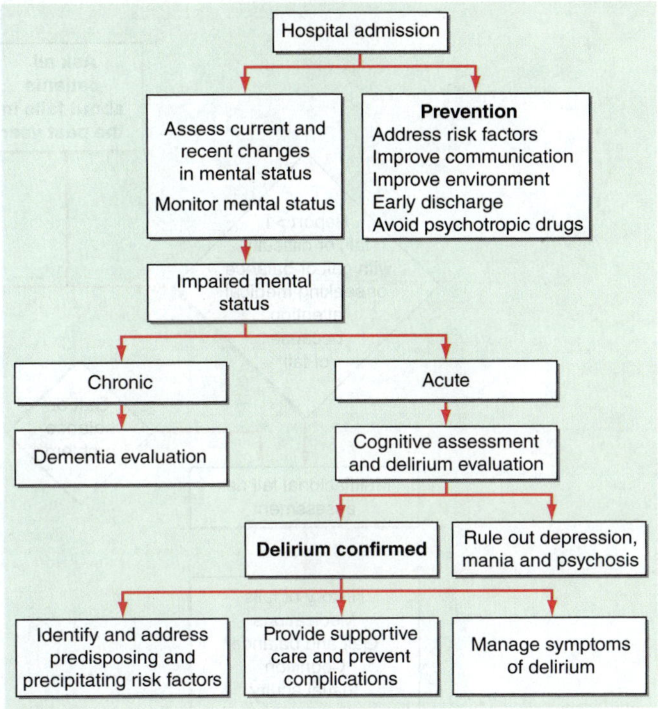

FIGURE 11-16 Algorithm depicting assessment and management of delirium in hospitalized older patients. *(Modified from SK Inouye: N Engl J Med 354:1157, 2006.)*

anesthesia; persistent pain; treatment with opiates, narcotics, or anticholinergics; sleep deprivation, immobilization; hypoxia; malnutrition; and metabolic and electrolyte derangements. Both the occurrence and the severity of delirium can be reduced by anticipatory screening and preventive strategies targeting the precipitating causes. The Confusion Assessment Method is a simple, validated tool for screening in the hospital setting. The three pillars of treatment are (1) immediate identification and treatment of precipitating factors, (2) withdrawal of drugs that may have promoted the onset of delirium, and (3) supportive care, including management of hypoxia, hydration and nutrition, mobilization, and environmental modifications. Whether patients who are cared for in special delirium units have better outcomes than those who are not is still in question. Physical restraints should be avoided because they tend to increase agitation and injury. Whenever possible, drug treatment should be avoided because it may prolong or aggravate delirium in some cases. The treatment of choice is low-dose haloperidol. It remains difficult to reduce delirium in patients with acute illness or other stressful conditions. Interventions based on dietary supplementation or careful use of pain medications and sedatives in pre- and postoperative older patients have been only partially successful.

Falls and Balance Disorders Unstable gait and falls are serious concerns in the older adult because they lead not only to injury but also to restricted activity, increased health care utilization, and even death. Like all geriatric syndromes, problems with balance and falls tend to be multifactorial and are strongly connected with the disrupted aging systems that contribute to frailty. Poor muscle strength, neural damage in the basal ganglia and cerebellum, diabetes, and peripheral neuropathy are all recognized risk factors for falls. Therefore, evaluation and management require a structured multisystem approach that spans the entire frailty spectrum and beyond. Accordingly, interventions to prevent or reduce instability and falls usually require a mix of medical, rehabilitative, and environmental modification approaches. Guidelines for the evaluation and management of falls, released by the American Geriatrics Society, recommend asking all older adults about falls and perceived gait instability (Fig. 11-17). Patients with a positive history of multiple falls as well as persons who have sustained one or more injurious falls should undergo an evaluation of gait and balance as well as a targeted history and physical examination to detect

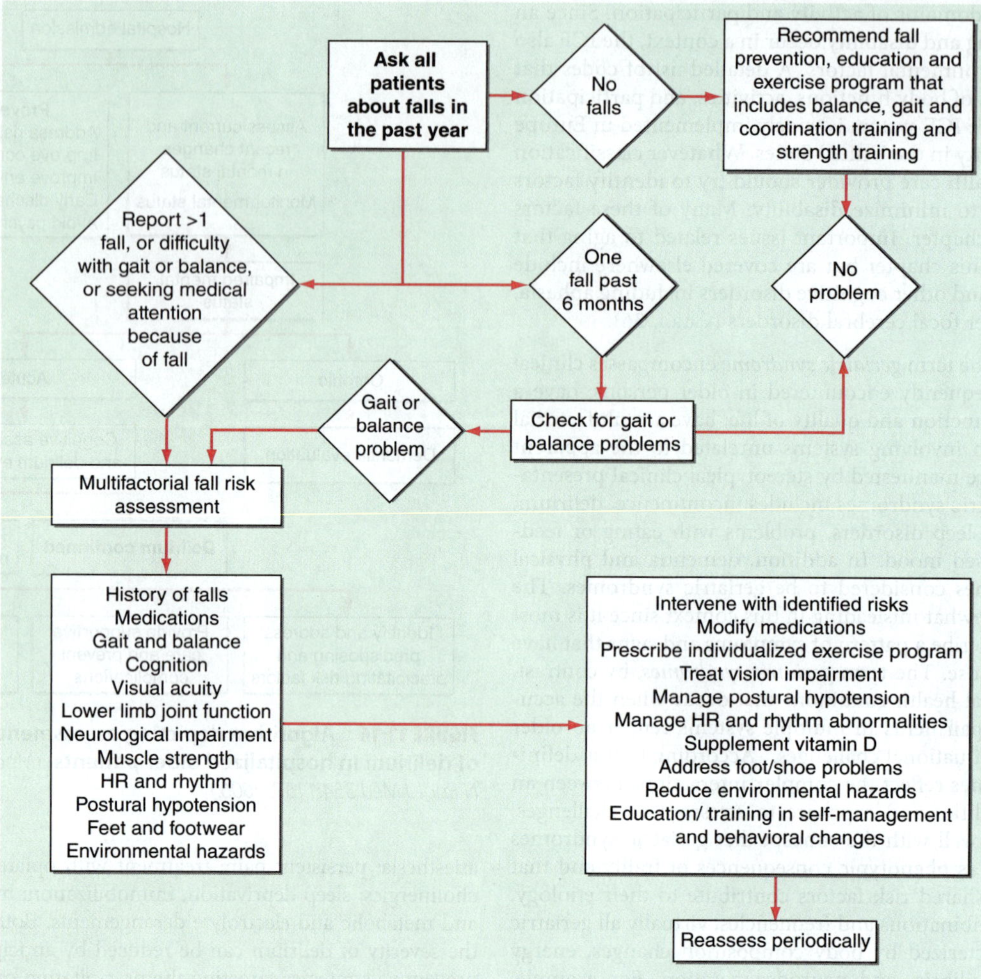

FIGURE 11-17 Algorithm depicting assessment and management of falls in older patients. HR, heart rate. *(From American Geriatrics Society and British Geriatrics Society: Clinical Practice Guideline for the Prevention of Falls in Older Persons. New York, American Geriatric Society, 2010.)*

sensory, nervous system, brain, cardiovascular, and musculoskeletal contributors. Interventions depend on the factors identified but often include medication adjustment, physical therapy, and home modifications. Meta-analyses of strategies to reduce the risk of falls have found that multifactorial risk assessment and management as well as individually targeted therapeutic exercise are effective. Supplementation with vitamin D at 800 IU daily may also help reduce falls, especially in older persons with low vitamin D levels.

Persistent Pain Pain from multiple sources is the most common symptom reported by older adults in primary care settings and is also common in acute-care, long-term-care, and palliative-care settings. Acute pain and cancer pain are beyond the scope of this chapter. Persistent pain results in restricted activity, depression, sleep disorders, and social isolation and increases the risk of adverse events due to medication. The most common causes of persistent pain are musculoskeletal problems, but neuropathic pain and ischemic pain occur frequently, and multiple concurrent causes are often found. Alterations in mechanical and structural elements of the skeleton commonly lead to secondary problems in other parts of the body, especially soft tissue or myofascial components. A structured history should elicit information about the quality, severity, and temporal patterns of pain. Physical examination should focus on the back and joints, on trigger points and periarticular areas, and on possible evidence of radicular neurologic patterns and peripheral vascular disease. Pharmacologic management should follow standard progressions, as recommended by the World Health Organization (Chap. 18), and adverse effects on the CNS, which are especially likely in this population, must be monitored. For persistent pain, regular analgesic schedules are appropriate and should be combined with nonpharmacologic approaches such as splints, physical exercise, heat, and other modalities. A variety of adjuvant analgesics such as antidepressants and anticonvulsants may be used; again, however, effects on reaction time and alertness may be dose limiting, especially in older persons with cognitive impairment. Joint or soft tissue injections may be helpful. Education of the patient and mutually agreed-upon goal setting are important since pain usually is not fully eliminated but rather is controlled to a tolerable level that maximizes function while minimizing adverse effects.

Urinary Incontinence Urinary incontinence—the involuntary leakage of urine—is highly prevalent among older persons (especially women) and has a profound negative impact on quality of life. Approximately 50% of American women will experience some form of urinary incontinence over a lifetime. Increasing age, white race, childbirth, obesity, and medical comorbidity are all risk factors for urinary incontinence. The three main clinical forms of urinary incontinence are as follows: (1) *Stress* incontinence is the failure of the sphincteric mechanism to remain closed when there is a sudden increase in intraabdominal pressure, such as a cough or sneeze. In women this condition is due to insufficient strength of the pelvic floor muscles, while in men it is almost exclusively secondary to prostate surgery. (2) *Urge* incontinence is the loss of urine accompanied by a sudden sensation of need to urinate and inability to control it and is due to detrusor muscle overactivity (lack of inhibition) caused by loss of neurologic control or local irritation. (3) *Overflow* incontinence is characterized by urinary dribbling, either constantly or for some period after urination. This condition is due to impaired detrusor contractility (due usually to denervation, for example, in

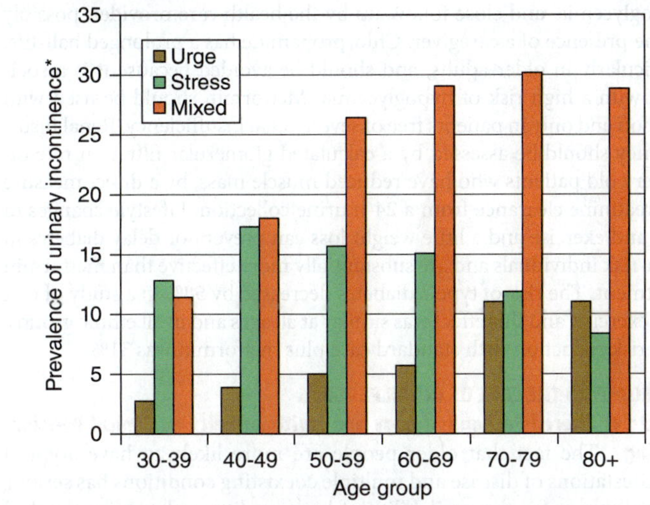

FIGURE 11-18 Rates of urge, stress, and mixed incontinence, by age group, in a sample of 3552 women. *Based on a sample of 3553 participants. *(From JL Melville et al: Arch Intern Med 165:537, 2005.)*

diabetes) or bladder outlet obstruction (prostate hypertrophy in men and cystocele in women). Thus, it is not surprising that the pathogenesis of urinary incontinence is connected to the disrupted aging systems that contribute to frailty, body composition changes (atrophy of the bladder and pelvic floor muscle), and neurodegeneration (both central and peripheral nervous systems). Frailty is a strong risk factor for urinary incontinence. Indeed, older women are more likely to have mixed (urge + stress) incontinence than any pure form (Fig. 11-18). In analogy with the other geriatric syndromes, urinary incontinence derives from a predisposing condition superimposed on a stressful precipitating factor. Accordingly, treatment of urinary incontinence should address both. The first line of treatment is bladder training associated with pelvic muscle exercise (Kegel exercises) that sometimes should be associated with electrical stimulation. Women with possible vaginal or uterine prolapse should be referred to a specialist. Urinary tract infections should be investigated and eventually treated. A long list of medications can precipitate urinary incontinence, including diuretics, antidepressants, sedative hypnotics, adrenergic agonists or blockers, anticholinergics, and calcium channel blockers. Whenever possible, these medications should be discontinued. Until recently, it was believed that oral or local estrogen treatment alleviated the symptoms of urinary incontinence in postmenopausal women, but this notion is now controversial. Antimuscarinic drugs such as tolterodine, darifenacin, and fesoterodine are modestly effective for mixed-etiology incontinence, but all of these drugs can affect cognition and so must be used with caution and with monitoring of cognitive status. In some cases, surgical treatment should be considered. Chronic catheterization has many adverse effects and should be limited to chronic urinary retention that cannot be managed in any other way. Bacteriuria always occurs and should be treated only if it is symptomatic. Bacterial communities isolated from the urine of women with urinary incontinence appear to differ with the type of incontinence; this observation suggests that the bladder microbiota may play a role in urinary incontinence. If so, this microbial population would be a potential target for treatment.

Undernutrition and Anorexia There is strong evidence that the healthy mammalian life span is greatly affected by changes in the activity of central nutrient-sensing mechanisms, especially those that involve the rapamycin (mTOR) network. Polymorphic variations in the gene that encodes mTOR in humans are associated with longevity; this association suggests that the role of nutrient signaling in healthy aging may be conserved in humans. Normal aging is associated with a decline in food intake that is more marked in men than in women. To some extent, food intake is reduced because energy demand declines as a result of the combination of a lower level of physical activity, a decline in lean body mass, and slowed rates of protein turnover. Other contributors to decreased food intake include losses of taste sensation, reduced stomach compliance, higher circulating levels of cholecystokinin, and, in men, low testosterone levels associated with increased leptin. When food intake decreases to a level below the reduced energy demand, the result is energy malnutrition.

Malnutrition in older persons should be considered a geriatric syndrome because it is the result of intrinsic susceptibility due to aging, complicated by multiple superimposed precipitating causes. Many older individuals tend to consume a monotonous diet that lacks sufficient fresh food, fruits, and vegetables, so that intake of important micronutrients is inadequate. Undernutrition in older people is associated with multiple adverse health consequences, including impaired muscle function, decreased bone mass, immune dysfunction, anemia, reduced cognitive function, poor wound healing, delayed recovery from surgery, and increased risk of falls, disability, and death. Despite these serious potential consequences, undernutrition often remains unrecognized until it is well advanced because weight loss tends to be ignored by both patients and physicians. Muscle wasting is a frequent feature of weight loss and malnutrition that is often associated with loss of subcutaneous fat. The main causes of weight loss are anorexia, cachexia, sarcopenia, malabsorption, hypermetabolism, and dehydration, almost always in various combinations. Many of these causes can be detected and corrected. Cancer accounts for only 10–15% of cases of weight loss and anorexia in older people. Other important causes include a recent move to a long-term-care setting, acute illness (often with inflammation), hospitalization with bed rest for as little as 1–2 days, depression, drugs that cause anorexia and nausea (e.g., digoxin and antibiotics), swallowing problems, oral infections, dental problems, gastrointestinal pathology, thyroid and other hormonal problems, poverty, and isolation, with reduced access to food. Weight loss may also result from dehydration, possibly related to excess sweating, diarrhea, vomiting, or reduced fluid intake. Early identification is paramount and requires careful weight monitoring. Patients or caregivers should be taught to record weight regularly at home, the patient should be weighed at each clinical encounter, and a record of serial weights should be maintained in the medical record. If malnutrition is suspected, formal assessment should begin with a standardized screening instrument such as the Mini Nutritional Assessment, the Malnutrition Universal Screening Tool, or the Simplified Nutritional Appetite Questionnaire. The Mini Nutritional Assessment includes questions on appetite, timing of eating, frequency of meals, and taste. Its sensitivity and specificity are >75% for future weight loss of ≥5% of body weight in older people. Many nutritional supplements are available, and their use should be initiated early to prevent more severe weight loss and its consequences. When an older patient has malnutrition, the diet should be liberalized and dietary restrictions should be lifted as much as possible. Nutritional supplements should be given between meals to avoid interference with food intake at mealtime. Limited evidence supports the use of any pharmacologic intervention to treat weight loss. The two antianorexic drugs most often prescribed in older persons are megesterol and dronabinol. Both can increase weight; however, the gain is mostly fat, not muscle, and both drugs have serious side effects. Dronabinol is an excellent drug for use in the palliative-care setting. There is little evidence that intentional weight loss in overweight older people prolongs life. Weight loss after the age of 70 should probably be limited to persons with extreme obesity and should always be medically supervised.

HOW THE AGING PHENOTYPE AFFECTS DISEASE PRESENTATION

Common diseases in older adults may have unexpected and atypical clinical features. Most age-related changes in clinical presentation, evolution, and response to treatment are due to interaction of disease pathophysiology with age-related system dysregulation. Some diseases, such as Parkinson's disease (PD) and diabetes, directly affect aging systems and therefore have a devastating impact on frailty and its consequences.

Parkinson's Disease (See also Chap. 449) Most cases of PD begin after the age of 60 years, and the incidence increases up to the age of ~80 years. Brain aging and PD have long been thought to be related. The nigrostriatal system deteriorates with aging, and many older persons tend to develop a mild form of movement disorder characterized by bradykinesia and stooped posture that mimics mild PD. It is interesting that, in PD, older age at presentation is associated with a more severe and rapid decline in gait, balance, posture, and cognition. These age-related motor and cognitive manifestations of PD tend to be poorly responsive to levodopa or dopamine agonist treatments, especially in the oldest old. In contrast, age at presentation does not correlate with the severity and progression of other classic PD symptoms, such as tremor, rigidity, and bradykinesia, nor does it affect the response of these symptoms to levodopa. The pattern of PD features in older persons suggests that late-life PD may reflect a failure of the normal cellular compensatory mechanisms in vulnerable brain regions and that this vulnerability is increased by age-related neurodegeneration, making PD symptoms particularly resistant to levodopa treatment. In addition to motor symptoms, older PD patients tend to have reduced muscle mass (sarcopenia), eating disorders, and poor levels of fitness. Accordingly, PD is a powerful risk factor for frailty and its consequences, including disability, comorbidity, falls, incontinence, chronic pain, and delirium. Use of levodopa and dopaminergic agonists by older PD patients requires complex dosing schedules; therefore, slow-release preparations are preferred. Both dopaminergic and anticholinergic agents increase the risk of confusion and hallucinations. Use of anticholinergic agents should generally be avoided. For dopaminergic agents, cognitive side effects can be dose limiting.

Diabetes (See also Chaps. 417–419) Both the incidence and the prevalence of diabetes mellitus increase with aging. Among persons ≥65 years old, the prevalence is ~12% (with higher figures among African Americans and Hispanics), reflecting the effects of population aging and the obesity epidemic. Diabetes affects all four main aging systems that contribute to frailty. Obesity, especially visceral obesity, is a strong risk factor for insulin resistance, the metabolic syndrome, and diabetes. Diabetes is associated with both reduced muscle mass and accelerated rates of muscle wasting. Diabetic patients have an elevated RMR and a poor degree of fitness. Diabetes is associated with multiple hormone dysregulation, a proinflammatory state, and excess oxidative stress. Finally, diabetes-induced neurodegeneration involves both the central and peripheral nervous systems. Given these characteristics, it is not surprising that patients with diabetes mellitus are more likely to be frail and at high risk of developing physical disability, depression, delirium, cognitive impairment, urinary incontinence, injurious falls, and persistent pain. Thus, the assessment of older diabetic patients should always include screening and risk factor evaluation for these conditions.

In young and adult patients, the main treatment goal has been strict glycemic control aimed at bringing the hemoglobin A1c level to within normal values (i.e., ≤6%). However, the risk/benefit ratio is optimized by the use of less aggressive glycemic targets. In fact, in the context of a randomized clinical trial, strict glycemic control was associated with a higher mortality rate. Thus, a more reasonable goal for hemoglobin A1c is 7% or slightly below. Treatment goals are altered further in frail older adults who have a high risk of complications of hypoglycemia and a life expectancy of <5 years. In these cases, an even less stringent target (e.g., 7–8%) should be considered, with A1c monitored every 6 or 12 months. Hypoglycemia is particularly difficult to identify in older diabetic patients because autonomic and nervous system symptoms occur at a lower blood sugar level than in younger diabetics, although the metabolic reactions and neurologic injury effects are similar in the two age groups. The autonomic symptoms of hypoglycemia are often masked by beta blockers. Frail older adults are at even higher risk for serious hypoglycemia than are healthier, higher-functioning older adults. In older patients with type 2 diabetes, a history of severe hypoglycemic episodes is associated with higher mortality risk, more severe microvascular complications, and greater risk of dementia. Thus, patients with suspected or documented episodes of hypoglycemia, especially those who are frail or disabled, need more liberal glucose-control goals, careful education about hypoglycemia, and close follow-up by the health care provider, possibly in the presence of a caregiver. Chlorpropamide has a prolonged half-life, particularly in older adults, and should be avoided because it is associated with a high risk of hypoglycemia. Metformin should be used with caution and only in patients free of severe renal insufficiency. Renal insufficiency should be assessed by a calculated glomerular filtration rate or, in very old patients who have reduced muscle mass, by a direct measure of creatinine clearance from a 24-h urine collection. Lifestyle changes in diet and exercise and a little weight loss can prevent or delay diabetes in high-risk individuals and are substantially more effective than metformin treatment. The risk of type 2 diabetes decreased by 58% in a study of diet and exercise, and this effect was similar at all ages and in all ethnic groups. The risk reduction with standard care plus metformin was 31%.

APPROACH TO THE CARE OF OLDER PERSONS

Effects of Altered Pathophysiology and Multimorbidity on Clinical Decision-Making The fact that older people are more likely to have atypical manifestations of disease and multiple coexisting conditions has serious consequences for the availability of high-quality evidence for medical practice and clinical decision-making. Randomized clinical trials—the basis for high-quality evidence—have tended to exclude older persons with atypical manifestations of disease, multimorbidity, or functional limitations. Across a wide range of conditions, the average age of a clinical trial participant is 20 years younger than the average age of the population with the condition. Clinical practice guidelines and care-quality metrics are focused on one condition at a time and tend not to consider the impact of comorbid conditions on the safety and feasibility of each set of recommendations. These disease-centric recommendations tend to result in fragmented care. Therefore, clinical decision-making with regard to an older person with multiple chronic conditions must be based on the weighing of several influential factors, including the patient's priorities and preferences, potential beneficial and harmful interactions among the several conditions and their treatments, life expectancy, and practical issues such as transportation, or ability to cooperate with the test or treatment.

Organization of Health Care for Older Adults The complex underlying physiology of aging leads to multiple coexisting medical problems and functional consequences that are often chronic, with recurrent exacerbations and remissions. Combined with the social consequences of aging (e.g., widowhood or lack of an available caregiver), these medical and functional factors mandate that older adults must sometimes use nonmedical services to meet functional needs. The end result of these medical, functional, and social factors is that older adults use many health care and social support services in a variety of settings. Thus, it is incumbent on the internist, whether a generalist or specialist, to be familiar with the scope of settings and services that are used by their patients.

For many settings, Medicare reimbursement requires a medical order based on specific indications, so the hospitalist or referring physician must be familiar with eligibility requirements. Table 11-5 summarizes the types of services and payment sources for common settings of care. Older adults who have experienced new disability during a hospitalization are eligible for rehabilitation services. Inpatient rehabilitation requires at least 3 h per day of active rehabilitative activity and is limited to specific diagnoses. More and more rehabilitative services are provided in postacute settings, where the required intensity of service is less stringent. Postacute settings are also used for complex nursing services such as provision and supervision of long-term parenteral medication use or wound care. Under current policy, Medicare covers postacute care only if there is an eligible medical, nursing, or rehabilitation service. Otherwise, nursing home care is not covered by Medicare and must be paid for with personal assets until all resources have been consumed, at which time Medicaid coverage becomes available.

Medicaid is a state–federal partnership whose greatest single expenditure is nursing home care. Thus, the need for chronic daily assistance with personal care in a nursing home consumes a large part of most state Medicaid budgets as well as personal assets. Accordingly, alternatives to chronic nursing-home care are of great interest to states, patients, and families. Some states have developed Medicaid-funded day-care programs, sometimes based on the Program for All-Inclusive

TABLE 11-5 CARE SETTINGS FOR OLDER PATIENTS

Setting	Services	Payment Source
Hospital acute care	Medical, surgical, and psychiatric services that cannot be provided in less complex settings	Medicare, Medicaid, and private insurance
Emergency room	Resuscitation, stabilization, triage, disposition	Medicare, Medicaid, and private insurance
Inpatient rehabilitation	Hospital-based residential program providing team-based, physician-supervised, intensive therapeutic rehabilitation for specific diagnoses	Medicare, Medicaid, and private insurance
Outpatient clinic	Chronic, urgent, and preventive services	Medicare, Medicaid, and private insurance
Postacute care	Medical, nursing, and rehabilitative services after hospitalization, often based in hospitals or nursing homes	Medicare up to 100 days with eligibility requirements
Long-term care	Residential program with daily nursing and aide care for persons who are dependent in self-care	Medicaid, private payment, long-term care insurance
Assisted living	Residential program with daily aide care and housing for persons who are dependent in household management	Private payment
Home health care	Nursing and rehabilitative services for episodes of care provided to persons in the community	Medicare, Medicaid
Day programs	Supervised settings providing nursing and aide care for scheduled hours	Private payment, Medicaid

Care of the Elderly (PACE) model. In this situation, older adults who are eligible for both Medicare and Medicaid and who are otherwise eligible for chronic nursing-home care can receive coordinated medical and functional services in conjunction with a day-care program.

For most older adults, a caregiver must be available to provide assistance on weeknights and weekends. Under current policy, home health services do not provide chronic functional assistance in the home but rather are targeted at episodes of care supplied by medical or rehabilitative services for older adults who are considered home bound. Some community agencies, whether private or public, can provide homemaker and home aide services to assist the home-bound older adult with functional needs, but there may be income requirements or expensive private payment may be needed.

Within the past decade, there has been tremendous growth in a broad spectrum of assisted-living settings. Such settings do not offer the degree of 24-h nursing supervision or personal aide care that is provided in traditional nursing homes, although distinctions are becoming blurred. Most assisted-living settings provide meals, medication supervision, and homemaking services, but they often require that residents be capable of transporting themselves to a congregate meal site. Moreover, most of these settings accept only private payment from residents and their families and thus are hard to access for older adults with limited resources. Some states are exploring coverage for lower-cost residential-care services such as family care homes.

Models of Care Coordination The complexity and fragmentation of care for older adults results in both increased costs and increased risk of iatrogenic complications such as missed diagnoses, adverse medication events, further worsening of function, and even death. These serious consequences have led to a strong interest in care coordination through teams of providers, with the goals to reduce unnecessary costs and to prevent adverse events. Table 11-6 lists examples of evidence-based models of care coordination that were recommended in a 2009

TABLE 11-6 EVIDENCE-BASED MODELS OF CARE COORDINATION FOR OLDER PATIENTS (INSTITUTE OF MEDICINE, 2009)

Model	Team Members	Services
Interdisciplinary primary care "medical home"	Primary care physician plus social worker, nurse, nurse practitioner, or other care coordinators	Coordination of medical and social needs across settings
Case management	Nurse or social worker	Education of and information dissemination to patients and families; in some cases, communication with providers and settings
Disease management	Nurse	Health education and follow-up support for specific chronic diseases
Preventive home visits	Physician, nurse, social worker, and others	Structured assessment of physical, mental, functional, and social status in the home setting, with recommendations for care and prevention
Comprehensive outpatient geriatric assessment and management	Physician, nurse, social worker, and sometimes others (e.g., pharmacist, rehabilitation therapist, psychologist)	Structured assessment of physical, mental, functional, and social status in the outpatient setting, with recommendations for care and prevention. Some programs also take responsibility for implementing the recommendations.
Pharmaceutical care management	Pharmacist	Review and recommendations, in any setting, regarding the total medication regimen
Chronic disease self-management	Nurse, health educator, or other health professional	Health education and coaching for specific chronic conditions
Prevention rehabilitation	Rehabilitation therapist	Anticipatory evaluation, therapeutic exercise, and assistive technology in the home or outpatient setting for older adults with physical disability
Caregiver services	Social worker, psychologist, or other health professional	Education, counseling, and resource referral for caregivers of older adults with chronic functional and mental health problems
Hospital discharge/transition coordination	Nurse, nurse practitioner	Care planning and education for patient and family before and after hospital discharge
Hospital at home	Physician, nurse, pharmacist	Diagnostic testing and medical treatments that can replace hospitalization or reduce length of hospital stay for target conditions
Nursing home care coordination	Nurse practitioner or physician assistant	Scheduled assessment and care planning as well as education for health workers in chronic-care settings
Hospital delirium comprehensive care	Physician, nurse	Prevention, screening, and management of delirium in the hospital setting
Comprehensive inpatient geriatric assessment and management	Physician, nurse, social worker, and sometimes others (e.g., pharmacist, rehabilitation therapist, psychologist)	Specialized inpatient settings such as acute care of the elderly (ACE) units or roving multidisciplinary teams that provide evaluation and recommendations for medical, mental health, functional, and social needs. ACE units and some teams take responsibility for implementation of recommendations.

Source: Reproduced with permission from C Boult et al: J Am Geriatr Soc 57:2328, 2009.

Institute of Medicine report. While not mentioned as a specific type of team care, modern information technology offers substantial promise in providing consistent, readily available information across settings and providers. All such team programs are targeted at prevention and management of chronic and complex problems. Evidence from clinical trials or quasi-experimental studies supports the benefit of each model, and for some models data are sufficient to support meta-analyses. The evidence for benefit is not always consistent between studies or types of care but includes some support for improved quality of care, quality of life, function, survival, and health care costs and use. Some models of care are disease-specific and focus on common chronic conditions such as diabetes mellitus, congestive heart failure, chronic obstructive pulmonary disease, and stroke. One challenge in the use of these models is that a majority of older adults will have multiple simultaneous conditions and thus will need services from multiple programs that may not communicate among themselves.

Most models of care are difficult to implement in today's health care system because nonphysician services are not reimbursed, nor is physician effort that is not incorporated into "face-to-face" time. Thus, several models have been developed largely by the Department of Veterans Affairs Health Care System, Medicare Managed Care providers, and other sponsoring agencies. Medicare has developed a series of demonstration projects that can expand the evidence base and serve policy makers. More recently, there has been an effort to promote coordinated care through Accountable Care Organizations and patient-centered "medical homes." However, the processes and outcomes of such care must evolve from disease-specific indicators to more general markers, such as optimizing functional status, focusing on outcomes that are important to patients, and minimizing inappropriate care.

SCREENING AND PREVENTION IN OLDER PERSONS

In older adults, prevention tests and interventions are less consistently recommended for all asymptomatic patients. The guidelines fail to address the influence of health status and life expectancy on recommendations, although the benefits of prevention are clearly affected by life expectancy. For example, in most types of cancer, screening provides no benefit in patients with a life expectancy of ≤5 years. More research is needed to build an appropriate evidence base for age- and life expectancy–adapted preventive services. Health behavior modification, especially increasing physical activity and improving nutrition, probably has the greatest potential to promote healthy aging.

Screening Tests

- Osteoporosis: Bone mineral density (BMD) should be measured at least once after the age of 65 years. There is little evidence that regular monitoring of BMD improves the prediction of fractures. Because of limitations in the precision of dual-energy x-ray absorptiometry, the minimal interval between evaluations should be 2–3 years.
- Hypertension: Blood pressure should be determined at least once a year or more often in patients with hypertension.
- Diabetes: Serum glucose and hemoglobin A1c should be checked every 3 years or more often in patients who are obese or hypertensive.
- Lipid disorders: A lipid panel should be done every 5 years or more often in patients with diabetes or any cardiovascular disease.
- Colorectal cancer: A fecal occult blood test and a sigmoidoscopy or colonoscopy should be done on a regular schedule up to the age of 75 years. No consensus guidelines exist for these tests >75 years of age.
- Breast cancer: Mammography should be done every 2 years between the ages of 50 and 74 years. No consensus guidelines exist for mammography after the age of 75 years.
- Cervical cancer: A Pap smear should be done every 3 years up to the age of 65 years.

Preventive Interventions

- Influenza: Immunize annually.
- Shingles: Administer herpes zoster vaccine once after the age of 50 years.
- Pneumonia: Administer pneumococcal vaccine once at the age of 65 years.
- Myocardial infarction: Prescribe daily aspirin for patients with prevalent cardiovascular disease or with a poor cardiovascular risk profile.
- Osteoporosis: Prescribe calcium at 1200 mg daily and vitamin D at ≥800 IU daily.

Exercise Rates of regular physical activity decrease with age and are lowest in older persons. This situation is unfortunate because increased physical activity has clear benefits in older adults, improving physical function, muscle strength, mood, sleep, and metabolic risk profile. Some studies suggest that exercise can improve cognition and prevent dementia, but this association is still controversial. Exercise programs, both aerobic and strength training, are feasible and beneficial even in very old and frail individuals. Regular, moderate-intensity exercise can reduce the rate of age-associated decline in physical function. The Centers for Disease Control and Prevention recommends that older persons should spend at least 150 min per week in moderate-intensity aerobic activity (e.g., brisk walking) and should engage in muscle-strengthening activities that work all major muscle groups (legs, hips, back, abdomen, chest, shoulders, and arms) at least 2 days a week. In the absence of contraindications, more intense and prolonged physical activity provides greater benefits. Frail and sedentary persons may need supervision, at least at the start of the exercise program, to avoid falls and exercise-related injuries.

Nutrition Older persons are particularly vulnerable to malnutrition, and many problems that affect older patients can be addressed by dietary modification. As mentioned above, nutrient sensing is the major factor associated with differential longevity in several animal models, including mammals. Treatment with rapamycin, the only pharmacologic intervention that has been associated with longevity, affects nutrient sensing. Nevertheless, there are almost no evidence-based guidelines for individualizing dietary modifications based on differing health outcomes in the elderly. Even when guidelines exist, older people tend to be poorly compliant with dietary recommendations. Basic principles of a healthy diet that are also valid for older persons are as follows:

- Encourage the consumption of fruits and vegetables; they are rich in micronutrients, mineral, and fibers. Whole grains are also a good source of fiber. Keep in mind that some of these foods are costly and thus less accessible to low-income persons.
- Emphasize that good hydration is essential. Fluid intake should be at least 1000 mL daily.
- Encourage the use of fat-free and low-fat dairy products, legumes, poultry, and lean meats. Encourage consumption of fish at least once a week, since there is strong epidemiologic evidence that fish consumption is associated with a lowered risk of Alzheimer's disease.
- Match intake of energy (calories) to overall energy needs in order to maintain a healthy weight and BMI (20–27). Recommend moderate (5–10%) caloric restriction only when the BMI is >27.
- Limit consumption of foods with high caloric density, high sugar content, and high salt content.
- Limit the intake of foods with a high content of saturated fatty acids and cholesterol.
- Limit alcohol consumption (one drink per day or less).
- Introduce vitamin D–fortified foods and/or vitamin D supplements into the diet. Older persons who have little exposure to UVB radiation are at risk of vitamin D insufficiency.
- Make sure that the diet includes adequate food-related intake of magnesium, vitamin A, and vitamin B_{12}.
- Monitor daily protein intake, which, in healthy older persons, should be in the range of 1.0–1.2 g/kg of body weight. Higher daily protein intake (i.e., ≥1.2–1.5 g/kg) is advised for those who are exercising or are affected by chronic diseases, especially if these conditions are associated with chronic inflammation. Older people with severe kidney disease (i.e., an estimated glomerular filtration rate of <30 mL/min per 1.73 m^2) who are not on dialysis should limit protein intake.

- For constipation, increase dietary fiber intake to 10–25 g/d and fluid intake to 1500 mL/d. A bulk laxative (methylcellulose or psyllium) can be added.

Novel Interventions to Modify Aging Processes Aging is a complex process with multiple manifestations at the molecular, cellular, organ, and whole-organism level. The nature of the aging process is still not fully understood, but aging and its effects may be modulated by appropriate interventions. Dietary and genetic alterations can increase healthy life span and prevent the development of dysregulated systems and the aging phenotype in laboratory model organisms. The mechanisms responsible for life span expansion are "food" sensors typically activated in situations of food shortage, such as IGF/insulin and the TOR (target of rapamycin) pathways. Accordingly, a reduction in food intake without malnutrition extends the life span by 10–50% in diverse organisms, from yeasts to rhesus monkeys. Mechanisms that mediate the effects of caloric restriction are under intensive study because they are potential targets for interventions aimed at counteracting the emergence of the aging phenotype and its deleterious effects in humans. For example, resveratrol, a natural compound found in grape skin that mimics some of the effects of dietary restriction, increases longevity and improves health in mice fed a high-fat diet but has little effect on mice fed a standard diet. Other compounds that potentially mimic caloric restriction are being developed and tested. A high prevalence of IGF-1 receptor gene mutation has been found in Ashkenazi Jewish centenarians and in other long-lived individuals, suggesting that the downregulation of IGF-1 signaling may promote human longevity. A 20-year period of 30% dietary restriction applied to adult rhesus monkeys was associated with reduced cardiovascular and cancer morbidity, reduced signs of aging, and greater longevity, although a second such study did not find increased longevity. In humans, dietary restriction is effective against obesity and reduces insulin resistance, inflammation, blood pressure, CRP level, and intima-media thickness of the carotid arteries. However, the beneficial effects of dietary restriction in humans are still controversial, and some potential negative effects have not been sufficiently studied. An interesting effect of caloric restriction in humans is mitochondrial biogenesis. Mitochondrial dysfunction has emerged as a potentially important underlying contributor to aging. Reduced expression of mitochondrial genes is a strongly conserved feature of aging across different species. Mitochondria are the machinery for chemical energy production, and brain and muscle are particularly susceptible to defective mitochondrial function. Thus, declining mitochondrial function may be a direct cause of at least three of the main dysregulated systems contributing to the phenotype of aging.

OTHER ASPECTS OF AGING

This chapter has touched on some of the fundamental aspects of human aging, focusing mostly on those that are relevant to the care of older patients. Many aspects of geriatric medicine have not been addressed because of space limitations. Valuable topics not considered include details of comprehensive geriatric assessment, depression and anxiety, hypertension, orthostatic hypotension, dementia, vision and hearing impairment, osteoporosis, palliative care, prostate disorders, foot problems, and women's health. Some of these topics are treated extensively elsewhere in this text, sometimes with comments on age-specific issues.

CONCLUSIONS

The universal process of aging is becoming better understood. There appear to be shared underlying cellular and molecular processes that induce widespread dysregulation in key systems. This dysregulation contributes to clinical manifestations of a frailty phenotype and can be used to understand how to evaluate and manage the older patient.

Acknowledgment

We would like to thank our colleagues who provided criticisms and suggestions for improvement of this chapter. We are particularly indebted to Dr. John Morley for his valuable suggestions regarding the section on undernutrition and anorexia.

12e The Safety and Quality of Health Care

David W. Bates

This is a digital-only chapter. It is available on the DVD that accompanies this book, as well as on Access Medicine/Harrison's Online, and the eBook and "app" editions of HPIM 19e.

Safety and quality are two of the central dimensions of health care. In recent years it has become easier to measure safety and quality, and it is increasingly clear that performance in both dimensions could be much better. The public is—with good justification—demanding measurement and accountability, and payment for services will increasingly be based on performance in these areas. Thus, physicians must learn about these two domains, how they can be improved, and the relative strengths and limitations of the current ability to measure them.

13e Primary Care in Low- and Middle-Income Countries

Tim Evans, Kumanan Rasanathan

This is a digital-only chapter. It is available on the DVD that accompanies this book, as well as on Access Medicine/Harrison's Online, and the eBook and "app" editions of HPIM 19e.

The twentieth century witnessed the rise of an unprecedented global health divide. Industrialized or high-income countries experienced rapid improvement in standards of living, nutrition, health, and health care. Meanwhile, in low- and middle-income countries with much less favorable conditions, health and health care progressed much more slowly. The scale of this divide is reflected in the current extremes of life expectancy at birth, with Japan at the high end (83 years) and Sierra Leone at the low end (47 years). This nearly 40-year difference reflects the daunting range of health challenges faced by low- and middle-income countries. These nations must deal not only with a complex mixture of diseases (both infectious and chronic) and illness-promoting conditions but also, and more fundamentally, with the fragility of the foundations underlying good health (e.g., sufficient food, water, sanitation, and education) and of the systems necessary for universal access to good-quality health care. In the last decades of the twentieth century, the need to bridge this global health divide and establish health equity was increasingly recognized. The Declaration of Alma Ata in 1978 crystallized a vision of justice in health, regardless of income, gender, ethnicity, or education, and called for "health for all by the year 2000" through primary health care. While much progress has been made since the declaration, at the end of the first decade and a half of the twenty-first century, much remains to be done to achieve global health equity.

This chapter looks first at the nature of the health challenges in low- and middle-income countries that underlie the health divide. It then outlines the values and principles of a primary health care approach, with a focus on primary care services. Next, the chapter reviews the experience of low- and middle-income countries in addressing health challenges through primary care and a primary health care approach. Finally, the chapter identifies how current challenges and global context provide an agenda and opportunities for the renewal of primary health care and primary care.

14e Complementary, Alternative, and Integrative Health Practices

Josephine P. Briggs

This is a digital-only chapter. It is available on the DVD that accompanies this book, as well as on Access Medicine/Harrison's Online, and the eBook and "app" editions of HPIM 19e.

The search for health includes many beliefs and practices that are outside conventional medicine. Physicians are important sources for information and guidance about health matters, but our patients also rely on a wide range of other sources including family and friends, cultural traditions, alternative practitioners, and increasingly the Internet, popular media, and advertising. It is essential for physicians to understand what patients are doing to seek health, as this understanding is important to harness potential benefits and to help patients avoid harm.

15e The Economics of Medical Care

Joseph P. Newhouse

This is a digital-only chapter. It is available on the DVD that accompanies this book, as well as on Access Medicine/Harrison's Online, and the eBook and "app" editions of HPIM 19e.

The purpose of this chapter is to explain to physicians how economists think about physicians' decision-making with regard to the treatment of patients. Economists' mode of thinking has shaped health care policy and institutions and thus the environment in which physicians practice, not only in the United States but in many other countries as well. It may prove useful for physicians to understand some aspects of the economists' way of thinking, even if it sometimes seems foreign or uncongenial.

16e Racial and Ethnic Disparities in Health Care

Joseph R. Betancourt, Alexander R. Green

This is a digital-only chapter. It is available on the DVD that accompanies this book, as well as on Access Medicine/Harrison's Online, and the eBook and "app" editions of HPIM 19e.

Over the course of its history, the United States has experienced dramatic improvements in overall health and life expectancy, largely as a result of initiatives in public health, health promotion, disease prevention, and chronic care management. Our ability to prevent, detect, and treat diseases in their early stages has allowed us to target and reduce rates of morbidity and mortality. Despite interventions that have improved the overall health of the majority of Americans, racial and ethnic minorities (blacks, Hispanics/Latinos, Native Americans/Alaskan Natives, Asian/Pacific Islanders) have benefited less from these advances than whites and have suffered poorer health outcomes from many major diseases, including cardiovascular disease, cancer, and diabetes. Research has revealed that minorities may receive less care and lower-quality care than whites, even when confounders such as stage of presentation, comorbidities, and health insurance are controlled. These differences in quality are called *racial and ethnic disparities in health care.* Addressing these disparities has taken on greater importance with the significant transformation of the U.S. health care system and the implementation of health care reform and value-based purchasing. The shift toward creating financial incentives and disincentives to achieve quality goals makes focusing on those who receive lower-quality care more important than ever before. This chapter will provide an overview of racial and ethnic disparities in health and health care, identify root causes, and provide key recommendations to address these disparities at both the clinical and health system levels.

17e Ethical Issues in Clinical Medicine

Bernard Lo, Christine Grady

This is a digital-only chapter. It is available on the DVD that accompanies this book, as well as on Access Medicine/Harrison's Online, and the eBook and "app" editions of HPIM 19e.

Twenty-first-century physicians face novel ethical dilemmas that can be perplexing and emotionally draining. For example, electronic medical records, handheld personal devices, and provision of care by interdisciplinary teams all hold the promise of more coordinated and comprehensive care but also raise new concerns about confidentiality, appropriate boundaries of the doctor–patient relationship, and responsibility. Chapter 1 puts the practice of medicine into a professional and historical context. The present chapter presents approaches and principles that physicians can use to address the ethical issues they encounter in their work. Physicians make ethical judgments about clinical situations every day. Traditional professional codes and ethical principles provide instructive guidance for physicians but need to be interpreted and applied to each situation. Physicians need to be prepared for lifelong learning about ethical issues and dilemmas as well as about new scientific and clinical developments. When struggling with difficult ethical issues, physicians may need to reevaluate their basic convictions, tolerate uncertainty, and maintain their integrity while respecting the opinions of others. Discussing perplexing ethical issues with other members of the health care team, ethics consultation services, or the hospital ethics committee can clarify issues and reveal strategies for resolution, including improving communication and dealing with strong or conflicting emotions.

SECTION 1 PAIN

18 Pain: Pathophysiology and Management

James P. Rathmell, Howard L. Fields

The province of medicine is to preserve and restore health and to relieve suffering. Understanding pain is essential to both of these goals. Because pain is universally understood as a signal of disease, it is the most common symptom that brings a patient to a physician's attention. The function of the pain sensory system is to protect the body and maintain homeostasis. It does this by detecting, localizing, and identifying potential or actual tissue-damaging processes. Because different diseases produce characteristic patterns of tissue damage, the quality, time course, and location of a patient's pain lend important diagnostic clues. It is the physician's responsibility to provide rapid and effective pain relief.

THE PAIN SENSORY SYSTEM

Pain is an unpleasant sensation localized to a part of the body. It is often described in terms of a penetrating or tissue-destructive process (e.g., stabbing, burning, twisting, tearing, squeezing) and/or of a bodily or emotional reaction (e.g., terrifying, nauseating, sickening). Furthermore, any pain of moderate or higher intensity is accompanied by anxiety and the urge to escape or terminate the feeling. These properties illustrate the duality of pain: it is both sensation and emotion. When it is acute, pain is characteristically associated with behavioral arousal and a stress response consisting of increased blood pressure, heart rate, pupil diameter, and plasma cortisol levels. In addition, local muscle contraction (e.g., limb flexion, abdominal wall rigidity) is often present.

PERIPHERAL MECHANISMS

The Primary Afferent Nociceptor A peripheral nerve consists of the axons of three different types of neurons: primary sensory afferents, motor neurons, and sympathetic postganglionic neurons (Fig. 18-1). The cell bodies of primary sensory afferents are located in the dorsal root ganglia within the vertebral foramina. The primary afferent axon has two branches: one projects centrally into the spinal cord and the other projects peripherally to innervate tissues. Primary afferents are classified by their diameter, degree of myelination, and conduction velocity. The largest diameter afferent fibers, A-beta (Aβ), respond maximally to light touch and/or moving stimuli; they are present primarily in nerves that innervate the skin. In normal individuals, the activity of these fibers does not produce pain. There are two other classes of primary afferent nerve fibers: the small diameter myelinated A-delta (Aδ) and the unmyelinated (C) axons (Fig. 18-1). These fibers are present in nerves to the skin and to deep somatic and visceral structures. Some tissues, such as the cornea, are innervated only by Aδ and C fiber afferents. Most Aδ and C fiber afferents respond maximally only to intense (painful) stimuli and produce the subjective experience of pain when they are electrically stimulated; this defines them as *primary afferent nociceptors* (*pain receptors*). The ability to detect painful stimuli is completely abolished when conduction in Aδ and C fiber axons is blocked.

Individual primary afferent nociceptors can respond to several different types of noxious stimuli. For example, most nociceptors respond to heat; intense cold; intense mechanical distortion, such as a pinch; changes in pH, particularly an acidic environment; and application of chemical irritants including adenosine triphosphate (ATP), serotonin, bradykinin, and histamine.

Sensitization When intense, repeated, or prolonged stimuli are applied to damaged or inflamed tissues, the threshold for activating primary afferent nociceptors is lowered, and the frequency of firing is higher for all stimulus intensities. Inflammatory mediators such as bradykinin, nerve-growth factor, some prostaglandins, and leukotrienes contribute to this process, which is called *sensitization*. Sensitization occurs at the level of the peripheral nerve terminal (*peripheral sensitization*) as well as at the level of the dorsal horn of the spinal cord (*central sensitization*). Peripheral sensitization occurs in damaged or inflamed tissues, when inflammatory mediators activate intracellular signal transduction in nociceptors, prompting an increase in the production, transport, and membrane insertion of chemically gated and voltage-gated ion channels. These changes increase the excitability of nociceptor terminals and lower their threshold for activation by mechanical, thermal, and chemical stimuli. Central sensitization occurs when activity, generated by nociceptors during inflammation, enhances the excitability of nerve cells in the dorsal horn of the spinal cord. Following injury and resultant sensitization, normally innocuous stimuli can produce pain (termed *allodynia*). Sensitization is a clinically important process that contributes to tenderness, soreness, and *hyperalgesia* (increased pain intensity in response to the same noxious stimulus; e.g., moderate pressure causes severe pain). A striking example of sensitization is

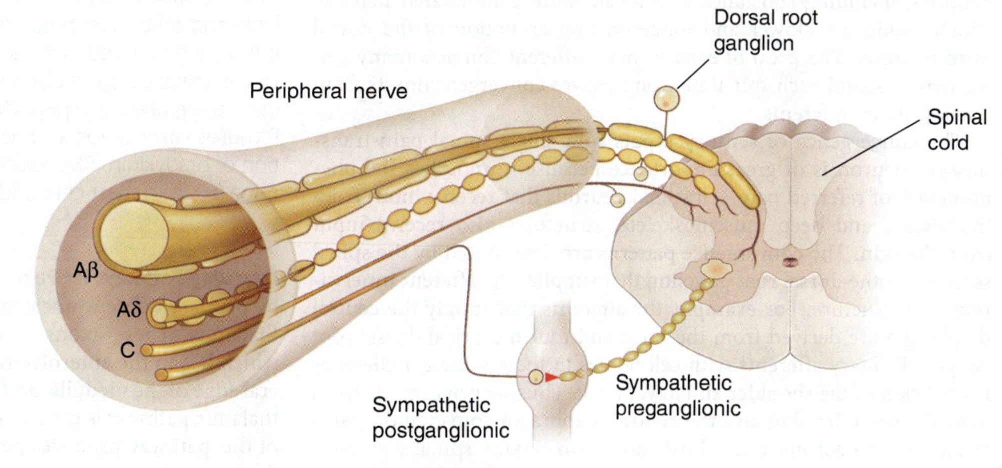

FIGURE 18-1 Components of a typical cutaneous nerve. There are two distinct functional categories of axons: primary afferents with cell bodies in the dorsal root ganglion, and sympathetic postganglionic fibers with cell bodies in the sympathetic ganglion. Primary afferents include those with large-diameter myelinated (Aβ), small-diameter myelinated (Aδ), and unmyelinated (C) axons. All sympathetic postganglionic fibers are unmyelinated.

sunburned skin, in which severe pain can be produced by a gentle slap on the back or a warm shower.

Sensitization is of particular importance for pain and tenderness in deep tissues. Viscera are normally relatively insensitive to noxious mechanical and thermal stimuli, although hollow viscera do generate significant discomfort when distended. In contrast, when affected by a disease process with an inflammatory component, deep structures such as joints or hollow viscera characteristically become exquisitely sensitive to mechanical stimulation.

A large proportion of Aδ and C fiber afferents innervating viscera are completely insensitive in normal noninjured, noninflamed tissue. That is, they cannot be activated by known mechanical or thermal stimuli and are not spontaneously active. However, in the presence of inflammatory mediators, these afferents become sensitive to mechanical stimuli. Such afferents have been termed *silent nociceptors*, and their characteristic properties may explain how, under pathologic conditions, the relatively insensitive deep structures can become the source of severe and debilitating pain and tenderness. Low pH, prostaglandins, leukotrienes, and other inflammatory mediators such as bradykinin play a significant role in sensitization.

Nociceptor-Induced Inflammation Primary afferent nociceptors also have a neuroeffector function. Most nociceptors contain polypeptide mediators that are released from their peripheral terminals when they are activated (Fig. 18-2). An example is substance P, an 11-amino-acid peptide. Substance P is released from primary afferent nociceptors and has multiple biologic activities. It is a potent vasodilator, degranulates mast cells, is a chemoattractant for leukocytes, and increases the production and release of inflammatory mediators. Interestingly, depletion of substance P from joints reduces the severity of experimental arthritis. Primary afferent nociceptors are not simply passive messengers of threats to tissue injury but also play an active role in tissue protection through these neuroeffector functions.

CENTRAL MECHANISMS

The Spinal Cord and Referred Pain The axons of primary afferent nociceptors enter the spinal cord via the dorsal root. They terminate in the dorsal horn of the spinal gray matter (Fig. 18-3). The terminals of primary afferent axons contact spinal neurons that transmit the pain signal to brain sites involved in pain perception. When primary afferents are activated by noxious stimuli, they release neurotransmitters from their terminals that excite the spinal cord neurons. The major neurotransmitter released is glutamate, which rapidly excites dorsal horn neurons. Primary afferent nociceptor terminals also release peptides, including substance P and calcitonin gene-related peptide, which produce a slower and longer-lasting excitation of the dorsal horn neurons. The axon of each primary afferent contacts many spinal neurons, and each spinal neuron receives convergent inputs from many primary afferents.

The convergence of sensory inputs to a single spinal pain-transmission neuron is of great importance because it underlies the phenomenon of referred pain. All spinal neurons that receive input from the viscera and deep musculoskeletal structures also receive input from the skin. The convergence patterns are determined by the spinal segment of the dorsal root ganglion that supplies the afferent innervation of a structure. For example, the afferents that supply the central diaphragm are derived from the third and fourth cervical dorsal root ganglia. Primary afferents with cell bodies in these same ganglia supply the skin of the shoulder and lower neck. Thus, sensory inputs from both the shoulder skin and the central diaphragm converge on pain-transmission neurons in the third and fourth cervical spinal segments. *Because of this convergence and the fact that the spinal neurons are most often activated by inputs from the skin, activity evoked in spinal neurons by input from deep structures is mislocalized by the patient to a place that roughly corresponds with the region of skin innervated by the same spinal segment.* Thus, inflammation near the central diaphragm is often reported as shoulder discomfort. This spatial displacement of pain sensation from the site of the injury that produces it is known as *referred pain*.

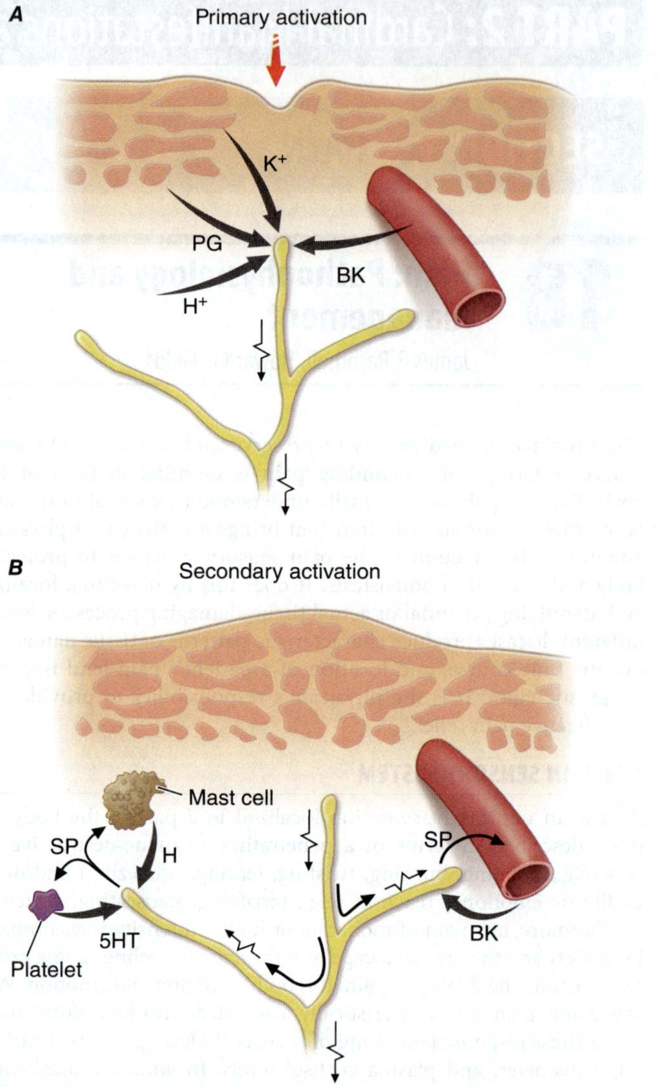

FIGURE 18-2 Events leading to activation, sensitization, and spread of sensitization of primary afferent nociceptor terminals. ***A.*** Direct activation by intense pressure and consequent cell damage. Cell damage induces lower pH (H^+) and leads to release of potassium (K^+) and to synthesis of prostaglandins (PG) and bradykinin (BK). Prostaglandins increase the sensitivity of the terminal to bradykinin and other pain-producing substances. ***B.*** Secondary activation. Impulses generated in the stimulated terminal propagate not only to the spinal cord but also into other terminal branches where they induce the release of peptides, including substance P (SP). Substance P causes vasodilation and neurogenic edema with further accumulation of bradykinin (BK). Substance P also causes the release of histamine (H) from mast cells and serotonin (5HT) from platelets.

Ascending Pathways for Pain A majority of spinal neurons contacted by primary afferent nociceptors send their axons to the contralateral thalamus. These axons form the contralateral spinothalamic tract, which lies in the anterolateral white matter of the spinal cord, the lateral edge of the medulla, and the lateral pons and midbrain. The spinothalamic pathway is crucial for pain sensation in humans. Interruption of this pathway produces permanent deficits in pain and temperature discrimination.

Spinothalamic tract axons ascend to several regions of the thalamus. There is tremendous divergence of the pain signal from these thalamic sites to several distinct areas of the cerebral cortex that subserve different aspects of the pain experience (Fig. 18-4). One of the thalamic projections is to the somatosensory cortex. This projection mediates the purely sensory aspects of pain, i.e., its location, intensity, and quality. Other thalamic neurons project to cortical regions that are linked

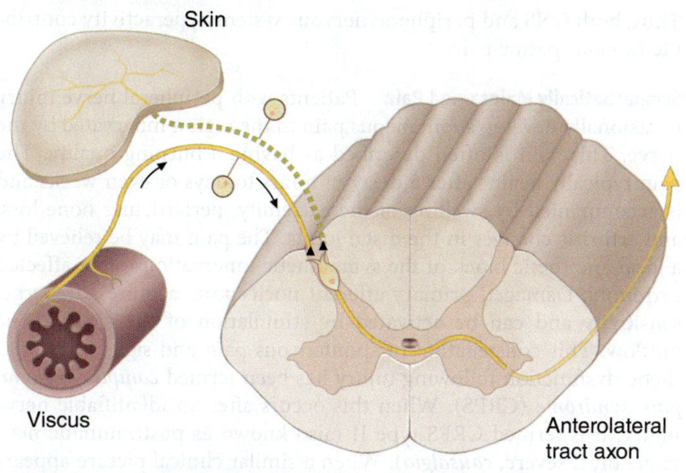

FIGURE 18-3 The convergence-projection hypothesis of referred pain. According to this hypothesis, visceral afferent nociceptors converge on the same pain-projection neurons as the afferents from the somatic structures in which the pain is perceived. The brain has no way of knowing the actual source of input and mistakenly "projects" the sensation to the somatic structure.

to emotional responses, such as the cingulate gyrus and other areas of the frontal lobes, including the insular cortex. These pathways to the frontal cortex subserve the affective or unpleasant emotional dimension of pain. This affective dimension of pain produces suffering and exerts potent control of behavior. Because of this dimension, fear is a constant companion of pain. As a consequence, injury or surgical lesions to areas of the frontal cortex activated by painful stimuli can diminish the emotional impact of pain while largely preserving the individual's ability to recognize noxious stimuli as painful.

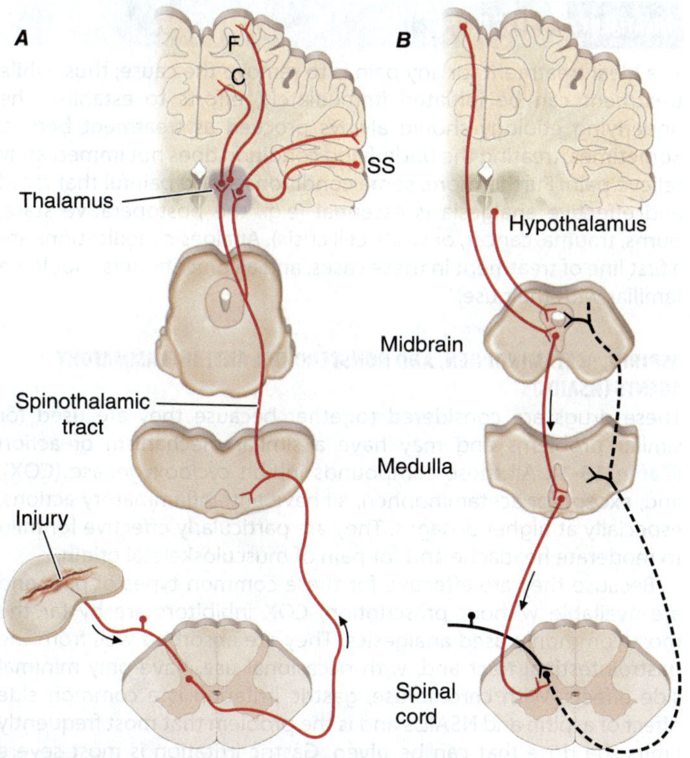

FIGURE 18-4 Pain transmission and modulatory pathways. ***A.*** Transmission system for nociceptive messages. Noxious stimuli activate the sensitive peripheral ending of the primary afferent nociceptor by the process of transduction. The message is then transmitted over the peripheral nerve to the spinal cord, where it synapses with cells of origin of the major ascending pain pathway, the spinothalamic tract. The message is relayed in the thalamus to the anterior cingulate (C), frontal insular (F), and somatosensory cortex (SS). ***B.*** Pain-modulation network. Inputs from frontal cortex and hypothalamus activate cells in the midbrain that control spinal pain-transmission cells via cells in the medulla.

PAIN MODULATION

The pain produced by injuries of similar magnitude is remarkably variable in different situations and in different individuals. For example, athletes have been known to sustain serious fractures with only minor pain, and Beecher's classic World War II survey revealed that many soldiers in battle were unbothered by injuries that would have produced agonizing pain in civilian patients. Furthermore, even the suggestion that a treatment will relieve pain can have a significant analgesic effect (the *placebo effect*). On the other hand, many patients find even minor injuries (such as venipuncture) frightening and unbearable, and the expectation of pain can induce pain even without a noxious stimulus. The suggestion that pain will worsen following administration of an inert substance can increase its perceived intensity (the *nocebo effect*).

The powerful effect of expectation and other psychological variables on the perceived intensity of pain is explained by brain circuits that modulate the activity of the pain-transmission pathways. One of these circuits has links to the hypothalamus, midbrain, and medulla, and it selectively controls spinal pain-transmission neurons through a descending pathway (Fig. 18-4).

Human brain-imaging studies have implicated this pain-modulating circuit in the pain-relieving effect of attention, suggestion, and opioid analgesic medications (Fig. 18-5). Furthermore, each of the component structures of the pathway contains opioid receptors and is sensitive to the direct application of opioid drugs. In animals, lesions of this descending modulatory system reduce the analgesic effect of systemically administered opioids such as morphine. Along with the opioid receptor, the component nuclei of this pain-modulating circuit contain endogenous opioid peptides such as the enkephalins and β-endorphin.

The most reliable way to activate this endogenous opioid-mediated modulating system is by suggestion of pain relief or by intense emotion directed away from the pain-causing injury (e.g., during severe threat or an athletic competition). In fact, pain-relieving endogenous opioids are released following surgical procedures and in patients given a placebo for pain relief.

Pain-modulating circuits can enhance as well as suppress pain. Both pain-inhibiting and pain-facilitating neurons in the medulla project to and control spinal pain-transmission neurons. Because pain-transmission neurons can be activated by modulatory neurons, it is theoretically possible to generate a pain signal with no peripheral noxious stimulus. In fact, human functional imaging studies have demonstrated increased activity in this circuit during migraine headaches. A central circuit that facilitates pain could account for the finding that pain can be induced by suggestion or enhanced by expectation and provides a framework for understanding how psychological factors can contribute to chronic pain.

NEUROPATHIC PAIN

Lesions of the peripheral or central nociceptive pathways typically result in a loss or impairment of pain sensation. Paradoxically, damage to or dysfunction of these pathways can also produce pain. For example, damage to peripheral nerves, as occurs in diabetic neuropathy, or to primary afferents, as in herpes zoster infection, can result in pain that is referred to the body region innervated by the damaged nerves. Pain may also be produced by damage to the central nervous system (CNS), for example, in some patients following trauma or vascular injury to the spinal cord, brainstem, or thalamic areas that contain central nociceptive pathways. Such neuropathic pains are often severe and are typically resistant to standard treatments for pain.

Neuropathic pain typically has an unusual burning, tingling, or electric shock–like quality and may be triggered by very light touch. These features are rare in other types of pain. On examination, a sensory deficit is characteristically present in the area of the patient's pain. *Hyperpathia*, a greatly exaggerated pain sensation to innocuous

Pattern of Brain Activity During Placebo Analgesia

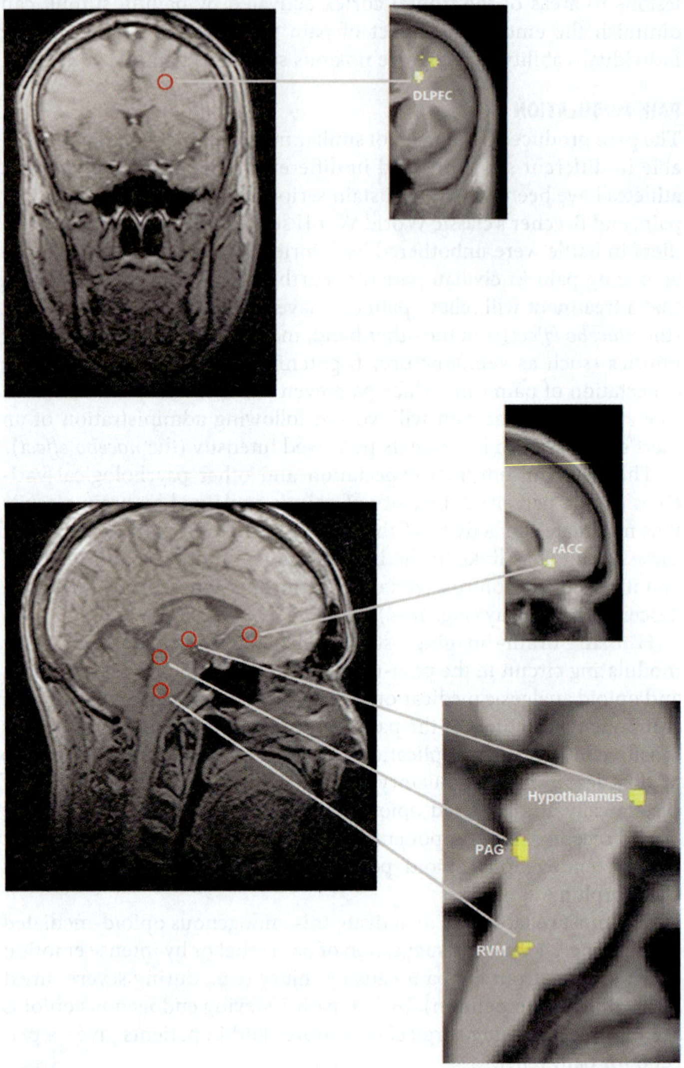

FIGURE 18-5 Functional magnetic resonance imaging (fMRI) demonstrates placebo-enhanced brain activity in anatomic regions correlating with the opioidergic descending pain control system. *Top panel:* Frontal fMRI image shows placebo-enhanced brain activity in the dorsal lateral prefrontal cortex (DLPFC). *Bottom panel:* Sagittal fMRI images show placebo-enhanced responses in the rostral anterior cingulate cortex (rACC), the rostral ventral medullae (RVM), the periaqueductal gray (PAG) area, and the hypothalamus. The placebo-enhanced activity in all areas was reduced by naloxone, demonstrating the link between the descending opioidergic system and the placebo analgesic response. *(Adapted with permission from F Eippert et al: Neuron 63:533, 2009.)*

or mild nociceptive stimuli, is also characteristic of neuropathic pain; patients often complain that the very lightest moving stimulus evokes exquisite pain (allodynia). In this regard, it is of clinical interest that a topical preparation of 5% lidocaine in patch form is effective for patients with postherpetic neuralgia who have prominent allodynia.

A variety of mechanisms contribute to neuropathic pain. As with sensitized primary afferent nociceptors, damaged primary afferents, including nociceptors, become highly sensitive to mechanical stimulation and may generate impulses in the absence of stimulation. Increased sensitivity and spontaneous activity are due, in part, to an increased concentration of sodium channels in the damaged nerve fiber. Damaged primary afferents may also develop sensitivity to norepinephrine. Interestingly, spinal cord pain-transmission neurons cut off from their normal input may also become spontaneously active. Thus, both CNS and peripheral nervous system hyperactivity contribute to neuropathic pain.

Sympathetically Maintained Pain Patients with peripheral nerve injury occasionally develop spontaneous pain in the region innervated by the nerve. This pain is often described as having a burning quality. The pain typically begins after a delay of hours to days or even weeks and is accompanied by swelling of the extremity, periarticular bone loss, and arthritic changes in the distal joints. The pain may be relieved by a local anesthetic block of the sympathetic innervation to the affected extremity. Damaged primary afferent nociceptors acquire adrenergic sensitivity and can be activated by stimulation of the sympathetic outflow. This constellation of spontaneous pain and signs of sympathetic dysfunction following injury has been termed *complex regional pain syndrome* (CRPS). When this occurs after an identifiable nerve injury, it is termed CRPS type II (also known as posttraumatic neuralgia or, if severe, *causalgia*). When a similar clinical picture appears without obvious nerve injury, it is termed CRPS type I (also known as *reflex sympathetic dystrophy*). CRPS can be produced by a variety of injuries, including fractures of bone, soft tissue trauma, myocardial infarction, and stroke (Chap. 446). CRPS type I typically resolves with symptomatic treatment; however, when it persists, detailed examination often reveals evidence of peripheral nerve injury. Although the pathophysiology of CRPS is poorly understood, the pain and the signs of inflammation, when acute, can be rapidly relieved by blocking the sympathetic nervous system. This implies that sympathetic activity can activate undamaged nociceptors when inflammation is present. Signs of sympathetic hyperactivity should be sought in patients with posttraumatic pain and inflammation and no other obvious explanation.

TREATMENT ACUTE PAIN

The ideal treatment for any pain is to remove the cause; thus, while treatment can be initiated immediately, efforts to establish the underlying etiology should always proceed as treatment begins. Sometimes, treating the underlying condition does not immediately relieve pain. Furthermore, some conditions are so painful that rapid and effective analgesia is essential (e.g., the postoperative state, burns, trauma, cancer, or sickle cell crisis). Analgesic medications are a first line of treatment in these cases, and all practitioners should be familiar with their use.

ASPIRIN, ACETAMINOPHEN, AND NONSTEROIDAL ANTI-INFLAMMATORY AGENTS (NSAIDs)

These drugs are considered together because they are used for similar problems and may have a similar mechanism of action (Table 18-1). All these compounds inhibit cyclooxygenase (COX), and, except for acetaminophen, all have anti-inflammatory actions, especially at higher dosages. They are particularly effective for mild to moderate headache and for pain of musculoskeletal origin.

Because they are effective for these common types of pain and are available without prescription, COX inhibitors are by far the most commonly used analgesics. They are absorbed well from the gastrointestinal tract and, with occasional use, have only minimal side effects. With chronic use, gastric irritation is a common side effect of aspirin and NSAIDs and is the problem that most frequently limits the dose that can be given. Gastric irritation is most severe with aspirin, which may cause erosion and ulceration of the gastric mucosa leading to bleeding or perforation. Because aspirin irreversibly acetylates platelet cyclooxygenase and thereby interferes with coagulation of the blood, gastrointestinal bleeding is a particular risk. Older age and history of gastrointestinal disease increase the risks of aspirin and NSAIDs. In addition to the well-known gastrointestinal toxicity of NSAIDs, nephrotoxicity is a significant problem for patients using these drugs on a chronic basis. Patients at risk for renal insufficiency, particularly those with significant contraction of their intravascular volume as occurs with chronic diuretic use or

TABLE 18-1 DRUGS FOR RELIEF OF PAIN

Generic Name	Dose, mg	Interval	Comments
Nonnarcotic analgesics: usual doses and intervals			
Acetylsalicylic acid	650 PO	q4h	Enteric-coated preparations available
Acetaminophen	650 PO	q4h	Side effects uncommon
Ibuprofen	400 PO	q4–6h	Available without prescription
Naproxen	250–500 PO	q12h	Delayed effects may be due to long half-life
Fenoprofen	200 PO	q4–6h	Contraindicated in renal disease
Indomethacin	25–50 PO	q8h	Gastrointestinal side effects common
Ketorolac	15–60 IM/IV	q4–6h	Available for parenteral use
Celecoxib	100–200 PO	q12–24h	Useful for arthritis
Valdecoxib	10–20 PO	q12–24h	Removed from U.S. market in 2005

Generic Name	Parenteral Dose, mg	PO Dose, mg	Comments
Narcotic analgesics: usual doses and intervals			
Codeine	30–60 q4h	30–60 q4h	Nausea common
Oxycodone	—	5–10 q4–6h	Usually available with acetaminophen or aspirin
Morphine	5 q4h	30 q4h	
Morphine sustained release	—	15–60 bid to tid	Oral slow-release preparation
Hydromorphone	1–2 q4h	2–4 q4h	Shorter acting than morphine sulfate
Levorphanol	2 q6–8h	4 q6–8h	Longer acting than morphine sulfate; absorbed well PO
Methadone	5–10 q6–8h	5–20 q6–8h	Delayed sedation due to long half-life; therapy should not be initiated with >40 mg/d, and dose escalation should be made no more frequently than every 3 days
Meperidine	50–100 q3–4h	300 q4h	Poorly absorbed PO; normeperidine is a toxic metabolite; routine use of this agent is not recommended
Butorphanol	—	1–2 q4h	Intranasal spray
Fentanyl	25–100 μg/h	—	72-h transdermal patch
Buprenorphine	5–20 μg/h		7-day transdermal patch
Buprenorphine	0.3 q6–8h		Parenteral administration
Tramadol	—	50–100 q4–6h	Mixed opioid/adrenergic action

	Uptake Blockade							
Generic Name	**5-HT**	**NE**	**Sedative Potency**	**Anticholinergic Potency**	**Orthostatic Hypotension**	**Cardiac Arrhythmia**	**Ave. Dose, mg/d**	**Range, mg/d**
Antidepressants[a]								
Doxepin	++	+	High	Moderate	Moderate	Less	200	75–400
Amitriptyline	++++	++	High	Highest	Moderate	Yes	150	25–300
Imipramine	++++	++	Moderate	Moderate	High	Yes	200	75–400
Nortriptyline	+++	++	Moderate	Moderate	Low	Yes	100	40–150
Desipramine	+++	++++	Low	Low	Low	Yes	150	50–300
Venlafaxine	+++	++	Low	None	None	No	150	75–400
Duloxetine	+++	+++	Low	None	None	No	40	30–60

Generic Name	PO Dose, mg	Interval	Generic Name	PO Dose, mg	Interval
Anticonvulsants and antiarrhythmics[a]					
Phenytoin	300	daily/qhs	Clonazepam	1	q6h
Carbamazepine	200–300	q6h	Gabapentin[b]	600–1200	q8h
Oxcarbazepine	300	bid	Pregabalin	150–600	bid

[a]Antidepressants, anticonvulsants, and antiarrhythmics have not been approved by the U.S. Food and Drug Administration (FDA) for the treatment of pain. [b]Gabapentin in doses up to 1800 mg/d is FDA approved for postherpetic neuralgia.

Abbreviations: 5-HT, serotonin; NE, norepinephrine.

acute hypovolemia, should be monitored closely. NSAIDs can also increase blood pressure in some individuals. Long-term treatment with NSAIDs requires regular blood pressure monitoring and treatment if necessary. Although toxic to the liver when taken in high doses, acetaminophen rarely produces gastric irritation and does not interfere with platelet function.

The introduction of parenteral forms of NSAIDs, ketorolac and diclofenac, extends the usefulness of this class of compounds in the management of acute severe pain. Both agents are sufficiently potent and rapid in onset to supplant opioids for many patients with acute severe headache and musculoskeletal pain.

There are two major classes of COX: COX-1 is constitutively expressed, and COX-2 is induced in the inflammatory state. COX-2–selective drugs have similar analgesic potency and produce less gastric irritation than the nonselective COX inhibitors. The use of COX-2–selective drugs does not appear to lower the risk of nephrotoxicity compared to nonselective NSAIDs. On the other hand, COX-2–selective drugs offer a significant benefit in the management of acute postoperative pain because they do not affect blood coagulation. Nonselective COX inhibitors are usually contraindicated postoperatively because they impair platelet-mediated blood clotting and are thus associated with increased bleeding at the operative site. COX-2 inhibitors, including celecoxib (Celebrex), are associated with increased cardiovascular risk. It appears that this is a class effect of NSAIDs, excluding aspirin. These drugs are contraindicated in patients in the immediate period after coronary artery bypass surgery and should be used with caution in elderly patients and those with a history of or significant risk factors for cardiovascular disease.

OPIOID ANALGESICS

Opioids are the most potent pain-relieving drugs currently available. Of all analgesics, they have the broadest range of efficacy and provide the most reliable and effective method for rapid pain relief. Although side effects are common, most are reversible: nausea, vomiting, pruritus, and constipation are the most frequent and bothersome side effects. Respiratory depression is uncommon at standard analgesic doses, but can be life-threatening. Opioid-related side effects can be reversed rapidly with the narcotic antagonist naloxone. Many physicians, nurses, and patients have a certain trepidation about using opioids that is based on an exaggerated fear of addiction. In fact, there is a vanishingly small chance of patients becoming addicted to narcotics as a result of their appropriate medical use. The physician should not hesitate to use opioid analgesics in patients with acute severe pain. Table 18-1 lists the most commonly used opioid analgesics.

Opioids produce analgesia by actions in the CNS. They activate pain-inhibitory neurons and directly inhibit pain-transmission neurons. Most of the commercially available opioid analgesics act at the same opioid receptor (μ-receptor), differing mainly in potency, speed of onset, duration of action, and optimal route of administration. Some side effects are due to accumulation of nonopioid metabolites that are unique to individual drugs. One striking example of this is normeperidine, a metabolite of meperidine. At higher doses of meperidine, typically greater than 1 g/d, accumulation of normeperidine can produce hyperexcitability and seizures that are not reversible with naloxone. Normeperidine accumulation is increased in patients with renal failure.

The most rapid pain relief is obtained by intravenous administration of opioids; relief with oral administration is significantly slower. Because of the potential for respiratory depression, patients with any form of respiratory compromise must be kept under close observation following opioid administration; an oxygen-saturation monitor may be useful, but only in a setting where the monitor is under constant surveillance. Opioid-induced respiratory depression is typically accompanied by sedation and a reduction in respiratory rate. A fall in oxygen saturation represents a critical level of respiratory depression and the need for immediate intervention to prevent life-threatening hypoxemia. Ventilatory assistance should be maintained until the opioid-induced respiratory depression has resolved. The opioid antagonist naloxone should be readily available whenever opioids are used at high doses or in patients with compromised pulmonary function. Opioid effects are dose-related, and there is great variability among patients in the doses that relieve pain and produce side effects. Synergistic respiratory depression is common when opioids are administered with other CNS depressants, most commonly the benzodiazepines. Because of this, initiation of therapy requires titration to optimal dose and interval. The most important principle is to provide adequate pain relief. This requires determining whether the drug has adequately relieved the pain and frequent reassessment to determine the optimal interval for dosing. *The most common error made by physicians in managing severe pain with opioids is to prescribe an inadequate dose. Because many patients are reluctant to complain, this practice leads to needless suffering.* In the absence of sedation at the expected time of peak effect, a physician should not hesitate to repeat the initial dose to achieve satisfactory pain relief.

An innovative approach to the problem of achieving adequate pain relief is the use of patient-controlled analgesia (PCA). PCA uses a microprocessor-controlled infusion device that can deliver a baseline continuous dose of an opioid drug as well as preprogrammed additional doses whenever the patient pushes a button. The patient can then titrate the dose to the optimal level. This approach is used most extensively for the management of postoperative pain, but there is no reason why it should not be used for any hospitalized patient with persistent severe pain. PCA is also used for short-term home care of patients with intractable pain, such as that caused by metastatic cancer.

It is important to understand that the PCA device delivers small, repeated doses to maintain pain relief; in patients with severe pain, the pain must first be brought under control with a loading dose before transitioning to the PCA device. The bolus dose of the drug (typically 1 mg of morphine, 0.2 mg of hydromorphone, or 10 μg of fentanyl) can then be delivered repeatedly as needed. To prevent overdosing, PCA devices are programmed with a lockout period after each demand dose is delivered (5–10 min) and a limit on the total dose delivered per hour. Although some have advocated the use of a simultaneous continuous or basal infusion of the PCA drug, this increases the risk of respiratory depression and has not been shown to increase the overall efficacy of the technique.

The availability of new routes of administration has extended the usefulness of opioid analgesics. Most important is the availability of spinal administration. Opioids can be infused through a spinal catheter placed either intrathecally or epidurally. By applying opioids directly to the spinal or epidural space adjacent to the spinal cord, regional analgesia can be obtained using relatively low total doses. Indeed, the dose required to produce effective localized analgesia when using morphine intrathecally (0.1–0.3 mg) is a fraction of that required to produce similar analgesia when administered intravenously (5–10 mg). In this way, side effects such as sedation, nausea, and respiratory depression can be minimized. This approach has been used extensively during labor and delivery and for postoperative pain relief following surgical procedures. Continuous intrathecal delivery via implanted spinal drug-delivery systems is now commonly used, particularly for the treatment of cancer-related pain that would require sedating doses for adequate pain control if given systemically. Opioids can also be given intranasally (butorphanol), rectally, and transdermally (fentanyl and buprenorphine), or through the oral mucosa (fentanyl), thus avoiding the discomfort of frequent injections in patients who cannot be given oral medication. The fentanyl and buprenorphine transdermal patches have the advantage of providing fairly steady plasma levels, which maximizes patient comfort.

Recent additions to the armamentarium for treating opioid-induced side effects are the peripherally acting opioid antagonists alvimopan (Entereg) and methylnaltrexone (Rellistor). Alvimopan is available as an orally administered agent that is restricted to the intestinal lumen by limited absorption; methylnaltrexone is available in a subcutaneously administered form that has virtually no penetration into the CNS. Both agents act by binding to peripheral μ-receptors, thereby inhibiting or reversing the effects of opioids at these peripheral sites. The action of both agents is restricted to receptor sites outside of the CNS; thus, these drugs can reverse the adverse effects of opioid analgesics that are mediated through their peripheral receptors without reversing their analgesic effects. Alvimopan has proven effective in lowering the duration of persistent ileus following abdominal surgery in patients receiving opioid analgesics for postoperative pain control. Methylnaltrexone has proven effective for relief of opioid-induced constipation in patients taking opioid analgesics on a chronic basis.

Opioid and COX Inhibitor Combinations When used in combination, opioids and COX inhibitors have additive effects. Because a lower dose of each can be used to achieve the same degree of pain relief and their side effects are nonadditive, such combinations are used to lower the severity of dose-related side effects. However, fixed-ratio combinations of an opioid with acetaminophen carry an important risk. Dose escalation as a result of increased severity of pain or decreased opioid effect as a result of tolerance may lead to ingestion of levels of acetaminophen that are toxic to the liver. Although acetaminophen-related hepatotoxicity is uncommon, it remains a significant cause for liver failure. Thus, many practitioners have moved away from the use of opioid-acetaminophen combination analgesics to avoid the risk of excessive acetaminophen exposure as the dose of the analgesic is escalated.

CHRONIC PAIN

Managing patients with chronic pain is intellectually and emotionally challenging. The patient's problem is often difficult or impossible to diagnose with certainty; such patients are demanding of the physician's time and often appear emotionally distraught. The traditional medical approach of seeking an obscure organic pathology is usually unhelpful. On the other hand, psychological evaluation and behaviorally based treatment paradigms are frequently helpful, particularly in the setting of a multidisciplinary pain-management center. Unfortunately, this approach, while effective, remains largely underused in current medical practice.

There are several factors that can cause, perpetuate, or exacerbate chronic pain. First, of course, the patient may simply have a disease that is characteristically painful for which there is presently no cure. Arthritis, cancer, chronic daily headaches, fibromyalgia, and diabetic neuropathy are examples of this. Second, there may be secondary perpetuating factors that are initiated by disease and persist after that disease has resolved. Examples include damaged sensory nerves, sympathetic efferent activity, and painful reflex muscle contraction (spasm). Finally, a variety of psychological conditions can exacerbate or even cause pain.

There are certain areas to which special attention should be paid in a patient's medical history. Because depression is the most common emotional disturbance in patients with chronic pain, patients should be questioned about their mood, appetite, sleep patterns, and daily activity. A simple standardized questionnaire, such as the Beck Depression Inventory, can be a useful screening device. It is important to remember that major depression is a common, treatable, and potentially fatal illness.

Other clues that a significant emotional disturbance is contributing to a patient's chronic pain complaint include pain that occurs in multiple, unrelated sites; a pattern of recurrent, but separate, pain problems beginning in childhood or adolescence; pain beginning at a time of emotional trauma, such as the loss of a parent or spouse; a history of physical or sexual abuse; and past or present substance abuse.

On examination, special attention should be paid to whether the patient guards the painful area and whether certain movements or postures are avoided because of pain. Discovering a mechanical component to the pain can be useful both diagnostically and therapeutically. Painful areas should be examined for deep tenderness, noting whether this is localized to muscle, ligamentous structures, or joints. Chronic myofascial pain is very common, and, in these patients, deep palpation may reveal highly localized trigger points that are firm bands or knots in muscle. Relief of the pain following injection of local anesthetic into these trigger points supports the diagnosis. A neuropathic component to the pain is indicated by evidence of nerve damage, such as sensory impairment, exquisitely sensitive skin (allodynia), weakness, and muscle atrophy, or loss of deep tendon reflexes. Evidence suggesting sympathetic nervous system involvement includes the presence of diffuse swelling, changes in skin color and temperature, and hypersensitive skin and joint tenderness compared with the normal side. Relief of the pain with a sympathetic block supports the diagnosis, but once the condition becomes chronic, the response to sympathetic blockade is of variable magnitude and duration; the role for repeated sympathetic blocks in the overall management of CRPS is not established.

A guiding principle in evaluating patients with chronic pain is to assess both emotional and organic factors before initiating therapy. Addressing these issues together, rather than waiting to address emotional issues after organic causes of pain have been ruled out, improves compliance in part because it assures patients that a psychological evaluation does not mean that the physician is questioning the validity of their complaint. Even when an organic cause for a patient's pain can be found, it is still wise to look for other factors. For example, a cancer patient with painful bony metastases may have additional pain due to nerve damage and may also be depressed. Optimal therapy requires that each of these factors be looked for and treated.

TREATMENT CHRONIC PAIN

Once the evaluation process has been completed and the likely causative and exacerbating factors identified, an explicit treatment plan should be developed. An important part of this process is to identify specific and realistic functional goals for therapy, such as getting a good night's sleep, being able to go shopping, or returning to work. A multidisciplinary approach that uses medications, counseling, physical therapy, nerve blocks, and even surgery may be required to improve the patient's quality of life. There are also some newer, relatively invasive procedures that can be helpful for some patients with intractable pain. These include image-guided interventions such as epidural injection of glucocorticoids for acute radicular pain and radiofrequency treatment of the facet joints for chronic facet-related back and neck pain. For patients with severe and persistent pain that is unresponsive to more conservative treatment, placement of electrodes within the spinal canal overlying the dorsal columns of the spinal cord (spinal cord stimulation) or implantation of intrathecal drug-delivery systems has shown significant benefit. The criteria for predicting which patients will respond to these procedures continue to evolve. They are generally reserved for patients who have not responded to conventional pharmacologic approaches. Referral to a multidisciplinary pain clinic for a full evaluation should precede any invasive procedure. Such referrals are clearly not necessary for all chronic pain patients. For some, pharmacologic management alone can provide adequate relief.

ANTIDEPRESSANT MEDICATIONS

The tricyclic antidepressants (TCAs), particularly nortriptyline and desipramine (Table 18-1), are useful for the management of chronic pain. Although developed for the treatment of depression, the TCAs have a spectrum of dose-related biologic activities that include analgesia in a variety of chronic clinical conditions. Although the mechanism is unknown, the analgesic effect of TCAs has a more rapid onset and occurs at a lower dose than is typically required for the treatment of depression. Furthermore, patients with chronic pain who are not depressed obtain pain relief with antidepressants. There is evidence that TCAs potentiate opioid analgesia, so they may be useful adjuncts for the treatment of severe persistent pain such as occurs with malignant tumors. Table 18-2 lists some of the painful conditions that respond to TCAs. TCAs are of particular value in the management of neuropathic pain such as occurs in diabetic neuropathy and postherpetic neuralgia, for which there are few other therapeutic options.

The TCAs that have been shown to relieve pain have significant side effects (Table 18-1; Chap. 466). Some of these side effects, such as orthostatic hypotension, drowsiness, cardiac conduction delay, memory impairment, constipation, and urinary retention,

TABLE 18-2 PAINFUL CONDITIONS THAT RESPOND TO TRICYCLIC ANTIDEPRESSANTS

Postherpetic neuralgia[a]
Diabetic neuropathy[a]
Tension headache[a]
Migraine headache[a]
Rheumatoid arthritis[a,b]
Chronic low back pain[b]
Cancer
Central poststroke pain

[a]Controlled trials demonstrate analgesia. [b]Controlled studies indicate benefit but not analgesia.

are particularly problematic in elderly patients, and several are additive to the side effects of opioid analgesics. The selective serotonin reuptake inhibitors such as fluoxetine (Prozac) have fewer and less serious side effects than TCAs, but they are much less effective for relieving pain. It is of interest that venlafaxine (Effexor) and duloxetine (Cymbalta), which are nontricyclic antidepressants that block both serotonin and norepinephrine reuptake, appear to retain most of the pain-relieving effect of TCAs with a side effect profile more like that of the selective serotonin reuptake inhibitors. These drugs may be particularly useful in patients who cannot tolerate the side effects of TCAs.

ANTICONVULSANTS AND ANTIARRHYTHMICS

These drugs are useful primarily for patients with neuropathic pain. Phenytoin (Dilantin) and carbamazepine (Tegretol) were first shown to relieve the pain of trigeminal neuralgia. This pain has a characteristic brief, shooting, electric shock–like quality. In fact, anticonvulsants seem to be particularly helpful for pains that have such a lancinating quality. Newer anticonvulsants, gabapentin (Neurontin) and pregabalin (Lyrica), are effective for a broad range of neuropathic pains. Furthermore, because of their favorable side effect profile, these newer anticonvulsants are often used as first-line agents.

CHRONIC OPIOID MEDICATION

The long-term use of opioids is accepted for patients with pain due to malignant disease. Although opioid use for chronic pain of nonmalignant origin is controversial, it is clear that, for many patients, opioids are the only option that produces meaningful pain relief. This is understandable because opioids are the most potent and have the broadest range of efficacy of any analgesic medications. Although addiction is rare in patients who first use opioids for pain relief, some degree of tolerance and physical dependence is likely with long-term use. Furthermore, animal studies suggest that long-term opioid therapy may worsen pain in some individuals. Therefore, before embarking on opioid therapy, other options should be explored, and the limitations and risks of opioids should be explained to the patient. It is also important to point out that some opioid analgesic medications have mixed agonist-antagonist properties (e.g., butorphanol and buprenorphine). From a practical standpoint, this means that they may worsen pain by inducing an abstinence syndrome in patients who are physically dependent on other opioid analgesics.

With long-term outpatient use of orally administered opioids, it is desirable to use long-acting compounds such as levorphanol, methadone, sustained-release morphine, or transdermal fentanyl (Table 18-1). The pharmacokinetic profiles of these drug preparations enable the maintenance of sustained analgesic blood levels, potentially minimizing side effects such as sedation that are associated with high peak plasma levels, and reducing the likelihood of rebound pain associated with a rapid fall in plasma opioid concentration. Although long-acting opioid preparations may provide superior pain relief in patients with a continuous pattern of ongoing pain, others suffer from intermittent severe episodic pain and experience superior pain control and fewer side effects with the periodic use of short-acting opioid analgesics. Constipation is a virtually universal side effect of opioid use and should be treated expectantly. As noted above in the discussion of acute pain treatment, a recent advance for patients is the development of peripherally acting opioid antagonists that can reverse the constipation associated with opioid use without interfering with analgesia.

Soon after the introduction of a controlled-release oxycodone formulation (OxyContin) in the late 1990s, a dramatic rise in emergency department visits and deaths associated with oxycodone ingestion appeared, focusing public attention on misuse of prescription pain medications. The magnitude of prescription opioid abuse has grown over the last decade, leading the Centers for Disease Control and Prevention to classify prescription opioid analgesic abuse as an epidemic. This appears to be due in large part to individuals using a prescription drug nonmedically, most often an opioid analgesic.

TABLE 18-3 GUIDELINES FOR SELECTING AND MONITORING PATIENTS RECEIVING CHRONIC OPIOID THERAPY (COT) FOR THE TREATMENT OF CHRONIC, NONCANCER PAIN

Patient Selection

- Conduct a history, physical examination, and appropriate testing, including an assessment of risk of substance abuse, misuse, or addiction.
- Consider a trial of COT if pain is moderate or severe, pain is having an adverse impact on function or quality of life, and potential therapeutic benefits outweigh potential harms.
- A benefit-to-harm evaluation, including a history, physical examination, and appropriate diagnostic testing, should be performed and documented before and on an ongoing basis during COT.

Informed Consent and Use of Management Plans

- Informed consent should be obtained. A continuing discussion with the patient regarding COT should include goals, expectations, potential risks, and alternatives to COT.
- Consider using a written COT management plan to document patient and clinician responsibilities and expectations and assist in patient education.

Initiation and Titration

- Initial treatment with opioids should be considered as a therapeutic trial to determine whether COT is appropriate.
- Opioid selection, initial dosing, and titration should be individualized according to the patient's health status, previous exposure to opioids, attainment of therapeutic goals, and predicted or observed harms.

Monitoring

- Reassess patients on COT periodically and as warranted by changing circumstances. Monitoring should include documentation of pain intensity and level of functioning, assessments of progress toward achieving therapeutic goals, presence of adverse events, and adherence to prescribed therapies.
- In patients on COT who are at high risk or who have engaged in aberrant drug-related behaviors, clinicians should periodically obtain urine drug screens or other information to confirm adherence to the COT plan of care.
- In patients on COT not at high risk and not known to have engaged in aberrant drug-related behaviors, clinicians should consider periodically obtaining urine drug screens or other information to confirm adherence to the COT plan of care.

Source: Adapted with permission from R Chou et al: J Pain 10:113, 2009.

Drug-induced deaths have rapidly risen and are now the second leading cause of death in Americans, just behind motor vehicle fatalities. In 2011, the Office of National Drug Control Policy established a multifaceted approach to address prescription drug abuse, including Prescription Drug Monitoring Programs that allow practitioners to determine if patients are receiving prescriptions from multiple providers and use of law enforcement to eliminate improper prescribing practices. This increased scrutiny leaves many practitioners hesitant to prescribe opioid analgesics, other than for brief periods to control pain associated with illness or injury. For now, the choice to begin chronic opioid therapy for a given patient is left to the individual practitioner. Pragmatic guidelines for properly selecting and monitoring patients receiving chronic opioid therapy are shown in Table 18-3.

TREATMENT OF NEUROPATHIC PAIN

It is important to individualize treatment for patients with neuropathic pain. Several general principles should guide therapy: the first is to move quickly to provide relief, and the second is to minimize drug side effects. For example, in patients with postherpetic neuralgia and significant cutaneous hypersensitivity, topical lidocaine (Lidoderm patches) can provide immediate relief without side effects. Anticonvulsants (gabapentin or pregabalin; see above) or antidepressants (nortriptyline, desipramine, duloxetine, or venlafaxine) can be used as first-line drugs for patients with neuropathic pain. Systemically administered antiarrhythmic drugs such as lidocaine and mexiletine are less likely to be effective; although intravenous infusion of lidocaine can provide analgesia for patients with different types of neuropathic pain, the relief is usually transient, typically lasting just hours after the cessation of the infusion.

The oral lidocaine congener mexiletine is poorly tolerated, producing frequent gastrointestinal adverse effects. There is no consensus on which class of drug should be used as a first-line treatment for any chronically painful condition. However, because relatively high doses of anticonvulsants are required for pain relief, sedation is very common. Sedation is also a problem with TCAs but is much less of a problem with serotonin/norepinephrine reuptake inhibitors (SNRIs; e.g., venlafaxine and duloxetine). Thus, in the elderly or in patients whose daily activities require high-level mental activity, these drugs should be considered the first line. In contrast, opioid medications should be used as a second- or third-line drug class. Although highly effective for many painful conditions, opioids are sedating, and their effect tends to lessen over time, leading to dose escalation and, occasionally, a worsening of pain due to physical dependence. Drugs of different classes can be used in combination to optimize pain control.

It is worth emphasizing that many patients, especially those with chronic pain, seek medical attention primarily because they are suffering and because only physicians can provide the medications required for pain relief. A primary responsibility of all physicians is to minimize the physical and emotional discomfort of their patients. Familiarity with pain mechanisms and analgesic medications is an important step toward accomplishing this aim.

19 Chest Discomfort

David A. Morrow

Chest discomfort is among the most common reasons for which patients present for medical attention at either an emergency department (ED) or an outpatient clinic. The evaluation of nontraumatic chest discomfort is inherently challenging owing to the broad variety of possible causes, a minority of which are life-threatening conditions that should not be missed. It is helpful to frame the initial diagnostic assessment and triage of patients with acute chest discomfort around three categories: (1) myocardial ischemia; (2) other cardiopulmonary causes (pericardial disease, aortic emergencies, and pulmonary conditions); and (3) non-cardiopulmonary causes. Although rapid identification of high-risk conditions is a priority of the initial assessment, strategies that incorporate routine liberal use of testing carry the potential for adverse effects of unnecessary investigations.

EPIDEMIOLOGY AND NATURAL HISTORY

Chest discomfort is the third most common reason for visits to the ED in the United States, resulting in 6 to 7 million emergency visits each year. More than 60% of patients with this presentation are hospitalized for further testing, and the rest undergo additional investigation in the ED. Fewer than 25% of evaluated patients are eventually diagnosed with acute coronary syndrome (ACS), with rates of 5–15% in most series of unselected populations. In the remainder, the most common diagnoses are gastrointestinal causes (Fig. 19-1), and fewer than 10% are other life-threatening cardiopulmonary conditions. In a large proportion of patients with transient acute chest discomfort, ACS or another acute cardiopulmonary cause is excluded but the cause is not determined. Therefore, the resources and time devoted to the evaluation of chest discomfort *in the absence of a severe cause* are substantial. Nevertheless, a disconcerting 2–6% of patients with chest discomfort of presumed non-ischemic etiology who are discharged from the ED are later deemed to have had a missed myocardial infarction (MI). Patients with a missed diagnosis of MI have a 30-day risk of death that is double that of their counterparts who are hospitalized.

The natural histories of ACS, acute pericardial diseases, pulmonary embolism, and aortic emergencies are discussed in Chaps. 288, 294 and 295, 300, and 301, respectively. In a study of more than 350,000 patients with unspecified presumed non-cardiopulmonary chest discomfort, the mortality rate 1 year after discharge was <2% and did not differ significantly from age-adjusted mortality in the general population. The estimated rate of major cardiovascular events through 30 days in patients with acute chest pain who had been stratified as low risk was 2.5% in a large population-based study that excluded patients with ST-segment elevation or definite noncardiac chest pain.

CAUSES OF CHEST DISCOMFORT

The major etiologies of chest discomfort are discussed in this section and summarized in Table 19-1. Additional elements of the history, physical examination, and diagnostic testing that aid in distinguishing these causes are discussed in a later section (see "Approach to the Patient").

MYOCARDIAL ISCHEMIA/INJURY

Myocardial ischemia causing chest discomfort, termed *angina pectoris*, is a primary clinical concern in patients presenting with chest symptoms. Myocardial ischemia is precipitated by an imbalance between myocardial oxygen requirements and myocardial oxygen supply, resulting in insufficient delivery of oxygen to meet the heart's metabolic demands. Myocardial oxygen consumption may be elevated by increases in heart rate, ventricular wall stress, and myocardial contractility, whereas myocardial oxygen supply is determined by coronary

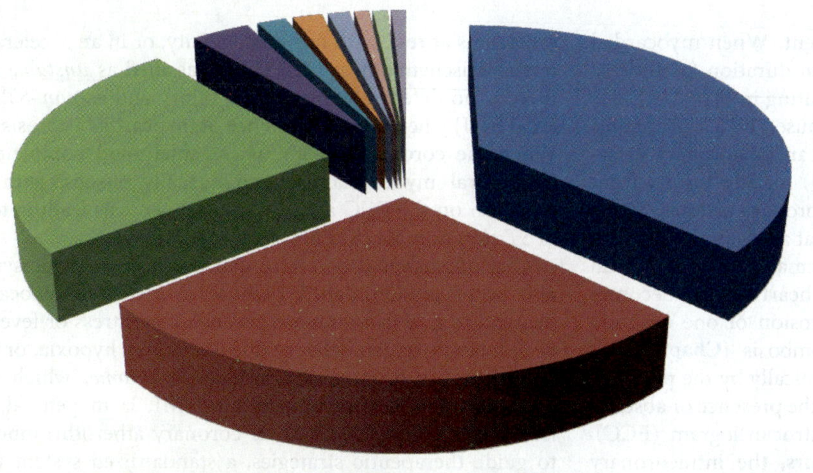

FIGURE 19-1 Distribution of final discharge diagnoses in patients with nontraumatic acute chest pain. *(Figure prepared from data in P Fruergaard et al: Eur Heart J 17:1028, 1996.)*

TABLE 19-1 TYPICAL CLINICAL FEATURES OF MAJOR CAUSES OF ACUTE CHEST DISCOMFORT

System	Condition	Onset/Duration	Quality	Location	Associated Features
Cardiopulmonary					
Cardiac	Myocardial ischemia	*Stable angina:* Precipitated by exertion, cold, or stress; 2–10 min *Unstable angina:* Increasing pattern or at rest *Myocardial infarction:* Usually >30 min	Pressure, tightness, squeezing, heaviness, burning	Retrosternal; often radiation to neck, jaw, shoulders, or arms; sometimes epigastric	S_4 gallop or mitral regurgitation murmur (rare) during pain; S_3 or rales if severe ischemia or complication of myocardial infarction
	Pericarditis	Variable; hours to days; may be episodic	Pleuritic, sharp	Retrosternal or toward cardiac apex; may radiate to left shoulder	May be relieved by sitting up and leaning forward; pericardial friction rub
Vascular	Acute aortic syndrome	Sudden onset of unrelenting pain	Tearing or ripping; knifelike	Anterior chest, often radiating to back, between shoulder blades	Associated with hypertension and/or underlying connective tissue disorder; murmur of aortic insufficiency; loss of peripheral pulses
	Pulmonary embolism	Sudden onset	Pleuritic; may manifest as heaviness with massive pulmonary embolism	Often lateral, on the side of the embolism	Dyspnea, tachypnea, tachycardia, and hypotension
	Pulmonary hypertension	Variable; often exertional	Pressure	Substernal	Dyspnea, signs of increased venous pressure
Pulmonary	Pneumonia or pleuritis	Variable	Pleuritic	Unilateral, often localized	Dyspnea, cough, fever, rales, occasional rub
	Spontaneous pneumothorax	Sudden onset	Pleuritic	Lateral to side of pneumothorax	Dyspnea, decreased breath sounds on side of pneumothorax
Non-cardiopulmonary					
Gastrointenstinal	Esophageal reflux	10–60 min	Burning	Substernal, epigastric	Worsened by postprandial recumbency; relieved by antacids
	Esophageal spasm	2–30 min	Pressure, tightness, burning	Retrosternal	Can closely mimic angina
	Peptic ulcer	Prolonged; 60–90 min after meals	Burning	Epigastric, substernal	Relieved with food or antacids
	Gallbladder disease	Prolonged	Aching or colicky	Epigastric, right upper quadrant; sometimes to the back	May follow meal
Neuromuscular	Costochondritis	Variable	Aching	Sternal	Sometimes swollen, tender, warm over joint; may be reproduced by localized pressure on examination
	Cervical disk disease	Variable; may be sudden	Aching; may include numbness	Arms and shoulders	May be exacerbated by movement of neck
	Trauma or strain	Usually constant	Aching	Localized to area of strain	Reproduced by movement or palpation
	Herpes zoster	Usually prolonged	Sharp or burning	Dermatomal distribution	Vesicular rash in area of discomfort
Psychological	Emotional and psychiatric conditions	Variable; may be fleeting or prolonged	Variable; often manifests as tightness and dyspnea with feeling of panic or doom	Variable; may be retrosternal	Situational factors may precipitate symptoms; history of panic attacks, depression

blood flow and coronary arterial oxygen content. When myocardial ischemia is sufficiently severe and prolonged in duration (as little as 20 min), irreversible cellular injury occurs, resulting in MI.

Ischemic heart disease is most commonly caused by atheromatous plaque that obstructs one or more of the epicardial coronary arteries. Stable ischemic heart disease (Chap. 293) usually results from the gradual atherosclerotic narrowing of the coronary arteries. *Stable angina* is characterized by ischemic episodes that are typically precipitated by a superimposed increase in oxygen demand during physical exertion and relieved upon resting. Ischemic heart disease becomes unstable most commonly when rupture or erosion of one or more atherosclerotic lesions triggers coronary thrombosis (Chap. 291e). Unstable ischemic heart disease is classified clinically by the presence or absence of detectable myocardial injury and the presence or absence of ST-segment elevation on the patient's electrocardiogram (ECG). When acute coronary atherothrombosis occurs, the intracoronary thrombus may be partially obstructive, generally leading to myocardial ischemia in the absence of ST-segment elevation. Marked by ischemic symptoms at rest, with minimal activity, or in an accelerating pattern, unstable ischemic heart disease is classified as *unstable angina* when there is no detectable myocardial injury and as *non–ST elevation MI* (NSTEMI) when there is evidence of myocardial necrosis (Chap. 294). When the coronary thrombus is acutely and completely occlusive, transmural myocardial ischemia usually ensues, with ST-segment elevation on the ECG and myocardial necrosis leading to a diagnosis of *ST elevation MI* (STEMI, see Chap. 295).

Clinicians should be aware that unstable ischemic symptoms may also occur predominantly because of increased myocardial oxygen demand (e.g., during intense psychological stress or fever) or because of decreased oxygen delivery due to anemia, hypoxia, or hypotension. However, the term *acute coronary syndrome*, which encompasses unstable angina, NSTEMI, and STEMI, is in general reserved for ischemia precipitated by acute coronary atherothrombosis. In order to guide therapeutic strategies, a standardized system for classification of MI has been expanded to discriminate MI resulting from acute coronary thrombosis (type 1) from MI occurring secondary to other imbalances of myocardial oxygen supply and demand (type 2; see Chap. 294).

Other contributors to stable and unstable ischemic heart disease, such as endothelial dysfunction, microvascular disease, and vasospasm, may exist alone or in combination with coronary atherosclerosis and may be the dominant cause of myocardial ischemia in some patients. Moreover, non-atherosclerotic processes, including congenital abnormalities of the coronary vessels, myocardial bridging, coronary arteritis, and radiation-induced coronary disease, can lead to coronary obstruction. In addition, conditions associated with extreme myocardial oxygen demand and impaired endocardial blood flow, such as aortic valve disease (Chap. 301), hypertrophic cardiomyopathy, or idiopathic dilated cardiomyopathy (Chap. 287), can precipitate myocardial ischemia in patients with or without underlying obstructive atherosclerosis.

Characteristics of Ischemic Chest Discomfort The clinical characteristics of angina pectoris, often referred to simply as "angina," are highly similar whether the ischemic discomfort is a manifestation of stable ischemic heart disease, unstable angina, or MI; the exceptions are differences in the pattern and duration of symptoms associated with these syndromes (Table 19-1). Heberden initially described angina as a sense of "strangling and anxiety." Chest discomfort characteristic of myocardial ischemia is typically described as aching, heavy, squeezing, crushing, or constricting. However, in a substantial minority of patients, the quality of discomfort is extremely vague and may be described as a mild tightness, or merely an uncomfortable feeling, that sometimes is experienced as numbness or a burning sensation. The site of the discomfort is usually retrosternal, but radiation is common and generally occurs down the ulnar surface of the left arm; the right arm, both arms, neck, jaw, or shoulders may also be involved. These and other characteristics of ischemic chest discomfort pertinent to discrimination from other causes of chest pain are discussed later in this chapter (see "Approach to the Patient").

Stable angina usually begins gradually and reaches its maximal intensity over a period of minutes before dissipating within several minutes with rest or with nitroglycerin. The discomfort typically occurs predictably at a characteristic level of exertion or psychological stress. By definition, unstable angina is manifest by self-limited anginal chest discomfort that is exertional but occurs at increased frequency with progressively lower intensity of physical activity or even at rest. Chest discomfort associated with MI is typically more severe, is prolonged (usually lasting ≥30 min), and is not relieved by rest.

Mechanisms of Cardiac Pain The neural pathways involved in ischemic cardiac pain are poorly understood. Ischemic episodes are thought to excite local chemosensitive and mechanoreceptive receptors that, in turn, stimulate release of adenosine, bradykinin, and other substances that activate the sensory ends of sympathetic and vagal afferent fibers. The afferent fibers traverse the nerves that connect to the upper five thoracic sympathetic ganglia and upper five distal thoracic roots of the spinal cord. From there, impulses are transmitted to the thalamus. Within the spinal cord, cardiac sympathetic afferent impulses may converge with impulses from somatic thoracic structures, and this convergence may be the basis for referred cardiac pain. In addition, cardiac vagal afferent fibers synapse in the nucleus tractus solitarius of the medulla and then descend to the upper cervical spinothalamic tract, and this route may contribute to anginal pain experienced in the neck and jaw.

OTHER CARDIOPULMONARY CAUSES

Pericardial and Other Myocardial Diseases (See also Chap. 288) Inflammation of the pericardium due to infectious or noninfectious causes can be responsible for acute or chronic chest discomfort. The visceral surface and most of the parietal surface of the pericardium are insensitive to pain. Therefore, the pain of pericarditis is thought to arise principally from associated pleural inflammation and is more common with infectious causes of pericarditis, which typically involve the pleura. Because of this pleural association, the discomfort of pericarditis is usually pleuritic pain that is exacerbated by breathing, coughing, or changes in position. Moreover, owing to the overlapping sensory supply of the central diaphragm via the phrenic nerve with somatic sensory fibers originating in the third to fifth cervical segments, the pain of pleural pericarditis is often referred to the shoulder and neck. Involvement of the pleural surface of the lateral diaphragm can lead to pain in the upper abdomen.

Acute inflammatory and other non-ischemic myocardial diseases can also produce chest discomfort. The symptoms of *Takotsubo (stress-related) cardiomyopathy* often start abruptly with chest pain and shortness of breath. This form of cardiomyopathy, in its most recognizable form, is triggered by an emotionally or physically stressful event and may mimic acute MI because of its commonly associated ECG abnormalities, including ST-segment elevation, and elevated biomarkers of myocardial injury. Observational studies support a predilection for women >50 years of age. The symptoms of acute myocarditis are highly varied. Chest discomfort may either originate with inflammatory injury of the myocardium or be due to severe increases in wall stress related to poor ventricular performance.

Diseases of the Aorta (See also Chap. 301) Acute aortic dissection (Fig. 19-1) is a less common cause of chest discomfort but is important because of the catastrophic natural history of certain subsets of cases when recognized late or left untreated. Acute aortic syndromes encompass a spectrum of acute aortic diseases related to disruption of the media of the aortic wall. *Aortic dissection* involves a tear in the aortic intima, resulting in separation of the media and creation of a separate "false" lumen. A *penetrating ulcer* has been described as ulceration of an aortic atheromatous plaque that extends through the intima and into the aortic media, with the potential to initiate an intramedial dissection or rupture into the adventitia. *Intramural hematoma* is an aortic wall hematoma with no demonstrable intimal flap, no radiologically apparent intimal tear, and no false lumen. Intramural hematoma can occur due to either rupture of the vasa vasorum or, less commonly, a penetrating ulcer.

Each of these subtypes of acute aortic syndrome typically presents with chest discomfort that is often severe, sudden in onset, and sometimes described as "tearing" in quality. Acute aortic syndromes involving the *ascending* aorta tend to cause pain in the midline of the anterior chest, whereas *descending* aortic syndromes most often present with pain in the back. Therefore, dissections that begin in the ascending aorta and extend to the descending aorta tend to cause pain in the front of the chest that extends toward the back, between the shoulder blades. Proximal aortic dissections that involve the ascending aorta (type A in the Stanford nomenclature) are at high risk for major complications that may influence the clinical presentation, including (1) compromise of the aortic ostia of the coronary arteries, resulting in MI; (2) disruption of the aortic valve, causing acute aortic insufficiency; and (3) rupture of the hematoma into the pericardial space, leading to pericardial tamponade.

Knowledge of the epidemiology of acute aortic syndromes can be helpful in maintaining awareness of this relatively uncommon group of disorders (estimated annual incidence, 3 cases per 100,000 population). Nontraumatic aortic dissections are very rare in the absence of hypertension or conditions associated with deterioration of the elastic or muscular components of the aortic media, including pregnancy, bicuspid aortic disease, or inherited connective tissue diseases, such as Marfan and Ehlers-Danlos syndromes.

Although aortic aneurysms are most often asymptomatic, thoracic aortic aneurysms can cause chest pain and other symptoms by compressing adjacent structures. This pain tends to be steady, deep, and occasionally severe. Aortitis, whether of noninfectious or infectious etiology, in the absence of aortic dissection is a rare cause of chest or back discomfort.

Pulmonary Conditions Pulmonary and pulmonary-vascular conditions that cause chest discomfort usually do so in conjunction with dyspnea and often produce symptoms that have a pleuritic nature.

PULMONARY EMBOLISM (See also Chap. 300) Pulmonary emboli (annual incidence, ~1 per 1000) can produce dyspnea and chest discomfort that is sudden in onset. Typically pleuritic in pattern, the chest discomfort associated with pulmonary embolism may result from (1) involvement of the pleural surface of the lung adjacent to a resultant pulmonary infarction; (2) distention of the pulmonary artery; or (3) possibly, right ventricular wall stress and/or subendocardial ischemia related to acute pulmonary hypertension. The pain associated with small pulmonary emboli is often lateral and pleuritic and is believed to be related to the first of these three possible mechanisms. In contrast, massive pulmonary emboli may cause severe substernal pain that may mimic an MI and that is plausibly attributed to the second and third of these potential mechanisms. Massive or submassive pulmonary embolism may also be associated with syncope, hypotension, and signs of right heart failure. Other typical characteristics that aid in the recognition of pulmonary embolism are discussed later in this chapter (see "Approach to the Patient").

PNEUMOTHORAX (See also Chap. 317) *Primary spontaneous pneumothorax* is a rare cause of chest discomfort, with an estimated annual incidence in the United States of 7 per 100,000 among men and <2 per 100,000 among women. Risk factors include male sex, smoking, family history, and Marfan syndrome. The symptoms are usually sudden in onset, and dyspnea may be mild; thus, presentation to medical attention is sometimes delayed. *Secondary spontaneous pneumothorax* may occur in patients with underlying lung disorders, such as chronic obstructive pulmonary disease, asthma, or cystic fibrosis, and usually produces symptoms that are more severe. Tension pneumothorax is a medical emergency caused by trapped intrathoracic air that precipitates hemodynamic collapse.

Other Pulmonary Parenchymal, Pleural, or Vascular Disease (See also Chaps. 304, 305, and 316) Most pulmonary diseases that produce chest pain, including pneumonia and malignancy, do so because of involvement of the pleura or surrounding structures. Pleurisy is typically described as a knifelike pain that is worsened by inspiration or coughing. In contrast, chronic pulmonary hypertension can manifest as chest pain that may be very similar to angina in its characteristics, suggesting right ventricular myocardial ischemia in some cases. Reactive airways diseases similarly can cause chest tightness associated with breathlessness rather than pleurisy.

NON-CARDIOPULMONARY CAUSES

Gastrointenstinal Conditions (See also Chap. 344) Gastrointestinal disorders are the most common cause of nontraumatic chest discomfort and often produce symptoms that are difficult to discern from more serious causes of chest pain, including myocardial ischemia. Esophageal disorders, in particular, may simulate angina in the character and location of the pain. Gastroesophageal reflux and disorders of esophageal motility are common and should be considered in the differential diagnosis of chest pain (Fig. 19-1 and Table 19-1). Acid reflux often causes a burning discomfort. The pain of esophageal spasm, in contrast, is commonly an intense, squeezing discomfort that is retrosternal in location and, like angina, may be relieved by nitroglycerin or dihydropyridine calcium channel antagonists. Chest pain can also result from injury to the esophagus, such as a Mallory-Weiss tear or even an esophageal rupture (Boerhaave syndrome) caused by severe vomiting. Peptic ulcer disease is most commonly epigastric in location but can radiate into the chest (Table 19-1).

Hepatobiliary disorders, including cholecystitis and biliary colic, may mimic acute cardiopulmonary diseases. Although the pain arising from these disorders usually localizes to the right upper quadrant of the abdomen, it is variable and may be felt in the epigastrium and radiate to the back and lower chest. This discomfort is sometimes referred to the scapula or may in rare cases be felt in the shoulder, suggesting diaphragmatic irritation. The pain is steady, usually lasts several hours, and subsides spontaneously, without symptoms between attacks. Pain resulting from pancreatitis is typically aching epigastric pain that radiates to the back.

Musculoskeletal and Other Causes (See also Chap. 393) Chest discomfort can be produced by any musculoskeletal disorder involving the chest wall or the nerves of the chest wall, neck, or upper limbs. Costochondritis causing tenderness of the costochondral junctions (*Tietze's syndrome*) is relatively common. Cervical radiculitis may manifest as a prolonged or constant aching discomfort in the upper chest and limbs. The pain may be exacerbated by motion of the neck. Occasionally, chest pain can be caused by compression of the brachial plexus by the cervical ribs, and tendinitis or bursitis involving the left shoulder may mimic the radiation of angina. Pain in a dermatomal distribution can also be caused by cramping of intercostal muscles or by herpes zoster (Chap. 217).

Emotional and Psychiatric Conditions As many as 10% of patients who present to emergency departments with acute chest discomfort have a panic disorder or related condition (Table 19-1). The symptoms may include chest tightness or aching that is associated with a sense of anxiety and difficulty breathing. The symptoms may be prolonged or fleeting.

APPROACH TO THE PATIENT: Chest Discomfort

Given the broad set of potential causes and the heterogeneous risk of serious complications in patients who present with acute nontraumatic chest discomfort, the priorities of the initial clinical encounter include assessment of (1) the patient's clinical stability and (2) the probability that the patient has an underlying cause of the discomfort that may be life-threatening. The high-risk conditions of principal concern are acute cardiopulmonary processes, including ACS, acute aortic syndrome, pulmonary embolism, tension pneumothorax, and pericarditis with tamponade. Among non-cardiopulmonary causes of chest pain, esophageal rupture likely holds the greatest urgency for diagnosis. Patients with these conditions may deteriorate rapidly despite initially appearing well. The remaining population with non-cardiopulmonary conditions has a more favorable prognosis during completion of the diagnostic work-up. A rapid targeted assessment for a serious cardiopulmonary cause is of particular relevance for patients with acute ongoing pain who have presented for emergency evaluation. Among patients presenting in the outpatient setting with chronic pain or pain that has resolved, a general diagnostic assessment is reasonably undertaken (see "Outpatient Evaluation of Chest Discomfort," below). A series of questions that can be used to structure the clinical evaluation of patients with chest discomfort is shown in Table 19-2.

TABLE 19-2 CONSIDERATIONS IN THE ASSESSMENT OF THE PATIENT WITH CHEST DISCOMFORT

1. Could the chest discomfort be due to an acute, potentially life-threatening condition that warrants urgent evaluation and management?			
Unstable ischemic heart disease	Aortic dissection	Pneumothorax	Pulmonary embolism
2. If not, could the discomfort be due to a chronic condition likely to lead to serious complications?			
Stable angina	Aortic stenosis	Pulmonary hypertension	
3. If not, could the discomfort be due to an acute condition that warrants specific treatment?			
Pericarditis	Pneumonia/ pleuritis	Herpes zoster	
4. If not, could the discomfort be due to another treatable chronic condition?			
Esophageal reflux		Cervical disk disease	
Esophageal spasm		Arthritis of the shoulder or spine	
Peptic ulcer disease		Costochondritis	
Gallbladder disease		Other musculoskeletal disorders	
Other gastrointestinal conditions		Anxiety state	

Source: Developed by Dr. Thomas H. Lee for the 18th edition of *Harrison's Principles of Internal Medicine.*

HISTORY

The evaluation of nontraumatic chest discomfort relies heavily on the clinical history and physical examination to direct subsequent diagnostic testing. The evaluating clinician should assess the quality, location (including radiation), and pattern (including onset and duration) of the pain as well as any provoking or alleviating factors. The presence of associated symptoms may also be useful in establishing a diagnosis.

Quality of Pain The quality of chest discomfort alone is never sufficient to establish a diagnosis. However, the characteristics of the pain are pivotal in formulating an initial clinical impression and assessing the likelihood of a serious cardiopulmonary process (Table 19-1), including acs in particular (Fig. 19-2). Pressure or tightness is consistent with a typical presentation of myocardial ischemic pain. Nevertheless, the clinician must remember that some patients with ischemic chest symptoms deny any "pain" but rather complain of dyspnea or a vague sense of anxiety. The severity of the discomfort has poor diagnostic accuracy. It is often helpful to ask about the similarity of the discomfort to previous definite ischemic symptoms. It is unusual for angina to be sharp, as in knifelike, stabbing, or pleuritic; however, patients sometimes use the word "sharp" to convey the intensity of discomfort rather than the quality. Pleuritic discomfort is suggestive of a process involving the pleura, including pericarditis, pulmonary embolism, or pulmonary parenchymal processes. Less frequently, the pain of pericarditis or massive pulmonary embolism is a steady severe pressure or aching that can be difficult to discriminate from myocardial ischemia. "Tearing" or "ripping" pain is often described by patients with acute aortic dissection. However, acute aortic emergencies also present commonly with severe, knifelike pain. A burning quality can suggest acid reflux or peptic ulcer disease but may also occur with myocardial ischemia. Esophageal pain, particularly with spasm, can be a severe squeezing discomfort identical to angina.

Location of Discomfort A substernal location with radiation to the neck, jaw, shoulder, or arms is typical of myocardial ischemic discomfort. Some patients present with aching in sites of radiated pain as their only symptoms of ischemia. However, pain that is highly localized—e.g., that which can be demarcated by the tip of one finger—is highly unusual for angina. A retrosternal location should prompt consideration of esophageal pain; however, other gastrointestinal conditions usually present with pain that is most intense in the abdomen or epigastrium, with possible radiation into the chest. Angina may also occur in an epigastric location. However, pain that occurs solely above the mandible or below the epigastrium is rarely angina. Severe pain radiating to the back, particularly between the shoulder blades, should prompt consideration of an acute aortic syndrome. Radiation to the trapezius ridge is characteristic of pericardial pain and does not usually occur with angina.

Pattern Myocardial ischemic discomfort usually builds over minutes and is exacerbated by activity and mitigated by rest. In contrast, pain that reaches its peak intensity immediately is more suggestive of aortic dissection, pulmonary embolism, or spontaneous pneumothorax. Pain that is fleeting (lasting only a few seconds) is rarely ischemic in origin. Similarly, pain that is constant in intensity for a prolonged period (many hours to days) is unlikely to represent myocardial ischemia if it occurs in the absence of other clinical consequences, such as abnormalities of the ECG, elevation of cardiac biomarkers, or clinical sequelae (e.g., heart failure or hypotension). Both myocardial ischemia and acid reflux may have their onset in the morning, the latter because of the absence of food to absorb gastric acid.

Provoking and Alleviating Factors Patients with myocardial ischemic pain usually prefer to rest, sit, or stop walking. However, clinicians should be aware of the phenomenon of "warm-up angina" in which some patients experience relief of angina as they continue at the same or even a greater level of exertion without symptoms (Chap. 293). Alterations in the intensity of pain with changes in position or movement of the upper extremities and neck are less likely with myocardial ischemia and suggest a musculoskeletal etiology. The pain of pericarditis, however, often is worse in the supine position and relieved by sitting upright and leaning forward. Gastroesophageal reflux may be exacerbated by alcohol, some foods, or by a reclined position. Relief can occur with sitting.

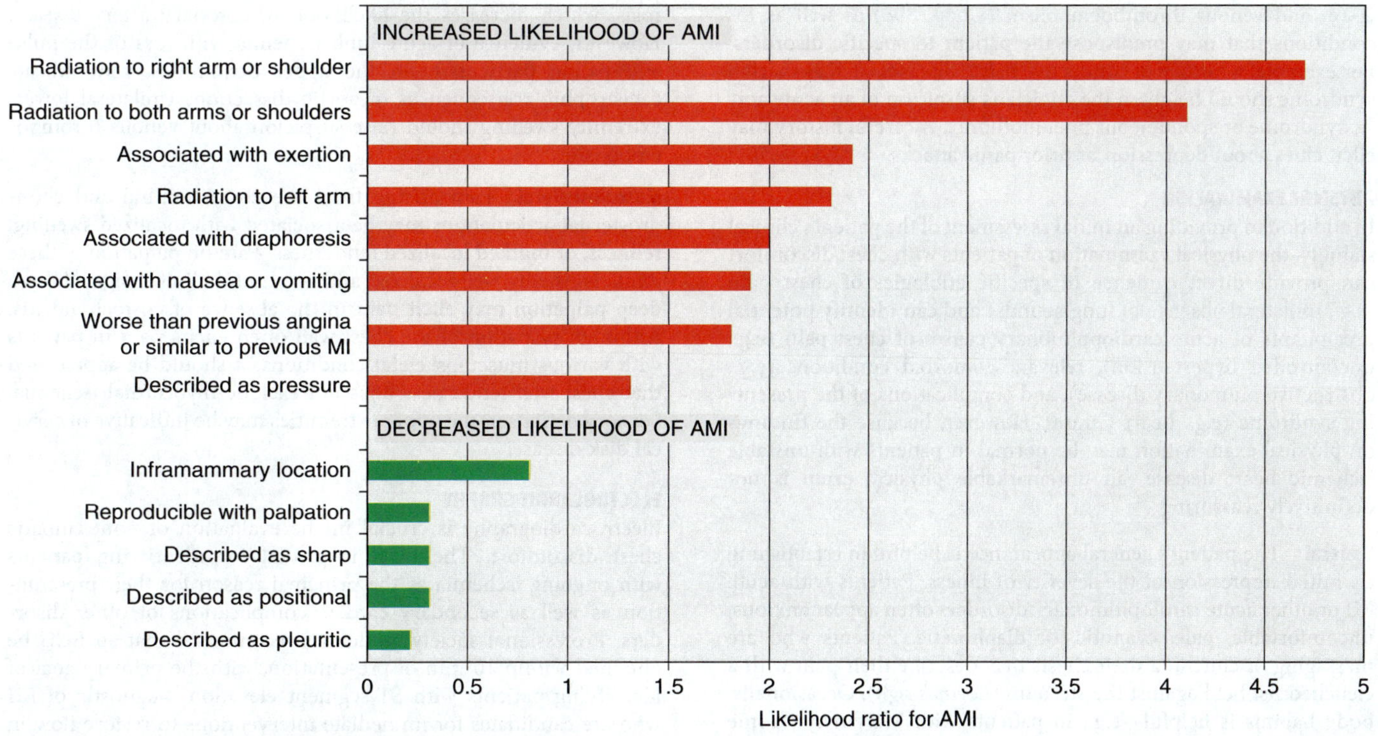

FIGURE 19-2 Association of chest pain characteristics with the probability of acute myocardial infarction (AMI). *(Figure prepared from data in CJ Swap, JT Nagurney: JAMA 294:2623, 2005.)*

Exacerbation by eating suggests a gastrointestinal etiology such as peptic ulcer disease, cholecystitis, or pancreatitis. Peptic ulcer disease tends to become symptomatic 60–90 min after meals. However, in the setting of severe coronary atherosclerosis, redistribution of blood flow to the splanchnic vasculature after eating can trigger postprandial angina. The discomfort of acid reflux and peptic ulcer disease is usually diminished promptly by acid-reducing therapies. In contrast with its impact in some patients with angina, physical exertion is very unlikely to alter symptoms from gastrointestinal causes of chest pain. Relief of chest discomfort within minutes after administration of nitroglycerin is suggestive of but not sufficiently sensitive or specific for a definitive diagnosis of myocardial ischemia. Esophageal spasm may also be relieved promptly with nitroglycerin. A delay of >10 min before relief is obtained after nitroglycerin suggests that the symptoms either are not caused by ischemia or are caused by severe ischemia, such as during acute MI.

Associated Symptoms Symptoms that accompany myocardial ischemia may include diaphoresis, dyspnea, nausea, fatigue, faintness, and eructations. In addition, these symptoms may exist in isolation as anginal equivalents (i.e., symptoms of myocardial ischemia other than typical angina), particularly in women and the elderly. Dyspnea may occur with multiple conditions considered in the differential diagnosis of chest pain and thus is not discriminative, but the presence of dyspnea is important because it suggests a cardiopulmonary etiology. Sudden onset of significant respiratory distress should lead to consideration of pulmonary embolism and spontaneous pneumothorax. Hemoptysis may occur with pulmonary embolism, or as blood-tinged frothy sputum in severe heart failure but usually points toward a pulmonary parenchymal etiology of chest symptoms. Presentation with syncope or pre-syncope should prompt consideration of hemodynamically significant pulmonary embolism or aortic dissection as well as ischemic arrhythmias. Although nausea and vomiting suggest a gastrointestinal disorder, these symptoms may occur in the setting of MI (more commonly inferior MI), presumably because of activation of the vagal reflex or stimulation of left ventricular receptors as part of the Bezold-Jarisch reflex.

Past Medical History The past medical history is useful in assessing the patient for risk factors for coronary atherosclerosis (Chap. 291e) and venous thromboembolism (Chap. 300) as well as for conditions that may predispose the patient to specific disorders. For example, a history of connective tissue diseases such as marfan syndrome should heighten the clinician's suspicion of an acute aortic syndrome or spontaneous pneumothorax. A careful history may elicit clues about depression or prior panic attacks.

PHYSICAL EXAMINATION

In addition to providing an initial assessment of the patient's clinical stability, the physical examination of patients with chest discomfort can provide direct evidence of specific etiologies of chest pain (e.g., unilateral absence of lung sounds) and can identify potential precipitants of acute cardiopulmonary causes of chest pain (e.g., uncontrolled hypertension), relevant comorbid conditions (e.g., obstructive pulmonary disease), and complications of the presenting syndrome (e.g., heart failure). However, because the findings on physical examination may be normal in patients with unstable ischemic heart disease, an unremarkable physical exam is not definitively reassuring.

General The patient's general appearance is helpful in establishing an initial impression of the severity of illness. Patients with acute MI or other acute cardiopulmonary disorders often appear anxious, uncomfortable, pale, cyanotic, or diaphoretic. Patients who are massaging or clutching their chests may describe their pain with a clenched fist held against the sternum (*Levine's sign*). Occasionally, body habitus is helpful—e.g., in patients with Marfan syndrome or the prototypical young, tall, thin man with spontaneous pneumothorax.

Vital Signs Significant tachycardia and hypotension are indicative of important hemodynamic consequences of the underlying cause of chest discomfort and should prompt a rapid survey for the most severe conditions, such as acute MI with cardiogenic shock, massive pulmonary embolism, pericarditis with tamponade, or tension pneumothorax. Acute aortic emergencies usually present with severe hypertension but may be associated with profound hypotension when there is coronary arterial compromise or dissection into the pericardium. Sinus tachycardia is an important manifestation of submassive pulmonary embolism. Tachypnea and hypoxemia point toward a pulmonary cause. The presence of low-grade fever is nonspecific because it may occur with MI and with thromboembolism in addition to infection.

Pulmonary Examination of the lungs may localize a primary pulmonary cause of chest discomfort, as in cases of pneumonia, asthma, or pneumothorax. Left ventricular dysfunction from severe ischemia/infarction as well as acute valvular complications of MI or aortic dissection can lead to pulmonary edema, which is an indicator of high risk.

Cardiac The jugular venous pulse is often normal in patients with acute myocardial ischemia but may reveal characteristic patterns with pericardial tamponade or acute right ventricular dysfunction (Chaps. 267 and 288). Cardiac auscultation may reveal a third or, more commonly, a fourth heart sound, reflecting myocardial systolic or diastolic dysfunction. Murmurs of mitral regurgitation or a harsh murmur of a ventricular-septal defect may indicate mechanical complications of STEMI. A murmur of aortic insufficiency may be a complication of proximal aortic dissection. Other murmurs may reveal underlying cardiac disorders contributory to ischemia (e.g., aortic stenosis or hypertrophic cardiomyopathy). Pericardial friction rubs reflect pericardial inflammation.

Abdominal Localizing tenderness on the abdominal exam is useful in identifying a gastrointestinal cause of the presenting syndrome. Abdominal findings are infrequent with purely acute cardiopulmonary problems, except in the case of underlying chronic cardiopulmonary disease or severe right ventricular dysfunction leading to hepatic congestion.

Vascular Pulse deficits may reflect underlying chronic atherosclerosis, which increases the likelihood of coronary artery disease. However, evidence of acute limb ischemia with loss of the pulse and pallor, particularly in the upper extremities, can indicate catastrophic consequences of aortic dissection. Unilateral lower-extremity swelling should raise suspicion about venous thromboembolism.

Musculoskeletal Pain arising from the costochondral and chondrosternal articulations may be associated with localized swelling, redness, or marked localized tenderness. Pain on palpation of these joints is usually well localized and is a useful clinical sign, though deep palpation may elicit pain in the absence of costochondritis. Although palpation of the chest wall often elicits pain in patients with various musculoskeletal conditions, it should be appreciated that chest wall tenderness does not exclude myocardial ischemia. Sensory deficits in the upper extremities may be indicative of cervical disk disease.

ELECTROCARDIOGRAPHY

Electrocardiography is crucial in the evaluation of nontraumatic chest discomfort. The ECG is pivotal for identifying patients with ongoing ischemia as the principal reason for their presentation as well as secondary cardiac complications of other disorders. Professional society guidelines recommend that an ECG be obtained within 10 min of presentation, with the primary goal of identifying patients with ST-segment elevation diagnostic of MI who are candidates for immediate interventions to restore flow in the occluded coronary artery. ST-segment depression and symmetric T-wave inversions at least 0.2 mV in depth are useful for detecting myocardial ischemia in the absence of STEMI and are also indicative of higher risk of death or recurrent ischemia. Serial performance of ECGs (every 30–60 min) is recommended in the ED evaluation of suspected ACS. In addition, an ECG with right-sided lead placement should be considered in patients with clinically suspected ischemia and a nondiagnostic standard 12-lead ECG. Despite the value of the resting ECG, its sensitivity for ischemia is poor—as low as 20% in some studies.

Abnormalities of the ST segment and T wave may occur in a variety of conditions, including pulmonary embolism, ventricular hypertrophy, acute and chronic pericarditis, myocarditis, electrolyte imbalance, and metabolic disorders. Notably, hyperventilation associated with panic disorder can also lead to nonspecific ST and T-wave abnormalities. Pulmonary embolism is most often associated with sinus tachycardia but can also lead to rightward shift of the ECG axis, manifesting as an S-wave in lead I, with a Q-wave and T-wave in lead III (Chaps. 268 and 300). In patients with ST-segment elevation, the presence of diffuse lead involvement not corresponding to a specific coronary anatomic distribution and PR-segment depression can aid in distinguishing pericarditis from acute MI.

CHEST RADIOGRAPHY

(See Chap. 308e) Plain radiography of the chest is performed routinely when patients present with acute chest discomfort and selectively when individuals who are being evaluated as outpatients have subacute or chronic pain. The chest radiograph is most useful for identifying pulmonary processes, such as pneumonia or pneumothorax. Findings are often unremarkable in patients with ACS, but pulmonary edema may be evident. Other specific findings include widening of the mediastinum in some patients with aortic dissection, Hampton's hump or Westermark's sign in patients with pulmonary embolism (Chaps. 300 and 308e), or pericardial calcification in chronic pericarditis.

CARDIAC BIOMARKERS

Laboratory testing in patients with acute chest pain is focused on the detection of myocardial injury. Such injury can be detected by the presence of circulating proteins released from damaged myocardial cells. Owing to the time necessary for this release, initial biomarkers of injury may be in the normal range, even in patients with STEMI. Because of superior cardiac tissue-specificity compared with creatine kinase MB, cardiac troponin is the preferred biomarker for the diagnosis of MI and should be measured in all patients with suspected ACS at presentation and repeated in 3–6 h. Testing after 6 h is required only when there is uncertainty regarding the onset of pain or when stuttering symptoms have occurred. It is not necessary or advisable to measure troponin in patients without suspicion of ACS unless this test is being used specifically for risk stratification (e.g., in pulmonary embolism or heart failure).

The development of cardiac troponin assays with progressively greater analytical sensitivity has facilitated detection of substantially lower blood concentrations of troponin than was previously possible. This evolution permits earlier detection of myocardial injury, enhances the overall accuracy of a diagnosis of MI, and improves risk stratification in suspected ACS. The greater negative predictive value of a negative troponin result with current-generation assays is an advantage in the evaluation of chest pain in the ED. Rapid rule-out protocols that use serial testing and changes in troponin concentration over as short a period as 1–2 h appear promising and remain under investigation. However, with these advantages has come a trade-off: myocardial injury is detected in a larger proportion of patients who have non-ACS cardiopulmonary conditions than with previous, less sensitive assays. This evolution in testing for myocardial necrosis has rendered other aspects of the clinical evaluation critical to the practitioner's determination of the probability that the symptoms represent ACS. In addition, observation of a change in cardiac troponin concentration between serial samples is useful in discriminating acute causes of myocardial injury from chronic elevation due to underlying structural heart disease, end-stage renal disease, or interfering antibodies. The diagnosis of MI is reserved for acute myocardial injury that is marked by a rising and/or falling pattern—with at least one value exceeding the 99th percentile reference limit—and that is caused by ischemia. Other non-ischemic insults, such as myocarditis, may result in myocardial injury but should not be labeled MI.

Other laboratory assessments may include the D-dimer test to aid in exclusion of pulmonary embolism (Chap. 300). Measurement of a B-type natriuretic peptide is useful when considered in conjunction with the clinical history and exam for the diagnosis of heart failure. B-type natriuretic peptides also provide prognostic information regarding patients with ACS and those with pulmonary embolism. Other putative biomarkers of acute myocardial ischemia or ACS, such as myeloperoxidase, have not been adopted in routine use.

INTEGRATIVE DECISION-AIDS

Multiple clinical algorithms have been developed to aid in decision-making during the evaluation and disposition of patients with acute nontraumatic chest pain. Such decision-aids have been derived on the basis of their capacity to estimate either of two closely related but not identical probabilities: (1) the probability of a final diagnosis of ACS and (2) the probability of major cardiac events during short-term follow-up. Such decision-aids are used most commonly to identify patients with a low clinical probability of ACS who are candidates either for early provocative testing for ischemia or for discharge from the ED. Goldman and Lee developed one of the first such decision-aids, using only the ECG and risk indicators—hypotension, pulmonary rales, and known ischemic heart disease—to categorize patients into four risk categories ranging from a <1% to a >16% probability of a major cardiovascular complication. The Acute Cardiac Ischemia Time-Insensitive Predictive Instrument (ACI-TIPI) combines age, sex, chest pain presence, and ST-segment abnormalities to define a probability of ACS. More recently developed decision-aids are shown in Fig. 19-3. Elements common to each of these tools are (1) symptoms typical for ACS; (2) older age; (3) risk factors for or known atherosclerosis; (4) ischemic ECG abnormalities; and (5) elevated cardiac troponin levels. Although, because of very low specificity, the overall diagnostic performance of such decision-aids is poor (area under the receiver operating curve, 0.55–0.65), they can help identify patients with a very low probability of ACS (e.g., <1%). Nevertheless, no such decision-aid (or single clinical factor) is sufficiently sensitive and well validated to use as a sole tool for clinical decision-making.

Clinicians should differentiate between the algorithms discussed above and risk scores derived for stratification of prognosis (e.g., the TIMI and GRACE risk scores, Chap. 295) in patients *who already have an established diagnosis of ACS*. The latter risk scores were not designed to be used for *diagnostic* assessment.

PROVOCATIVE TESTING FOR ISCHEMIA

Exercise electrocardiography ("stress testing") is commonly employed for completion of risk stratification of patients who have undergone an initial evaluation that has not revealed a specific cause of chest discomfort and has identified them as being at low or selectively intermediate risk of ACS. Early exercise testing is safe in patients without high-risk findings after 8–12 h of observation and can assist in refining their prognostic assessment. For example, of low-risk patients who underwent exercise testing in the first 48 h after presentation, those without evidence of ischemia had a 2% rate of cardiac events through 6 months, whereas the rate was 15% among patients with either clear evidence of ischemia or an equivocal result. Patients who are unable to exercise may undergo pharmacological stress testing with either nuclear perfusion imaging or echocardiography. Notably, some experts have deemed the routine use of stress testing for low-risk patients unsupported by direct clinical evidence and a potentially unnecessary source of cost.

Professional society guidelines identify ongoing chest pain as a contraindication to stress testing. In selected patients with persistent pain and nondiagnostic ECG and biomarker data, resting

HEART Score		
History	Highly suspicious Moderately suspicious Slightly suspicious	2 1 0
ECG	Significant ST-depression Non-specific abnormality Normal	2 1 0
Age	≥65 y 45–<65 y <45 y	2 1 0
Risk factors	≥3 risk factors 1–2 risk factors None	2 1 0
Troponin (serial)	≥3 × 99th percentile 1–<3 × 99th percentile ≤99th percentile	2 1 0
	TOTAL	
	Low-risk: 0–3 **Not low risk:** ≥4	

North American Chest Pain Rule	
High Risk Criteria	**Y/N**
Typical symptoms for ischemia	
ECG: acute ischemic changes	
Age ≥50 y	
Known coronary artery disease	
Troponin (serial) >99th percentile	
Low-risk: All No **Not Low-risk:** Any Yes	

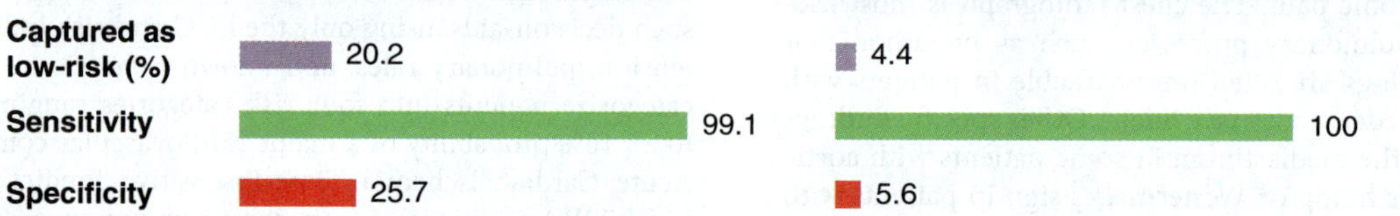

FIGURE 19-3 Examples of decision-aids used in conjunction with serial measurement of cardiac troponin for evaluation of acute chest pain. *(Figure prepared from data in SA Mahler et al: Int J Cardiol 168:795, 2013.)*

myocardial perfusion images can be obtained; the absence of any perfusion abnormality substantially reduces the likelihood of coronary artery disease. In some centers, early myocardial perfusion imaging is performed as part of a routine strategy for evaluating patients at low or intermediate risk of ACS in parallel with other testing. Management of patients with normal perfusion images can be expedited with earlier discharge and outpatient stress testing, if indicated. Those with abnormal rest perfusion imaging, which cannot discriminate between old or new myocardial defects, must undergo additional in-hospital evaluation.

OTHER NONINVASIVE STUDIES

Other noninvasive imaging studies of the chest can be used selectively to provide additional diagnostic and prognostic information on patients with chest discomfort.

Echocardiography Echocardiography is not necessarily routine in patients with chest discomfort. However, in patients with an uncertain diagnosis, particularly those with nondiagnostic ST elevation, ongoing symptoms, or hemodynamic instability, detection of abnormal regional wall motion provides evidence of possible ischemic dysfunction. Echocardiography is diagnostic in patients with mechanical complications of MI or in patients with pericardial tamponade. Transthoracic echocardiography is poorly sensitive for aortic dissection, although an intimal flap may sometimes be detected in the ascending aorta.

CT Angiography (See Chap. 270e) CT angiography is emerging as a modality for the evaluation of patients with acute chest discomfort. Coronary CT angiography is a sensitive technique for detection of obstructive coronary disease, particularly in the proximal third of the major epicardial coronary arteries. CT appears to enhance the speed to disposition of patients with a low-intermediate probability for ACS; its major strength being the negative predictive value of a finding of no significant disease. In addition, contrast-enhanced CT can detect focal areas of myocardial injury in the acute setting as decreased areas of enhancement. At the same time, CT angiography can exclude aortic dissection, pericardial effusion, and pulmonary embolism. Balancing factors in the consideration of the emerging role of coronary CT angiography in low-risk patients are radiation exposure and additional testing prompted by nondiagnostic abnormal results.

MRI (See Chap. 270e) Cardiac magnetic resonance (CMR) imaging is an evolving, versatile technique for structural and functional evaluation of the heart and the vasculature of the chest. CMR accurately measures ventricular dimensions and function and can be performed as a modality for pharmacologic stress perfusion imaging. Gadolinium-enhanced CMR can provide early detection of MI, defining areas of myocardial necrosis accurately, and can delineate patterns of myocardial disease that are often useful in discriminating ischemic from non-ischemic myocardial injury. Although usually not practical for the urgent evaluation of acute chest discomfort, CMR can be a useful modality for cardiac structural evaluation of patients with elevated cardiac troponin levels in the absence of definite coronary artery disease. CMR coronary angiography is in its early stages. MRI also permits highly accurate assessment for aortic dissection but is infrequently used as the first test because CT and transesophageal echocardiography are usually more practical.

CRITICAL PATHWAYS FOR ACUTE CHEST DISCOMFORT

Because of the challenges inherent in reliably identifying the small proportion of patients with serious causes of acute chest discomfort while not exposing the larger number of low-risk patients to unnecessary testing and extended ED or hospital evaluations, many medical centers have adopted critical pathways to expedite the assessment and management of patients with nontraumatic chest pain, often in dedicated chest pain units. Such pathways are generally aimed at

(1) rapid identification, triage, and treatment of high-risk cardiopulmonary conditions (e.g., STEMI); (2) accurate identification of low-risk patients who can be safely observed in units with less intensive monitoring, undergo early exercise testing, or be discharged home; and (3) through more efficient and systematic accelerated diagnostic protocols, safe reduction in costs associated with overuse of testing and unnecessary hospitalizations. In some studies, provision of protocol-driven care in chest pain units has decreased costs and overall duration of hospital evaluation with no detectable excess of adverse clinical outcomes.

OUTPATIENT EVALUATION OF CHEST DISCOMFORT

Chest pain is common in outpatient practice, with a lifetime prevalence of 20–40% in the general population. More than 25% of patients with MI have had a related visit with a primary care physician in the previous month. The diagnostic principles are the same as in the ED. However, the pretest probability of an acute cardiopulmonary cause is significantly lower. Therefore, testing paradigms are less intense, with an emphasis on the history, physical examination, and ECG. Moreover, decision-aids developed for settings with a high prevalence of significant cardiopulmonary disease have lower positive predictive value when applied in the practitioner's office. However, in general, if the level of clinical suspicion of ACS is sufficiently high to consider troponin testing, the patient should be referred to the ED for evaluation.

20 Abdominal Pain

Danny O. Jacobs, William Silen

Correctly interpreting acute abdominal pain can be quite challenging. Few clinical situations require greater judgment, because the most catastrophic of events may be forecast by the subtlest of symptoms and signs. In every instance, the clinician must distinguish those conditions that require urgent intervention from those that do not and can best be managed nonoperatively. A meticulously executed, detailed history and physical examination are critically important for focusing the differential diagnosis, where necessary, and allowing the diagnostic evaluation to proceed expeditiously (Table 20-1).

The etiologic classification in Table 20-2, although not complete, provides a useful framework for evaluating patients with abdominal pain.

The most common causes of abdominal pain on admission are acute appendicitis, nonspecific abdominal pain, pain of urologic origin, and intestinal obstruction. A diagnosis of "acute or surgical abdomen" is not acceptable because of its often misleading and erroneous connotations. Most patients who present with acute abdominal pain will have self-limited disease processes. However, it is important to remember that pain severity does not necessarily correlate with the severity of the underlying condition. The most obvious of "acute abdomens" may not require operative intervention, and the mildest of abdominal pains may herald an urgently correctable lesion. Any patient with abdominal pain of recent onset requires early and thorough evaluation and accurate diagnosis.

TABLE 20-1 SOME KEY COMPONENTS OF THE PATIENT'S HISTORY

Age
Time and mode of onset of the pain
Pain characteristics
Duration of symptoms
Location of pain and sites of radiation
Associated symptoms and their relationship to the pain
Nausea, emesis, and anorexia
Diarrhea, constipation, or other changes in bowel habits
Menstrual history

SOME MECHANISMS OF PAIN ORIGINATING IN THE ABDOMEN

Inflammation of the Parietal Peritoneum The pain of parietal peritoneal inflammation is steady and aching in character and is located directly over the inflamed area, its exact reference being possible because it is transmitted by somatic nerves supplying the parietal peritoneum. The intensity of the pain is dependent on the type and amount of material to which the peritoneal surfaces are exposed in a given time period. For example , the sudden release into the peritoneal cavity of a small quantity of *sterile* acid gastric juice causes much more pain than the same amount of grossly contaminated neutral feces. Enzymatically active pancreatic juice incites more pain and inflammation than does the same amount of sterile bile containing no potent enzymes. Blood is normally only a mild irritant and the response to urine can be bland, so exposure of blood and urine to the peritoneal cavity may go unnoticed unless it is sudden and massive. Bacterial contamination, such as may occur with pelvic inflammatory disease or perforated distal intestine, causes low-intensity pain until multiplication causes a significant amount of inflammatory mediators to be released. Patients with perforated upper gastrointestinal ulcers may present entirely differently depending on how quickly gastric juices enter the peritoneal cavity. Thus, the rate at which any inflammatory material irritates the peritoneum is important.

The pain of peritoneal inflammation is invariably accentuated by pressure or changes in tension of the peritoneum, whether produced by palpation or by movement such as with coughing or sneezing. The patient with peritonitis characteristically lies quietly in bed, preferring to avoid motion, in contrast to the patient with colic, who may be thrashing in discomfort.

Another characteristic feature of peritoneal irritation is tonic reflex spasm of the abdominal musculature, localized to the involved body segment. Its intensity depends on the integrity of the nervous system, the location of the inflammatory process, and the rate at which it develops. Spasm over a perforated retrocecal appendix or perforation into the lesser peritoneal sac may be minimal or absent because of the protective effect of overlying viscera. Catastrophic abdominal emergencies may be associated with minimal or no detectable pain or muscle spasm in obtunded, seriously ill, debilitated, immunosuppressed, or psychotic patients. A slowly developing process also often greatly attenuates the degree of muscle spasm.

Obstruction of Hollow Viscera Intraluminal obstruction classically elicits intermittent or colicky abdominal pain that is not as well localized as the pain of parietal peritoneal irritation. However, the absence of cramping discomfort should not be misleading because distention of a hollow viscus may also produce steady pain with only rare paroxysms.

Small-bowel obstruction often presents as poorly localized, intermittent periumbilical or supraumbilical pain. As the intestine progressively dilates and loses muscular tone, the colicky nature of the pain may diminish. With superimposed strangulating obstruction, pain may spread to the lower lumbar region if there is traction on the root of the mesentery. The colicky pain of colonic obstruction is of lesser intensity, is commonly located in the infraumbilical area, and may often radiate to the lumbar region.

Sudden distention of the biliary tree produces a steady rather than colicky type of pain; hence, the term *biliary colic* is misleading. Acute distention of the gallbladder usually causes pain in the right upper quadrant with radiation to the right posterior region of the thorax or to the tip of the right scapula, but it is also not uncommonly found near the midline. Distention of the common bile duct often causes epigastric pain that may radiate to the upper lumbar region. Considerable variation is common, however, so that differentiation between these may be impossible. The typical subscapular pain or lumbar radiation is frequently absent. Gradual dilatation of the biliary tree, as can occur with carcinoma of the head of the pancreas, may cause no pain

TABLE 20-2 SOME IMPORTANT CAUSES OF ABDOMINAL PAIN

Pain Originating in the Abdomen	
Parietal peritoneal inflammation	Vascular disturbances
Bacterial contamination	Embolism or thrombosis
Perforated appendix or other perforated viscus	Vascular rupture
Pelvic inflammatory disease	Pressure or torsional occlusion
Chemical irritation	Sickle cell anemia
Perforated ulcer	Abdominal wall
Pancreatitis	Distortion or traction of mesentery
Mittelschmerz	Trauma or infection of muscles
Mechanical obstruction of hollow viscera	Distension of visceral surfaces, e.g., by hemorrhage
Obstruction of the small or large intestine	Hepatic or renal capsules
Obstruction of the biliary tree	Inflammation
Obstruction of the ureter	Appendicitis
	Typhoid fever
	Neutropenic enterocolitis or "typhlitis"
Pain Referred from Extraabdominal Source	
Cardiothoracic	Pleurodynia
Acute myocardial infarction	Pneumothorax
Myocarditis, endocarditis, pericarditis	Empyema
Congestive heart failure	Esophageal disease, including spasm, rupture, or inflammation
Pneumonia (especially lower lobes)	Genitalia
Pulmonary embolus	Torsion of the testis
Metabolic Causes	
Diabetes	Acute adrenal insufficiency
Uremia	Familial Mediterranean fever
Hyperlipidemia	Porphyria
Hyperparathyroidism	C1 esterase inhibitor deficiency (angioneurotic edema)
Neurologic/Psychiatric Causes	
Herpes zoster	Spinal cord or nerve root compression
Tabes dorsalis	Functional disorders
Causalgia	Psychiatric disorders
Radiculitis from infection or arthritis	
Toxic Causes	
Lead poisoning	
Insect or animal envenomation	
Black widow spider bites	
Snake bites	
Uncertain Mechanisms	
Narcotic withdrawal	
Heat stroke	

or only a mild aching sensation in the epigastrium or right upper quadrant. The pain of distention of the pancreatic ducts is similar to that described for distention of the common bile duct but, in addition, is very frequently accentuated by recumbency and relieved by the upright position.

Obstruction of the urinary bladder usually causes dull, low-intensity pain in the suprapubic region. Restlessness without specific complaint of pain may be the only sign of a distended bladder in an obtunded patient. In contrast, acute obstruction of the intravesicular portion of the ureter is characterized by severe suprapubic and flank pain that radiates to the penis, scrotum, or inner aspect of the upper thigh. Obstruction of the ureteropelvic junction manifests as pain near the costovertebral angle, whereas obstruction of the remainder of the ureter is associated with flank pain that often extends into the same side of the abdomen.

Vascular Disturbances A frequent misconception is that pain due to intraabdominal vascular disturbances is sudden and catastrophic in nature. Certain disease processes, such as embolism or thrombosis of the superior mesenteric artery or impending rupture of an abdominal aortic aneurysm, can certainly be associated with diffuse, severe pain. Yet, just as frequently, the patient with occlusion of the superior mesenteric artery only has mild continuous or cramping diffuse pain for 2 or 3 days before vascular collapse or findings of peritoneal inflammation appear. The early, seemingly insignificant discomfort is caused by hyperperistalsis rather than peritoneal inflammation. Indeed, absence of tenderness and rigidity in the presence of continuous, diffuse pain (e.g., "pain out of proportion to physical findings") in a patient likely to have vascular disease is quite characteristic of occlusion of the superior mesenteric artery. Abdominal pain with radiation to the sacral region, flank, or genitalia should always signal the possible presence of a rupturing abdominal aortic aneurysm. This pain may persist over a period of several days before rupture and collapse occur.

Abdominal Wall Pain arising from the abdominal wall is usually constant and aching. Movement, prolonged standing, and pressure accentuate the discomfort and associated muscle spasm. In the case of hematoma of the rectus sheath, now most frequently encountered in association with anticoagulant therapy, a mass may be present in the lower quadrants of the abdomen. Simultaneous involvement of muscles in other parts of the body usually serves to differentiate myositis of the abdominal wall from other processes that might cause pain in the same region.

REFERRED PAIN IN ABDOMINAL DISEASE

Pain referred to the abdomen from the thorax , spine, or genitalia may present a vexing diagnostic challenge because diseases of the upper part of the abdominal cavity such as acute cholecystitis or perforated ulcer may be associated with intrathoracic complications. A most important, yet often forgotten, dictum is that the possibility of intrathoracic disease must be considered in every patient with abdominal pain, especially if the pain is in the upper abdomen.

Systematic questioning and examination directed toward detecting myocardial or pulmonary infarction, pneumonia, pericarditis, or esophageal disease (the intrathoracic diseases that most often masquerade as abdominal emergencies) will often provide sufficient clues to establish the proper diagnosis. Diaphragmatic pleuritis resulting from pneumonia or pulmonary infarction may cause pain in the right upper quadrant and pain in the supraclavicular area, the latter radiation to be distinguished from the referred subscapular pain caused by acute distention of the extrahepatic biliary tree. The ultimate decision as to the origin of abdominal pain may require deliberate and planned observation over a period of several hours, during which repeated questioning and examination will provide the diagnosis or suggest the appropriate studies.

Referred pain of thoracic origin is often accompanied by splinting of the involved hemithorax with respiratory lag and decrease in excursion more marked than that seen in the presence of intraabdominal disease. In addition, apparent abdominal muscle spasm caused by referred pain will diminish during the inspiratory phase of respiration, whereas it persists throughout both respiratory phases if it is of abdominal origin. Palpation over the area of referred pain in the abdomen also does not usually accentuate the pain and, in many instances, actually seems to relieve it.

Thoracic disease and abdominal disease frequently coexist and may be difficult or impossible to differentiate. For example, the patient with known biliary tract disease often has epigastric pain during myocardial infarction, or biliary colic may be referred to the precordium or left shoulder in a patient who has suffered previously from angina pectoris. **For an explanation of the radiation of pain to a previously diseased area, see Chap. 18.**

Referred pain from the spine, which usually involves compression or irritation of nerve roots, is characteristically intensified by certain motions such as cough, sneeze, or strain and is associated with hyperesthesia over the involved dermatomes. Pain referred to the abdomen from the testes or seminal vesicles is generally accentuated by the slightest pressure on either of these organs. The abdominal discomfort experienced is of dull, aching character and is poorly localized.

METABOLIC ABDOMINAL CRISES

Pain of metabolic origin may simulate almost any other type of intraabdominal disease. Several mechanisms may be at work. In certain instances, such as hyperlipidemia, the metabolic disease itself may be accompanied by an intraabdominal process such as pancreatitis, which can lead to unnecessary laparotomy unless recognized. C1 esterase deficiency associated with angioneurotic edema is often associated with episodes of severe abdominal pain. Whenever the cause of abdominal pain is obscure, a metabolic origin always must be considered. Abdominal pain is also the hallmark of familial Mediterranean fever (Chap. 392).

The problem of differential diagnosis is often not readily resolved. The pain of porphyria and of lead colic is usually difficult to distinguish from that of intestinal obstruction, because severe hyperperistalsis is a prominent feature of both. The pain of uremia or diabetes is nonspecific, and the pain and tenderness frequently shift in location and intensity. Diabetic acidosis may be precipitated by acute appendicitis or intestinal obstruction, so if prompt resolution of the abdominal pain does not result from correction of the metabolic abnormalities, an underlying organic problem should be suspected. Black widow spider bites produce intense pain and rigidity of the abdominal muscles and back, an area infrequently involved in intraabdominal disease.

IMMUNOCOMPROMISE

Evaluating and diagnosing causes of abdominal pain in immunosuppressed or otherwise immunocompromised patients is very difficult. This includes those who have undergone organ transplantation; who are receiving immunosuppressive treatments for autoimmune diseases, chemotherapy, or glucocorticoids; who have AIDS; and who are very old. In these circumstances, normal physiologic responses may be absent or masked. In addition, unusual infections may cause abdominal pain where the etiologic agents include cytomegalovirus, mycobacteria, protozoa, and fungi. These pathogens may affect all gastrointestinal organs, including the gallbladder, liver, and pancreas, as well as the gastrointestinal tract, causing occult or overtly symptomatic perforations of the latter. Splenic abscesses due to *Candida* or *Salmonella* infection should also be considered, especially when evaluating patients with left upper quadrant or left flank pain. Acalculous cholecystitis is a relative common complication in patients with AIDS, where it is often associated with cryptosporidiosis or cytomegalovirus infection.

Neutropenic enterocolitis is often identified as a cause of abdominal pain and fever in some patients with bone marrow suppression due to chemotherapy. Acute graft-versus-host disease should be considered. Optimal management of these patients may require meticulous follow-up including serial examinations to be certain that surgical intervention is not required to treat an underlying disease process.

NEUROGENIC CAUSES

Diseases that injure sensory nerves may cause causalgic pain. It has a burning character and is usually limited to the distribution of a given peripheral nerve. Normal nonpainful stimuli such as touch or a change in temperature may be causalgic and may frequently be present even at rest. The demonstration of irregularly spaced cutaneous pain spots may be the only indication that an old nerve injury exists. Even though the pain may be precipitated by gentle palpation, rigidity of the abdominal muscles is absent, and the respirations are not disturbed. Distention of the abdomen is uncommon, and the pain has no relationship to the intake of food.

Pain arising from spinal nerves or roots comes and goes suddenly and is of a lancinating type (Chap. 22). It may be caused by herpes zoster, impingement by arthritis, tumors, a herniated nucleus pulposus, diabetes , or syphilis. It is not associated with food intake, abdominal distention, or changes in respiration. Severe muscle spasm, as in the gastric crises of tabes dorsalis, is common but is either relieved or not accentuated by abdominal palpation. The pain is made worse by movement of the spine and is usually confined to a few dermatomes. Hyperesthesia is very common.

Pain due to functional causes conforms to none of the aforementioned patterns. Mechanisms of disease are not clearly established. Irritable bowel syndrome (IBS) is a functional gastrointestinal disorder characterized by abdominal pain and altered bowel habits. The diagnosis is made on the basis of clinical criteria (Chap. 352) and after exclusion of demonstrable structural abnormalities. The episodes of abdominal pain are often brought on by stress, and the pain varies considerably in type and location. Nausea and vomiting are rare. Localized tenderness and muscle spasm are inconsistent or absent. The causes of IBS or related functional disorders are not known.

APPROACH TO THE PATIENT: **Abdominal Pain**

Few abdominal conditions require such urgent operative intervention that an orderly approach need be abandoned, no matter how ill the patient. Only patients with exsanguinating intraabdominal hemorrhage (e.g., ruptured aneurysm) must be rushed to the operating room immediately, but in such instances, only a few minutes are required to assess the critical nature of the problem. Under these circumstances, all obstacles must be swept aside, adequate venous access for fluid replacement obtained, and the operation begun. Many of these patients have died in the radiology department or the emergency room while awaiting unnecessary examinations such as electrocardiograms or computed tomography (CT) scans. *There are no contraindications to operation when massive intraabdominal hemorrhage is present.* Fortunately, this situation is relatively rare. This statement does not necessarily apply to patients with intraluminal gastrointestinal hemorrhage, who can often be managed by other means (Chap. 57). Nothing will supplant an orderly, painstakingly *detailed history,* which is far more valuable than any laboratory or radiographic examination. This kind of history is laborious and time-consuming, making it not especially popular, even though a reasonably accurate diagnosis can be made on the basis of the history alone in the majority of cases.

In cases of *acute* abdominal pain, a diagnosis is readily established in most instances, whereas success is not so frequent in patients with *chronic* pain. IBS is one of the most common causes of abdominal pain and must always be kept in mind (Chap. 352). The location of the pain can assist in narrowing the differential diagnosis (Table 20-3); however, the *chronological sequence of events* in the patient's history is often more important than the pain's location. If the examiner is sufficiently open-minded and unhurried, asks the proper questions, and listens, the patient will usually provide the diagnosis. Careful attention should be paid to the extraabdominal regions. Narcotics or analgesics should *not* be withheld until a definitive diagnosis or a definitive plan has been formulated; obfuscation of the diagnosis by adequate analgesia is unlikely.

An accurate menstrual history in a female patient is essential. It is important to remember that normal anatomic relationships can be significantly altered by the gravid uterus. Abdominal and pelvic pain may occur during pregnancy due to conditions that do not require surgery. Lastly, some otherwise noteworthy laboratory values (e.g., leukocytosis) may represent the normal physiologic changes of pregnancy.

In the examination, simple critical inspection of the patient, e.g., of facies, position in bed, and respiratory activity, provides valuable clues. The amount of information to be gleaned is directly proportional to the *gentleness* and thoroughness of the examiner. Once a patient with peritoneal inflammation has been examined brusquely, accurate assessment by the next examiner becomes almost impossible. Eliciting rebound tenderness by sudden release of a deeply palpating hand in a patient with suspected peritonitis is cruel and unnecessary. The same information can be obtained by gentle percussion of the abdomen (rebound tenderness on a miniature scale), a maneuver that can be far more precise and localizing. Asking the patient to cough will elicit true rebound tenderness without the need for placing a hand on the abdomen. Furthermore, the forceful demonstration of rebound tenderness will startle and induce protective spasm in a nervous or worried patient in whom true rebound tenderness is not present. A palpable gallbladder will be missed if palpation is so aggressive that voluntary muscle spasm becomes superimposed on involuntary muscular rigidity. As with history taking, sufficient time should be spent in the examination. Abdominal signs may be minimal but nevertheless, if accompanied by consistent symptoms, may be exceptionally meaningful. Abdominal signs may be virtually or totally absent in cases of pelvic peritonitis, so careful *pelvic and rectal examinations are mandatory in every patient with abdominal pain.* Tenderness on pelvic or rectal examination in the absence of other abdominal signs can be caused by operative indications such as perforated appendicitis, diverticulitis, twisted ovarian cyst, and many others. Much attention has been paid to the presence or absence of peristaltic sounds, their quality, and their frequency. Auscultation of the abdomen is one of the least revealing aspects of the physical examination of a patient with abdominal pain. Catastrophes such as a strangulating small intestinal obstruction or perforated appendicitis may occur in the presence of normal peristaltic sounds. Conversely, when the proximal part of the intestine above obstruction becomes markedly distended and edematous, peristaltic sounds may lose the characteristics of borborygmi and become weak or absent, even when peritonitis is not present. It is usually the severe chemical peritonitis of sudden onset that is associated with the truly silent abdomen.

Laboratory examinations may be valuable in assessing the patient with abdominal pain, yet, with few exceptions, they rarely establish a diagnosis. Leukocytosis should never be the single deciding factor as to whether or not operation is indicated. A white blood cell count >20,000/μL may be observed with perforation of a viscus, but pancreatitis, acute cholecystitis, pelvic inflammatory disease, and intestinal infarction may also be associated with marked leukocytosis. A normal white blood cell count is not rare in cases of perforation of abdominal viscera. The diagnosis of anemia may be more helpful than the white blood cell count, especially when combined with the history.

The urinalysis may reveal the state of hydration or rule out severe renal disease, diabetes, or urinary infection. Blood urea nitrogen, glucose, and serum bilirubin levels may be helpful. Serum amylase levels may be increased by many diseases other than pancreatitis, e.g., perforated ulcer, strangulating intestinal obstruction, and acute cholecystitis; thus, elevations of serum amylase do not rule out the need for an operation.

Plain and upright or lateral decubitus radiographs of the abdomen may be of value in cases of intestinal obstruction, perforated ulcer, and a variety of other conditions. They are usually unnecessary in patients with acute appendicitis or strangulated external hernias. In rare instances, barium or water-soluble contrast study of the upper part of the gastrointestinal tract may demonstrate partial intestinal obstruction that may elude diagnosis by other means. If there is any question of obstruction of the colon, oral administration of barium sulfate should be avoided. On the other hand, in

TABLE 20-3 DIFFERENTIAL DIAGNOSES OF ABDOMINAL PAIN BY LOCATION

Right Upper Quadrant	Epigastric	Left Upper Quadrant
Cholecystitis	Peptic ulcer disease	Splenic infarct
Cholangitis	Gastritis	Splenic rupture
Pancreatitis	GERD	Splenic abscess
Pneumonia/empyema	Pancreatitis	Gastritis
Pleurisy/pleurodynia	Myocardial infarction	Gastric ulcer
Subdiaphragmatic abscess	Pericarditis	Pancreatitis
Hepatitis	Ruptured aortic aneurysm	Subdiaphragmatic abscess
Budd-Chiari syndrome	Esophagitis	
Right Lower Quadrant	**Periumbilical**	**Left Lower Quadrant**
Appendicitis	Early appendicitis	Diverticulitis
Salpingitis	Gastroenteritis	Salpingitis
Inguinal hernia	Bowel obstruction	Inguinal hernia
Ectopic pregnancy	Ruptured aortic aneurysm	Ectopic pregnancy
Nephrolithiasis		Nephrolithiasis
Inflammatory bowel disease		Irritable bowel syndrome
Mesenteric lymphadenitis		Inflammatory bowel disease
Typhlitis		
Diffuse Nonlocalized Pain		
Gastroenteritis	Malaria	
Mesenteric ischemia	Familial Mediterranean fever	
Bowel obstruction	Metabolic diseases	
Irritable bowel syndrome	Psychiatric disease	
Peritonitis		
Diabetes		

Abbreviation: GERD, gastroesophageal reflux disease.

cases of suspected colonic obstruction (without perforation), a contrast enema may be diagnostic.

In the absence of trauma, peritoneal lavage has been replaced as a diagnostic tool by CT scanning and laparoscopy. Ultrasonography has proved to be useful in detecting an enlarged gallbladder or pancreas, the presence of gallstones, an enlarged ovary, or a tubal pregnancy. Laparoscopy is especially helpful in diagnosing pelvic conditions, such as ovarian cysts, tubal pregnancies, salpingitis, and acute appendicitis.

Radioisotopic hepatobiliary iminodiacetic acid scans (HIDAs) may help differentiate acute cholecystitis or biliary colic from acute pancreatitis. A CT scan may demonstrate an enlarged pancreas, ruptured spleen, or thickened colonic or appendiceal wall and streaking of the mesocolon or mesoappendix characteristic of diverticulitis or appendicitis.

Sometimes, even under the best circumstances with all available aids and with the greatest of clinical skill, a definitive diagnosis cannot be established at the time of the initial examination. Nevertheless, even in the absence of a clear anatomic diagnosis, it may be abundantly clear to an experienced and thoughtful physician and surgeon that operation is indicated on clinical grounds alone. Should that decision be questionable, watchful waiting with repeated questioning and examination will often elucidate the true nature of the illness and indicate the proper course of action.

21 Headache

Peter J. Goadsby, Neil H. Raskin

Headache is among the most common reasons patients seek medical attention, on a global basis being responsible for more disability than any other neurologic problem. Diagnosis and management are based on a careful clinical approach augmented by an understanding of the anatomy, physiology, and pharmacology of the nervous system pathways mediating the various headache syndromes. This chapter will focus on the general approach to a patient with headache; migraine and other primary headache disorders are discussed in Chap. 447.

GENERAL PRINCIPLES

A classification system developed by the International Headache Society (*www.ihs-headache.org/*) characterizes headache as primary or secondary (Table 21-1). *Primary headaches* are those in which headache and its associated features are the disorder in itself, whereas *secondary headaches* are those caused by exogenous disorders (Headache Classification Committee of the International Headache Society, 2013). Primary headache often results in considerable disability and a decrease in the patient's quality of life. Mild secondary headache, such as that seen in association with upper respiratory tract infections, is common but rarely worrisome. Life-threatening headache is relatively uncommon, but vigilance is required in order to recognize and appropriately treat such patients.

TABLE 21-1 COMMON CAUSES OF HEADACHE

Primary Headache		Secondary Headache	
Type	**%**	**Type**	**%**
Tension-type	69	Systemic infection	63
Migraine	16	Head injury	4
Idiopathic stabbing	2	Vascular disorders	1
Exertional	1	Subarachnoid hemorrhage	<1
Cluster	0.1	Brain tumor	0.1

Source: After J Olesen et al: *The Headaches*. Philadelphia, Lippincott Williams & Wilkins, 2005.

ANATOMY AND PHYSIOLOGY OF HEADACHE

Pain usually occurs when peripheral nociceptors are stimulated in response to tissue injury, visceral distension, or other factors (Chap. 18). In such situations, pain perception is a normal physiologic response mediated by a healthy nervous system. Pain can also result when pain-producing pathways of the peripheral or central nervous system (CNS) are damaged or activated inappropriately. Headache may originate from either or both mechanisms. Relatively few cranial structures are pain-producing; these include the scalp, middle meningeal artery, dural sinuses, falx cerebri, and proximal segments of the large pial arteries. The ventricular ependyma, choroid plexus, pial veins, and much of the brain parenchyma are not pain-producing.

The key structures involved in primary headache appear to be the following:

- The large intracranial vessels and dura mater and the peripheral terminals of the trigeminal nerve that innervate these structures
- The caudal portion of the trigeminal nucleus, which extends into the dorsal horns of the upper cervical spinal cord and receives input from the first and second cervical nerve roots (the trigeminocervical complex)
- Rostral pain-processing regions, such as the ventroposteromedial thalamus and the cortex
- The pain-modulatory systems in the brain that modulate input from trigeminal nociceptors at all levels of the pain-processing pathways and influence vegetative functions, such as hypothalamus and brainstem structures

The innervation of the large intracranial vessels and dura mater by the trigeminal nerve is known as the *trigeminovascular system*. Cranial autonomic symptoms, such as *lacrimation, conjunctival injection, nasal congestion, rhinorrhea, periorbital swelling, aural fullness*, and *ptosis*, are prominent in the trigeminal autonomic cephalalgias, including cluster headache and paroxysmal hemicrania, and may also be seen in migraine, even in children. These autonomic symptoms reflect activation of cranial parasympathetic pathways, and functional imaging studies indicate that vascular changes in migraine and cluster headache, when present, are similarly driven by these cranial autonomic systems. Moreover, they can often be mistaken for symptoms or signs of cranial sinus inflammation, which is thus overdiagnosed and inappropriately managed. Migraine and other primary headache types are not "vascular headaches"; these disorders do not reliably manifest vascular changes, and treatment outcomes cannot be predicted by vascular effects. Migraine is a brain disorder and is best understood and managed as such.

CLINICAL EVALUATION OF ACUTE, NEW-ONSET HEADACHE

The patient who presents with a new, severe headache has a differential diagnosis that is quite different from the patient with recurrent headaches over many years. In new-onset and severe headache, the probability of finding a potentially serious cause is considerably greater than in recurrent headache. Patients with recent onset of pain require prompt evaluation and appropriate treatment. Serious causes to be considered include meningitis, subarachnoid hemorrhage, epidural or subdural hematoma, glaucoma, tumor, and purulent sinusitis. When worrisome symptoms and signs are present (Table 21-2), rapid diagnosis and management are critical.

A careful neurologic examination is an essential first step in the evaluation. In most cases, patients with an abnormal examination or a history of recent-onset headache should be evaluated by a computed tomography (CT) or magnetic resonance imaging (MRI) study. As an initial screening procedure for intracranial pathology in this setting, CT and MRI methods appear to be equally sensitive. In some circumstances, a lumbar puncture (LP) is also required, unless a benign etiology can be otherwise established. A general evaluation of acute headache might include cranial arteries by palpation; cervical spine by

TABLE 21-2 HEADACHE SYMPTOMS THAT SUGGEST A SERIOUS UNDERLYING DISORDER

Sudden-onset headache
First severe headache
"Worst" headache ever
Vomiting that precedes headache
Subacute worsening over days or weeks
Pain induced by bending, lifting, cough
Pain that disturbs sleep or presents immediately upon awakening
Known systemic illness
Onset after age 55
Fever or unexplained systemic signs
Abnormal neurologic examination
Pain associated with local tenderness, e.g., region of temporal artery

the effect of passive movement of the head and by imaging; the investigation of cardiovascular and renal status by blood pressure monitoring and urine examination; and eyes by funduscopy, intraocular pressure measurement, and refraction.

The psychological state of the patient should also be evaluated because a relationship exists between head pain and depression. This is intended to identify comorbidity rather than provide an explanation for the headache, because troublesome headache is seldom simply caused by mood change. Although it is notable that medicines with antidepressant actions are also effective in the prophylactic treatment of both tension-type headache and migraine, each symptom must be treated optimally.

Underlying recurrent headache disorders may be activated by pain that follows otologic or endodontic surgical procedures. Thus, pain about the head as the result of diseased tissue or trauma may reawaken an otherwise quiescent migraine syndrome. Treatment of the headache is largely ineffective until the cause of the primary problem is addressed.

Serious underlying conditions that are associated with headache are described below. Brain tumor is a rare cause of headache and even less commonly a cause of severe pain. The vast majority of patients presenting with severe headache have a benign cause.

SECONDARY HEADACHE

The management of secondary headache focuses on diagnosis and treatment of the underlying condition.

MENINGITIS

Acute, severe headache with stiff neck and fever suggests meningitis. LP is mandatory. Often there is striking accentuation of pain with eye movement. Meningitis can be easily mistaken for migraine in that the cardinal symptoms of pounding headache, photophobia, nausea, and vomiting are frequently present, perhaps reflecting the underlying biology of some of the patients.

Meningitis is discussed in Chaps. 164 and 165.

INTRACRANIAL HEMORRHAGE

Acute, severe headache with stiff neck but without fever suggests subarachnoid hemorrhage. A ruptured aneurysm, arteriovenous malformation, or intraparenchymal hemorrhage may also present with headache alone. Rarely, if the hemorrhage is small or below the foramen magnum, the head CT scan can be normal. Therefore, LP may be required to definitively diagnose subarachnoid hemorrhage.

Intracranial hemorrhage is discussed in Chap. 330.

BRAIN TUMOR

Approximately 30% of patients with brain tumors consider headache to be their chief complaint. The head pain is usually nondescript—an intermittent deep, dull aching of moderate intensity, which may worsen with exertion or change in position and may be associated with nausea and vomiting. This pattern of symptoms results from migraine far more often than from brain tumor. The headache of brain tumor disturbs sleep in about 10% of patients. Vomiting that precedes the appearance of headache by weeks is highly characteristic of posterior fossa brain tumors. A history of amenorrhea or galactorrhea should lead one to question whether a prolactin-secreting pituitary adenoma (or the polycystic ovary syndrome) is the source of headache. Headache arising de novo in a patient with known malignancy suggests either cerebral metastases or carcinomatous meningitis, or both. Head pain appearing abruptly after bending, lifting, or coughing can be due to a posterior fossa mass, a Chiari malformation, or low cerebrospinal fluid (CSF) volume.

Brain tumors are discussed in Chap. 118.

TEMPORAL ARTERITIS

(See also Chaps. 39 and 385) Temporal (giant cell) arteritis is an inflammatory disorder of arteries that frequently involves the extracranial carotid circulation. It is a common disorder of the elderly; its annual incidence is 77 per 100,000 individuals age 50 and older. The average age of onset is 70 years, and women account for 65% of cases. About half of patients with untreated temporal arteritis develop blindness due to involvement of the ophthalmic artery and its branches; indeed, the ischemic optic neuropathy induced by giant cell arteritis is the major cause of rapidly developing bilateral blindness in patients >60 years. Because treatment with glucocorticoids is effective in preventing this complication, prompt recognition of the disorder is important.

Typical presenting symptoms include headache, polymyalgia rheumatica (Chap. 385), jaw claudication, fever, and weight loss. Headache is the dominant symptom and often appears in association with malaise and muscle aches. Head pain may be unilateral or bilateral and is located temporally in 50% of patients but may involve any and all aspects of the cranium. Pain usually appears gradually over a few hours before peak intensity is reached; occasionally, it is explosive in onset. The quality of pain is only seldom throbbing; it is almost invariably described as dull and boring, with superimposed episodic stabbing pains similar to the sharp pains that appear in migraine. Most patients can recognize that the origin of their head pain is superficial, external to the skull, rather than originating deep within the cranium (the pain site for migraineurs). Scalp tenderness is present, often to a marked degree; brushing the hair or resting the head on a pillow may be impossible because of pain. Headache is usually worse at night and often aggravated by exposure to cold. Additional findings may include reddened, tender nodules or red streaking of the skin overlying the temporal arteries, and tenderness of the temporal or, less commonly, the occipital arteries.

The erythrocyte sedimentation rate (ESR) is often, although not always, elevated; a normal ESR does not exclude giant cell arteritis. A temporal artery biopsy followed by immediate treatment with prednisone 80 mg daily for the first 4–6 weeks should be initiated when clinical suspicion is high. The prevalence of migraine among the elderly is substantial, considerably higher than that of giant cell arteritis. Migraineurs often report amelioration of their headaches with prednisone; thus, caution must be used when interpreting the therapeutic response.

GLAUCOMA

Glaucoma may present with a prostrating headache associated with nausea and vomiting. The headache often starts with severe eye pain. On physical examination, the eye is often red with a fixed, moderately dilated pupil.

Glaucoma is discussed in Chap. 39.

PRIMARY HEADACHE DISORDERS

Primary headaches are disorders in which headache and associated features occur in the absence of any exogenous cause. The most common are migraine, tension-type headache, and the trigeminal autonomic cephalalgias, notably cluster headache. These entities are discussed in detail in Chap. 447.

TABLE 21-3 CLASSIFICATION OF CHRONIC DAILY HEADACHE

Primary		
>4 h Daily	**<4 h Daily**	**Secondary**
Chronic migraine[a]	Chronic cluster headache[b]	Posttraumatic Head injury Iatrogenic Postinfectious
Chronic tension-type headache[a]	Chronic paroxysmal hemicrania	Inflammatory, such as Giant cell arteritis Sarcoidosis Behçet's syndrome
Hemicrania continua[a]	SUNCT/SUNA	Chronic CNS infection
New daily persistent headache[a]	Hypnic headache	Medication-overuse headache[a]

[a]May be complicated by medication overuse. [b]Some patients may have headache >4 h/d.

Abbreviations: CNS, central nervous system; SUNA, short-lasting *u*nilateral *n*euralgiform headache *a*ttacks with cranial autonomic symptoms; SUNCT, short-lasting *u*nilateral *n*euralgiform headache attacks with *c*onjunctival injection and *t*earing.

CHRONIC DAILY HEADACHE

The broad diagnosis of chronic daily headache (CDH) can be applied when a patient experiences headache on 15 days or more per month. CDH is not a single entity; it encompasses a number of different headache syndromes, both primary and secondary (Table 21-3). In aggregate, this group presents considerable disability and is thus specially dealt with here. Population-based estimates suggest that about 4% of adults have daily or near-daily headache.

APPROACH TO THE PATIENT: Chronic Daily Headache

The first step in the management of patients with CDH is to diagnose any secondary headache and treat that problem (Table 21-3). This can sometimes be a challenge where the underlying cause triggers a worsening of a primary headache. For patients with primary headaches, diagnosis of the headache type will guide therapy. Preventive treatments such as tricyclics, either amitriptyline or nortriptyline at doses up to 1 mg/kg, are very useful in patients with CDH arising from migraine or tension-type headache or where the secondary cause has activated the underlying primary headache. Tricyclics are started in low doses (10–25 mg) daily and may be given 12 h before the expected time of awakening in order to avoid excess morning sleepiness. Anticonvulsants, such as topiramate, valproate, flunarizine (not available in the United States), and candesartan are also useful in migraine.

MANAGEMENT OF MEDICALLY INTRACTABLE DISABLING PRIMARY CHRONIC DAILY HEADACHE

The management of medically intractable headache is difficult. Currently there are a number of promising neuromodulatory approaches, such as occipital nerve stimulation, which appears to modulate thalamic processing in migraine, and has also shown promise in chronic cluster headache, short-lasting unilateral neuralgiform headache attacks with cranial autonomic symptoms (SUNA), short-lasting unilateral neuralgiform headache attacks with conjunctival injection and tearing (SUNCT), and hemicrania continua (Chap. 447). Single-pulse transcranial magnetic stimulation is in use in Europe and is approved for migraine with aura in the United States. Other modalities are discussed in Chap. 447.

MEDICATION-OVERUSE HEADACHE

Overuse of analgesic medication for headache can aggravate headache frequency, markedly impair the effect of preventive medicines, and induce a state of refractory daily or near-daily headache called *medication-overuse headache*. A proportion of patients who stop taking analgesics will experience substantial improvement in the severity and frequency of their headache. However, even after cessation of analgesic use, many patients continue to have headache, although they may feel clinically improved in some way, especially if they have been using opioids or barbiturates regularly. The residual symptoms probably represent the underlying primary headache disorder, and most commonly, this issue occurs in patients prone to migraine.

Management of Medication Overuse: Outpatients For patients who overuse medications, it is essential that analgesic use be reduced and eliminated. One approach is to reduce the medication dose by 10% every 1–2 weeks. Immediate cessation of analgesic use is possible for some patients, provided there is no contraindication. Both approaches are facilitated by the use of a medication diary maintained during the month or two before cessation; this helps to identify the scope of the problem. A small dose of a nonsteroidal anti-inflammatory drug (NSAID) such as naproxen, 500 mg bid, if tolerated, will help relieve residual pain as analgesic use is reduced. NSAID overuse is not usually a problem for patients with daily headache when a NSAID with a longer half-life is taken once or twice daily; however, overuse problems may develop with more frequent dosing schedules or shorter acting NSAIDS. Once the patient has substantially reduced analgesic use, a preventive medication should be introduced. It must be emphasized that *preventives generally do not work in the presence of analgesic overuse*. The most common cause of unresponsiveness to treatment is the use of a preventive when analgesics continue to be used regularly. For some patients, discontinuing analgesics is very difficult; often the best approach is to directly inform the patient that some degree of pain is inevitable during this initial period.

Management of Medication Overuse: Inpatients Some patients will require hospitalization for detoxification. Such patients have typically failed efforts at outpatient withdrawal or have a significant medical condition, such as diabetes mellitus, which would complicate withdrawal as an outpatient. Following admission to the hospital, acute medications are withdrawn completely on the first day, in the absence of a contraindication. Antiemetics and fluids are administered as required; clonidine is used for opioid withdrawal symptoms. For acute intolerable pain during the waking hours, aspirin, 1 g IV (not approved in United States), is useful. IM chlorpromazine can be helpful at night; patients must be adequately hydrated. Three to 5 days into the admission, as the effect of the withdrawn substance wears off, a course of IV dihydroergotamine (DHE) can be used. DHE, administered every 8 h for 5 consecutive days, can induce a significant remission that allows a preventive treatment to be established. 5-HT_3 antagonists, such as ondansetron or granisetron, or the neurokinin receptor antagonist, aprepitant, may be required with DHE to prevent significant nausea, and domperidone (not approved in the United States) orally or by suppository can be very helpful. Avoiding sedating or otherwise side effect prone antiemetics is helpful.

NEW DAILY PERSISTENT HEADACHE

New daily persistent headache (NDPH) is a clinically distinct syndrome; its causes are listed in Table 21-4.

TABLE 21-4 DIFFERENTIAL DIAGNOSIS OF NEW DAILY PERSISTENT HEADACHE

Primary	Secondary
Migrainous-type	Subarachnoid hemorrhage
Featureless (tension-type)	Low cerebrospinal fluid (CSF) volume headache
	Raised CSF pressure headache
	Posttraumatic headache[a]
	Chronic meningitis

[a]Includes postinfectious forms.

Clinical Presentation The patient with NDPH presents with headache on most if not all days, and the patient can clearly, and often vividly, recall the moment of onset. The headache usually begins abruptly, but onset may be more gradual; evolution over 3 days has been proposed as the upper limit for this syndrome. Patients typically recall the exact day and circumstances of the onset of headache; the new, persistent head pain does not remit. The first priority is to distinguish between a primary and a secondary cause of this syndrome. Subarachnoid hemorrhage is the most serious of the secondary causes and must be excluded either by history or appropriate investigation (Chap. 330).

Secondary NDPH • ***LOW CSF VOLUME HEADACHE*** In these syndromes, head pain is positional: it begins when the patient sits or stands upright and resolves upon reclining. The pain, which is occipitofrontal, is usually a dull ache but may be throbbing. Patients with chronic low CSF volume headache typically present with a history of headache from one day to the next that is generally not present on waking but worsens during the day. Recumbency usually improves the headache within minutes, and it can take only minutes to an hour for the pain to return when the patient resumes an upright position.

The most common cause of headache due to persistent low CSF volume is CSF leak following LP. Post-LP headache usually begins within 48 h but may be delayed for up to 12 days. Its incidence is between 10 and 30%. Beverages with caffeine may provide temporary relief. Besides LP, index events may include epidural injection or a vigorous Valsalva maneuver, such as from lifting, straining, coughing, clearing the eustachian tubes in an airplane, or multiple orgasms. Spontaneous CSF leaks are well recognized, and the diagnosis should be considered whenever the headache history is typical, even when there is no obvious index event. As time passes from the index event, the postural nature may become less apparent; cases in which the index event occurred several years before the eventual diagnosis have been recognized. Symptoms appear to result from low volume rather than low pressure: although low CSF pressures, typically 0–50 mmH_2O, are usually identified, a pressure as high as 140 mmH_2O has been noted with a documented leak.

Postural orthostatic tachycardia syndrome (POTS; Chap. 454) can present with orthostatic headache similar to low CSF volume headache and is a diagnosis that needs consideration in this setting.

When imaging is indicated to identify the source of a presumed leak, an MRI with gadolinium is the initial study of choice (Fig. 21-1). A striking pattern of diffuse meningeal enhancement is so typical that in the appropriate clinical context the diagnosis is established. Chiari malformations may sometimes be noted on MRI; in such cases, surgery to decompress the posterior fossa usually worsens the headache. Spinal MRI with T2 weighting may reveal a leak, and spinal MRI may demonstrate spinal meningeal cysts whose role in these syndromes is yet to be elucidated. The source of CSF leakage may be identified by spinal MRI with appropriate sequences, by CT, or increasingly by MR myelography. Less used now, ^{111}In-DTPA CSF studies in the absence of a directly identified site of leakage, may demonstrate early emptying of ^{111}In-DTPA tracer into the bladder or slow progress of tracer across the brain suggesting a CSF leak.

Initial treatment for low CSF volume headache is bed rest. For patients with persistent pain, IV caffeine (500 mg in 500 mL of saline administered over 2 h) can be very effective. An electrocardiogram (ECG) to screen for arrhythmia should be performed before administration. It is reasonable to administer at least two infusions of caffeine before embarking on additional tests to identify the source of the CSF leak. Because IV caffeine is safe and can be curative, it spares many patients the need for further investigations. If unsuccessful, an abdominal binder may be helpful. If a leak can be identified, an autologous blood patch is usually curative. A blood patch is also effective for post-LP headache; in this setting, the location is empirically determined to be the site of the LP. In patients with intractable pain, oral theophylline is a useful alternative; however, its effect is less rapid than caffeine.

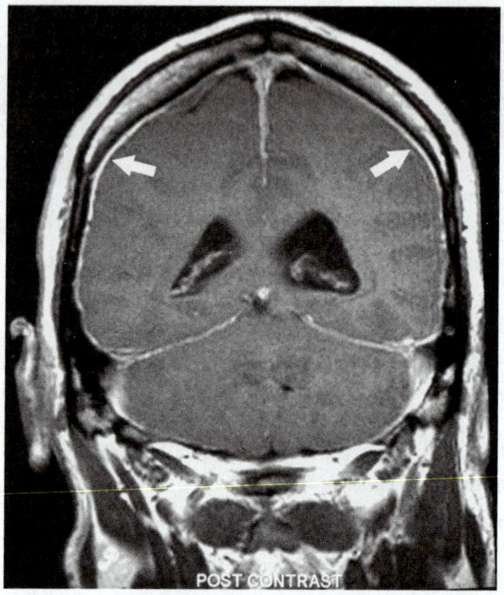

FIGURE 21-1 Magnetic resonance image showing diffuse meningeal enhancement after gadolinium administration in a patient with low cerebrospinal fluid (CSF) volume headache.

RAISED CSF PRESSURE HEADACHE Raised CSF pressure is well recognized as a cause of headache. Brain imaging can often reveal the cause, such as a space-occupying lesion. NDPH due to raised CSF pressure can be the presenting symptom for patients with idiopathic intracranial hypertension (pseudotumor cerebri) without visual problems, particularly when the fundi are normal. Persistently raised intracranial pressure can trigger chronic migraine. These patients typically present with a history of generalized headache that is present on waking and improves as the day goes on. It is generally worse with recumbency. Visual obscurations are frequent. The diagnosis is relatively straightforward when papilledema is present, but the possibility must be considered even in patients without funduscopic changes. Formal visual field testing should be performed even in the absence of overt ophthalmic involvement. Headache on rising in the morning or nocturnal headache is also characteristic of obstructive sleep apnea or poorly controlled hypertension.

Evaluation of patients suspected to have raised CSF pressure requires brain imaging. It is most efficient to obtain an MRI, including an MR venogram, as the initial study. If there are no contraindications, the CSF pressure should be measured by LP; this should be done when the patient is symptomatic so that both the pressure and the response to removal of 20–30 mL of CSF can be determined. An elevated opening pressure and improvement in headache following removal of CSF are diagnostic.

Initial treatment is with acetazolamide (250–500 mg bid); the headache may improve within weeks. If ineffective, topiramate is the next treatment of choice; it has many actions that may be useful in this setting, including carbonic anhydrase inhibition, weight loss, and neuronal membrane stabilization, likely mediated via effects on phosphorylation pathways. Severely disabled patients who do not respond to medical treatment require intracranial pressure monitoring and may require shunting.

POSTTRAUMATIC HEADACHE A traumatic event can trigger a headache process that lasts for many months or years after the event. The term *trauma* is used in a very broad sense: headache can develop following an injury to the head, but it can also develop after an infectious episode, typically viral meningitis, a flulike illness, or a parasitic infection. Complaints of dizziness, vertigo, and impaired memory can accompany the headache. Symptoms may remit after several weeks or persist for months and even years after the injury. Typically the neurologic examination is normal and CT or MRI studies are unrevealing. Chronic subdural hematoma may on occasion mimic this disorder. Posttraumatic headache may also be seen after carotid dissection and subarachnoid hemorrhage and after intracranial surgery. The underlying theme appears to be that a traumatic event involving the pain-producing meninges can trigger a headache process that lasts for many years.

OTHER CAUSES In one series, one-third of patients with NDPH reported headache beginning after a transient flulike illness characterized by fever, neck stiffness, photophobia, and marked malaise. Evaluation typically reveals no apparent cause for the headache. There is no convincing evidence that persistent Epstein-Barr virus infection plays a role in NDPH. A complicating factor is that many patients undergo LP during the acute illness; iatrogenic low CSF volume headache must be considered in these cases.

TREATMENT Treatment is largely empirical. Tricyclic antidepressants, notably amitriptyline, and anticonvulsants, such as topiramate, valproate, and gabapentin, have been used with reported benefit. The monoamine oxidase inhibitor phenelzine may also be useful in carefully selected patients. The headache usually resolves within 3–5 years, but it can be quite disabling.

PRIMARY CARE AND HEADACHE MANAGEMENT

Most patients with headache will be seen first in a primary care setting. The task of the primary care physician is to identify the very few worrisome secondary headaches from the very great majority of primary and less troublesome secondary headaches (Table 21-2).

Absent any warning signs, a reasonable approach is to treat when a diagnosis is established. As a general rule, the investigation should focus on identifying worrisome causes of headache or on gaining confidence if no primary headache diagnosis can be made.

After treatment has been initiated, follow-up care is essential to identify whether progress has been made against the headache complaint. Not all headaches will respond to treatment, but, in general, worrisome headaches will progress and will be easier to identify.

When a primary care physician feels the diagnosis is a primary headache disorder, it is worth noting that more than 90% of patients who present to primary care with a complaint of headache will have migraine (Chap. 447).

In general, patients who do not have a clear diagnosis, have a primary headache disorder other than migraine or tension-type headache, or are unresponsive to two or more standard therapies for the considered headache type should be considered for referral to a specialist. In a practical sense, the threshold for referral is also determined by the experience of the primary care physician in headache medicine and the availability of secondary care options.

22 Back and Neck Pain

John W. Engstrom, Richard A. Deyo

The importance of back and neck pain in our society is underscored by the following: (1) the cost of back pain in the United States exceeds $100 billion annually; approximately one-third of these costs are direct health care expenses, and two-thirds are indirect costs resulting from loss of wages and productivity; (2) back symptoms are the most common cause of disability in those <45 years; (3) low back pain is the second most common reason for visiting a physician in the United States; and (4) 70% of persons will have back pain at some point in their lives.

ANATOMY OF THE SPINE

The anterior spine consists of cylindrical vertebral bodies separated by intervertebral disks and held together by the anterior and posterior longitudinal ligaments. The intervertebral disks are composed of a central gelatinous nucleus pulposus surrounded by a tough cartilaginous ring, the annulus fibrosis. Disks are responsible for 25% of spinal column length and allow the bony vertebrae to move easily upon each other (Figs. 22-1 and 22-2). Desiccation of the nucleus pulposus and degeneration of the annulus fibrosus increase with age and result in loss of disk height. The disks are largest in the cervical and lumbar regions where movements of the spine are greatest. The anterior spine absorbs the shock of bodily movements such as walking and running and, with the posterior spine, protects the spinal cord and nerve roots in the spinal canal.

The posterior spine consists of the vertebral arches and processes. Each arch consists of paired cylindrical pedicles anteriorly and paired lamina posteriorly. The vertebral arch also gives rise to two transverse processes laterally, one spinous process posteriorly, plus two superior and two inferior articular facets. The apposition of a superior and inferior facet constitutes a *facet joint*. The posterior spine provides an anchor for the attachment of muscles and ligaments. The contraction of muscles attached to the spinous and transverse processes and lamina works like a system of pulleys and levers that results in flexion, extension, and lateral bending movements of the spine.

Nerve root injury (*radiculopathy*) is a common cause of neck, arm, low back, buttock, and leg pain (see Figs. 31-2 and 31-3). The nerve roots exit at a level above their respective vertebral bodies in the cervical region (e.g., the C7 nerve root exits at the C6-C7 level) and below their respective vertebral bodies in the thoracic and lumbar regions (e.g., the T1 nerve root exits at the T1-T2 level). The cervical nerve roots follow a short intraspinal course before exiting. By contrast, because the spinal cord ends at the vertebral L1 or L2 level, the lumbar nerve roots follow a long intraspinal course and can be injured anywhere from the upper lumbar spine to their exit at the intervertebral foramen. For example, disk herniation at the L4-L5 level can produce not only L5 root compression, but also compression of the traversing S1 nerve root (Fig. 22-3). The lumbar nerve roots are mobile in the spinal canal, but eventually pass through the narrow *lateral recess* of the spinal canal and *intervertebral foramen* (Figs. 22-2 and 22-3). Neuroimaging of the spine must include both sagittal and axial views to assess possible compression in either the lateral recess or intervertebral foramen.

Pain-sensitive structures of the spine include the periosteum of the vertebrae, dura, facet joints, annulus fibrosus of the intervertebral disk, epidural veins and arteries, and the longitudinal ligaments. Disease of these diverse structures may explain many cases of back pain without nerve root compression. Under normal circumstances, the nucleus pulposus of the intervertebral disk is not pain sensitive.

APPROACH TO THE PATIENT: Back Pain

TYPES OF BACK PAIN

Delineating the type of pain reported by the patient is the essential first step. Attention is also focused on identification of risk factors for a serious underlying etiology. The most frequent causes of back pain are radiculopathy, fracture, tumor, infection, or referred pain from visceral structures (Table 22-1).

Local pain is caused by injury to pain-sensitive structures that compress or irritate sensory nerve endings. The site of the pain is near the affected part of the back.

Pain referred to the back may arise from abdominal or pelvic viscera. The pain is usually described as primarily abdominal or pelvic, accompanied by back pain and usually unaffected by posture. The patient may occasionally complain of back pain only.

Pain of spine origin may be located in the back or referred to the buttocks or legs. Diseases affecting the upper lumbar spine tend to refer pain to the lumbar region, groin, or anterior thighs. Diseases affecting the lower lumbar spine tend to produce pain referred to the buttocks, posterior thighs, calves, or feet. Referred pain can explain pain syndromes that cross multiple dermatomes without evidence of nerve root compression.

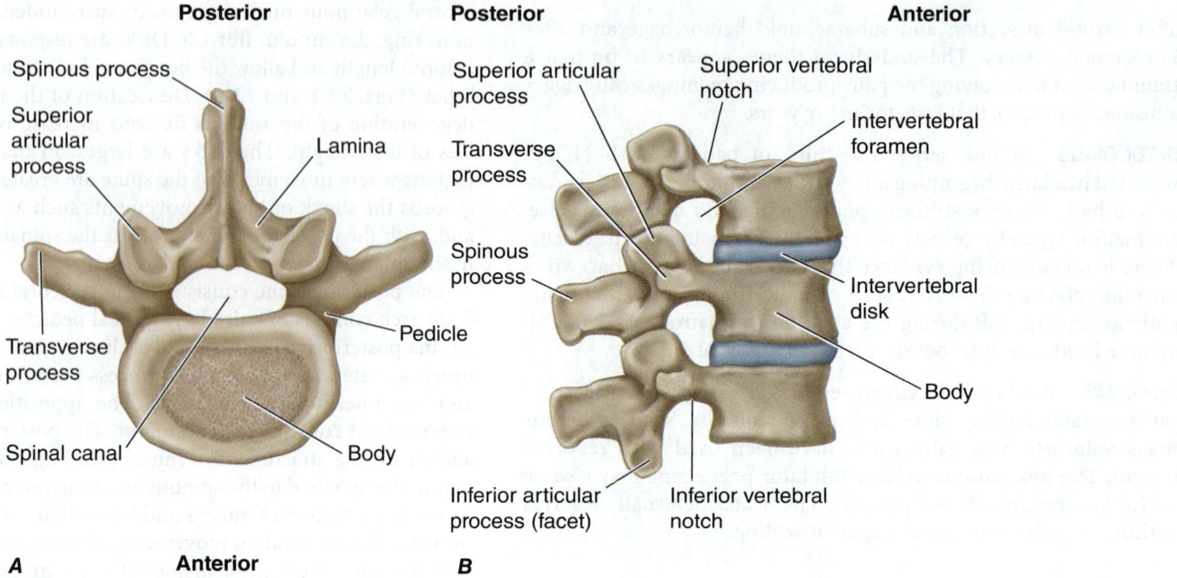

FIGURE 22-1 **Vertebral anatomy.** *(From A Gauthier Cornuelle, DH Gronefeld: Radiographic Anatomy Positioning. New York, McGraw-Hill, 1998; with permission.)*

Radicular pain is typically sharp and radiates from the low back to a leg within the territory of a nerve root (see "Lumbar Disk Disease," below). Coughing, sneezing, or voluntary contraction of abdominal muscles (lifting heavy objects or straining at stool) may elicit the radiating pain. The pain may increase in postures that stretch the nerves and nerve roots. Sitting with the leg outstretched places traction on the sciatic nerve and L5 and S1 roots because the nerve passes posterior to the hip. The femoral nerve (L2, L3, and L4 roots) passes anterior to the hip and is not stretched by sitting.

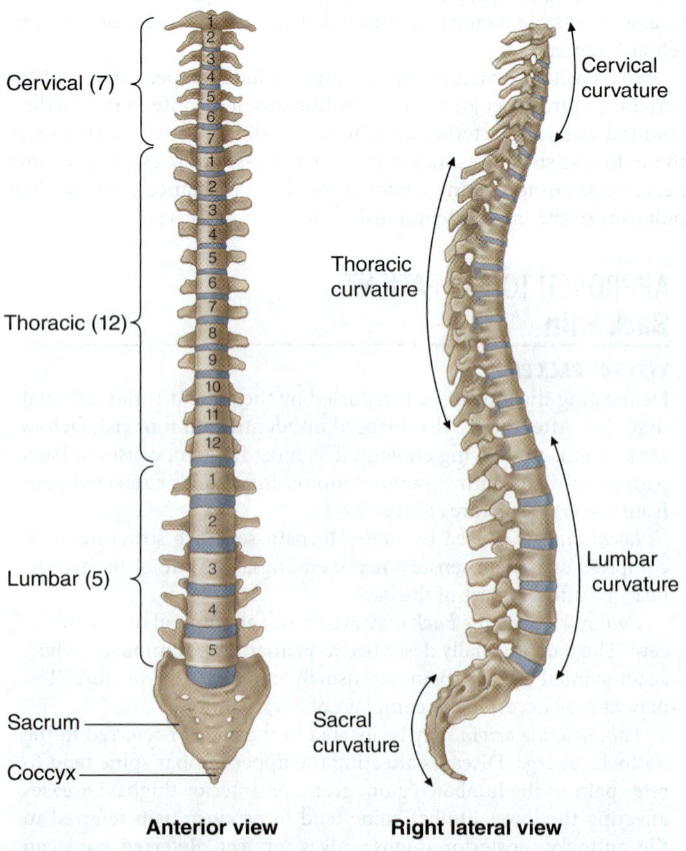

FIGURE 22-2 **Spinal column.** *(From A Gauthier Cornuelle, DH Gronefeld: Radiographic Anatomy Positioning. New York, McGraw-Hill, 1998; with permission.)*

The description of the pain alone often fails to distinguish between referred pain and radiculopathy, although a burning or electric quality favors radiculopathy.

Pain associated with muscle spasm, although of obscure origin, is commonly associated with many spine disorders. The spasms are accompanied by abnormal posture, tense paraspinal muscles, and dull or achy pain in the paraspinal region.

Knowledge of the circumstances associated with the onset of back pain is important when weighing possible serious underlying causes for the pain. Some patients involved in accidents or work-related injuries may exaggerate their pain for the purpose of compensation or for psychological reasons.

EXAMINATION OF THE BACK

A physical examination that includes the abdomen and rectum is advisable. Back pain referred from visceral organs may be reproduced during palpation of the abdomen (pancreatitis, abdominal aortic aneurysm [AAA]) or percussion over the costovertebral angles (pyelonephritis).

The normal spine has a cervical and lumbar lordosis and a thoracic kyphosis. Exaggeration of these normal alignments may result in hyperkyphosis of the thoracic spine or hyperlordosis of the lumbar spine. Inspection may reveal a lateral curvature of the spine (scoliosis). An asymmetry in the prominence of the paraspinal muscles suggests muscle spasm. Spine pain reproduced by palpation over the spinous process reflects injury of the affected vertebrae or adjacent pain-sensitive structures.

Forward bending is often limited by paraspinal muscle spasm; the latter may flatten the usual lumbar lordosis. Flexion at the hips is normal in patients with lumbar spine disease, but flexion of the lumbar spine is limited and sometimes painful. Lateral bending to the side opposite the injured spinal element may stretch the damaged tissues, worsen pain, and limit motion. Hyperextension of the spine (with the patient prone or standing) is limited when nerve root compression, facet joint pathology, or other bony spine disease is present.

Pain from hip disease may mimic the pain of lumbar spine disease. Hip pain can be reproduced by internal and external rotation at the hip with the knee and hip in flexion or by compressing the heel with the examiner's palm while the leg is extended (heel percussion sign).

The *straight leg-raising (SLR)* maneuver is a simple bedside test for nerve root disease. With the patient supine, passive flexion of the extended leg at the hip stretches the L5 and S1 nerve roots and

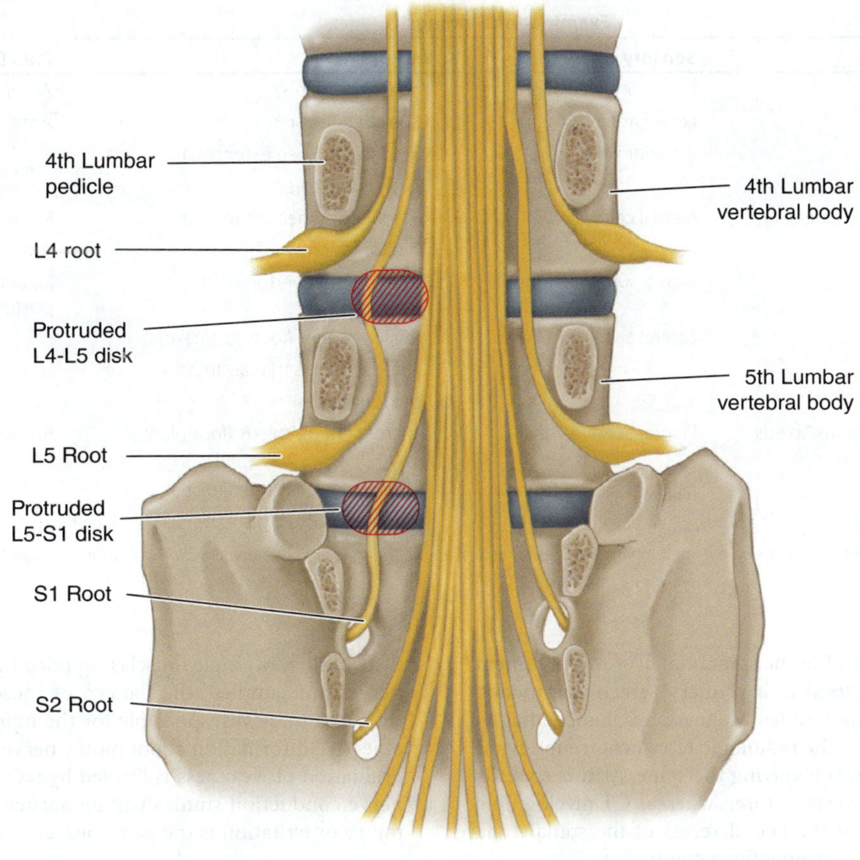

FIGURE 22-3 Compression of L5 and S1 roots by herniated disks. *(From AH Ropper, MA Samuels: Adams and Victor's Principles of Neurology, 9th ed. New York, McGraw-Hill, 2009; with permission.)*

the sciatic nerve. Passive dorsiflexion of the foot during the maneuver adds to the stretch. In healthy individuals, flexion to at least 80° is normally possible without causing pain, although a tight, stretching sensation in the hamstring muscles is common. The SLR test is positive if the maneuver reproduces the patient's usual back or limb pain. Eliciting the SLR sign in both the supine and sitting positions can help determine if the finding is reproducible. The patient may describe pain in the low back, buttocks, posterior thigh, or lower leg, but the *key feature is reproduction of the patient's usual pain.*

TABLE 22-1 ACUTE LOW BACK PAIN: RISK FACTORS FOR AN IMPORTANT STRUCTURAL CAUSE

History
Pain worse at rest or at night
Prior history of cancer
History of chronic infection (especially lung, urinary tract, skin)
History of trauma
Incontinence
Age >70 years
Intravenous drug use
Glucocorticoid use
History of a rapidly progressive neurologic deficit
Examination
Unexplained fever
Unexplained weight loss
Percussion tenderness over the spine
Abdominal, rectal, or pelvic mass
Internal/external rotation of the leg at the hip; heel percussion sign
Straight leg- or reverse straight leg–raising signs
Progressive focal neurologic deficit

The *crossed SLR sign* is present when flexion of one leg reproduces the usual pain in the opposite leg or buttocks. In disk herniation, the crossed SLR sign is less sensitive but more specific than the SLR sign. The *reverse SLR sign* is elicited by standing the patient next to the examination table and passively extending each leg with the knee fully extended. This maneuver, which stretches the L2-L4 nerve roots, lumbosacral plexus, and femoral nerve, is considered positive if the patient's usual back or limb pain is reproduced. For all of these tests, the nerve or nerve root lesion is always on the side of the pain.

The neurologic examination includes a search for focal weakness or muscle atrophy, focal reflex changes, diminished sensation in the legs, or signs of spinal cord injury. The examiner should be alert to the possibility of breakaway weakness, defined as fluctuations in the maximum power generated during muscle testing. Breakaway weakness may be due to pain or a combination of pain and an underlying true weakness. Breakaway weakness without pain is almost always due to a lack of effort. In uncertain cases, electromyography (EMG) can determine if true weakness due to nerve tissue injury is present. Findings with specific lumbosacral nerve root lesions are shown in Table 22-2 and are discussed below.

LABORATORY, IMAGING, AND EMG STUDIES

Laboratory studies are rarely needed for the initial evaluation of nonspecific acute (<3 months in duration) low back pain (ALBP). Risk factors for a serious underlying cause and for infection, tumor, or fracture, in particular, should be sought by history and exam. If risk factors are present (Table 22-1), then laboratory studies (complete blood count [CBC], erythrocyte sedimentation rate [ESR], urinalysis) are indicated. If risk factors are absent, then management is conservative (see "Treatment," below)

Computed tomography (CT) scanning is superior to routine x-rays for the detection of fractures involving posterior spine structures, craniocervical and cervicothoracic junctions, C1 and C2

TABLE 22-2 LUMBOSACRAL RADICULOPATHY: NEUROLOGIC FEATURES

Lumbosacral Nerve Roots	Examination Findings: Reflex	Sensory	Motor	Pain Distribution
L2[a]	—	Upper anterior thigh	Psoas (hip flexors)	Anterior thigh
L3[a]	—	Lower anterior thigh	Psoas (hip flexors)	Anterior thigh, knee
		Anterior knee	Quadriceps (knee extensors)	
			Thigh adductors	
L4[a]	Quadriceps (knee)	Medial calf	Quadriceps (knee extensors)[b]	Knee, medial calf
			Thigh adductors	Anterolateral thigh
L5[c]	—	Dorsal surface—foot	Peronei (foot evertors)[b]	Lateral calf, dorsal foot, posterolateral thigh, buttocks
		Lateral calf	Tibialis anterior (foot dorsiflexors)	
			Gluteus medius (hip abductors)	
			Toe dorsiflexors	
S1[c]	Gastrocnemius/soleus (ankle)	Plantar surface—foot	Gastrocnemius/soleus (foot plantar flexors)[b]	Bottom foot, posterior calf, posterior thigh, buttocks
		Lateral aspect—foot	Abductor hallucis (toe flexors)[b]	
			Gluteus maximus (hip extensors)	

[a]Reverse straight leg–raising sign present—see "Examination of the Back." [b]These muscles receive the majority of innervation from this root. [c]Straight leg–raising sign present—see "Examination of the Back."

vertebrae, bone fragments within the spinal canal, or misalignment. CT scans are increasingly used as a primary screening modality for moderate to severe acute trauma. Magnetic resonance imaging (MRI) or CT myelography is the radiologic test of choice for evaluation of most serious diseases involving the spine. MRI is superior for the definition of soft tissue structures, whereas CT myelography provides optimal imaging of the lateral recess of the spinal canal and is better tolerated by claustrophobic patients.

Annual population surveys in the United States suggest that patients with back pain have reported progressively worse functional limitations in recent years, rather than progressive improvements, despite rapid increases in spine imaging, opioid prescribing, injections, and spine surgery. This suggests that more selective use of diagnostic and treatment modalities may be appropriate.

Spine imaging often reveals abnormalities of dubious clinical relevance that may alarm clinicians and patients alike and prompt further testing and unnecessary therapy. Both randomized trials and observational studies have suggested such a "cascade effect" of imaging may create a gateway to other unnecessary care. Based in part on such evidence, the American College of Physicians has made parsimonious spine imaging a high priority in its "Choosing Wisely" campaign, aimed at reducing unnecessary care. Successful efforts to reduce unnecessary imaging have typically been multifaceted. Some include physician education by clinical leaders and computerized decision support, to identify any recent relevant imaging tests and require approved indications for ordering an imaging test. Other strategies have included audit and feedback regarding individual rates of ordering and indications, and more rapid access to physical therapy or consultation for patients without imaging indications.

When imaging tests are reported, it may be useful to indicate that certain degenerative findings are common in normal, pain-free individuals. In an observational study, this strategy was associated with lower rates of repeat imaging, opioid therapy, and physical therapy referral.

Electrodiagnostic studies can be used to assess the functional integrity of the peripheral nervous system (Chap. 442e). Sensory nerve conduction studies are normal when focal sensory loss confirmed by examination is due to nerve root damage because the nerve roots are proximal to the nerve cell bodies in the dorsal root ganglia. Injury to nerve tissue distal to the dorsal root ganglion (e.g., plexus or peripheral nerve) results in reduced sensory nerve signals. Needle EMG complements nerve conduction studies by detecting denervation or reinnervation changes in a myotomal (segmental) distribution. Multiple muscles supplied by different nerve roots and nerves are sampled; the pattern of muscle involvement indicates the nerve root(s) responsible for the injury. Needle EMG provides objective information about motor nerve fiber injury when clinical evaluation of weakness is limited by pain or poor effort. EMG and nerve conduction studies will be normal when sensory nerve root injury or irritation is the pain source.

CAUSES OF BACK PAIN

(Table 22-3)

LUMBAR DISK DISEASE

This is a common cause of acute, chronic, or recurrent low back and leg pain (Figs. 22-3 and 22-4). Disk disease is most likely to occur at the L4-L5 or L5-S1 levels, but upper lumbar levels are involved occasionally. The cause is often unknown, but the risk is increased in overweight individuals. Disk herniation is unusual prior to age 20 years and is rare in the fibrotic disks of the elderly. Complex genetic factors may play a role in predisposing some patients to disk disease. The pain may be located in the low back only or referred to a leg, buttock, or hip. A sneeze, cough, or trivial movement may cause the nucleus pulposus to prolapse, pushing the frayed and weakened annulus posteriorly. With severe disk disease, the nucleus may protrude through the annulus (herniation) or become extruded to lie as a free fragment in the spinal canal.

The mechanism by which intervertebral disk injury causes back pain is controversial. The inner annulus fibrosus and nucleus pulposus are normally devoid of innervation. Inflammation and production of proinflammatory cytokines within a ruptured nucleus pulposus may trigger or perpetuate back pain. Ingrowth of nociceptive (pain) nerve fibers into inner portions of a diseased disk may be responsible for some chronic "diskogenic" pain. Nerve root injury (radiculopathy) from disk herniation is usually due to inflammation, but lateral herniation may produce compression in the lateral recess or at the intervertebral foramen.

A ruptured disk may be asymptomatic or cause back pain, abnormal posture, limitation of spine motion (particularly flexion), a focal neurologic deficit, or radicular pain. A dermatomal pattern of sensory loss or a reduced or absent deep tendon reflex is more suggestive of a specific root lesion than is the pattern of pain. Motor findings (focal weakness, muscle atrophy, or fasciculations) occur less frequently than focal sensory or reflex changes. Symptoms and signs are usually unilateral, but bilateral involvement does occur with large central disk herniations that compress multiple roots or cause inflammation of

TABLE 22-3 CAUSES OF BACK OR NECK PAIN

Lumbar Disk Disease
Degenerative Spine Disease
Lumbar spinal stenosis without or with neurogenic claudication
Intervertebral foraminal or lateral recess narrowing
Disk-osteophyte complex
Facet or uncovertebral joint hypertrophy
Lateral disk protrusion
Spondylosis (osteoarthritis) and spondylolisthesis
Spine Infection
Vertebral osteomyelitis
Spinal epidural abscess
Septic disk (diskitis)
Meningitis
Lumbar arachnoiditis
Neoplasms—Metastatic, Hematologic, Primary Bone Tumors
Fractures
Trauma/falls, motor vehicle accidents
Atraumatic fractures: osteoporosis, neoplastic infiltration, osteomyelitis
Minor Trauma
Strain or sprain
Whiplash injury
Metabolic Spine Disease
Osteoporosis—hyperparathyroidism, immobility
Osteosclerosis (e.g., Paget's disease)
Congenital/Developmental
Spondylolysis
Kyphoscoliosis
Spina bifida occulta
Tethered spinal cord
Autoimmune Inflammatory Arthritis
Other Causes of Back Pain
Referred pain from visceral disease (e.g., abdominal aortic aneurysm)
Postural
Psychiatric, malingering, chronic pain syndromes

nerve roots within the spinal canal. Clinical manifestations of specific nerve root lesions are summarized in Table 22-2.

The differential diagnosis covers a variety of serious and treatable conditions, including epidural abscess, hematoma, fracture, or tumor.

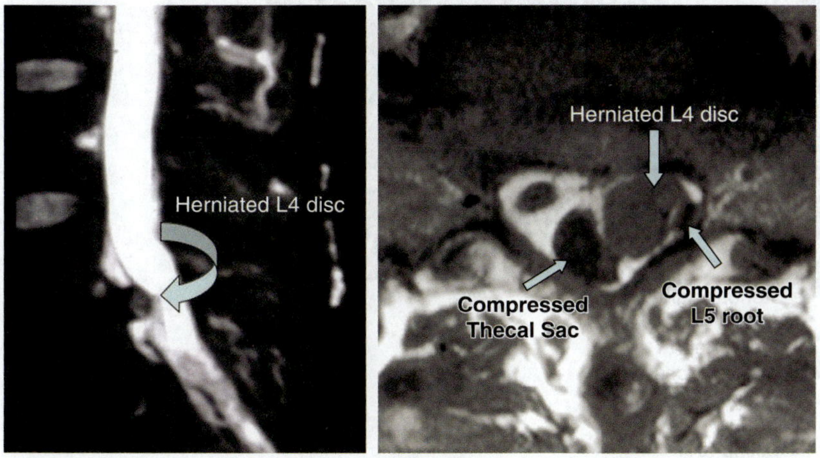

FIGURE 22-4 Left L5 radiculopathy. ***A.*** Sagittal T2-weighted image on the left reveals disk herniation at the L4-L5 level. ***B.*** Axial T1-weighted image shows paracentral disk herniation with displacement of the thecal sac medially and the left L5 nerve root posteriorly in the left lateral recess.

Fever, constant pain uninfluenced by position, sphincter abnormalities, or signs of spinal cord disease suggest an etiology other than lumbar disk disease. Absence of ankle reflexes can be a normal finding in persons older than age 60 years or a sign of bilateral S1 radiculopathy. An absent deep tendon reflex or focal sensory loss may indicate injury to a nerve root, but other sites of injury along the nerve must also be considered. For example, an absent knee reflex may be due to a femoral neuropathy or an L4 nerve root injury. A loss of sensation over the foot and lateral lower calf may result from a peroneal or lateral sciatic neuropathy or an L5 nerve root injury. Focal muscle atrophy may reflect injury to the anterior horn cells of the spinal cord, a nerve root, peripheral nerve, or disuse.

A lumbar spine MRI scan or CT myelogram is necessary to establish the location and type of pathology. Spine MRIs yield exquisite views of intraspinal and adjacent soft tissue anatomy. Bony lesions of the lateral recess or intervertebral foramen are optimally visualized by CT myelography. The correlation of neuroradiologic findings to symptoms, particularly pain, is not simple. Contrast-enhancing tears in the annulus fibrosus or disk protrusions are widely accepted as common sources of back pain; however, studies have found that many asymptomatic adults have similar findings. Asymptomatic disk protrusions are also common and may enhance with contrast. Furthermore, in patients with known disk herniation treated either medically or surgically, persistence of the herniation 10 years later had no relationship to the clinical outcome. In summary, MRI findings of disk protrusion, tears in the annulus fibrosus, or hypertrophic facet joints are common incidental findings that, by themselves, should not dictate management decisions for patients with back pain.

The diagnosis of nerve root injury is most secure when the history, examination, results of imaging studies, and the EMG are concordant. The correlation between CT and EMG for localization of nerve root injury is between 65 and 73%. Up to one-third of asymptomatic adults have a lumbar disk protrusion detected by CT or MRI scans.

Management of lumbar disk disease is discussed below.

Cauda equina syndrome (CES) signifies an injury of multiple lumbosacral nerve roots within the spinal canal distal to the termination of the spinal cord at L1-L2. Low back pain, weakness and areflexia in the legs, saddle anesthesia, or loss of bladder function may occur. The problem must be distinguished from disorders of the lower spinal cord (conus medullaris syndrome), acute transverse myelitis (Chap. 456), and Guillain-Barré syndrome (Chap. 460). Combined involvement of the conus medullaris and cauda equina can occur. CES is commonly due to a ruptured lumbosacral intervertebral disk, lumbosacral spine fracture, hematoma within the spinal canal (e.g., following lumbar puncture in patients with coagulopathy), compressive tumor, or other mass lesion. Treatment options include surgical decompression, sometimes urgently in an attempt to restore or preserve motor or sphincter function, or radiotherapy for metastatic tumors (Chap. 118).

DEGENERATIVE CONDITIONS

Lumbar spinal stenosis (LSS) describes a narrowed lumbar spinal canal and is frequently asymptomatic. Typical is *neurogenic claudication*, consisting of back and buttock or leg pain induced by walking or standing and relieved by sitting. Symptoms in the legs are usually bilateral. Unlike vascular claudication, symptoms are often provoked by standing without walking. Unlike lumbar disk disease, symptoms are usually relieved by sitting. Patients with neurogenic claudication can often walk much farther when leaning over a shopping cart and can pedal a stationary bike with ease while sitting. These flexed positions increase the anteroposterior spinal canal diameter and reduce intraspinal venous hypertension, resulting in pain relief. Focal weakness, sensory loss, or reflex changes may occur when spinal stenosis is associated with neural foraminal narrowing and radiculopathy. Severe neurologic deficits, including paralysis and urinary incontinence, occur only rarely.

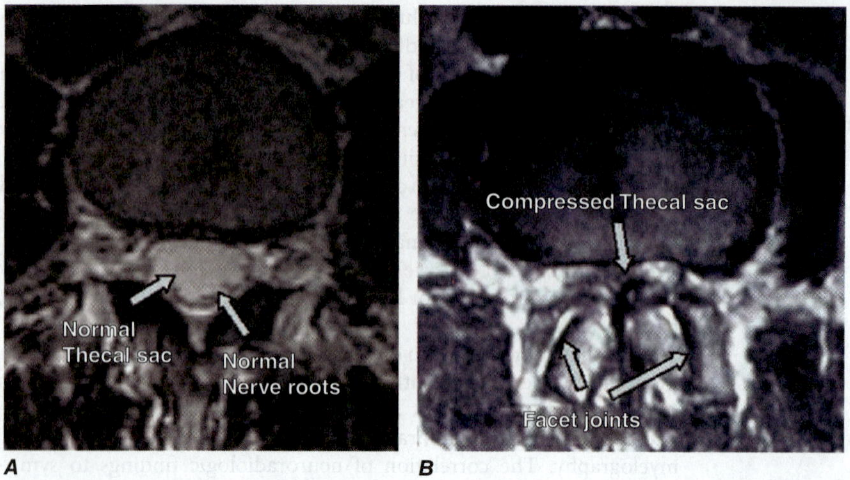

FIGURE 22-5 Axial T2-weighted images of the lumbar spine. ***A.*** The image shows a normal thecal sac within the lumbar spinal canal. The thecal sac is bright. The lumbar roots are dark punctuate dots in the posterior thecal sac with the patient supine. ***B.*** The thecal sac is not well visualized due to severe lumbar spinal canal stenosis, partially the result of hypertrophic facet joints.

LSS by itself is frequently asymptomatic, and the correlation between the severity of symptoms and degree of stenosis of the spinal canal is variable. LSS can be acquired (75%), congenital, or both. Congenital forms (achondroplasia, idiopathic) are characterized by short, thick pedicles that produce both spinal canal and lateral recess stenosis. Acquired factors that contribute to spinal stenosis include degenerative diseases (spondylosis, spondylolisthesis, scoliosis), trauma, spine surgery, metabolic or endocrine disorders (epidural lipomatosis, osteoporosis, acromegaly, renal osteodystrophy, hypoparathyroidism), and Paget's disease. MRI provides the best definition of the abnormal anatomy (Fig. 22-5).

Conservative treatment of symptomatic LSS includes nonsteroidal anti-inflammatory drugs (NSAIDs), acetaminophen, exercise programs, and symptomatic treatment of acute pain episodes. There is insufficient evidence to support the routine use of epidural glucocorticoid injections. Surgical therapy is considered when medical therapy does not relieve symptoms sufficiently to allow for resumption of activities of daily living or when focal neurologic signs are present. Most patients with neurogenic claudication who are treated medically do not improve over time. Surgical management can produce significant relief of back and leg pain within 6 weeks, and pain relief persists for at least 2 years. However, up to one-quarter develop recurrent stenosis at the same spinal level or an adjacent level 7–10 years after the initial surgery; recurrent symptoms usually respond to a second surgical decompression.

Neural foraminal narrowing with radiculopathy is a common consequence of osteoarthritic processes that cause lumbar spinal stenosis (Figs. 22-1 and 22-6), including osteophytes, lateral disk protrusion, calcified disk-osteophytes, facet joint hypertrophy, uncovertebral joint hypertrophy (cervical spine), congenitally shortened pedicles, or, frequently, a combination of these processes. Neoplasms (primary or metastatic), fractures, infections (epidural abscess), or hematomas are other considerations. These conditions can produce unilateral nerve root symptoms or signs due to compression at the intervertebral foramen or in the lateral recess; symptoms are indistinguishable from disk-related radiculopathy, but treatment may differ depending on the specific etiology. The history and neurologic examination alone cannot distinguish between these possibilities. A spine neuroimaging (CT or MRI) procedure is required to identify the anatomic cause. Neurologic findings from the examination and EMG can help direct the attention of the radiologist to specific nerve roots, especially on axial images. For *facet joint hypertrophy,* surgical foraminotomy produces long-term relief of leg and back pain in 80–90% of patients. The usefulness of therapeutic facet joint blocks for pain is controversial. Medical causes of lumbar or cervical radiculopathy unrelated to anatomic spine disease include infections

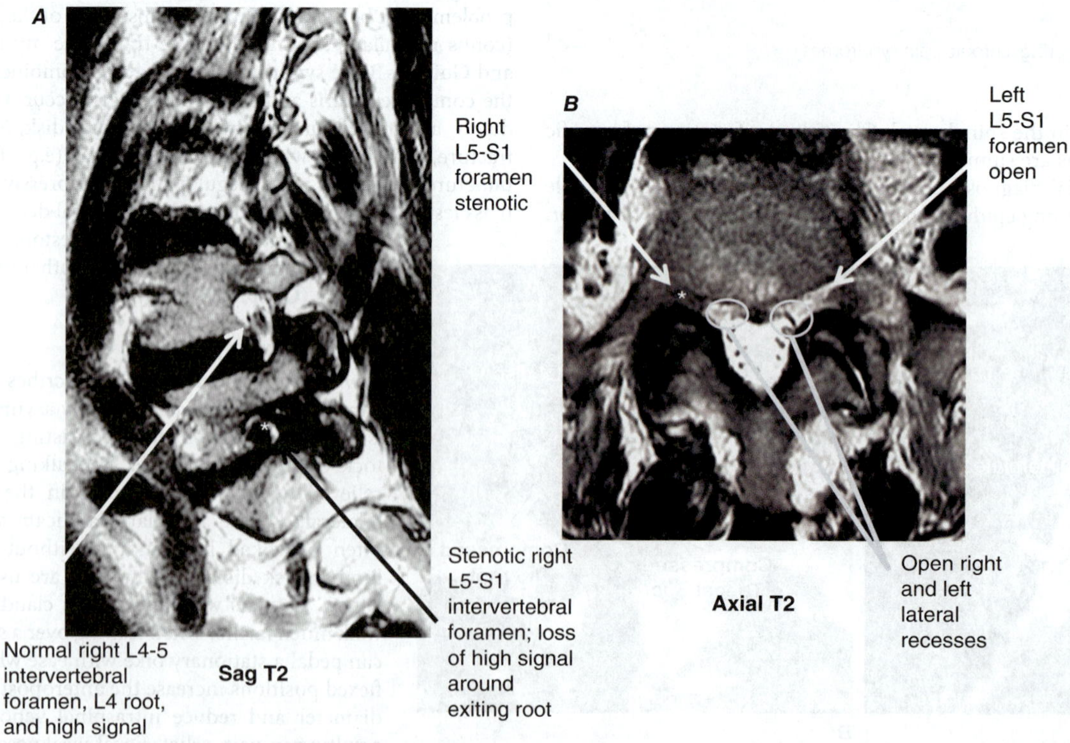

FIGURE 22-6 Right L5 radiculopathy. ***A.*** Sagittal T2-weighted image. There is normal high signal around the exiting right L4 nerve root in the right neural foramen at L4-L5; effacement of the high signal in the right L5-S1 foramen is present one level caudal on the right at L5-S1. ***B.*** Axial T2-weighted image. The lateral recesses are normal bilaterally; the intervertebral foramen is normal on the left, but severely stenotic on the right. *Severe right L5-S1 foraminal stenosis.

(e.g., herpes zoster, Lyme disease), carcinomatous meningitis, and root avulsion or traction (severe trauma).

SPONDYLOSIS AND SPONDYLOLISTHESIS

Spondylosis, or osteoarthritic spine disease, typically occurs in later life and primarily involves the cervical and lumbosacral spine. Patients often complain of back pain that increases with movement, is associated with stiffness, and is better when inactive. The relationship between clinical symptoms and radiologic findings is usually not straightforward. Pain may be prominent when x-ray, CT, or MRI findings are minimal, and prominent degenerative spine disease can be seen in asymptomatic patients. Osteophytes or combined disk-osteophytes may cause or contribute to central spinal canal stenosis, lateral recess stenosis, or neural foraminal narrowing.

Spondylolisthesis is the anterior slippage of the vertebral body, pedicles, and superior articular facets, leaving the posterior elements behind. Spondylolisthesis can be associated with spondylolysis, congenital anomalies, degenerative spine disease, or other causes of mechanical weakness of the pars (e.g., infection, osteoporosis, tumor, trauma, prior surgery). The slippage may be asymptomatic or may cause low back pain and hamstring tightness, nerve root injury (the L5 root most frequently), symptomatic spinal stenosis, or CES in severe cases. Tenderness may be elicited near the segment that has "slipped" forward (most often L4 on L5 or occasionally L5 on S1). Focal anterolisthesis or retrolisthesis can occur at any cervical or lumbar level and be the source of neck or low back pain. Plain x-rays with the neck or low back in flexion and extension will reveal the movement at the abnormal spinal segment. Surgery is considered for pain symptoms that do not respond to conservative measures (e.g., rest, physical therapy) and in cases with progressive neurologic deficit, postural deformity, slippage >50%, or scoliosis.

NEOPLASMS

Back pain is the most common neurologic symptom in patients with systemic cancer and is the presenting symptom in 20%. The cause is usually vertebral body metastasis but can also result from spread of cancer through the intervertebral foramen (especially with lymphoma), from carcinomatous meningitis, or from metastasis to the spinal cord. Cancer-related back pain tends to be constant, dull, unrelieved by rest, and worse at night. By contrast, mechanical low back pain usually improves with rest. MRI, CT, and CT myelography are the studies of choice when spinal metastasis is suspected. Once a metastasis is found, imaging of the entire spine reveals additional tumor deposits in one-third of patients. MRI is preferred for soft tissue definition, but the most rapidly available imaging modality is best because the patient's condition may worsen quickly without intervention. Fewer than 5% of patients who are nonambulatory at the time of diagnosis ever regain the ability to walk; thus, early diagnosis is crucial. The management of spinal metastasis is discussed in detail in Chap. 118.

INFECTIONS/INFLAMMATION

Vertebral osteomyelitis is often caused by staphylococci, but other bacteria or tuberculosis (Pott's disease) may be responsible. The primary source of infection is usually the urinary tract, skin, or lungs. Intravenous drug use is a well-recognized risk factor. Whenever pyogenic osteomyelitis is found, the possibility of bacterial endocarditis should be considered. Back pain unrelieved by rest, spine tenderness over the involved spine segment, and an elevated ESR are the most common findings in vertebral osteomyelitis. Fever or an elevated white blood cell count is found in a minority of patients. MRI and CT are sensitive and specific for early detection of osteomyelitis; CT may be more readily available in emergency settings and better tolerated by some patients with severe back pain. The intervertebral disk can also be affected by infection (diskitis) and, very rarely, by tumor.

Spinal epidural abscess (Chap. 456) presents with back pain (aggravated by movement or palpation), fever, radiculopathy, or signs of spinal cord compression. The subacute development of two or more of these findings should increase the index of suspicion for spinal epidural abscess. The abscess may track over multiple spinal levels and is best delineated by spine MRI.

Lumbar adhesive arachnoiditis with radiculopathy is due to fibrosis following inflammation within the subarachnoid space. The fibrosis results in nerve root adhesions and presents as back and leg pain associated with focal motor, sensory, or reflex changes. Causes of arachnoiditis include multiple lumbar operations, chronic spinal infections (especially tuberculosis in the developing world), spinal cord injury, intrathecal hemorrhage, myelography (rare), intrathecal injections (glucocorticoids, anesthetics, or other agents), and foreign bodies. The MRI shows clumped nerve roots or loculations of cerebrospinal fluid within the thecal sac. Clumped nerve roots may also occur with demyelinating polyneuropathy or neoplastic infiltration. Treatment is usually unsatisfactory. Microsurgical lysis of adhesions, dorsal rhizotomy, dorsal root ganglionectomy, and epidural glucocorticoids have been tried, but outcomes have been poor. Dorsal column stimulation for pain relief has produced varying results.

TRAUMA

A patient complaining of back pain and an inability to move the legs may have a spine fracture or dislocation; with fractures above L1 the spinal cord is at risk for compression. Care must be taken to avoid further damage to the spinal cord or nerve roots by immobilizing the back or neck pending the results of radiologic studies. Vertebral fractures frequently occur in the absence of trauma in association with osteoporosis, glucocorticoid use, osteomyelitis, or neoplastic infiltration.

Sprains and Strains The terms *low back sprain*, *strain*, and *mechanically induced muscle spasm* refer to minor, self-limited injuries associated with lifting a heavy object, a fall, or a sudden deceleration such as in an automobile accident. These terms are used loosely and do not clearly describe a specific anatomic lesion. The pain is usually confined to the lower back, and there is no radiation to the buttocks or legs. Patients with paraspinal muscle spasm often assume unusual postures.

Traumatic Vertebral Fractures Most traumatic fractures of the lumbar vertebral bodies result from injuries producing anterior wedging or compression. With severe trauma, the patient may sustain a fracture-dislocation or a "burst" fracture involving the vertebral body and posterior elements. Traumatic vertebral fractures are caused by falls from a height, sudden deceleration in an automobile accident, or direct injury. Neurologic impairment is common, and early surgical treatment is indicated. In victims of blunt trauma, CT scans of the chest, abdomen, or pelvis can be reformatted to detect associated vertebral fractures.

METABOLIC CAUSES

Osteoporosis and Osteosclerosis Immobilization, osteomalacia, the postmenopausal state, renal disease, multiple myeloma, hyperparathyroidism, hyperthyroidism, metastatic carcinoma, or glucocorticoid use may accelerate osteoporosis and weaken the vertebral body, leading to compression fractures and pain. Up to two-thirds of compression fractures seen on radiologic imaging are asymptomatic. The most common nontraumatic vertebral body fractures are due to postmenopausal or senile osteoporosis (Chap. 425). The risk of an additional vertebral fracture at 1 year following a first vertebral fracture is 20%. The presence of fever, weight loss, fracture at a level above T4, or the conditions described above should increase suspicion for a cause other than senile osteoporosis. The sole manifestation of a compression fracture may be localized back or radicular pain exacerbated by movement and often reproduced by palpation over the spinous process of the affected vertebra.

Relief of acute pain can often be achieved with acetaminophen or a combination of opioids and acetaminophen. The role of NSAIDs is controversial. Both pain and disability are improved with bracing. Antiresorptive drugs, especially bisphosphonates (e.g., alendronate), have been shown to reduce the risk of osteoporotic fractures and are the preferred treatment to prevent additional fractures. Less than one-third of patients with prior compression fractures are adequately treated for osteoporosis despite the increased risk for future fractures; even fewer at-risk patients without a history of fracture are adequately treated. Given the negative results of sham-controlled studies of percutaneous vertebroplasty (PVP) and of kyphoplasty for osteoporotic compression fractures associated with debilitating pain, these procedures are not routinely recommended.

Osteosclerosis, an abnormally increased bone density often due to Paget's disease, is readily identifiable on routine x-ray studies and can sometimes be a source of back pain. It may be associated with an isolated increase in alkaline phosphatase in an otherwise healthy older person. Spinal cord or nerve root compression can result from bony encroachment. The diagnosis of Paget's disease as the cause of a patient's back pain is a diagnosis of exclusion.

For further discussion of these bone disorders, see Chaps. 424, 425, and 426e.

AUTOIMMUNE INFLAMMATORY ARTHRITIS

Autoimmune inflammatory disease of the spine can present with the insidious onset of low back, buttock, or neck pain. Examples include rheumatoid arthritis (Chap 380), ankylosing spondylitis, reactive arthritis, psoriatic arthritis, or inflammatory bowel disease (Chap. 384).

CONGENITAL ANOMALIES OF THE LUMBAR SPINE

Spondylolysis is a bony defect in the vertebral pars interarticularis (a segment near the junction of the pedicle with the lamina); the cause is usually a stress microfracture in a congenitally abnormal segment. It occurs in up to 6% of adolescents. The defect (usually bilateral) is best visualized on plain x-rays, CT scan, or bone scan and is frequently asymptomatic. Symptoms may occur in the setting of a single injury, repeated minor injuries, or during a growth spurt. Spondylolysis is the most common cause of persistent low back pain in adolescents and is often associated with sports-related activities.

Scoliosis refers to an abnormal curvature in the coronal (lateral) plane of the spine. With *kyphoscoliosis,* there is, in addition, a forward curvature of the spine. The abnormal curvature may be congenital due to abnormal spine development, acquired in adulthood due to degenerative spine disease, or occasionally progressive due to neuromuscular disease. The deformity can progress until ambulation or pulmonary function is compromised.

Spina bifida occulta is a failure of closure of one or several vertebral arches posteriorly; the meninges and spinal cord are normal. A dimple or small lipoma may overlie the defect. Most cases are asymptomatic and discovered incidentally during an evaluation for back pain.

Tethered cord syndrome usually presents as a progressive cauda equina disorder (see below), although myelopathy may also be the initial manifestation. The patient is often a young adult who complains of perineal or perianal pain, sometimes following minor trauma. MRI studies reveal a low-lying conus (below L1 and L2) and a short and thickened filum terminale.

REFERRED PAIN FROM VISCERAL DISEASE

Diseases of the thorax, abdomen, or pelvis may refer pain to the posterior portion of the spinal segment that innervates the diseased organ. Occasionally, back pain may be the first and only manifestation. Upper abdominal diseases generally refer pain to the lower thoracic or upper lumbar region (eighth thoracic to the first and second lumbar vertebrae), lower abdominal diseases to the midlumbar region (second to fourth lumbar vertebrae), and pelvic diseases to the sacral region. Local signs (pain with spine palpation, paraspinal muscle spasm) are absent, and little or no pain accompanies routine movements of the spine.

Low Thoracic or Lumbar Pain with Abdominal Disease Tumors of the posterior wall of the stomach or duodenum typically produce epigastric pain (Chaps. 109 and 348), but midline back or paraspinal pain may occur if retroperitoneal extension is present. Fatty foods occasionally induce back pain associated with biliary disease. Diseases of the pancreas can produce right or left paraspinal back pain. Pathology in retroperitoneal structures (hemorrhage, tumors, pyelonephritis) can produce paraspinal pain that radiates to the lower abdomen, groin, or anterior thighs. A mass in the iliopsoas region can produce unilateral lumbar pain with radiation toward the groin, labia, or testicle. The sudden appearance of lumbar pain in a patient receiving anticoagulants suggests retroperitoneal hemorrhage.

Isolated low back pain occurs in some patients with a contained rupture of an abdominal aortic aneurysm (AAA). The classic clinical triad of abdominal pain, shock, and back pain occurs in <20% of patients. The typical patient at risk is an elderly male smoker with back pain. The diagnosis may be missed because the symptoms and signs can be nonspecific. Misdiagnoses include nonspecific back pain, diverticulitis, renal colic, sepsis, and myocardial infarction. A careful abdominal examination revealing a pulsatile mass (present in 50–75% of patients) is an important physical finding. Patients with suspected AAA should be evaluated with abdominal ultrasound, CT, or MRI (Chap. 301).

Sacral Pain with Gynecologic and Urologic Disease Pelvic organs rarely cause low back pain, except for gynecologic disorders involving the uterosacral ligaments. The pain is referred to the sacral region. Endometriosis or uterine cancers may invade the uterosacral ligaments. Pain associated with endometriosis is typically premenstrual and often continues until it merges with menstrual pain. Uterine malposition may cause uterosacral ligament traction (retroversion, descensus, and prolapse) or produce sacral pain after prolonged standing.

Menstrual pain may be felt in the sacral region sometimes with poorly localized, cramping pain radiating down the legs. Pain due to neoplastic infiltration of nerves is typically continuous, progressive in severity, and unrelieved by rest at night. Less commonly, radiation therapy of pelvic tumors may produce sacral pain from late radiation necrosis of tissue. Low back pain that radiates into one or both thighs is common in the last weeks of pregnancy.

Urologic sources of lumbosacral back pain include chronic prostatitis, prostate cancer with spinal metastasis (Chap. 115), and diseases of the kidney or ureter. Lesions of the bladder and testes do not often produce back pain. Infectious, inflammatory, or neoplastic renal diseases may produce ipsilateral lumbosacral pain, as can renal artery or vein thrombosis. Paraspinal lumbar pain may be a symptom of ureteral obstruction due to nephrolithiasis.

OTHER CAUSES OF BACK PAIN

Postural Back Pain There is a group of patients with nonspecific chronic low back pain (CLBP) in whom no specific anatomic lesion can be found despite exhaustive investigation. These individuals complain of vague, diffuse back pain with prolonged sitting or standing that is relieved by rest. Exercises to strengthen the paraspinal and abdominal muscles are sometimes helpful.

Psychiatric Disease CLBP may be encountered in patients who seek financial compensation; in malingerers; or in those with concurrent substance abuse. Many patients with CLBP have a history of psychiatric illness (depression, anxiety states) or childhood trauma (physical or sexual abuse) that antedates the onset of back pain. Preoperative psychological assessment has been used to exclude patients with marked psychological impairments that predict a poor surgical outcome from spine surgery.

IDIOPATHIC

The cause of low back pain occasionally remains unclear. Some patients have had multiple operations for disk disease but have persistent pain and disability. The original indications for surgery may have been questionable, with back pain only, no definite neurologic signs, or a minor disk bulge noted on CT or MRI. Scoring systems based on neurologic signs, psychological factors, physiologic studies, and imaging studies have been devised to minimize the likelihood of unsuccessful surgery.

TREATMENT BACK PAIN

HEALTH CARE FOR POPULATIONS OF BACK PAIN PATIENTS: A CLINICAL CARE SYSTEMS VIEW

There are increasing pressures to contain health care costs, especially when expensive care is not based on sound evidence. Physicians, patients, the insurance industry, and government providers of health care will need to work together to ensure cost-effective care for patients with back pain.

Surveys in the United States indicate that patients with back pain have reported progressively worse functional limitations in recent years, despite rapid increases in spine imaging, opioid prescribing, injections, and spine surgery. This suggests that more selective use of diagnostic and treatment modalities may be appropriate.

Spine imaging often reveals abnormalities of dubious clinical relevance that may alarm clinicians and patients and prompt further testing and unnecessary therapy. Both randomized trials and observational studies have suggested a "cascade effect" of imaging, which may create a gateway to other unnecessary care. Based in part on such evidence, the American College of Physicians has made parsimonious spine imaging a high priority in its "Choosing Wisely" campaign, aimed at reducing unnecessary care. Successful efforts to reduce unnecessary imaging have included physician education by clinical leaders, computerized decision support to identify recent imaging tests and eliminate duplication, and requiring an approved indication to order an imaging test. Other strategies have included audit and feedback regarding individual practitioners' rates of ordering and indications and facilitating rapid access to physical therapy for patients who do not need imaging. When imaging tests are reported, it may also be useful to routinely note that some degenerative findings are common in normal, pain-free individuals. In an observational study, this strategy was associated with lower rates of repeat imaging, opioid therapy, and referral for physical therapy.

Mounting evidence of morbidities from long-term opioid therapy (including overdose, dependency, addiction, falls, fractures, accident risk, and sexual dysfunction) has prompted efforts to reduce use for chronic pain, including back pain (Chap. 18). Safety may be improved with automated reminders for high doses, early refills, or overlapping opioid and benzodiazepine prescriptions. Greater access to alternative treatments for chronic pain, such as tailored exercise programs and cognitive-behavioral therapy, may also reduce opioid prescribing.

The high cost, wide geographic variations, and rapidly increasing rates of spinal fusion surgery have prompted scrutiny over appropriate indications. Some insurance carriers have begun to limit coverage for the most controversial indications, such as low back pain without radiculopathy. Finally, educating patients and the public about the risks of imaging and excessive therapy may be necessary. A successful media campaign in Australia provides a successful model for this approach.

ALBP WITHOUT RADICULOPATHY

ALBP is defined as pain of <3 months in duration. Full recovery can be expected in more than 85% of adults with ALBP without leg pain. Most have purely "mechanical" symptoms (i.e., pain that is aggravated by motion and relieved by rest).

The initial assessment excludes serious causes of spine pathology that require urgent intervention including infection, cancer, or trauma. Risk factors for a serious cause of ALBP are shown in Table 22-1. Laboratory and imaging studies are unnecessary if risk factors are absent. CT, MRI, or plain spine films are rarely indicated in the first month of symptoms unless a spine fracture, tumor, or infection is suspected.

The prognosis is generally excellent. Many patients do not seek medical care and improve on their own. Even among those seen in primary care, two-thirds report being substantially improved after 7 weeks. This spontaneous improvement can mislead clinicians and researchers about the efficacy of treatment interventions unless subjected to rigorous prospective trials. Many treatments commonly used in the past but now known to be ineffective, including bed rest, lumbar traction, and coccygectomy, have been largely abandoned.

Clinicians should reassure patients that improvement is very likely and instruct them in self-care. Education is an important part of treatment. Satisfaction and the likelihood of follow-up increase when patients are educated about prognosis, treatment methods, activity modifications, and strategies to prevent future exacerbations. Patients who report that they did not receive an adequate explanation for their symptoms are likely to request further diagnostic tests. In general, bed rest should be avoided for relief of severe symptoms or kept to a day or two at most. Several randomized trials suggest that bed rest does not hasten the pace of recovery. In general, the best activity recommendation is for early resumption of normal physical activity, avoiding only strenuous manual labor. Possible advantages of early ambulation for ALBP include maintenance of cardiovascular conditioning, improved disk and cartilage nutrition, improved bone and muscle strength, and increased endorphin levels. Specific back exercises or early vigorous exercise have not shown benefits for acute back pain, but may be useful for chronic pain. Use of heating pads or blankets is sometimes helpful.

Evidence-based guidelines recommend over-the-counter medicines such as acetaminophen and NSAIDs as first-line options for treatment of ALBP. In otherwise healthy patients, a trial of acetaminophen can be followed by NSAIDs for time-limited periods. In theory, the anti-inflammatory effects of NSAIDs might provide an advantage over acetaminophen to suppress inflammatory changes that accompany many causes of ALBP, but in practice, there is no clinical evidence to support the superiority of NSAIDs. The risk of renal and gastrointestinal toxicity with NSAIDs is increased in patients with preexisting medical comorbidities (e.g., renal insufficiency, cirrhosis, prior gastrointestinal hemorrhage, use of anticoagulants or steroids, heart failure). Skeletal muscle relaxants, such as cyclobenzaprine or methocarbamol, may be useful, but sedation is a common side effect. Limiting the use of muscle relaxants to nighttime only may be an option for patients with back pain that interferes with sleep.

There is no good evidence to support the use of opioid analgesics or tramadol as first-line therapy for ALBP. Their use is best reserved for patients who cannot tolerate acetaminophen or NSAIDs or for those with severe refractory pain. As with muscle relaxants, these drugs are often sedating, so it may be useful to prescribe them at nighttime only. Side effects of short-term opioid use include nausea, constipation, and pruritus; risks of long-term opioid use include hypersensitivity to pain, hypogonadism, and dependency. Falls, fractures, driving accidents, and fecal impaction are other risks. Clinical efficacy of opioids beyond 16 weeks of use is unproven.

There is no evidence to support use of oral or injected glucocorticoids for ALBP without radiculopathy. Similarly, therapies for neuropathic pain, such as gabapentin or tricyclic antidepressants, are not indicated for ALBP.

Nonpharmacologic treatments for ALBP include spinal manipulation, exercise, physical therapy, massage, acupuncture, transcutaneous electrical nerve stimulation, and ultrasound. Spinal manipulation appears to be roughly equivalent to conventional medical treatments and may be a useful alternative for patients who wish to avoid or who cannot tolerate drug therapy. There is little evidence to support the use of physical therapy, massage, acupuncture, laser therapy, therapeutic ultrasound, corsets, or lumbar traction. Although important for chronic pain, back exercises for ALBP are generally not supported by clinical evidence. There is no convincing evidence regarding the value of ice or heat applications for ABLP; however, many patients report temporary symptomatic relief from ice or frozen gel packs, and heat may produce a short-term reduction in pain after the first week. Patients often report improved satisfaction with the care that they receive when they actively participate in the selection of symptomatic approaches that are tried.

CLBP WITHOUT RADICULOPATHY

CLBP is defined as pain lasting >12 weeks; it accounts for 50% of total back pain costs. Risk factors include obesity, female gender, older age, prior history of back pain, restricted spinal mobility, pain radiating into a leg, high levels of psychological distress, poor self-rated health, minimal physical activity, smoking, job dissatisfaction, and widespread pain. In general, the same treatments that are recommended for ALBP can be useful for patients with CLBP. In this setting, however, the long-term benefit of opioid therapy or muscle relaxants is less clear.

Evidence supports the use of exercise therapy, and this can be one of the mainstays of treatment for CLBP. Effective regimens have generally included a combination of gradually increasing aerobic exercise, strengthening exercises, and stretching exercises. Motivating patients is sometimes challenging, and in this setting, a program of supervised exercise can improve compliance. In general, activity tolerance is the primary goal, while pain relief is secondary. Supervised intensive physical exercise or "work hardening" regimens have been effective in returning some patients to work, improving walking distance, and reducing pain. In addition, some forms of yoga have been evaluated in randomized trials and may be helpful for patients who are interested. A long-term benefit of spinal manipulation or massage for CLBP is unproven.

Medications for CLBP may include acetaminophen, NSAIDs, and tricyclic antidepressants. Trials of tricyclics suggest benefit even for patients without evidence of depression. Trials do not support the efficacy of selective serotonin reuptake inhibitors (SSRIs) for CLBP. However, depression is common among patients with chronic pain and should be appropriately treated.

Cognitive-behavioral therapy is based on evidence that psychological and social factors, as well as somatic pathology, are important in the genesis of chronic pain and disability. Cognitive-behavioral therapy includes efforts to identify and modify patients' thinking about their pain and disability. A systematic review concluded that such treatments are more effective than a waiting list control group for short-term pain relief; however, long-term results remain unclear. Behavioral treatments may have effects similar in magnitude to exercise therapy.

Back pain is the most frequent reason for seeking complementary and alternative treatments. The most common of these for back pain are spinal manipulation, acupuncture, and massage. The role of most complementary and alternative medicine approaches remains unclear. Biofeedback has not been studied rigorously. There is no convincing evidence that either spinal manipulation or transcutaneous electrical nerve stimulation (TENS) is effective in treating CLBP. Rigorous recent trials of acupuncture suggest that true acupuncture is not superior to sham acupuncture, but that both may offer an advantage over routine care. Whether this is due entirely to placebo effects provided even by sham acupuncture is uncertain. Some trials of massage therapy have been encouraging, but this has been less well studied than spinal manipulation or acupuncture.

Various injections, including epidural glucocorticoid injections, facet joint injections, and trigger point injections, have been used for treating CLBP. However, in the absence of radiculopathy, there is no evidence that these approaches are effective.

Injection studies are sometimes used diagnostically to help determine the anatomic source of back pain. The use of discography to provide evidence that a specific disk is the pain generator is not recommended. Pain relief following a glucocorticoid injection into a facet is commonly used as evidence that the facet joint is the pain source; however, the possibility that the response was a placebo effect or due to systemic absorption of the glucocorticoids is difficult to exclude.

Another category of intervention for chronic back pain is electrothermal and radiofrequency therapy. Intradiskal therapy has been proposed using both types of energy to thermocoagulate and destroy nerves in the intervertebral disk, using specially designed catheters or electrodes. Current evidence does not support the use of these intradiskal therapies.

Radiofrequency denervation is sometimes used to destroy nerves that are thought to mediate pain, and this technique has been used for facet joint pain (with the target nerve being the medial branch of the primary dorsal ramus), for back pain thought to arise from the intervertebral disk (ramus communicans), and radicular back pain (dorsal root ganglia). A few small trials have produced conflicting results for facet joint and diskogenic pain. A trial in patients with chronic radicular pain found no difference between radiofrequency denervation of the dorsal root ganglia and sham treatment. These interventional therapies have not been studied in sufficient detail to draw conclusions of their value for CLBP.

Surgical intervention for CLBP without radiculopathy has been evaluated in a small number of randomized trials, all conducted in Europe. Each of these studies included patients with back pain and a degenerative disk, but no sciatica. Three of the four trials concluded that lumbar fusion surgery was no more effective than highly structured, rigorous rehabilitation combined with cognitive-behavioral therapy. The fourth trial found an advantage of fusion surgery over haphazard "usual care," which appeared to be less effective than the structured rehabilitation in other trials. Given conflicting evidence, indications for surgery for CLBP without radiculopathy have remained controversial. Both U.S. and British guidelines suggest considering referral for an opinion on spinal fusion for people who have completed an optimal nonsurgical treatment program (including combined physical and psychological treatment) and who have persistent severe back pain for which they would consider surgery.

Lumbar disk replacement with prosthetic disks is U.S. Food and Drug Administration approved for uncomplicated patients needing single-level surgery at the L3-S1 levels. The disks are generally designed as metal plates with a polyethylene cushion sandwiched in between. The trials that led to approval of these devices compared them to spine fusion and concluded that the artificial disks were "not inferior." Serious complications are somewhat more likely with the artificial disk. This treatment remains controversial for CLBP.

Intensive multidisciplinary rehabilitation programs may involve daily or frequent physical therapy, exercise, cognitive-behavioral therapy, a workplace evaluation, and other interventions. For patients who have not responded to other approaches, such programs appear to offer some benefit. Systematic reviews suggest that the evidence is limited and benefits are incremental.

Some observers have raised concern that CLBP may often be overtreated. For CLBP without radiculopathy, new British guidelines explicitly recommend against use of SSRIs, any type of injection, TENS, lumbar supports, traction, radiofrequency facet joint denervation, intradiskal electrothermal therapy, or intradiskal radiofrequency thermocoagulation. These treatments are also not recommended in guidelines from the American College of Physicians and the American Pain Society. On the other hand, exercise therapy and treatment of depression appear to be useful and underused.

LOW BACK PAIN WITH RADICULOPATHY

A common cause of back pain with radiculopathy is a herniated disk with nerve root impingement, resulting in back pain with radiation down the leg. The term sciatica is used when the leg pain radiates posteriorly in a sciatic or L5/S1 distribution. The prognosis for acute low back and leg pain with radiculopathy due to disk herniation is generally favorable, with most patients showing substantial improvement over months. Serial imaging studies suggest spontaneous regression of the herniated portion of the disk in two-thirds of patients over 6 months. Nonetheless, there are several important treatment options to provide symptomatic relief while this natural healing process unfolds.

Resumption of normal activity is recommended. Randomized trial evidence suggests that bed rest is ineffective for treating sciatica as well as back pain alone. Acetaminophen and NSAIDs are useful for pain relief, although severe pain may require short courses of opioid analgesics.

Epidural glucocorticoid injections have a role in providing temporary symptom relief for sciatica due to a herniated disk. However, there does not appear to be a benefit in terms of reducing subsequent surgical interventions. Diagnostic nerve root blocks have been advocated to determine if pain originates from a specific nerve root. However, improvement may result even when the nerve root is not responsible for the pain; this may occur as a placebo effect, from a pain-generating lesion located distally along the peripheral nerve, or from effects of systemic absorption. The utility of diagnostic nerve root blocks remains a subject of debate.

Surgical intervention is indicated for patients who have progressive motor weakness due to nerve root injury demonstrated on clinical examination or EMG. Urgent surgery is recommended for patients who have evidence of CES or spinal cord compression, generally suggested by bowel or bladder dysfunction, diminished sensation in a saddle distribution, a sensory level on the trunk, and bilateral leg weakness or spasticity.

Surgery is also an important option for patients who have disabling radicular pain despite optimal conservative treatment. Sciatica is perhaps the most common reason for recommending spine surgery. Because patients with a herniated disk and sciatica generally experience rapid improvement over a matter of weeks, most experts do not recommend considering surgery unless the patient has failed to respond to 6–8 weeks of maximum nonsurgical management. For patients who have not improved, randomized trials indicate that, compared to nonsurgical treatment, surgery results in more rapid pain relief. However, after the first year or two of follow-up, patients with sciatica appear to have much the same level of pain relief and functional improvement with or without surgery. Thus, both treatment approaches are reasonable, and patient preferences and needs (e.g., rapid return to employment) strongly influence decision making. Some patients will want the fastest possible relief and find surgical risks acceptable. Others will be more risk-averse and more tolerant of symptoms and will choose watchful waiting if they understand that improvement is likely in the end.

The usual surgical procedure is a partial hemilaminectomy with excision of the prolapsed disk (diskectomy). Fusion of the involved lumbar segments should be considered only if significant spinal instability is present (i.e., degenerative spondylolisthesis). The costs associated with lumbar interbody fusion have increased dramatically in recent years. There are no large prospective, randomized trials comparing fusion to other types of surgical intervention. In one study, patients with persistent low back pain despite an initial diskectomy fared no better with spine fusion than with a conservative regimen of cognitive intervention and exercise. Artificial disks have been in use in Europe for the past decade; their utility remains controversial in the United States.

PAIN IN THE NECK AND SHOULDER

Neck pain, which usually arises from diseases of the cervical spine and soft tissues of the neck, is common. Neck pain arising from the cervical spine is typically precipitated by movement and may be accompanied by focal tenderness and limitation of motion. Many of the prior comments made regarding causes of low back pain also apply to disorders of the cervical spine. The text below will emphasize differences. Pain arising from the brachial plexus, shoulder, or peripheral nerves can be confused with cervical spine disease (Table 22-4), but the history and examination usually identify a more distal origin for the pain. Cervical spine trauma, disk disease, or spondylosis with intervertebral foraminal narrowing may be asymptomatic or painful and can produce a myelopathy, radiculopathy, or both. The same risk factors for serious causes of low back pain also apply to neck pain with the additional feature that neurologic signs of myelopathy (incontinence, sensory level, spastic legs) may also occur. Lhermitte's sign, an electrical shock down the spine with neck flexion, suggests involvement of the cervical spinal cord.

TRAUMA TO THE CERVICAL SPINE

Trauma to the cervical spine (fractures, subluxation) places the spinal cord at risk for compression. Motor vehicle accidents, violent crimes, or falls account for 87% of cervical spinal cord injuries (Chap. 456). Immediate immobilization of the neck is essential to minimize further spinal cord injury from movement of unstable cervical spine segments. The decision to obtain imaging should be based on the nature of the injury. The NEXUS low-risk criteria established that normally alert patients without palpation tenderness in the midline; intoxication; neurologic deficits; or painful distracting injuries were very unlikely to have sustained a clinically significant traumatic injury to the cervical spine. The Canadian C-spine rule recommends that imaging should be obtained following neck region trauma if the patient is >65 years old or has limb paresthesias or if there was a dangerous mechanism for the injury (e.g., bicycle collision with tree or parked car, fall from height >3 feet or five stairs, diving accident). These guidelines are helpful but must be tailored to individual circumstances; for example, patients with advanced osteoporosis, glucocorticoid use, or cancer may warrant imaging after even mild trauma. A CT scan is the diagnostic procedure of choice for detection of acute fractures following severe trauma; plain x-rays can be used for lesser degrees of trauma. When traumatic injury to the vertebral arteries or cervical spinal cord is suspected, visualization by MRI with magnetic resonance angiography is preferred.

Whiplash injury is due to rapid flexion and extension of the neck, usually in automobile accidents. The exact mechanism of the injury is unclear. This diagnosis should not be applied to patients with fractures, disk herniation, head injury, focal neurologic findings, or altered consciousness. Up to 50% of persons reporting whiplash injury acutely have persistent neck pain 1 year later. Once personal

TABLE 22-4 CERVICAL RADICULOPATHY: NEUROLOGIC FEATURES

Cervical Nerve Roots	Examination Findings			Pain Distribution
	Reflex	Sensory	Motor	
C5	Biceps	Lateral deltoid	Rhomboids[a] (elbow extends backward with hand on hip)	Lateral arm, medial scapula
			Infraspinatus[a] (arm rotates externally with elbow flexed at the side)	
			Deltoid[a] (arm raised laterally 30–45° from the side)	
C6	Biceps	Thumb/index finger;	Biceps[a] (arm flexed at the elbow in supination)	Lateral forearm, thumb/index fingers
		Dorsal hand/lateral forearm	Pronator teres (forearm pronated)	
C7	Triceps	Middle fingers	Triceps[a] (forearm extension, flexed at elbow)	Posterior arm, dorsal forearm, dorsal hand
		Dorsal forearm	Wrist/finger extensors[a]	
C8	Finger flexors	Palmar surface of little finger	Abductor pollicis brevis (abduction of thumb)	Fourth and fifth fingers, medial hand and forearm
		Medial hand and forearm	First dorsal interosseous (abduction of index finger)	
			Abductor digiti minimi (abduction of little finger)	
T1	Finger flexors	Axilla and medial arm	Abductor pollicis brevis (abduction of thumb)	Medial arm, axilla
			First dorsal interosseous (abduction of index finger)	
			Abductor digiti minimi (abduction of little finger)	

[a]These muscles receive the majority of innervation from this root.

compensation for pain and suffering was removed from the Australian health care system, the prognosis for recovery at 1 year from whiplash injury improved also. Imaging of the cervical spine is not cost-effective acutely but is useful to detect disk herniations when symptoms persist for >6 weeks following the injury. Severe initial symptoms have been associated with a poor long-term outcome.

CERVICAL DISK DISEASE

Herniation of a lower cervical disk is a common cause of pain or tingling in the neck, shoulder, arm, or hand. Neck pain, stiffness, and a range of motion limited by pain are the usual manifestations. Herniated cervical disks are responsible for ~25% of cervical radiculopathies. Extension and lateral rotation of the neck narrow the ipsilateral intervertebral foramen and may reproduce radicular symptoms (Spurling's sign). In young adults, acute nerve root compression from a ruptured cervical disk is often due to trauma. Cervical disk herniations are usually posterolateral near the lateral recess. Typical patterns of reflex, sensory, and motor changes that accompany cervical nerve root lesions are summarized in Table 22-4. Although the classic patterns are clinically helpful, there are numerous exceptions because (1) there is overlap in sensory function between adjacent nerve roots, (2) symptoms and signs may be evident in only part of the injured nerve root territory, and (3) the location of pain is the most variable of the clinical features.

CERVICAL SPONDYLOSIS

Osteoarthritis of the cervical spine may produce neck pain that radiates into the back of the head, shoulders, or arms, or may be the source of headaches in the posterior occipital region (supplied by the C2-C4 nerve roots). Osteophytes, disk protrusions, or hypertrophic facet or uncovertebral joints may alone or in combination compress one or several nerve roots at the intervertebral foramina; these causes together account for 75% of cervical radiculopathies. The roots most commonly affected are C7 and C6. Narrowing of the spinal canal by osteophytes, ossification of the posterior longitudinal ligament (OPLL), or a large central disk may compress the cervical spinal cord and produce signs of radiculopathy and myelopathy in combination (myeloradiculopathy). When little or no neck pain accompanies cervical cord involvement, other diagnoses to be considered include amyotrophic lateral sclerosis (Chap. 452), multiple sclerosis (Chap. 458), spinal cord tumors, or syringomyelia (Chap. 456). The possibility of cervical spondylosis should be considered even when the patient presents with symptoms or signs in the legs only. MRI is the study of choice to define anatomic abnormalities of soft tissues in the cervical region including the spinal cord, but plain CT is adequate to assess bony spurs, foraminal narrowing, lateral recess stenosis, or OPLL. EMG and nerve conduction studies can localize and assess the severity of nerve root injury.

OTHER CAUSES OF NECK PAIN

Rheumatoid arthritis (RA) (Chap. 380) of the cervical facet joints produces neck pain, stiffness, and limitation of motion. Synovitis of the atlantoaxial joint (C1-C2; Fig. 22-2) may damage the transverse ligament of the atlas, producing forward displacement of the atlas on the axis (atlantoaxial subluxation). Radiologic evidence of atlantoaxial subluxation occurs in up to 30% of patients with RA. The degree of subluxation correlates with the severity of erosive disease. When subluxation is present, careful assessment is important to identify early signs of myelopathy. Occasional patients develop high spinal cord compression leading to quadriparesis, respiratory insufficiency, and death. Surgery should be considered when myelopathy or spinal instability is present. MRI is the imaging modality of choice. *Ankylosing spondylitis* can cause neck pain and less commonly atlantoaxial subluxation; surgery may be required to prevent spinal cord compression.

Acute *herpes zoster* can presents as acute posterior occipital or neck pain prior to the outbreak of vesicles. *Neoplasms* metastatic to the cervical spine, *infections* (osteomyelitis and epidural abscess), and *metabolic bone diseases* may be the cause of neck pain, as discussed above among causes of low back pain. Neck pain may also be referred from the heart with coronary artery ischemia (cervical angina syndrome).

THORACIC OUTLET SYNDROMES

The thoracic outlet contains the first rib, the subclavian artery and vein, the brachial plexus, the clavicle, and the lung apex. Injury to these structures may result in postural or movement-induced pain around the shoulder and supraclavicular region, classified as follows.

True neurogenic thoracic outlet syndrome (TOS) is an uncommon disorder resulting from compression of the lower trunk of the brachial plexus or ventral rami of the C8 or T1 nerve roots, caused most often by an anomalous band of tissue connecting an elongate transverse process at C7 with the first rib. Pain is mild or may be absent. Signs include weakness and wasting of intrinsic muscles of the hand and diminished sensation on the palmar aspect of the fifth digit. An anteroposterior cervical spine x-ray will show an elongate C7 transverse process (an anatomic marker for the anomalous cartilaginous band), and EMG and nerve conduction studies confirm the diagnosis. Treatment consists of surgical resection of the anomalous band. The weakness and wasting of intrinsic hand muscles typically does not improve, but surgery halts the insidious progression of weakness.

Arterial TOS results from compression of the subclavian artery by a cervical rib, resulting in poststenotic dilatation of the artery and in some cases secondary thrombus formation. Blood pressure is reduced in the affected limb, and signs of emboli may be present in the hand. Neurologic signs are absent. Ultrasound can confirm the diagnosis noninvasively. Treatment is with thrombolysis or anticoagulation (with or without embolectomy) and surgical excision of the cervical rib compressing the subclavian artery.

Venous TOS is due to subclavian vein thrombosis resulting in swelling of the arm and pain. The vein may be compressed by a cervical rib or anomalous scalene muscle. Venography is the diagnostic test of choice.

Disputed TOS accounts for 95% of patients diagnosed with TOS; chronic arm and shoulder pain are prominent and of unclear cause. The lack of sensitive and specific findings on physical examination or specific markers for this condition results in diagnostic uncertainty. The role of surgery in disputed TOS is controversial. Multidisciplinary pain management is a conservative approach, although treatment is often unsuccessful.

BRACHIAL PLEXUS AND NERVES

Pain from injury to the brachial plexus or peripheral nerves of the arm can occasionally mimic referred pain of cervical spine origin including cervical radiculopathy. Neoplastic infiltration of the lower trunk of the brachial plexus may produce shoulder or supraclavicular pain radiating down the arm, numbness of the fourth and fifth fingers or medial forearm, and weakness of intrinsic hand muscles innervated by the ulnar and median nerves. Delayed radiation injury may produce similar findings, although pain is less often present and almost always less severe. A Pancoast tumor of the lung (Chap. 107) is another cause and should be considered, especially when a concurrent Horner's syndrome is present. *Suprascapular neuropathy* may produce severe shoulder pain, weakness, and wasting of the supraspinatus and infraspinatus muscles. *Acute brachial neuritis* is often confused with radiculopathy; the acute onset of severe shoulder or scapular pain is followed typically over days by weakness of the proximal arm and shoulder girdle muscles innervated by the upper brachial plexus. The onset may be preceded by an infection, vaccination, or minor surgical procedure. The long thoracic nerve may be affected resulting in a winged scapula. Brachial neuritis may also present as an isolated paralysis of the diaphragm with or without involvement of other nerves of the upper limb. Recovery may take up to 3 years.

Occasional cases of carpal tunnel syndrome produce pain and paresthesias extending into the forearm, arm, and shoulder resembling a C5 or C6 root lesion. Lesions of the radial or ulnar nerve can mimic a radiculopathy at C7 or C8, respectively. EMG and nerve conduction studies can accurately localize lesions to the nerve roots, brachial plexus, or peripheral nerves.

For further discussion of peripheral nerve disorders, see Chap. 459.

SHOULDER

Pain arising from the shoulder can on occasion mimic pain from the spine. If symptoms and signs of radiculopathy are absent, then the differential diagnosis includes mechanical shoulder pain (tendonitis, bursitis, rotator cuff tear, dislocation, adhesive capsulitis, or rotator cuff impingement under the acromion) and referred pain (subdiaphragmatic irritation, angina, Pancoast tumor). Mechanical pain is often worse at night, associated with local shoulder tenderness and aggravated by passive abduction, internal rotation, or extension of the arm. Pain from shoulder disease may radiate into the arm or hand, but focal neurologic signs (sensory, motor, or reflex changes) are absent.

TREATMENT NECK PAIN WITHOUT RADICULOPATHY

The evidence regarding treatment for neck pain is less complete than that for low back pain, but the approach is remarkably similar in many respects. As with low back pain, spontaneous improvement is the norm for acute neck pain. The usual goals of therapy are to promote a rapid return to normal function and provide symptom relief while healing proceeds.

The evidence in support of nonsurgical treatments for whiplash-associated disorders is generally of limited quality and neither supports nor refutes the common treatments used for symptom relief. Gentle mobilization of the cervical spine combined with exercise programs may be beneficial. Evidence is insufficient to recommend for or against the routine use of acupuncture, cervical traction, TENS, ultrasound, diathermy, or massage. Some patients obtain modest relief using a soft neck collar; there is little risk or cost.

For patients with neck pain unassociated with trauma, supervised exercise with or without mobilization appears to be effective. Exercises often include shoulder rolls and neck stretches. The evidence for the use of muscle relaxants, analgesics, and NSAIDs in acute and chronic neck pain is of lower quality and less consistent than for low back pain.

Low-level laser therapy directed at areas of tenderness, local acupuncture points, or a grid of predetermined points is a controversial approach to the treatment of neck pain. A 2009 meta-analysis suggested that this treatment may provide greater pain relief than sham therapy for both acute and chronic neck pain, but comparison to other conservative and less expensive treatment measures is needed.

Although some surgical studies have proposed a role for anterior diskectomy and fusion in patients with neck pain, these studies generally have not been rigorously conducted. A systematic review suggested that there was no valid clinical evidence to support either cervical fusion or cervical disk arthroplasty in patients with neck pain without radiculopathy. Similarly, there is no evidence to support radiofrequency neurotomy or cervical facet injections for neck pain without radiculopathy.

TREATMENT NECK PAIN WITH RADICULOPATHY

The natural history of neck pain with acute radiculopathy due to disk disease is favorable, and many patients will improve without specific therapy. Although there are no randomized trials of NSAIDs for neck pain, a course of NSAIDs, acetaminophen, or both, with or without muscle relaxants, is reasonable as initial therapy. Other nonsurgical treatments are commonly used, including opioid analgesics, oral glucocorticoids, cervical traction, and immobilization with a hard or soft cervical collar. However, there are no randomized trials that establish the effectiveness of these treatments. Soft cervical collars can be modestly helpful by limiting spontaneous and reflex neck movements that exacerbate pain.

As for lumbar radiculopathy, epidural glucocorticoids appear to provide short-term symptom relief in cervical radiculopathy, but rigorous studies addressing this question have not been conducted. If cervical radiculopathy is due to bony compression from cervical spondylosis with foraminal narrowing, periodic follow-up to assess for progression is indicated and consideration of surgical decompression is reasonable.

Surgical treatment can produce rapid pain relief, although it is unclear whether long-term outcomes are improved over nonsurgical therapy. Indications for cervical disk surgery include a progressive radicular motor deficit, functionally limiting pain that fails to respond to conservative management, or spinal cord compression.

Surgical treatments include anterior cervical diskectomy alone, laminectomy with diskectomy, or diskectomy with fusion. The risk of subsequent radiculopathy or myelopathy at cervical segments adjacent to a fusion is ~3% per year and 26% per decade. Although this risk is sometimes portrayed as a late complication of surgery, it may also reflect the natural history of degenerative cervical disk disease.

SECTION 2 ALTERATIONS IN BODY TEMPERATURE

23 Fever

Charles A. Dinarello, Reuven Porat

Body temperature is controlled by the hypothalamus. Neurons in both the preoptic anterior hypothalamus and the posterior hypothalamus receive two kinds of signals: one from peripheral nerves that transmit information from warmth/cold receptors in the skin and the other from the temperature of the blood bathing the region. These two types of signals are integrated by the thermoregulatory center of the hypothalamus to maintain normal temperature. In a neutral temperature environment, the human metabolic rate produces more heat than is necessary to maintain the core body temperature in the range of 36.5–37.5°C (97.7–99.5°F).

A normal body temperature is ordinarily maintained despite environmental variations because the hypothalamic thermoregulatory center balances the excess heat production derived from metabolic activity in muscle and the liver with heat dissipation from the skin and lungs. According to studies of healthy individuals 18–40 years of age, the mean oral temperature is 36.8° ± 0.4°C (98.2° ± 0.7°F), with low levels at 6 A.M. and higher levels at 4–6 P.M. The maximal normal oral temperature is 37.2°C (98.9°F) at 6 A.M. and 37.7°C (99.9°F) at 4 P.M.; these values define the 99th percentile for healthy individuals. In light of these studies, *an A.M. temperature of >37.2°C (>98.9°F) or a P.M. temperature of >37.7°C (>99.9°F) would define a fever*. The normal daily temperature variation is typically 0.5°C (0.9°F). However, in some individuals recovering from a febrile illness, this daily variation can be as great as 1.0°C. During a febrile illness, the diurnal variation is usually maintained, but at higher, febrile levels. The daily temperature variation appears to be fixed in early childhood; in contrast, elderly individuals can exhibit a reduced ability to develop fever, with only a modest fever even in severe infections.

Rectal temperatures are generally 0.4°C (0.7°F) higher than oral readings. The lower oral readings are probably attributable to mouth breathing, which is a factor in patients with respiratory infections and rapid breathing. Lower-esophageal temperatures closely reflect core temperature. Tympanic membrane thermometers measure radiant heat from the tympanic membrane and nearby ear canal and display that absolute value (*unadjusted mode*) or a value automatically calculated from the absolute reading on the basis of nomograms relating the radiant temperature measured to actual core temperatures obtained in clinical studies (*adjusted mode*). These measurements, although convenient, may be more variable than directly determined oral or rectal values. Studies in adults show that readings are lower with unadjusted-mode than with adjusted-mode tympanic membrane thermometers and that unadjusted-mode tympanic membrane values are 0.8°C (1.6°F) lower than rectal temperatures.

In women who menstruate, the A.M. temperature is generally lower in the 2 weeks before ovulation; it then rises by ~0.6°C (1°F) with ovulation and remains at that level until menses occur. Body temperature can be elevated in the postprandial state. Pregnancy and endocrinologic dysfunction also affect body temperature.

FEVER VERSUS HYPERTHERMIA

Fever is an elevation of body temperature that exceeds the normal daily variation and occurs *in conjunction with an increase in the hypothalamic set point* (e.g., from 37°C to 39°C). This shift of the set point from "normothermic" to febrile levels very much resembles the resetting of the home thermostat to a higher level in order to raise the ambient temperature in a room. Once the hypothalamic set point is raised, neurons in the vasomotor center are activated and vasoconstriction commences. The individual first notices vasoconstriction in the hands and feet. Shunting of blood away from the periphery to the internal organs essentially decreases heat loss from the skin, and the person feels cold. For most fevers, body temperature increases by 1–2°C. Shivering, which increases heat production from the muscles, may begin at this time; however, shivering is not required if heat conservation mechanisms raise blood temperature sufficiently. Nonshivering heat production from the liver also contributes to increasing core temperature. Behavioral adjustments (e.g., putting on more clothing or bedding) help raise body temperature by decreasing heat loss.

The processes of heat conservation (vasoconstriction) and heat production (shivering and increased nonshivering thermogenesis) continue until the temperature of the blood bathing the hypothalamic neurons matches the new thermostat setting. Once that point is reached, the hypothalamus maintains the temperature at the febrile level by the same mechanisms of heat balance that function in the afebrile state. When the hypothalamic set point is again reset downward (in response to either a reduction in the concentration of pyrogens or the use of antipyretics), the processes of heat loss through vasodilation and sweating are initiated. Loss of heat by sweating and vasodilation continues until the blood temperature at the hypothalamic level matches the lower setting. Behavioral changes (e.g., removal of clothing) facilitate heat loss.

A fever of >41.5°C (>106.7°F) is called *hyperpyrexia*. This extraordinarily high fever can develop in patients with severe infections but most commonly occurs in patients with central nervous system (CNS) hemorrhages. In the preantibiotic era, fever due to a variety of infectious diseases rarely exceeded 106°F, and there has been speculation that this natural "thermal ceiling" is mediated by neuropeptides functioning as central antipyretics.

In rare cases, the hypothalamic set point is elevated as a result of local trauma, hemorrhage, tumor, or intrinsic hypothalamic malfunction. The term *hypothalamic fever* is sometimes used to describe elevated temperature caused by abnormal hypothalamic function. However, most patients with hypothalamic damage have *sub*normal, not *supra*normal, body temperatures.

Although most patients with elevated body temperature have fever, there are circumstances in which elevated temperature represents not fever but *hyperthermia* (*heat stroke*). Hyperthermia is characterized by an uncontrolled increase in body temperature that exceeds the body's ability to lose heat. The setting of the hypothalamic thermoregulatory center is unchanged. In contrast to fever in infections, hyperthermia does not involve pyrogenic molecules. Exogenous heat exposure and endogenous heat production are two mechanisms by which hyperthermia can result in dangerously high internal temperatures. Excessive heat production can easily cause hyperthermia despite physiologic and behavioral control of body temperature. For example, work or exercise in hot environments can produce heat faster than peripheral mechanisms can lose it. **For a detailed discussion of hyperthermia, see Chap. 479e.**

It is important to distinguish between fever and hyperthermia since hyperthermia can be rapidly fatal and characteristically does not respond to antipyretics. In an emergency situation, however, making this distinction can be difficult. For example, in systemic sepsis, fever (hyperpyrexia) can be rapid in onset, and temperatures can exceed 40.5°C (104.9°F). Hyperthermia is often diagnosed on the basis of the events immediately preceding the elevation of core temperature—e.g., heat exposure or treatment with drugs that interfere with thermoregulation. In patients with heat stroke syndromes and in those taking drugs that block sweating, the skin is hot but dry, whereas in fever the skin can be cold as a consequence of vasoconstriction. Antipyretics do not reduce the elevated temperature in hyperthermia, whereas in fever—and even in hyperpyrexia—adequate doses of either aspirin or acetaminophen usually result in some decrease in body temperature.

PATHOGENESIS OF FEVER

PYROGENS

The term *pyrogen* (Greek *pyro*, "fire") is used to describe any substance that causes fever. *Exogenous* pyrogens are derived from outside the patient; most are microbial products, microbial toxins, or whole microorganisms (including viruses). The classic example of an exogenous pyrogen is the lipopolysaccharide (endotoxin) produced by all gram-negative bacteria. Pyrogenic products of gram-positive organisms include the enterotoxins of *Staphylococcus aureus* and the groups A and B streptococcal toxins, also called *superantigens*. One staphylococcal toxin of clinical importance is that associated with isolates of *S. aureus* from patients with toxic shock syndrome. These products of staphylococci and streptococci cause fever in experimental animals when injected intravenously at concentrations of 1–10 μg/kg. Endotoxin is a highly pyrogenic molecule in humans: when injected intravenously into volunteers, a dose of 2–3 ng/kg produces fever, leukocytosis, acute-phase proteins, and generalized symptoms of malaise.

PYROGENIC CYTOKINES

Cytokines are small proteins (molecular mass, 10,000–20,000 Da) that regulate immune, inflammatory, and hematopoietic processes. For example, the elevated leukocytosis seen in several infections with an absolute neutrophilia is attributable to the cytokines interleukin (IL) 1 and IL-6. Some cytokines also cause fever; formerly referred to as *endogenous pyrogens*, they are now called *pyrogenic cytokines*. The pyrogenic cytokines include IL-1, IL-6, tumor necrosis factor (TNF), and ciliary neurotropic factor, a member of the IL-6 family. Interferons (IFNs), particularly IFN-α, also are pyrogenic cytokines; fever is a prominent side effect of IFN-α used in the treatment of hepatitis. Each pyrogenic cytokine is encoded by a separate gene, and each has been shown to cause fever in laboratory animals and in humans. When injected into humans at low doses (10–100 ng/kg), IL-1 and TNF produce fever; in contrast, for IL-6, a dose of 1–10 μg/kg is required for fever production.

A wide spectrum of bacterial and fungal products induce the synthesis and release of pyrogenic cytokines. However, fever can be a manifestation of disease in the absence of microbial infection. For example, inflammatory processes, trauma, tissue necrosis, and antigen-antibody complexes induce the production of IL-1, TNF, and/or IL-6; individually or in combination, these cytokines trigger the hypothalamus to raise the set point to febrile levels.

ELEVATION OF THE HYPOTHALAMIC SET POINT BY CYTOKINES

During fever, levels of prostaglandin E_2 (PGE_2) are elevated in hypothalamic tissue and the third cerebral ventricle. The concentrations of PGE_2 are highest near the circumventricular vascular organs (organum vasculosum of lamina terminalis)—networks of enlarged capillaries surrounding the hypothalamic regulatory centers. Destruction of these organs reduces the ability of pyrogens to produce fever. Most studies in animals have failed to show, however, that pyrogenic cytokines pass from the circulation into the brain itself. Thus, it appears that both exogenous pyrogens and pyrogenic cytokines interact with the endothelium of these capillaries and that this interaction is the first step in initiating fever—i.e., in raising the set point to febrile levels.

The key events in the production of fever are illustrated in Fig. 23-1. Myeloid and endothelial cells are the primary cell types that produce pyrogenic cytokines. Pyrogenic cytokines such as IL-1, IL-6, and TNF are released from these cells and enter the systemic circulation. Although these circulating cytokines lead to fever by inducing the synthesis of PGE_2, they also induce PGE_2 in peripheral tissues. The increase in PGE_2 in the periphery accounts for the nonspecific myalgias and arthralgias that often accompany fever. It is thought that some systemic PGE_2 escapes destruction by the lung and gains access to the hypothalamus via the internal carotid. However, it is the elevation of PGE_2 in the brain that starts the process of raising the hypothalamic set point for core temperature.

There are four receptors for PGE_2, and each signals the cell in different ways. Of the four receptors, the third (EP-3) is essential for fever: when the gene for this receptor is deleted in mice, no fever follows the injection of IL-1 or endotoxin. Deletion of the other PGE_2 receptor genes leaves the fever mechanism intact. Although PGE_2 is essential for fever, it is not a neurotransmitter. Rather, the release of PGE_2 from the brain side of the hypothalamic endothelium triggers the PGE_2 receptor on glial cells, and this stimulation results in the rapid release of cyclic adenosine 5′-monophosphate (cAMP), which is a neurotransmitter. As shown in Fig. 23-1, the release of cAMP from glial cells activates neuronal endings from the thermoregulatory center that extend into the area. The elevation of cAMP is thought to account for changes in the hypothalamic set point either directly or indirectly (by inducing the release of neurotransmitters). Distinct receptors for microbial products are located on the hypothalamic endothelium. These receptors are called *Toll-like receptors* and are similar in many ways to IL-1 receptors. IL-1 receptors and Toll-like receptors share the same signal-transducing mechanism. Thus, the direct activation of Toll-like receptors or IL-1 receptors results in PGE_2 production and fever.

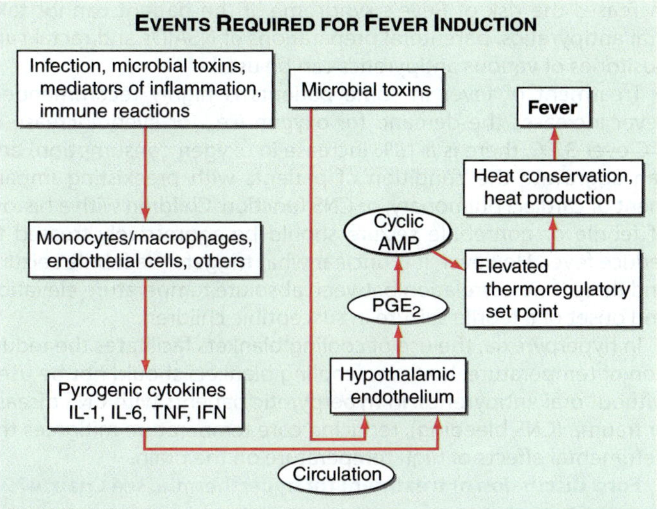

FIGURE 23-1 Chronology of events required for the induction of fever. AMP, adenosine 5′-monophosphate; IFN, interferon; IL, interleukin; PGE_2, prostaglandin E_2; TNF, tumor necrosis factor.

PRODUCTION OF CYTOKINES IN THE CNS

Cytokines produced in the brain may account for the hyperpyrexia of CNS hemorrhage, trauma, or infection. Viral infections of the CNS induce microglial and possibly neuronal production of IL-1, TNF, and IL-6. In experimental animals, the concentration of a cytokine required to cause fever is several orders of magnitude lower with direct injection into the brain substance or brain ventricles than with systemic injection. Therefore, cytokines produced in the CNS can raise the hypothalamic set point, bypassing the circumventricular organs. CNS cytokines likely account for the hyperpyrexia of CNS hemorrhage, trauma, or infection.

APPROACH TO THE PATIENT: Fever

PHYSICAL EXAMINATION

The chronology of events preceding fever, including exposure to other infected individuals or to vectors of disease, should be ascertained. Electronic devices for measuring oral, tympanic membrane, or rectal temperatures are reliable, but the same site should be used consistently to monitor a febrile disease. Moreover, physicians should be aware that newborns, elderly patients, patients with chronic liver or renal failure, and patients taking glucocorticoids or being treated with an anticytokine may have active infection in the absence of fever due to a blunted febrile response.

LABORATORY TESTS

The workup should include a complete blood count; a differential count should be performed manually or with an instrument sensitive to the identification of juvenile or band forms, toxic granulations, and Döhle bodies, which are suggestive of bacterial infection. Neutropenia may be present with some viral infections.

Measurement of circulating cytokines in patients with fever is not helpful since levels of cytokines such as IL-1 and TNF in the circulation often are below the detection limit of the assay or do not coincide with fever. However, in patients with low-grade fevers or possible disease, the most valuable measurements are the C-reactive protein level and the erythrocyte sedimentation rate. These markers of inflammatory processes are particularly helpful in detecting occult disease. Measurement of circulating IL-6 is useful because IL-6 induces C-reactive protein. Acute-phase reactants are discussed in Chap. 325.

FEVER IN PATIENTS RECEIVING ANTICYTOKINE THERAPY

Patients receiving long-term treatment with anticytokine-based regimens are at a disadvantage because of lowered host defense against infection. Even when the results of tests for latent *Mycobacterium tuberculosis* infection are negative, active tuberculosis can develop in patients receiving anti-TNF therapy. With the increasing use of anticytokines to reduce the activity of IL-1, IL-6, IL-12, or TNF in patients with Crohn's disease, rheumatoid arthritis, or psoriasis, the possibility that these therapies blunt the febrile response must be kept in mind.

The blocking of cytokine activity has the distinct clinical drawback of lowering the level of host defenses against both routine bacterial and opportunistic infections. The opportunistic infections reported in patients treated with agents that neutralize TNF-α are similar to those reported in the HIV-1-infected population (e.g., a new infection with or reactivation of *Mycobacterium tuberculosis*, with dissemination).

In nearly all reported cases of infection associated with anticytokine therapy, fever is among the presenting signs. However, the extent to which the febrile response is blunted in these patients remains unknown. A similar situation is seen in patients receiving high-dose glucocorticoid therapy or anti-inflammatory agents such as ibuprofen. Therefore, low-grade fever is of considerable concern in patients receiving anticytokine therapies. The physician should conduct an early and rigorous diagnostic evaluation in these patients.

TREATMENT FEVER

THE DECISION TO TREAT FEVER

Most fevers are associated with self-limited infections, such as common viral diseases. The use of antipyretics is not contraindicated in these infections: no significant clinical evidence indicates either that antipyretics delay the resolution of viral or bacterial infections or that fever facilitates recovery from infection or acts as an adjuvant to the immune system. In short, treatment of fever and its symptoms with routine antipyretics does no harm and does not slow the resolution of common viral and bacterial infections.

However, in bacterial infections, the withholding of antipyretic therapy can be helpful in evaluating the effectiveness of a particular antibiotic, especially in the absence of positive cultures of the infecting organism, and the routine use of antipyretics can mask an inadequately treated bacterial infection. Withholding antipyretics in some cases may facilitate the diagnosis of an unusual febrile disease. Temperature-pulse dissociation (*relative bradycardia*) occurs in typhoid fever, brucellosis, leptospirosis, some drug-induced fevers, and factitious fever. As stated earlier, in newborns, elderly patients, patients with chronic liver or kidney failure, and patients taking glucocorticoids, fever may not be present despite infection. Hypothermia can develop in patients with septic shock.

Some infections have characteristic patterns in which febrile episodes are separated by intervals of normal temperature. For example, *Plasmodium vivax* causes fever every third day, whereas fever occurs every fourth day with *P. malariae*. Another relapsing fever is related to *Borrelia* infection, with days of fever followed by a several-day afebrile period and then a relapse into additional days of fever. In the Pel-Ebstein pattern, fever lasting 3–10 days is followed by afebrile periods of 3–10 days; this pattern can be classic for Hodgkin's disease and other lymphomas. In cyclic neutropenia, fevers occur every 21 days and accompany the neutropenia. There is no periodicity of fever in patients with familial Mediterranean fever. However, these patterns have limited or no diagnostic value compared with specific and rapid laboratory tests.

ANTICYTOKINE THERAPY TO REDUCE FEVER IN AUTOIMMUNE AND AUTOINFLAMMATORY DISEASES

Recurrent fever is documented at some point in most autoimmune diseases and nearly all autoinflammatory diseases. Although fever can be a manifestation of autoimmune diseases, recurrent fevers are characteristic of autoinflammatory diseases (Table 23-1), including adult and juvenile Still's disease, familial Mediterranean fever, and hyper-IgD syndrome. In addition to recurrent fevers, neutrophilia and serosal inflammation characterize autoinflammatory diseases. The fevers associated with these illnesses are dramatically reduced by blocking of IL-1β activity. Anticytokines therefore reduce fever in autoimmune and autoinflammatory diseases. Although fevers in autoinflammatory diseases are mediated by IL-1β, patients also respond to antipyretics.

TABLE 23-1 AUTOINFLAMMATORY DISEASES IN WHICH FEVER IS CHARACTERISTIC

Adult and juvenile Still's disease
Cryopyrin-associated periodic syndromes (CAPS)
Familial Mediterranean fever
Hyper-IgD syndrome
Behçet's syndrome
Macrophage activation syndrome
Normocomplementemic urticarial vasculitis
Antisynthetase myositis
PAPA[a] syndrome
Blau syndrome
Gouty arthritis

[a]Pyogenic arthritis, pyoderma gangrenosum, and acne.

MECHANISMS OF ANTIPYRETIC AGENTS

The reduction of fever by lowering of the elevated hypothalamic set point is a direct function of reduction of the PGE_2 level in the thermoregulatory center. The synthesis of PGE_2 depends on the constitutively expressed enzyme cyclooxygenase. The substrate for cyclooxygenase is arachidonic acid released from the cell membrane, and this release is the rate-limiting step in the synthesis of PGE_2. Therefore, inhibitors of cyclooxygenase are potent antipyretics. The antipyretic potency of various drugs is directly correlated with the inhibition of brain cyclooxygenase. Acetaminophen is a poor cyclooxygenase inhibitor in peripheral tissue and lacks noteworthy anti-inflammatory activity; in the brain, however, acetaminophen is oxidized by the p450 cytochrome system, and the oxidized form inhibits cyclooxygenase activity. Moreover, in the brain, the inhibition of another enzyme, COX-3, by acetaminophen may account for the antipyretic effect of this agent. However, COX-3 is not found outside the CNS.

Oral aspirin and acetaminophen are equally effective in reducing fever in humans. Nonsteroidal anti-inflammatory drugs (NSAIDs) such as ibuprofen and specific inhibitors of COX-2 also are excellent antipyretics. Chronic, high-dose therapy with antipyretics such as aspirin or any NSAID does not reduce normal core body temperature. Thus, PGE_2 appears to play no role in normal thermoregulation.

As effective antipyretics, glucocorticoids act at two levels. First, similar to the cyclooxygenase inhibitors, glucocorticoids reduce PGE_2 synthesis by inhibiting the activity of phospholipase A_2, which is needed to release arachidonic acid from the cell membrane. Second, glucocorticoids block the transcription of the mRNA for the pyrogenic cytokines. Limited experimental evidence indicates that ibuprofen and COX-2 inhibitors reduce IL-1-induced IL-6 production and may contribute to the antipyretic activity of NSAIDs.

REGIMENS FOR THE TREATMENT OF FEVER

The objectives in treating fever are first to reduce the elevated hypothalamic set point and second to facilitate heat loss. Reducing fever with antipyretics also reduces systemic symptoms of headache, myalgias, and arthralgias.

Oral aspirin and NSAIDs effectively reduce fever but can adversely affect platelets and the gastrointestinal tract. Therefore, acetaminophen is preferred as an antipyretic. In children, acetaminophen or oral ibuprofen must be used because aspirin increases the risk of Reye's syndrome. If the patient cannot take oral antipyretics, parenteral preparations of NSAIDs and rectal suppositories of various antipyretics can be used.

Treatment of fever in some patients is highly recommended. Fever increases the demand for oxygen (i.e., for every increase of 1°C over 37°C, there is a 13% increase in oxygen consumption) and can aggravate the condition of patients with preexisting impairment of cardiac, pulmonary, or CNS function. Children with a history of febrile or nonfebrile seizure should be aggressively treated to reduce fever. However, it is unclear what triggers the febrile seizure, and there is no correlation between absolute temperature elevation and onset of a febrile seizure in susceptible children.

In hyperpyrexia, the use of cooling blankets facilitates the reduction of temperature; however, cooling blankets should not be used without oral antipyretics. In hyperpyretic patients with CNS disease or trauma (CNS bleeding), reducing core temperature mitigates the detrimental effects of high temperature on the brain.

For a discussion of treatment for hyperthermia, see Chap. 479e.

24 Fever and Rash

Elaine T. Kaye, Kenneth M. Kaye

The acutely ill patient with fever and rash may present a diagnostic challenge for physicians. However, the distinctive appearance of an eruption in concert with a clinical syndrome can facilitate a prompt diagnosis and the institution of life-saving therapy or critical infection-control interventions. **Representative images of many of the rashes discussed in this chapter are included in Chap. 25e.**

APPROACH TO THE PATIENT: Fever and Rash

A thorough history of patients with fever and rash includes the following relevant information: immune status, medications taken within the previous month, specific travel history, immunization status, exposure to domestic pets and other animals, history of animal (including arthropod) bites, recent dietary exposures, existence of cardiac abnormalities, presence of prosthetic material, recent exposure to ill individuals, and exposure to sexually transmitted diseases. The history should also include the site of onset of the rash and its direction and rate of spread.

A thorough physical examination entails close attention to the rash, with an assessment and precise definition of its salient features. First, it is critical to determine what *type* of lesions make up the eruption. *Macules* are flat lesions defined by an area of changed color (i.e., a blanchable erythema). *Papules* are raised, solid lesions <5 mm in diameter; *plaques* are lesions >5 mm in diameter with a flat, plateau-like surface; and *nodules* are lesions >5 mm in diameter with a more rounded configuration. *Wheals* (urticaria, hives) are papules or plaques that are pale pink and may appear annular (ringlike) as they enlarge; classic (nonvasculitic) wheals are transient, lasting only 24 h in any defined area. *Vesicles* (<5 mm) and *bullae* (>5 mm) are circumscribed, elevated lesions containing fluid. *Pustules* are raised lesions containing purulent exudate; vesicular processes such as varicella or herpes simplex may evolve to pustules. *Nonpalpable purpura* is a flat lesion that is due to bleeding into the skin. If <3 mm in diameter, the purpuric lesions are termed *petechiae*; if >3 mm, they are termed *ecchymoses*. *Palpable purpura* is a raised lesion that is due to inflammation of the vessel wall (vasculitis) with subsequent hemorrhage. An *ulcer* is a defect in the skin extending at least into the upper layer of the dermis, and an *eschar* (tâche noire) is a necrotic lesion covered with a black crust.

Other pertinent features of rashes include their *configuration* (i.e., annular or target), the *arrangement* of their lesions, and their *distribution* (i.e., central or peripheral).

For further discussion, see Chaps. 70, 72, and 147.

CLASSIFICATION OF RASH

This chapter reviews rashes that reflect systemic disease, but it does not include localized skin eruptions (i.e., cellulitis, impetigo) that may also be associated with fever (Chap. 156). The chapter is not intended to be all-inclusive, but it covers the most important and most common diseases associated with fever and rash. Rashes are classified herein on the basis of lesion morphology and distribution. For practical purposes, this classification system is based on the most typical disease presentations. However, morphology may vary as rashes evolve, and the presentation of diseases with rashes is subject to many variations (Chap. 72). For instance, the classic petechial rash of Rocky Mountain spotted fever (Chap. 211) may initially consist of blanchable erythematous macules distributed peripherally; at times, however, the rash associated with this disease may not be predominantly acral, or no rash may develop at all.

Diseases with fever and rash may be classified by type of eruption: centrally distributed maculopapular, peripheral, confluent desquamative erythematous, vesiculobullous, urticaria-like, nodular, purpuric, ulcerated, or with eschars. Diseases are listed by these categories in Table 24-1, and many are highlighted in the text. However, for a more detailed discussion of each disease associated with a rash, the reader is referred to the chapter dealing with that specific disease. **(Reference chapters are cited in the text and listed in Table 24-1.)**

CENTRALLY DISTRIBUTED MACULOPAPULAR ERUPTIONS

Centrally distributed rashes, in which lesions are primarily truncal, are the most common type of eruption. The rash of *rubeola* (measles) starts at the hairline 2–3 days into the illness and moves down the body, typically sparing the palms and soles (Chap. 229). It begins as discrete erythematous lesions, which become confluent as the rash spreads. Koplik's spots (1- to 2-mm white or bluish lesions with an erythematous halo on the buccal mucosa) are pathognomonic for measles and are generally seen during the first 2 days of symptoms. They should not be confused with Fordyce's spots (ectopic sebaceous glands), which have no erythematous halos and are found in the mouth of healthy individuals. Koplik's spots may briefly overlap with the measles exanthem.

Rubella (German measles) also spreads from the hairline downward; unlike that of measles, however, the rash of rubella tends to clear from originally affected areas as it migrates, and it may be pruritic (Chap. 230e). Forchheimer spots (palatal petechiae) may develop but are nonspecific because they also develop in *infectious mononucleosis* (Chap. 218) and *scarlet fever* (Chap. 173). Postauricular and suboccipital adenopathy and arthritis are common among adults with rubella. Exposure of pregnant women to ill individuals should be avoided, as rubella causes severe congenital abnormalities. Numerous strains of *enteroviruses* (Chap. 228), primarily echoviruses and coxsackieviruses, cause nonspecific syndromes of fever and eruptions that may mimic rubella or measles. Patients with *infectious mononucleosis* caused by Epstein-Barr virus (Chap. 218) or with *primary HIV infection* (Chap. 226) may exhibit pharyngitis, lymphadenopathy, and a nonspecific maculopapular exanthem.

The rash of *erythema infectiosum* (fifth disease), which is caused by human parvovirus B19, primarily affects children 3–12 years old; it develops after fever has resolved as a bright blanchable erythema on the cheeks ("slapped cheeks") with perioral pallor (Chap. 221). A more diffuse rash (often pruritic) appears the next day on the trunk and extremities and then rapidly develops into a lacy reticular eruption that may wax and wane (especially with temperature change) over 3 weeks. Adults with fifth disease often have arthritis, and fetal hydrops can develop in association with this condition in pregnant women.

Exanthem subitum (roseola) is caused by human herpesvirus 6 and is most common among children <3 years of age (Chap. 219). As in erythema infectiosum, the rash usually appears after fever has subsided. It consists of 2- to 3-mm rose-pink macules and papules that coalesce only rarely, occur initially on the trunk and sometimes on the extremities (sparing the face), and fade within 2 days.

Although drug reactions have many manifestations, including urticaria, exanthematous *drug-induced eruptions* (Chap. 74) are most common and are often difficult to distinguish from viral exanthems. Eruptions elicited by drugs are usually more intensely erythematous and pruritic than viral exanthems, but this distinction is not reliable. A history of new medications and an absence of prostration may help to distinguish a drug-related rash from an eruption of another etiology. Rashes may persist for up to two weeks after administration of the offending agent is discontinued. Certain populations are more prone than others to drug rashes. Of HIV-infected patients, 50–60% develop a rash in response to sulfa drugs; 90% of patients with mononucleosis due to Epstein-Barr virus develop a rash when given ampicillin.

Rickettsial illnesses (Chap. 211) should be considered in the evaluation of individuals with centrally distributed maculopapular eruptions. The usual setting for *epidemic typhus* is a site of war or natural disaster in which people are exposed to body lice. *Endemic typhus* or *leptospirosis* (the latter caused by a spirochete) (Chap. 208) may be

TABLE 24-1 DISEASES ASSOCIATED WITH FEVER AND RASH

Disease	Etiology	Description	Group Affected/ Epidemiologic Factors	Clinical Syndrome	Chapter
Centrally Distributed Maculopapular Eruptions					
Acute meningococcemia[a]	—	—	—	—	180
Drug reaction with eosinophilia and systemic symptoms (DRESS) (also termed drug-induced hypersensitivity syndrome; DIHS)[b]	—	—	—	—	74
Rubeola (measles, first disease)	Paramyxovirus	Discrete lesions that become confluent as rash spreads from hairline downward, usually sparing palms and soles; lasts ≥3 days; Koplik's spots	Nonimmune individuals	Cough, conjunctivitis, coryza, severe prostration	229
Rubella (German measles, third disease)	Togavirus	Spreads from hairline downward, clearing as it spreads; Forschheimer spots	Nonimmune individuals	Adenopathy, arthritis	230e
Erythema infectiosum (fifth disease)	Human parvovirus B19	Bright-red "slapped-cheeks" appearance followed by lacy reticular rash that waxes and wanes over 3 weeks; rarely, papular-purpuric "gloves-and-socks" syndrome on hands and feet	Most common among children 3–12 years old; occurs in winter and spring	Mild fever; arthritis in adults; rash following resolution of fever	221
Exanthem subitum (roseola, sixth disease)	Human herpesvirus 6	Diffuse maculopapular eruption over trunk and neck; resolves within 2 days	Usually affects children <3 years old	Rash following resolution of fever; similar to Boston exanthem (echovirus 16); febrile seizures may occur	219
Primary HIV infection	HIV	Nonspecific diffuse macules and papules; less commonly, urticarial or vesicular oral or genital ulcers	Individuals recently infected with HIV	Pharyngitis, adenopathy, arthralgias	226
Infectious mononucleosis	Epstein-Barr virus	Diffuse maculopapular eruption (5% of cases; 90% if ampicillin is given); urticaria, petechiae in some cases; periorbital edema (50%); palatal petechiae (25%)	Adolescents, young adults	Hepatosplenomegaly, pharyngitis, cervical lymphadenopathy, atypical lymphocytosis, heterophile antibody	218
Other viral exanthems	Echoviruses 2, 4, 9, 11, 16, 19, 25; coxsackieviruses A9, B1, B5; etc.	Wide range of skin findings that may mimic rubella or measles	Affect children more commonly than adults	Nonspecific viral syndromes	228
Exanthematous drug-induced eruption	Drugs (antibiotics, anticonvulsants, diuretics, etc.)	Intensely pruritic, bright-red macules and papules, symmetric on trunk and extremities; may become confluent	Occurs 2–3 days after exposure in previously sensitized individuals; otherwise, after 2–3 weeks (but can occur anytime, even shortly after drug is discontinued)	Variable findings: fever and eosinophilia	74
Epidemic typhus	*Rickettsia prowazekii*	Maculopapular eruption appearing in axillae, spreading to trunk and later to extremities; usually spares face, palms, soles; evolves from blanchable macules to confluent eruption with petechiae; rash evanescent in recrudescent typhus (Brill-Zinsser disease)	Exposure to body lice; occurrence of recrudescent typhus as relapse after 30–50 years	Headache, myalgias; mortality rates 10–40% if untreated; milder clinical presentation in recrudescent form	211
Endemic (murine) typhus	*Rickettsia typhi*	Maculopapular eruption, usually sparing palms, soles	Exposure to rat or cat fleas	Headache, myalgias	211
Scrub typhus	*Orientia tsutsugamushi*	Diffuse macular rash starting on trunk; eschar at site of mite bite	Endemic in South Pacific, Australia, Asia; transmitted by mites	Headache, myalgias, regional adenopathy; mortality rates up to 30% if untreated	211
Rickettsial spotted fevers	*Rickettsia conorii* (boutonneuse fever), *Rickettsia australis* (North Queensland tick typhus), *Rickettsia sibirica* (Siberian tick typhus), and others	Eschar common at bite site; maculopapular (rarely, vesicular and petechial) eruption on proximal extremities, spreading to trunk and face	Exposure to ticks; *R. conorii* in Mediterranean region, India, Africa; *R. australis* in Australia; *R. sibirica* in Siberia, Mongolia	Headache, myalgias, regional adenopathy	211

(Continued)

TABLE 24-1 DISEASES ASSOCIATED WITH FEVER AND RASH (*CONTINUED*)

Disease	Etiology	Description	Group Affected/ Epidemiologic Factors	Clinical Syndrome	Chapter
Centrally Distributed Maculopapular Eruptions (*Continued*)					
Human monocytotropic ehrlichiosis[c]	*Ehrlichia chaffeensis*	Maculopapular eruption (40% of cases), involves trunk and extremities; may be petechial	Tick-borne; most common in U.S. Southeast, southern Midwest, and mid-Atlantic regions	Headache, myalgias, leukopenia	211
Leptospirosis	*Leptospira interrogans*	Maculopapular eruption; conjunctivitis; scleral hemorrhage in some cases	Exposure to water contaminated with animal urine	Myalgias; aseptic meningitis; *fulminant form*: icterohemorrhagic fever (Weil's disease)	208
Lyme disease	*Borrelia burgdorferi* (sole cause in U.S.), *Borrelia afzelii, Borrelia garinii*	Papule expanding to erythematous annular lesion with central clearing (erythema migrans; average diameter, 15 cm), sometimes with concentric rings, sometimes with indurated or vesicular center; multiple secondary erythema migrans lesions in some cases	Bite of *Ixodes* tick vector	Headache, myalgias, chills, photophobia occurring acutely; CNS disease, myocardial disease, arthritis weeks to months later in some cases	210
Southern tick-associated rash illness (STARI, Master's disease)	Unknown (possibly *Borrelia lonestari* or other *Borrelia* spirochetes)	Similar to erythema migrans of Lyme disease with several differences, including: multiple secondary lesions less likely; lesions tending to be smaller (average diameter, ~8 cm); central clearing more likely	Bite of tick vector *Amblyomma americanum* (Lone Star tick); often found in regions where Lyme disease is uncommon, including southern United States	Compared with Lyme disease: fewer constitutional symptoms, tick bite more likely to be recalled; other Lyme disease sequelae lacking	210
Typhoid fever	*Salmonella typhi*	Transient, blanchable erythematous macules and papules, 2–4 mm, usually on trunk (rose spots)	Ingestion of contaminated food or water (rare in U.S.)	Variable abdominal pain and diarrhea; headache, myalgias, hepatosplenomegaly	190
Dengue fever[d]	Dengue virus (4 serotypes; flaviviruses)	Rash in 50% of cases; initially diffuse flushing; midway through illness, onset of maculopapular rash, which begins on trunk and spreads centrifugally to extremities and face; pruritus, hyperesthesia in some cases; after defervescence, petechiae on extremities in some cases	Occurs in tropics and subtropics; transmitted by mosquito	Headache, musculoskeletal pain ("breakbone fever"); leukopenia; occasionally biphasic ("saddleback") fever	233
Rat-bite fever (sodoku)	*Spirillum minus*	Eschar at bite site; then blotchy violaceous or red-brown rash involving trunk and extremities	Rat bite; primarily found in Asia; rare in U.S.	Regional adenopathy; recurrent fevers if untreated	167e
Relapsing fever	*Borrelia* species	Central rash at end of febrile episode; petechiae in some cases	Exposure to ticks or body lice	Recurrent fever, headache, myalgias, hepatosplenomegaly	209
Erythema marginatum (rheumatic fever)	Group A *Streptococcus*	Erythematous annular papules and plaques occurring as polycyclic lesions in waves over trunk, proximal extremities; evolving and resolving within hours	Patients with rheumatic fever	Pharyngitis preceding polyarthritis, carditis, subcutaneous nodules, chorea	381
Systemic lupus erythematosus (SLE)	Autoimmune disease	Macular and papular erythema, often in sun-exposed areas; discoid lupus lesions (local atrophy, scale, pigmentary changes); periungual telangiectasis; malar rash; vasculitis sometimes causing urticaria, palpable purpura; oral erosions in some cases	Most common in young to middle-aged women; flares precipitated by sun exposure	Arthritis; cardiac, pulmonary, renal, hematologic, and vasculitic disease	378
Still's disease	Autoimmune disease	Transient 2- to 5-mm erythematous papules appearing at height of fever on trunk, proximal extremities; lesions evanescent	Children and young adults	High spiking fever, polyarthritis, splenomegaly; erythrocyte sedimentation rate, >100 mm/h	398
African trypanosomiasis	*Trypanosoma brucei rhodesiense/ gambiense*	Blotchy or annular erythematous macular and papular rash (trypanid), primarily on trunk; pruritus; chancre at site of tsetse fly bite may precede rash by several weeks	Tsetse fly bite in eastern (*T. brucei rhodesiense*) or western (*T. brucei gambiense*) Africa	Hemolymphatic disease followed by meningoencephalitis; Winterbottom's sign (posterior cervical lymphadenopathy) (*T. brucei gambiense*)	252
Arcanobacterial pharyngitis	*Arcanobacterium (Corynebacterium) haemolyticum*	Diffuse, erythematous, maculopapular eruption involving trunk and proximal extremities; may desquamate	Children and young adults	Exudative pharyngitis, lymphadenopathy	175
West Nile fever	West Nile virus	Maculopapular eruption involving the trunk, extremities, and head or neck; rash in 20–50% of cases	Mosquito bite; rarely, blood transfusion or transplanted organ	Headache, weakness, malaise, myalgias, neuroinvasive disease (encephalitis, meningitis, flaccid paralysis)	233

(*Continued*)

TABLE 24-1 DISEASES ASSOCIATED WITH FEVER AND RASH (*CONTINUED*)

Disease	Etiology	Description	Group Affected/ Epidemiologic Factors	Clinical Syndrome	Chapter
Peripheral Eruptions					
Chronic meningococcemia, disseminated gonococcal infection,[a] human parvovirus B19 infection[e]	—	—	—	—	180, 181, 221
Rocky Mountain spotted fever	*Rickettsia rickettsii*	Rash beginning on wrists and ankles and spreading centripetally; appears on palms and soles later in disease; lesion evolution from blanchable macules to petechiae	Tick vector; widespread but more common in southeastern and south-west-central U.S.	Headache, myalgias, abdominal pain; mortality rates up to 40% if untreated	211
Secondary syphilis	*Treponema pallidum*	Coincident primary chancre in 10% of cases; copper-colored, scaly papular eruption, diffuse but prominent on palms and soles; rash never vesicular in adults; condyloma latum, mucous patches, and alopecia in some cases	Sexually transmitted	Fever, constitutional symptoms	206
Chikungunya fever	Chikungunya virus	Maculopapular eruption; prominent on upper extremities and face, but can also occur on trunk and lower extremities	*Aedes aegypti* and *A. albopictus* mosquito bites; primarily in Africa and Indian Ocean region	Severe polyarticular, migratory arthralgias, especially involving small joints (e.g., hands, wrists, ankles)	233
Hand-foot-and-mouth disease	Coxsackievirus A16 most common cause	Tender vesicles, erosions in mouth; 0.25-cm papules on hands and feet with rim of erythema evolving into tender vesicles	Summer and fall; primarily children <10 years old; multiple family members	Transient fever	228
Erythema multiforme (EM)	Infection, drugs, idiopathic causes	Target lesions (central erythema surrounded by area of clearing and another rim of erythema) up to 2 cm; symmetric on knees, elbows, palms, soles; spreads centripetally; papular, sometimes vesicular; when extensive and involving mucous membranes, termed *EM major*	Herpes simplex virus or *Mycoplasma pneumoniae* infection; drug intake (i.e., sulfa, phenytoin, penicillin)	50% of patients <20 years old; fever more common in most severe form, EM major, which can be confused with Stevens-Johnson syndrome (but EM major lacks prominent skin sloughing)	—[f]
Rat-bite fever (Haverhill fever)	*Streptobacillus moniliformis*	Maculopapular eruption over palms, soles, and extremities; tends to be more severe at joints; eruption sometimes becoming generalized; may be purpuric; may desquamate	Rat bite, ingestion of contaminated food	Myalgias; arthritis (50%); fever recurrence in some cases	167e
Bacterial endocarditis	*Streptococcus*, *Staphylococcus*, etc.	*Subacute course*: Osler's nodes (tender pink nodules on finger or toe pads); petechiae on skin and mucosa; splinter hemorrhages. *Acute course* (e.g., *Staphylococcus aureus*): Janeway lesions (painless erythematous or hemorrhagic macules, usually on palms and soles)	Abnormal heart valve (e.g., viridans group streptococci), intravenous drug use	New or changing heart murmur	155
Confluent Desquamative Erythemas					
Scarlet fever (second disease)	Group A *Streptococcus* (pyrogenic exotoxins A, B, C)	Diffuse blanchable erythema beginning on face and spreading to trunk and extremities; circumoral pallor; "sandpaper" texture to skin; accentuation of linear erythema in skin folds (Pastia's lines); enanthem of white evolving into red "strawberry" tongue; desquamation in second week	Most common among children 2–10 years old; usually follows group A streptococcal pharyngitis	Fever, pharyngitis, headache	173
Kawasaki disease	Idiopathic causes	Rash similar to scarlet fever (scarlatiniform) or EM; fissuring of lips, strawberry tongue; conjunctivitis; edema of hands, feet; desquamation later in disease	Children <8 years old	Cervical adenopathy, pharyngitis, coronary artery vasculitis	72, 385
Streptococcal toxic shock syndrome	Group A *Streptococcus* (associated with pyrogenic exotoxin A and/or B or certain M types)	When present, rash often scarlatiniform	May occur in setting of severe group A streptococcal infections (e.g., necrotizing fasciitis, bacteremia, pneumonia)	Multiorgan failure, hypotension; mortality rate 30%	173
Staphylococcal toxic shock syndrome	*S. aureus* (toxic shock syndrome toxin 1, enterotoxins B and others)	Diffuse erythema involving palms; pronounced erythema of mucosal surfaces; conjunctivitis; desquamation 7–10 days into illness	Colonization with toxin-producing *S. aureus*	Fever >39°C (>102°F), hypotension, multiorgan dysfunction	172

(Continued)

TABLE 24-1 DISEASES ASSOCIATED WITH FEVER AND RASH (*CONTINUED*)

Disease	Etiology	Description	Group Affected/ Epidemiologic Factors	Clinical Syndrome	Chapter
Confluent Desquamative Erythemas (*Continued*)					
Staphylococcal scalded-skin syndrome	*S. aureus*, phage group II	Diffuse tender erythema, often with bullae and desquamation; Nikolsky's sign	Colonization with toxin-producing *S. aureus*; occurs in children <10 years old (termed *Ritter's disease* in neonates) or adults with renal dysfunction	Irritability; nasal or conjunctival secretions	172
Exfoliative erythroderma syndrome	Underlying psoriasis, eczema, drug eruption, mycosis fungoides	Diffuse erythema (often scaling) interspersed with lesions of underlying condition	Usually occurs in adults over age 50; more common among men	Fever, chills (i.e., difficulty with thermoregulation); lymphadenopathy	72, 74
DRESS (DIHS)	Aromatic anticonvulsants; other drugs, including sulfonamides, minocycline	Maculopapular eruption (mimicking exanthematous drug rash), sometimes progressing to exfoliative erythroderma; profound edema, especially facial; pustules may occur	Individuals genetically unable to detoxify arene oxides (anticonvulsants), patients with slow *N*-acetylating capacity (sulfonamides)	Lymphadenopathy, multiorgan failure (especially hepatic), eosinophilia, atypical lymphocytes; mimics sepsis	74
Stevens-Johnson syndrome (SJS), toxic epidermal necrolysis (TEN)	Drugs (80% of cases; often allopurinol, anticonvulsants, antibiotics), infection, idiopathic	Erythematous and purpuric macules, sometimes targetoid, or diffuse erythema progressing to bullae, with sloughing and necrosis of entire epidermis; Nikolsky's sign; involves mucosal surfaces; TEN (>30% epidermal necrosis) is maximal form; SJS involves <10% of epidermis; SJS/TEN overlap involves 10–30% of epidermis	Uncommon among children; more common among patients with HIV infection, SLE, certain HLA types, or slow acetylators	Dehydration, sepsis sometimes resulting from lack of normal skin integrity; mortality rates up to 30%	74
Vesiculobullous or Pustular Eruptions					
Hand-foot-and-mouth syndrome[g]; staphylococcal scalded-skin syndrome; TEN[b]; DRESS[b]	—	—	—	—	—[f]
Varicella (chickenpox)	VZV	Macules (2–3 mm) evolving into papules, then vesicles (sometimes umbilicated), on an erythematous base ("dewdrops on a rose petal"); pustules then forming and crusting; lesions appearing in crops; may involve scalp, mouth; intensely pruritic	Usually affects children; 10% of adults susceptible; most common in late winter and spring; incidence down by 90% in U.S. as a result of varicella vaccination	Malaise; generally mild disease in healthy children; more severe disease with complications in adults and immunocompromised children	217
Pseudomonas "hot-tub" folliculitis	*Pseudomonas aeruginosa*	Pruritic erythematous follicular, papular, vesicular, or pustular lesions that may involve axillae, buttocks, abdomen, and especially areas occluded by bathing suits; can manifest as tender isolated nodules on palmar or plantar surfaces (the latter designated "*Pseudomonas* hot-foot syndrome")	Bathers in hot tubs or swimming pools; occurs in outbreaks	Earache, sore eyes and/or throat; fever may be absent; generally self-limited	189
Variola (smallpox)	Variola major virus	Red macules on tongue and palate evolving to papules and vesicles; skin macules evolving to papules, then vesicles, then pustules over 1 week, with subsequent lesion crusting; lesions initially appearing on face and spreading centrifugally from trunk to extremities; differs from varicella in that (1) skin lesions in any given area are at same stage of development and (2) there is a prominent distribution of lesions on face and extremities (including palms, soles)	Nonimmune individuals exposed to smallpox	Prodrome of fever, headache, backache, myalgias; vomiting in 50% of cases	261e
Primary herpes simplex virus (HSV) infection	HSV	Erythema rapidly followed by hallmark painful *grouped vesicles* that may evolve into pustules that ulcerate, especially on mucosal surfaces; lesions at site of inoculation: commonly gingivostomatitis for HSV-1 and genital lesions for HSV-2; recurrent disease milder (e.g., herpes labialis does not involve oral mucosa)	Primary infection most common among children and young adults for HSV-1 and among sexually active young adults for HSV-2; no fever in recurrent infection	Regional lymphadenopathy	216

(*Continued*)

TABLE 24-1 DISEASES ASSOCIATED WITH FEVER AND RASH (*CONTINUED*)

Disease	Etiology	Description	Group Affected/ Epidemiologic Factors	Clinical Syndrome	Chapter
Vesiculobullous or Pustular Eruptions (*Continued*)					
Disseminated herpesvirus infection	Varicella-zoster virus (VZV) or HSV	Generalized vesicles that can evolve to pustules and ulcerations; individual lesions similar for VZV and HSV. *Zoster cutaneous dissemination*: >25 lesions extending outside involved dermatome. *HSV*: extensive, progressive mucocutaneous lesions that may occur in absence of dissemination, sometimes disseminate in eczematous skin (eczema herpeticum); HSV visceral dissemination may occur with only localized mucocutaneous disease; in disseminated neonatal disease, skin lesions diagnostically helpful when present, but rash absent in a substantial minority of cases	Patients with immunosuppression, eczema; neonates	Visceral organ involvement (e.g., liver, lungs) in some cases; neonatal disease particularly severe	164, 216, 217
Rickettsialpox	*Rickettsia akari*	Eschar found at site of mite bite; generalized rash involving face, trunk, extremities; may involve palms and soles; <100 papules and plaques (2–10 mm); tops of lesions developing vesicles that may evolve into pustules	Seen in urban settings; transmitted by mouse mites	Headache, myalgias, regional adenopathy; mild disease	211
Acute generalized eruptive pustulosis	Drugs (mostly anticonvulsants or antimicrobials); also viral	Tiny sterile nonfollicular pustules on erythematous, edematous skin; begins on face and in body folds, then becomes generalized	Appears 2–21 days after start of drug therapy, depending on whether patient has been sensitized	Acute fever, pruritus, leukocytosis	74
Disseminated *Vibrio vulnificus* infection	*V. vulnificus*	Erythematous lesions evolving into hemorrhagic bullae and then into necrotic ulcers	Patients with cirrhosis, diabetes, renal failure; exposure by ingestion of contaminated saltwater, seafood	Hypotension; mortality rate 50%	193
Ecthyma gangrenosum	*P. aeruginosa*, other gram-negative rods, fungi	Indurated plaque evolving into hemorrhagic bulla or pustule that sloughs, resulting in eschar formation; erythematous halo; most common in axillary, groin, perianal regions	Usually affects neutropenic patients; occurs in up to 28% of individuals with *Pseudomonas* bacteremia	Clinical signs of sepsis	189
Urticaria-Like Eruptions					
Urticarial vasculitis	Serum sickness, often due to infection (including hepatitis B viral, enteroviral, parasitic), drugs; connective tissue disease	Erythematous, edematous "urticaria-like" plaques, pruritic or burning; unlike urticaria: typical lesion duration >24 h (up to 5 days) and lack of complete lesion blanching with compression due to hemorrhage	Patients with serum sickness (including hepatitis B), connective tissue disease	Fever variable; arthralgias/arthritis	385[f]
Nodular Eruptions					
Disseminated infection	Fungal infections (e.g., candidiasis, histoplasmosis, cryptococcosis, sporotrichosis, coccidioidomycosis); mycobacteria	Subcutaneous nodules (up to 3 cm); fluctuance, draining common with mycobacteria; necrotic nodules (extremities, periorbital or nasal regions) common with *Aspergillus*, *Mucor*	Immunocompromised hosts (i.e., bone marrow transplant recipients, patients undergoing chemotherapy, HIV-infected patients, alcoholics)	Features vary with organism	—[f]
Erythema nodosum (septal panniculitis)	Infections (e.g., streptococcal, fungal, mycobacterial, yersinial); drugs (e.g., sulfas, penicillins, oral contraceptives); sarcoidosis; idiopathic causes	Large, violaceous, nonulcerative, subcutaneous nodules; exquisitely tender; usually on lower legs but also on upper extremities	More common among girls and women 15–30 years old	Arthralgias (50%); features vary with associated condition	—[f]
Sweet syndrome (acute febrile neutrophilic dermatosis)	Yersiniae; upper respiratory infection; inflammatory bowel disease; pregnancy; malignancy (usually hematologic); drugs (G-CSF)	Tender red or blue edematous nodules giving impression of vesiculation; usually on face, neck, upper extremities; when on lower extremities, may mimic erythema nodosum	More common among women and among persons 30–60 years old; 20% of cases associated with malignancy (men and women equally affected in this group)	Headache, arthralgias, leukocytosis	72

(*Continued*)

TABLE 24-1 DISEASES ASSOCIATED WITH FEVER AND RASH (*CONTINUED*)

Disease	Etiology	Description	Group Affected/ Epidemiologic Factors	Clinical Syndrome	Chapter
Nodular Eruption (*Continued*)					
Bacillary angiomatosis	*Bartonella henselae*, *B. quintana*	Many forms, including erythematous, smooth vascular nodules; friable, exophytic lesions; erythematous plaques (may be dry, scaly); subcutaneous nodules (may be erythematous)	Immunosuppressed individuals, especially those with advanced HIV infection	Peliosis of liver and spleen in some cases; lesions sometimes involving multiple organs; bacteremia	197
Purpuric Eruptions					
Rocky Mountain spotted fever, rat-bite fever, endocarditis[g]; epidemic typhus[e]; dengue fever[d,e]; human parvovirus B19 infection[e]	—	—	—	—	—[f]
Acute meningococcemia	*Neisseria meningitidis*	Initially pink maculopapular lesions evolving into petechiae; petechiae rapidly becoming numerous, sometimes enlarging and becoming vesicular; trunk, extremities most commonly involved; may appear on face, hands, feet; may include purpura fulminans (see below) reflecting DIC	Most common among children, individuals with asplenia or terminal complement component deficiency (C5–C8)	Hypotension, meningitis (sometimes preceded by upper respiratory infection)	180
Purpura fulminans	Severe DIC	Large ecchymoses with sharply irregular shapes evolving into hemorrhagic bullae and then into black necrotic lesions	Individuals with sepsis (e.g., involving *N. meningitidis*), malignancy, or massive trauma; asplenic patients at high risk for sepsis	Hypotension	180, 325
Chronic meningococcemia	*N. meningitidis*	Variety of recurrent eruptions, including pink maculopapular; nodular (usually on lower extremities); petechial (sometimes developing vesicular centers); purpuric areas with pale blue-gray centers	Individuals with complement deficiencies	Fevers, sometimes intermittent; arthritis, myalgias, headache	180
Disseminated gonococcal infection	*Neisseria gonorrhoeae*	Papules (1–5 mm) evolving over 1–2 days into hemorrhagic pustules with gray necrotic centers; hemorrhagic bullae occurring rarely; lesions (usually <40) distributed peripherally near joints (more commonly on upper extremities)	Sexually active individuals (more often females), some with complement deficiency	Low-grade fever, tenosynovitis, arthritis	181
Enteroviral petechial rash	Usually echovirus 9 or coxsackievirus A9	Disseminated petechial lesions (may also be maculopapular, vesicular, or urticarial)	Often occurs in outbreaks	Pharyngitis, headache; aseptic meningitis with echovirus 9	228
Viral hemorrhagic fever	Arboviruses (including dengue) and arenaviruses	Petechial rash	Residence in or travel to endemic areas, other virus exposure	Triad of fever, shock, hemorrhage from mucosa or gastrointestinal tract	233, 234
Thrombotic thrombocytopenic purpura/ hemolytic-uremic syndrome	Idiopathic, bloody diarrhea caused by Shiga toxin–generating bacteria (e.g., *Escherichia coli* O157:H7), deficiency in ADAMTS13 (cleaves von Willebrand factor), drugs (e.g., quinine, chemotherapy, immunosuppression)	Petechiae	Individuals with *E. coli* O157:H7 gastroenteritis (especially children), cancer chemotherapy, HIV infection, autoimmune diseases, pregnant/postpartum women	Fever (not always present), microangiopathic hemolytic anemia, thrombocytopenia, renal dysfunction, neurologic dysfunction; coagulation studies normal	72, 129, 140, 186, 191
Cutaneous small-vessel vasculitis (leukocytoclastic vasculitis)	Infections (including that caused by group A *Streptococcus*, viral hepatitis), drugs, idiopathic causes	Palpable purpuric lesions appearing in crops on legs or other dependent areas; may become vesicular or ulcerative	Occurs in a wide spectrum of diseases, including connective tissue disease, cryoglobulinemia, malignancy, Henoch-Schönlein purpura (HSP); more common among children	Fever (not always present), malaise, arthralgias, myalgias; systemic vasculitis in some cases; renal, joint, and gastrointestinal involvement common in HSP	72
Eruptions with Ulcers and/or Eschars					
Scrub typhus, rickettsial spotted fevers, rat-bite fever[e]; rickettsialpox, ecthyma gangrenosum[h]	—	—	—	—	—[f]

(*Continued*)

TABLE 24-1 DISEASES ASSOCIATED WITH FEVER AND RASH (*CONTINUED*)

Disease	Etiology	Description	Group Affected/ Epidemiologic Factors	Clinical Syndrome	Chapter
Eruptions with Ulcers and/or Eschars (*Continued*)					
Tularemia	*Francisella tularensis*	Ulceroglandular form: erythematous, tender papule evolves into necrotic, tender ulcer with raised borders; in 35% of cases, eruptions (maculopapular, vesiculopapular, acneiform, or urticarial; erythema nodosum; or EM) may occur	Exposure to ticks, biting flies, infected animals	Fever, headache, lymphadenopathy	195
Anthrax	*Bacillus anthracis*	Pruritic papule enlarging and evolving into a 1- by 3-cm painless ulcer surrounded by vesicles and then developing a central eschar with edema; residual scar	Exposure to infected animals or animal products, other exposure to anthrax spores	Lymphadenopathy, headache	261e

[a]See "Purpuric Eruptions." [b]See "Confluent Desquamative Erythemas." [c]In human granulocytotropic ehrlichiosis or anaplasmosis (caused by *Anaplasma phagocytophila;* most common in the upper midwestern and northeastern United States), rash is rare. [d]See "Viral hemorrhagic fever" under "Purpuric Eruptions" for dengue hemorrhagic fever/dengue shock syndrome. [e]See "Centrally Distributed Maculopapular Eruptions." [f]See etiology-specific chapters. [g]See "Peripheral Eruptions." [h]See "Vesiculobullous or Pustular Eruptions."

Abbreviations: CNS, central nervous system; DIC, disseminated intravascular coagulation; G-CSF, granulocyte colony-stimulating factor; HLA, human leukocyte antigen.

seen in urban environments where rodents proliferate. Outside the United States, other rickettsial diseases cause a spotted-fever syndrome and should be considered in residents of or travelers to endemic areas. Similarly, *typhoid fever*, a nonrickettsial disease caused by *Salmonella typhi* (Chap. 190), is usually acquired during travel outside the United States. *Dengue fever*, caused by a mosquito-transmitted flavivirus, occurs in tropical and subtropical regions of the world (Chap. 233).

Some centrally distributed maculopapular eruptions have distinctive features. Erythema migrans, the rash of *Lyme disease* (Chap. 210), typically manifests as single or multiple annular plaques. Untreated erythema migrans lesions usually fade within a month but may persist for more than a year. *Southern tick-associated rash illness* (STARI) (Chap. 210) has an erythema migrans–like rash but is less severe than Lyme disease and often occurs in regions where Lyme is not endemic. *Erythema marginatum*, the rash of *acute rheumatic fever* (Chap. 381), has a distinctive pattern of enlarging and shifting transient annular lesions.

Collagen vascular diseases may cause fever and rash. Patients with *systemic lupus erythematosus* (Chap. 378) typically develop a sharply defined, erythematous eruption in a butterfly distribution on the cheeks (malar rash) as well as many other skin manifestations. *Still's disease* (Chap. 398) presents as an evanescent, salmon-colored rash on the trunk and proximal extremities that coincides with fever spikes.

PERIPHERAL ERUPTIONS

These rashes are alike in that they are most prominent peripherally or begin in peripheral (acral) areas before spreading centripetally. Early diagnosis and therapy are critical in *Rocky Mountain spotted fever* (Chap. 211) because of its grave prognosis if untreated. Lesions evolve from macular to petechial, start on the wrists and ankles, spread centripetally, and appear on the palms and soles only later in the disease. The rash of *secondary syphilis* (Chap. 206), which may be generalized but is prominent on the palms and soles, should be considered in the differential diagnosis of pityriasis rosea, especially in sexually active patients. *Chikungunya fever* (Chap. 233), which is transmitted by mosquito bite in Africa and the Indian Ocean region, is associated with a maculopapular eruption and severe polyarticular small-joint arthralgias. *Hand-foot-and-mouth disease* (Chap. 228), most commonly caused by coxsackievirus A16, is distinguished by tender vesicles distributed peripherally and in the mouth; outbreaks commonly occur within families. The classic target lesions of *erythema multiforme* appear symmetrically on the elbows, knees, palms, soles, and face. In severe cases, these lesions spread diffusely and involve mucosal surfaces. Lesions may develop on the hands and feet in *endocarditis* (Chap. 155).

CONFLUENT DESQUAMATIVE ERYTHEMAS

These eruptions consist of diffuse erythema frequently followed by desquamation. The eruptions caused by group A *Streptococcus* or *Staphylococcus aureus* are toxin-mediated. *Scarlet fever* (Chap. 173) usually follows pharyngitis; patients have a facial flush, a "strawberry" tongue, and accentuated petechiae in body folds (Pastia's lines). *Kawasaki disease* (Chaps. 72 and 385) presents in the pediatric population as fissuring of the lips, a strawberry tongue, conjunctivitis, adenopathy, and sometimes cardiac abnormalities. *Streptococcal toxic shock syndrome* (Chap. 173) manifests with hypotension, multiorgan failure, and, often, a severe group A streptococcal infection (e.g., necrotizing fasciitis). *Staphylococcal toxic shock syndrome* (Chap. 172) also presents with hypotension and multiorgan failure, but usually only *S. aureus* colonization—not a severe *S. aureus* infection—is documented. *Staphylococcal scalded-skin syndrome* (Chap. 172) is seen primarily in children and in immunocompromised adults. Generalized erythema is often evident during the prodrome of fever and malaise; profound tenderness of the skin is distinctive. In the exfoliative stage, the skin can be induced to form bullae with light lateral pressure (Nikolsky's sign). In a mild form, a scarlatiniform eruption mimics scarlet fever, but the patient does not exhibit a strawberry tongue or circumoral pallor. In contrast to the staphylococcal scalded-skin syndrome, in which the cleavage plane is superficial in the epidermis, *toxic epidermal necrolysis* (Chap. 74), a maximal variant of *Stevens-Johnson syndrome*, involves sloughing of the entire epidermis, resulting in severe disease. *Exfoliative erythroderma syndrome* (Chaps. 72 and 74) is a serious reaction associated with systemic toxicity that is often due to eczema, psoriasis, a drug reaction, or mycosis fungoides. *Drug rash with eosinophilia and systemic symptoms (DRESS)*, often due to antiepileptic and antibiotic agents (Chap. 74), initially appears similar to an exanthematous drug reaction but may progress to exfoliative erythroderma; it is accompanied by multi-organ failure and has an associated mortality rate of ~10%.

VESICULOBULLOUS OR PUSTULAR ERUPTIONS

Varicella (Chap. 217) is highly contagious, often occurring in winter or spring. At any point in time, within a given region of the body, varicella lesions are in different stages of development. In immunocompromised hosts, varicella vesicles may lack the characteristic erythematous base or may appear hemorrhagic. Lesions of *Pseudomonas "hot-tub" folliculitis* (Chap. 189) are also pruritic and may appear similar to those of varicella. However, hot-tub folliculitis generally occurs in outbreaks after bathing in hot tubs or swimming pools, and lesions occur in regions occluded by bathing suits. Lesions of *variola (smallpox)* (Chap. 261e) also appear similar to those of varicella but are all at the same stage of development in a given region of the body. Variola lesions are most prominent on the face and extremities, while varicella lesions are most prominent on the trunk. *Herpes simplex virus infection* (Chap. 216) is characterized by hallmark grouped vesicles on an erythematous base. Primary herpes infection is accompanied by fever and toxicity, while recurrent disease is milder. *Rickettsialpox* (Chap. 211) is often documented in urban settings and is characterized by vesicles followed by pustules. It can be distinguished from varicella by an eschar at the site of the mouse-mite bite and the papule/plaque base of each vesicle. *Acute generalized eruptive pustulosis* should be considered in individuals who are acutely febrile and are taking new medications, especially anticonvulsant or antimicrobial agents (Chap. 74). Disseminated *Vibrio vulnificus* infection (Chap. 193) or *ecthyma gangrenosum* due to *Pseudomonas aeruginosa* (Chap. 189) should be considered in immunosuppressed individuals with sepsis and hemorrhagic bullae.

URTICARIA-LIKE ERUPTIONS

Individuals with classic urticaria ("hives") usually have a hypersensitivity reaction without associated fever. In the presence of fever, urticaria-like eruptions are most often due to *urticarial vasculitis* (Chap. 385). Unlike individual lesions of classic urticaria, which last up to 24 h, these lesions may last 3–5 days. Etiologies include serum sickness (often induced by drugs such as penicillins, sulfas, salicylates, or barbiturates), connective-tissue disease (e.g., systemic lupus erythematosus or Sjögren's syndrome), and infection (e.g., with hepatitis B virus, enteroviruses, or parasites). Malignancy, especially lymphoma, may be associated with fever and chronic urticaria (Chap. 72).

NODULAR ERUPTIONS

In immunocompromised hosts, nodular lesions often represent disseminated infection. Patients with disseminated *candidiasis* (often due to *Candida tropicalis*) may have a triad of fever, myalgias, and eruptive nodules (Chap. 240). Disseminated *cryptococcosis* lesions (Chap. 239) may resemble molluscum contagiosum (Chap. 220e). Necrosis of nodules should raise the suspicion of *aspergillosis* (Chap. 241) or *mucormycosis* (Chap. 242). *Erythema nodosum* presents with exquisitely tender nodules on the lower extremities. *Sweet syndrome* (Chap. 72) should be considered in individuals with multiple nodules and plaques, often so edematous that they give the appearance of vesicles or bullae. Sweet syndrome may occur in individuals with infection, inflammatory bowel disease, or malignancy and can also be induced by drugs.

PURPURIC ERUPTIONS

Acute meningococcemia (Chap. 180) classically presents in children as a petechial eruption, but initial lesions may appear as blanchable macules or urticaria. Rocky Mountain spotted fever should be considered in the differential diagnosis of acute meningococcemia. *Echovirus 9 infection* (Chap. 228) may mimic acute meningococcemia; patients should be treated as if they have bacterial sepsis because prompt differentiation of these conditions may be impossible. Large ecchymotic areas of *purpura fulminans* (Chaps. 180 and 325) reflect severe underlying disseminated intravascular coagulation, which may be due to infectious or noninfectious causes. The lesions of *chronic meningococcemia* (Chap. 180) may have a variety of morphologies, including petechial. Purpuric nodules may develop on the legs and resemble erythema nodosum but lack its exquisite tenderness. Lesions of *disseminated gonococcemia* (Chap. 181) are distinctive, sparse, countable hemorrhagic pustules, usually located near joints. The lesions of chronic meningococcemia and those of gonococcemia may be indistinguishable in terms of appearance and distribution. *Viral hemorrhagic fever* (Chaps. 233 and 234) should be considered in patients with an appropriate travel history and a petechial rash. *Thrombotic thrombocytopenic purpura* (Chaps. 72, 129, and 140) and *hemolytic-uremic syndrome* (Chaps. 140, 186, and 191) are closely related and are noninfectious causes of fever and petechiae. *Cutaneous small-vessel vasculitis* (*leukocytoclastic vasculitis*) typically manifests as palpable purpura and has a wide variety of causes (Chap. 72).

ERUPTIONS WITH ULCERS OR ESCHARS

The presence of an ulcer or eschar in the setting of a more widespread eruption can provide an important diagnostic clue. For example, the presence of an eschar may suggest the diagnosis of *scrub typhus* or *rickettsialpox* (Chap. 211) in the appropriate setting. In other illnesses (e.g., anthrax) (Chap. 261e), an ulcer or eschar may be the only skin manifestation.

25e Atlas of Rashes Associated with Fever

Kenneth M. Kaye, Elaine T. Kaye

This is a digital-only chapter. It is available on the DVD that accompanies this book, as well as on Access Medicine/Harrison's Online, and the eBook and "app" editions of HPIM 19e.

Given the extremely broad differential diagnosis, the presentation of a patient with fever and rash often poses a thorny diagnostic challenge for even the most astute and experienced clinician. Rapid narrowing of the differential by prompt recognition of a rash's key features can result in appropriate and sometimes life-saving therapy. This atlas presents high-quality images of a variety of rashes that have an infectious etiology and are commonly associated with fever.

26 Fever of Unknown Origin

Chantal P. Bleeker-Rovers, Jos W. M. van der Meer

DEFINITION

Clinicians commonly refer to any febrile illness without an initially obvious etiology as *fever of unknown origin* (FUO). Most febrile illnesses either resolve before a diagnosis can be made or develop distinguishing characteristics that lead to a diagnosis. The term *FUO* should be reserved for prolonged febrile illnesses without an established etiology despite intensive evaluation and diagnostic testing. This chapter focuses on classic FUO in the adult patient.

FUO was originally defined by Petersdorf and Beeson in 1961 as an illness of >3 weeks' duration with fever of ≥38.3°C (101°F) on two occasions and an uncertain diagnosis despite 1 week of inpatient evaluation. Nowadays, most patients with FUO are hospitalized if their clinical condition requires it, but not for diagnostic purposes only; thus the in-hospital evaluation requirement has been eliminated from the definition. The definition of FUO has been further modified by the exclusion of immunocompromised patients, whose workup requires an entirely different diagnostic and therapeutic approach. For the optimal comparison of patients with FUO in different geographic areas, it has been proposed that the quantitative criterion (diagnosis uncertain after 1 week of evaluation) be changed to a qualitative criterion that requires the performance of a specific list of investigations. Accordingly, FUO is now defined as:

1. Fever >38.3°C (101°F) on at least two occasions
2. Illness duration of ≥3 weeks
3. No known immunocompromised state
4. Diagnosis that remains uncertain after a thorough history-taking, physical examination, and the following obligatory investigations: determination of erythrocyte sedimentation rate (ESR) and C-reactive protein (CRP) level; platelet count; leukocyte count and differential; measurement of levels of hemoglobin, electrolytes, creatinine, total protein, alkaline phosphatase, alanine aminotransferase, aspartate aminotransferase, lactate dehydrogenase, creatine kinase, ferritin, antinuclear antibodies, and rheumatoid factor; protein electrophoresis; urinalysis; blood cultures (n = 3); urine culture; chest x-ray; abdominal ultrasonography; and tuberculin skin test (TST).

ETIOLOGY AND EPIDEMIOLOGY

The range of FUO etiologies has evolved over time as a result of changes in the spectrum of diseases causing FUO, the widespread

TABLE 26-1 ETIOLOGY OF FEVER OF UNKNOWN ORIGIN (FUO) OVER THE PAST 20 YEARS: FINDINGS FROM LARGE FUO STUDIES

		Percentage of Cases Due to Indicated Cause				
First Author (Country, Year of Publication)	**No. of Patients (Recruitment Period)**	**Infections**	**Noninfectious Inflammatory Diseases**	**Neoplasms**	**Miscellaneous**	**Unknown**
Western Countries						
De Kleijn et al. (Netherlands, 1997)	167 (1992–1994)	26	24	13	8	30
Vanderschueren et al. (Belgium, 2003)	185 (1990–1999)	11	18	10	8	53
Zenone et al. (France, 2006)	144 (1999–2005)	23	26	10	15	26
Bleeker-Rovers (Netherlands, 2007)	73 (2003–2005)	16	22	7	4	51
Mansueto et al. (Italy, 2008)	91 (1991–2002)	32	12	14	10	32
Efstathiou et al. (Greece, 2010)	112 (2001–2007)	30	33	11	5	21
Total	**772**	**22**	**23**	**11**	**9**	**36**
Other Geographic Locations						
Tabak et al. (Turkey, 2003)	117 (1984–2001)	34	29	19	4	14
Saltoglu et al. (Turkey, 2004)	87 (1994–2002)	59	18	14	2	7
Ergonul et al. (Turkey, 2005)	80 (1993–1999)	52	16	18	3	11
Chin et al. (Taiwan, 2006)	94 (2001–2002)	57	7	9	9	18
Colpan et al. (Turkey, 2007)	71 (2001–2004)	45	27	14	6	9
Hu et al. (China, 2008)	142 (2002–2003)	36	32	13	5	14
Kucukardali et al. (Turkey, 2008)	154 (2003–2004)	34	31	14	5	16
Ali-Eldin et al. (Egypt, 2011)	93 (2009–2010)	42	15	30	0	12
Total	**838**	**43**	**23**	**16**	**4**	**13**

use of antibiotics, and the availability of new diagnostic techniques. The proportion of cases caused by intraabdominal abscesses and tumors, for example, has decreased because of earlier detection by CT and ultrasound. In addition, infective endocarditis is a less frequent cause because blood culture and echocardiographic techniques have improved. Conversely, some diagnoses, such as acute HIV infection, were unknown four decades ago.

Table 26-1 summarizes the findings of several large studies on FUO conducted over the past 20 years. In general, infection accounts for about 20–25% of cases of FUO in Western countries; next in frequency are neoplasms and noninfectious inflammatory diseases (NIIDs), the latter including "collagen or rheumatic diseases," vasculitis syndromes, and granulomatous disorders. In geographic areas outside the West, infections are a much more common cause of FUO (43% vs 22%), while the proportions of cases due to NIIDs and neoplasms are similar. Up to 50% of cases caused by infections in patients with FUO outside Western nations are due to tuberculosis, which is a less common cause in the United States and Western Europe. The number of FUO patients diagnosed with NIIDs probably will not decrease in the near future, as fever may precede more typical manifestations or serologic evidence by months in these diseases. Moreover, many NIIDs can be diagnosed only after prolonged observation and exclusion of other diseases.

In the West, the percentage of undiagnosed cases of FUO has increased in more recent studies. An important factor contributing to the seemingly high diagnostic failure rate is that a diagnosis is more often being established before 3 weeks have elapsed, given that patients with fever tend to seek medical advice earlier and better diagnostic techniques, such as CT and MRI, are widely available; therefore, only the cases that are more difficult to diagnose continue to meet the criteria for FUO. Furthermore, most patients who have FUO without a diagnosis currently do well, and thus a less aggressive diagnostic approach may be used in clinically stable patients once diseases with immediate therapeutic or prognostic consequences have been ruled out to a reasonable extent. This factor may be especially relevant to patients with recurrent fever who are asymptomatic in between febrile episodes. In patients with recurrent fever (defined as repeated episodes of fever interspersed with fever-free intervals of at least 2 weeks and apparent remission of the underlying disease), the chance of attaining an etiologic diagnosis is <50%.

DIFFERENTIAL DIAGNOSIS

The differential diagnosis for FUO is extensive, but it is important to remember that FUO is far more often caused by an atypical presentation of a rather common disease than by a very rare disease. Table 26-2 presents an overview of possible causes of FUO. An atypical presentation of endocarditis, diverticulitis, vertebral osteomyelitis, and extrapulmonary tuberculosis are the more common infectious disease diagnoses. Q fever and Whipple's disease are quite rare but should always be kept in mind as a cause of FUO since the presenting symptoms

TABLE 26-2 ALL REPORTED CAUSES OF FUO[a]

Infections	
Bacterial, nonspecific	Abdominal abscess, adnexitis, apical granuloma, appendicitis, cholangitis, cholecystitis, diverticulitis, endocarditis, endometritis, epidural abscess, infected vascular catheter, infected joint prosthesis, infected vascular prosthesis, infectious arthritis, infective myonecrosis, intracranial abscess, liver abscess, lung abscess, malakoplakia, mastoiditis, mediastinitis, mycotic aneurysm, osteomyelitis, pelvic inflammatory disease, prostatitis, pyelonephritis, pylephlebitis, renal abscess, septic phlebitis, sinusitis, spondylodiscitis, xanthogranulomatous urinary tract infection
Bacterial, specific	Actinomycosis, atypical mycobacterial infection, bartonellosis, brucellosis, *Campylobacter* infection, *Chlamydia pneumoniae* infection, chronic meningococcemia, ehrlichiosis, gonococcemia, legionellosis, leptospirosis, listeriosis, louse-borne relapsing fever (*Borrelia recurrentis*), Lyme disease, melioidosis (*Pseudomonas pseudomallei*), *Mycoplasma* infection, nocardiosis, psittacosis, Q fever (*Coxiella burnetii*), rickettsiosis, *Spirillum minor* infection, *Streptobacillus moniliformis* infection, syphilis, tick-borne relapsing fever (*Borrelia duttonii*), tuberculosis, tularemia, typhoid fever and other salmonelloses, Whipple's disease (*Tropheryma whipplei*), yersiniosis
Fungal	Aspergillosis, blastomycosis, candidiasis, coccidioidomycosis, cryptococcosis, histoplasmosis, *Malassezia furfur* infection, paracoccidioidomycosis, *Pneumocystis jirovecii* pneumonia, sporotrichosis, zygomycosis
Parasitic	Amebiasis, babesiosis, echinococcosis, fascioliasis, malaria, schistosomiasis, strongyloidiasis, toxocariasis, toxoplasmosis, trichinellosis, trypanosomiasis, visceral leishmaniasis
Viral	Colorado tick fever, coxsackievirus infection, cytomegalovirus infection, dengue, Epstein-Barr virus infection, hantavirus infection, hepatitis (A, B, C, D, E), herpes simplex, HIV infection, human herpesvirus 6 infection, parvovirus infection, West Nile virus infection
Noninfectious Inflammatory Diseases	
Systemic rheumatic and autoimmune diseases	Ankylosing spondylitis, antiphospholipid syndrome, autoimmune hemolytic anemia, autoimmune hepatitis, Behçet's disease, cryoglobulinemia, dermatomyositis, Felty syndrome, gout, mixed connective-tissue disease, polymyositis, pseudogout, reactive arthritis, relapsing polychondritis, rheumatic fever, rheumatoid arthritis, Sjögren's syndrome, systemic lupus erythematosus, Vogt-Koyanagi-Harada syndrome
Vasculitis	Allergic vasculitis, Churg-Strauss syndrome, giant cell vasculitis/polymyalgia rheumatica, granulomatosis with polyangiitis, hypersensitivity vasculitis, Kawasaki's disease, polyarteritis nodosa, Takayasu arteritis, urticarial vasculitis
Granulomatous diseases	Idiopathic granulomatous hepatitis, sarcoidosis
Autoinflammatory syndromes	Adult-onset Still's disease, Blau syndrome, CAPS[b] (cryopyrin-associated periodic syndromes), Crohn's disease, DIRA (deficiency of the interleukin 1 receptor antagonist), familial Mediterranean fever, hemophagocytic syndrome, hyper-IgD syndrome (HIDS, also known as mevalonate kinase deficiency), juvenile idiopathic arthritis, PAPA syndrome (pyogenic sterile arthritis, pyoderma gangrenosum, and acne), PFAPA syndrome (periodic fever, aphthous stomatitis, pharyngitis, adenitis), recurrent idiopathic pericarditis, SAPHO (synovitis, acne, pustulosis, hyperostosis, osteomyelitis), Schnitzler's syndrome, TRAPS (tumor necrosis factor receptor–associated periodic syndrome)
Neoplasms	
Hematologic malignancies	Amyloidosis, angioimmunoblastic lymphoma, Castleman's disease, Hodgkin's disease, hypereosinophilic syndrome, leukemia, lymphomatoid granulomatosis, malignant histiocytosis, multiple myeloma, myelodysplastic syndrome, myelofibrosis, non-Hodgkin's lymphoma, plasmacytoma, systemic mastocytosis, vaso-occlusive crisis in sickle cell disease
Solid tumors	Most solid tumors and metastases can cause fever. Those most commonly causing FUO are breast, colon, hepatocellular, lung, pancreatic, and renal cell carcinomas.
Benign tumors	Angiomyolipoma, cavernous hemangioma of the liver, craniopharyngioma, necrosis of dermoid tumor in Gardner's syndrome
Miscellaneous	
	ADEM (acute disseminated encephalomyelitis), adrenal insufficiency, aneurysms, anomalous thoracic duct, aortic dissection, aortic-enteral fistula, aseptic meningitis (Mollaret's syndrome), atrial myxoma, brewer's yeast ingestion, Caroli disease, cholesterol emboli, cirrhosis, complex partial status epilepticus, cyclic neutropenia, drug fever, Erdheim-Chester disease, extrinsic allergic alveolitis, Fabry's disease, factitious disease, fire-eater's lung, fraudulent fever, Gaucher's disease, Hamman-Rich syndrome (acute interstitial pneumonia), Hashimoto's encephalopathy, hematoma, hypersensitivity pneumonitis, hypertriglyceridemia, hypothalamic hypopituitarism, idiopathic normal-pressure hydrocephalus, inflammatory pseudotumor, Kikuchi's disease, linear IgA dermatosis, mesenteric fibromatosis, metal fume fever, milk protein allergy, myotonic dystrophy, nonbacterial osteitis, organic dust toxic syndrome, panniculitis, POEMS (polyneuropathy, organomegaly, endocrinopathy, monoclonal protein, skin changes), polymer fume fever, post–cardiac injury syndrome, primary biliary cirrhosis, primary hyperparathyroidism, pulmonary embolism, pyoderma gangrenosum, retroperitoneal fibrosis, Rosai-Dorfman disease, sclerosing mesenteritis, silicone embolization, subacute thyroiditis (de Quervain's), Sweet syndrome (acute febrile neutrophilic dermatosis), thrombosis, tubulointerstitial nephritis and uveitis syndrome (TINU), ulcerative colitis
Thermoregulatory Disorders	
Central	Brain tumor, cerebrovascular accident, encephalitis, hypothalamic dysfunction
Peripheral	Anhidrotic ectodermal dysplasia, exercise-induced hyperthermia, hyperthyroidism, pheochromocytoma

[a]This table includes all causes of FUO that have been described in the literature. [b]CAPS includes chronic infantile neurologic cutaneous and articular syndrome (CINCA, also known as neonatal-onset multisystem inflammatory disease, or NOMID), familial cold autoinflammatory syndrome (FCAS), and Muckle-Wells syndrome.

can be nonspecific. Serologic testing for Q fever, which results from exposure to animals or animal products, should be performed when the patient lives in a rural area or has a history of heart valve disease, an aortic aneurysm, or a vascular prosthesis. In patients with unexplained symptoms localized to the central nervous system (CNS), gastrointestinal tract, or joints, polymerase chain reaction (PCR) testing for *Tropheryma whipplei* should be performed. Travel to or (former) residence in tropical countries or the American Southwest should lead to consideration of infectious diseases such as malaria, leishmaniasis, histoplasmosis, or coccidioidomycosis. Fever with signs of endocarditis and negative blood culture results poses a special problem. Culture-negative endocarditis may be due to difficult-to-culture bacteria such as nutritionally variant bacteria, HACEK organisms (*Haemophilus parainfluenzae*, *H. paraphrophilus*, *Aggregatibacter* species [*actinomycetemcomitans*, *aphrophilus*], *Cardiobacterium* species [*hominis*, *valvarum*], *Eikenella corrodens*, and *Kingella kingae*; discussed below),

Coxiella burnetii (as indicated above), *T. whipplei*, and *Bartonella* species. Marantic endocarditis is a sterile thrombotic disease that occurs as a paraneoplastic phenomenon, especially with adenocarcinomas. Sterile endocarditis is also seen in the context of systemic lupus erythematosus and antiphospholipid syndrome.

Of the NIIDs, large-vessel vasculitis, polymyalgia rheumatica, sarcoidosis, familial Mediterranean fever, and adult-onset Still's disease are rather common diagnoses in patients with FUO. The hereditary autoinflammatory syndromes are very rare and usually present in young patients. Schnitzler's syndrome, which can present at any age, is uncommon but can often be diagnosed easily in a patient with FUO who presents with urticaria, bone pain, and monoclonal gammopathy.

Although most tumors can present with fever, malignant lymphoma is by far the most common diagnosis of FUO among the neoplasms. Sometimes the fever even precedes lymphadenopathy detectable by physical examination.

Apart from drug-induced fever and exercise-induced hyperthermia, none of the miscellaneous causes of fever is found very frequently in patients with FUO. Virtually all drugs can cause fever, even that commencing after long-term use. *Drug-induced fever*, including DRESS (drug reaction with eosinophilia and systemic symptoms; Fig. 25e-49), is often accompanied by eosinophilia and also by lymphadenopathy, which can be extensive. More common causes of drug-induced fever are allopurinol, carbamazepine, lamotrigine, phenytoin, sulfasalazine, furosemide, antimicrobial drugs (especially sulfonamides, minocycline, vancomycin, β-lactam antibiotics, and isoniazid), some cardiovascular drugs (e.g., quinidine), and some antiretroviral drugs (e.g., nevirapine). *Exercise-induced hyperthermia* (Chap. 479e) is characterized by an elevated body temperature that is associated with moderate to strenuous exercise lasting from half an hour up to several hours without an increase in CRP level or ESR; typically these patients sweat during the temperature elevation. *Factitious fever* (fever artificially induced by the patient—for example, by IV injection of contaminated water) should be considered in all patients but is more common among young women in health care professions. In *fraudulent fever*, the patient is normothermic but manipulates the thermometer. Simultaneous measurements at different body sites (rectum, ear, mouth) should rapidly identify this diagnosis. Another clue to fraudulent fever is a dissociation between pulse rate and temperature.

Previous studies of FUO have shown that a diagnosis is more likely in elderly patients than in younger age groups. In many cases, FUO in the elderly results from an atypical manifestation of a common disease, among which giant cell arteritis and polymyalgia rheumatica are most frequently involved. Tuberculosis is the most common infectious disease associated with FUO in elderly patients, occurring much more often than in younger patients. As many of these diseases are treatable, it is well worth pursuing the cause of fever in elderly patients.

APPROACH TO THE PATIENT: **Fever of Unknown Origin**

FIRST-STAGE DIAGNOSTIC TESTS

Figure 26-1 shows a structured approach to patients presenting with FUO. The most important step in the diagnostic workup is the search for potentially diagnostic clues (PDCs) through complete and repeated history-taking and physical examination and the obligatory investigations listed above. *PDCs* are defined as all localizing signs, symptoms, and abnormalities potentially pointing toward a diagnosis. Although PDCs are often misleading, only with their help can a concise list of probable diagnoses be made. The history should include information about the fever pattern (continuous or recurrent) and duration, previous medical history, present and recent drug use, family history, sexual history, country of origin, recent and remote travel, unusual environmental exposures associated with travel or hobbies, and animal contacts. A complete physical examination should be performed, with special attention to the eyes, lymph nodes, temporal arteries, liver, spleen, sites of previous surgery, entire skin surface, and mucous membranes. Before further diagnostic tests are initiated, antibiotic and glucocorticoid treatment, which can mask many diseases, should be stopped. For example, blood and other cultures are not reliable when samples are obtained during antibiotic treatment, and the size of enlarged lymph nodes usually decreases during glucocorticoid treatment, regardless of the cause of the lymphadenopathy. Despite the high number of false-positive ultrasounds and the relatively low sensitivity of chest x-rays, the performance of these simple, low-cost diagnostic tests remains obligatory in all patients with FUO in order to separate cases that are caused by easily diagnosed diseases from those that are not. Abdominal ultrasound is preferred to abdominal CT as an obligatory test because of relatively low cost, lack of radiation burden, and absence of side effects.

Only rarely do biochemical tests (beyond the obligatory tests needed to classify a patient's fever as FUO) lead directly to a definitive diagnosis in the absence of PDCs. The diagnostic yield of immunologic serology other than that included in the obligatory tests is relatively low. These tests more often yield false-positive rather than true-positive results and are of little use without PDCs pointing to specific immunologic disorders. Given the absence of specific symptoms in many patients and the relatively low cost of the test, investigation of cryoglobulins appears to be a valuable screening test in patients with FUO.

Multiple blood samples should be cultured in the laboratory long enough to ensure ample growth time for any fastidious organisms, such as HACEK organisms. It is critical to inform the laboratory of the intent to test for unusual organisms. Specialized media should be used when the history suggests uncommon microorganisms, such as *Histoplasma* or *Legionella*. Performing more than three blood cultures or more than one urine culture is useless in patients with FUO in the absence of PDCs (e.g., a high level of clinical suspicion of endocarditis). Repeating blood or urine cultures is useful only when previously cultured samples were collected during antibiotic treatment or within 1 week after its discontinuation. FUO with headache should prompt microbiologic examination of cerebrospinal fluid (CSF) for organisms including herpes simplex virus (HSV; especially HSV-2), *Cryptococcus neoformans*, and *Mycobacterium tuberculosis*. In CNS tuberculosis, the CSF typically has elevated protein and lowered glucose concentrations, with a mononuclear pleocytosis. CSF protein levels range from 100 to 500 mg/dL in most patients, the CSF glucose concentration is <45 mg/dL in 80% of cases, and the usual CSF cell count is between 100 and 500 cells/μL.

Microbiologic serology should not be included in the diagnostic workup in patients without PDCs for specific infections. A TST is included in the obligatory investigations, but it may yield false-negative results in patients with miliary tuberculosis, malnutrition, or immunosuppression. Although the interferon γ release assay is less influenced by prior vaccination with bacille Calmette-Guérin or by infection with nontuberculous mycobacteria, its sensitivity is similar to that of the TST; a negative TST or interferon γ release assay therefore does not exclude a diagnosis of tuberculosis. Miliary tuberculosis is especially difficult to diagnose. Granulomatous disease in liver or bone marrow biopsy samples, for example, should always lead to a (re)consideration of this diagnosis. If miliary tuberculosis is suspected, liver biopsy for acid-fast smear, culture, and PCR probably still has the highest diagnostic yield; however, biopsies of bone marrow, lymph nodes, or other involved organs also can be considered.

The diagnostic yield of echocardiography, sinus radiography, radiologic or endoscopic evaluation of the gastrointestinal tract, and bronchoscopy is very low in the absence of PDCs. Therefore, these tests should not be used as screening procedures.

After identification of all PDCs retrieved from the history, physical examination, and obligatory tests, a limited list of the most probable diagnoses should be made. Since most investigations are helpful only for patients who have PDCs for the diagnoses sought, further diagnostic procedures should be limited to specific investigations aimed at confirming or excluding diseases on this list. In FUO, the

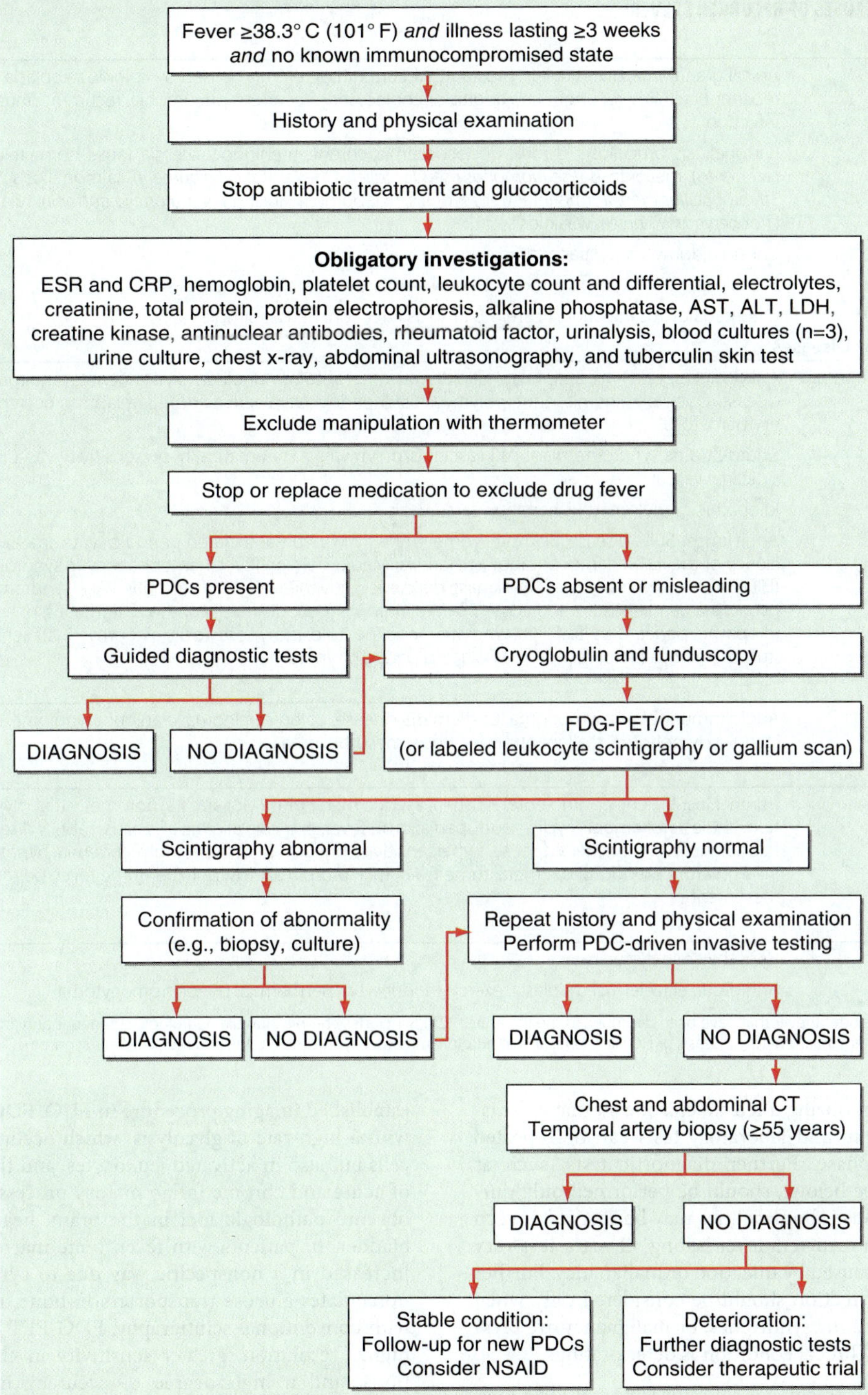

FIGURE 26-1 Structured approach to patients with FUO. ALT, alanine aminotransferase; AST, aspartate aminotransferase; CRP, C-reactive protein; ESR, erythrocyte sedimentation rate; FDG-PET/CT, ^{18}F-fluorodeoxyglucose positron emission tomography combined with low-dose computed tomography; LDH, lactate dehydrogenase; PDCs, potentially diagnostic clues (all localizing signs, symptoms, and abnormalities potentially pointing toward a diagnosis); NSAID, nonsteroidal anti-inflammatory drug.

diagnostic pointers are numerous and diverse but may be missed on initial examination, often being detected only by a very careful examination performed subsequently. In the absence of PDCs, the history and physical examination should therefore be repeated regularly. One of the first steps should be to rule out factitious or fraudulent fever, particularly in patients without signs of inflammation in laboratory tests. All medications, including nonprescription drugs and nutritional supplements, should be discontinued early in the evaluation to exclude drug fever. If fever persists beyond 72 h after discontinuation of the suspected drug, it is unlikely that this drug is the cause. In patients without PDCs or with only misleading PDCs, funduscopy by an ophthalmologist may be useful in the early stage of the diagnostic workup. When the first-stage diagnostic tests do not lead to a diagnosis, scintigraphy should be performed, especially when the ESR or CRP level is elevated.

Recurrent Fever In patients with recurrent fever, the diagnostic workup should consist of thorough history-taking, physical examination, and obligatory tests. The search for PDCs should be directed to clues matching known recurrent syndromes (Table 26-3). Patients

TABLE 26-3 ALL REPORTED CAUSES OF RECURRENT FEVER[a]

Infections	
Bacterial, nonspecific	Apical granuloma, diverticulitis, prostatitis, recurrent bacteremia caused by colonic neoplasia or persistent focal infection, recurrent cellulitis, recurrent cholangitis or cholecystitis, recurrent pneumonia, recurrent sinusitis, recurrent urinary tract infection
Bacterial, specific	Bartonellosis, brucellosis, chronic gonococcemia, chronic meningococcemia, louse-borne relapsing fever (*Borrelia recurrentis*), melioidosis (*Pseudomonas pseudomallei*), Q fever (*Coxiella burnetii*), salmonellosis, *Spirillum minor* infection, *Streptobacillus moniliformis* infection, syphilis, tick-borne relapsing fever (*Borrelia duttonii*), tularemia, Whipple's disease (*Tropheryma whipplei*), yersiniosis
Fungal	Coccidioidomycosis, paracoccidioidomycosis
Parasitic	Babesiosis, malaria, toxoplasmosis, trypanosomiasis, visceral leishmaniasis
Viral	Cytomegalovirus infection, Epstein-Barr virus infection, herpes simplex
Noninfectious Inflammatory Diseases	
Systemic rheumatic and autoimmune diseases	Ankylosing spondylitis, antiphospholipid syndrome, autoimmune hemolytic anemia, autoimmune hepatitis, Behçet's disease, cryoglobulinemia, gout, polymyositis, pseudogout, reactive arthritis, relapsing polychondritis, systemic lupus erythematosus
Vasculitis	Churg-Strauss syndrome, giant cell vasculitis/polymyalgia rheumatica, hypersensitivity vasculitis, polyarteritis nodosa, urticarial vasculitis
Granulomatous diseases	Idiopathic granulomatous hepatitis, sarcoidosis
Autoinflammatory syndromes	Adult-onset Still's disease, Blau syndrome, CAPS[b] (cryopyrin-associated periodic syndrome), Crohn's disease, DIRA (deficiency of the IL-1 receptor antagonist), familial Mediterranean fever, hemophagocytic syndrome, hyper-IgD syndrome (HIDS, also known as mevalonate kinase deficiency), juvenile idiopathic arthritis, PAPA syndrome (pyogenic sterile arthritis, pyoderma gangrenosum, and acne), PFAPA syndrome (periodic fever, aphthous stomatitis, pharyngitis, adenitis), recurrent idiopathic pericarditis, SAPHO (synovitis, acne, pustulosis, hyperostosis, osteomyelitis), Schnitzler's syndrome, TRAPS (tumor necrosis factor receptor–associated periodic syndrome)
Neoplasms	
	Angioimmunoblastic lymphoma, Castleman's disease, colon carcinoma, craniopharyngioma, Hodgkin's disease, non-Hodgkin lymphoma, malignant histiocytosis, mesothelioma
Miscellaneous	
	Adrenal insufficiency, aortic-enteral fistula, aseptic meningitis (Mollaret's syndrome), atrial myxoma, brewer's yeast ingestion, cholesterol emboli, cyclic neutropenia, drug fever, extrinsic allergic alveolitis, Fabry's disease, factitious disease, fraudulent fever, Gaucher's disease, hypersensitivity pneumonitis, hypertriglyceridemia, hypothalamic hypopituitarism, inflammatory pseudotumor, metal fume fever, milk protein allergy, polymer fume fever, pulmonary embolism, sclerosing mesenteritis
Thermoregulatory Disorders	
Central	Hypothalamic dysfunction
Peripheral	Anhidrotic ectodermal dysplasia, exercise-induced hyperthermia, pheochromocytoma

[a]This table includes all causes of recurrent fever that have been described in the literature. [b]CAPS includes chronic infantile neurologic cutaneous and articular syndrome (CINCA, also known as neonatal-onset multisystem inflammatory disease, or NOMID), familial cold autoinflammatory syndrome (FCAS), and Muckle-Wells syndrome.

should be asked to return during a febrile episode so that the history, physical examination, and laboratory tests can be repeated during a symptomatic phase. Further diagnostic tests, such as scintigraphic imaging (see below), should be performed only during a febrile episode because abnormalities may be absent between episodes. In patients with recurrent fever lasting >2 years, it is very unlikely that the fever is caused by infection or malignancy. Further diagnostic tests in that direction should be considered only when PDCs for infections, vasculitis syndromes, or malignancy are present or when the patient's clinical condition is deteriorating.

Scintigraphy Scintigraphic imaging is a noninvasive method allowing delineation of foci in all parts of the body on the basis of functional changes in tissues. This procedure plays an important role in the diagnosis of patients with FUO in clinical practice. Conventional scintigraphic methods used in clinical practice are ^{67}Ga-citrate scintigraphy and ^{111}In- or ^{99m}Tc-labeled leukocyte scintigraphy. Focal infectious and inflammatory processes can also be detected by several radiologic techniques, such as CT, MRI, and ultrasound. However, because of the lack of substantial pathologic changes in the early phase, infectious and inflammatory foci cannot be detected at this time. Furthermore, distinguishing active infectious or inflammatory lesions from residual changes due to cured processes or surgery remains critical. Finally, CT and MRI routinely provide information only on part of the body, while scintigraphy readily allows whole-body imaging.

Fluorodeoxyglucose Positron Emission Tomography ^{18}F-fluorodeoxyglucose (FDG) positron emission tomography (PET) has become an established imaging procedure in FUO. FDG accumulates in tissues with a high rate of glycolysis, which occurs not only in malignant cells but also in activated leukocytes, and thus permits the imaging of acute and chronic inflammatory processes. Normal uptake may obscure pathologic foci in the brain, heart, bowel, kidneys, and bladder. In patients with fever, bone marrow uptake is frequently increased in a nonspecific way due to cytokine activation, which upregulates glucose transporters in bone marrow cells. Compared with conventional scintigraphy, FDG-PET offers the advantages of higher resolution, greater sensitivity in chronic low-grade infections, and a high degree of accuracy in the central skeleton. Furthermore, vascular uptake of FDG is increased in patients with vasculitis. The mechanisms responsible for FDG uptake do not allow differentiation among infection, sterile inflammation, and malignancy. However, in patients with FUO, since all of these disorders are causes of FUO, FDG-PET can be used to guide additional diagnostic tests (e.g., targeted biopsies) that may yield the final diagnosis. Improved anatomic resolution by direct integration with CT (FDG-PET/CT) has further improved the accuracy of this modality.

Overall rates of helpfulness in final diagnosis of FUO are 40% for FDG-PET and 54% for FDG-PET/CT. In one study, FDG-PET was never helpful in diagnosing FUO in patients with a normal CRP level and a normal ESR. In two prospective studies in patients with FUO, FDG-PET was superior to ^{67}Ga-citrate scintigraphy, with a similar or better diagnostic yield and results that were available within hours instead of days. In one study, the sensitivity of FDG-PET was greater than that of ^{111}In-granulocyte scintigraphy (86% vs 20%) in patients with FUO.

Although scintigraphic techniques do not directly provide a definitive diagnosis, they often identify the anatomic location of a particular ongoing metabolic process and, with the help of other techniques such as biopsy and culture, facilitate timely diagnosis and treatment. Pathologic FDG uptake is quickly eradicated by treatment with glucocorticoids in many diseases, including vasculitis and lymphoma; therefore, glucocorticoid use should be stopped or postponed until after FDG-PET is performed. Results reported in the literature and the advantages offered by FDG-PET indicate that conventional scintigraphic techniques should be replaced by FDG-PET/CT in the investigation of patients with FUO at institutions where this technique is available. FDG-PET/CT is a relatively expensive procedure whose availability is still limited compared with that of CT and conventional scintigraphy. Nevertheless, FDG-PET/CT can be cost-effective in the FUO diagnostic workup if used at an early stage, helping to establish an early diagnosis, reducing days of hospitalization for diagnostic purposes, and obviating unnecessary and unhelpful tests.

LATER-STAGE DIAGNOSTIC TESTS

In some cases, more invasive tests are appropriate. Abnormalities found with scintigraphic techniques often need to be confirmed by pathology and/or culture of biopsy specimens. If lymphadenopathy is found, lymph node biopsy is necessary, even when the affected lymph nodes are hard to reach. In the case of skin lesions, skin biopsy should be undertaken. In one study, pulmonary wedge excision, histologic examination of an excised tonsil, and biopsy of the peritoneum were performed in light of PDCs or abnormal FDG-PET results and yielded a diagnosis.

If no diagnosis is reached despite scintigraphic and PDC-driven histologic investigations or culture, second-stage screening diagnostic tests should be considered (Fig. 26-1). In three studies, the diagnostic yield of screening chest and abdominal CT in patients with FUO was ~20%. The specificity of chest CT was ~80%, but that of abdominal CT varied between 63% and 80%. Despite the relatively limited specificity of abdominal CT and the probably limited additional value of chest CT after normal FDG-PET, chest and abdominal CT may be used as screening procedures at a later stage of the diagnostic protocol because of their noninvasive nature and high sensitivity. Bone marrow aspiration is seldom useful in the absence of PDCs for bone marrow disorders. With addition of FDG-PET, which is very sensitive in detecting lymphoma, carcinoma, and osteomyelitis, the value of bone marrow biopsy as a screening procedure is probably further reduced. Several studies have shown a high prevalence of giant cell arteritis among patients with FUO, with rates up to 17% among elderly patients. Giant cell arteritis often involves large arteries and in most cases can be diagnosed by FDG-PET. However, temporal artery biopsy is still recommended for patients ≥55 years of age in a later stage of the diagnostic protocol: FDG-PET will not be useful in vasculitis limited to the temporal arteries because of the small diameter of these vessels and the high levels of FDG uptake in the brain that overlies them. In the past, liver biopsies have often been performed as a screening procedure in patients with FUO. In each of two recent studies, liver biopsy as part of the later stage of a screening diagnostic protocol was helpful in only one patient. Moreover, abnormal liver tests are not predictive of a diagnostic liver biopsy in FUO. Liver biopsy is an invasive procedure that carries the possibility of complications and even death. Therefore, it should not be used for screening purposes in patients with FUO except in those with PDCs for liver disease.

In patients with unexplained fever after all of the above procedures, the last step in the diagnostic workup—with only a marginal diagnostic yield—comes at an extraordinarily high cost in terms of both expense and discomfort for the patient. Repetition of a thorough history-taking and physical examination and review of laboratory results and imaging studies (including those from other hospitals) are recommended. Diagnostic delay often results from a failure to recognize PDCs in the available information. In these patients with persisting FUO, waiting for new PDCs to appear probably is better than ordering more screening investigations. Only when a patient's condition deteriorates without providing new PDCs should a further diagnostic workup be performed.

TREATMENT FEVER OF UNKNOWN ORIGIN

Empirical therapeutic trials with antibiotics, glucocorticoids, or antituberculous agents should be avoided in FUO except when a patient's condition is rapidly deteriorating after the aforementioned diagnostic tests have failed to provide a definite diagnosis.

ANTIBIOTICS AND ANTITUBERCULOUS THERAPY

Antibiotic or antituberculous therapy may irrevocably diminish the ability to culture fastidious bacteria or mycobacteria. However, hemodynamic instability or neutropenia is a good indication for empirical antibiotic therapy. If the TST is positive or if granulomatous disease is present with anergy and sarcoidosis seems unlikely, a therapeutic trial for tuberculosis should be started. Especially in miliary tuberculosis, it may be very difficult to obtain a rapid diagnosis. If the fever does not respond after 6 weeks of empirical antituberculous treatment, another diagnosis should be considered.

COLCHICINE, NONSTEROIDAL ANTI-INFLAMMATORY DRUGS, AND GLUCOCORTICOIDS

Colchicine is highly effective in preventing attacks of familial Mediterranean fever but is not always effective once an attack is well under way. When familial Mediterranean fever is suspected, the response to colchicine is not a completely reliable diagnostic tool in the acute phase, but with colchicine treatment most patients show remarkable improvements in the frequency and severity of subsequent febrile episodes within weeks to months. If the fever persists and the source remains elusive after completion of the later-stage investigations, supportive treatment with nonsteroidal anti-inflammatory drugs (NSAIDs) can be helpful. The response of adult-onset Still's disease to NSAIDs is dramatic in some cases. The effects of glucocorticoids on giant cell arteritis and polymyalgia rheumatica are equally impressive. Early empirical trials with glucocorticoids, however, decrease the chances of reaching a diagnosis for which more specific and sometimes life-saving treatment might be more appropriate, such as malignant lymphoma. The ability of NSAIDs and glucocorticoids to mask fever while permitting the spread of infection or lymphoma dictates that their use should be avoided unless infectious diseases and malignant lymphoma have been largely ruled out and inflammatory disease is probable and is likely to be debilitating or threatening.

ANAKINRA

Interleukin (IL) 1 is a key cytokine in local and systemic inflammation and the febrile response. The availability of specific IL-1-targeting agents has revealed a pathologic role of IL-1-mediated inflammation in a growing list of diseases. Anakinra, a recombinant form of the naturally occurring IL-1 receptor antagonist (IL-1Ra), blocks the activity of both IL-1α and IL-1β. Anakinra is extremely effective in the treatment of many autoinflammatory syndromes, such as familial Mediterranean fever, cryopyrin-associated periodic syndrome, tumor necrosis factor receptor–associated periodic syndrome, hyper-IgD syndrome, and Schnitzler's syndrome. There is a growing list of other chronic inflammatory disorders in which the reduction of IL-1 activity can be highly effective. A therapeutic trial with anakinra can be considered in patients whose FUO has not been diagnosed after later-stage diagnostic tests. Although most chronic inflammatory conditions without a known basis can be controlled with glucocorticoids, monotherapy with IL-1 blockade can provide improved control without the metabolic, immunologic, and gastrointestinal side effects of glucocorticoid administration.

PROGNOSIS

FUO-related mortality rates have continuously declined over recent decades. The majority of fevers are caused by treatable diseases, and the risk of death related to FUO is, of course, dependent on the underlying disease. In a study by our group (Table 26-1), none of 37 FUO patients without a diagnosis died during a follow-up period of at least 6 months; 4 of 36 patients with a diagnosis died during follow-up due to infection ($n = 1$) or malignancy ($n = 3$). Other studies have also shown that malignancy accounts for most FUO-related deaths. Non-Hodgkin's lymphoma carries a disproportionately high death toll. In nonmalignant FUO, fatality rates are very low. The good outcome in patients without a diagnosis confirms that potentially lethal occult diseases are very unusual and that empirical therapy with antibiotics, antituberculous agents, or glucocorticoids is rarely required in stable patients. In less affluent regions, infectious diseases are still a major cause of FUO, and outcomes may be different.

SECTION 3 NERVOUS SYSTEM DYSFUNCTION

27 Syncope

Roy Freeman

Syncope is a transient, self-limited loss of consciousness due to acute global impairment of cerebral blood flow. The onset is rapid, duration brief, and recovery spontaneous and complete. Other causes of transient loss of consciousness need to be distinguished from syncope; these include seizures, vertebrobasilar ischemia, hypoxemia, and hypoglycemia. A syncopal prodrome (*presyncope*) is common, although loss of consciousness may occur without any warning symptoms. Typical presyncopal symptoms include dizziness, lightheadedness or faintness, weakness, fatigue, and visual and auditory disturbances. The causes of syncope can be divided into three general categories: (1) neurally mediated syncope (also called *reflex or vasovagal syncope*), (2) orthostatic hypotension, and (3) cardiac syncope.

Neurally mediated syncope comprises a heterogeneous group of functional disorders that are characterized by a transient change in the reflexes responsible for maintaining cardiovascular homeostasis. Episodic vasodilation (or loss of vasoconstrictor tone) and bradycardia occur in varying combinations, resulting in temporary failure of blood pressure control. In contrast, in patients with orthostatic hypotension due to autonomic failure, these cardiovascular homeostatic reflexes are chronically impaired. Cardiac syncope may be due to arrhythmias or structural cardiac diseases that cause a decrease in cardiac output. The clinical features, underlying pathophysiologic mechanisms, therapeutic interventions, and prognoses differ markedly among these three causes.

EPIDEMIOLOGY AND NATURAL HISTORY

Syncope is a common presenting problem, accounting for approximately 3% of all emergency room visits and 1% of all hospital admissions. The annual cost for syncope-related hospitalization in the United States is ~$2.4 billion. Syncope has a lifetime cumulative incidence of up to 35% in the general population. The peak incidence in the young occurs between ages 10 and 30 years, with a median peak around 15 years. Neurally mediated syncope is the etiology in the vast majority of these cases. In elderly adults, there is a sharp rise in the incidence of syncope after 70 years.

In population-based studies, neurally mediated syncope is the most common cause of syncope. The incidence is slightly higher in females than males. In young subjects, there is often a family history in first-degree relatives. Cardiovascular disease due to structural disease or arrhythmias is the next most common cause in most series, particularly in emergency room settings and in older patients. Orthostatic hypotension also increases in prevalence with age because of the reduced baroreflex responsiveness, decreased cardiac compliance, and attenuation of the vestibulosympathetic reflex associated with aging. In the elderly, orthostatic hypotension is substantially more common in institutionalized (54–68%) than community-dwelling (6%) individuals, an observation most likely explained by the greater prevalence of predisposing neurologic disorders, physiologic impairment, and vasoactive medication use among institutionalized patients.

TABLE 27-1 HIGH-RISK FEATURES INDICATING HOSPITALIZATION OR INTENSIVE EVALUATION OF SYNCOPE

Chest pain suggesting coronary ischemia
Features of congestive heart failure
Moderate or severe valvular disease
Moderate or severe structural cardiac disease
Electrocardiographic features of ischemia
History of ventricular arrhythmias
Prolonged QT interval (>500 ms)
Repetitive sinoatrial block or sinus pauses
Persistent sinus bradycardia
Bi- or trifascicular block or intraventricular conduction delay with QRS duration≥120 ms
Atrial fibrillation
Nonsustained ventricular tachycardia
Family history of sudden death
Preexcitation syndromes
Brugada pattern on ECG
Palpitations at time of syncope
Syncope at rest or during exercise

The prognosis after a single syncopal event for all age groups is generally benign. In particular, syncope of noncardiac and unexplained origin in younger individuals has an excellent prognosis; life expectancy is unaffected. By contrast, syncope due to a cardiac cause, either structural heart disease or primary arrhythmic disease, is associated with an increased risk of sudden cardiac death and mortality from other causes. Similarly, mortality rate is increased in individuals with syncope due to orthostatic hypotension related to age and the associated comorbid conditions (Table 27-1).

PATHOPHYSIOLOGY

The upright posture imposes a unique physiologic stress upon humans; most, although not all, syncopal episodes occur from a standing position. Standing results in pooling of 500–1000 mL of blood in the lower extremities and splanchnic circulation. There is a decrease in venous return to the heart and reduced ventricular filling that result in diminished cardiac output and blood pressure. These hemodynamic changes provoke a compensatory reflex response, initiated by the baroreceptors in the carotid sinus and aortic arch, resulting in increased sympathetic outflow and decreased vagal nerve activity (Fig. 27-1). The reflex increases peripheral resistance, venous return to the heart, and cardiac output and thus limits the fall in blood pressure. If this response fails, as is the case chronically in orthostatic hypotension and transiently in neurally mediated syncope, cerebral hypoperfusion occurs.

Syncope is a consequence of global cerebral hypoperfusion and thus represents a failure of cerebral blood flow autoregulatory mechanisms.

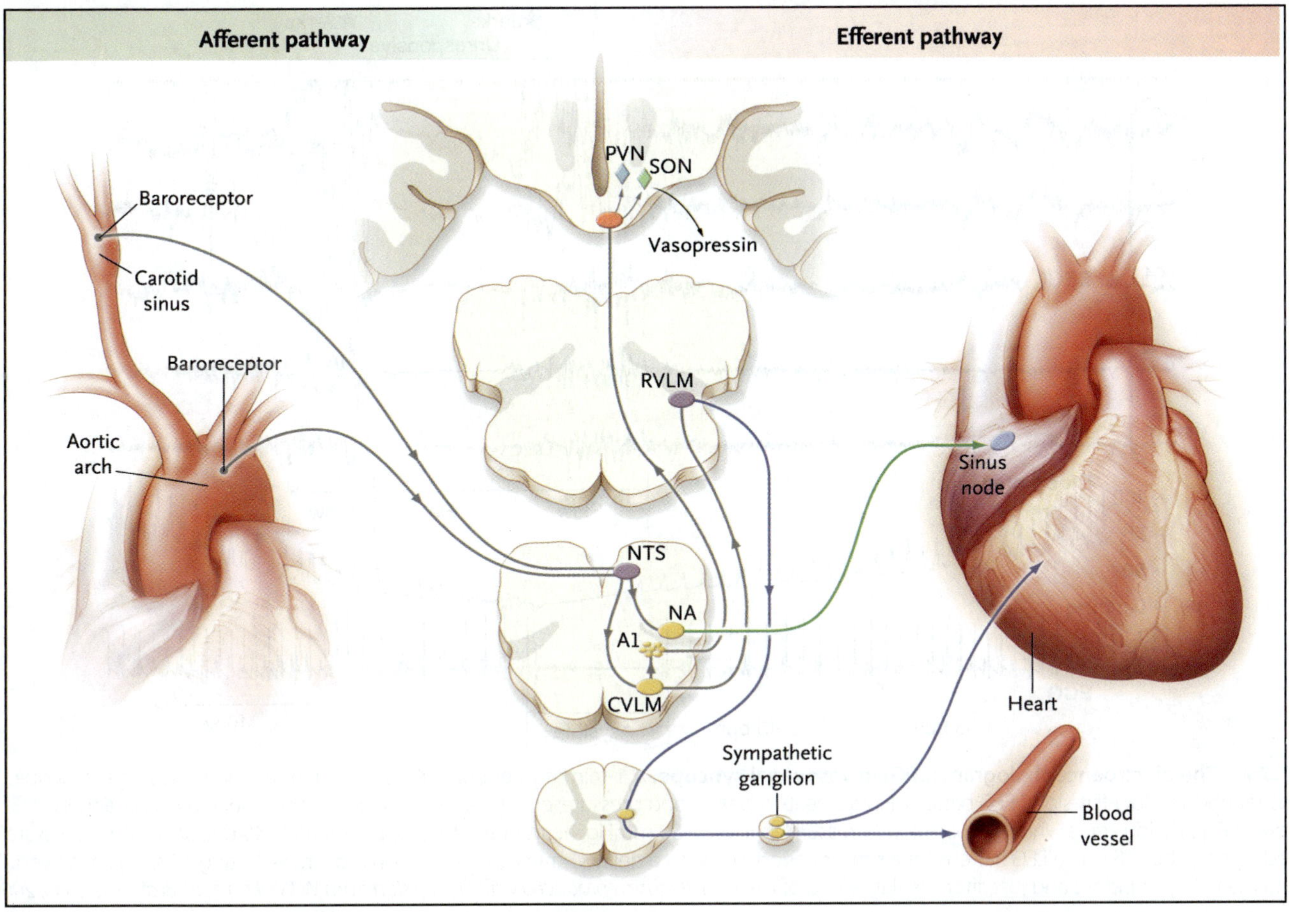

FIGURE 27-1 The baroreflex. A decrease in arterial pressure unloads the baroreceptors—the terminals of afferent fibers of the glossopharyngeal and vagus nerves—that are situated in the carotid sinus and aortic arch. This leads to a reduction in the afferent impulses that are relayed from these mechanoreceptors through the glossopharyngeal and vagus nerves to the nucleus of the tractus solitarius (NTS) in the dorsomedial medulla. The reduced baroreceptor afferent activity produces a decrease in vagal nerve input to the sinus node that is mediated via connections of the NTS to the nucleus ambiguus (NA). There is an increase in sympathetic efferent activity that is mediated by the NTS projections to the caudal ventrolateral medulla (CVLM) (an excitatory pathway) and from there to the rostral ventrolateral medulla (RVLM) (an inhibitory pathway). The activation of RVLM presympathetic neurons in response to hypotension is thus predominantly due to disinhibition. In response to a sustained fall in blood pressure, vasopressin release is mediated by projections from the A1 noradrenergic cell group in the ventrolateral medulla. This projection activates vasopressin-synthesizing neurons in the magnocellular portion of the paraventricular nucleus (PVN) and the supraoptic nucleus (SON) of the hypothalamus. *Blue* denotes sympathetic neurons, and *green* denotes parasympathetic neurons. *(From R Freeman: N Engl J Med 358:615, 2008.)*

Myogenic factors, local metabolites, and to a lesser extent autonomic neurovascular control are responsible for the autoregulation of cerebral blood flow (Chap. 330). The latency of the autoregulatory response is 5–10 s. Typically cerebral blood flow ranges from 50 to 60 mL/min per 100 g brain tissue and remains relatively constant over perfusion pressures ranging from 50 to 150 mmHg. Cessation of blood flow for 6–8 s will result in loss of consciousness, while impairment of consciousness ensues when blood flow decreases to 25 mL/min per 100 g brain tissue.

From the clinical standpoint, a fall in systemic systolic blood pressure to ~50 mmHg or lower will result in syncope. A decrease in cardiac output and/or systemic vascular resistance—the determinants of blood pressure—thus underlies the pathophysiology of syncope. Common causes of impaired cardiac output include decreased effective circulating blood volume; increased thoracic pressure; massive pulmonary embolus; cardiac brady- and tachyarrhythmias; valvular heart disease; and myocardial dysfunction. Systemic vascular resistance may be decreased by central and peripheral autonomic nervous system diseases, sympatholytic medications, and transiently during neurally mediated syncope. Increased cerebral vascular resistance, most frequently due to hypocarbia induced by hyperventilation, may also contribute to the pathophysiology of syncope.

Two patterns of electroencephalographic (EEG) changes occur in syncopal subjects. The first is a "slow-flat-slow" pattern (Fig. 27-2) in which normal background activity is replaced with high-amplitude slow delta waves. This is followed by sudden flattening of the EEG—a cessation or attenuation of cortical activity—followed by the return of slow waves, and then normal activity. A second pattern, the "slow pattern," is characterized by increasing and decreasing slow wave activity only. The EEG flattening that occurs in the slow-flat-slow pattern is a marker of more severe cerebral hypoperfusion. Despite the presence of myoclonic movements and other motor activity during some syncopal events, EEG seizure discharges are not detected.

CLASSIFICATION

NEURALLY MEDIATED SYNCOPE

Neurally mediated (reflex; vasovagal) syncope is the final pathway of a complex central and peripheral nervous system reflex arc. There is a sudden, transient change in autonomic efferent activity with increased parasympathetic outflow, plus sympathoinhibition (the vasodepressor response), resulting in bradycardia, vasodilation, and/or reduced vasoconstrictor tone. The resulting fall in systemic blood pressure can then reduce cerebral blood flow to below the compensatory limits of autoregulation (Fig. 27-3). In order to elicit neutrally mediated syncope, a functioning autonomic nervous system is necessary, in contrast to syncope resulting from autonomic failure (discussed below).

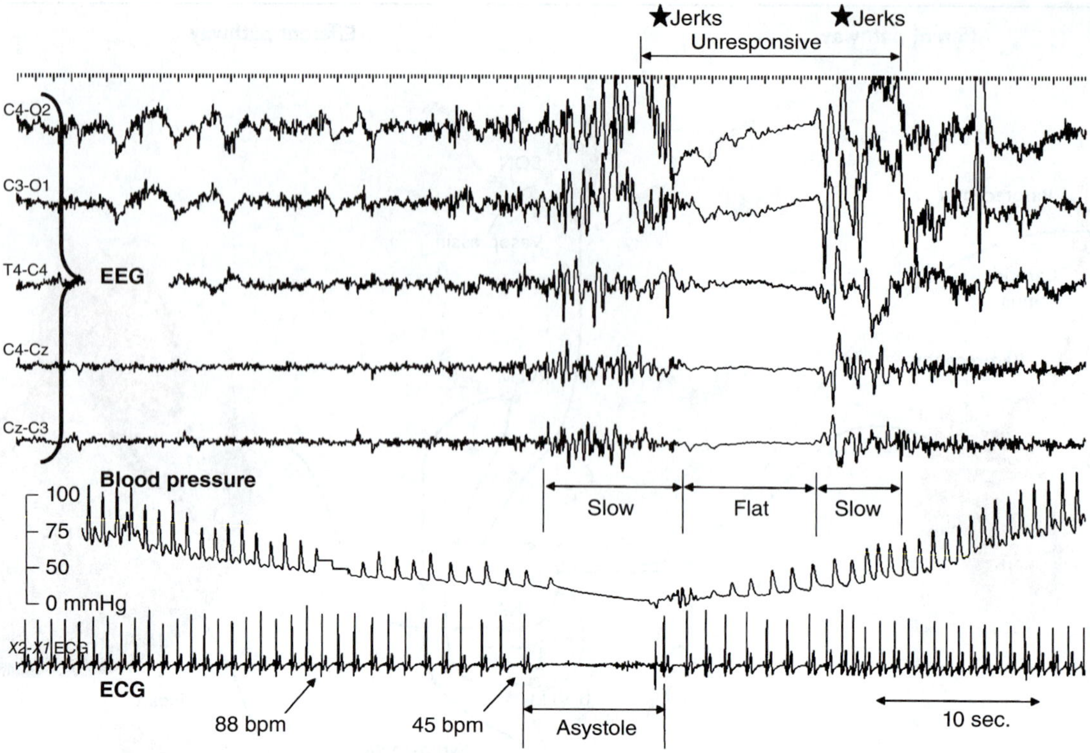

FIGURE 27-2 The electroencephalogram (EEG) in vasovagal syncope. A 1-min segment of a tilt-table test with typical vasovagal syncope demonstrating the "slow-flat-slow" EEG pattern. Finger beat-to-beat blood pressure, electrocardiogram (ECG), and selected EEG channels are shown. EEG slowing starts when systolic blood pressure drops to ~50 mmHg; heart rate is then approximately 45 beats/min (bpm). Asystole occurred, lasting about 8 s. The EEG flattens for a similar period, but with a delay. A transient loss of consciousness, lasting 14 s, was observed. There were muscle jerks just before and just after the flat period of the EEG. *(Figure reproduced with permission from W Wieling et al: Brain 132:2630, 2009.)*

Multiple triggers of the afferent limb of the reflex arc can result in neutrally mediated syncope. In some situations, these can be clearly defined, e.g., the carotid sinus, the gastrointestinal tract, or the bladder. Often, however, the trigger is less easily recognized and the cause is multifactorial. Under these circumstances, it is likely that different afferent pathways converge on the central autonomic network within the medulla that integrates the neural impulses and mediates the vasodepressor-bradycardic response.

Classification of Neurally Mediated Syncope Neurally mediated syncope may be subdivided based on the afferent pathway and provocative trigger. Vasovagal syncope (the common faint) is provoked by intense emotion, pain, and/or orthostatic stress, whereas the situational reflex syncopes have specific localized stimuli that provoke the reflex vasodilation and bradycardia that leads to syncope. The underlying mechanisms have been identified and pathophysiology delineated for most of these situational reflex syncopes. The afferent trigger may originate in the pulmonary system, gastrointestinal system, urogenital system, heart, and carotid artery (Table 27-2). Hyperventilation leading to hypocarbia and cerebral vasoconstriction, and raised intrathoracic pressure that impairs venous return to the heart, play a central role in many of the situational reflex syncopes. The afferent pathway of the reflex arc differs among these disorders, but the efferent response via the vagus and sympathetic pathways is similar.

Alternately, neurally mediated syncope may be subdivided based on the predominant efferent pathway. Vasodepressor syncope describes syncope predominantly due to efferent, sympathetic, vasoconstrictor failure; cardioinhibitory syncope describes syncope predominantly associated with bradycardia or asystole due

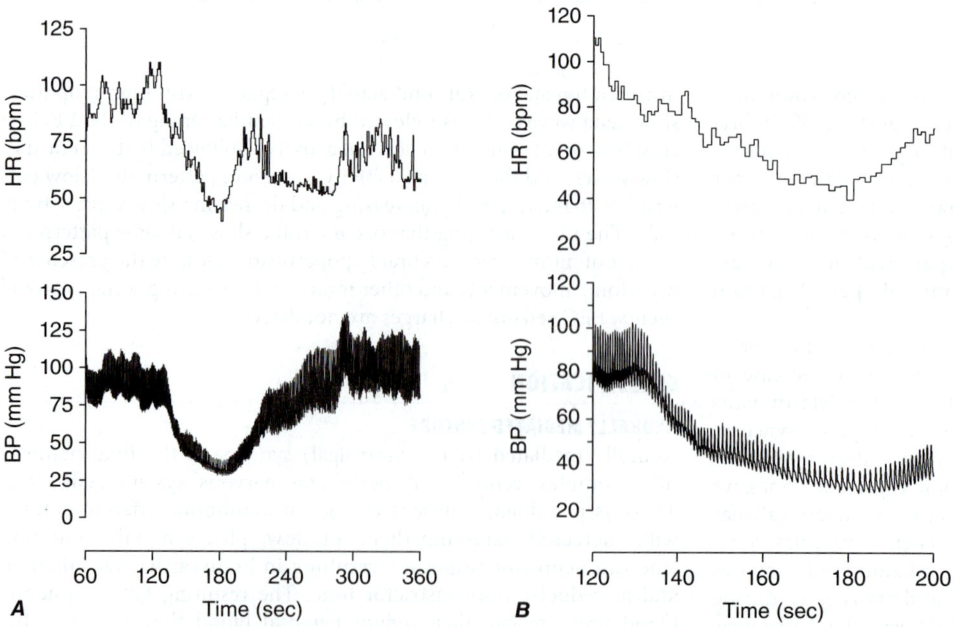

FIGURE 27-3 ***A.*** The paroxysmal hypotensive-bradycardic response that is characteristic of neurally mediated syncope. Noninvasive beat-to-beat blood pressure and heart rate are shown over 5 min (from 60 to 360 s) of an upright tilt on a tilt table. ***B.*** The same tracing expanded to show 80 s of the episode (from 80 to 200 s). BP, blood pressure; bpm, beats per minute; HR, heart rate.

TABLE 27-2 CAUSES OF SYNCOPE

A. Neurally Mediated Syncope

Vasovagal syncope

Provoked fear, pain, anxiety, intense emotion, sight of blood, unpleasant sights and odors, orthostatic stress

Situational reflex syncope

Pulmonary

Cough syncope, wind instrument player's syncope, weightlifter's syncope, "mess trick"[a] and "fainting lark,"[b] sneeze syncope, airway instrumentation

Urogenital

Postmicturition syncope, urogenital tract instrumentation, prostatic massage

Gastrointestinal

Swallow syncope, glossopharyngeal neuralgia, esophageal stimulation, gastrointestinal tract instrumentation, rectal examination, defecation syncope

Cardiac

Bezold-Jarisch reflex, cardiac outflow obstruction

Carotid sinus

Carotid sinus sensitivity, carotid sinus massage

Ocular

Ocular pressure, ocular examination, ocular surgery

B. Orthostatic Hypotension

Primary autonomic failure due to idiopathic central and peripheral neurodegenerative diseases—the "synucleinopathies"

Lewy body diseases

Parkinson's disease

Lewy body dementia

Pure autonomic failure

Multiple system atrophy (the Shy-Drager syndrome)

Secondary autonomic failure due to autonomic peripheral neuropathies

Diabetes

Hereditary amyloidosis (familial amyloid polyneuropathy)

Primary amyloidosis (AL amyloidosis; immunoglobulin light chain associated)

Hereditary sensory and autonomic neuropathies (HSAN) (especially type III—familial dysautonomia)

Idiopathic immune-mediated autonomic neuropathy

Autoimmune autonomic ganglionopathy

Sjögren's syndrome

Paraneoplastic autonomic neuropathy

HIV neuropathy

Postprandial hypotension

Iatrogenic (drug-induced)

Volume depletion

C. Cardiac Syncope

Arrhythmias

Sinus node dysfunction

Atrioventricular dysfunction

Supraventricular tachycardias

Ventricular tachycardias

Inherited channelopathies

Cardiac structural disease

Valvular disease

Myocardial ischemia

Obstructive and other cardiomyopathies

Atrial myxoma

Pericardial effusions and tamponade

[a]Hyperventilation for ~1 minute, followed by sudden chest compression. [b]Hyperventilation (~20 breaths) in a squatting position, rapid rise to standing, then Valsalva.

to increased vagal outflow; and mixed syncope describes syncope in which there are both vagal and sympathetic reflex changes.

Features of Neurally Mediated Syncope In addition to symptoms of orthostatic intolerance such as dizziness, lightheadedness, and fatigue, premonitory features of autonomic activation may be present in patients with neurally mediated syncope. These include diaphoresis, pallor, palpitations, nausea, hyperventilation, and yawning. During the syncopal event, proximal and distal myoclonus (typically arrhythmic and multifocal) may occur, raising the possibility of epilepsy. The eyes typically remain open and usually deviate upward. Pupils are usually dilated. Roving eye movements may occur. Grunting, moaning, snorting, and stertorous breathing may be present. Urinary incontinence may occur. Fecal incontinence is very rare. Postictal confusion is also rare, although visual and auditory hallucinations and near death and out-of-body experiences are sometimes reported.

Although some predisposing factors and provocative stimuli are well established (for example, motionless upright posture, warm ambient temperature, intravascular volume depletion, alcohol ingestion, hypoxemia, anemia, pain, the sight of blood, venipuncture, and intense emotion), the underlying basis for the widely different thresholds for syncope among individuals exposed to the same provocative stimulus is not known. A genetic basis for neurally mediated syncope may exist; several studies have reported an increased incidence of syncope in first-degree relatives of fainters, but no gene or genetic marker has been identified, and environmental, social, and cultural factors have not been excluded by these studies.

TREATMENT NEURALLY MEDIATED SYNCOPE

Reassurance, avoidance of provocative stimuli, and plasma volume expansion with fluid and salt are the cornerstones of the management of neurally mediated syncope. Isometric counterpressure maneuvers of the limbs (leg crossing or handgrip and arm tensing) may raise blood pressure by increasing central blood volume and cardiac output. By maintaining pressure in the autoregulatory zone, these maneuvers avoid or delay the onset of syncope. Randomized controlled trials support this intervention.

Fludrocortisone, vasoconstricting agents, and beta-adrenoreceptor antagonists are widely used by experts to treat refractory patients, although there is no consistent evidence from randomized controlled trials for any pharmacotherapy to treat neurally mediated syncope. Because vasodilation is the dominant pathophysiologic syncopal mechanism in most patients, use of a cardiac pacemaker is rarely beneficial. Possible exceptions are older patients (>40 years) in whom syncope is associated with asystole or severe bradycardia and patients with prominent cardioinhibition due to carotid sinus syndrome. In these patients, dual-chamber pacing may be helpful.

ORTHOSTATIC HYPOTENSION

Orthostatic hypotension, defined as a reduction in systolic blood pressure of at least 20 mmHg or diastolic blood pressure of at least 10 mmHg within 3 min of standing or head-up tilt on a tilt table, is a manifestation of sympathetic vasoconstrictor (autonomic) failure (Fig. 27-4). In many (but not all) cases, there is no compensatory increase in heart rate despite hypotension; with partial autonomic failure, heart rate may increase to some degree but is insufficient to maintain cardiac output. A variant of orthostatic hypotension is "delayed" orthostatic hypotension, which occurs beyond 3 min of standing; this may reflect a mild or early form of sympathetic adrenergic dysfunction. In some cases, orthostatic hypotension occurs within 15 s of standing (so-called "initial" orthostatic hypotension), a finding that may reflect a transient mismatch between cardiac output and peripheral vascular resistance and does not represent autonomic failure.

Characteristic symptoms of orthostatic hypotension include lightheadedness, dizziness, and presyncope (near-faintness) occurring in response to sudden postural change. However, symptoms may be

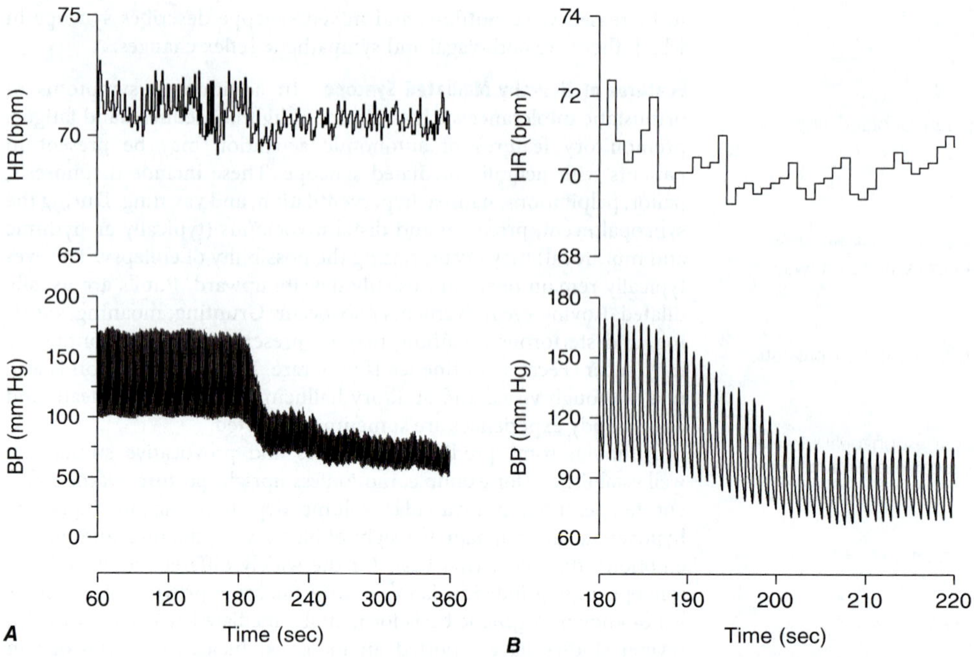

FIGURE 27-4 ***A.*** The gradual fall in blood pressure without a compensatory heart rate increase that is characteristic of orthostatic hypotension due to autonomic failure. Blood pressure and heart rate are shown over 5 min (from 60 to 360 s) of an upright tilt on a tilt table. ***B.*** The same tracing expanded to show 40 s of the episode (from 180 to 220 s). BP, blood pressure; bpm, beats per minute; HR, heart rate.

absent or nonspecific, such as generalized weakness, fatigue, cognitive slowing, leg buckling, or headache. Visual blurring may occur, likely due to retinal or occipital lobe ischemia. Neck pain, typically in the suboccipital, posterior cervical, and shoulder region (the "coat-hanger headache"), most likely due to neck muscle ischemia, may be the only symptom. Patients may report orthostatic dyspnea (thought to reflect ventilation-perfusion mismatch due to inadequate perfusion of ventilated lung apices) or angina (attributed to impaired myocardial perfusion even with normal coronary arteries). Symptoms may be exacerbated by exertion, prolonged standing, increased ambient temperature, or meals. Syncope is usually preceded by warning symptoms, but may occur suddenly, suggesting the possibility of a seizure or cardiac cause.

Supine hypertension is common in patients with orthostatic hypotension due to autonomic failure, affecting over 50% of patients in some series. Orthostatic hypotension may present after initiation of therapy for hypertension, and supine hypertension may follow treatment of orthostatic hypotension. However, in other cases, the association of the two conditions is unrelated to therapy; it may in part be explained by baroreflex dysfunction in the presence of residual sympathetic outflow, particularly in patients with central autonomic degeneration.

Causes of Neurogenic Orthostatic Hypotension Causes of neurogenic orthostatic hypotension include central and peripheral autonomic nervous system dysfunction (Chap. 454). Autonomic dysfunction of other organ systems (including the bladder, bowels, sexual organs, and sudomotor system) of varying severity frequently accompanies orthostatic hypotension in these disorders (Table 27-2).

The primary autonomic degenerative disorders are multiple system atrophy (the Shy-Drager syndrome; Chap. 454), Parkinson's disease (Chap. 449), dementia with Lewy bodies (Chap. 448), and pure autonomic failure (Chap. 454). These are often grouped together as "synucleinopathies" due to the presence of alpha-synuclein, a small protein that precipitates predominantly in the cytoplasm of neurons in the Lewy body disorders (Parkinson's disease, dementia with Lewy bodies, and pure autonomic failure) and in the glia in multiple system atrophy.

Peripheral autonomic dysfunction may also accompany small-fiber peripheral neuropathies such as those seen in diabetes, amyloid, immune-mediated neuropathies, hereditary sensory and autonomic neuropathies (HSAN; particularly HSAN type III, familial dysautonomia), and inflammatory neuropathies (Chaps. 459 and 460). Less frequently, orthostatic hypotension is associated with the peripheral neuropathies that accompany vitamin B_{12} deficiency, neurotoxic exposure, HIV and other infections, and porphyria.

Patients with autonomic failure and the elderly are susceptible to falls in blood pressure associated with meals. The magnitude of the blood pressure fall is exacerbated by large meals, meals high in carbohydrate, and alcohol intake. The mechanism of postprandial syncope is not fully elucidated.

Orthostatic hypotension is often iatrogenic. Drugs from several classes may lower peripheral resistance (e.g., alpha-adrenoreceptor antagonists used to treat hypertension and prostatic hypertrophy; antihypertensive agents of several classes; nitrates and other vasodilators; tricyclic agents and phenothiazines). Iatrogenic volume depletion due to diuresis and volume depletion due to medical causes (hemorrhage, vomiting, diarrhea, or decreased fluid intake) may also result in decreased effective circulatory volume, orthostatic hypotension, and syncope.

TREATMENT ORTHOSTATIC HYPOTENSION

The first step is to remove reversible causes—usually vasoactive medications (Table 454-6). Next, nonpharmacologic interventions should be introduced. These interventions include patient education regarding staged moves from supine to upright; warnings about the hypotensive effects of large meals; instructions about the isometric counterpressure maneuvers that increase intravascular pressure (see above); and raising the head of the bed to reduce supine hypertension. Intravascular volume should be expanded by increasing dietary fluid and salt. If these nonpharmacologic measures fail, pharmacologic intervention with fludrocortisone acetate and vasoconstricting agents such as midodrine, L-dihydroxyphenylserine, and pseudoephedrine should be introduced. Some patients with intractable symptoms require additional therapy with supplementary agents that include pyridostigmine, yohimbine, desmopressin acetate (DDAVP), and erythropoietin (Chap. 454).

CARDIAC SYNCOPE

Cardiac (or cardiovascular) syncope is caused by arrhythmias and structural heart disease. These may occur in combination because structural disease renders the heart more vulnerable to abnormal electrical activity.

Arrhythmias Bradyarrhythmias that cause syncope include those due to severe sinus node dysfunction (e.g., sinus arrest or sinoatrial block) and atrioventricular (AV) block (e.g., Mobitz type II, high-grade, and complete AV block). The bradyarrhythmias due to sinus node dysfunction are often associated with an atrial tachyarrhythmia, a disorder known as the tachycardia-bradycardia syndrome. A prolonged pause following the termination of a tachycardic episode is a frequent cause of syncope in patients with the tachycardia-bradycardia syndrome. Medications of several classes may also cause bradyarrhythmias of sufficient severity to cause syncope. Syncope due to bradycardia or asystole is referred to as a Stokes-Adams attack.

Ventricular tachyarrhythmias frequently cause syncope. The likelihood of syncope with ventricular tachycardia is in part dependent on the ventricular rate; rates below 200 beats/min are less likely to cause syncope. The compromised hemodynamic function during ventricular tachycardia is caused by ineffective ventricular contraction, reduced diastolic filling due to abbreviated filling periods, loss of AV synchrony, and concurrent myocardial ischemia.

Several disorders associated with cardiac electrophysiologic instability and arrhythmogenesis are due to mutations in ion channel subunit genes. These include the long QT syndrome, Brugada syndrome, and catecholaminergic polymorphic ventricular tachycardia. The long QT syndrome is a genetically heterogeneous disorder associated with prolonged cardiac repolarization and a predisposition to ventricular arrhythmias. Syncope and sudden death in patients with long QT syndrome result from a unique polymorphic ventricular tachycardia called *torsades des pointes* that degenerates into ventricular fibrillation. The long QT syndrome has been linked to genes encoding K^+ channel α-subunits, K^+ channel β-subunits, voltage-gated Na^+ channel, and a scaffolding protein, ankyrin B (ANK2). Brugada syndrome is characterized by idiopathic ventricular fibrillation in association with right ventricular electrocardiogram (ECG) abnormalities without structural heart disease. This disorder is also genetically heterogeneous, although it is most frequently linked to mutations in the Na^+ channel α-subunit, SCN5A. Catecholaminergic polymorphic tachycardia is an inherited, genetically heterogeneous disorder associated with exercise- or stress-induced ventricular arrhythmias, syncope, or sudden death. Acquired QT interval prolongation, most commonly due to drugs, may also result in ventricular arrhythmias and syncope. **These disorders are discussed in detail in Chap. 277.**

Structural Disease Structural heart disease (e.g., valvular disease, myocardial ischemia, hypertrophic and other cardiomyopathies, cardiac masses such as atrial myxoma, and pericardial effusions) may lead to syncope by compromising cardiac output. Structural disease may also contribute to other pathophysiologic mechanisms of syncope. For example, cardiac structural disease may predispose to arrhythmogenesis; aggressive treatment of cardiac failure with diuretics and/or vasodilators may lead to orthostatic hypotension; and inappropriate reflex vasodilation may occur with structural disorders such as aortic stenosis and hypertrophic cardiomyopathy, possibly provoked by increased ventricular contractility.

TREATMENT CARDIAC SYNCOPE

Treatment of cardiac disease depends on the underlying disorder. Therapies for arrhythmias include cardiac pacing for sinus node disease and AV block, and ablation, antiarrhythmic drugs, and cardioverter-defibrillators for atrial and ventricular tachyarrhythmias. These disorders are best managed by physicians with specialized skills in this area.

APPROACH TO THE PATIENT: Syncope

DIFFERENTIAL DIAGNOSIS

Syncope is easily diagnosed when the characteristic features are present; however, several disorders with transient real or apparent loss of consciousness may create diagnostic confusion.

Generalized and partial seizures may be confused with syncope; however, there are a number of differentiating features. Whereas tonic-clonic movements are the hallmark of a generalized seizure, myoclonic and other movements also may occur in up to 90% of syncopal episodes. Myoclonic jerks associated with syncope may be multifocal or generalized. They are typically arrhythmic and of short duration (<30 s). Mild flexor and extensor posturing also may occur. Partial or partial-complex seizures with secondary generalization are usually preceded by an aura, commonly an unpleasant smell; fear; anxiety; abdominal discomfort; or other visceral sensations. These phenomena should be differentiated from the premonitory features of syncope.

Autonomic manifestations of seizures (autonomic epilepsy) may provide a more difficult diagnostic challenge. Autonomic seizures have cardiovascular, gastrointestinal, pulmonary, urogenital, pupillary, and cutaneous manifestations that are similar to the premonitory features of syncope. Furthermore, the cardiovascular manifestations of autonomic epilepsy include clinically significant tachycardias and bradycardias that may be of sufficient magnitude to cause loss of consciousness. The presence of accompanying non-autonomic auras may help differentiate these episodes from syncope.

Loss of consciousness associated with a seizure usually lasts longer than 5 min and is associated with prolonged postictal drowsiness and disorientation, whereas reorientation occurs almost immediately after a syncopal event. Muscle aches may occur after both syncope and seizures, although they tend to last longer and be more severe following a seizure. Seizures, unlike syncope, are rarely provoked by emotions or pain. Incontinence of urine may occur with both seizures and syncope; however, fecal incontinence occurs very rarely with syncope.

Hypoglycemia may cause transient loss of consciousness, typically in individuals with type 1 or type 2 diabetes treated with insulin. The clinical features associated with impending or actual hypoglycemia include tremor, palpitations, anxiety, diaphoresis, hunger, and paresthesias. These symptoms are due to autonomic activation to counter the falling blood glucose. Hunger, in particular, is not a typical premonitory feature of syncope. Hypoglycemia also impairs neuronal function, leading to fatigue, weakness, dizziness, and cognitive and behavioral symptoms. Diagnostic difficulties may occur in individuals in strict glycemic control; repeated hypoglycemia impairs the counterregulatory response and leads to a loss of the characteristic warning symptoms that are the hallmark of hypoglycemia.

Patients with cataplexy experience an abrupt partial or complete loss of muscular tone triggered by strong emotions, typically anger or laughter. Unlike syncope, consciousness is maintained throughout the attacks, which typically last between 30 s and 2 min. There are no premonitory symptoms. Cataplexy occurs in 60–75% of patients with narcolepsy.

The clinical interview and interrogation of eyewitnesses usually allow differentiation of syncope from falls due to vestibular dysfunction, cerebellar disease, extrapyramidal system dysfunction, and other gait disorders. If the fall is accompanied by head trauma, a postconcussive syndrome, amnesia for the precipitating events, and/or the presence of loss of consciousness may contribute to diagnostic difficulty.

Apparent loss of consciousness can be a manifestation of psychiatric disorders such as generalized anxiety, panic disorders, major depression, and somatization disorder. These possibilities should be considered in individuals who faint frequently without prodromal symptoms. Such patients are rarely injured despite numerous falls. There are no clinically significant hemodynamic changes concurrent with these episodes. In contrast, transient loss of consciousness due to vasovagal syncope precipitated by fear, stress, anxiety, and emotional distress is accompanied by hypotension, bradycardia, or both.

INITIAL EVALUATION

The goals of the initial evaluation are to determine whether the transient loss of consciousness was due to syncope; to identify the cause; and to assess risk for future episodes and serious harm (Table 27-1). The initial evaluation should include a detailed history, thorough questioning of eyewitnesses, and a complete physical and neurologic examination. Blood pressure and heart rate should be measured in the supine position and after 3 min of standing to determine whether orthostatic hypotension is present. An ECG should be performed if there is suspicion of syncope due to an arrhythmia or underlying cardiac disease. Relevant electrocardiographic abnormalities include bradyarrhythmias or tachyarrhythmias, AV block, ischemia, old myocardial infarction, long QT syndrome, and bundle branch block. This initial assessment will lead to the identification of a cause of syncope in approximately

50% of patients and also allows stratification of patients at risk for cardiac mortality.

Laboratory Tests Baseline laboratory blood tests are rarely helpful in identifying the cause of syncope. Blood tests should be performed when specific disorders, e.g., myocardial infarction, anemia, and secondary autonomic failure, are suspected (Table 27-2).

Autonomic Nervous System Testing (Chap. 454) Autonomic testing, including tilt-table testing, can be performed in specialized centers. Autonomic testing is helpful to uncover objective evidence of autonomic failure and also to demonstrate a predisposition to neurally mediated syncope. Autonomic testing includes assessments of parasympathetic autonomic nervous system function (e.g., heart rate variability to deep respiration and a Valsalva maneuver), sympathetic cholinergic function (e.g., thermoregulatory sweat response and quantitative sudomotor axon reflex test), and sympathetic adrenergic function (e.g., blood pressure response to a Valsalva maneuver and a tilt-table test with beat-to-beat blood pressure measurement). The hemodynamic abnormalities demonstrated on tilt-table test (Figs. 27-3 and 27-4) may be useful in distinguishing orthostatic hypotension due to autonomic failure from the hypotensive bradycardic response of neurally mediated syncope. Similarly, the tilt-table test may help identify patients with syncope due to immediate or delayed orthostatic hypotension.

Carotid sinus massage should be considered in patients with symptoms suggestive of carotid sinus syncope and in patients over age 50 years with recurrent syncope of unknown etiology. This test should only be carried out under continuous ECG and blood pressure monitoring and should be avoided in patients with carotid bruits, plaques, or stenosis.

Cardiac Evaluation ECG monitoring is indicated for patients with a high pretest probability of arrhythmia causing syncope. Patients should be monitored in hospital if the likelihood of a life-threatening arrhythmia is high, e.g., patients with severe structural or coronary artery disease, nonsustained ventricular tachycardia, trifascicular heart block, prolonged QT interval, Brugada syndrome ECG pattern, or family history of sudden cardiac death (Table 27-1). Outpatient Holter monitoring is recommended for patients who experience frequent syncopal episodes (one or more per week), whereas loop recorders, which continually record and erase cardiac rhythm, are indicated for patients with suspected arrhythmias with low risk of sudden cardiac death. Loop recorders may be external (recommended for evaluation of episodes that occur at a frequency of greater than one per month) or implantable (if syncope occurs less frequently).

Echocardiography should be performed in patients with a history of cardiac disease or if abnormalities are found on physical examination or the ECG. Echocardiographic diagnoses that may be responsible for syncope include aortic stenosis, hypertrophic cardiomyopathy, cardiac tumors, aortic dissection, and pericardial tamponade. Echocardiography also has a role in risk stratification based on the left ventricular ejection fraction.

Treadmill exercise testing with ECG and blood pressure monitoring should be performed in patients who have experienced syncope during or shortly after exercise. Treadmill testing may help identify exercise-induced arrhythmias (e.g., tachycardia-related AV block) and exercise-induced exaggerated vasodilation.

Electrophysiologic studies are indicated in patients with structural heart disease and ECG abnormalities in whom noninvasive investigations have failed to yield a diagnosis. Electrophysiologic studies have low sensitivity and specificity and should only be performed when a high pretest probability exists. Currently, this test is rarely performed to evaluate patients with syncope.

Psychiatric Evaluation Screening for psychiatric disorders may be appropriate in patients with recurrent unexplained syncope episodes. Tilt-table testing, with demonstration of symptoms in the absence of hemodynamic change, may be useful in reproducing syncope in patients with suspected psychogenic syncope.

28 Dizziness and Vertigo

Mark F. Walker, Robert B. Daroff

Dizziness is an imprecise symptom used to describe a variety of sensations that include vertigo, light-headedness, faintness, and imbalance. When used to describe a sense of spinning or other motion, dizziness is designated as *vertigo*. Vertigo may be physiologic, occurring during or after a sustained head rotation, or it may be pathologic, due to vestibular dysfunction. The term *light-headedness* is commonly applied to presyncopal sensations due to brain hypoperfusion but also may refer to disequilibrium and imbalance. A challenge to diagnosis is that patients often have difficulty distinguishing among these various symptoms, and the words they choose do not reliably indicate the underlying etiology.

There are a number of potential causes of dizziness. Vascular disorders cause presyncopal dizziness as a result of cardiac dysrhythmia, orthostatic hypotension, medication effects, or other causes. Such presyncopal sensations vary in duration; they may increase in severity until loss of consciousness occurs, or they may resolve before loss of consciousness if the cerebral ischemia is corrected. Faintness and syncope, which are discussed in detail in Chap. 27, should always be considered when one is evaluating patients with brief episodes of dizziness or dizziness that occurs with upright posture.

Vestibular causes of dizziness (vertigo or imbalance) may be due to peripheral lesions that affect the labyrinths or vestibular nerves or to involvement of the central vestibular pathways. They may be paroxysmal or due to a fixed unilateral or bilateral vestibular deficit. Acute unilateral lesions cause vertigo due to a sudden imbalance in vestibular inputs from the two labyrinths. Bilateral lesions cause imbalance and instability of vision (*oscillopsia*) when the head moves. Other causes of dizziness include nonvestibular imbalance and gait disorders (e.g., loss of proprioception from sensory neuropathy, parkinsonism) and anxiety.

When evaluating patients with dizziness, questions to consider include the following: (1) Is it dangerous (e.g., arrhythmia, transient ischemic attack/stroke)? (2) Is it vestibular? (3) If vestibular, is it peripheral or central? A careful history and examination often provide sufficient information to answer these questions and determine whether additional studies or referral to a specialist is necessary.

APPROACH TO THE PATIENT: Dizziness

HISTORY

When a patient presents with dizziness, the first step is to delineate more precisely the nature of the symptom. In the case of vestibular disorders, the physical symptoms depend on whether the lesion is unilateral or bilateral, and whether it is acute or chronic and progressive. Vertigo, an illusion of self or environmental motion, implies asymmetry of vestibular inputs from the two labyrinths or in their central pathways that is usually acute. Symmetric bilateral vestibular hypofunction causes imbalance but no vertigo. Because of the ambiguity in patients' descriptions of their symptoms, diagnosis based simply on symptom characteristics is typically unreliable. The history should focus closely on other features, including whether this is the first attack, the duration of this and any prior episodes, provoking factors, and accompanying symptoms.

Dizziness can be divided into episodes that last for seconds, minutes, hours, or days. Common causes of brief dizziness (seconds) include benign paroxysmal positional vertigo (BPPV) and orthostatic hypotension, both of which typically are provoked by changes in head and body position. Attacks of vestibular migraine and Ménière's disease often last hours. When episodes are of intermediate duration (minutes), transient ischemic attacks of the posterior circulation should be considered, although migraine and a number of other causes are also possible.

Symptoms that accompany vertigo may be helpful in distinguishing peripheral vestibular lesions from central causes. Unilateral hearing loss and other aural symptoms (ear pain, pressure, fullness) typically point to a peripheral cause. Because the auditory pathways quickly become bilateral upon entering the brainstem, central lesions are unlikely to cause unilateral hearing loss, unless the lesion lies near the root entry zone of the auditory nerve. Symptoms such as double vision, numbness, and limb ataxia suggest a brainstem or cerebellar lesion.

EXAMINATION

Because dizziness and imbalance can be a manifestation of a variety of neurologic disorders, the neurologic examination is important in the evaluation of these patients. Particular focus should be given to assessment of eye movements, vestibular function, and hearing. The range of eye movements and whether they are equal in each eye should be observed. Peripheral eye movement disorders (e.g., cranial neuropathies, eye muscle weakness) are usually disconjugate (different in the two eyes). One should check pursuit (the ability to follow a smoothly moving target) and saccades (the ability to look back and forth accurately between two targets). Poor pursuit or inaccurate (dysmetric) saccades usually indicates central pathology, often involving the cerebellum. Finally, one should look for spontaneous nystagmus, an involuntary back-and-forth movement of the eyes. Nystagmus is most often of the jerk type, in which a slow drift (slow phase) in one direction alternates with a rapid saccadic movement (quick phase or fast phase) in the opposite direction that resets the position of the eyes in the orbits. Except in the case of acute vestibulopathy (e.g., vestibular neuritis), if primary position nystagmus is easily seen in the light, it is probably due to a central cause. Two forms of nystagmus that are characteristic of lesions of the cerebellar pathways are vertical nystagmus with downward fast phases (downbeat nystagmus) and horizontal nystagmus that changes direction with gaze (gaze-evoked nystagmus). By contrast, peripheral lesions typically cause unidirectional horizontal nystagmus. Use of Frenzel eyeglasses (self-illuminated goggles with convex lenses that blur the patient's vision but allow the examiner to see the eyes greatly magnified) can aid in the detection of peripheral vestibular nystagmus, because they reduce the patient's ability to use visual fixation to suppress nystagmus. Table 28-1 outlines key findings that help distinguish peripheral from central causes of vertigo.

The most useful bedside test of peripheral vestibular function is the head impulse test, in which the vestibuloocular reflex (VOR) is assessed with small-amplitude (~20 degrees) rapid head rotations. While the patient fixates on a target, the head is rotated to the left or right. If the VOR is deficient, the rotation is followed by a catch-up saccade in the opposite direction (e.g., a leftward saccade after a rightward rotation). The head impulse test can identify both unilateral (catch-up saccades after rotations toward the weak side) and bilateral vestibular hypofunction (catch-up saccades after rotations in both directions).

All patients with episodic dizziness, especially if provoked by positional change, should be tested with the Dix-Hallpike maneuver. The patient begins in a sitting position with the head turned 45 degrees; holding the back of the head, the examiner then lowers the patient into a supine position with the head extended backward by about 20 degrees while watching the eyes. Posterior canal BPPV can be diagnosed confidently if transient upbeating-torsional nystagmus is seen. If no nystagmus is observed after 15–20 s, the patient is raised to the sitting position, and the procedure is repeated with the head turned to the other side. Again, Frenzel goggles may improve the sensitivity of the test.

Dynamic visual acuity is a functional test that can be useful in assessing vestibular function. Visual acuity is measured with the head still and when the head is rotated back and forth by the examiner (about 1–2 Hz). A drop in visual acuity during head motion of more than one line on a near card or Snellen chart is abnormal and indicates vestibular dysfunction.

ANCILLARY TESTING

The choice of ancillary tests should be guided by the history and examination findings. Audiometry should be performed whenever a vestibular disorder is suspected. Unilateral sensorineural hearing loss supports a peripheral disorder (e.g., vestibular schwannoma). Predominantly low-frequency hearing loss is characteristic of Ménière's disease. Electronystagmography or videonystagmography includes recordings of spontaneous nystagmus (if present) and measurement of positional nystagmus. Caloric testing assesses the responses of the two horizontal semicircular canals. The test battery often includes recording of saccades and pursuit to assess central ocular motor function. Neuroimaging is important if a central vestibular disorder is suspected. In addition, patients with unexplained unilateral hearing loss or vestibular hypofunction should undergo magnetic resonance imaging (MRI) of the internal auditory canals, including administration of gadolinium, to rule out a schwannoma.

TABLE 28-1 FEATURES OF PERIPHERAL AND CENTRAL VERTIGO

- Nystagmus from an acute peripheral lesion is unidirectional, with fast phases beating away from the ear with the lesion. Nystagmus that changes direction with gaze is due to a central lesion.
- Transient mixed vertical-torsional nystagmus occurs in BPPV, but pure vertical or pure torsional nystagmus is a central sign.
- Nystagmus from a peripheral lesion may be inhibited by visual fixation, whereas central nystagmus is not suppressed.
- Absence of a head impulse sign in a patient with acute prolonged vertigo should suggest a central cause.
- Unilateral hearing loss suggests peripheral vertigo. Findings such as diplopia, dysarthria, and limb ataxia suggest a central disorder.

DIFFERENTIAL DIAGNOSIS AND TREATMENT

Treatment of vestibular symptoms should be driven by the underlying diagnosis. Simply treating dizziness with vestibular suppressant medications is often not helpful and may make the symptoms worse and prolong recovery. The diagnostic and specific treatment approaches for the most commonly encountered vestibular disorders are discussed below.

ACUTE PROLONGED VERTIGO (VESTIBULAR NEURITIS)

An acute unilateral vestibular lesion causes constant vertigo, nausea, vomiting, oscillopsia (motion of the visual scene), and imbalance. These symptoms are due to a sudden asymmetry of inputs from the two labyrinths or in their central connections, simulating a continuous rotation of the head. Unlike BPPV, continuous vertigo persists even when the head remains still.

When a patient presents with an acute vestibular syndrome, the most important question is whether the lesion is central (e.g., a cerebellar or brainstem infarct or hemorrhage), which may be life-threatening, or peripheral, affecting the vestibular nerve or labyrinth (vestibular neuritis). Attention should be given to any symptoms or signs that point to central dysfunction (diplopia, weakness or numbness, dysarthria). The pattern of spontaneous nystagmus, if present, may be helpful (Table 28-1). If the head impulse test is normal, an acute peripheral vestibular lesion is unlikely. A central lesion cannot always be excluded with certainty based on symptoms and examination alone; thus, older patients with vascular risk factors who present with an acute vestibular syndrome should be evaluated for the possibility of stroke even when there are no specific findings that indicate a central lesion.

Most patients with vestibular neuritis recover spontaneously, but glucocorticoids can improve outcome if administered within 3 days of symptom onset. Antiviral medications are of no proven benefit and are not typically given unless there is evidence to suggest herpes zoster oticus (Ramsay Hunt syndrome). Vestibular suppressant medications may reduce acute symptoms but should be avoided after the first several days because they may impede central compensation and recovery. Patients should be encouraged to resume a normal level of activity as soon as possible, and directed vestibular rehabilitation therapy may accelerate improvement.

BENIGN PAROXYSMAL POSITIONAL VERTIGO

BPPV is a common cause of recurrent vertigo. Episodes are brief (<1 min and typically 15–20 s) and are always provoked by changes in head position relative to gravity, such as lying down, rolling over in bed, rising from a supine position, and extending the head to look upward. The attacks are caused by free-floating otoconia (calcium carbonate crystals) that have been dislodged from the utricular macula and have moved into one of the semicircular canals, usually the posterior canal. When head position changes, gravity causes the otoconia to move within the canal, producing vertigo and nystagmus. With posterior canal BPPV, the nystagmus beats upward and torsionally (the upper poles of the eyes beat toward the affected lower ear). Less commonly, the otoconia enter the horizontal canal, resulting in a horizontal nystagmus when the patient is lying with either ear down. Superior (also called anterior) canal involvement is rare. BPPV is treated with repositioning maneuvers that use gravity to remove the otoconia from the semicircular canal. For posterior canal BPPV, the Epley maneuver (Fig. 28-1) is the most commonly used procedure. For more refractory cases of BPPV, patients can be taught a variant of this maneuver that they can perform alone at home. A demonstration of the Epley maneuver is available online (*http://www.dizziness-and-balance.com/disorders/bppv/bppv.html*).

VESTIBULAR MIGRAINE

Vestibular symptoms occur frequently in migraineurs, sometimes as a headache aura but usually independent of headache. The duration of vertigo may be from minutes to hours, and some patients also experience more prolonged periods of disequilibrium (lasting days to weeks). Motion sensitivity and sensitivity to visual motion (e.g., movies) are common in patients with vestibular migraine. Although data from controlled studies are generally lacking, vestibular migraine typically is treated with medications that are used for prophylaxis of migraine headaches. Antiemetics may be helpful to relieve symptoms at the time of an attack.

MÉNIÈRE'S DISEASE

Attacks of Ménière's disease consist of vertigo and hearing loss, as well as pain, pressure, and/or fullness in the affected ear. The low-frequency hearing loss and aural symptoms are key features that distinguish Ménière's disease from other peripheral vestibulopathies and from vestibular migraine. Audiometry at the time of an attack shows a characteristic asymmetric low-frequency hearing loss; hearing commonly improves between attacks, although permanent hearing loss may eventually occur. Ménière's disease is thought to be due to excess fluid (endolymph) in the inner ear; hence the term *endolymphatic hydrops*. Patients suspected of having Ménière's disease should be referred to an otolaryngologist for further evaluation. Diuretics and sodium restriction are the initial treatments. If attacks persist, injections of gentamicin into the middle ear are typically the next line of therapy. Full ablative procedures (vestibular nerve section, labyrinthectomy) are seldom required.

VESTIBULAR SCHWANNOMA

Vestibular schwannomas (sometimes termed *acoustic neuromas*) and other tumors at the cerebellopontine angle cause slowly progressive unilateral sensorineural hearing loss and vestibular hypofunction. These patients typically do not have vertigo, because the gradual vestibular deficit is compensated centrally as it develops. The diagnosis often is not made until there is sufficient hearing loss to be noticed. The examination will show a deficient response to the head impulse test when the head is rotated toward the affected side. As noted above, patients with unexplained unilateral sensorineural hearing loss or vestibular hypofunction require MRI of the internal auditory canals to look for a schwannoma.

BILATERAL VESTIBULAR HYPOFUNCTION

Patients with bilateral loss of vestibular function also typically do not have vertigo, because vestibular function is lost on both sides simultaneously, and there is no asymmetry of vestibular input. Symptoms include loss of balance, particularly in the dark, where vestibular input is most critical, and oscillopsia during head movement, such as while walking or riding in a car. Bilateral vestibular hypofunction may be (1) idiopathic and progressive, (2) part of a neurodegenerative disorder, or (3) iatrogenic, due to medication ototoxicity (most commonly

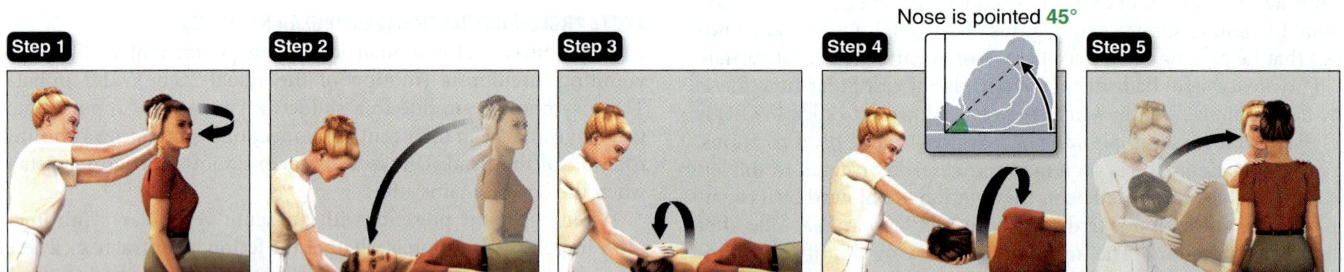

FIGURE 28-1 Modified Epley maneuver for treatment of benign paroxysmal positional vertigo of the right (*top panels*) and left (*bottom panels*) posterior semicircular canals. **Step 1.** With the patient seated, turn the head 45 degrees toward the affected ear. **Step 2.** Keeping the head turned, lower the patient to the head-hanging position and hold for at least 30 s and until nystagmus disappears. **Step 3.** Without lifting the head, turn it 90 degrees toward the other side. Hold for another 30 s. **Step 4.** Rotate the patient onto her side while turning the head another 90 degrees, so that the nose is pointed down 45 degrees. Hold again for 30 s. **Step 5.** Have the patient sit up on the side of the table. After a brief rest, the maneuver should be repeated to confirm successful treatment. *(Figure adapted from http://www.dizziness-and-balance.com/disorders/bppv/movies/Epley-480x640.avi.)*

gentamicin or other aminoglycoside antibiotics). Other causes include bilateral vestibular schwannomas (neurofibromatosis type 2), autoimmune disease, superficial siderosis, and meningeal-based infection or tumor. It also may occur in patients with peripheral polyneuropathy; in these patients, both vestibular loss and impaired proprioception may contribute to poor balance. Finally, unilateral processes such as vestibular neuritis and Ménière's disease may involve both ears sequentially, resulting in bilateral vestibulopathy.

Examination findings include diminished *dynamic visual acuity* (see above) due to loss of stable vision when the head is moving, abnormal head impulse responses in both directions, and a Romberg sign. Responses to caloric testing are reduced. Patients with bilateral vestibular hypofunction should be referred for vestibular rehabilitation therapy. Vestibular suppressant medications should not be used, as they will increase the imbalance. Evaluation by a neurologist is important not only to confirm the diagnosis but also to consider any other associated neurologic abnormalities that may clarify the etiology.

CENTRAL VESTIBULAR DISORDERS

Central lesions causing vertigo typically involve vestibular pathways in the brainstem and/or cerebellum. They may be due to discrete lesions, such as from ischemic or hemorrhagic stroke (Chap. 446), demyelination (Chap. 458), or tumors (Chap. 118), or they may be due to neurodegenerative conditions that include the vestibulocerebellum (Chap. 448). Subacute cerebellar degeneration may be due to immune, including paraneoplastic, processes (Chaps. 122 and 450). Table 28-1 outlines important features of the history and examination that help to identify central vestibular disorders. Acute central vertigo is a medical emergency, due to the possibility of life-threatening stroke or hemorrhage. All patients with suspected central vestibular disorders should undergo brain MRI, and the patient should be referred for full neurologic evaluation.

PSYCHOSOMATIC DIZZINESS/VERTIGO

Psychological factors play an important role in chronic dizziness. First, dizziness may be a somatic manifestation of a psychiatric condition such as major depression, anxiety, or panic disorder (Chap. 465e). Second, patients may develop anxiety and autonomic symptoms as a consequence or comorbidity of an independent vestibular disorder. One particular form of this has been termed variously *phobic postural vertigo*, *psychophysiologic vertigo*, or *chronic subjective dizziness*. These patients have a chronic feeling (months or longer) of dizziness and disequilibrium, an increased sensitivity to self-motion and visual motion (e.g., movies), and a particular intensification of symptoms when moving through complex visual environments such as supermarkets (visual vertigo). Although there may be a past history of an acute vestibular disorder (e.g., vestibular neuritis), the neurootologic examination and vestibular testing are normal or indicative of a compensated vestibular deficit, indicating that the ongoing subjective dizziness cannot be explained by a primary vestibular disorder. Anxiety disorders are particularly common in patients with chronic dizziness and contribute substantially to the morbidity. Thus, treatment with antianxiety medications (selective serotonin reuptake inhibitors [SSRIs]) and cognitive-behavioral therapy may be helpful. Vestibular rehabilitation therapy is also sometimes beneficial. Vestibular suppressant medications generally should be avoided. This condition should be suspected when the patient states, "My dizziness is so bad, I'm afraid to leave my house" (agoraphobia).

TREATMENT VERTIGO

Table 28-2 provides a list of commonly used medications for suppression of vertigo. As noted, these medications should be reserved for short-term control of active vertigo, such as during the first few days of acute vestibular neuritis, or for acute attacks of Ménière's disease. They are less helpful for chronic dizziness and, as previously stated, may hinder central compensation. An exception is that benzodiazepines may attenuate psychosomatic dizziness and the associated anxiety, although SSRIs are generally preferable in such patients.

TABLE 28-2 TREATMENT OF VERTIGO

Agent[a]	Dose[b]
Antihistamines	
Meclizine	25–50 mg 3 times daily
Dimenhydrinate	50 mg 1–2 times daily
Promethazine	25 mg 2–3 times daily (also can be given rectally and IM)
Benzodiazepines	
Diazepam	2.5 mg 1–3 times daily
Clonazepam	0.25 mg 1–3 times daily
Anticholinergic	
Scopolamine transdermal[c]	Patch
Physical therapy	
Repositioning maneuvers[d]	
Vestibular rehabilitation	
Other	
Diuretics and/or low-sodium (1000 mg/d) diet[e]	
Antimigrainous drugs[f]	
Methylprednisolone[g]	100 mg daily days 1–3; 80 mg daily days 4–6; 60 mg daily days 7–9; 40 mg daily days 10–12; 20 mg daily days 13–15; 10 mg daily days 16–18, 20, 22
Selective serotonin reuptake inhibitors[h]	

[a]All listed drugs are approved by the U.S. Food and Drug Administration, but most are not approved for the treatment of vertigo. [b]Usual oral (unless otherwise stated) starting dose in adults; a higher maintenance dose can be reached by a gradual increase. [c]For motion sickness only. [d]For benign paroxysmal positional vertigo. [e]For Ménière's disease. [f]For vestibular migraine. [g]For acute vestibular neuritis (started within 3 days of onset). [h]For psychosomatic vertigo.

Vestibular rehabilitation therapy promotes central adaptation processes that compensate for vestibular loss and also may help habituate motion sensitivity and other symptoms of psychosomatic dizziness. The general approach is to use a graded series of exercises that progressively challenge gaze stabilization and balance.

29 Fatigue

Jeffrey M. Gelfand, Vanja C. Douglas

Fatigue is one of the most common symptoms in clinical medicine. It is a prominent manifestation of a number of systemic, neurologic, and psychiatric syndromes, although a precise cause will not be identified in a substantial minority of patients. Fatigue refers to an inherently subjective human experience of physical and mental weariness, sluggishness, and exhaustion. In the context of clinical medicine, fatigue is most typically and practically defined as difficulty initiating or maintaining voluntary mental or physical activity. Nearly everyone who has ever been ill with a self-limited infection has experienced this near-universal symptomatology, and fatigue is usually brought to medical attention only when it is either of unclear cause or the severity is out of proportion with what would be expected for the associated trigger. *Fatigue* should be distinguished from *muscle weakness*, a reduction of neuromuscular power (Chap. 30); most patients complaining of fatigue are not truly weak when direct muscle power is tested. By definition, fatigue is also distinct from *somnolence* and *dyspnea on exertion*, although patients may use the word fatigue to describe those two symptoms. The task facing clinicians when a patient presents with fatigue is to identify an underlying cause if one exists and to develop a therapeutic alliance, the goal of which is to spare patients expensive and fruitless diagnostic workups and steer them toward effective therapy.

EPIDEMIOLOGY AND GLOBAL CONSIDERATIONS

Variability in the definitions of fatigue and the survey instruments used in different studies makes it difficult to arrive at precise figures about the global burden of fatigue. The point prevalence of fatigue was 6.7% and the lifetime prevalence was 25% in a large National Institute of Mental Health survey of the U.S. general population. In primary care clinics in Europe and the United States, between 10 and 25% of patients surveyed endorsed symptoms of prolonged (present for >1 month) or chronic (present for >6 months) fatigue, but fatigue was the primary reason for seeking medical attention in only a minority of patients. In a community survey of women in India, 12% reported chronic fatigue. By contrast, the prevalence of chronic fatigue syndrome, as defined by the U.S. Centers for Disease Control and Prevention, is low (Chap. 464e).

DIFFERENTIAL DIAGNOSIS

Psychiatric Disease Fatigue is a common somatic manifestation of many major psychiatric syndromes, including depression, anxiety, and somatoform disorders. Psychiatric symptoms are reported in more than three-quarters of patients with unexplained chronic fatigue. Even in patients with systemic or neurologic syndromes in which fatigue is independently recognized as a manifestation of disease, comorbid psychiatric symptoms or disease may still be an important source of interaction.

Neurologic Disease Patients complaining of fatigue often say they feel weak, but upon careful examination, objective muscle weakness is rarely discernible. If found, muscle weakness must then be localized to the central nervous system, peripheral nervous system, neuromuscular junction, or muscle and the appropriate follow-up studies obtained (Chap. 30). *Fatigability* of muscle power is a cardinal manifestation of some neuromuscular disorders such as myasthenia gravis and can be distinguished from *fatigue* by finding clinically apparent diminution of the amount of force that a muscle generates upon repeated contraction (Chap. 461). Fatigue is one of the most common and bothersome symptoms reported in multiple sclerosis (MS) (Chap. 458), affecting nearly 90% of patients; fatigue in MS can persist between MS attacks and does not necessarily correlate with magnetic resonance imaging (MRI) disease activity. Fatigue is also increasingly identified as a troublesome feature of many other neurodegenerative diseases, including Parkinson's disease, central dysautonomias, and amyotrophic lateral sclerosis. Poststroke fatigue is a well-described but poorly understood entity with a widely varying prevalence. Episodic fatigue can be a premonitory symptom of migraine. Fatigue is also a frequent result of traumatic brain injury, often occurring in association with depression and sleep disorders.

Sleep Disorders Obstructive sleep apnea is an important cause of excessive daytime sleepiness in association with fatigue and should be investigated using overnight polysomnography, particularly in those with prominent snoring, obesity, or other predictors of obstructive sleep apnea (Chap. 319). Whether the cumulative sleep deprivation that is common in modern society contributes to clinically apparent fatigue is not known (Chap. 38).

Endocrine Disorders Fatigue, sometimes in association with true muscle weakness, can be a heralding symptom of hypothyroidism, particularly in the context of hair loss, dry skin, cold intolerance, constipation, and weight gain. Fatigue in association with heat intolerance, sweating, and palpitations is typical of hyperthyroidism. Adrenal insufficiency can also manifest with unexplained fatigue as a primary or prominent symptom, often in association with anorexia, weight loss, nausea, myalgias, and arthralgias; hyponatremia and hyperkalemia may be present at time of diagnosis. Mild hypercalcemia can cause fatigue, which may be relatively vague, whereas severe hypercalcemia can lead to lethargy, stupor, and coma. Both hypoglycemia and hyperglycemia can cause lethargy, often in association with confusion; chronic diabetes, particularly type 1 diabetes, is also associated with fatigue independent of glucose levels. Fatigue may also accompany Cushing's disease, hypoaldosteronism, and hypogonadism.

Liver and Kidney Disease Both chronic liver failure and chronic kidney disease can cause fatigue. Over 80% of hemodialysis patients complain of fatigue, which makes this one of the most common patient-reported symptoms in chronic kidney disease.

Obesity Obesity is associated with fatigue and sleepiness independent of the presence of obstructive sleep apnea. Obese patients undergoing bariatric surgery experience improvement in daytime sleepiness sooner than would be expected if the improvement were solely the result of weight loss and resolution of sleep apnea. A number of other factors common in obese patients are likely contributors as well, including depression, physical inactivity, and diabetes.

Malnutrition Although fatigue can be a presenting feature of malnutrition, nutritional status may also be an important comorbidity and contributor to fatigue in other chronic illnesses, including cancer-associated fatigue.

Infection Both acute and chronic infections commonly lead to fatigue as part of the broader infectious syndrome. Evaluation for undiagnosed infection as the cause of unexplained fatigue, and particularly prolonged or chronic fatigue, should be guided by the history, physical examination, and infectious risk factors, with particular attention to risk for tuberculosis, HIV, chronic hepatitis B and C, and endocarditis. Infectious mononucleosis may cause prolonged fatigue that persists for weeks to months following the acute illness, but infection with the Epstein-Barr virus is only very rarely the cause of unexplained chronic fatigue.

Drugs Many medications, drug use, drug withdrawal, and chronic alcohol use can all lead to fatigue. Medications that are more likely to be causative in this context include antidepressants, antipsychotics, anxiolytics, opiates, antispasticity agents, antiseizure agents, and beta blockers.

Cardiovascular and Pulmonary Fatigue is one of the most taxing patient-reported symptoms of congestive heart failure and chronic obstructive pulmonary disease and negatively affects quality of life.

Malignancy Fatigue, particularly in association with unexplained unintended weight loss, can be a sign of occult malignancy, but this is only rarely identified as causative in patients with unexplained chronic fatigue in the absence of other telltale signs or symptoms. Cancer-related fatigue is experienced by 40% of patients at time of diagnosis and greater than 80% of patients later in the disease course.

Hematologic Chronic or progressive anemia may present with fatigue, sometimes in association with exertional tachycardia and breathlessness. Anemia may also contribute to fatigue in chronic illness. Low serum ferritin in the absence of anemia may also cause fatigue that is reversible with iron replacement.

Systemic Inflammatory/Rheumatologic Disorders Fatigue is a prominent complaint in many chronic inflammatory disorders, including systemic lupus erythematosus, polymyalgia rheumatica, rheumatoid arthritis, inflammatory bowel disease, antineutrophil cytoplasmic antibody (ANCA)–associated vasculitis, sarcoidosis, and Sjögren's syndrome, but is not usually an isolated symptom.

Pregnancy Fatigue is very commonly reported by women during all stages of pregnancy and postpartum.

Disorders of Unclear Cause Chronic fatigue syndrome (Chap. 464e) and fibromyalgia (Chap. 396) incorporate chronic fatigue as part of the syndromic definition when present in association with a number of other inclusion and exclusion criteria, as discussed in detail in their respective chapters. The pathophysiology of each is unknown. Idiopathic chronic fatigue is used to describe the syndrome of unexplained chronic fatigue in the absence of enough additional clinical features to meet the diagnostic criteria for chronic fatigue syndrome.

APPROACH TO THE PATIENT: Fatigue

A detailed history focusing on the quality, pattern, time-course, associated symptoms, and alleviating factors of fatigue is critical in defining the syndrome, determining whether fatigue is the appropriate designation, determining whether the symptoms are acute or chronic, and determining whether fatigue is primarily mental, physical, or both in order to direct further evaluation and treatment. The review of systems should attempt to distinguish fatigue from excessive daytime sleepiness, dyspnea on exertion, exercise intolerance, and muscle weakness. The presence of fever, chills, night sweats, or weight loss should raise suspicion for an occult infection or malignancy. A careful review of prescription, over-the-counter, herbal, and recreational drug and alcohol use is mandatory. Circumstances surrounding the onset of symptoms and potential triggers should be investigated. The social history is important, with attention paid to job stress and work hours, the social support network, and domestic affairs including a screen for intimate partner violence. Sleep habits and sleep hygiene should be questioned. The impact of fatigue on daily functioning is important to understand the patient's experience and gauge recovery and the success of treatment.

The physical examination of patients with fatigue is guided by the history and differential diagnosis. A detailed mental status examination should be performed with particular attention to symptoms of depression and anxiety. A formal neurologic examination is required to determine whether objective muscle weakness is present. This is usually a straightforward exercise, although occasionally patients with fatigue have difficulty sustaining effort against resistance and sometimes report that generating full power requires substantial mental effort. On confrontational testing, they are able to generate full power for only a brief period before suddenly giving way to the examiner. This type of weakness is often referred to as *breakaway weakness* and may or may not be associated with pain. This is contrasted with weakness due to lesions in the motor tracts or lower motor unit, in which the patient's resistance can be overcome in a smooth and steady fashion and full power can never be generated. Occasionally, a patient may demonstrate fatigable weakness, in which power is full when first tested but becomes weak upon repeat evaluation without interval rest. Fatigable weakness, which usually indicates a problem of neuromuscular transmission, never has the sudden breakaway quality that one occasionally observes in patients with fatigue. If the presence or absence of muscle weakness cannot be determined with the physical examination, electromyography with nerve conductions studies can be a helpful ancillary test.

The general physical examination should screen for signs of cardiopulmonary disease, malignancy, lymphadenopathy, organomegaly, infection, liver failure, kidney disease, malnutrition, endocrine abnormalities, and connective tissue disease. Although the diagnostic yield of the general physical examination may be relatively low in the context of evaluation of unexplained chronic fatigue, elucidating the cause of 2% of cases in one prospective analysis, the yield of a detailed neuropsychiatric and mental status evaluation is likely to be much higher, revealing a potential explanation for fatigue in up to 75–80% of patients in some series. Furthermore, the rite of physical examination demonstrates a thorough and systematic approach to the patient's complaint and helps build trust and a therapeutic alliance.

Laboratory testing is likely to identify the cause of chronic fatigue in only about 5% of cases. Beyond a few standard screening tests, laboratory evaluation should be guided by the history and physical examination; extensive testing is more likely to lead to false-positive results that require explanation and unnecessary investigation and should be avoided in lieu of frequent clinical follow-up. A reasonable approach to screening includes a complete blood count with differential (to screen for anemia, infection, and malignancy), electrolytes (including sodium, potassium, and calcium), glucose, renal function, liver function, and thyroid function. Testing for HIV and adrenal function can also be considered. Published guidelines defining chronic fatigue syndrome also recommend an erythrocyte sedimentation rate (ESR) as part of the evaluation for mimics, but unless the value is very high, such nonspecific testing in the absence of other features is unlikely to clarify the situation. Routine screening with an antinuclear antibody (ANA) test is also unlikely to be informative in isolation and is frequently positive at low titers in otherwise healthy adults. Additional unfocused studies, such as whole-body imaging scans, are usually not indicated; in addition to their inconvenience, potential risk, and cost, they often reveal unrelated incidental findings that can prolong the workup unnecessarily.

TREATMENT FATIGUE

The first priority of treatment is to address the underlying disorder or disorders that account for fatigue, because this can be curative in select contexts and palliative in others. Unfortunately, in many chronic illnesses, fatigue may be refractory to traditional disease-modifying therapies, and it is important in such cases to evaluate for other potential contributors, because the cause may be multifactorial. Antidepressant treatment (Chap. 466) may be helpful for treatment of chronic fatigue when symptoms of depression are present and may be most effective in the context of a multimodal approach. However, antidepressants can also cause fatigue and should be discontinued if they are not clearly effective. Cognitive-behavioral therapy has also been demonstrated to be helpful in the context of chronic fatigue syndrome as well as cancer-associated fatigue. Graded exercise therapy in which physical exercise, most typically walking, is gradually increased with attention to target heart rates to avoid overexertion, was shown to modestly improve walking times and self-reported fatigue measures in patients in the United Kingdom with chronic fatigue syndrome in the large 2011 randomized controlled PACE trial. Psychostimulants such as amphetamines, modafinil, and armodafinil can help increase alertness and concentration and reduce excessive daytime sleepiness in certain clinical contexts, which may in turn help with symptoms of fatigue in a minority of patients, but they have generally proven to be unhelpful in randomized trials for treating fatigue in posttraumatic brain injury, Parkinson's disease, and MS.

Development of more effective therapy for fatigue is hampered by limited knowledge of the biologic basis of this symptom. Tentative data suggests that proinflammatory cytokines, such as interleukin 1β and tumor necrosis factor α, might mediate fatigue in some patients; thus, cytokine antagonists represent one possible future approach.

PROGNOSIS

Acute fatigue significant enough to require medical evaluation is more likely to lead to an identifiable medical, neurologic, or psychiatric cause than unexplained chronic fatigue. Evaluation of unexplained chronic fatigue most commonly leads to diagnosis of a psychiatric condition or remains unexplained. Identification of a previously undiagnosed serious or life-threatening culprit etiology is rare on longitudinal follow-up in patients with unexplained chronic fatigue. Complete resolution of unexplained chronic fatigue is uncommon, at least over the short term, but multidisciplinary treatment approaches can lead to symptomatic improvements that can substantially improve quality of life.

30 Neurologic Causes of Weakness and Paralysis

Michael J. Aminoff

Normal motor function involves integrated muscle activity that is modulated by the activity of the cerebral cortex, basal ganglia, cerebellum, red nucleus, brainstem reticular formation, lateral vestibular nucleus, and spinal cord. Motor system dysfunction leads to weakness or paralysis, discussed in this chapter, or to ataxia (Chap. 450) or abnormal movements (Chap. 449). *Weakness* is a reduction in the power that can be exerted by one or more muscles. It must be distinguished from increased *fatigability* (i.e., the inability to sustain the performance of an activity that should be normal for a person of the same age, sex, and size), limitation in function due to pain or articular stiffness, or impaired motor activity because severe *proprioceptive sensory loss* prevents adequate feedback information about the direction and power of movements. It is also distinct from *bradykinesia* (in which increased time is required for full power to be exerted) and *apraxia*, a disorder of planning and initiating a skilled or learned movement unrelated to a significant motor or sensory deficit (Chap. 36).

Paralysis or the suffix "-plegia" indicates weakness so severe that a muscle cannot be contracted at all, whereas *paresis* refers to less severe weakness. The prefix "hemi-" refers to one-half of the body, "para-" to both legs, and "quadri-" to all four limbs.

The *distribution* of weakness helps to localize the underlying lesion. Weakness from involvement of upper motor neurons occurs particularly in the extensors and abductors of the upper limb and the flexors of the lower limb. Lower motor neuron weakness depends on whether involvement is at the level of the anterior horn cells, nerve root, limb plexus, or peripheral nerve—only muscles supplied by the affected structure are weak. Myopathic weakness is generally most marked in proximal muscles. Weakness from impaired neuromuscular transmission has no specific pattern of involvement.

Weakness often is accompanied by other neurologic abnormalities that help indicate the site of the responsible lesion (Table 30-1).

Tone is the resistance of a muscle to passive stretch. Increased tone may be of several types. *Spasticity* is the increase in tone associated with disease of upper motor neurons. It is velocity-dependent, has a sudden release after reaching a maximum (the "clasp-knife" phenomenon), and predominantly affects the antigravity muscles (i.e., upper-limb flexors and lower-limb extensors). *Rigidity* is hypertonia that is present throughout the range of motion (a "lead pipe" or "plastic" stiffness) and affects flexors and extensors equally; it sometimes has a cogwheel quality that is enhanced by voluntary movement of the contralateral limb (reinforcement). Rigidity occurs with certain extrapyramidal disorders, such as Parkinson's disease. *Paratonia* (or *gegenhalten*) is increased tone that varies irregularly in a manner seemingly related to the degree of relaxation, is present throughout the range of motion, and affects flexors and extensors equally; it usually results from disease of the frontal lobes. Weakness with *decreased tone* (*flaccidity*) or normal tone occurs with disorders of *motor units*. A motor unit consists of a single lower motor neuron and all the muscle fibers that it innervates.

Muscle bulk generally is not affected by upper motor neuron lesions, although mild disuse atrophy eventually may occur. By contrast, atrophy is often conspicuous when a lower motor neuron lesion is responsible for weakness and also may occur with advanced muscle disease.

Muscle stretch (tendon) reflexes are usually increased with upper motor neuron lesions, but may be decreased or absent for a variable period immediately after onset of an acute lesion. Hyperreflexia is usually—but not invariably—accompanied by loss of *cutaneous reflexes* (such as superficial abdominals; Chap. 437) and, in particular, by an extensor plantar (Babinski) response. The muscle stretch reflexes are depressed with lower motor neuron lesions directly involving specific reflex arcs. They generally are preserved in patients with myopathic weakness except in advanced stages, when they sometimes are attenuated. In disorders of the neuromuscular junction, reflex responses may be affected by preceding voluntary activity of affected muscles; such activity may lead to enhancement of initially depressed reflexes in Lambert-Eaton myasthenic syndrome and, conversely, to depression of initially normal reflexes in myasthenia gravis (Chap. 461).

The distinction of *neuropathic* (lower motor neuron) from *myopathic* weakness is sometimes difficult clinically, although distal weakness is likely to be neuropathic, and symmetric proximal weakness myopathic. *Fasciculations* (visible or palpable twitch within a muscle due to the spontaneous discharge of a motor unit) and early atrophy indicate that weakness is neuropathic.

PATHOGENESIS

Upper Motor Neuron Weakness Lesions of the upper motor neurons or their descending axons to the spinal cord (Fig. 30-1) produce weakness through decreased activation of lower motor neurons. In general, distal muscle groups are affected more severely than proximal ones, and axial movements are spared unless the lesion is severe and bilateral. Spasticity is typical but may not be present acutely. Rapid repetitive movements are slowed and coarse, but normal rhythmicity is maintained. With corticobulbar involvement, weakness occurs in the lower face and tongue; extraocular, upper facial, pharyngeal, and jaw muscles are typically spared. Bilateral corticobulbar lesions produce a *pseudobulbar palsy*: dysarthria, dysphagia, dysphonia, and emotional lability accompany bilateral facial weakness and a brisk jaw jerk. Electromyogram (EMG) (Chap. 442e) shows that with weakness of the upper motor neuron type, motor units have a diminished maximal discharge frequency.

Lower Motor Neuron Weakness This pattern results from disorders of lower motor neurons in the brainstem motor nuclei and the anterior horn of the spinal cord or from dysfunction of the axons of these neurons as they pass to skeletal muscle (Fig. 30-2). Weakness is due to a decrease in the number of muscle fibers that can be activated through a loss of α motor neurons or disruption of their connections to muscle. Loss of γ motor neurons does not cause weakness but decreases tension on the muscle spindles, which decreases muscle tone and attenuates the stretch reflexes. An absent stretch reflex suggests involvement of spindle afferent fibers.

When a motor unit becomes diseased, especially in anterior horn cell diseases, it may discharge spontaneously, producing *fasciculations*. When α motor neurons or their axons degenerate, the denervated muscle fibers also may discharge spontaneously. These single muscle

TABLE 30-1 SIGNS THAT DISTINGUISH THE ORIGIN OF WEAKNESS

Sign	Upper Motor Neuron	Lower Motor Neuron	Myopathic	Psychogenic
Atrophy	None	Severe	Mild	None
Fasciculations	None	Common	None	None
Tone	Spastic	Decreased	Normal/decreased	Variable/paratonia
Distribution of weakness	Pyramidal/regional	Distal/segmental	Proximal	Variable/inconsistent with daily activities
Muscle stretch reflexes	Hyperactive	Hypoactive/absent	Normal/hypoactive	Normal
Babinski sign	Present	Absent	Absent	Absent

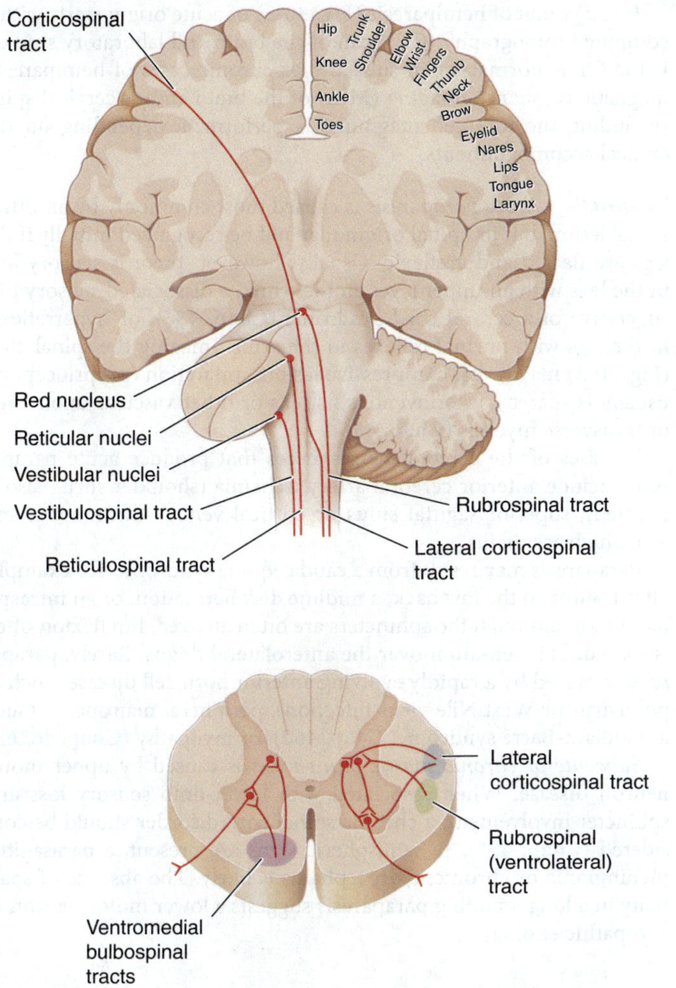

FIGURE 30-1 The corticospinal and bulbospinal upper motor neuron pathways. Upper motor neurons have their cell bodies in layer V of the primary motor cortex (the precentral gyrus, or Brodmann's area 4) and in the premotor and supplemental motor cortex (area 6). The upper motor neurons in the primary motor cortex are somatotopically organized (right side of figure).

Axons of the upper motor neurons descend through the subcortical white matter and the posterior limb of the internal capsule. Axons of the *pyramidal* or *corticospinal system* descend through the brainstem in the cerebral peduncle of the midbrain, the basis pontis, and the medullary pyramids. At the cervicomedullary junction, most corticospinal axons decussate into the contralateral corticospinal tract of the lateral spinal cord, but 10–30% remain ipsilateral in the anterior spinal cord. Corticospinal neurons synapse on premotor interneurons, but some—especially in the cervical enlargement and those connecting with motor neurons to distal limb muscles—make direct monosynaptic connections with lower motor neurons. They innervate most densely the lower motor neurons of hand muscles and are involved in the execution of learned, fine movements. Corticobulbar neurons are similar to corticospinal neurons but innervate brainstem motor nuclei.

Bulbospinal upper motor neurons influence strength and tone but are not part of the pyramidal system. The descending *ventromedial bulbospinal pathways* originate in the tectum of the midbrain (tectospinal pathway), the vestibular nuclei (vestibulospinal pathway), and the reticular formation (reticulospinal pathway). These pathways influence axial and proximal muscles and are involved in the maintenance of posture and integrated movements of the limbs and trunk. The descending *ventrolateral bulbospinal pathways,* which originate predominantly in the red nucleus (rubrospinal pathway), facilitate distal limb muscles. The bulbospinal system sometimes is referred to as the *extrapyramidal upper motor neuron system.* In all figures, nerve cell bodies and axon terminals are shown, respectively, as closed circles and forks.

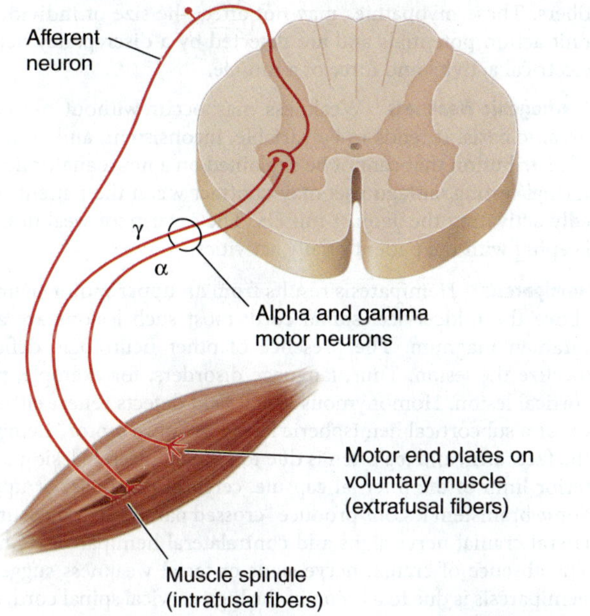

FIGURE 30-2 Lower motor neurons are divided into α and γ types. The larger α motor neurons are more numerous and innervate the extrafusal muscle fibers of the motor unit. Loss of α motor neurons or disruption of their axons produces lower motor neuron weakness. The smaller, less numerous γ motor neurons innervate the intrafusal muscle fibers of the muscle spindle and contribute to normal tone and stretch reflexes. The α motor neuron receives direct excitatory input from corticomotoneurons and primary muscle spindle afferents. The α and γ motor neurons also receive excitatory input from other descending upper motor neuron pathways, segmental sensory inputs, and interneurons. The α motor neurons receive direct inhibition from Renshaw cell interneurons, and other interneurons indirectly inhibit the α and γ motor neurons.

A muscle stretch (tendon) reflex requires the function of all the illustrated structures. A tap on a tendon stretches muscle spindles (which are tonically activated by γ motor neurons) and activates the primary spindle afferent neurons. These neurons stimulate the α motor neurons in the spinal cord, producing a brief muscle contraction, which is the familiar tendon reflex.

fiber discharges, or *fibrillation potentials,* cannot be seen but can be recorded with EMG. Weakness leads to delayed or reduced recruitment of motor units, with fewer than normal activated at a particular discharge frequency.

Neuromuscular Junction Weakness Disorders of the neuromuscular junctions produce weakness of variable degree and distribution. The number of muscle fibers that are activated varies over time, depending on the state of rest of the neuromuscular junctions. Strength is influenced by preceding activity of the affected muscle. In myasthenia gravis, for example, sustained or repeated contractions of affected muscle decline in strength despite continuing effort (Chap. 461). Thus, fatigable weakness is suggestive of disorders of the neuromuscular junction, which cause functional loss of muscle fibers due to failure of their activation.

Myopathic Weakness Myopathic weakness is produced by a decrease in the number or contractile force of muscle fibers activated within motor units. With muscular dystrophies, inflammatory myopathies, or myopathies with muscle fiber necrosis, the number of muscle fibers is reduced within many motor units. On EMG, the size of each motor unit action potential is decreased, and motor units must be recruited more rapidly than normal to produce the desired power. Some myopathies produce weakness through loss of contractile force of muscle fibers or through relatively selective involvement of type II (fast) fibers. These myopathies may not affect the size of individual motor unit action potentials and are detected by a discrepancy between the electrical activity and force of a muscle.

Psychogenic Weakness Weakness may occur without a recognizable organic basis. It tends to be variable, inconsistent, and with a pattern of distribution that cannot be explained on a neuroanatomic basis. On formal testing, antagonists may contract when the patient is supposedly activating the agonist muscle. The severity of weakness is out of keeping with the patient's daily activities.

Hemiparesis Hemiparesis results from an upper motor neuron lesion above the midcervical spinal cord; most such lesions are above the foramen magnum. The presence of other neurologic deficits helps localize the lesion. Thus, language disorders, for example, point to a cortical lesion. Homonymous visual field defects reflect either a cortical or a subcortical hemispheric lesion. A "pure motor" hemiparesis of the face, arm, and leg often is due to a small, discrete lesion in the posterior limb of the internal capsule, cerebral peduncle, or upper pons. Some brainstem lesions produce "crossed paralyses," consisting of ipsilateral cranial nerve signs and contralateral hemiparesis (Chap. 446). The absence of cranial nerve signs or facial weakness suggests that a hemiparesis is due to a lesion in the high cervical spinal cord, especially if associated with the Brown-Séquard syndrome (Chap. 456).

Acute or episodic hemiparesis usually results from focal structural lesions, particularly rapidly expanding lesions, or an inflammatory process. *Subacute hemiparesis* that evolves over days or weeks may relate to subdural hematoma, infectious or inflammatory disorders (e.g., cerebral abscess, fungal granuloma or meningitis, parasitic infection, multiple sclerosis, sarcoidosis), or primary and metastatic neoplasms. AIDS may present with subacute hemiparesis due to toxoplasmosis or primary central nervous system (CNS) lymphoma. *Chronic hemiparesis* that evolves over months usually is due to a neoplasm or vascular malformation, a chronic subdural hematoma, or a degenerative disease.

Investigation of hemiparesis (Fig. 30-3) of acute origin starts with a computed tomography (CT) scan of the brain and laboratory studies. If the CT is normal, or in subacute or chronic cases of hemiparesis, magnetic resonance imaging (MRI) of the brain and/or cervical spine (including the foramen magnum) is performed, depending on the clinical accompaniments.

Paraparesis *Acute paraparesis* is caused most commonly by an intraspinal lesion, but its spinal origin may not be recognized initially if the legs are flaccid and areflexic. Usually, however, there is sensory loss in the legs with an upper level on the trunk, a dissociated sensory loss suggestive of a central cord syndrome (Chap. 456), or hyperreflexia in the legs with normal reflexes in the arms. Imaging the spinal cord (Fig. 30-3) may reveal compressive lesions, infarction (proprioception usually is spared), arteriovenous fistulas or other vascular anomalies, or transverse myelitis (Chap. 456).

Diseases of the cerebral hemispheres that produce acute paraparesis include anterior cerebral artery ischemia (shoulder shrug also is affected), superior sagittal sinus or cortical venous thrombosis, and acute hydrocephalus.

Paraparesis may result from a cauda equina syndrome, for example, after trauma to the low back, a midline disk herniation, or an intraspinal tumor; although the sphincters are often affected, hip flexion often is spared, as is sensation over the anterolateral thighs. Rarely, paraparesis is caused by a rapidly evolving anterior horn cell disease (such as poliovirus or West Nile virus infection), peripheral neuropathy (such as Guillain-Barré syndrome; Chap. 460), or myopathy (Chap. 462e).

Subacute or chronic spastic paraparesis is caused by upper motor neuron disease. When associated with lower-limb sensory loss and sphincter involvement, a chronic spinal cord disorder should be considered (Chap. 456). If hemispheric signs are present, a parasagittal meningioma or chronic hydrocephalus is likely. The absence of spasticity in a long-standing paraparesis suggests a lower motor neuron or myopathic etiology.

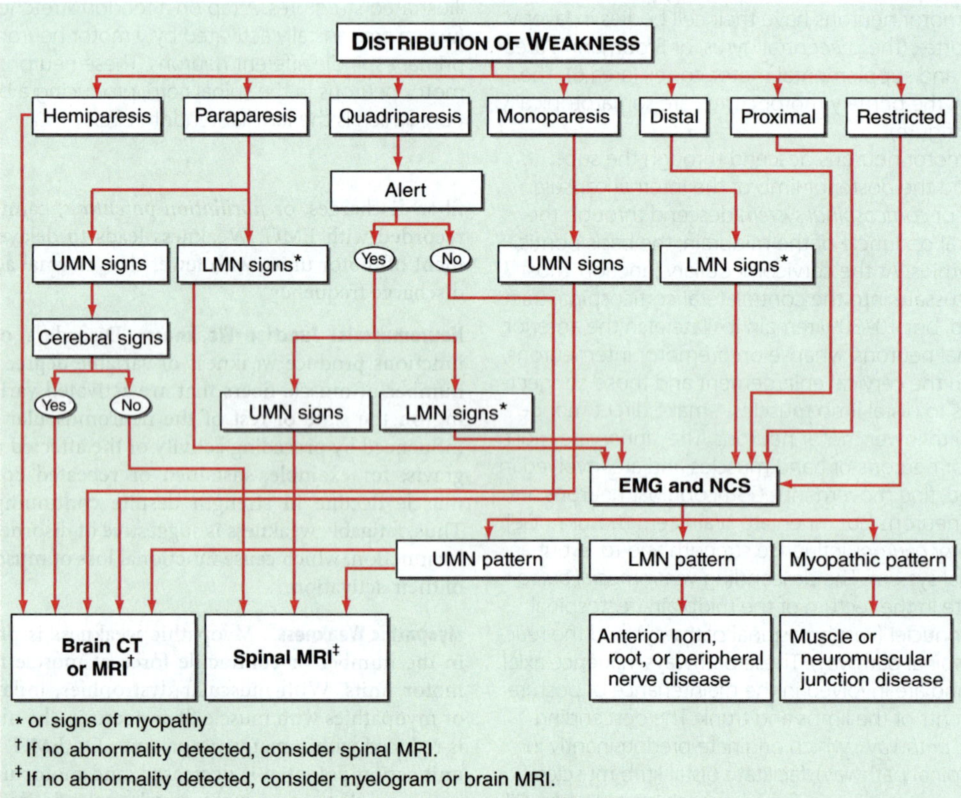

FIGURE 30-3 An algorithm for the initial workup of a patient with weakness. CT, computed tomography; EMG, electromyography; LMN, lower motor neuron; MRI, magnetic resonance imaging; NCS, nerve conduction studies; UMN, upper motor neuron.

Investigations typically begin with spinal MRI, but when upper motor neuron signs are associated with drowsiness, confusion, seizures, or other hemispheric signs, brain MRI should also be performed, sometimes as the initial investigation. Electrophysiologic studies are diagnostically helpful when clinical findings suggest an underlying neuromuscular disorder.

Quadriparesis or Generalized Weakness Generalized weakness may be due to disorders of the CNS or the motor unit. Although the terms often are used interchangeably, *quadriparesis* is commonly used when an upper motor neuron cause is suspected, and *generalized weakness* is used when a disease of the motor units is likely. Weakness from CNS disorders usually is associated with changes in consciousness or cognition and accompanied by spasticity, hyperreflexia, and sensory disturbances. Most neuromuscular causes of generalized weakness are associated with normal mental function, hypotonia, and hypoactive muscle stretch reflexes. The major causes of intermittent weakness are listed in Table 30-2. A patient with generalized fatigability without objective weakness may have the chronic fatigue syndrome (Chap. 464e).

ACUTE QUADRIPARESIS Quadriparesis with onset over minutes may result from disorders of upper motor neurons (such as from anoxia, hypotension, brainstem or cervical cord ischemia, trauma, and systemic metabolic abnormalities) or muscle (electrolyte disturbances, certain inborn errors of muscle energy metabolism, toxins, and periodic paralyses). Onset over hours to weeks may, in addition to these disorders, be due to lower motor neuron disorders such as Guillain-Barré syndrome (Chap. 460).

In obtunded patients, evaluation begins with a CT scan of the brain. If upper motor neuron signs are present but the patient is alert, the initial test is usually an MRI of the cervical cord. If weakness is lower motor neuron, myopathic, or uncertain in origin, the clinical approach begins with blood studies to determine the level of muscle enzymes and electrolytes and with EMG and nerve conduction studies.

SUBACUTE OR CHRONIC QUADRIPARESIS Quadriparesis due to upper motor neuron disease may develop over weeks to years from chronic myelopathies, multiple sclerosis, brain or spinal tumors, chronic subdural hematomas, and various metabolic, toxic, and infectious disorders. It may also result from lower motor neuron disease, a chronic neuropathy (in which weakness is often most profound distally), or myopathic weakness (typically proximal).

When *quadriparesis* develops acutely in obtunded patients, evaluation begins with a CT scan of the brain. If upper motor neuron signs have developed acutely but the patient is alert, the initial test is usually an MRI of the cervical cord. When onset has been gradual, disorders of the cerebral hemispheres, brainstem, and cervical spinal cord can usually be distinguished clinically, and imaging is directed first at the clinically suspected site of pathology. If weakness is lower motor neuron, myopathic, or uncertain in origin, laboratory studies to determine the levels of muscle enzymes and electrolytes, and EMG and nerve conduction studies help to localize the pathologic process.

TABLE 30-2 CAUSES OF EPISODIC GENERALIZED WEAKNESS

1. Electrolyte disturbances, e.g., hypokalemia, hyperkalemia, hypercalcemia, hypernatremia, hyponatremia, hypophosphatemia, hypermagnesemia
2. Muscle disorders
   a. Channelopathies (periodic paralyses)
   b. Metabolic defects of muscle (impaired carbohydrate or fatty acid utilization; abnormal mitochondrial function)
3. Neuromuscular junction disorders
   a. Myasthenia gravis
   b. Lambert-Eaton myasthenic syndrome
4. Central nervous system disorders
   a. Transient ischemic attacks of the brainstem
   b. Transient global cerebral ischemia
   c. Multiple sclerosis
5. Lack of voluntary effort
   a. Anxiety
   b. Pain or discomfort
   c. Somatization disorder

Monoparesis Monoparesis usually is due to lower motor neuron disease, with or without associated sensory involvement. Upper motor neuron weakness occasionally presents as a monoparesis of distal and nonantigravity muscles. Myopathic weakness rarely is limited to one limb.

ACUTE MONOPARESIS If weakness is predominantly distal and of upper motor neuron type and is not associated with sensory impairment or pain, focal cortical ischemia is likely (Chap. 446); diagnostic possibilities are similar to those for acute hemiparesis. Sensory loss and pain usually accompany acute lower motor neuron weakness; the weakness commonly localizes to a single nerve root or peripheral nerve, but occasionally reflects plexus involvement. If lower motor neuron weakness is likely, evaluation begins with EMG and nerve conduction studies.

SUBACUTE OR CHRONIC MONOPARESIS Weakness and atrophy that develop over weeks or months are usually of lower motor neuron origin. When associated with sensory symptoms, a peripheral cause (nerve, root, or plexus) is likely; otherwise, anterior horn cell disease should be considered. In either case, an electrodiagnostic study is indicated. If weakness is of the upper motor neuron type, a discrete cortical (precentral gyrus) or cord lesion may be responsible, and appropriate imaging is performed.

Distal Weakness Involvement of two or more limbs distally suggests lower motor neuron or peripheral nerve disease. Acute distal lower-limb weakness results occasionally from an acute toxic polyneuropathy or cauda equina syndrome. Distal symmetric weakness usually develops over weeks, months, or years and, when associated with numbness, is due to peripheral neuropathy (Chap. 459). Anterior horn cell disease may begin distally but is typically asymmetric and without accompanying numbness (Chap. 452). Rarely, myopathies present with distal weakness (Chap. 462e). Electrodiagnostic studies help localize the disorder (Fig. 30-3).

Proximal Weakness Myopathy often produces symmetric weakness of the pelvic or shoulder girdle muscles (Chap. 462e). Diseases of the neuromuscular junction, such as myasthenia gravis (Chap. 461), may present with symmetric proximal weakness often associated with ptosis, diplopia, or bulbar weakness and fluctuating in severity during the day. In anterior horn cell disease, proximal weakness is usually asymmetric, but it may be symmetric if familial. Numbness does not occur with any of these diseases. The evaluation usually begins with determination of the serum creatine kinase level and electrophysiologic studies.

Weakness in a Restricted Distribution Weakness may not fit any of these patterns, being limited, for example, to the extraocular, hemifacial, bulbar, or respiratory muscles. If it is unilateral, restricted weakness usually is due to lower motor neuron or peripheral nerve disease, such as in a facial palsy. Weakness of part of a limb is commonly due to a peripheral nerve lesion such as an entrapment neuropathy. Relatively symmetric weakness of extraocular or bulbar muscles frequently is due to a myopathy (Chap. 462e) or neuromuscular junction disorder (Chap. 461). Bilateral facial palsy with areflexia suggests Guillain-Barré syndrome (Chap. 460). Worsening of relatively symmetric weakness with fatigue is characteristic of neuromuscular junction disorders. Asymmetric bulbar weakness usually is due to motor neuron disease. Weakness limited to respiratory muscles is uncommon and usually is due to motor neuron disease, myasthenia gravis, or polymyositis/dermatomyositis (Chap. 388).

31 Numbness, Tingling, and Sensory Loss

Michael J. Aminoff

Normal somatic sensation reflects a continuous monitoring process, little of which reaches consciousness under ordinary conditions. By contrast, disordered sensation, particularly when experienced as painful, is alarming and dominates the patient's attention. Physicians should be able to recognize abnormal sensations by how they are described, know their type and likely site of origin, and understand their implications. Pain is considered separately in Chap. 18.

POSITIVE AND NEGATIVE SYMPTOMS

Abnormal sensory symptoms can be divided into two categories: positive and negative. The prototypical positive symptom is tingling (pins and needles); other positive sensory phenomena include itch and altered sensations that are described as pricking, bandlike, lightning-like shooting feelings (lancinations), aching, knifelike, twisting, drawing, pulling, tightening, burning, searing, electrical, or raw feelings. Such symptoms are often painful.

Positive phenomena usually result from trains of impulses generated at sites of lowered threshold or heightened excitability along a peripheral or central sensory pathway. The nature and severity of the abnormal sensation depend on the number, rate, timing, and distribution of ectopic impulses and the type and function of nervous tissue in which they arise. Because positive phenomena represent excessive activity in sensory pathways, they are not necessarily associated with a sensory deficit (loss) on examination.

Negative phenomena represent loss of sensory function and are characterized by diminished or absent feeling that often is experienced as numbness and by abnormal findings on sensory examination. In disorders affecting peripheral sensation, at least one-half the afferent axons innervating a particular site are probably lost or functionless before a sensory deficit can be demonstrated by clinical examination. If the rate of loss is slow, however, lack of cutaneous feeling may be unnoticed by the patient and difficult to demonstrate on examination, even though few sensory fibers are functioning; if it is rapid, both positive and negative phenomena are usually conspicuous. Subclinical degrees of sensory dysfunction may be revealed by sensory nerve conduction studies or somatosensory evoked potentials (Chap. 442e).

Whereas sensory symptoms may be either positive or negative, sensory signs on examination are always a measure of negative phenomena.

TERMINOLOGY

Paresthesias and dysesthesias are general terms used to denote positive sensory symptoms. The term *paresthesias* typically refers to tingling or pins-and-needles sensations but may include a wide variety of other abnormal sensations, except pain; it sometimes implies that the abnormal sensations are perceived spontaneously. The more general term *dysesthesias* denotes all types of abnormal sensations, including painful ones, regardless of whether a stimulus is evident.

Another set of terms refers to sensory abnormalities found on examination. *Hypesthesia* or *hypoesthesia* refers to a reduction of cutaneous sensation to a specific type of testing such as pressure, light touch, and warm or cold stimuli; *anesthesia*, to a complete absence of skin sensation to the same stimuli plus pinprick; and *hypalgesia* or *analgesia*, to reduced or absent pain perception (nociception). *Hyperesthesia* means pain or increased sensitivity in response to touch. Similarly, *allodynia* describes the situation in which a nonpainful stimulus, once perceived, is experienced as painful, even excruciating. An example is elicitation of a painful sensation by application of a vibrating tuning fork. *Hyperalgesia* denotes severe pain in response to a mildly noxious stimulus, and *hyperpathia*, a broad term, encompasses all the phenomena described by hyperesthesia, allodynia, and hyperalgesia. With hyperpathia, the threshold for a sensory stimulus is increased and perception is delayed, but once felt, it is unduly painful.

Disorders of deep sensation arising from muscle spindles, tendons, and joints affect proprioception (position sense). Manifestations include imbalance (particularly with eyes closed or in the dark), clumsiness of precision movements, and unsteadiness of gait, which are referred to collectively as *sensory ataxia*. Other findings on examination usually, but not invariably, include reduced or absent joint position and vibratory sensibility and absent deep tendon reflexes in the affected limbs. The Romberg sign is positive, which means that the patient sways markedly or topples when asked to stand with feet close together and eyes closed. In severe states of deafferentation involving deep sensation, the patient cannot walk or stand unaided or even sit unsupported. Continuous involuntary movements (*pseudoathetosis*) of the outstretched hands and fingers occur, particularly with eyes closed.

ANATOMY OF SENSATION

Cutaneous receptors are classified by the type of stimulus that optimally excites them. They consist of naked nerve endings (nociceptors, which respond to tissue-damaging stimuli, and thermoreceptors, which respond to noninjurious thermal stimuli) and encapsulated terminals (several types of mechanoreceptor, activated by physical deformation of the skin). Each type of receptor has its own set of sensitivities to specific stimuli, size and distinctness of receptive fields, and adaptational qualities.

Afferent fibers in peripheral nerve trunks traverse the dorsal roots and enter the dorsal horn of the spinal cord (Fig. 31-1). From there, the polysynaptic projections of the smaller fibers (unmyelinated and small myelinated), which subserve mainly nociception, itch, temperature sensibility, and touch, cross and ascend in the opposite anterior and lateral columns of the spinal cord, through the brainstem, to the ventral posterolateral (VPL) nucleus of the thalamus and ultimately project to the postcentral gyrus of the parietal cortex (Chap. 18). This is the *spinothalamic pathway* or *anterolateral system*. The larger fibers, which subserve tactile and position sense and kinesthesia, project rostrally in the posterior and posterolateral columns on the same side of the spinal cord and make their first synapse in the gracile or cuneate nucleus of the lower medulla. Axons of second-order neurons decussate and ascend in the medial lemniscus located medially in the medulla and in the tegmentum of the pons and midbrain and synapse in the VPL nucleus; third-order neurons project to parietal cortex as well as to other cortical areas. This large-fiber system is referred to as the *posterior column–medial lemniscal pathway* (lemniscal, for short). Although the fiber types and functions that make up the spinothalamic and lemniscal systems are relatively well known, many other fibers, particularly those associated with touch, pressure, and position sense, ascend in a diffusely distributed pattern both ipsilaterally and contralaterally in the anterolateral quadrants of the spinal cord. This explains why a complete lesion of the posterior columns of the spinal cord may be associated with little sensory deficit on examination.

Nerve conduction studies and nerve biopsy are important means of investigating the peripheral nervous system, but they do not evaluate the function or structure of cutaneous receptors and free nerve endings or of unmyelinated or thinly myelinated nerve fibers in the nerve trunks. Skin biopsy can be used to evaluate these structures in the dermis and epidermis.

CLINICAL EXAMINATION OF SENSATION

The main components of the sensory examination are tests of primary sensation (pain, touch, vibration, joint position, and thermal sensation) (Table 31-1). The examiner must depend on patient responses, and this complicates interpretation. Further, examination may be limited in some patients. In a stuporous patient, for example, sensory examination is reduced to observing the briskness of withdrawal in response to a pinch or another noxious stimulus. Comparison of responses on the two sides of the body is essential. In an alert but uncooperative patient, it may not be possible to examine cutaneous sensation, but some idea of proprioceptive function may be gained by noting the patient's best performance of movements requiring balance and precision.

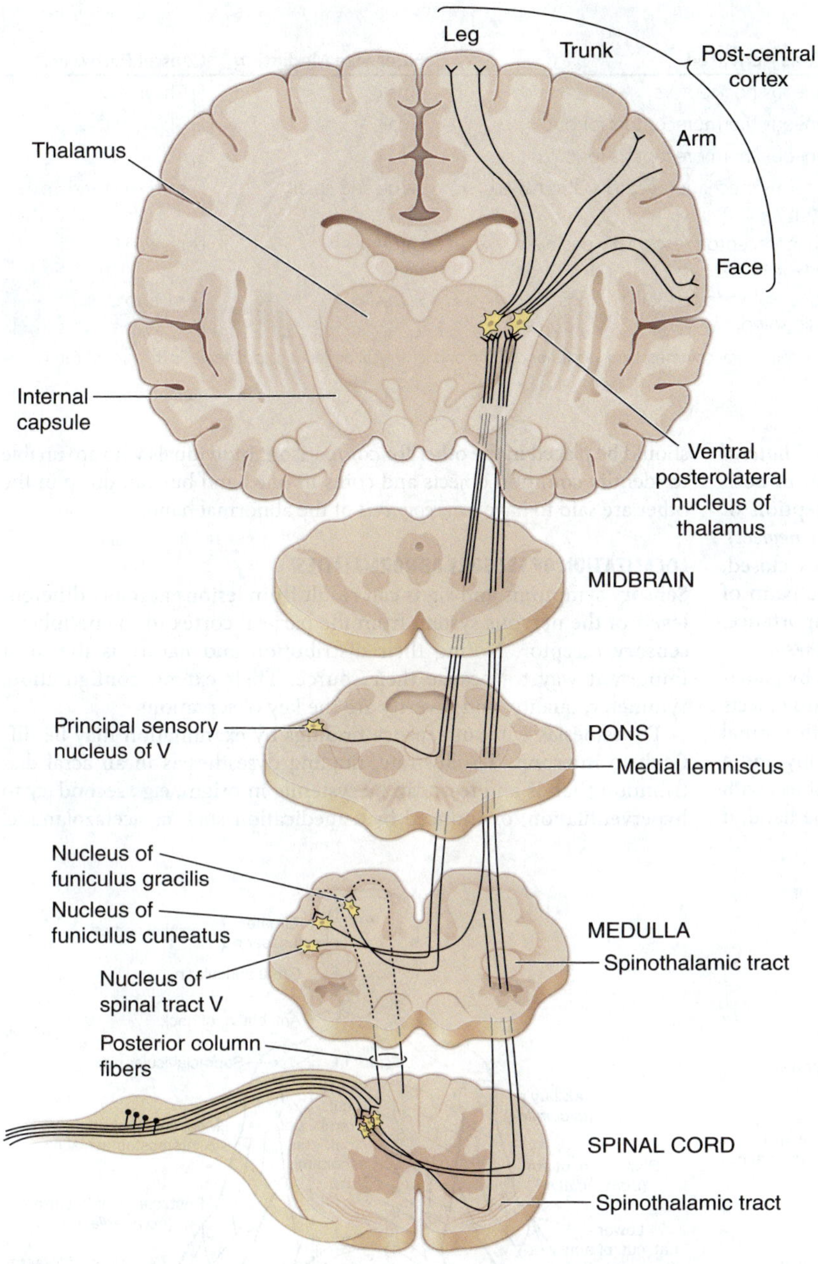

FIGURE 31-1 The main somatosensory pathways. The spinothalamic tract (pain, thermal sense) and the posterior column–lemniscal system (touch, pressure, joint position) are shown. Offshoots from the ascending anterolateral fasciculus (spinothalamic tract) to nuclei in the medulla, pons, and mesencephalon and nuclear terminations of the tract are indicated. *(From AH Ropper, MA Samuels: Adams and Victor's Principles of Neurology, 9th ed. New York, McGraw-Hill, 2009.)*

Primary Sensation The sense of pain usually is tested with a clean pin, which is then discarded. The patient is asked to close the eyes and focus on the pricking or unpleasant quality of the stimulus, not just the pressure or touch sensation elicited. Areas of hypalgesia should be mapped by proceeding radially from the most hypalgesic site. Temperature sensation to both hot and cold is best tested with small containers filled with water of the desired temperature. An alternative way to test cold sensation is to touch a metal object, such as a tuning fork at room temperature, to the skin. For testing warm temperatures, the tuning fork or another metal object may be held under warm water of the desired temperature and then used. The appreciation of both cold and warmth should be tested because different receptors respond to each. Touch usually is tested with a wisp of cotton or a fine camel hair brush, minimizing pressure on the skin. In general, it is better to avoid testing touch on hairy skin because of the profusion of the sensory endings that surround each hair follicle. The patient is tested with the eyes closed and should indicate as soon as the stimulus is perceived, indicating its location.

Joint position testing is a measure of proprioception. With the patient's eyes closed, joint position is tested in the distal interphalangeal joint of the great toe and fingers. The digit is held by its sides, distal to the joint being tested, and moved passively while more proximal joints are stabilized—the patient indicates the change in position or direction of movement. If errors are made, more proximal joints are tested. A test of proximal joint position sense, primarily at the shoulder, is performed by asking the patient to bring the two index fingers together with arms extended and eyes closed. Normal individuals can do this accurately, with errors of 1 cm or less.

The sense of vibration is tested with an oscillating tuning fork that vibrates at 128 Hz. Vibration is tested over bony points, beginning distally; in the feet, it is tested over the dorsal surface of the distal phalanx of the big toes and at the malleoli of the ankles, and in the hands, it is tested dorsally at the distal phalanx of the fingers. If abnormalities are found, more proximal sites should be examined. Vibratory thresholds at the same site in the patient and the examiner may be compared for control purposes.

Quantitative Sensory Testing Effective sensory testing devices are commercially available. Quantitative sensory testing is particularly useful for serial evaluation of cutaneous sensation in clinical trials. Threshold testing for touch and vibratory and thermal sensation is the most widely used application.

Cortical Sensation The most commonly used tests of cortical function are two-point discrimination, touch localization, and bilateral simultaneous stimulation and tests for graphesthesia and stereognosis. Abnormalities of these sensory tests, in the presence of normal primary sensation in an alert cooperative patient, signify a lesion of the parietal cortex or thalamocortical projections. If primary sensation is altered, these cortical discriminative functions usually will be abnormal also. Comparisons should always be made between analogous sites on the two sides of the body because the deficit with a specific parietal lesion is likely to be unilateral.

Two-point discrimination is tested with special calipers, the points of which may be set from 2 mm to several centimeters apart and then applied simultaneously to the test site. On the fingertips, a normal individual can distinguish about a 3-mm separation of points.

Touch localization is performed by light pressure for an instant with the examiner's fingertip or a wisp of cotton wool; the patient,

In patients with sensory complaints, testing should begin in the center of the affected region and proceed radially until sensation is perceived as normal. The distribution of any abnormality is defined and compared to root and peripheral nerve territories (Figs. 31-2 and 31-3). Some patients present with sensory symptoms that do not fit an anatomic localization and are accompanied by either no abnormalities or gross inconsistencies on examination. The examiner should consider whether the sensory symptoms are a disguised request for help with psychologic or situational problems. Sensory examination of a patient who has no neurologic complaints can be brief and consist of pinprick, touch, and vibration testing in the hands and feet plus evaluation of stance and gait, including the Romberg maneuver (Chap. 438). Evaluation of stance and gait also tests the integrity of motor and cerebellar systems.

TABLE 31-1 TESTING PRIMARY SENSATION

Sense	Test Device	Endings Activated	Fiber Size Mediating	Central Pathway
Pain	Pinprick	Cutaneous nociceptors	Small	SpTh, also D
Temperature, heat	Warm metal object	Cutaneous thermoreceptors for hot	Small	SpTh
Temperature, cold	Cold metal object	Cutaneous thermoreceptors for cold	Small	SpTh
Touch	Cotton wisp, fine brush	Cutaneous mechanoreceptors, also naked endings	Large and small	Lem, also D and SpTh
Vibration	Tuning fork, 128 Hz	Mechanoreceptors, especially pacinian corpuscles	Large	Lem, also D
Joint position	Passive movement of specific joints	Joint capsule and tendon endings, muscle spindles	Large	Lem, also D

Abbreviations: D, diffuse ascending projections in ipsilateral and contralateral anterolateral columns; Lem, posterior column and lemniscal projection, ipsilateral; SpTh, spinothalamic projection, contralateral.

whose eyes are closed, is required to identify the site of touch. *Bilateral simultaneous stimulation* at analogous sites (e.g., the dorsum of both hands) can be carried out to determine whether the perception of touch is extinguished consistently on one side (*extinction* or *neglect*). *Graphesthesia* refers to the capacity to recognize, with eyes closed, letters or numbers drawn by the examiner's fingertip on the palm of the hand. Once again, interside comparison is of prime importance. Inability to recognize numbers or letters is termed *agraphesthesia*.

Stereognosis refers to the ability to identify common objects by palpation, recognizing their shape, texture, and size. Common standard objects such as keys, paper clips, and coins are best used. Patients with normal stereognosis should be able to distinguish a dime from a penny and a nickel from a quarter without looking. Patients should feel the object with only one hand at a time. If they are unable to identify it in one hand, it should be placed in the other for comparison. Individuals who are unable to identify common objects and coins in one hand but can do so in the other are said to have *astereognosis* of the abnormal hand.

LOCALIZATION OF SENSORY ABNORMALITIES

Sensory symptoms and signs can result from lesions at many different levels of the nervous system from the parietal cortex to the peripheral sensory receptor. Noting their distribution and nature is the most important way to localize their source. Their extent, configuration, symmetry, quality, and severity are the key observations.

Dysesthesias without sensory findings by examination may be difficult to interpret. To illustrate, tingling dysesthesias in an acral distribution (hands and feet) can be systemic in origin, e.g., secondary to hyperventilation, or induced by a medication such as acetazolamide.

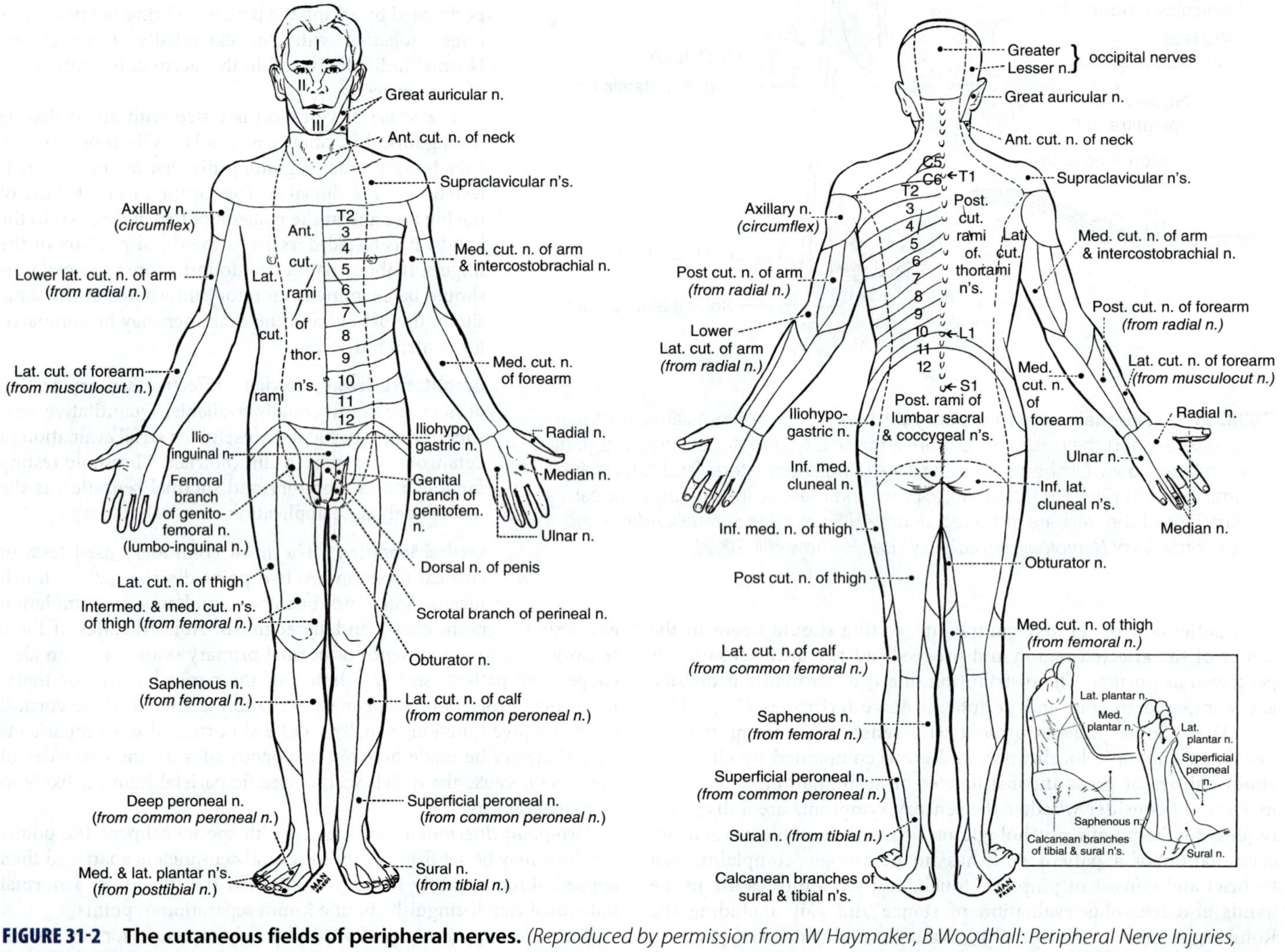

FIGURE 31-2 The cutaneous fields of peripheral nerves. *(Reproduced by permission from W Haymaker, B Woodhall: Peripheral Nerve Injuries, 2nd ed. Philadelphia, Saunders, 1953.)*

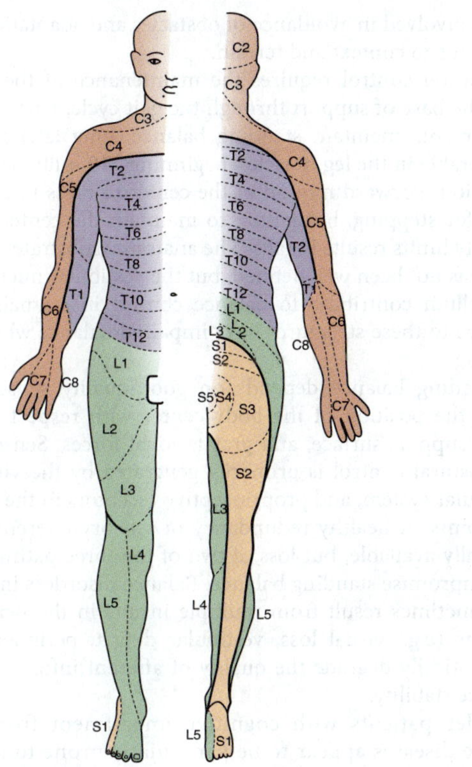

FIGURE 31-3 Distribution of the sensory spinal roots on the surface of the body (dermatomes). *(From D Sinclair: Mechanisms of Cutaneous Sensation. Oxford, UK, Oxford University Press, 1981; with permission from Dr. David Sinclair.)*

Distal dysesthesias can also be an early event in an evolving polyneuropathy or may herald a myelopathy, such as from vitamin B_{12} deficiency. Sometimes distal dysesthesias have no definable basis. In contrast, dysesthesias that correspond in distribution to that of a particular peripheral nerve structure denote a lesion at that site. For instance, dysesthesias restricted to the fifth digit and the adjacent one-half of the fourth finger on one hand reliably point to disorder of the ulnar nerve, most commonly at the elbow.

Nerve and Root In focal nerve trunk lesions, sensory abnormalities are readily mapped and generally have discrete boundaries (Figs. 31-2 and 31-3). Root ("radicular") lesions frequently are accompanied by deep, aching pain along the course of the related nerve trunk. With compression of a fifth lumbar (L5) or first sacral (S1) root, as from a ruptured intervertebral disk, sciatica (radicular pain relating to the sciatic nerve trunk) is a common manifestation (Chap. 22). With a lesion affecting a single root, sensory deficits may be minimal or absent because adjacent root territories overlap extensively.

Isolated mononeuropathies may cause symptoms beyond the territory supplied by the affected nerve, but abnormalities on examination typically are confined to appropriate anatomic boundaries. In multiple mononeuropathies, symptoms and signs occur in discrete territories supplied by different individual nerves and—as more nerves are affected—may simulate a polyneuropathy if deficits become confluent. With polyneuropathies, sensory deficits are generally graded, distal, and symmetric in distribution (Chap. 459). Dysesthesias, followed by numbness, begin in the toes and ascend symmetrically. When dysesthesias reach the knees, they usually also have appeared in the fingertips. The process is nerve length–dependent, and the deficit is often described as "stocking-glove" in type. Involvement of both hands and feet also occurs with lesions of the upper cervical cord or the brainstem, but an upper level of the sensory disturbance may then be found on the trunk and other evidence of a central lesion may be present, such as sphincter involvement or signs of an upper motor neuron lesion (Chap. 30). Although most polyneuropathies are pansensory and affect all modalities of sensation, selective sensory dysfunction according to nerve fiber size may occur. Small-fiber polyneuropathies are characterized by burning, painful dysesthesias with reduced pinprick and thermal sensation but with sparing of proprioception, motor function, and deep tendon reflexes. Touch is involved variably; when it is spared, the sensory pattern is referred to as exhibiting *sensory dissociation*. Sensory dissociation may occur also with spinal cord lesions as well as small-fiber neuropathies. Large-fiber polyneuropathies are characterized by vibration and position sense deficits, imbalance, absent tendon reflexes, and variable motor dysfunction but preservation of most cutaneous sensation. Dysesthesias, if present at all, tend to be tingling or bandlike in quality.

Sensory neuronopathy (or ganglionopathy) is characterized by widespread but asymmetric sensory loss occurring in a non-length-dependent manner so that it may occur proximally or distally and in the arms, legs, or both. Pain and numbness progress to sensory ataxia and impairment of all sensory modalities with time. This condition is usually paraneoplastic or idiopathic in origin (Chaps. 122 and 459) or related to an autoimmune disease, particularly Sjögren's syndrome.

Spinal Cord (See also Chap. 456) If the spinal cord is transected, all sensation is lost below the level of transection. Bladder and bowel function also are lost, as is motor function. Lateral hemisection of the spinal cord produces the Brown-Séquard syndrome, with absent pain and temperature sensation contralaterally and loss of proprioceptive sensation and power ipsilaterally below the lesion (see Figs. 31-1 and 456-1).

Numbness or paresthesias in both feet may arise from a spinal cord lesion; this is especially likely when the upper level of the sensory loss extends to the trunk. When all extremities are affected, the lesion is probably in the cervical region or brainstem unless a peripheral neuropathy is responsible. The presence of upper motor neuron signs (Chap. 30) supports a central lesion; a hyperesthetic band on the trunk may suggest the level of involvement.

A dissociated sensory loss can reflect spinothalamic tract involvement in the spinal cord, especially if the deficit is unilateral and has an upper level on the torso. Bilateral spinothalamic tract involvement occurs with lesions affecting the center of the spinal cord, such as in syringomyelia. There is a dissociated sensory loss with impairment of pinprick and temperature appreciation but relative preservation of light touch, position sense, and vibration appreciation.

Dysfunction of the posterior columns in the spinal cord or of the posterior root entry zone may lead to a bandlike sensation around the trunk or a feeling of tight pressure in one or more limbs. Flexion of the neck sometimes leads to an electric shock–like sensation that radiates down the back and into the legs (Lhermitte's sign) in patients with a cervical lesion affecting the posterior columns, such as from multiple sclerosis, cervical spondylosis, or recent irradiation to the cervical region.

Brainstem Crossed patterns of sensory disturbance, in which one side of the face and the opposite side of the body are affected, localize to the lateral medulla. Here a small lesion may damage both the ipsilateral descending trigeminal tract and the ascending spinothalamic fibers subserving the opposite arm, leg, and hemitorso (see "Lateral medullary syndrome" in Fig. 446-10). A lesion in the tegmentum of the pons and midbrain, where the lemniscal and spinothalamic tracts merge, causes pansensory loss contralaterally.

Thalamus Hemisensory disturbance with tingling numbness from head to foot is often thalamic in origin but also can arise from the anterior parietal region. If abrupt in onset, the lesion is likely to be due to a small stroke (lacunar infarction), particularly if localized to the thalamus. Occasionally, with lesions affecting the VPL nucleus or adjacent white matter, a syndrome of thalamic pain, also called *Déjerine-Roussy syndrome*, may ensue. The persistent, unrelenting unilateral pain often is described in dramatic terms.

Cortex With lesions of the parietal lobe involving either the cortex or the subjacent white matter, the most prominent symptoms are contralateral hemineglect, hemi-inattention, and a tendency not to use the affected hand and arm. On cortical sensory testing (e.g., two-point discrimination, graphesthesia), abnormalities are often found but primary sensation is usually intact. Anterior parietal infarction may present as a pseudothalamic syndrome with contralateral loss of primary sensation from head to toe. Dysesthesias or a sense of numbness and, rarely, a painful state may also occur.

Focal Sensory Seizures These seizures generally are due to lesions in the area of the postcentral or precentral gyrus. The principal symptom of focal sensory seizures is tingling, but additional, more complex sensations may occur, such as a rushing feeling, a sense of warmth, or a sense of movement without detectable motion. Symptoms typically are unilateral; commonly begin in the arm or hand, face, or foot; and often spread in a manner that reflects the cortical representation of different bodily parts, as in a Jacksonian march. Their duration is variable; seizures may be transient, lasting only for seconds, or persist for an hour or more. Focal motor features may supervene, often becoming generalized with loss of consciousness and tonic-clonic jerking.

ACKNOWLEDGMENT

Arthur Asbury authored or co-authored this chapter in earlier editions of this book.

32 Gait and Balance Disorders

Lewis Sudarsky

PREVALENCE, MORBIDITY, AND MORTALITY

Gait and balance problems are common in the elderly and contribute to the risk of falls and injury. Gait disorders have been described in 15% of individuals older than 65. By age 80 one person in four will use a mechanical aid to assist with ambulation. Among those 85 and older, the prevalence of gait abnormality approaches 40%. In epidemiologic studies, gait disorders are consistently identified as a major risk factor for falls and injury.

A substantial number of older persons report insecure balance and experience falls and fear of falling. Prospective studies indicate that 30% of those older than 65 fall each year. The proportion is even higher in frail elderly and nursing home patients. Each year, 8% of individuals older than 75 suffer a serious fall-related injury. Hip fractures result in hospitalization, can lead to nursing home admission, and are associated with an increased mortality risk in the subsequent year. For each person who is physically disabled, there are others whose functional independence is limited by anxiety and fear of falling. Nearly one in five elderly individuals voluntarily restricts his or her activity because of fear of falling. With loss of ambulation, the quality of life diminishes, and rates of morbidity and mortality increase.

ANATOMY AND PHYSIOLOGY

An upright bipedal gait depends on the successful integration of postural control and locomotion. These functions are widely distributed in the central nervous system. The biomechanics of bipedal walking are complex, and the performance is easily compromised by a neurologic deficit at any level. Command and control centers in the brainstem, cerebellum, and forebrain modify the action of spinal pattern generators to promote stepping. While a form of "fictive locomotion" can be elicited from quadrupedal animals after spinal transection, this capacity is limited in primates. Step generation in primates is dependent on locomotor centers in the pontine tegmentum, midbrain, and subthalamic region. Locomotor synergies are executed through the reticular formation and descending pathways in the ventromedial spinal cord. Cerebral control provides a goal and purpose for walking and is involved in avoidance of obstacles and adaptation of locomotor programs to context and terrain.

Postural control requires the maintenance of the center of mass over the base of support through the gait cycle. Unconscious postural adjustments maintain standing balance: long latency responses are measurable in the leg muscles, beginning 110 milliseconds after a perturbation. Forward motion of the center of mass provides propulsive force for stepping, but failure to maintain the center of mass within stability limits results in falls. The anatomic substrate for dynamic balance has not been well defined, but the vestibular nucleus and midline cerebellum contribute to balance control in animals. Patients with damage to these structures have impaired balance while standing and walking.

Standing balance depends on good-quality sensory information about the position of the body center with respect to the environment, support surface, and gravitational forces. Sensory information for postural control is primarily generated by the visual system, the vestibular system, and proprioceptive receptors in the muscle spindles and joints. A healthy redundancy of sensory afferent information is generally available, but loss of two of the three pathways is sufficient to compromise standing balance. Balance disorders in older individuals sometimes result from multiple insults in the peripheral sensory systems (e.g., visual loss, vestibular deficit, peripheral neuropathy) that critically degrade the quality of afferent information needed for balance stability.

Older patients with cognitive impairment from neurodegenerative diseases appear to be particularly prone to falls and injury. There is a growing body of literature on the use of attentional resources to manage gait and balance. Walking is generally considered to be unconscious and automatic, but the ability to walk while attending to a cognitive task (*dual-task walking*) may be compromised in frail elderly individuals with a history of falls. Older patients with deficits in executive function may have particular difficulty in managing the attentional resources needed for dynamic balance when distracted.

DISORDERS OF GAIT

Disorders of gait may be attributed to frailty, fatigue, arthritis, and orthopedic deformity, but neurologic causes are disabling and important to address. The heterogeneity of gait disorders observed in clinical practice reflects the large network of neural systems involved in the task. Walking is vulnerable to neurologic disease at every level. Gait disorders have been classified descriptively on the basis of abnormal physiology and biomechanics. One problem with this approach is that many failing gaits look fundamentally similar. This overlap reflects common patterns of adaptation to threatened balance stability and declining performance. *The gait disorder observed clinically must be viewed as the product of a neurologic deficit and a functional adaptation.* Unique features of the failing gait are often overwhelmed by the adaptive response. Some common patterns of abnormal gait are summarized next. Gait disorders can also be classified by etiology (Table 32-1).

TABLE 32-1 ETIOLOGY OF GAIT DISORDERS

Etiology	No. of Cases	Percent
Sensory deficits	22	18.3
Myelopathy	20	16.7
Multiple infarcts	18	15.0
Parkinsonism	14	11.7
Cerebellar degeneration	8	6.7
Hydrocephalus	8	6.7
Toxic/metabolic causes	3	2.5
Psychogenic causes	4	3.3
Other	6	5.0
Unknown causes	17	14.2
Total	120	100

Source: Reproduced with permission from J Masdeu, L Sudarsky, L Wolfson: *Gait Disorders of Aging*. Lippincott Raven, 1997.

CAUTIOUS GAIT

The term *cautious gait* is used to describe the patient who walks with an abbreviated stride and lowered center of mass, as if walking on a slippery surface. This disorder is both common and nonspecific. It is, in essence, an adaptation to a perceived postural threat. There may be an associated fear of falling. This disorder can be observed in more than one-third of older patients with gait impairment. Physical therapy often improves walking to the degree that follow-up observation may reveal a more specific underlying disorder.

STIFF-LEGGED GAIT

Spastic gait is characterized by stiffness in the legs, an imbalance of muscle tone, and a tendency to circumduct and scuff the feet. The disorder reflects compromise of corticospinal command and overactivity of spinal reflexes. The patient may walk on the toes. In extreme instances, the legs cross due to increased tone in the adductors. Upper motor neuron signs are present on physical examination. Shoes often reflect an uneven pattern of wear across the outside. The disorder may be cerebral or spinal in origin.

Myelopathy from cervical spondylosis is a common cause of spastic or spastic-ataxic gait in the elderly. Demyelinating disease and trauma are the leading causes of myelopathy in younger patients. In chronic progressive myelopathy of unknown cause, a workup with laboratory and imaging tests may establish a diagnosis. A family history should suggest hereditary spastic paraplegia (Chap. 452); genetic testing is now available for some of the common mutations responsible for this disorder. Tropical spastic paraparesis related to the retrovirus human T-cell lymphotropic virus 1 (HTLV-1) is endemic in parts of the Caribbean and South America. A structural lesion, such as a tumor or a spinal vascular malformation, should be excluded with appropriate testing. **Spinal cord disorders are discussed in detail in Chap. 456.**

With cerebral spasticity, asymmetry is common, the upper extremities are usually involved, and dysarthria is often an associated feature. Common causes include vascular disease (stroke), multiple sclerosis, and perinatal injury to the nervous system (cerebral palsy).

Other stiff-legged gaits include dystonia (Chap. 449) and stiff-person syndrome (Chap. 122). Dystonia is a disorder characterized by sustained muscle contractions resulting in repetitive twisting movements and abnormal posture. It often has a genetic basis. Dystonic spasms can produce plantar flexion and inversion of the feet, sometimes with torsion of the trunk. In autoimmune stiff-person syndrome, exaggerated lordosis of the lumbar spine and overactivation of antagonist muscles restrict trunk and lower-limb movement and result in a wooden or fixed posture.

PARKINSONISM AND FREEZING GAIT

Parkinson's disease (Chap. 449) is common, affecting 1% of the population >55 years of age. The stooped posture and shuffling gait are characteristic and distinctive features. Patients sometimes accelerate (festinate) with walking, display retropulsion, or exhibit a tendency to turn en bloc. A National Institutes of Health workshop defined freezing of gait as "brief, episodic absence of forward progression of the feet, despite the intention to walk." Gait freezing occurs in 26% of Parkinson's patients by the end of 5 years and develops in most such patients eventually. Postural instability and falling occur as the disease progresses; some falls are precipitated by freezing of gait.

Freezing of gait is even more common in some Parkinson's-related neurodegenerative disorders, such as progressive supranuclear palsy, multiple-system atrophy, and corticobasal degeneration. Patients with these disorders frequently present with axial stiffness, postural instability, and a shuffling, freezing gait while lacking the characteristic pill-rolling tremor of Parkinson's disease. Falls within the first year suggest the possibility of progressive supranuclear palsy.

Hyperkinetic movement disorders also produce characteristic and recognizable disturbances in gait. In Huntington's disease (Chap. 449), the unpredictable occurrence of choreic movements gives the gait a dancing quality. Tardive dyskinesia is the cause of many odd, stereotypic gait disorders seen in patients chronically exposed to antipsychotics and other drugs that block the D_2 dopamine receptor.

FRONTAL GAIT DISORDER

Frontal gait disorder, sometimes known as *gait apraxia*, is common in the elderly and has a variety of causes. The term is used to describe a shuffling, freezing gait with imbalance and other signs of higher cerebral dysfunction. Typical features include a wide base of support, a short stride, shuffling along the floor, and difficulty with starts and turns. Many patients exhibit a difficulty with gait initiation that is descriptively characterized as the "slipping clutch" syndrome or gait ignition failure. The term *lower-body parkinsonism* is also used to describe such patients. Strength is generally preserved, and patients are able to make stepping movements when not standing and maintaining their balance at the same time. This disorder is best considered a higher-level motor control disorder, as opposed to an apraxia (Chap. 36).

The most common cause of frontal gait disorder is vascular disease, particularly subcortical small-vessel disease. Lesions are frequently found in the deep frontal white matter and centrum ovale. Gait disorder may be the salient feature in hypertensive patients with ischemic lesions of the deep-hemisphere white matter (*Binswanger's disease*). The clinical syndrome includes mental changes (variable in degree), dysarthria, pseudobulbar affect (emotional disinhibition), increased tone, and hyperreflexia in the lower limbs.

Communicating hydrocephalus in adults also presents with a gait disorder of this type. Other features of the diagnostic triad (mental changes, incontinence) may be absent in the initial stages. MRI demonstrates ventricular enlargement, an enlarged flow void about the aqueduct, and a variable degree of periventricular white-matter change. A lumbar puncture or dynamic test is necessary to confirm hydrocephalus.

CEREBELLAR GAIT ATAXIA

Disorders of the cerebellum have a dramatic impact on gait and balance. Cerebellar gait ataxia is characterized by a wide base of support, lateral instability of the trunk, erratic foot placement, and decompensation of balance when attempting to walk on a narrow base. Difficulty maintaining balance when turning is often an early feature. Patients are unable to walk tandem heel to toe and display truncal sway in narrow-based or tandem stance. They show considerable variation in their tendency to fall in daily life.

Causes of cerebellar ataxia in older patients include stroke, trauma, tumor, and neurodegenerative disease such as multiple-system atrophy (Chaps. 449 and 454) and various forms of hereditary cerebellar degeneration (Chap. 450). A short expansion at the site of the fragile X mutation (*fragile X pre-mutation*) has been associated with gait ataxia in older men. Alcoholic cerebellar degeneration can be screened by history and often confirmed by MRI. In patients with ataxia, MRI demonstrates the extent and topography of cerebellar atrophy.

SENSORY ATAXIA

As reviewed earlier in this chapter, balance depends on high-quality afferent information from the visual and the vestibular systems and proprioception. When this information is lost or degraded, balance during locomotion is impaired and instability results. The sensory ataxia of tabetic neurosyphilis is a classic example. The contemporary equivalent is the patient with neuropathy affecting large fibers. Vitamin B_{12} deficiency is a treatable cause of large-fiber sensory loss in the spinal cord and peripheral nervous system. Joint position and vibration sense are diminished in the lower limbs. The stance in such patients is destabilized by eye closure; they often look down at their feet when walking and do poorly in the dark. Table 32-2 compares sensory ataxia with cerebellar ataxia and frontal gait disorder. Some frail older patients exhibit a syndrome of imbalance from the combined effect of multiple sensory deficits. Such patients have disturbances in proprioception, vision, and vestibular sense that impair postural support.

NEUROMUSCULAR DISEASE

Patients with neuromuscular disease often have an abnormal gait, occasionally as a presenting feature. With distal weakness (peripheral neuropathy), the step height is increased to compensate for footdrop, and the sole of the foot may slap on the floor during weight acceptance. Neuropathy may be associated with a degree of sensory imbalance, as described earlier. Patients with myopathy or muscular dystrophy more

TABLE 32-2 FEATURES OF CEREBELLAR ATAXIA, SENSORY ATAXIA, AND FRONTAL GAIT DISORDERS

Feature	Cerebellar Ataxia	Sensory Ataxia	Frontal Gait
Base of support	Wide-based	Narrow base, looks down	Wide-based
Velocity	Variable	Slow	Very slow
Stride	Irregular, lurching	Regular with path deviation	Short, shuffling
Romberg test	+/–	Unsteady, falls	+/–
Heel → shin	Abnormal	+/–	Normal
Initiation	Normal	Normal	Hesitant
Turns	Unsteady	+/–	Hesitant, multistep
Postural instability	+	+++	++++ Poor postural synergies rising from a chair
Falls	Late event	Frequent	Frequent

typically exhibit proximal weakness. Weakness of the hip girdle may result in some degree of excess pelvic sway during locomotion.

TOXIC AND METABOLIC DISORDERS

Alcohol intoxication is the most common cause of acute walking difficulty. Chronic toxicity from medications and metabolic disturbances can impair motor function and gait. Mental status changes may be found, and examination may reveal asterixis or myoclonus. Static equilibrium is disturbed, and such patients are easily thrown off balance. Disequilibrium is particularly evident in patients with chronic renal disease and those with hepatic failure, in whom asterixis may impair postural support. Sedative drugs, especially neuroleptics and long-acting benzodiazepines, affect postural control and increase the risk for falls. These disorders are especially important to recognize because they are often treatable.

PSYCHOGENIC GAIT DISORDER

Psychogenic disorders are common in neurologic practice, and the presentation often involves gait. Some patients with extreme anxiety or phobia walk with exaggerated caution with abduction of the arms, as if walking on ice. This inappropriately overcautious gait differs in degree from the gait of the patient who is insecure and making adjustments for imbalance. Depressed patients exhibit primarily slowness, a manifestation of psychomotor retardation, and lack of purpose in their stride. Hysterical gait disorders are among the most spectacular encountered. Odd gyrations of posture with wastage of muscular energy (astasia–abasia), extreme slow motion, and dramatic fluctuations over time may be observed in patients with somatoform disorders and conversion reactions.

APPROACH TO THE PATIENT: Slowly Progressive Disorder of Gait

When reviewing the history, it is helpful to inquire about the onset and progression of disability. Initial awareness of an unsteady gait often follows a fall. Stepwise evolution or sudden progression suggests vascular disease. Gait disorder may be associated with urinary urgency and incontinence, particularly in patients with cervical spine disease or hydrocephalus. It is always important to review the use of alcohol and medications that affect gait and balance. Information on localization derived from the neurologic examination can be helpful in narrowing the list of possible diagnoses.

Gait observation provides an immediate sense of the patient's degree of disability. Arthritic and antalgic gaits are recognized by observation, though neurologic and orthopedic problems may coexist. Characteristic patterns of abnormality are sometimes seen, though, as stated previously, failing gaits often look fundamentally similar. Cadence (steps per minute), velocity, and stride length can be recorded by timing a patient over a fixed distance. Watching the patient rise from a chair provides a good functional assessment of balance.

Brain imaging studies may be informative in patients with an undiagnosed disorder of gait. MRI is sensitive for cerebral lesions of vascular or demyelinating disease and is a good screening test for occult hydrocephalus. Patients with recurrent falls are at risk for subdural hematoma. As mentioned earlier, many elderly patients with gait and balance difficulty have white matter abnormalities in the periventricular region and centrum semiovale. While these lesions may be an incidental finding, a substantial burden of white matter disease will ultimately impact cerebral control of locomotion.

DISORDERS OF BALANCE

DEFINITION, ETIOLOGY, AND MANIFESTATIONS

Balance is the ability to maintain equilibrium—a state in which opposing physical forces cancel one another out. In physiology, this term is taken to mean the ability to control the center of mass with respect to gravity and the support surface. In reality, people are not consciously aware of their center of mass, but everyone (particularly gymnasts, figure skaters, and platform divers, for example) move so as to manage it. Disorders of balance present as difficulty maintaining posture while standing and walking and as a subjective sense of disequilibrium, which is a form of dizziness.

The cerebellum and vestibular system organize antigravity responses needed to maintain an upright posture. These responses are physiologically complex, and the anatomic representation they entail is not well understood. Failure, resulting in disequilibrium, can occur at several levels: cerebellar, vestibular, somatosensory, and higher-level disequilibrium.

Patients with *cerebellar* ataxia do not generally complain of dizziness, though balance is visibly impaired. Neurologic examination reveals a variety of cerebellar signs. Postural compensation may prevent falls early on, but falls are inevitable with disease progression. The progression of neurodegenerative ataxia is often measured by the number of years to loss of stable ambulation.

Vestibular disorders (Chap. 28) have symptoms and signs that fall into three categories: (1) vertigo (the subjective inappropriate perception or illusion of movement); (2) nystagmus (involuntary eye movements); and (3) impaired standing balance. Not every patient has all manifestations. Patients with vestibular deficits related to ototoxic drugs may lack vertigo or obvious nystagmus, but their balance is impaired on standing and walking, and they cannot navigate in the dark. Laboratory testing is available to investigate vestibular deficits.

Somatosensory deficits also produce imbalance and falls. There is often a subjective sense of insecure balance and fear of falling. Postural control is compromised by eye closure (*Romberg's sign*); these patients also have difficulty navigating in the dark. A dramatic example is provided by the patient with autoimmune subacute sensory neuropathy, which is sometimes a paraneoplastic disorder (Chap. 122). Compensatory strategies enable such patients to walk in the virtual absence of proprioception, but the task requires active visual monitoring.

Patients with *higher-level disorders of equilibrium* have difficulty maintaining balance in daily life and may present with falls. Their awareness of balance impairment may be reduced. Patients taking sedating medications are in this category. In prospective studies, dementia and sedating medications substantially increase the risk for falls.

FALLS

Falls are common in the elderly; 30% of people older than 65 who are living in the community fall each year. Modest changes in balance function have been described in fit older individuals as a result of normal aging. Subtle deficits in sensory systems, attention, and motor reaction time contribute to the risk, and environmental hazards abound. Many falls by older adults are episodes of tripping or slipping, often designated *mechanical falls.* A fall is not a neurologic problem per se, but there are events for which neurologic evaluation is appropriate.

It is important to distinguish falls associated with loss of consciousness (syncope, seizure), which require appropriate evaluation and intervention (Chaps. 27 and 445). In most prospective studies, a small subset of individuals experience a large number of fall events. These individuals with recurrent falls often have gait and balance issues that need to be addressed.

Fall Patterns: The Event Description The history of a fall is often problematic or incomplete, and the underlying mechanism or cause may be difficult to establish in retrospect. The patient and family may have limited information about what triggered the fall. Injuries can complicate the physical examination. While there is no standard nosology of falls, some common clinical patterns may emerge and provide a clue.

DROP ATTACKS AND COLLAPSING FALLS Drop attacks are sudden collapsing falls without loss of consciousness. Patients who collapse from lack of postural tone present a diagnostic challenge. Patients may report that their legs just "gave out" underneath them; their families may describe these patients as "collapsing in a heap." Orthostatic hypotension may be a factor in some such falls, and this possibility should be thoroughly evaluated. Rarely, a colloid cyst of the third ventricle can present with intermittent obstruction of the foramen of Monro, with a consequent drop attack. While collapsing falls are more common among older patients with vascular risk factors, they should not be confused with vertebrobasilar ischemic attacks.

TOPPLING FALLS Some patients maintain tone in antigravity muscles but fall over like a tree trunk, as if postural defenses had disengaged. There may be a consistent direction to such falls. The patient with cerebellar pathology may lean and topple over toward the side of the lesion. Patients with lesions of the vestibular system or its central pathways may experience lateral pulsion and toppling falls. Patients with progressive supranuclear palsy often fall over backward. Falls of this nature occur in patients with advanced Parkinson's disease once postural instability has developed.

FALLS DUE TO GAIT FREEZING Another fall pattern in Parkinson's disease and related disorders is the fall due to freezing of gait. The feet stick to the floor and the center of mass keeps moving, resulting in a disequilibrium from which the patient has difficulty recovering. This sequence of events can result in a forward fall. Gait freezing can also occur as the patient attempts to turn and change direction. Similarly, patients with Parkinson's disease and festinating gait may find their feet unable to keep up and may thus fall forward.

FALLS RELATED TO SENSORY LOSS Patients with somatosensory, visual, or vestibular deficits are prone to falls. These patients have particular difficulty dealing with poor illumination or walking on uneven ground. They often report subjective imbalance, apprehension, and fear of falling. Deficits in joint position and vibration sense are apparent on physical examination. These patients may be especially responsive to a rehabilitation-based intervention.

WEAKNESS AND FRAILTY Patients who lack strength in antigravity muscles have difficulty rising from a chair, tire easily when walking, and have difficulty maintaining their balance after a perturbation. These patients are often unable to get up after a fall and may have to remain on the floor for a prolonged period until help arrives. Deconditioning of this sort is often treatable. Resistance strength training can increase muscle mass and leg strength, even for people in their eighties and nineties.

RISK FACTORS FOR FALLS

The most productive approach is to identify the high-risk patient prospectively, before there is a serious injury. Patients at particular risk include hospitalized patients with mental status changes, nursing home residents, patients with dementia, and those taking medications that compromise attention and alertness. Patients with Parkinson's disease and other gait disorders are also at increased risk. (Table 32-3) summarizes a meta-analysis of prospective studies establishing the principal risk factors for falls. It is often possible to address and mitigate some of the major risk factors. Medication overuse may be the most important remediable risk factor for falls.

TABLE 32-3 META-ANALYSIS OF RISK FACTORS FOR FALLS: SUMMARY OF 16 CONTROLLED STUDIES

Risk Factor	Mean RR (OR)	Range
Weakness	4.9	1.9–10.3
Balance deficit	3.2	1.6–5.4
Gait disorder	3.0	1.7–4.8
Visual deficit	2.8	1.1–7.4
Mobility limitation	2.5	1.0–5.3
Cognitive impairment	2.4	2.0–4.7
Impaired functional status	2.0	1.0–3.1
Postural hypotension	1.9	1.0–3.4

Abbreviations: OR, odds ratio from retrospective studies; RR, relative risk from prospective studies.

Source: Reproduced with permission from J Masdeu, L Sudarsky, L Wolfson: *Gait Disorders of Aging*. Lippincott Raven, 1997.

TREATMENT INTERVENTIONS TO REDUCE THE RISK OF FALLS AND INJURY

Efforts should be made to define the etiology of the gait disorder and the mechanism underlying the falls by a given patient. Orthostatic changes in blood pressure and pulse should be recorded. Rising from a chair and walking should be evaluated for safety. Specific treatment may be possible once a diagnosis is established. Therapeutic intervention is often recommended for older patients at substantial risk for falls, even if no neurologic disease is identified. A home visit to look for environmental hazards can be helpful. A variety of modifications may be recommended to improve safety, including improved lighting and the installation of grab bars and nonslip surfaces.

Rehabilitative interventions aim to improve muscle strength and balance stability and to make the patient more resistant to injury. High-intensity resistance strength training with weights and machines is useful to improve muscle mass, even in frail older patients. Improvements realized in posture and gait should translate to reduced risk of falls and injury. Sensory balance training is another approach to improving balance stability. Measurable gains can be made in a few weeks of training, and benefits can be maintained over 6 months by a 10- to 20-min home exercise program. This strategy is particularly successful in patients with vestibular and somatosensory balance disorders. A Tai Chi exercise program has been demonstrated to reduce the risk of falls and injury in patients with Parkinson's disease.

33e Video Library of Gait Disorders

Gail Kang, Nicholas B. Galifianakis, Michael D. Geschwind

This is a digital-only chapter. It is available on the DVD that accompanies this book, as well as on Access Medicine/Harrison's Online, and the eBook and "app" editions of HPIM 19e.

Problems with gait and balance are major causes of falls, accidents, and resulting disability, especially in later life, and are often harbingers of neurologic disease. Early diagnosis is essential, especially for treatable conditions, because it may permit the institution of prophylactic measures to prevent dangerous falls and also to reverse or ameliorate the underlying cause. In this video, examples of gait disorders due to Parkinson's disease, other extrapyramidal disorders, and ataxias, as well as other common gait disorders, are presented.

34 Confusion and Delirium

S. Andrew Josephson, Bruce L. Miller

Confusion, a mental and behavioral state of reduced comprehension, coherence, and capacity to reason, is one of the most common problems encountered in medicine, accounting for a large number of emergency department visits, hospital admissions, and inpatient consultations. *Delirium*, a term used to describe an acute confusional state, remains a major cause of morbidity and mortality, costing over $150 billion dollars yearly in health care costs in the United States alone. Despite increased efforts targeting awareness of this condition, delirium often goes unrecognized in the face of evidence that it is usually the cognitive manifestation of serious underlying medical or neurologic illness.

CLINICAL FEATURES OF DELIRIUM

A multitude of terms are used to describe patients with delirium, including *encephalopathy, acute brain failure, acute confusional state,* and *postoperative* or *intensive care unit (ICU) psychosis.* Delirium has many clinical manifestations, but is defined as a relatively acute decline in cognition that fluctuates over hours or days. The hallmark of delirium is a deficit of attention, although all cognitive domains—including memory, executive function, visuospatial tasks, and language—are variably involved. Associated symptoms that may be present in some cases include altered sleep-wake cycles, perceptual disturbances such as hallucinations or delusions, affect changes, and autonomic findings that include heart rate and blood pressure instability.

Delirium is a clinical diagnosis that is made only at the bedside. Two subtypes have been described—hyperactive and hypoactive—based on differential psychomotor features. The cognitive syndrome associated with severe alcohol withdrawal (i.e., "delirium tremens") remains the classic example of the hyperactive subtype, featuring prominent hallucinations, agitation, and hyperarousal, often accompanied by life-threatening autonomic instability. In striking contrast is the hypoactive subtype, exemplified by benzodiazepine intoxication, in which patients are withdrawn and quiet, with prominent apathy and psychomotor slowing.

This dichotomy between subtypes of delirium is a useful construct, but patients often fall somewhere along a spectrum between the hyperactive and hypoactive extremes, sometimes fluctuating from one to the other. Therefore, clinicians must recognize this broad range of presentations of delirium to identify all patients with this potentially reversible cognitive disturbance. Hyperactive patients are often easily recognized by their characteristic severe agitation, tremor, hallucinations, and autonomic instability. Patients who are quietly hypoactive are more often overlooked on the medical wards and in the ICU.

The reversibility of delirium is emphasized because many etiologies, such as systemic infection and medication effects, can be treated easily. The long-term cognitive effects of delirium remain largely unknown. Some episodes of delirium continue for weeks, months, or even years. The persistence of delirium in some patients and its high recurrence rate may be due to inadequate initial treatment of the underlying etiology. In other instances, delirium appears to cause permanent neuronal damage and cognitive decline. Even if an episode of delirium completely resolves, there may be lingering effects of the disorder; a patient's recall of events after delirium varies widely, ranging from complete amnesia to repeated re-experiencing of the frightening period of confusion, similar to what is seen in patients with posttraumatic stress disorder.

RISK FACTORS

An effective primary prevention strategy for delirium begins with identification of patients at high risk for this disorder, including those preparing for elective surgery or being admitted to the hospital. Although no single validated scoring system has been widely accepted as a screen for asymptomatic patients, there are multiple well-established risk factors for delirium.

The two most consistently identified risks are older age and baseline cognitive dysfunction. Individuals who are over age 65 or exhibit low scores on standardized tests of cognition develop delirium upon hospitalization at a rate approaching 50%. Whether age and baseline cognitive dysfunction are truly independent risk factors is uncertain. Other predisposing factors include sensory deprivation, such as preexisting hearing and visual impairment, as well as indices for poor overall health, including baseline immobility, malnutrition, and underlying medical or neurologic illness.

In-hospital risks for delirium include the use of bladder catheterization, physical restraints, sleep and sensory deprivation, and the addition of three or more new medications. Avoiding such risks remains a key component of delirium prevention as well as treatment. Surgical and anesthetic risk factors for the development of postoperative delirium include specific procedures such as those involving cardiopulmonary bypass, inadequate or excessive treatment of pain in the immediate postoperative period, and perhaps specific agents such as inhalational anesthetics.

The relationship between delirium and dementia (Chap. 448) is complicated by significant overlap between the two conditions, and it is not always simple to distinguish between them. Dementia and preexisting cognitive dysfunction serve as major risk factors for delirium, and at least two-thirds of cases of delirium occur in patients with coexisting underlying dementia. A form of dementia with parkinsonism, termed *dementia with Lewy bodies*, is characterized by a fluctuating course, prominent visual hallucinations, parkinsonism, and an attentional deficit that clinically resembles hyperactive delirium; patients with this condition are particularly vulnerable to delirium. Delirium in the elderly often reflects an insult to the brain that is vulnerable due to an underlying neurodegenerative condition. Therefore, the development of delirium sometimes heralds the onset of a previously unrecognized brain disorder.

EPIDEMIOLOGY

Delirium is common, but its reported incidence has varied widely with the criteria used to define this disorder. Estimates of delirium in hospitalized patients range from 18 to 64%, with higher rates reported for elderly patients and patients undergoing hip surgery. Older patients in the ICU have especially high rates of delirium that approach 75%. The condition is not recognized in up to one-third of delirious inpatients, and the diagnosis is especially problematic in the ICU environment, where cognitive dysfunction is often difficult to appreciate in the setting of serious systemic illness and sedation. Delirium in the ICU should be viewed as an important manifestation of organ dysfunction not unlike liver, kidney, or heart failure. Outside the acute hospital setting, delirium occurs in nearly one-quarter of patients in nursing homes and in 50 to 80% of those at the end of life. These estimates emphasize the remarkably high frequency of this cognitive syndrome in older patients, a population expected to grow in the upcoming decades.

Until recently, an episode of delirium was viewed as a transient condition that carried a benign prognosis. It is now recognized as a disorder with a substantial morbidity rate and increased mortality rate and often represents the first manifestation of a serious underlying illness. Recent estimates of in-hospital mortality rates among delirious patients have ranged from 25 to 33%, a rate similar to that of patients with sepsis. Patients with an in-hospital episode of delirium have a fivefold higher mortality rate in the months after their illness compared with age-matched nondelirious hospitalized patients. Delirious hospitalized patients have a longer length of stay, are more likely to be discharged to a nursing home, and are more likely to experience subsequent episodes of delirium and cognitive decline; as a result, this condition has enormous economic implications.

PATHOGENESIS

The pathogenesis and anatomy of delirium are incompletely understood. The attentional deficit that serves as the neuropsychological hallmark of delirium has a diffuse localization within the brainstem, thalamus, prefrontal cortex, and parietal lobes. Rarely, focal lesions such as ischemic strokes have led to delirium in otherwise healthy persons; right parietal and medial dorsal thalamic lesions have been reported most commonly, pointing to the importance of these areas to delirium pathogenesis. In most cases, delirium results from widespread disturbances in cortical and subcortical regions rather than a focal neuroanatomic cause. Electroencephalogram (EEG) data in persons with delirium usually show symmetric slowing, a nonspecific finding that supports diffuse cerebral dysfunction.

Multiple neurotransmitter abnormalities, proinflammatory factors, and specific genes likely play a role in the pathogenesis of delirium. Deficiency of acetylcholine may play a key role, and medications with anticholinergic properties also can precipitate delirium. Dementia patients are susceptible to episodes of delirium, and those with Alzheimer's pathology and dementia with Lewy bodies or Parkinson's disease dementia are known to have a chronic cholinergic deficiency state due to degeneration of acetylcholine-producing neurons in the basal forebrain. Additionally, other neurotransmitters are also likely to be involved in this diffuse cerebral disorder. For example, increases in dopamine can also lead to delirium. Patients with Parkinson's disease treated with dopaminergic medications can develop a delirium-like state that features visual hallucinations, fluctuations, and confusion.

Not all individuals exposed to the same insult will develop signs of delirium. A low dose of an anticholinergic medication may have no cognitive effects on a healthy young adult but produce a florid delirium in an elderly person with known underlying dementia, although even healthy young persons develop delirium with very high doses of anticholinergic medications. This concept of delirium developing as the result of an insult in predisposed individuals is currently the most widely accepted pathogenic construct. Therefore, if a previously healthy individual with no known history of cognitive illness develops delirium in the setting of a relatively minor insult such as elective surgery or hospitalization, an unrecognized underlying neurologic illness such as a neurodegenerative disease, multiple previous strokes, or another diffuse cerebral cause should be considered. In this context, delirium can be viewed as a "stress test for the brain" whereby exposure to known inciting factors such as systemic infection and offending drugs can unmask a decreased cerebral reserve and herald a serious underlying and potentially treatable illness.

TABLE 34-1 THE CONFUSION ASSESSMENT METHOD (CAM) DIAGNOSTIC ALGORITHM[a]

The diagnosis of delirium requires the presence of features 1 and 2 and of *either* feature 3 or 4.

Feature 1. Acute onset and fluctuating course

This feature is satisfied by positive responses to the following questions: Is there evidence of an acute change in mental status from the patient's baseline? Did the (abnormal) behavior fluctuate during the day, that is, tend to come and go, or did it increase and decrease in severity?

Feature 2. Inattention

This feature is satisfied by a positive response to the following question: Did the patient have difficulty focusing attention, for example, being easily distractible, or have difficulty keeping track of what was being said?

Feature 3. Disorganized thinking

This feature is satisfied by a positive response to the following question: Was the patient's thinking disorganized or incoherent, such as rambling or irrelevant conversation, unclear or illogical flow of ideas, or unpredictable switching from subject to subject?

Feature 4. Altered level of consciousness

This feature is satisfied by any answer other than "alert" to the following question: Overall, how would you rate the patient's level of consciousness: alert (normal), vigilant (hyperalert), lethargic (drowsy, easily aroused), stupor (difficult to arouse), or coma (unarousable)?

[a]Information is usually obtained from a reliable reporter, such as a family member, caregiver, or nurse.

Source: Modified from SK Inouye et al: Clarifying confusion: The Confusion Assessment Method. A new method for detection of delirium. Ann Intern Med 113:941, 1990.

APPROACH TO THE PATIENT: Delirium

Because the diagnosis of delirium is clinical and is made at the bedside, a careful history and physical examination are necessary in evaluating patients with possible confusional states. Screening tools can aid physicians and nurses in identifying patients with delirium, including the Confusion Assessment Method (CAM) (Table 34-1); the Organic Brain Syndrome Scale; the Delirium Rating Scale; and, in the ICU, the ICU version of the CAM and the Delirium Detection Score. Using the well-validated CAM, a diagnosis of delirium is made if there is (1) an acute onset and fluctuating course and (2) inattention accompanied by either (3) disorganized thinking or (4) an altered level of consciousness. These scales may not identify the full spectrum of patients with delirium, and all patients who are acutely confused should be presumed delirious regardless of their presentation due to the wide variety of possible clinical features. A course that fluctuates over hours or days and may worsen at night (termed *sundowning*) is typical but not essential for the diagnosis. Observation of the patient usually will reveal an altered level of consciousness or a deficit of attention. Other features that are sometimes present include alteration of sleep-wake cycles, thought disturbances such as hallucinations or delusions, autonomic instability, and changes in affect.

HISTORY

It may be difficult to elicit an accurate history in delirious patients who have altered levels of consciousness or impaired attention. Information from a collateral source such as a spouse or another family member is therefore invaluable. The three most important pieces of history are the patient's baseline cognitive function, the time course of the present illness, and current medications.

Premorbid cognitive function can be assessed through the collateral source or, if needed, via a review of outpatient records. Delirium by definition represents a change that is relatively acute, usually over hours to days, from a cognitive baseline. As a result, an acute confusional state is nearly impossible to diagnose without some knowledge of baseline cognitive function. Without this information, many patients with dementia or depression may be mistaken as delirious during a single initial evaluation. Patients with a more hypoactive, apathetic presentation with psychomotor slowing may be identified as being different from baseline only through conversations with family members. A number of validated instruments have been shown to diagnose cognitive dysfunction accurately using a collateral source, including the modified Blessed Dementia Rating Scale and the Clinical Dementia Rating (CDR). Baseline cognitive impairment is common in patients with delirium. Even when no such history of cognitive impairment is elicited, there should still be a high suspicion for a previously unrecognized underlying neurologic disorder.

Establishing the time course of cognitive change is important not only to make a diagnosis of delirium but also to correlate the onset of the illness with potentially treatable etiologies such as recent medication changes or symptoms of systemic infection.

Medications remain a common cause of delirium, especially compounds with anticholinergic or sedative properties. It is estimated that nearly one-third of all cases of delirium are secondary to medications, especially in the elderly. Medication histories should include all prescription as well as over-the-counter and herbal substances taken by the patient and any recent changes in dosing or formulation, including substitution of generics for brand-name medications.

Other important elements of the history include screening for symptoms of organ failure or systemic infection, which often contributes to delirium in the elderly. A history of illicit drug use, alcoholism, or toxin exposure is common in younger delirious patients. Finally, asking the patient and collateral source about other symptoms that may accompany delirium, such as depression, may help identify potential therapeutic targets.

PHYSICAL EXAMINATION

The general physical examination in a delirious patient should include careful screening for signs of infection such as fever, tachypnea, pulmonary consolidation, heart murmur, and stiff neck. The patient's fluid status should be assessed; both dehydration and fluid overload with resultant hypoxemia have been associated with delirium, and each is usually easily rectified. The appearance of the skin can be helpful, showing jaundice in hepatic encephalopathy, cyanosis in hypoxemia, or needle tracks in patients using intravenous drugs.

The neurologic examination requires a careful assessment of mental status. Patients with delirium often present with a fluctuating course; therefore, the diagnosis can be missed when one relies on a single time point of evaluation. Some but not all patients exhibit the characteristic pattern of sundowning, a worsening of their condition in the evening. In these cases, assessment only during morning rounds may be falsely reassuring.

An altered level of consciousness ranging from hyperarousal to lethargy to coma is present in most patients with delirium and can be assessed easily at the bedside. In a patient with a relatively normal level of consciousness, a screen for an attentional deficit is in order, because this deficit is the classic neuropsychological hallmark of delirium. Attention can be assessed while taking a history from the patient. Tangential speech, a fragmentary flow of ideas, or inability to follow complex commands often signifies an attentional problem. There are formal neuropsychological tests to assess attention, but a simple bedside test of digit span forward is quick and fairly sensitive. In this task, patients are asked to repeat successively longer random strings of digits beginning with two digits in a row, said to the patient at 1-second intervals. Healthy adults can repeat a string of five to seven digits before faltering; a digit span of four or less usually indicates an attentional deficit unless hearing or language barriers are present, and many patients with delirium have digit spans of three or fewer digits.

More formal neuropsychological testing can be helpful in assessing a delirious patient, but it is usually too cumbersome and time-consuming in the inpatient setting. A Mini-Mental State Examination (MMSE) provides information regarding orientation, language, and visuospatial skills; however, performance of many tasks on the MMSE, including the spelling of "world" backward and serial subtraction of digits, will be impaired by delirious patients' attentional deficits, rendering the test unreliable.

The remainder of the screening neurologic examination should focus on identifying new focal neurologic deficits. Focal strokes or mass lesions in isolation are rarely the cause of delirium, but patients with underlying extensive cerebrovascular disease or neurodegenerative conditions may not be able to cognitively tolerate even relatively small new insults. Patients should be screened for other signs of neurodegenerative conditions such as parkinsonism, which is seen not only in idiopathic Parkinson's disease but also in other dementing conditions such as Alzheimer's disease, dementia with Lewy bodies, and progressive supranuclear palsy. The presence of multifocal myoclonus or asterixis on the motor examination is nonspecific but usually indicates a metabolic or toxic etiology of the delirium.

ETIOLOGY

Some etiologies can be easily discerned through a careful history and physical examination, whereas others require confirmation with laboratory studies, imaging, or other ancillary tests. A large, diverse group of insults can lead to delirium, and the cause in many patients is often multifactorial. Common etiologies are listed in Table 34-2.

Prescribed, over-the-counter, and herbal medications all can precipitate delirium. Drugs with anticholinergic properties, narcotics, and benzodiazepines are particularly common offenders, but nearly any compound can lead to cognitive dysfunction in a predisposed patient. Whereas an elderly patient with baseline dementia may become delirious upon exposure to a relatively low dose of a medication, less susceptible individuals may become delirious only with very high doses of the same medication. This observation emphasizes the importance of correlating the timing of recent medication changes, including dose and formulation, with the onset of cognitive dysfunction.

In younger patients, illicit drugs and toxins are common causes of delirium. In addition to more classic drugs of abuse, the recent rise in availability of methylenedioxymethamphetamine (MDMA, ecstasy), γ-hydroxybutyrate (GHB), "bath salts," synthetic cannabis, and the phencyclidine (PCP)-like agent ketamine, has led to an increase in delirious young persons presenting to acute care settings (Chap. 469e). Many common prescription drugs such as oral

TABLE 34-2 COMMON ETIOLOGIES OF DELIRIUM

Toxins
Prescription medications: especially those with anticholinergic properties, narcotics, and benzodiazepines
Drugs of abuse: alcohol intoxication and alcohol withdrawal, opiates, ecstasy, LSD, GHB, PCP, ketamine, cocaine, "bath salts," marijuana and its synthetic forms
Poisons: inhalants, carbon monoxide, ethylene glycol, pesticides
Metabolic conditions
Electrolyte disturbances: hypoglycemia, hyperglycemia, hyponatremia, hypernatremia, hypercalcemia, hypocalcemia, hypomagnesemia
Hypothermia and hyperthermia
Pulmonary failure: hypoxemia and hypercarbia
Liver failure/hepatic encephalopathy
Renal failure/uremia
Cardiac failure
Vitamin deficiencies: B_{12}, thiamine, folate, niacin
Dehydration and malnutrition
Anemia
Infections
Systemic infections: urinary tract infections, pneumonia, skin and soft tissue infections, sepsis
CNS infections: meningitis, encephalitis, brain abscess
Endocrine conditions
Hyperthyroidism, hypothyroidism
Hyperparathyroidism
Adrenal insufficiency
Cerebrovascular disorders
Global hypoperfusion states
Hypertensive encephalopathy
Focal ischemic strokes and hemorrhages (rare): especially nondominant parietal and thalamic lesions
Autoimmune disorders
CNS vasculitis
Cerebral lupus
Neurologic paraneoplastic syndromes
Seizure-related disorders
Nonconvulsive status epilepticus
Intermittent seizures with prolonged postictal states
Neoplastic disorders
Diffuse metastases to the brain
Gliomatosis cerebri
Carcinomatous meningitis
CNS lymphoma
Hospitalization
Terminal end-of-life delirium

Abbreviations: CNS, central nervous system; GHB, γ-hydroxybutyrate; LSD, lysergic acid diethylamide; PCP, phencyclidine.

narcotics and benzodiazepines are often abused and readily available on the street. Alcohol abuse leading to high serum levels causes confusion, but more commonly, it is withdrawal from alcohol that leads to a hyperactive delirium. Alcohol and benzodiazepine withdrawal should be considered in all cases of delirium because even patients who drink only a few servings of alcohol every day can experience relatively severe withdrawal symptoms upon hospitalization.

Metabolic abnormalities such as electrolyte disturbances of sodium, calcium, magnesium, or glucose can cause delirium, and mild derangements can lead to substantial cognitive disturbances in susceptible individuals. Other common metabolic etiologies include liver and renal failure, hypercarbia and hypoxemia, vitamin deficiencies of thiamine and B_{12}, autoimmune disorders including central nervous system (CNS) vasculitis, and endocrinopathies such as thyroid and adrenal disorders.

Systemic infections often cause delirium, especially in the elderly. A common scenario involves the development of an acute cognitive decline in the setting of a urinary tract infection in a patient with baseline dementia. Pneumonia, skin infections such as cellulitis, and frank sepsis also lead to delirium. This so-called septic encephalopathy, often seen in the ICU, is probably due to the release of proinflammatory cytokines and their diffuse cerebral effects. CNS infections such as meningitis, encephalitis, and abscess are less common etiologies of delirium; however, in light of the high mortality rates associated with these conditions when they are not treated quickly, clinicians must always maintain a high index of suspicion.

In some susceptible individuals, exposure to the unfamiliar environment of a hospital itself can lead to delirium. This etiology usually occurs as part of a multifactorial delirium and should be considered a diagnosis of exclusion after all other causes have been thoroughly investigated. Many primary prevention and treatment strategies for delirium involve relatively simple methods to address the aspects of the inpatient setting that are most confusing.

Cerebrovascular etiologies of delirium are usually due to global hypoperfusion in the setting of systemic hypotension from heart failure, septic shock, dehydration, or anemia. Focal strokes in the right parietal lobe and medial dorsal thalamus rarely can lead to a delirious state. A more common scenario involves a new focal stroke or hemorrhage causing confusion in a patient who has decreased cerebral reserve. In these individuals, it is sometimes difficult to distinguish between cognitive dysfunction resulting from the new neurovascular insult itself and delirium due to the infectious, metabolic, and pharmacologic complications that can accompany hospitalization after stroke.

Because a fluctuating course often is seen in delirium, intermittent seizures may be overlooked when one is considering potential etiologies. Both nonconvulsive status epilepticus and recurrent focal or generalized seizures followed by postictal confusion can cause delirium; EEG remains essential for this diagnosis. Seizure activity spreading from an electrical focus in a mass or infarct can explain global cognitive dysfunction caused by relatively small lesions.

It is very common for patients to experience delirium at the end of life in palliative care settings. This condition, sometimes described as *terminal restlessness*, must be identified and treated aggressively because it is an important cause of patient and family discomfort at the end of life. It should be remembered that these patients also may be suffering from more common etiologies of delirium such as systemic infection.

LABORATORY AND DIAGNOSTIC EVALUATION

A cost-effective approach to the diagnostic evaluation of delirium allows the history and physical examination to guide further tests. No established algorithm for workup will fit all delirious patients due to the staggering number of potential etiologies, but one stepwise approach is detailed in Table 34-3. If a clear precipitant is identified, such as an offending medication, further testing may not be required. If, however, no likely etiology is uncovered with initial evaluation, an aggressive search for an underlying cause should be initiated.

Basic screening labs, including a complete blood count, electrolyte panel, and tests of liver and renal function, should be obtained in all patients with delirium. In elderly patients, screening for systemic infection, including chest radiography, urinalysis and culture, and possibly blood cultures, is important. In younger individuals, serum and urine drug and toxicology screening may be appropriate early in the workup. Additional laboratory tests addressing other autoimmune, endocrinologic, metabolic, and infectious etiologies should be reserved for patients in whom the diagnosis remains unclear after initial testing.

Multiple studies have demonstrated that brain imaging in patients with delirium is often unhelpful. If, however, the initial workup is unrevealing, most clinicians quickly move toward imaging of the brain to exclude structural causes. A noncontrast computed tomography (CT) scan can identify large masses and hemorrhages but is otherwise unlikely to help determine an etiology of delirium. The ability of magnetic resonance imaging (MRI) to identify most acute ischemic strokes as well as to provide neuroanatomic detail that gives clues to possible infectious, inflammatory, neurodegenerative, and neoplastic conditions makes it the test of choice. Because MRI techniques are limited by availability, speed of imaging, patient cooperation, and contraindications, many clinicians begin with CT scanning and proceed to MRI if the etiology of delirium remains elusive.

TABLE 34-3 STEPWISE EVALUATION OF A PATIENT WITH DELIRIUM

Initial evaluation
History with special attention to medications (including over-the-counter and herbals)
General physical examination and neurologic examination
Complete blood count
Electrolyte panel including calcium, magnesium, phosphorus
Liver function tests, including albumin
Renal function tests
First-tier further evaluation guided by initial evaluation
Systemic infection screen
Urinalysis and culture
Chest radiograph
Blood cultures
Electrocardiogram
Arterial blood gas
Serum and/or urine toxicology screen (perform earlier in young persons)
Brain imaging with MRI with diffusion and gadolinium (preferred) or CT
Suspected CNS infection: lumbar puncture after brain imaging
Suspected seizure-related etiology: electroencephalogram (EEG) (if high suspicion, should be performed immediately)
Second-tier further evaluation
Vitamin levels: B_{12}, folate, thiamine
Endocrinologic laboratories: thyroid-stimulating hormone (TSH) and free T_4; cortisol
Serum ammonia
Sedimentation rate
Autoimmune serologies: antinuclear antibodies (ANA), complement levels; p-ANCA, c-ANCA. consider paraneoplastic serologies
Infectious serologies: rapid plasmin reagin (RPR); fungal and viral serologies if high suspicion; HIV antibody
Lumbar puncture (if not already performed)
Brain MRI with and without gadolinium (if not already performed)

Abbreviations: c-ANCA, cytoplasmic antineutrophil cytoplasmic antibody; CNS, central nervous system; CT, computed tomography; MRI, magnetic resonance imaging; p-ANCA, perinuclear antineutrophil cytoplasmic antibody.

Lumbar puncture (LP) must be obtained immediately after appropriate neuroimaging in all patients in whom CNS infection is suspected. Spinal fluid examination can also be useful in identifying inflammatory and neoplastic conditions. As a result, LP should be considered in any delirious patient with a negative workup. EEG does not have a routine role in the workup of delirium, but it remains invaluable if seizure-related etiologies are considered.

TREATMENT DELIRIUM

Management of delirium begins with treatment of the underlying inciting factor (e.g., patients with systemic infections should be given appropriate antibiotics, and underlying electrolyte disturbances judiciously corrected). These treatments often lead to prompt resolution of delirium. Blindly targeting the symptoms of delirium pharmacologically only serves to prolong the time patients remain in the confused state and may mask important diagnostic information.

Relatively simple methods of supportive care can be highly effective in treating patients with delirium. Reorientation by the nursing staff and family combined with visible clocks, calendars, and outside-facing windows can reduce confusion. Sensory isolation should be prevented by providing glasses and hearing aids to patients who need them. Sundowning can be addressed to a large extent through vigilance to appropriate sleep-wake cycles. During the day, a well-lit room should be accompanied by activities or exercises to prevent napping. At night, a quiet, dark environment with limited interruptions by staff can assure proper rest. These sleep-wake cycle interventions are especially important in the ICU setting as the usual constant 24-h activity commonly provokes delirium. Attempting to mimic the home environment as much as possible also has been shown to help treat and even prevent delirium. Visits from friends and family throughout the day minimize the anxiety associated with the constant flow of new faces of staff and physicians. Allowing hospitalized patients to have access to home bedding, clothing, and nightstand objects makes the hospital environment less foreign and therefore less confusing. Simple standard nursing practices such as maintaining proper nutrition and volume status as well as managing incontinence and skin breakdown also help alleviate discomfort and resulting confusion.

In some instances, patients pose a threat to their own safety or to the safety of staff members, and acute management is required. Bed alarms and personal sitters are more effective and much less disorienting than physical restraints. Chemical restraints should be avoided, but only when necessary, very-low-dose typical or atypical antipsychotic medications administered on an as-needed basis are effective. The recent association of antipsychotic use in the elderly with increased mortality rates underscores the importance of using these medications judiciously and only as a last resort. Benzodiazepines often worsen confusion through their sedative properties. Although many clinicians still use benzodiazepines to treat acute confusion, their use should be limited to cases in which delirium is caused by alcohol or benzodiazepine withdrawal.

PREVENTION

In light of the high morbidity associated with delirium and the tremendously increased health care costs that accompany it, development of an effective strategy to prevent delirium in hospitalized patients is extremely important. Successful identification of high-risk patients is the first step, followed by initiation of appropriate interventions. Simple standardized protocols used to manage risk factors for delirium, including sleep-wake cycle reversal, immobility, visual impairment, hearing impairment, sleep deprivation, and dehydration, have been shown to be effective. Recent trials in the ICU have focused both on identifying sedatives, such as dexmedetomidine, that are less likely to lead to delirium in critically ill patients and on developing protocols for daily awakenings in which infusions of sedative medications are interrupted and the patient is reorientated by the staff. All hospitals and health care systems should work toward decreasing the incidence of delirium.

35 Dementia

William W. Seeley, Bruce L. Miller

Dementia, a syndrome with many causes, affects >5 million people in the United States and results in a total annual health care cost between $157 and $215 billion. Dementia is defined as an acquired deterioration in cognitive abilities that impairs the successful performance of activities of daily living. Episodic memory, the ability to recall events specific in time and place, is the cognitive function most commonly lost; 10% of persons age >70 years and 20–40% of individuals age >85 years have clinically identifiable memory loss. In addition to memory, dementia may erode other mental faculties, including language, visuospatial, praxis, calculation, judgment, and problem-solving abilities. Neuropsychiatric and social deficits also arise in many dementia syndromes, manifesting as depression, apathy, anxiety, hallucinations, delusions, agitation, insomnia, sleep disturbances, compulsions, or disinhibition. The clinical course may be slowly progressive, as in Alzheimer's disease (AD); static, as in anoxic encephalopathy; or may fluctuate from day to day or minute to minute, as in dementia with Lewy bodies. Most patients with AD, the most prevalent form of dementia, begin with episodic memory impairment, although in other dementias, such as frontotemporal dementia, memory loss is not typically a presenting feature. **Focal cerebral disorders are discussed in Chap. 36 and illustrated in a video library in Chap. 37e; the pathogenesis of AD and related disorders is discussed in Chap. 448.**

FUNCTIONAL ANATOMY OF THE DEMENTIAS

Dementia syndromes result from the disruption of specific large-scale neuronal networks; the location and severity of synaptic and neuronal loss combine to produce the clinical features (Chap. 36). Behavior, mood, and attention are modulated by ascending noradrenergic, serotonergic, and dopaminergic pathways, whereas cholinergic signaling is critical for attention and memory functions. The dementias differ in the relative neurotransmitter deficit profiles; accordingly, accurate diagnosis guides effective pharmacologic therapy.

AD begins in the entorhinal region of the medial temporal lobe, spreads to the hippocampus, and then moves to lateral and posterior temporal and parietal neocortex, eventually causing a more widespread degeneration. *Vascular dementia* is associated with focal damage in a variable patchwork of cortical and subcortical regions or white matter tracts that disconnect nodes within distributed networks. In keeping with its anatomy, AD typically presents with episodic memory loss accompanied later by aphasia or navigational problems. In contrast, dementias that begin in frontal or subcortical regions, such as *frontotemporal dementia* (FTD) or *Huntington's disease* (HD), are less likely to begin with memory problems and more likely to present with difficulties with judgment, mood, executive control, movement, and behavior.

Lesions of frontal-striatal[1] pathways produce specific and predictable effects on behavior. The dorsolateral prefrontal cortex has connections with a central band of the caudate nucleus. Lesions of either the caudate or dorsolateral prefrontal cortex, or their connecting white matter pathways, may result in executive dysfunction, manifesting as poor organization and planning, decreased cognitive flexibility, and impaired working memory. The lateral orbital frontal cortex connects with the ventromedial caudate, and lesions of this system cause impulsiveness, distractibility, and disinhibition. The anterior cingulate cortex and adjacent medial prefrontal cortex project to the nucleus accumbens, and interruption of this system produces apathy, poverty of speech, emotional blunting, or even akinetic mutism. All corticostriatal systems also include topographically organized projections through the globus pallidus and thalamus, and damage to these nodes

[1]The striatum comprises the caudate/putamen.

can likewise reproduce the clinical syndrome of cortical or striatal injury.

THE CAUSES OF DEMENTIA

The single strongest risk factor for dementia is increasing age. The prevalence of disabling memory loss increases with each decade over age 50 and is usually associated with the microscopic changes of AD at autopsy. Yet some centenarians have intact memory function and no evidence of clinically significant dementia. Whether dementia is an inevitable consequence of normal human aging remains controversial.

The many causes of dementia are listed in Table 35-1. The frequency of each condition depends on the age group under study, access of the group to medical care, country of origin, and perhaps racial or ethnic background. AD is the most common cause of dementia in Western countries, accounting for more than half of all patients. Vascular disease is considered the second most frequent cause for dementia and is particularly common in elderly patients or populations with limited access to medical care, where vascular risk factors are undertreated. Often, vascular brain injury is mixed with neurodegenerative disorders, making it difficult, even for the neuropathologist, to estimate the contribution of cerebrovascular disease to the cognitive disorder in an individual patient. Dementias associated with Parkinson's disease (PD) (Chap. 449) are common and may develop years after onset of a parkinsonian disorder, as seen with PD-related dementia (PDD), or can occur concurrently with or preceding the motor syndrome, as in dementia with Lewy bodies (DLB). In patients under the age of 65, FTD rivals AD as the most common cause of dementia. Chronic intoxications, including those resulting from alcohol and prescription drugs, are an important and often treatable cause of dementia. Other disorders listed in Table 35-1 are uncommon but important because many are reversible. The classification of dementing illnesses into reversible and irreversible disorders is a useful approach to differential diagnosis. When effective treatments for the neurodegenerative conditions emerge, this dichotomy will become obsolete.

TABLE 35-1 DIFFERENTIAL DIAGNOSIS OF DEMENTIA

Most Common Causes of Dementia	
Alzheimer's disease	Alcoholism[a]
Vascular dementia	PDD/LBD spectrum
Multi-infarct	Drug/medication intoxication[a]
Diffuse white matter disease (Binswanger's)	
Less Common Causes of Dementia	
Vitamin deficiencies	Toxic disorders
Thiamine (B_1): Wernicke's encephalopathy[a]	Drug, medication, and narcotic poisoning[a]
B_{12} (subacute combined degeneration)[a]	Heavy metal intoxication[a]
	Organic toxins
Nicotinic acid (pellagra)[a]	Psychiatric
Endocrine and other organ failure	Depression (pseudodementia)[a]
Hypothyroidism[a]	Schizophrenia[a]
Adrenal insufficiency and Cushing's syndrome[a]	Conversion disorder[a]
	Degenerative disorders
Hypo- and hyperparathyroidism[a]	Huntington's disease
Renal failure[a]	Multisystem atrophy
Liver failure[a]	Hereditary ataxias (some forms)
Pulmonary failure[a]	Frontotemporal lobar degeneration spectrum
Chronic infections	
HIV	Multiple sclerosis
Neurosyphilis[a]	Adult Down's syndrome with Alzheimer's disease
Papovavirus (JC virus) (progressive multifocal leukoencephalopathy)	ALS-parkinsonism-dementia complex of Guam
Tuberculosis, fungal, and protozoal[a]	
Whipple's disease[a]	Prion (Creutzfeldt-Jakob and Gerstmann-Sträussler-Scheinker diseases)
Head trauma and diffuse brain damage	
Chronic traumatic encephalopathy	Miscellaneous
Chronic subdural hematoma[a]	Sarcoidosis[a]
Postanoxia	Vasculitis[a]
Postencephalitis	CADASIL, etc.
Normal-pressure hydrocephalus[a]	Acute intermittent porphyria[a]
Intracranial hypotension	Recurrent nonconvulsive seizures[a]
Neoplastic	Additional conditions in children or adolescents
Primary brain tumor[a]	Pantothenate kinase–associated neurodegeneration
Metastatic brain tumor[a]	
Paraneoplastic/autoimmune limbic encephalitis[a]	Subacute sclerosing panencephalitis
	Metabolic disorders (e.g., Wilson's and Leigh's diseases, leukodystrophies, lipid storage diseases, mitochondrial mutations)

[a]Potentially reversible dementia.

Abbreviations: ALS, amyotrophic lateral sclerosis; CADASIL, cerebral autosomal dominant arteriopathy with subcortical infarcts and leukoencephalopathy; LBD, Lewy body disease; PDD, Parkinson's disease dementia.

In a study of 1000 persons attending a memory disorders clinic, 19% had a potentially reversible cause of the cognitive impairment and 23% had a potentially reversible concomitant condition that may have contributed to the patient's impairment. The three most common potentially reversible diagnoses were depression, normal pressure hydrocephalus (NPH), and alcohol dependence; medication side effects are also common and should be considered in every patient (Table 35-1).

Subtle cumulative decline in episodic memory is a common part of aging. This frustrating experience, often the source of jokes and humor, is referred to as *benign forgetfulness of the elderly. Benign* means that it is not so progressive or serious that it impairs reasonably successful and productive daily functioning, although the distinction between benign and more significant memory loss can be difficult to make. At age 85, the average person is able to learn and recall approximately one-half of the items (e.g., words on a list) that he or she could at age 18. A measurable cognitive problem that does not seriously disrupt daily activities is often referred to as *mild cognitive impairment* (MCI). Factors that predict progression from MCI to an AD dementia include a prominent memory deficit, family history of dementia, presence of an apolipoprotein ε4 (Apo ε4) allele, small hippocampal volumes, an AD-like signature of cortical atrophy, low cerebrospinal fluid Aβ, and elevated tau or evidence of brain amyloid deposition on positron emission tomography (PET) imaging.

The major degenerative dementias include AD, DLB, FTD and related disorders, HD, and prion diseases, including Creutzfeldt-Jakob disease (CJD). These disorders are all associated with the abnormal aggregation of a specific protein: $A\beta_{42}$ and tau in AD; α-synuclein in DLB; tau, TAR DNA-binding protein of 43 kDa (TDP-43), or *fu*sed in *s*arcoma (FUS) in FTD; huntingtin in HD; and misfolded prion protein (PrP^{sc}) in CJD (Table 35-2).

APPROACH TO THE PATIENT: Dementias

Three major issues should be kept at the forefront: (1) What is the best fit for a clinical diagnosis? (2) What component of the dementia syndrome is treatable or reversible? (3) Can the physician help to alleviate the burden on caregivers? A broad overview of the approach to dementia is shown in Table 35-3. The major degenerative dementias can usually be distinguished by the initial symptoms; neuropsychological, neuropsychiatric, and neurologic findings; and neuroimaging features (Table 35-4).

HISTORY

The history should concentrate on the onset, duration, and tempo of progression. An acute or subacute onset of confusion may be due to delirium (Chap. 34) and should trigger the search for intoxication, infection, or metabolic derangement. An elderly person

TABLE 35-2 THE MOLECULAR BASIS FOR DEGENERATIVE DEMENTIA

Dementia	Molecular Basis	Causal Genes (Chromosome)	Susceptibility Genes	Pathologic Findings
AD	Aβ/tau	*APP* (21), *PS-1* (14), *PS-2* (1) (<2% carry these mutations, most often in *PS-1*)	*Apo ε4* (19)	Amyloid plaques, neurofibrillary tangles, and neuropil threads
FTD	Tau	*MAPT* exon and intron mutations (17) (about 10% of familial cases)	H1 *MAPT* haplotype	Tau neuronal and glial inclusions varying in morphology and distribution
	TDP-43	*GRN* (10% of familial cases), *C9ORF72* (20–30% of familial cases), rare *VCP*, very rare *TARDBP*		TDP-43 neuronal and glial inclusions varying in morphology and distribution
	FUS	Very rare *FUS*		FUS neuronal and glial inclusions varying in morphology and distribution
DLB	α-Synuclein	Very rare *SNCA* (4)	Unknown	α-Synuclein neuronal inclusions (Lewy bodies)
CJD	PrP^{SC}	*PRNP* (20) (up to 15% of patients carry these dominant mutations)	Codon 129 homozygosity for methionine or valine	PrP^{SC} deposition, panlaminar spongiosis

Abbreviations: AD, Alzheimer's disease; CJD, Creutzfeldt-Jakob disease; DLB, dementia with Lewy bodies; FTD, frontotemporal dementia.

with slowly progressive memory loss over several years is likely to suffer from AD. Nearly 75% of patients with AD begin with memory symptoms, but other early symptoms include difficulty with managing money, driving, shopping, following instructions, finding words, or navigating. Personality change, disinhibition, and weight gain or compulsive eating suggest FTD, not AD. FTD is also suggested by prominent apathy, compulsivity, loss of empathy for others, or progressive loss of speech fluency or single-word comprehension and by a relative sparing of memory and visuospatial abilities. The diagnosis of DLB is suggested by early visual hallucinations; parkinsonism; proneness to delirium or sensitivity to psychoactive medications; rapid eye movement (REM) behavior disorder (RBD; the loss of skeletal muscle paralysis during dreaming); or Capgras syndrome, the delusion that a familiar person has been replaced by an impostor.

A history of stroke with irregular stepwise progression suggests vascular dementia. Vascular dementia is also commonly seen in the setting of hypertension, atrial fibrillation, peripheral vascular disease, and diabetes. In patients suffering from cerebrovascular disease, it can be difficult to determine whether the dementia is due to AD, vascular disease, or a mixture of the two because many of the risk factors for vascular dementia, including diabetes, high cholesterol, elevated homocysteine, and low exercise, are also putative risk factors for AD. Moreover, many patients with a major vascular contribution to their dementia lack a history of stepwise decline. Rapid progression with motor rigidity and myoclonus suggests CJD (Chap. 453e). Seizures may indicate strokes or neoplasm but also occur in AD, particularly early-age-of-onset AD. Gait disturbance is common in vascular dementia, PD/DLB, or NPH. A history of high-risk sexual behaviors or intravenous drug use

TABLE 35-3 EVALUATION OF THE PATIENT WITH DEMENTIA

Routine Evaluation	Optional Focused Tests	Occasionally Helpful Tests
History	Psychometric testing	EEG
Physical examination	Chest x-ray	Parathyroid function
Laboratory tests	Lumbar puncture	Adrenal function
Thyroid function (TSH)	Liver function	Urine heavy metals
Vitamin B_{12}	Renal function	RBC sedimentation rate
Complete blood count	Urine toxin screen	Angiogram
Electrolytes	HIV	Brain biopsy
CT/MRI	Apolipoprotein E	SPECT
	RPR or VDRL	PET
		Lab screen for autoantibodies
Diagnostic Categories		
Reversible Causes	**Irreversible/Degenerative Dementias**	**Psychiatric Disorders**
Examples	Examples	Depression
Hypothyroidism	Alzheimer's	Schizophrenia
Thiamine deficiency	Frontotemporal dementia	Conversion reaction
Vitamin B_{12} deficiency	Huntington's	
Normal-pressure hydrocephalus	Dementia with Lewy bodies	
Subdural hematoma	Vascular	
Chronic infection	Leukoencephalopathies	
Brain tumor	Parkinson's	
Drug intoxication		
Autoimmune encephalopathy		

Associated Treatable Conditions

Depression	Agitation
Seizures	Caregiver "burnout"
Insomnia	Drug side effects

Abbreviations: CT, computed tomography; EEG, electroencephalogram; MRI, magnetic resonance imaging; PET, positron emission tomography; RBC, red blood cell; RPR, rapid plasma reagin (test); SPECT, single-photon emission computed tomography; TSH, thyroid-stimulating hormone; VDRL, Venereal Disease Research Laboratory (test for syphilis).

TABLE 35-4 CLINICAL DIFFERENTIATION OF THE MAJOR DEMENTIAS

Disease	First Symptom	Mental Status	Neuropsychiatry	Neurology	Imaging
AD	Memory loss	Episodic memory loss	Irritability, anxiety, depression	Initially normal	Entorhinal cortex and hippocampal atrophy
FTD	Apathy; poor judgment/insight, speech/language; hyperorality	Frontal/executive and/or language; spares drawing	Apathy, disinhibition, overeating, compulsivity	May have vertical gaze palsy, axial rigidity, dystonia, alien hand, or MND	Frontal, insular, and/or temporal atrophy; usually spares posterior parietal lobe
DLB	Visual hallucinations, REM sleep behavior disorder, delirium, Capgras syndrome, parkinsonism	Drawing and frontal/executive; spares memory; delirium-prone	Visual hallucinations, depression, sleep disorder, delusions	Parkinsonism	Posterior parietal atrophy; hippocampi larger than in AD
CJD	Dementia, mood, anxiety, movement disorders	Variable, frontal/executive, focal cortical, memory	Depression, anxiety, psychosis in some	Myoclonus, rigidity, parkinsonism	Cortical ribboning and basal ganglia or thalamus hyperintensity on diffusion/FLAIR MRI
Vascular	Often but not always sudden; variable; apathy, falls, focal weakness	Frontal/executive, cognitive slowing; can spare memory	Apathy, delusions, anxiety	Usually motor slowing, spasticity; can be normal	Cortical and/or subcortical infarctions, confluent white matter disease

Abbreviations: AD, Alzheimer's disease; CBD, cortical basal degeneration; CJD, Creutzfeldt-Jakob disease; DLB, dementia with Lewy bodies; FLAIR, fluid-attenuated inversion recovery; FTD, frontotemporal dementia; MND, motor neuron disease; MRI, magnetic resonance imaging; PSP, progressive supranuclear palsy; REM, rapid eye movement.

should trigger a search for central nervous system (CNS) infection, especially HIV or syphilis. A history of recurrent head trauma could indicate chronic subdural hematoma, chronic traumatic encephalopathy (a progressive dementia best characterized in contact sport athletes such as boxers and American football players), intracranial hypotension, or NPH. Subacute onset of severe amnesia and psychosis with mesial temporal T2/fluid-attenuated inversion recovery (FLAIR) hyperintensities on magnetic resonance imaging (MRI) should raise concern for paraneoplastic limbic encephalitis, especially in a long-term smoker or other patients at risk for cancer. Related autoimmune conditions, such as voltage-gated potassium channel (VGKC)- or N-methyl-D-aspartate (NMDA)-receptor antibody-mediated encephalopathy, can present with a similar tempo and imaging signature with or without characteristic motor manifestations such as myokymia (anti-VGKC) and faciobrachial dystonic seizures (anti-NMDA). Alcohol abuse creates risk for malnutrition and thiamine deficiency. Veganism, bowel irradiation, an autoimmune diathesis, a remote history of gastric surgery, and chronic antihistamine therapy for dyspepsia or gastroesophageal reflux predispose to B_{12} deficiency. Certain occupations, such as working in a battery or chemical factory, might indicate heavy metal intoxication. Careful review of medication intake, especially for sedatives and analgesics, may raise the issue of chronic drug intoxication. An autosomal dominant family history is found in HD and in familial forms of AD, FTD, DLB, or prion disorders. A history of mood disorders, the recent death of a loved one, or depressive signs, such as insomnia or weight loss, raise the possibility of depression-related cognitive impairments.

PHYSICAL AND NEUROLOGIC EXAMINATION

A thorough general and neurologic examination is essential to document dementia, to look for other signs of nervous system involvement, and to search for clues suggesting a systemic disease that might be responsible for the cognitive disorder. Typical AD spares motor systems until later in the course. In contrast, FTD patients often develop axial rigidity, supranuclear gaze palsy, or a motor neuron disease reminiscent of amyotrophic lateral sclerosis (ALS). In DLB, the initial symptoms may include the new onset of a parkinsonian syndrome (resting tremor, cogwheel rigidity, bradykinesia, festinating gait), but DLB often starts with visual hallucinations or dementia. Symptoms referable to the lower brainstem (RBD, gastrointestinal or autonomic problems) may arise years or even decades before parkinsonism or dementia. Corticobasal syndrome (CBS) features asymmetric akinesia and rigidity, dystonia, myoclonus, alien limb phenomena, pyramidal signs, and prefrontal deficits such as nonfluent aphasia with or without motor speech impairment, executive dysfunction, apraxia, or a behavioral disorder. Progressive supranuclear palsy (PSP) is associated with unexplained falls, axial rigidity, dysphagia, and vertical gaze deficits. CJD is suggested by the presence of diffuse rigidity, an akinetic-mute state, and prominent, often startle-sensitive myoclonus.

Hemiparesis or other focal neurologic deficits suggest vascular dementia or brain tumor. Dementia with a myelopathy and peripheral neuropathy suggests vitamin B_{12} deficiency. Peripheral neuropathy could also indicate another vitamin deficiency, heavy metal intoxication, thyroid dysfunction, Lyme disease, or vasculitis. Dry, cool skin, hair loss, and bradycardia suggest hypothyroidism. Fluctuating confusion associated with repetitive stereotyped movements may indicate ongoing limbic, temporal, or frontal seizures. In the elderly, hearing impairment or visual loss may produce confusion and disorientation misinterpreted as dementia. Profound bilateral sensorineural hearing loss in a younger patient with short stature or myopathy, however, should raise concern for a mitochondrial disorder.

COGNITIVE AND NEUROPSYCHIATRIC EXAMINATION

Brief screening tools such as the Mini-Mental State Examination (MMSE), the Montreal Cognitive Assessment (MOCA), and Cognistat can be used to capture dementia and follow progression. None of these tests is highly sensitive to early-stage dementia or discriminates between dementia syndromes. The MMSE is a 30 point test of cognitive function, with each correct answer being scored as 1 point. It includes tests in the areas of: orientation (e.g., identify season/date/month/year/floor/hospital/town/state/country); registration (e.g., name and restate 3 objects); recall (e.g., remember the same three objects 5 minutes later); and language (e.g., name pencil and watch; repeat "no if's and's or but's"; follow a 3-step command; obey a written command; and write a sentence and copy a design). In most patients with MCI and some with clinically apparent AD, bedside screening tests may be normal, and a more challenging and comprehensive set of neuropsychological tests will be required. When the etiology for the dementia syndrome remains in doubt, a specially tailored evaluation should be performed that includes tasks of working and episodic memory, executive function, language, and visuospatial and perceptual abilities. In AD, the early deficits involve episodic memory, category generation ("name as many animals as you can in 1 minute"), and visuoconstructive ability. Usually deficits in verbal or visual episodic memory are the first neuropsychological abnormalities detected, and tasks that require the patient to recall a long list of words or a series of pictures after a predetermined delay will demonstrate deficits in most patients. In FTD, the earliest deficits on cognitive testing involve executive control or language (speech or naming) function, but some patients lack either finding despite profound social-emotional deficits. PDD or DLB patients have more severe deficits in visuospatial function but do better on episodic memory tasks than patients with AD. Patients with vascular dementia often demonstrate a mixture of executive control and visuospatial deficits, with prominent psychomotor slowing. In delirium, the most prominent deficits involve attention, working memory, and executive function, making the assessment of other cognitive domains challenging and often uninformative.

A functional assessment should also be performed to help the physician determine the day-to-day impact of the disorder on the patient's memory, community affairs, hobbies, judgment, dressing, and eating. Knowledge of the patient's functional abilities will help the clinician and the family to organize a therapeutic approach.

Neuropsychiatric assessment is important for diagnosis, prognosis, and treatment. In the early stages of AD, mild depressive features, social withdrawal, and irritability or anxiety are the most prominent psychiatric changes, but patients often maintain core social graces into the middle or late stages, when delusions, agitation, and sleep disturbance may emerge. In FTD, dramatic personality change with apathy, overeating, compulsions, disinhibition, euphoria, and loss of empathy are early and common. DLB is associated with visual hallucinations, delusions related to person or place identity, RBD, and excessive daytime sleepiness. Dramatic fluctuations occur not only in cognition but also in arousal. Vascular dementia can present with psychiatric symptoms such as depression, anxiety, delusions, disinhibition, or apathy.

LABORATORY TESTS

The choice of laboratory tests in the evaluation of dementia is complex and should be tailored to the individual patient. The physician must take measures to avoid missing a reversible or treatable cause, yet no single treatable etiology is common; thus, a screen must use multiple tests, each of which has a low yield. Cost/benefit ratios are difficult to assess, and many laboratory screening algorithms for dementia discourage multiple tests. Nevertheless, even a test with only a 1–2% positive rate is worth undertaking if the alternative is missing a treatable cause of dementia. Table 35-3 lists most screening tests for dementia. The American Academy of Neurology recommends the routine measurement of a complete blood count, electrolytes, renal and thyroid function, a vitamin B_{12} level, and a neuroimaging study (computed tomography [CT] or MRI).

Neuroimaging studies, especially MRI, help to rule out primary and metastatic neoplasms, locate areas of infarction or inflammation, detect subdural hematomas, and suggest NPH or diffuse white matter disease. They also help to establish a regional pattern of atrophy. Support for the diagnosis of AD includes hippocampal atrophy in addition to posterior-predominant cortical atrophy (Fig. 35-1). Focal frontal, insular, and/or anterior temporal atrophy suggests FTD (Chap. 448). DLB often features less prominent atrophy, with greater involvement of amygdala than hippocampus. In CJD, magnetic resonance (MR) diffusion-weighted imaging reveals restricted diffusion within the cortical ribbon and basal ganglia in most patients. Extensive white matter abnormalities correlate with a vascular etiology (Fig. 35-2). Communicating hydrocephalus with vertex effacement (crowding of dorsal convexity gyri/sulci), gaping Sylvian fissures despite minimal cortical atrophy, and additional features shown in Fig. 35-3 suggest NPH. Single-photon emission computed tomography (SPECT) and PET scanning show temporal-parietal hypoperfusion or hypometabolism in AD and frontotemporal deficits in FTD, but these changes often reflect atrophy and can therefore be detected with MRI alone in many patients. Recently, amyloid imaging has shown promise for the diagnosis of AD, and Pittsburgh Compound-B (PiB) (not available outside of research settings) and ^{18}F-AV-45 (florbetapir; approved by the U.S. Food and Drug Administration in 2013) are reliable radioligands for detecting brain amyloid associated with amyloid angiopathy or neuritic plaques of AD (Fig. 35-4). Because these abnormalities can be seen in cognitively normal older persons, however (~25% of individuals at age 65), amyloid imaging may also detect preclinical or incidental AD in patients lacking an AD-like dementia syndrome. Currently, the main clinical value of amyloid imaging is to exclude AD as the likely cause of dementia in patients who have negative scans. Once disease-modifying therapies become available, use of these biomarkers may help to identify treatment

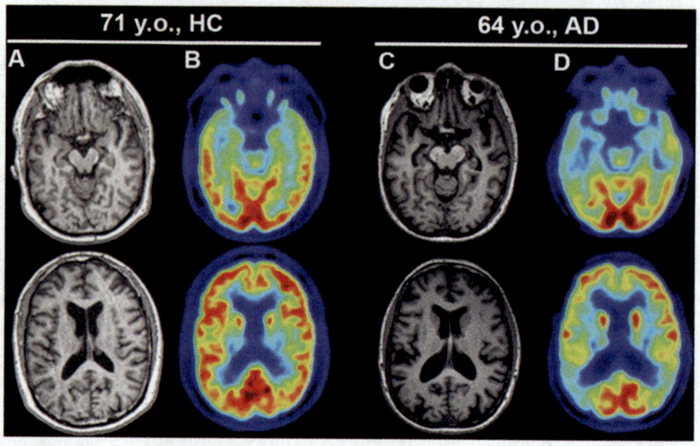

FIGURE 35-1 Alzheimer's disease (AD). Axial T1-weighted magnetic resonance images of a healthy 71-year-old (***A***) and a 64-year-old with AD (***C***). Note the reduction in medial temporal lobe volume in the patient with AD. Fluorodeoxyglucose positron emission tomography scans of the same individuals (***B*** and ***D***) demonstrate reduced glucose metabolism in the posterior temporoparietal regions bilaterally in AD, a typical finding in this condition. HC, healthy control. *(Images courtesy of Gil Rabinovici, University of California, San Francisco and William Jagust, University of California, Berkeley.)*

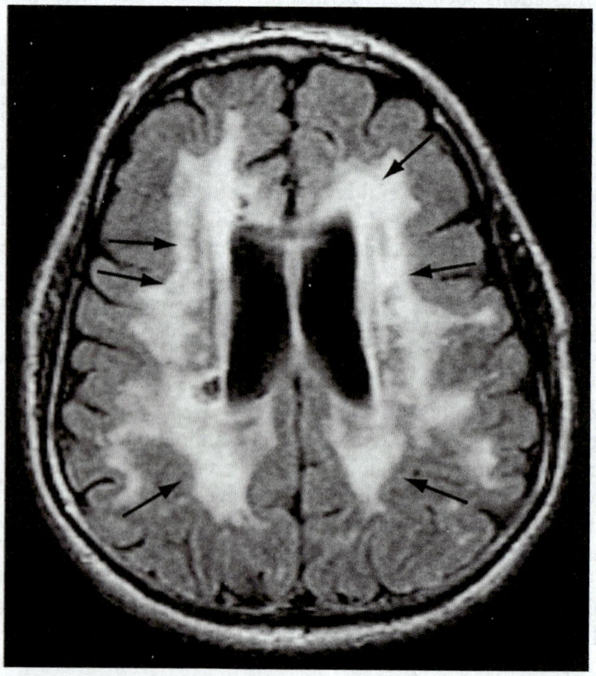

FIGURE 35-2 Diffuse white matter disease. Axial fluid-attenuated inversion recovery (FLAIR) magnetic resonance image through the lateral ventricles reveals multiple areas of hyperintensity (*arrows*) involving the periventricular white matter as well as the corona radiata and striatum. Although seen in some individuals with normal cognition, this appearance is more pronounced in patients with dementia of a vascular etiology.

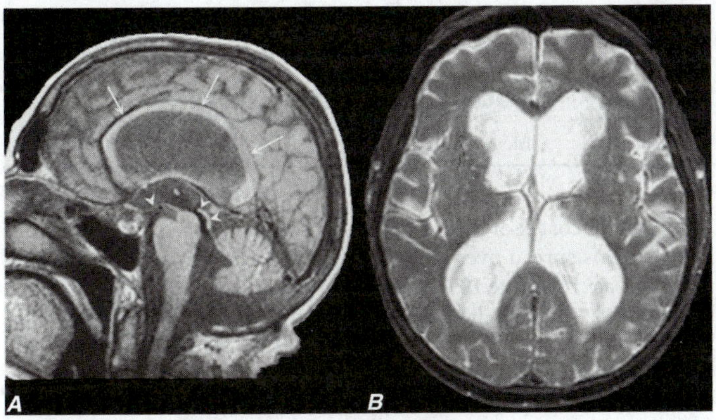

FIGURE 35-3 Normal-pressure hydrocephalus. *A.* Sagittal T1-weighted magnetic resonance image (MRI) demonstrates dilation of the lateral ventricle and stretching of the corpus callosum (*arrows*), depression of the floor of the third ventricle (*single arrowhead*), and enlargement of the aqueduct (*double arrowheads*). Note the diffuse dilation of the lateral, third, and fourth ventricles with a patent aqueduct, typical of communicating hydrocephalus. ***B.*** Axial T2-weighted MRIs demonstrate dilation of the lateral ventricles. This patient underwent successful ventriculoperitoneal shunting.

candidates before irreversible brain injury has occurred. In the meantime, the significance of detecting brain amyloid in an asymptomatic elder remains a topic of vigorous investigation. Similarly, MRI perfusion and structural/functional connectivity methods are being explored as potential treatment-monitoring strategies.

Lumbar puncture need not be done routinely in the evaluation of dementia, but it is indicated when CNS infection or inflammation are credible diagnostic possibilities. Cerebrospinal fluid (CSF) levels of $A\beta_{42}$ and tau proteins show differing patterns with the various dementias, and the presence of low $A\beta_{42}$ and mildly elevated CSF tau is highly suggestive of AD. The routine use of lumbar puncture in the diagnosis of dementia is debated, but the sensitivity and specificity of AD diagnostic measures are not yet high enough to warrant routine use. Formal psychometric testing helps to document the severity of cognitive disturbance, suggest psychogenic causes, and provide a more formal method for following the disease course. Electroencephalogram (EEG) is not routinely used but can help to suggest CJD (repetitive bursts of diffuse high-amplitude sharp waves, or "periodic complexes") or an underlying nonconvulsive seizure disorder (epileptiform discharges). Brain biopsy (including meninges) is not advised except to diagnose vasculitis, potentially treatable neoplasms, or unusual infections when the diagnosis is uncertain. Systemic disorders with CNS manifestations, such as sarcoidosis, can usually be confirmed through biopsy of lymph node or solid organ rather than brain. MR angiography should be considered when cerebral vasculitis or cerebral venous thrombosis is a possible cause of the dementia.

TREATMENT DEMENTIA

The major goals of dementia management are to treat reversible causes and to provide comfort and support to the patient and caregivers. Treatment of underlying causes includes thyroid replacement for hypothyroidism; vitamin therapy for thiamine or B_{12} deficiency or for elevated serum homocysteine; antimicrobials for opportunistic infections or antiretrovirals for HIV; ventricular shunting for NPH; or appropriate surgical, radiation, and/or chemotherapeutic treatment for CNS neoplasms. Removal of cognition-impairing drugs or medications is frequently useful. If the patient's cognitive complaints stem from a psychiatric disorder, vigorous treatment of this condition should seek to eliminate the cognitive complaint or confirm that it persists despite adequate resolution of the mood or anxiety symptoms. Patients with degenerative diseases may also be depressed or anxious, and those aspects of their condition often respond to therapy. Antidepressants, such as selective serotonin reuptake inhibitors (SSRIs) or serotonin-norepinephrine reuptake inhibitors (SNRIs) (Chap. 465e), which feature anxiolytic properties but few cognitive side effects, provide the mainstay of treatment when necessary. Anticonvulsants are used to control seizures. Levetiracetam may be particularly useful, but there have as yet been no randomized trials for treatment of AD-associated seizures.

Agitation, hallucinations, delusions, and confusion are difficult to treat. These behavioral problems represent major causes for nursing home placement and institutionalization. Before treating these behaviors with medications, the clinician should aggressively seek out modifiable environmental or metabolic factors. Hunger, lack of exercise, toothache, constipation, urinary tract or respiratory infection, electrolyte imbalance, and drug toxicity all represent easily correctable causes that can be remedied without psychoactive drugs. Drugs such as phenothiazines and benzodiazepines may ameliorate the behavior problems but have untoward side effects such as sedation, rigidity, dyskinesia, and occasionally paradoxical disinhibition (benzodiazepines). Despite their unfavorable side effect profile, second-generation antipsychotics such as quetiapine (starting dose, 12.5–25 mg daily) can be used for patients with agitation, aggression, and

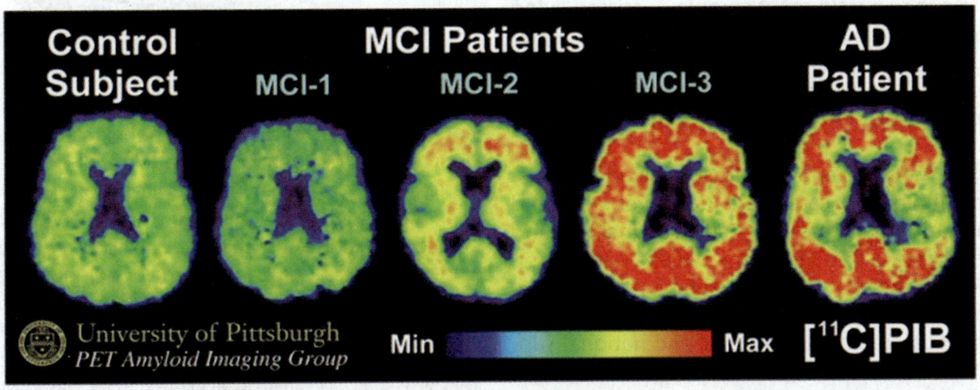

FIGURE 35-4 Positron emission tomography (PET) images obtained with the amyloid-imaging agent Pittsburgh Compound-B ([^{11}C]PIB) in a normal control (*left*); three different patients with mild cognitive impairment (MCI; *center*); and a patient with mild Alzheimer's disease (AD; *right*). Some MCI patients have control-like levels of amyloid, some have AD-like levels of amyloid, and some have intermediate levels. *(Images courtesy of William Klunk and Chester Mathis, University of Pittsburgh.)*

psychosis, although the risk profile for these compounds is significant. When patients do not respond to treatment, it is usually a mistake to advance to higher doses or to use anticholinergic drugs or sedatives (such as barbiturates or benzodiazepines). It is important to recognize and treat depression; treatment can begin with a low dose of an SSRI (e.g., escitalopram, starting dose 5 mg daily, target dose 5–10 mg daily) while monitoring for efficacy and toxicity. Sometimes apathy, visual hallucinations, depression, and other psychiatric symptoms respond to the cholinesterase inhibitors, especially in DLB, obviating the need for other more toxic therapies.

Cholinesterase inhibitors are being used to treat AD (donepezil, rivastigmine, galantamine) and PDD (rivastigmine). Recent work has focused on developing antibodies against $A\beta_{42}$ as a treatment for AD. Although the initial randomized controlled trials failed, there was some evidence for efficacy in the mildest patient groups. Therefore, researchers have begun to focus on patients with very mild disease and asymptomatic individuals at risk for AD, such as those who carry autosomal dominantly inherited genetic mutations or healthy elders with CSF or amyloid imaging biomarker evidence supporting presymptomatic AD. Memantine proves useful when treating some patients with moderate to severe AD; its major benefit relates to decreasing caregiver burden, most likely by decreasing resistance to dressing and grooming support. In moderate to severe AD, the combination of memantine and a cholinesterase inhibitor delayed nursing home placement in several studies, although other studies have not supported the efficacy of adding memantine to the regimen.

A proactive strategy has been shown to reduce the occurrence of delirium in hospitalized patients. This strategy includes frequent orientation, cognitive activities, sleep-enhancement measures, vision and hearing aids, and correction of dehydration.

Nondrug behavior therapy has an important place in dementia management. The primary goals are to make the patient's life comfortable, uncomplicated, and safe. Preparing lists, schedules, calendars, and labels can be helpful in the early stages. It is also useful to stress familiar routines, walks, and simple physical exercises. For many demented patients, memory for events is worse than their ability to carry out routine activities, and they may still be able to take part in activities such as walking, bowling, dancing, singing, bingo, and golf. Demented patients often object to losing control over familiar tasks such as driving, cooking, and handling finances. Attempts to help or take over may be greeted with complaints, depression, or anger. Hostile responses on the part of the caregiver are counterproductive and sometimes even harmful. Reassurance, distraction, and calm positive statements are more productive in this setting. Eventually, tasks such as finances and driving must be assumed by others, and the patient will conform and adjust. Safety is an important issue that includes not only driving but controlling the kitchen, bathroom, and sleeping area environments, as well as stairways. These areas need to be monitored, supervised, and made as safe as possible. A move to a retirement complex, assisted-living center, or nursing home can initially increase confusion and agitation. Repeated reassurance, reorientation, and careful introduction to the new personnel will help to smooth the process. Providing activities that are known to be enjoyable to the patient can be of considerable benefit.

The clinician must pay special attention to frustration and depression among family members and caregivers. Caregiver guilt and burnout are common. Family members often feel overwhelmed and helpless and may vent their frustrations on the patient, each other, and health care providers. Caregivers should be encouraged to take advantage of day-care facilities and respite services. Education and counseling about dementia are important. Local and national support groups, such as the Alzheimer's Association (*www.alz.org*), can provide considerable help.

36 Aphasia, Memory Loss, and Other Focal Cerebral Disorders

M.-Marsel Mesulam

The cerebral cortex of the human brain contains approximately 20 billion neurons spread over an area of 2.5 m^2. The primary sensory and motor areas constitute 10% of the cerebral cortex. The rest is subsumed by modality-selective, heteromodal, paralimbic, and limbic areas collectively known as the *association cortex* (Fig. 36-1). The association cortex mediates the integrative processes that subserve cognition, emotion, and comportment. A systematic testing of these mental functions is necessary for the effective clinical assessment of the association cortex and its diseases. According to current thinking, there are no centers for "hearing words," "perceiving space," or "storing memories."

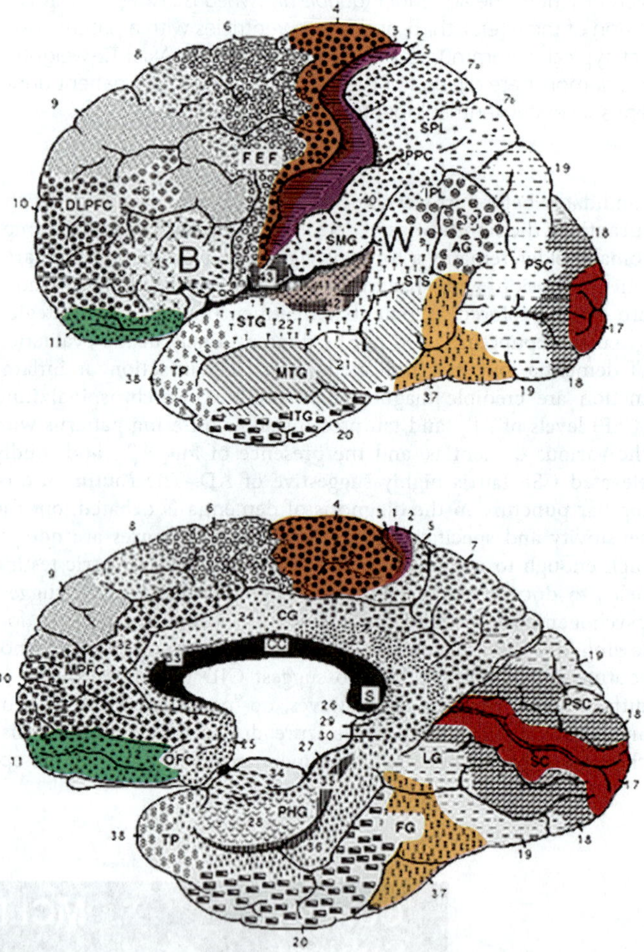

FIGURE 36-1 Lateral (*top*) and medial (*bottom*) views of the cerebral hemispheres. The numbers refer to the Brodmann cytoarchitectonic designations. Area 17 corresponds to the primary visual cortex, 41–42 to the primary auditory cortex, 1–3 to the primary somatosensory cortex, and 4 to the primary motor cortex. The rest of the cerebral cortex contains association areas. AG, angular gyrus; B, Broca's area; CC, corpus callosum; CG, cingulate gyrus; DLPFC, dorsolateral prefrontal cortex; FEF, frontal eye fields (premotor cortex); FG, fusiform gyrus; IPL, inferior parietal lobule; ITG, inferior temporal gyrus; LG, lingual gyrus; MPFC, medial prefrontal cortex; MTG, middle temporal gyrus; OFC, orbitofrontal cortex; PHG, parahippocampal gyrus; PPC, posterior parietal cortex; PSC, peristriate cortex; SC, striate cortex; SMG, supramarginal gyrus; SPL, superior parietal lobule; STG, superior temporal gyrus; STS, superior temporal sulcus; TP, temporopolar cortex; W, Wernicke's area.

Cognitive and behavioral functions (domains) are coordinated by intersecting *large-scale neural networks* that contain interconnected cortical and subcortical components. Five anatomically defined large-scale networks are most relevant to clinical practice: (1) a perisylvian network for language, (2) a parietofrontal network for spatial orientation, (3) an occipitotemporal network for face and object recognition, (4) a limbic network for retentive memory, and (5) a prefrontal network for the executive control of cognition and comportment.

THE LEFT PERISYLVIAN NETWORK FOR APHASIAS

The areas that are critical for language make up a distributed network located along the perisylvian region of the *left* hemisphere. One hub, located in the inferior frontal gyrus, is known as Broca's area. Damage to this region impairs phonology, fluency, and the grammatical structure of sentences. The location of a second hub, known as *Wernicke's area*, is less clearly settled but is traditionally thought to include the posterior parts of the temporal lobe. Cerebrovascular accidents that damage this area interfere with the ability to understand spoken or written sentences as well as the ability to express thoughts through meaningful words and statements. These two hubs are interconnected with each other and with surrounding parts of the frontal, parietal, and temporal lobes. Damage to this network gives rise to language impairments known as aphasia. Aphasia should be diagnosed only when there are deficits in the formal aspects of language, such as word finding, word choice, comprehension, spelling, or grammar. Dysarthria and mutism do not by themselves lead to a diagnosis of aphasia. In approximately 90% of right-handers and 60% of left-handers, aphasia occurs only after lesions of the left hemisphere.

CLINICAL EXAMINATION

The clinical examination of language should include the assessment of naming, spontaneous speech, comprehension, repetition, reading, and writing. A deficit of naming (*anomia*) is the single most common finding in aphasic patients. When asked to name a common object, the patient may fail to come up with the appropriate word, may provide a circumlocutious description of the object ("the thing for writing"), or may come up with the wrong word (*paraphasia*). If the patient offers an incorrect but related word ("pen" for "pencil"), the naming error is known as a *semantic paraphasia*; if the word approximates the correct answer but is phonetically inaccurate ("plentil" for "pencil"), it is known as a *phonemic paraphasia*. In most anomias, the patient cannot retrieve the appropriate name when shown an object but can point to the appropriate object when the name is provided by the examiner. This is known as a one-way (or retrieval-based) naming deficit. A two-way (comprehension-based) naming deficit exists if the patient can neither provide nor recognize the correct name. *Spontaneous speech* is described as "fluent" if it maintains appropriate output volume, phrase length, and melody or as "nonfluent" if it is sparse and halting and average utterance length is below four words. The examiner also should note the integrity of *grammar* as manifested by word order (syntax), tenses, suffixes, prefixes, plurals, and possessives. *Comprehension* can be tested by assessing the patient's ability to follow conversation, asking yes-no questions ("Can a dog fly?" "Does it snow in summer?"), asking the patient to point to appropriate objects ("Where is the source of illumination in this room?"), or asking for verbal definitions of single words. *Repetition* is assessed by asking the patient to repeat single words, short sentences, or strings of words such as "No ifs, ands, or buts." The testing of repetition with tongue twisters such as "hippopotamus" and "Irish constabulary" provides a better assessment of dysarthria and palilalia than of aphasia. It is important to make sure that the number of words does not exceed the patient's attention span. Otherwise, the failure of repetition becomes a reflection of the narrowed attention span (working memory) rather than an indication of an aphasic deficit. *Reading* should be assessed for deficits in reading aloud as well as comprehension. *Alexia* describes an inability to either read aloud or comprehend single words and simple sentences; *agraphia* (or dysgraphia) is used to describe an acquired deficit in spelling.

Aphasias can arise acutely in cerebrovascular accidents (CVAs) or gradually in neurodegenerative diseases. The syndromes listed in Table 36-1 are most applicable to the former group, where gray matter and white matter at the lesion site are abruptly and jointly destroyed. Progressive neurodegenerative diseases can have cellular, laminar, and regional specificity, giving rise to a different set of aphasias that will be described separately. The syndromes outlined below are idealizations and rarely occur in pure form.

Wernicke's Aphasia Comprehension is impaired for spoken and written words and sentences. Language output is fluent but is highly paraphasic and circumlocutious. Paraphasic errors may lead to strings of neologisms, which lead to "jargon aphasia." Speech contains few substantive nouns. The output is therefore voluminous but uninformative. For example, a patient attempts to describe how his wife accidentally threw away something important, perhaps his dentures: "We don't need it anymore, she says. And with it when that was downstairs was my teeth-tick … a … den … dentith … my dentist. And they happened to be in that bag … see? …Where my two … two little pieces of dentist that I use … that I … all gone. If she throws the whole thing away … visit some friends of hers and she can't throw them away."

Gestures and pantomime do not improve communication. The patient may not realize that his or her language is incomprehensible and may appear angry and impatient when the examiner fails to decipher the meaning of a severely paraphasic statement. In some patients this type of aphasia can be associated with severe agitation and paranoia. The ability to follow commands aimed at axial musculature may be preserved. The dissociation between the failure to understand simple questions ("What is your name?") in a patient who rapidly closes his or her eyes, sits up, or rolls over when asked to do so is characteristic of Wernicke's aphasia and helps differentiate it from

TABLE 36-1 CLINICAL FEATURES OF APHASIAS AND RELATED CONDITIONS COMMONLY SEEN IN CEREBROVASCULAR ACCIDENTS

	Comprehension	Repetition of Spoken Language	Naming	Fluency
Wernicke's	Impaired	Impaired	Impaired	Preserved or increased
Broca's	Preserved (except grammar)	Impaired	Impaired	Decreased
Global	Impaired	Impaired	Impaired	Decreased
Conduction	Preserved	Impaired	Impaired	Preserved
Nonfluent (anterior) transcortical	Preserved	Preserved	Impaired	Impaired
Fluent (posterior) transcortical	Impaired	Preserved	Impaired	Preserved
Isolation	Impaired	Echolalia	Impaired	No purposeful speech
Anomic	Preserved	Preserved	Impaired	Preserved except for word-finding pauses
Pure word deafness	Impaired only for spoken language	Impaired	Preserved	Preserved
Pure alexia	Impaired only for reading	Preserved	Preserved	Preserved

deafness, psychiatric disease, or malingering. Patients with Wernicke's aphasia cannot express their thoughts in meaning-appropriate words and cannot decode the meaning of words in any modality of input. This aphasia therefore has expressive as well as receptive components. Repetition, naming, reading, and writing also are impaired.

The lesion site most commonly associated with Wernicke's aphasia is the posterior portion of the language network. An embolus to the inferior division of the middle cerebral artery, to the posterior temporal or angular branches in particular, is the most common etiology (Chap. 446). Intracerebral hemorrhage, head trauma, and neoplasm are other causes of Wernicke's aphasia. A coexisting right hemianopia or superior quadrantanopia is common, and mild right nasolabial flattening may be found, but otherwise, the examination is often unrevealing. The paraphasic, neologistic speech in an agitated patient with an otherwise unremarkable neurologic examination may lead to the suspicion of a primary psychiatric disorder such as schizophrenia or mania, but the other components characteristic of acquired aphasia and the absence of prior psychiatric disease usually settle the issue. Prognosis for recovery of language function is guarded.

Broca's Aphasia Speech is nonfluent, labored, interrupted by many word-finding pauses, and usually dysarthric. It is impoverished in function words but enriched in meaning-appropriate nouns. Abnormal word order and the inappropriate deployment of *bound morphemes* (word endings used to denote tenses, possessives, or plurals) lead to a characteristic agrammatism. Speech is telegraphic and pithy but quite informative. In the following passage, a patient with Broca's aphasia describes his medical history: "I see … the dotor, dotor sent me … Bosson. Go to hospital. Dotor … kept me beside. Two, tee days, doctor send me home."

Output may be reduced to a grunt or single word ("yes" or "no"), which is emitted with different intonations in an attempt to express approval or disapproval. In addition to fluency, naming and repetition are impaired. Comprehension of spoken language is intact except for syntactically difficult sentences with a passive voice structure or embedded clauses, indicating that Broca's aphasia is not just an "expressive" or "motor" disorder and that it also may involve a comprehension deficit in decoding syntax. Patients with Broca's aphasia can be tearful, easily frustrated, and profoundly depressed. Insight into their condition is preserved, in contrast to Wernicke's aphasia. Even when spontaneous speech is severely dysarthric, the patient may be able to display a relatively normal articulation of words when singing. This dissociation has been used to develop specific therapeutic approaches (melodic intonation therapy) for Broca's aphasia. Additional neurologic deficits include right facial weakness, hemiparesis or hemiplegia, and a buccofacial apraxia characterized by an inability to carry out motor commands involving oropharyngeal and facial musculature (e.g., patients are unable to demonstrate how to blow out a match or suck through a straw). The cause is most often infarction of Broca's area (the inferior frontal convolution; "B" in Fig. 36-1) and surrounding anterior perisylvian and insular cortex due to occlusion of the superior division of the middle cerebral artery (Chap. 446). Mass lesions, including tumor, intracerebral hemorrhage, and abscess, also may be responsible. When the cause of Broca's aphasia is stroke, recovery of language function generally peaks within 2 to 6 months, after which time further progress is limited. Speech therapy is more successful than in Wernicke's aphasia.

Conduction Aphasia Speech output is fluent but contains many phonemic paraphasias, comprehension of spoken language is intact, and repetition is severely impaired. Naming elicits phonemic paraphasias, and spelling is impaired. Reading aloud is impaired, but reading comprehension is preserved. The lesion sites spare the functionality of Broca's and Wernicke's areas but may induce a disconnection between the two. Occasionally, a transient Wernicke's aphasia may rapidly resolve into a conduction aphasia. The paraphasic output in conduction aphasia interferes with the ability to express meaning, but this deficit is not nearly as severe as the one displayed by patients with Wernicke's aphasia. Associated neurologic signs in conduction aphasia vary according to the primary lesion site.

Transcortical Aphasias: Fluent and Nonfluent Clinical features of *fluent (posterior) transcortical aphasia* are similar to those of Wernicke's aphasia, but repetition is intact. The lesion site disconnects the intact core of the language network from other temporoparietal association areas. Associated neurologic findings may include hemianopia. Cerebrovascular lesions (e.g., infarctions in the posterior watershed zone) and neoplasms that involve the temporoparietal cortex posterior to Wernicke's area are common causes. The features of *nonfluent (anterior) transcortical aphasia* are similar to those of Broca's aphasia, but repetition is intact and agrammatism is less pronounced. The neurologic examination may be otherwise intact, but a right hemiparesis also can exist. The lesion site disconnects the intact language network from prefrontal areas of the brain and usually involves the anterior watershed zone between anterior and middle cerebral artery territories or the supplementary motor cortex in the territory of the anterior cerebral artery.

Global and Isolation Aphasias *Global aphasia* represents the combined dysfunction of Broca's and Wernicke's areas and usually results from strokes that involve the entire middle cerebral artery distribution in the left hemisphere. Speech output is nonfluent, and comprehension of language is severely impaired. Related signs include right hemiplegia, hemisensory loss, and homonymous hemianopia. *Isolation aphasia* represents a combination of the two transcortical aphasias. Comprehension is severely impaired, and there is no purposeful speech output. The patient may parrot fragments of heard conversations (*echolalia*), indicating that the neural mechanisms for repetition are at least partially intact. This condition represents the pathologic function of the language network when it is isolated from other regions of the brain. Broca's and Wernicke's areas tend to be spared, but there is damage to the surrounding frontal, parietal, and temporal cortex. Lesions are patchy and can be associated with anoxia, carbon monoxide poisoning, or complete watershed zone infarctions.

Anomic Aphasia This form of aphasia may be considered the "minimal dysfunction" syndrome of the language network. Articulation, comprehension, and repetition are intact, but confrontation naming, word finding, and spelling are impaired. Word-finding pauses are uncommon, so language output is fluent but paraphasic, circumlocutious, and uninformative. The lesion sites can be anywhere within the left hemisphere language network, including the middle and inferior temporal gyri. *Anomic aphasia is the single most common language disturbance seen in head trauma, metabolic encephalopathy, and Alzheimer's disease.*

Pure Word Deafness The most common causes are either bilateral or left-sided middle cerebral artery (MCA) strokes affecting the superior temporal gyrus. The net effect of the underlying lesion is to interrupt the flow of information from the auditory association cortex to the language network. Patients have no difficulty understanding written language and can express themselves well in spoken or written language. They have no difficulty interpreting and reacting to environmental sounds since primary auditory cortex and auditory association areas of the right hemisphere are spared. Because auditory information cannot be conveyed to the language network, however, it cannot be decoded into neural word representations, and the patient reacts to speech as if it were in an alien tongue that cannot be deciphered. Patients cannot repeat spoken language but have no difficulty naming objects. In time, patients with pure word deafness teach themselves lipreading and may appear to have improved. There may be no additional neurologic findings, but agitated paranoid reactions are common in the acute stages. Cerebrovascular lesions are the most common cause.

Pure Alexia Without Agraphia This is the visual equivalent of pure word deafness. The lesions (usually a combination of damage to the left occipital cortex and to a posterior sector of the corpus callosum—the splenium) interrupt the flow of visual input into the language network. There is usually a right hemianopia, but the core language network remains unaffected. The patient can understand and produce spoken language, name objects in the left visual hemifield, repeat, and write. However, the patient acts as if illiterate when asked to read even the simplest sentence because the visual information from the written words (presented to the intact left visual hemifield) cannot reach the language network. Objects in the left hemifield may be named accurately because they activate nonvisual associations in the right hemisphere, which in turn can access the language network through transcallosal pathways anterior to the splenium. Patients with this syndrome also may lose the ability to name colors, although they can match colors. This is known as a *color anomia*. The most common etiology of pure alexia is a vascular lesion in the territory of the posterior cerebral artery or an infiltrating neoplasm in the left occipital cortex that involves the optic radiations as well as the crossing fibers of the splenium. Because the posterior cerebral artery also supplies medial temporal components of the limbic system, a patient with pure alexia also may experience an amnesia, but this is usually transient because the limbic lesion is unilateral.

Apraxia and Aphemia *Apraxia* designates a complex motor deficit that cannot be attributed to pyramidal, extrapyramidal, cerebellar, or sensory dysfunction and that does not arise from the patient's failure to understand the nature of the task. *Apraxia of speech* is used to designate articulatory abnormalities in the duration, fluidity, and stress of syllables that make up words. Intoning the words may improve articulation. It can arise with CVAs in the posterior part of Broca's area or in the course of frontotemporal lobar degeneration (FTLD) with tauopathy. *Aphemia* is a severe form of acute speech apraxia that presents with severely impaired fluency (often mutism). Recovery is the rule and involves an intermediate stage of hoarse whispering. Writing, reading, and comprehension are intact, and so this is not a true aphasic syndrome. CVAs in parts of Broca's area or subcortical lesions that undercut its connections with other parts of the brain may be present. Occasionally, the lesion site is on the medial aspects of the frontal lobes and may involve the supplementary motor cortex of the left hemisphere. *Ideomotor apraxia* is diagnosed when commands to perform a specific motor act ("cough," "blow out a match") or pantomime the use of a common tool (a comb, hammer, straw, or toothbrush) in the absence of the real object cannot be followed. The patient's ability to comprehend the command is ascertained by demonstrating multiple movements and establishing that the correct one can be recognized. Some patients with this type of apraxia can imitate the appropriate movement (when it is demonstrated by the examiner) and show no impairment when handed the real object, indicating that the sensorimotor mechanisms necessary for the movement are intact. Some forms of ideomotor apraxia represent a disconnection of the language network from pyramidal motor systems so that commands to execute complex movements are understood but cannot be conveyed to the appropriate motor areas. *Buccofacial apraxia* involves apraxic deficits in movements of the face and mouth. *Limb apraxia* encompasses apraxic deficits in movements of the arms and legs. Ideomotor apraxia almost always is caused by lesions in the left hemisphere and is commonly associated with aphasic syndromes, especially Broca's aphasia and conduction aphasia. Because the handling of real objects is not impaired, ideomotor apraxia by itself causes no major limitation of daily living activities. Patients with lesions of the anterior corpus callosum can display ideomotor apraxia confined to the left side of the body, a sign known as *sympathetic dyspraxia*. A severe form of sympathetic dyspraxia, known as the *alien hand* syndrome, is characterized by additional features of motor disinhibition on the left hand. *Ideational apraxia* refers to a deficit in the sequencing of goal-directed movements in patients who have no difficulty executing the individual components of the sequence. For example, when the patient is asked to pick up a pen and write, the sequence of uncapping the pen, placing the cap at the opposite end, turning the point toward the writing surface, and writing may be disrupted, and the patient may be seen trying to write with the wrong end of the pen or even with the removed cap. These motor sequencing problems usually are seen in the context of confusional states and dementias rather than focal lesions associated with aphasic conditions. *Limb-kinetic apraxia* involves clumsiness in the use of tools or objects that cannot be attributed to sensory, pyramidal, extrapyramidal, or cerebellar dysfunction. This condition can emerge in the context of focal premotor cortex lesions or *corticobasal degeneration*.

Gerstmann's Syndrome The combination of *acalculia* (impairment of simple arithmetic), *dysgraphia* (impaired writing), *finger anomia* (an inability to name individual fingers such as the index and thumb), and *right-left confusion* (an inability to tell whether a hand, foot, or arm of the patient or examiner is on the right or left side of the body) is known as Gerstmann's syndrome. In making this diagnosis, it is important to establish that the finger and left-right naming deficits are not part of a more generalized anomia and that the patient is not otherwise aphasic. When Gerstmann's syndrome arises acutely and in isolation, it is commonly associated with damage to the inferior parietal lobule (especially the angular gyrus) in the left hemisphere.

Pragmatics and Prosody *Pragmatics* refers to aspects of language that communicate attitude, affect, and the figurative rather than literal aspects of a message (e.g., "green thumb" does not refer to the actual color of the finger). One component of pragmatics, *prosody,* refers to variations of melodic stress and intonation that influence attitude and the inferential aspect of verbal messages. For example, the two statements "He *is* clever." and "He is *clever*?" contain an identical word choice and syntax but convey vastly different messages because of differences in the intonation with which the statements are uttered. Damage to right hemisphere regions corresponding to Broca's area impairs the ability to introduce meaning-appropriate prosody into spoken language. The patient produces grammatically correct language with accurate word choice, but the statements are uttered in a monotone that interferes with the ability to convey the intended stress and affect. Patients with this type of *aprosodia* give the mistaken impression of being depressed or indifferent. Other aspects of pragmatics, especially the ability to infer the figurative aspect of a message, become impaired by damage to the right hemisphere or frontal lobes.

Subcortical Aphasia Damage to subcortical components of the language network (e.g., the striatum and thalamus of the left hemisphere) also can lead to aphasia. The resulting syndromes contain combinations of deficits in the various aspects of language but rarely fit the specific patterns described in Table 36-1. In a patient with a CVA, an anomic aphasia accompanied by dysarthria or a fluent aphasia with hemiparesis should raise the suspicion of a subcortical lesion site.

Progressive Aphasias Aphasias caused by major cerebrovascular accidents start suddenly and display maximal deficits at the onset. These are the "classic" aphasias described above. Aphasias caused by neurodegenerative diseases have an insidious onset and relentless progression. The neuropathology can be selective not only for gray matter but also for specific layers and cell types. The clinico-anatomic patterns are therefore different from those described in Table 36-1.

CLINICAL PRESENTATION AND DIAGNOSIS OF PRIMARY PROGRESSIVE APHASIA (PPA) Several neurodegenerative syndromes, such as typical Alzheimer-type (amnestic) and frontal-type (behavioral) dementias, can also undermine language as the disease progresses. In these cases, the aphasia is an ancillary component of the overall syndrome. When a neurodegenerative language disorder arises in relative isolation and becomes the primary concern that brings the patient to medical attention, a diagnosis of PPA is made.

LANGUAGE IN PPA The impairments of language in PPA have slightly different patterns from those seen in CVA-caused aphasias. Three major subtypes of PPA can be recognized. The *agrammatic variant* is characterized by consistently low fluency and impaired grammar but intact word comprehension. It most closely resembles Broca's aphasia or anterior transcortical aphasia but usually lacks the right hemiparesis or dysarthria and has more profound impairments of grammar. Peak sites of neuronal loss (gray matter atrophy) include the left inferior frontal gyrus where Broca's area is located. The neuropathology is usually an FTLD with tauopathy but can also be an atypical form of Alzheimer's disease (AD) pathology. The *semantic variant* is characterized by preserved fluency and syntax but poor single-word comprehension and profound two-way naming impairments. This kind of aphasia is not seen with CVAs. It differs from Wernicke's aphasia or posterior transcortical aphasia because speech is usually informative, repetition is intact, and comprehension of conversation is relatively preserved, as long as the meaning is not too dependent on words that the patient fails to understand. Peak atrophy sites are located in the left anterior temporal lobe, indicating that this part of the brain plays a critical role in the comprehension of words, especially words that denote concrete objects. The neuropathology is frequently an FTLD with abnormal precipitates of the 43-kDa transactive response DNA-binding protein TDP-43. The *logopenic variant* is characterized by preserved syntax and comprehension but frequent and severe word-finding pauses, anomia, circumlocutions, and simplifications during spontaneous speech. Peak atrophy sites are located in the temporoparietal junction and posterior temporal lobe, partially overlapping with traditional location of Wernicke's area. However, the comprehension impairment of *Wernicke's aphasia* is absent, perhaps because the underlying white matter, frequently damaged by cerebrovascular accidents, remains relatively intact in PPA. In contrast to Broca's aphasia or agrammatic PPA, the interruption of fluency is variable so that speech may appear entirely normal if the patient is allowed to engage in small talk. Logopenic PPA resembles the anomic aphasia of Table 36-1 but usually has longer and more frequent word-finding pauses. Patients may also have poor phrase and word repetition, in which case the aphasia resembles the *conduction aphasia* in Table 36-1. Of all PPA subtypes, this is the one most commonly associated with the pathology of AD, but FTLD can also be the cause. In addition to these three major subtypes, PPA can also present in the form of *pure word deafness* or *Gerstmann's syndrome*.

THE PARIETOFRONTAL NETWORK FOR NEGLECT AND RELATED CONDITIONS

Adaptive spatial orientation is subserved by a large-scale network containing three major cortical components. The *cingulate cortex* provides access to a motivational mapping of the extrapersonal space, the *posterior parietal cortex* to a sensorimotor representation of salient extrapersonal events, and the *frontal eye fields* to motor strategies for attentional behaviors (Fig. 36-2). Subcortical components of this network include the striatum and the thalamus. Damage to this network can undermine the distribution of attention within the extrapersonal space, giving rise to hemispatial neglect, simultanagnosia and object finding failures. The integration of egocentric (self-centered) with allocentric (object-centered) coordinates can also be disrupted, giving rise to impairments in route finding, the ability to avoid obstacles, and the ability to dress.

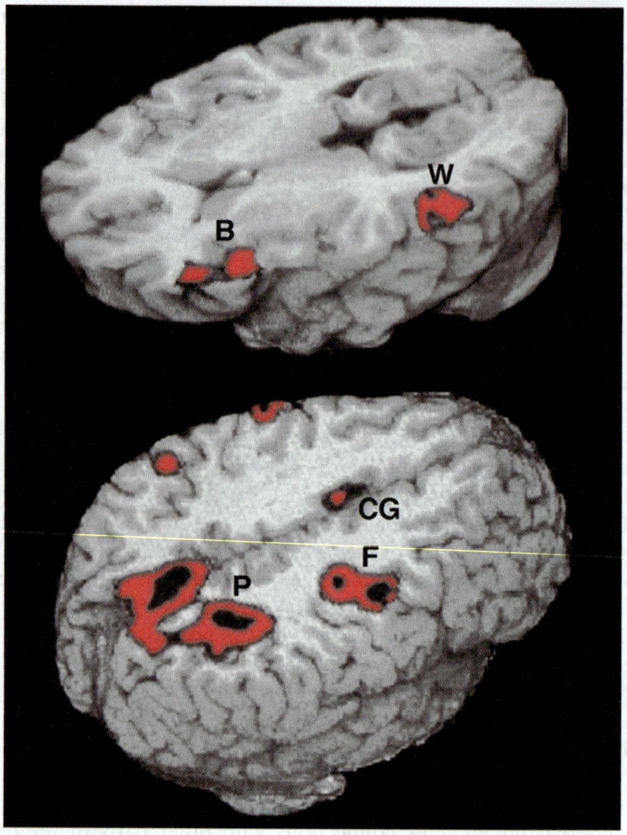

FIGURE 36-2 Functional magnetic resonance imaging of language and spatial attention in neurologically intact subjects. The red and black areas show regions of task-related significant activation. (*Top*) The subjects were asked to determine if two words were synonymous. This language task led to the simultaneous activation of the two epicenters of the language network, Broca's area (B) and Wernicke's area (W). The activations are exclusively in the left hemisphere. (*Bottom*) The subjects were asked to shift spatial attention to a peripheral target. This task led to the simultaneous activation of the three epicenters of the attentional network: the posterior parietal cortex (P), the frontal eye fields (F), and the cingulate gyrus (CG). The activations are predominantly in the right hemisphere. *(Courtesy of Darren Gitelman, MD; with permission.)*

HEMISPATIAL NEGLECT

Contralesional hemispatial neglect represents one outcome of damage to the cortical or subcortical components of this network. *The traditional view that hemispatial neglect always denotes a parietal lobe lesion is inaccurate.* According to one model of spatial cognition, the right hemisphere directs attention within the *entire* extrapersonal space, whereas the left hemisphere directs attention mostly within the contralateral right hemispace. Consequently, left hemisphere lesions do not give rise to much contralesional neglect because the global attentional mechanisms of the right hemisphere can compensate for the loss of the *contralaterally* directed attentional functions of the left hemisphere. Right hemisphere lesions, however, give rise to severe contralesional left hemispatial neglect because the unaffected left hemisphere does not contain ipsilateral attentional mechanisms. This model is consistent with clinical experience, which shows that contralesional neglect is more common, more severe, and longer lasting after damage to the right hemisphere than after damage to the left hemisphere. Severe neglect for the right hemispace is rare, even in left-handers with left hemisphere lesions.

Clinical Examination Patients with severe neglect may fail to dress, shave, or groom the left side of the body; fail to eat food placed on the left side of the tray; and fail to read the left half of sentences. When asked to copy a simple line drawing, the patient fails to copy detail on the left, and when the patient is asked to write, there is a tendency to leave an unusually wide margin on the left. Two bedside tests that are useful in assessing neglect are *simultaneous bilateral stimulation* and *visual target cancellation*. In the former, the examiner provides either unilateral or simultaneous bilateral stimulation in the visual, auditory, and tactile modalities. After right hemisphere injury, patients who have no difficulty detecting unilateral stimuli on either side experience the bilaterally presented stimulus as coming only from the right. This phenomenon is known as *extinction* and is a manifestation of the sensory-representational aspect of hemispatial neglect. In the target detection task, targets (e.g., A's) are interspersed with foils (e.g., other letters of the alphabet) on a 21.5- to 28.0-cm (8.5 to 11 in.) sheet of paper, and the patient is asked to circle all the targets. A failure to detect targets on the left is a manifestation of the exploratory (motor) deficit in hemispatial neglect (Fig. 36-3A). Hemianopia is not by itself sufficient to cause the target detection failure because the patient is free to turn the head and eyes to the left. Target detection failures therefore reflect a distortion of spatial attention, not just of sensory input. Some patients with neglect also may deny the existence of hemiparesis and may even deny ownership of the paralyzed limb, a condition known as *anosognosia*.

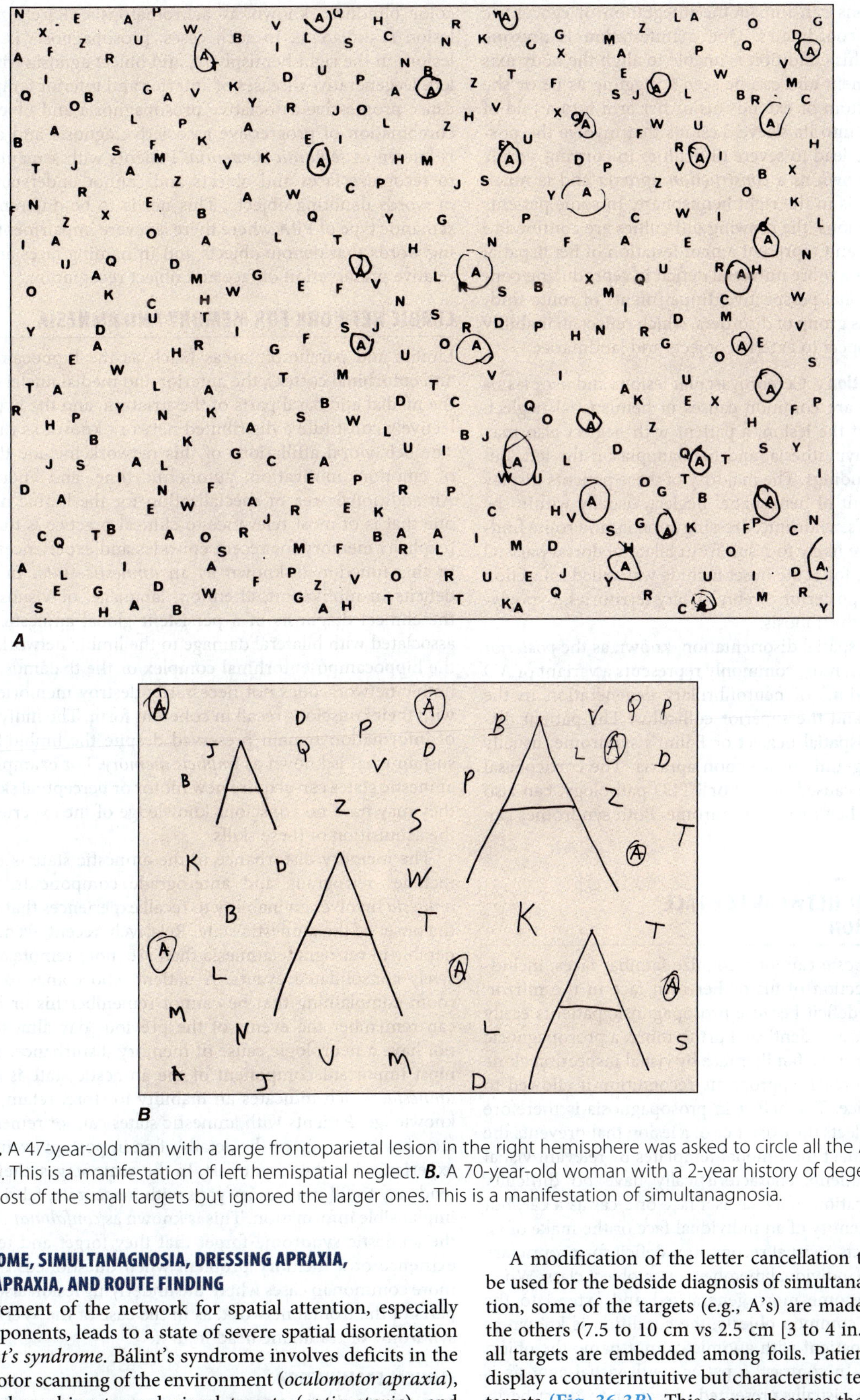

FIGURE 36-3 ***A.*** A 47-year-old man with a large frontoparietal lesion in the right hemisphere was asked to circle all the A's. Only targets on the right are circled. This is a manifestation of left hemispatial neglect. ***B.*** A 70-year-old woman with a 2-year history of degenerative dementia was able to circle most of the small targets but ignored the larger ones. This is a manifestation of simultanagnosia.

BÁLINT'S SYNDROME, SIMULTANAGNOSIA, DRESSING APRAXIA, CONSTRUCTION APRAXIA, AND ROUTE FINDING

Bilateral involvement of the network for spatial attention, especially its parietal components, leads to a state of severe spatial disorientation known as *Bálint's syndrome.* Bálint's syndrome involves deficits in the orderly visuomotor scanning of the environment (*oculomotor apraxia*), accurate manual reaching toward visual targets (*optic ataxia*), and the ability to integrate visual information in the center of gaze with more peripheral information (*simultanagnosia*). A patient with simultanagnosia "misses the forest for the trees." For example, a patient who is shown a table lamp and asked to name the object may look at its circular base and call it an ashtray. Some patients with simultanagnosia report that objects they look at may vanish suddenly, probably indicating an inability to look back at the original point of gaze after brief saccadic displacements. Movement and distracting stimuli greatly exacerbate the difficulties of visual perception. Simultanagnosia can occur without the other two components of Bálint's syndrome.

A modification of the letter cancellation task described above can be used for the bedside diagnosis of simultanagnosia. In this modification, some of the targets (e.g., A's) are made to be much larger than the others (7.5 to 10 cm vs 2.5 cm [3 to 4 in. vs 1 in.] in height), and all targets are embedded among foils. Patients with simultanagnosia display a counterintuitive but characteristic tendency to miss the larger targets (Fig. 36-3B). This occurs because the information needed for the identification of the larger targets cannot be confined to the immediate line of gaze and requires the integration of visual information across multiple fixation points. The greater difficulty in the detection of the larger targets also indicates that poor acuity is not responsible for the impairment of visual function and that the problem is central rather than peripheral. The test shown in Fig. 36-3B is not by itself sufficient to diagnose simultanagnosia because some patients with a frontal network syndrome may omit the large letters, perhaps because they lack the mental flexibility needed to realize that the two types of targets are symbolically identical despite being superficially different.

Bilateral parietal lesions can impair the integration of egocentric with allocentric spatial coordinates. One manifestation is *dressing apraxia*. A patient with this condition is unable to align the body axis with the axis of the garment and can be seen struggling as he or she holds a coat from its bottom or extends his or her arm into a fold of the garment rather than into its sleeve. Lesions that involve the posterior parietal cortex also lead to severe difficulties in copying simple line drawings. This is known as a *construction apraxia* and is much more severe if the lesion is in the right hemisphere. In some patients with right hemisphere lesions, the drawing difficulties are confined to the left side of the figure and represent a manifestation of hemispatial neglect; in others, there is a more universal deficit in reproducing contours and three-dimensional perspective. Impairments of route finding can be included in this group of disorders, which reflect an inability to orient the self with respect to external objects and landmarks.

Causes of Spatial Disorientation Cerebrovascular lesions and neoplasms in the right hemisphere are common causes of hemispatial neglect. Depending on the site of the lesion, a patient with neglect also may have hemiparesis, hemihypesthesia, and hemianopia on the left, but these are not invariant findings. The majority of these patients display considerable improvement of hemispatial neglect, usually within the first several weeks. Bálint's syndrome, dressing apraxia, and route finding impairments are more likely to result from bilateral dorsal parietal lesions; common settings for acute onset include watershed infarction between the middle and posterior cerebral artery territories, hypoglycemia, and sagittal sinus thrombosis.

A progressive form of spatial disorientation, known as the *posterior cortical atrophy* syndrome, most commonly represents a variant of AD with unusual concentrations of neurofibrillary degeneration in the parieto-occipital cortex and the superior colliculus. The patient displays a progressive hemispatial neglect or Bálint's syndrome, usually accompanied by dressing and construction apraxia. The corticobasal syndrome, which can be caused by AD or FTLD pathology, can also lead to a progressive left hemineglect syndrome. Both syndromes can impair route finding.

THE OCCIPITOTEMPORAL NETWORK FOR FACE AND OBJECT RECOGNITION

A patient with *prosopagnosia* cannot recognize familiar faces, including, sometimes, the reflection of his or her own face in the mirror. This is not a perceptual deficit because prosopagnosic patients easily can tell whether two faces are identical. Furthermore, a prosopagnosic patient who cannot recognize a familiar face by visual inspection alone can use auditory cues to reach appropriate recognition if allowed to listen to the person's voice. The deficit in prosopagnosia is therefore modality-specific and reflects the existence of a lesion that prevents the activation of otherwise intact multimodal templates by relevant visual input. Prosopagnosic patients characteristically have no difficulty with the generic identification of a face as a face or a car as a car, but may not recognize the identity of an individual face or the make of an individual car. This reflects a visual recognition deficit for proprietary features that characterize individual members of an object class. When recognition problems become more generalized and extend to the generic identification of common objects, the condition is known as *visual object agnosia*. A patient with anomia cannot name the object but can describe its use. In contrast, a patient with visual agnosia is unable either to name a visually presented object or to describe its use. Face and object recognition disorders also can result from the simultanagnosia of Bálint's syndrome, in which case they are known as *apperceptive* agnosias as opposed to the *associative* agnosias that result from inferior temporal lobe lesions.

CAUSES

The characteristic lesions in prosopagnosia and visual object agnosia of acute onset consist of bilateral infarctions in the territory of the posterior cerebral arteries. Associated deficits can include visual field defects (especially superior quadrantanopias) and a centrally based color blindness known as achromatopsia. Rarely, the responsible lesion is unilateral. In such cases, prosopagnosia is associated with lesions in the right hemisphere, and object agnosia with lesions in the left. Degenerative diseases of anterior and inferior temporal cortex can cause progressive associative prosopagnosia and object agnosia. The combination of progressive associative agnosia and a fluent aphasia is known as *semantic dementia*. Patients with semantic dementia fail to recognize faces and objects and cannot understand the meaning of words denoting objects. This needs to be differentiated from the semantic type of PPA where there is severe impairment in understanding words that denote objects and in naming faces and objects but a relative preservation of face and object recognition.

LIMBIC NETWORK FOR MEMORY AND AMNESIA

Limbic and paralimbic areas (such as the hippocampus, amygdala, and entorhinal cortex), the anterior and medial nuclei of the thalamus, the medial and basal parts of the striatum, and the hypothalamus collectively constitute a distributed network known as the *limbic system*. The behavioral affiliations of this network include the coordination of emotion, motivation, autonomic tone, and endocrine function. An additional area of specialization for the limbic network and the one that is of most relevance to clinical practice is that of declarative (explicit) memory for recent episodes and experiences. A disturbance in this function is known as an *amnestic state*. In the absence of deficits in motivation, attention, language, or visuospatial function, the clinical diagnosis of a persistent global amnestic state is always associated with bilateral damage to the limbic network, usually within the hippocampo-entorhinal complex or the thalamus. Damage to the limbic network does not necessarily destroy memories but interferes with their conscious recall in coherent form. The individual fragments of information remain preserved despite the limbic lesions and can sustain what is known as *implicit memory*. For example, patients with amnestic states can acquire new motor or perceptual skills even though they may have no conscious knowledge of the experiences that led to the acquisition of these skills.

The memory disturbance in the amnestic state is multimodal and includes retrograde and anterograde components. The *retrograde amnesia* involves an inability to recall experiences that occurred before the onset of the amnestic state. Relatively recent events are more vulnerable to retrograde amnesia than are more remote and more extensively consolidated events. A patient who comes to the emergency room complaining that he cannot remember his or her identity but can remember the events of the previous day almost certainly does not have a neurologic cause of memory disturbance. The second and most important component of the amnestic state is the *anterograde amnesia*, which indicates an inability to store, retain, and recall new knowledge. Patients with amnestic states cannot remember what they ate a few hours ago or the details of an important event they may have experienced in the recent past. In the acute stages, there also may be a tendency to fill in memory gaps with inaccurate, fabricated, and often implausible information. This is known as *confabulation*. Patients with the amnestic syndrome forget that they forget and tend to deny the existence of a memory problem when questioned. Confabulation is more common in cases where the underlying lesion also interferes with parts of the frontal network, as in the case of the Wernicke-Korsakoff syndrome or traumatic head injury.

CLINICAL EXAMINATION

A patient with an amnestic state is almost always disoriented, especially to time, and has little knowledge of current news. The anterograde component of an amnestic state can be tested with a list of four to five words read aloud by the examiner up to five times or until the patient can immediately repeat the entire list without an intervening delay. The next phase of the recall occurs after a period of 5 to 10 min during which the patient is engaged in other tasks. Amnestic patients fail this phase of the task and may even forget that they were given a list of words to remember. Accurate recognition of the words by multiple choice in a patient who cannot recall them indicates a less severe memory disturbance that affects mostly the retrieval stage of memory.

The retrograde component of an amnesia can be assessed with questions related to autobiographical or historic events. The anterograde component of amnestic states is usually much more prominent than the retrograde component. In rare instances, occasionally associated with temporal lobe epilepsy or herpes simplex encephalitis, the retrograde component may dominate. Confusional states caused by toxic-metabolic encephalopathies and some types of frontal lobe damage lead to secondary memory impairments, especially at the stages of encoding and retrieval, even in the absence of limbic lesions. This sort of memory impairment can be differentiated from the amnestic state by the presence of additional impairments in the attention-related tasks described below in the section on the frontal lobes.

CAUSES, INCLUDING ALZHEIMER'S DISEASE

Neurologic diseases that give rise to an amnestic state include tumors (of the sphenoid wing, posterior corpus callosum, thalamus, or medial temporal lobe), infarctions (in the territories of the anterior or posterior cerebral arteries), head trauma, herpes simplex encephalitis, Wernicke-Korsakoff encephalopathy, paraneoplastic limbic encephalitis, and degenerative dementias such as AD and Pick's disease. The one common denominator of all these diseases is the presence of bilateral lesions within one or more components in the limbic network. Occasionally, unilateral left-sided hippocampal lesions can give rise to an amnestic state, but the memory disorder tends to be transient. Depending on the nature and distribution of the underlying neurologic disease, the patient also may have visual field deficits, eye movement limitations, or cerebellar findings. AD and its prodromal state of mild cognitive impairment (MCI) are the most common causes of progressive memory impairments. The predilection of the entorhinal cortex and hippocampus for early neurofibrillary degeneration by typical AD pathology is responsible for the initially selective impairment of episodic memory. In time, additional impairments in language, attention, and visuospatial skills emerge as the neurofibrillary degeneration spreads to additional neocortical areas.

Transient global amnesia is a distinctive syndrome usually seen in late middle age. Patients become acutely disoriented and repeatedly ask who they are, where they are, and what they are doing. The spell is characterized by anterograde amnesia (inability to retain new information) and a retrograde amnesia for relatively recent events that occurred before the onset. The syndrome usually resolves within 24 to 48 h and is followed by the filling in of the period affected by the retrograde amnesia, although there is persistent loss of memory for the events that occurred during the ictus. Recurrences are noted in approximately 20% of patients. Migraine, temporal lobe seizures, and perfusion abnormalities in the posterior cerebral territory have been postulated as causes of transient global amnesia. The absence of associated neurologic findings occasionally may lead to the incorrect diagnosis of a psychiatric disorder.

THE PREFRONTAL NETWORK FOR EXECUTIVE FUNCTION AND BEHAVIOR

The frontal lobes can be subdivided into motor-premotor, dorsolateral prefrontal, medial prefrontal, and orbitofrontal components. The terms *frontal lobe syndrome* and *prefrontal cortex* refer only to the last three of these four components. These are the parts of the cerebral cortex that show the greatest phylogenetic expansion in primates, especially in humans. The dorsolateral prefrontal, medial prefrontal, and orbitofrontal areas, along with the subcortical structures with which they are interconnected (i.e., the head of the caudate and the dorsomedial nucleus of the thalamus), collectively make up a large-scale network that coordinates exceedingly complex aspects of human cognition and behavior.

The prefrontal network plays an important role in behaviors that require multitasking and the integration of thought with emotion. Cognitive operations impaired by prefrontal cortex lesions often are referred to as "executive functions." The most common clinical manifestations of damage to the prefrontal network take the form of two relatively distinct syndromes. In the *frontal abulic syndrome*, the patient shows a loss of initiative, creativity, and curiosity and displays a pervasive emotional blandness, apathy, and lack of empathy. In the *frontal disinhibition syndrome*, the patient becomes socially disinhibited and shows severe impairments of judgment, insight, foresight, and the ability to mind rules of conduct. The dissociation between intact intellectual function and a total lack of even rudimentary common sense is striking. Despite the preservation of all essential memory functions, the patient cannot learn from experience and continues to display inappropriate behaviors without appearing to feel emotional pain, guilt, or regret when those behaviors repeatedly lead to disastrous consequences. The impairments may emerge only in real-life situations when behavior is under minimal external control and may not be apparent within the structured environment of the medical office. Testing judgment by asking patients what they would do if they detected a fire in a theater or found a stamped and addressed envelope on the road is not very informative because patients who answer these questions wisely in the office may still act very foolishly in real-life settings. The physician must therefore be prepared to make a diagnosis of frontal lobe disease based on historic information alone even when the mental state is quite intact in the office examination.

CLINICAL EXAMINATION

The emergence of developmentally primitive reflexes, also known as frontal release signs, such as grasping (elicited by stroking the palm) and sucking (elicited by stroking the lips) are seen primarily in patients with large structural lesions that extend into the premotor components of the frontal lobes or in the context of metabolic encephalopathies. The vast majority of patients with prefrontal lesions and frontal lobe behavioral syndromes do not display these reflexes. Damage to the frontal lobe disrupts a variety of attention-related functions, including working memory (the transient online holding and manipulation of information), concentration span, the scanning and retrieval of stored information, the inhibition of immediate but inappropriate responses, and mental flexibility. Digit span (which should be seven forward and five reverse) is decreased, reflecting poor working memory; the recitation of the months of the year in reverse order (which should take less than 15 s) is slowed as another indication of poor working memory; and the fluency in producing words starting with the letter a, f, or s that can be generated in 1 min (normally ≥12 per letter) is diminished even in nonaphasic patients, indicating an impairment in the ability to search and retrieve information from long-term stores. In "go–no go" tasks (where the instruction is to raise the finger upon hearing one tap but keep it still upon hearing two taps), the patient shows a characteristic inability to inhibit the response to the "no go" stimulus. Mental flexibility (tested by the ability to shift from one criterion to another in sorting or matching tasks) is impoverished; distractibility by irrelevant stimuli is increased; and there is a pronounced tendency for impersistence and perseveration. The ability for abstracting similarities and interpreting proverbs is also undermined.

The attentional deficits disrupt the orderly registration and retrieval of new information and lead to *secondary* memory deficits. The distinction of the underlying neural mechanisms is illustrated by the observation that severely amnestic patients who cannot remember events that occurred a few minutes ago may have intact if not superior working memory capacity as shown in tests of digit span.

CAUSES: TRAUMA, NEOPLASM, AND FRONTOTEMPORAL DEMENTIA

The abulic syndrome tends to be associated with damage in dorsolateral or dorsomedial prefrontal cortex, and the disinhibition syndrome with damage in orbitofrontal or ventromedial cortex. These syndromes tend to arise almost exclusively after bilateral lesions. Unilateral lesions confined to the prefrontal cortex may remain silent until the pathology spreads to the other side; this explains why thromboembolic CVA is an unusual cause of the frontal lobe syndrome. Common settings for frontal lobe syndromes include head trauma, ruptured aneurysms, hydrocephalus, tumors (including metastases, glioblastoma, and falx or olfactory groove meningiomas), and focal degenerative diseases. A major clinical form of FTLD known as the behavioral variant of frontotemporal dementia (bvFTD) causes a progressive frontal lobe syndrome. The behavioral changes can range from apathy to shoplifting, compulsive gambling, sexual indiscretions, remarkable lack of common sense, new ritualistic behaviors, and alterations in dietary preferences, usually leading to increased taste for sweets or rigid attachment to specific food items. In many patients with AD, neurofibrillary degeneration eventually spreads to prefrontal cortex and gives rise to components of the frontal lobe syndrome, but almost always on a background of severe memory impairment. Rarely, the bvFTD syndrome can arise in isolation in the context of an atypical form of AD pathology.

Lesions in the caudate nucleus or in the dorsomedial nucleus of the thalamus (subcortical components of the prefrontal network) also can produce a frontal lobe syndrome. This is one reason why the changes in mental state associated with degenerative basal ganglia diseases such as Parkinson's disease and Huntington's disease display components of the frontal lobe syndrome. Bilateral multifocal lesions of the cerebral hemispheres, none of which are individually large enough to cause specific cognitive deficits such as aphasia and neglect, can collectively interfere with the connectivity and therefore integrating (executive) function of the prefrontal cortex. A frontal lobe syndrome is therefore the single most common behavioral profile associated with a variety of bilateral multifocal brain diseases, including metabolic encephalopathy, multiple sclerosis, and vitamin B_{12} deficiency, among others. Many patients with the clinical diagnosis of a frontal lobe syndrome tend to have lesions that do not involve prefrontal cortex but involve either the subcortical components of the prefrontal network or its connections with other parts of the brain. To avoid making a diagnosis of "frontal lobe syndrome" in a patient with no evidence of frontal cortex disease, it is advisable to use the diagnostic term *frontal network syndrome*, with the understanding that the responsible lesions can lie anywhere within this distributed network. A patient with frontal lobe disease raises potential dilemmas in differential diagnosis: the abulia and blandness may be misinterpreted as depression, and the disinhibition as idiopathic mania or acting out. Appropriate intervention may be delayed while a treatable tumor keeps expanding.

CARING FOR PATIENTS WITH DEFICITS OF HIGHER CEREBRAL FUNCTION

Brain damage may cause a dissociation between feeling states and their expression so that a patient who may superficially appear jocular could still be suffering from an underlying depression that needs to be treated. If neuroleptics become absolutely necessary for the control of agitation, atypical neuroleptics are preferable because of their lower extrapyramidal side effects. Treatment with neuroleptics in elderly patients with dementia requires weighing the potential benefits against the potentially serious side effects.

Spontaneous improvement of cognitive deficits due to acute neurologic lesions is common. It is most rapid in the first few weeks but may continue for up to 2 years, especially in young individuals with single brain lesions. Some of the initial deficits appear to arise from remote dysfunction (diaschisis) in parts of the brain that are interconnected with the site of initial injury. Improvement in these patients may reflect, at least in part, a normalization of the remote dysfunction. Other mechanisms may involve functional reorganization in surviving neurons adjacent to the injury or the compensatory use of homologous structures, e.g., the right superior temporal gyrus with recovery from Wernicke's aphasia. Cognitive rehabilitation procedures have been used in the treatment of higher cortical deficits. There are few controlled studies, but some show a benefit of rehabilitation in the recovery from hemispatial neglect and aphasia. Determining driving competence is challenging, especially in the early stages of dementing diseases. The diagnosis of a neurodegenerative disease is not by itself sufficient for asking the patient to stop driving. An on-the-road driving test and reports from family members may help time decisions related to this very important activity.

Some of the deficits described in this chapter are so complex that they may bewilder not only the patient and family but also the physician. It is imperative to carry out a systematic clinical evaluation to characterize the nature of the deficits and explain them in lay terms to the patient and family. An enlightened approach to patients with damage to the cerebral cortex requires an understanding of the principles that link neural networks to higher cerebral functions in health and disease.

37e Primary Progressive Aphasia, Memory Loss, and Other Focal Cerebral Disorders

Maria Luisa Gorno-Tempini, Jennifer Ogar, Joel Kramer, Bruce L. Miller, Gil Rabinovici, Maria Carmela Tartaglia

This is a digital-only chapter. It is available on the DVD that accompanies this book, as well as on Access Medicine/Harrison's Online, and the eBook and "app" editions of HPIM 19e.

Language and memory are essential human functions. For the experienced clinician, the recognition of different types of language and memory disturbances often provides essential clues to the anatomic localization and diagnosis of neurologic disorders. This video illustrates classic disorders of language and speech (including the aphasias), memory (the amnesias), and other disorders of cognition that are commonly encountered in clinical practice.

38 Sleep Disorders

Charles A. Czeisler, Thomas E. Scammell, Clifford B. Saper

Disturbed sleep is among the most frequent health complaints that physicians encounter. More than one-half of adults in the United States experience at least intermittent sleep disturbance, and only 30% of adult Americans report consistently obtaining a sufficient amount of sleep. The Institute of Medicine has estimated that 50–70 million Americans suffer from a chronic disorder of sleep and wakefulness, which can adversely affect daytime functioning as well as physical and mental health. Over the last 20 years, the field of sleep medicine has emerged as a distinct specialty in response to the impact of sleep disorders and sleep deficiency on overall health.

PHYSIOLOGY OF SLEEP AND WAKEFULNESS

Given the opportunity, most healthy young adults will sleep 7–8 h per night, although the timing, duration, and internal structure of sleep vary among individuals. In the United States, adults tend to have one consolidated sleep episode each night, although in some cultures sleep may be divided into a mid-afternoon nap and a shortened night sleep. This pattern changes considerably over the life span, as infants and young children sleep considerably more than older people.

The stages of human sleep are defined on the basis of characteristic patterns in the electroencephalogram (EEG), the electrooculogram (EOG—a measure of eye-movement activity), and the surface electromyogram (EMG) measured on the chin, neck, and legs. The continuous recording of these electrophysiologic parameters to define sleep and wakefulness is termed *polysomnography*.

Polysomnographic profiles define two basic states of sleep: (1) rapid eye movement (REM) sleep and (2) non–rapid eye movement (NREM) sleep. NREM sleep is further subdivided into three stages: N1,

N2, and N3, characterized by increasing arousal threshold and slowing of the cortical EEG. REM sleep is characterized by a low-amplitude, mixed-frequency EEG similar to that of NREM stage N1 sleep. The EOG shows bursts of rapid eye movements similar to those seen during eyes-open wakefulness. EMG activity is absent in nearly all skeletal muscles, reflecting the brainstem-mediated muscle atonia that is characteristic of REM sleep.

ORGANIZATION OF HUMAN SLEEP

Normal nocturnal sleep in adults displays a consistent organization from night to night (Fig. 38-1). After sleep onset, sleep usually progresses through NREM stages N1–N3 sleep within 45–60 min. NREM stage N3 sleep (also known as slow-wave sleep) predominates in the first third of the night and comprises 15–25% of total nocturnal sleep time in young adults. Sleep deprivation increases the rapidity of sleep onset and both the intensity and amount of slow-wave sleep.

The first REM sleep episode usually occurs in the second hour of sleep. NREM and REM sleep alternate through the night with an average period of 90–110 min (the "ultradian" sleep cycle). Overall, in a healthy young adult, REM sleep constitutes 20–25% of total sleep, and NREM stages N1 and N2 constitute 50–60%.

Age has a profound impact on sleep state organization (Fig. 38-1). N3 sleep is most intense and prominent during childhood, decreasing with puberty and across the second and third decades of life. N3 sleep declines during adulthood to the point where it may be completely absent in older adults. The remaining NREM sleep becomes more fragmented, with many more frequent awakenings from NREM sleep. It is the increased frequency of awakenings, rather than a decreased ability to fall back asleep, that accounts for the increased wakefulness during the sleep episode in older people. While REM sleep may account for 50% of total sleep time in infancy, the percentage falls off sharply over the first postnatal year as a mature REM-NREM cycle develops; thereafter, REM sleep occupies about 25% of total sleep time.

Sleep deprivation degrades cognitive performance, particularly on tests that require continual vigilance. Paradoxically, older people are less vulnerable to the neurobehavioral performance impairment induced by acute sleep deprivation than young adults, maintaining their reaction time and sustaining vigilance with fewer lapses of attention. However, it is more difficult for older adults to obtain recovery sleep after staying awake all night, as the ability to sleep during the daytime declines with age.

After sleep deprivation, NREM sleep is generally recovered first, followed by REM sleep. However, because REM sleep tends to be most prominent in the second half of the night, sleep truncation (e.g., by an alarm clock) results in selective REM sleep deprivation. This may increase REM sleep pressure to the point where the first REM sleep may occur much earlier in the nightly sleep episode. Because several disorders (see below) also cause sleep fragmentation, it is important that the patient have sufficient sleep opportunity (at least 8 h per night) for several nights prior to a diagnostic polysomnogram.

There is growing evidence that sleep deficiency in humans may cause glucose intolerance and contribute to the development of diabetes, obesity, and the metabolic syndrome, as well as impaired immune responses, accelerated atherosclerosis, and increased risk of cardiac disease and stroke. For these reasons, the Institute of Medicine declared sleep deficiency and sleep disorders "an unmet public health problem."

WAKE AND SLEEP ARE REGULATED BY BRAIN CIRCUITS

Two principal neural systems govern the expression of the sleep and wakefulness. The ascending arousal system, illustrated in green in Fig. 38-2, consists of clusters of nerve cells extending from the upper pons to the hypothalamus and basal forebrain that activate the cerebral cortex, thalamus (which is necessary to relay sensory information to the cortex), and other forebrain regions. The ascending arousal neurons use monoamines (norepinephrine, dopamine, serotonin, and histamine), glutamate, or acetylcholine as neurotransmitters to activate their target neurons. Additional arousal-promoting neurons in the hypothalamus use the peptide neurotransmitter orexin (also known as hypocretin, shown in blue) to reinforce activity in the other arousal cell groups.

Damage to the arousal system at the level of the rostral pons and lower midbrain causes coma, indicating that the ascending arousal influence from this level is critical in maintaining wakefulness. Damage to the hypothalamic branch of the arousal system causes profound sleepiness, but usually not coma. Specific loss of the orexin neurons produces the sleep disorder narcolepsy (see below).

The arousal system is turned off during sleep by inhibitory inputs from cell groups in the sleep-promoting system, shown in Fig. 38-2 in red. These neurons in the preoptic area, lateral hypothalamus, and pons use γ-aminobutyric acid (GABA) to inhibit the arousal system. Many sleep-promoting neurons are themselves inhibited by inputs from the arousal system. This mutual inhibition between the arousal- and sleep-promoting systems forms a neural circuit akin to what electrical engineers call a "flip-flop switch." A switch of this type tends to promote rapid transitions between the on (wake) and off (sleep) states, while avoiding intermediate states. The relatively rapid transitions between waking and sleeping states, as seen in the EEG of humans and animals, is consistent with this model.

Neurons in the ventrolateral preoptic nucleus, one of the key sleep-promoting sites, are lost during normal human aging, correlating with reduced ability to maintain sleep (sleep fragmentation). The ventrolateral preoptic neurons are also injured in Alzheimer's disease, which may in part account for the poor sleep quality in those patients.

Transitions between NREM and REM sleep appear to be governed by a similar switch in the brainstem. GABAergic REM-Off neurons have been identified in the lower midbrain that inhibit REM-On neurons in the upper pons. The REM-On group contains both GABAergic neurons that inhibit the REM-Off group (thus satisfying the conditions for a REM flip-flop switch) as well as glutamatergic neurons that project widely in the central nervous system (CNS) to cause the key phenomena associated with REM sleep. REM-On neurons that project to the medulla and spinal cord activate inhibitory (GABA and glycine-containing) interneurons, which in turn hyperpolarize the motor neurons, producing the atonia of REM sleep. REM-On neurons that project to the forebrain may be important in producing dreams.

The REM sleep switch receives cholinergic input, which favors transitions to REM sleep, and monoaminergic (norepinephrine and serotonin) input that prevents REM sleep. As a result, drugs that

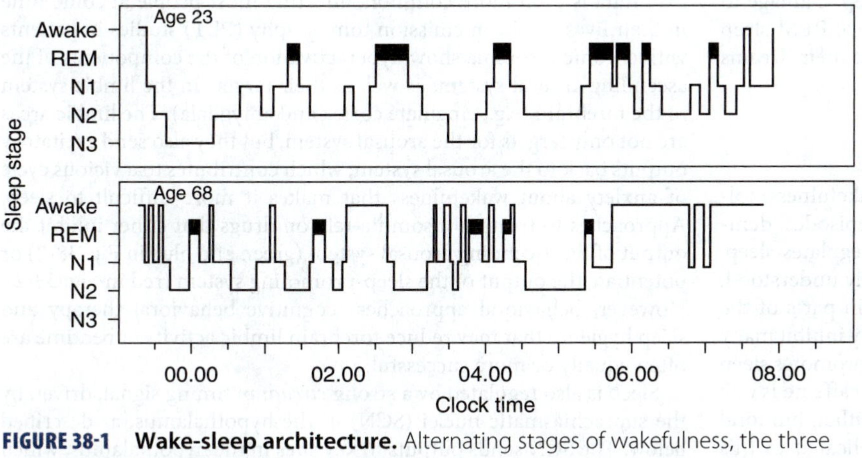

FIGURE 38-1 Wake-sleep architecture. Alternating stages of wakefulness, the three stages of NREM sleep (N1–N3), and REM sleep (*solid bars*) occur over the course of the night for representative young and older adult men. Characteristic features of sleep in older people include reduction of N3 slow-wave sleep, frequent spontaneous awakenings, early sleep onset, and early morning awakening. NREM, non–rapid eye movement; REM, rapid eye movement. *(From the Division of Sleep and Circadian Disorders, Brigham and Women's Hospital.)*

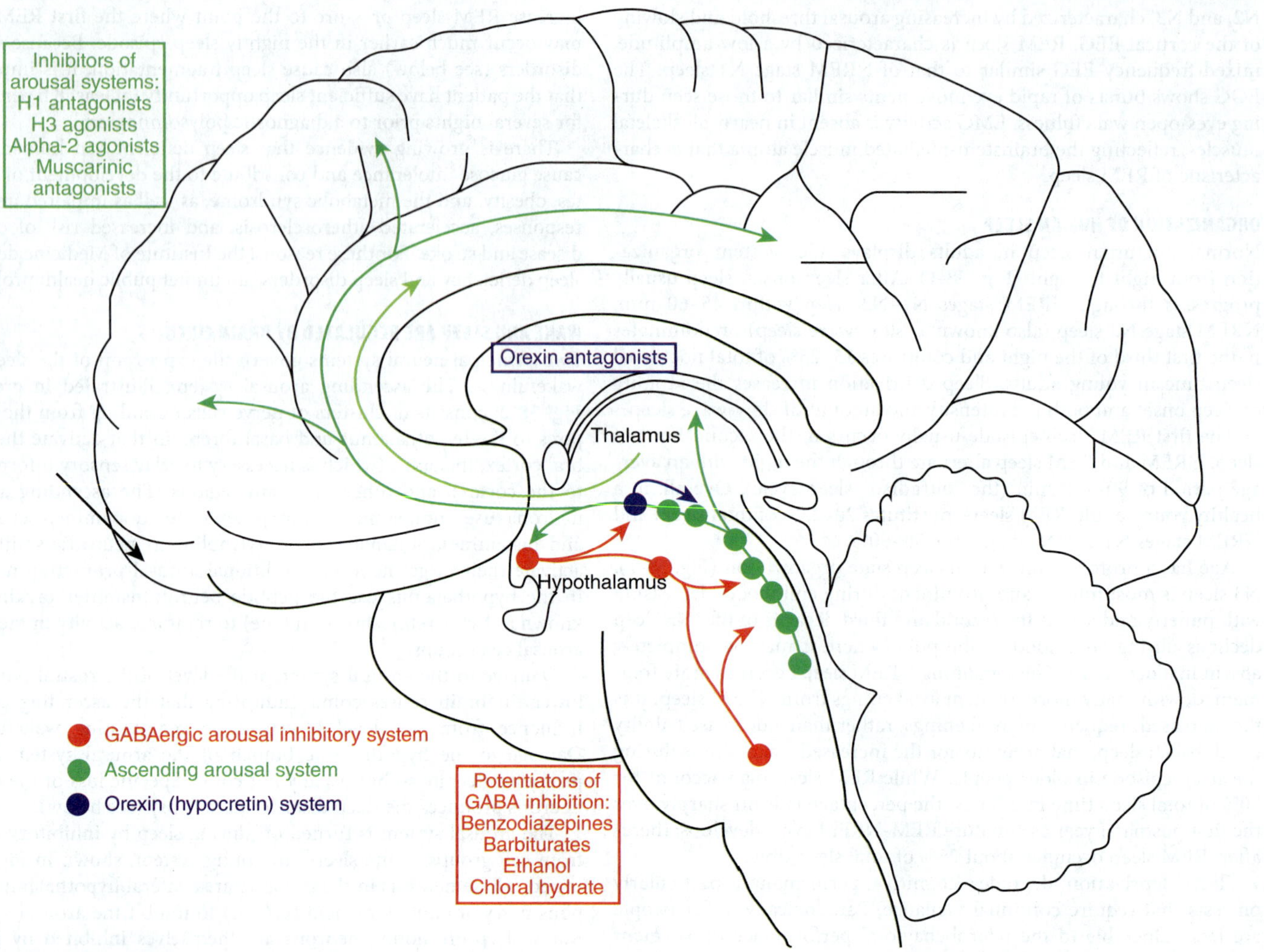

FIGURE 38-2 Relationship of drugs for insomnia with wake-sleep systems. The arousal system in the brain (*green*) includes monoaminergic, glutamatergic, and cholinergic neurons in the brainstem that activate neurons in the hypothalamus, thalamus, basal forebrain, and cerebral cortex. Orexin neurons (*blue*) in the hypothalamus, which are lost in narcolepsy, reinforce and stabilize arousal by activating other components of the arousal system. The sleep-promoting system (*red*) consists of GABAergic neurons in the preoptic area, lateral hypothalamus, and brainstem that inhibit the components of the arousal system, thus allowing sleep to occur. Drugs used to treat insomnia include those that block the effects of arousal system neurotransmitters (*green and blue*) and those that enhance the effects of γ-aminobutyric acid (GABA) produced by the sleep system (*red*).

increase monoamine tone (e.g., serotonin or norepinephrine reuptake inhibitors) tend to reduce the amount of REM sleep. Damage to the neurons that promote REM sleep atonia can produce REM sleep behavior disorder, a condition in which patients act out their dreams (see below).

SLEEP-WAKE CYCLES ARE DRIVEN BY HOMEOSTATIC, ALLOSTATIC, AND CIRCADIAN INPUTS

The gradual increase in sleep drive with prolonged wakefulness, followed by deeper slow-wave sleep and prolonged sleep episodes, demonstrates that there is a *homeostatic* mechanism that regulates sleep. The neurochemistry of sleep homeostasis is only partially understood, but with prolonged wakefulness, adenosine levels rise in parts of the brain. Adenosine may act through A1 receptors to directly inhibit many arousal-promoting brain regions. In addition, adenosine promotes sleep through A2a receptors; inhibition of these receptors by caffeine is one of the chief ways in which people fight sleepiness. Other humoral factors, such as prostaglandin D_2, have also been implicated in this process. Both adenosine and prostaglandin D_2 activate the sleep-promoting neurons in the ventrolateral preoptic nucleus.

Allostasis is the physiologic response to a threat that cannot be managed by homeostatic mechanisms (e.g., the presence of physical danger or psychological threat). These stress responses can severely impact the need for and ability to sleep. For example, insomnia is very common in patients with anxiety and other psychiatric disorders. Stress-induced insomnia is even more common, affecting most people at some time in their lives. Positron emission tomography (PET) studies in patients with chronic insomnia show hyperactivation of the components of the ascending arousal system, as well as their targets in the limbic system in the forebrain (e.g., cingulate cortex and amygdala). The limbic areas are not only targets for the arousal system, but they also send excitatory outputs back to the arousal system, which contributes to a vicious cycle of anxiety about wakefulness that makes it more difficult to sleep. Approaches to treating insomnia rely on drugs that either inhibit the output of the ascending arousal system (green and blue in Fig. 38-2) or potentiate the output of the sleep-promoting system (red in Fig. 38-2). However, behavioral approaches (cognitive behavioral therapy and sleep hygiene) that may reduce forebrain limbic activity at bedtime are often equally or more successful.

Sleep is also regulated by a strong *circadian* timing signal, driven by the suprachiasmatic nuclei (SCN) of the hypothalamus, as described below. The SCN sends outputs to key sites in the hypothalamus, which impose 24-h rhythms on a wide range of behaviors and body systems, including the wake-sleep cycle.

PHYSIOLOGY OF CIRCADIAN RHYTHMICITY

The wake-sleep cycle is the most evident of many 24-h rhythms in humans. Prominent daily variations also occur in endocrine, thermoregulatory, cardiac, pulmonary, renal, immune, gastrointestinal, and neurobehavioral functions. At the molecular level, endogenous circadian rhythmicity is driven by self-sustaining transcriptional/translational feedback loops. In evaluating daily rhythms in humans, it is important to distinguish between diurnal components passively evoked by periodic environmental or behavioral changes (e.g., the increase in blood pressure and heart rate that occurs upon assumption of the upright posture) and circadian rhythms actively driven by an endogenous oscillatory process (e.g., the circadian variations in adrenal cortisol and pineal melatonin secretion that persist across a variety of environmental and behavioral conditions).

While it is now recognized that most cells in the body have circadian clocks that regulate diverse physiologic processes, most of these disparate clocks are unable to maintain the synchronization with each other that is required to produce useful 24-h rhythms aligned with the external light-dark cycle. The neurons in the SCN are interconnected with one another in such a way as to produce a near-24-h synchronous rhythm of neural activity that is then transmitted to the rest of the body. Bilateral destruction of the SCN results in a loss of most endogenous circadian rhythms including wake-sleep behavior and rhythms in endocrine and metabolic systems. The genetically determined period of this endogenous neural oscillator, which averages ~24.15 h in humans, is normally synchronized to the 24-h period of the environmental light-dark cycle through direct input from intrinsically photosensitive ganglion cells in the retina to the SCN. Humans are exquisitely sensitive to the resetting effects of light, particularly the shorter wavelengths (~460–500 nm) of the visible spectrum. Small differences in circadian period contribute to variations in diurnal preference in young adults (with the circadian period shorter in those who typically go to bed and rise earlier compared to those who typically go to bed and wake up later), whereas changes in homeostatic sleep regulation may underlie the age-related tendency toward earlier sleep-wake timing.

The timing and internal architecture of sleep are directly coupled to the output of the endogenous circadian pacemaker. Paradoxically, the endogenous circadian rhythm for wake propensity peaks just before the habitual bedtime, whereas that of sleep propensity peaks near the habitual wake time. These rhythms are thus timed to oppose the rise of sleep tendency throughout the usual waking day and the decline of sleep propensity during the habitual sleep episode, respectively. Misalignment of the endogenous circadian pacemaker with the desired wake-sleep cycle can, therefore, induce insomnia, decreased alertness, and impaired performance evident in night-shift workers and airline travelers.

BEHAVIORAL AND PHYSIOLOGIC CORRELATES OF SLEEP STATES AND STAGES

Polysomnographic staging of sleep correlates with behavioral changes during specific states and stages. During the transitional state (stage N1) between wakefulness and deeper sleep, individuals may respond to faint auditory or visual signals. Formation of short-term memories is inhibited at the onset of NREM stage N1 sleep, which may explain why individuals aroused from that transitional sleep stage frequently lack situational awareness. After sleep deprivation, such transitions may intrude upon behavioral wakefulness notwithstanding attempts to remain continuously awake (see "Shift-Work Disorder," below).

Awakenings from REM sleep are associated with recall of vivid dream imagery over 80% of the time, especially later in the night. Imagery may also be reported after NREM sleep interruptions. Certain disorders may occur during specific sleep stages and are described below under "Parasomnias." These include sleepwalking, night terrors, and enuresis (bed wetting), which occur most commonly in children during deep (N3) NREM sleep, and REM sleep behavior disorder, which occurs mainly among older men who fail to maintain full atonia during REM sleep, and often call out, thrash around, or even act out entire dreams.

All major physiologic systems are influenced by sleep. Blood pressure and heart rate decrease during NREM sleep, particularly during N3 sleep. During REM sleep, bursts of eye movements are associated with large variations in both blood pressure and heart rate mediated by the autonomic nervous system. Cardiac dysrhythmias may occur selectively during REM sleep. Respiratory function also changes. In comparison to relaxed wakefulness, respiratory rate becomes slower but more regular during NREM sleep (especially N3 sleep) and becomes irregular during bursts of eye movements in REM sleep. Decreases in minute ventilation during NREM sleep are out of proportion to the decrease in metabolic rate, resulting in a slightly higher P_{CO_2}.

Endocrine function also varies with sleep. N3 sleep is associated with secretion of growth hormone in men, while sleep in general is associated with augmented secretion of prolactin in both men and women. Sleep has a complex effect on the secretion of luteinizing hormone (LH): during puberty, sleep is associated with increased LH secretion, whereas sleep in the postpubertal female inhibits LH secretion in the early follicular phase of the menstrual cycle. Sleep onset (and probably N3 sleep) is associated with inhibition of thyroid-stimulating hormone and of the adrenocorticotropic hormone–cortisol axis, an effect that is superimposed on the prominent circadian rhythms in the two systems.

The pineal hormone melatonin is secreted predominantly at night in both day- and night-active species, reflecting the direct modulation of pineal activity by a circuitous neural pathway that links the SCN to the sympathetic nervous system, which innervates the pineal gland. Melatonin secretion does not require sleep, but melatonin secretion is inhibited by ambient light, an effect mediated by the neural connection from the retina to the pineal gland via the SCN. Sleep efficiency is highest when the sleep episode coincides with endogenous melatonin secretion. Administration of exogenous melatonin can hasten sleep onset and increase sleep efficiency when administered at a time when endogenous melatonin levels are low, such as in the afternoon or evening or at the desired bedtime in patients with delayed sleep-wake phase disorder, but it does not increase sleep efficiency if administered when endogenous melatonin levels are elevated. This may explain why melatonin is often ineffective in the treatment of patients with primary insomnia.

Sleep is accompanied by alterations of thermoregulatory function. NREM sleep is associated with an increase in the firing of warm-responsive neurons in the preoptic area and a fall in body temperature; conversely, skin warming without increasing core body temperature has been found to increase NREM sleep. REM sleep is associated with reduced thermoregulatory responsiveness.

DISORDERS OF SLEEP AND WAKEFULNESS

APPROACH TO THE PATIENT: Sleep Disorders

Patients may seek help from a physician because of: (1) sleepiness or tiredness during the day; (2) difficulty initiating or maintaining sleep at night (insomnia); or (3) unusual behaviors during sleep itself (parasomnias).

Obtaining a careful history is essential. In particular, the duration, severity, and consistency of the symptoms are important, along with the patient's estimate of the consequences of the sleep disorder on waking function. Information from a bed partner or family member is often helpful because some patients may be unaware of symptoms such as heavy snoring or may underreport symptoms such as falling asleep at work or while driving. Physicians should inquire about when the patient typically goes to bed, when they fall asleep and wake up, whether they awaken during sleep, whether they feel rested in the morning, and whether they nap during the day. Depending on the primary complaint, it may be useful to ask about snoring, witnessed apneas, restless sensations in the legs, movements during sleep, depression, anxiety, and behaviors around the sleep episode. The physical exam may provide evidence of a small airway, large tonsils, or a neurologic or medical disorder that contributes to the main complaint.

It is important to remember that, rarely, seizures may occur exclusively during sleep, mimicking a primary sleep disorder; such sleep-related seizures typically occur during episodes of NREM sleep and may take the form of generalized tonic-clonic movements (sometimes with urinary incontinence or tongue biting) or stereotyped movements in partial complex epilepsy (Chap. 445).

It is often helpful for the patient to complete a daily sleep log for 1–2 weeks to define the timing and amounts of sleep. When relevant, the log can also include information on levels of alertness, work times, and drug and alcohol use, including caffeine and hypnotics.

Polysomnography is necessary for the diagnosis of several disorders such as sleep apnea, narcolepsy, and periodic limb movement disorder. A conventional polysomnogram performed in a clinical sleep laboratory allows measurement of sleep stages, respiratory effort and airflow, oxygen saturation, limb movements, heart rhythm, and additional parameters. A home sleep test usually focuses on just respiratory measures and is helpful in patients with a moderate to high likelihood of having obstructive sleep apnea. The multiple sleep latency test (MSLT) is used to measure a patient's propensity to sleep during the day and can provide crucial evidence for diagnosing narcolepsy and some other causes of sleepiness. The maintenance of wakefulness test is used to measure a patient's ability to sustain wakefulness during the daytime and can provide important evidence for evaluating the efficacy of therapies for improving sleepiness in conditions such as narcolepsy and obstructive sleep apnea.

EVALUATION OF DAYTIME SLEEPINESS

Up to 25% of the adult population has persistent daytime sleepiness that impairs an individual's ability to perform optimally in school, at work, while driving, and in other conditions that require alertness. Sleepy students often have trouble staying alert and performing well in school, and sleepy adults struggle to stay awake and focused on their work. More than half of Americans have fallen asleep while driving. An estimated 1.2 million motor vehicle crashes per year are due to drowsy drivers, causing about 20% of all serious crash injuries and deaths. One needn't fall asleep to have an accident, as the inattention and slowed responses of drowsy drivers are a major contributor. Reaction time is equally impaired by 24 h of sleep loss as by a blood alcohol concentration of 0.10 g/dL.

Identifying and quantifying sleepiness can be challenging. First, patients may describe themselves as "sleepy," "fatigued," or "tired," and the meanings of these words may differ between patients. For clinical purposes, it is best to use the term "sleepiness" to describe a propensity to fall asleep; whereas "fatigue" is best used to describe a feeling of low physical or mental energy but without a tendency to actually sleep. Sleepiness is usually most evident when the patient is sedentary, whereas fatigue may interfere with more active pursuits. Sleepiness generally occurs with disorders that reduce the quality or quantity of sleep or that interfere with the neural mechanisms of arousal, whereas fatigue is more common in inflammatory disorders such as cancer, multiple sclerosis (Chap. 458), fibromyalgia (Chap. 396), chronic fatigue syndrome (Chap. 464e), or endocrine deficiencies such as hypothyroidism (Chap. 405) or Addison's disease (Chap. 406). Second, sleepiness can affect judgment in a manner analogous to ethanol, such that patients may have limited insight into the condition and the extent of their functional impairment. Finally, patients may be reluctant to admit that sleepiness is a problem because they may have become unfamiliar with feeling fully alert and because sleepiness is sometimes viewed pejoratively as reflecting poor motivation or bad sleep habits.

Table 38-1 outlines the diagnostic and therapeutic approach to the patient with a complaint of excessive daytime sleepiness.

To determine the extent and impact of sleepiness on daytime function, it is helpful to ask patients about the occurrence of sleep episodes during normal waking hours, both intentional and unintentional. Specific areas to be addressed include the occurrence of inadvertent sleep episodes while driving or in other safety-related settings, sleepiness while at work or school (and the relationship of sleepiness to work and school performance), and the effect of sleepiness on social and family life. Standardized questionnaires such as the Epworth Sleepiness Scale are often used clinically to measure sleepiness.

Eliciting a history of daytime sleepiness is usually adequate, but objective quantification is sometimes necessary. The MSLT measures a patient's propensity to sleep under quiet conditions. The test is performed after an overnight polysomnogram to establish that the patient has had an adequate amount of good-quality nighttime sleep. The MSLT consists of five 20-min nap opportunities every 2 h across the day. The patient is instructed to try to fall asleep, and the major endpoints are the average latency to sleep and the occurrence of REM sleep during the naps. An average sleep latency across the naps of less than 8 min is considered objective evidence of excessive daytime sleepiness. REM sleep normally occurs only during the nighttime sleep episode, and the occurrence of REM sleep in two or more of the MSLT naps provides support for the diagnosis of narcolepsy.

For the safety of the individual and the general public, physicians have a responsibility to help manage issues around driving in patients with sleepiness. Legal reporting requirements vary from state to state, but at a minimum, physicians should inform sleepy patients about their increased risk of having an accident and advise such patients not to drive a motor vehicle until the sleepiness has been treated effectively. This discussion is especially important for professional drivers, and it should be documented in the patient's medical record.

INSUFFICIENT SLEEP

Insufficient sleep is probably the most common cause of excessive daytime sleepiness. The average adult needs 7.5–8 h of sleep, but on

TABLE 38-1 EVALUATION OF THE PATIENT WITH EXCESSIVE DAYTIME SLEEPINESS

Findings on History and Physical Examination	Diagnostic Evaluation	Diagnosis	Therapy
Difficulty waking in the morning, rebound sleep on weekends and vacations with improvement in sleepiness	Sleep log	Insufficient sleep	Sleep education and behavioral modification to increase amount of sleep
Obesity, snoring, hypertension	Polysomnogram	Obstructive sleep apnea (Chap. 319)	Continuous positive airway pressure; upper airway surgery (e.g., uvulopalatopharyngoplasty); dental appliance; weight loss
Cataplexy, hypnogogic hallucinations, sleep paralysis	Polysomnogram and multiple sleep latency test	Narcolepsy	Stimulants (e.g., modafinil, methylphenidate); REM sleep-suppressing antidepressants (e.g., venlafaxine); sodium oxybate
Restless legs, kicking movements during sleep	Assessment for predisposing medical conditions (e.g., iron deficiency or renal failure)	Restless legs syndrome with or without periodic limb movements	Treatment of predisposing condition if possible; dopamine agonists (e.g., pramipexole, ropinirole)
Sedating medications, stimulant withdrawal, head trauma, systemic inflammation, Parkinson's disease and other neurodegenerative disorders, hypothyroidism, encephalopathy	Thorough medical history and exam including detailed neurologic exam	Sleepiness due to a drug or medical condition	Change medications, treat underlying condition, consider stimulants

PART 2 Cardinal Manifestations and Presentation of Diseases

weeknights, the average U.S. adult gets only 6.75 h of sleep. Only 30% of the U.S. adult population reports consistently obtaining sufficient sleep. Insufficient sleep is especially common among shift workers, individuals working multiple jobs, and people in lower socioeconomic groups. Most teenagers need ≥9 h of sleep, but many fail to get enough sleep because of circadian phase delay, or social pressures to stay up late coupled with early school start times. Late evening light exposure, television viewing, video-gaming, social media, texting, and smartphone use often delay bedtimes despite the fixed, early wake times required for work or school. As is typical with any disorder that causes sleepiness, individuals with chronically insufficient sleep may feel inattentive, irritable, unmotivated, and depressed, and have difficulty with school, work, and driving. Individuals differ in their optimal amount of sleep, and it can be helpful to ask how much sleep the patient obtains on a quiet vacation when he or she can sleep without restrictions. Some patients may think that a short amount of sleep is normal or advantageous, and they may not appreciate their biological need for more sleep, especially if coffee and other stimulants mask the sleepiness. A 2-week sleep log documenting the timing of sleep and daily level of alertness is diagnostically useful and provides helpful feedback for the patient. Extending sleep to the optimal amount on a regular basis can resolve the sleepiness and other symptoms. As with any lifestyle change, extending sleep requires commitment and adjustments, but the improvements in daytime alertness make this change worthwhile.

SLEEP APNEA SYNDROMES

Respiratory dysfunction during sleep is a common, serious cause of excessive daytime sleepiness as well as of disturbed nocturnal sleep. At least 24% of middle-aged men and 9% of middle-aged women in the United States have a reduction or cessation of breathing dozens or more times each night during sleep, with 9% of men and 4% of women doing so more than a hundred times per night. These episodes may be due to an occlusion of the airway (*obstructive sleep apnea*), absence of respiratory effort (*central sleep apnea*), or a combination of these factors (*mixed sleep apnea*). Failure to recognize and treat these conditions appropriately may lead to impairment of daytime alertness, increased risk of sleep-related motor vehicle crashes, depression, hypertension, myocardial infarction, diabetes, stroke, and increased mortality. Sleep apnea is particularly prevalent in overweight men and in the elderly, yet it is estimated to go undiagnosed in most affected individuals. This is unfortunate because several effective treatments are available. **Readers are referred to Chap. 319 for a comprehensive review of the diagnosis and treatment of patients with sleep apnea.**

NARCOLEPSY

Narcolepsy is characterized by difficulty sustaining wakefulness, poor regulation of REM sleep, and disturbed nocturnal sleep. All patients with narcolepsy have excessive daytime sleepiness. This sleepiness is often severe, but in some, it is mild. In contrast to patients with disrupted sleep (e.g., sleep apnea), people with narcolepsy usually feel well rested upon awakening and then feel tired throughout much of the day. In addition, they often experience symptoms related to an intrusion of REM sleep characteristics. REM sleep is characterized by dreaming and muscle paralysis, and people with narcolepsy can have: (1) sudden muscle weakness without a loss of consciousness, which is usually triggered by strong emotions (cataplexy; Video 38-1); (2) dream-like hallucinations at sleep onset (hypnagogic hallucinations) or upon awakening (hypnopompic hallucinations); and (3) muscle paralysis upon awakening (sleep paralysis). With severe cataplexy, an individual may be laughing at a joke and then suddenly collapse to the ground, immobile but awake for 1–2 min. With milder episodes, patients may have mild weakness of the face or neck. Narcolepsy is one of the more common causes of chronic sleepiness and affects about 1 in 2000 people in the United States. Narcolepsy typically begins between age 10 and 20; once established, the disease persists for life.

Narcolepsy is caused by loss of the hypothalamic neurons that produce the orexin neuropeptides (also known as hypocretins). Research in mice and dogs first demonstrated that a loss of orexin signaling due to null mutations of either the orexin neuropeptides or one of the orexin receptors causes sleepiness and cataplexy nearly identical to that seen in people with narcolepsy. Although genetic mutations rarely cause human narcolepsy, researchers soon discovered that patients with narcolepsy had very low or undetectable levels of orexins in their cerebrospinal fluid, and autopsy studies showed a nearly complete loss of the orexin-producing neurons in the hypothalamus. The orexins normally promote long episodes of wakefulness and suppress REM sleep, and thus, loss of orexin signaling results in frequent intrusions of sleep during the usual waking episode, with REM sleep and fragments of REM sleep at any time of day (Fig. 38-3).

Extensive evidence suggests that an autoimmune process likely causes this selective loss of the orexin-producing neurons. Certain human leukocyte antigens (HLAs) can increase the risk of autoimmune disorders (Chap. 373e), and narcolepsy has the strongest known HLA association. HLA DQB1*06:02 is found in about 90% of people with narcolepsy, whereas it occurs in only 12–25% of the general population. Researchers now hypothesize that in people with DQB1*06:02, an immune response against influenza, *Streptococcus*, or other infections may also damage the orexin-producing neurons through a process of molecular mimicry. This mechanism may account for the 8- to 12-fold increase in new cases of narcolepsy among children in Europe who received a particular brand of H1N1 influenza A vaccine (Pandemrix).

On rare occasions, narcolepsy can occur with neurologic disorders such as tumors or strokes that directly damage the orexin-producing neurons in the hypothalamus or their projections.

Diagnosis Narcolepsy is most commonly diagnosed by the history of chronic sleepiness plus cataplexy or other symptoms. Many disorders can cause feelings of weakness, but with true cataplexy, patients will describe definite functional weakness (e.g., slurred speech, dropping a cup, slumping into a chair) that has consistent emotional triggers such as heartfelt mirth when laughing at a great joke, happy surprise at unexpectedly seeing a friend, or intense anger. Cataplexy occurs in about half of all narcolepsy patients and is diagnostically very helpful because it occurs in almost no other disorder. In contrast, occasional hypnagogic hallucinations and sleep paralysis occur in about 20% of the general population, and these symptoms are not as diagnostically specific.

When narcolepsy is suspected, the diagnosis should be firmly established with a polysomnogram followed by an MSLT. The

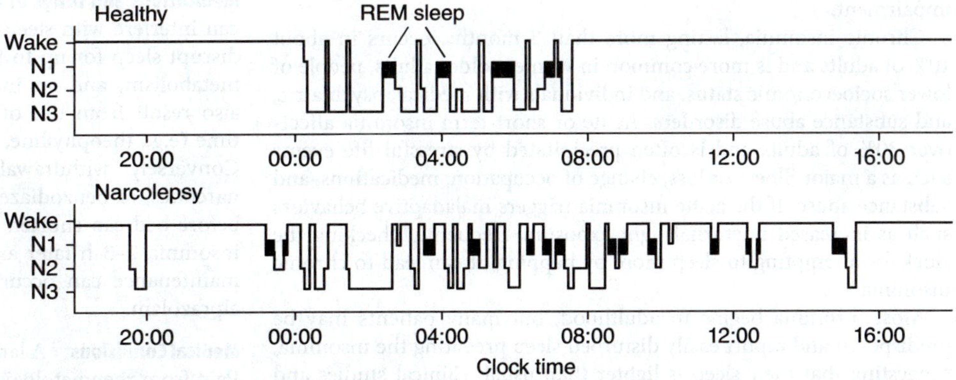

FIGURE 38-3 Polysomnographic recordings of a healthy individual and a patient with narcolepsy. The individual with narcolepsy enters rapid eye movement (REM) sleep quickly at night and has moderately fragmented sleep. During the day, the healthy subject stays awake from 8:00 AM until midnight, but the patient with narcolepsy dozes off frequently, with many daytime naps that include REM sleep.

polysomnogram helps rule out other possible causes of sleepiness such as sleep apnea, and the MSLT provides essential, objective evidence of sleepiness plus REM sleep dysregulation. Across the five naps of the MSLT, most patients with narcolepsy will fall asleep in less than 8 min on average, and they will have episodes of REM sleep in at least two of the naps. Abnormal regulation of REM sleep is also manifested by the appearance of REM sleep within 15 min of sleep onset at night, which is rare in healthy individuals sleeping at their habitual bedtime. Stimulants should be stopped 1 week before the MSLT and antidepressants should be stopped 3 weeks prior, because these medications can affect the MSLT. In addition, patients should be encouraged to obtain a fully adequate amount of sleep each night for the week prior to the test to eliminate any effects of insufficient sleep.

TREATMENT NARCOLEPSY

The treatment of narcolepsy is symptomatic. Most patients with narcolepsy feel more alert after sleep, and they should be encouraged to get adequate sleep each night and to take a 15- to 20-min nap in the afternoon. This nap may be sufficient for some patients with mild narcolepsy, but most also require treatment with wake-promoting medications. Modafinil is used quite often because it has fewer side effects than amphetamines and a relatively long half-life; for most patients, 200–400 mg each morning is very effective. Methylphenidate (10–20 mg bid) or dextroamphetamine (10 mg bid) are often effective, but sympathomimetic side effects, anxiety, and the potential for abuse can be concerns. These medications are available in slow-release formulations, extending their duration of action and allowing easier dosing. Sodium oxybate (gamma hydroxybutyrate) is given twice each night and is often very valuable in improving alertness, but it can produce excessive sedation, nausea, and confusion.

Cataplexy is usually much improved with antidepressants that increase noradrenergic or serotonergic tone because these medications strongly suppress REM sleep and cataplexy. Venlafaxine (37.5–150 mg each morning) and fluoxetine (10–40 mg each morning) are often quite effective. The tricyclic antidepressants, such as protriptyline (10–40 mg/d) or clomipramine (25–50 mg/d) are potent suppressors of cataplexy, but their anticholinergic effects, including sedation and dry mouth, make them less attractive.[1] Sodium oxybate, given at bedtime and 3–4 h later, is also very helpful in reducing cataplexy.

EVALUATION OF INSOMNIA

Insomnia is the complaint of poor sleep and usually presents as difficulty initiating or maintaining sleep. People with insomnia are dissatisfied with their sleep and feel that it impairs their ability to function well in work, school, and social situations. Affected individuals often experience fatigue, decreased mood, irritability, malaise, and cognitive impairment.

Chronic insomnia, lasting more than 3 months, occurs in about 10% of adults and is more common in women, older adults, people of lower socioeconomic status, and individuals with medical, psychiatric, and substance abuse disorders. Acute or short-term insomnia affects over 30% of adults and is often precipitated by stressful life events such as a major illness or loss, change of occupation, medications, and substance abuse. If the acute insomnia triggers maladaptive behaviors such as increased nocturnal light exposure, frequently checking the clock, or attempting to sleep more by napping, it can lead to chronic insomnia.

Most insomnia begins in adulthood, but many patients may be predisposed and report easily disturbed sleep predating the insomnia, suggesting that their sleep is lighter than usual. Clinical studies and animal models indicate that insomnia is associated with activation during sleep of brain areas normally active only during wakefulness. The polysomnogram is rarely used in the evaluation of insomnia, as it typically confirms the patient's subjective report of long latency to sleep and numerous awakenings but usually adds little new information. Many patients with insomnia have increased fast (beta) activity in the EEG during sleep; this fast activity is normally present only during wakefulness, which may explain why some patients report feeling awake for much of the night. The MSLT is rarely used in the evaluation of insomnia because, despite their feelings of low energy, most people with insomnia do not easily fall asleep during the day, and on the MSLT, their average sleep latencies are usually longer than normal.

Many factors can contribute to insomnia, and obtaining a careful history is essential so one can select therapies targeting the underlying factors. The assessment should focus on identifying predisposing, precipitating, and perpetuating factors.

Psychophysiologic Factors Many patients with insomnia have negative expectations and conditioned arousal that interfere with sleep. These individuals may worry about their insomnia during the day and have increasing anxiety as bedtime approaches if they anticipate a poor night of sleep. While attempting to sleep, they may frequently check the clock, which only heightens anxiety and frustration. They may find it easier to sleep in a new environment rather than their bedroom, as it lacks the negative associations.

Inadequate Sleep Hygiene Patients with insomnia sometimes develop counterproductive behaviors that contribute to their insomnia. These can include daytime napping that reduces sleep drive at night; an irregular sleep-wake schedule that disrupts their circadian rhythms; use of wake-promoting substances (e.g., caffeine, tobacco) too close to bedtime; engaging in alerting or stressful activities close to bedtime (e.g., arguing with a partner, work-related emailing and texting while in bed, sleeping with a smartphone or tablet at the bedside); and routinely using the bedroom for activities other than sleep or sex (e.g., TV, work), so the bedroom becomes associated with arousing or stressful feelings.

Psychiatric Conditions About 80% of patients with psychiatric disorders have sleep complaints, and about half of all chronic insomnia occurs in association with a psychiatric disorder. Depression is classically associated with early morning awakening, but it can also interfere with the onset and maintenance of sleep. Mania and hypomania can disrupt sleep and often are associated with substantial reductions in the total amount of sleep. Anxiety disorders can lead to racing thoughts and rumination that interfere with sleep and can be very problematic if the patient's mind becomes active midway through the night. Panic attacks can occur during sleep and need to be distinguished from other parasomnias. Insomnia is common in schizophrenia and other psychoses, often resulting in fragmented sleep, less deep NREM sleep, and sometimes reversal of the day-night sleep pattern.

Medications and Drugs of Abuse A wide variety of psychoactive drugs can interfere with sleep. Caffeine, which has a half-life of 6–9 h, can disrupt sleep for up to 8–14 h, depending on the dose, variations in metabolism, and an individual's caffeine sensitivity. Insomnia can also result from use of prescription medications too close to bedtime (e.g., theophylline, stimulants, antidepressants, glucocorticoids). Conversely, withdrawal of sedating medications such as alcohol, narcotics, or benzodiazepines can cause insomnia. Alcohol taken just before bed can shorten sleep latency, but it often produces rebound insomnia 2–3 h later as it wears off. This same problem with sleep maintenance can occur with short-acting benzodiazepines such as alprazolam.

Medical Conditions A large number of medical conditions disrupt sleep. Pain from rheumatologic disorders or a painful neuropathy commonly disrupts sleep. Some patients may sleep poorly because of respiratory conditions such as asthma, chronic obstructive pulmonary disease, cystic fibrosis, congestive heart failure, or restrictive lung disease, and some of these disorders are worse at night in bed due to circadian variations in airway resistance and postural changes that can result in

[1]No antidepressant has been approved by the U.S. Food and Drug Administration (FDA) for treating narcolepsy.

paroxysmal nocturnal dyspnea. Many women experience poor sleep with the hormonal changes of menopause. Gastroesophageal reflux is also a common cause of difficulty sleeping.

Neurologic Disorders Dementia (Chap. 35) is often associated with poor sleep, probably due to a variety of factors, including napping during the day, altered circadian rhythms, and perhaps a weakened output of the brain's sleep-promoting mechanisms. In fact, insomnia and nighttime wandering are some of the most common causes for institutionalization of patients with dementia, because they place a larger burden on caregivers. Conversely, in cognitively intact elderly men, fragmented sleep and poor sleep quality are associated with subsequent cognitive decline. Patients with Parkinson's disease may sleep poorly due to rigidity, dementia, and other factors. Fatal familial insomnia is a very rare neurodegenerative condition caused by mutations in the prion protein gene, and although insomnia is a common early symptom, most patients present with other obvious neurologic signs such dementia, myoclonus, dysarthria, or autonomic dysfunction.

TREATMENT INSOMNIA

Treatment of insomnia improves quality of life and can promote long-term health. With improved sleep, patients often report less daytime fatigue, improved cognition, and more energy. Treating the insomnia can also improve the comorbid disease. For example, management of insomnia at the time of diagnosis of major depression often improves the response to antidepressants and reduces the risk of relapse. Sleep loss can heighten the perception of pain, so a similar approach is warranted in acute and chronic pain management.

The treatment plan should target all putative contributing factors: establish good sleep hygiene, treat medical disorders, use behavioral therapies for anxiety and negative conditioning, and use pharmacotherapy and/or psychotherapy for psychiatric disorders. Behavioral therapies should be the first-line treatment, followed by judicious use of sleep-promoting medications if needed.

TREATMENT OF MEDICAL AND PSYCHIATRIC DISEASE

If the history suggests that a medical or psychiatric disease contributes to the insomnia, then it should be addressed by, for example, treating the pain, improving breathing, and switching or adjusting the timing of medications.

IMPROVE SLEEP HYGIENE

Attention should be paid to improving sleep hygiene and avoiding counterproductive, arousing behaviors before bedtime. Patients should establish a regular bedtime and wake time, even on weekends, to help synchronize their circadian rhythms and sleep patterns. The amount of time allocated for sleep should not be more than their actual total amount of sleep. In the 30 min before bedtime, patients should establish a relaxing "wind-down" routine that can include a warm bath, listening to music, meditation, or other relaxation techniques. The bedroom should be off-limits to computers, televisions, radios, smartphones, videogames, and tablets. Once in bed, patients should try to avoid thinking about anything stressful or arousing such as problems with relationships or work. If they cannot fall asleep within 20 min, it often helps to get out of bed and read or listen to relaxing music in dim light as a form of distraction from any anxiety, but artificial light, including light from a television, cell phone, or computer, should be avoided, because light itself suppresses melatonin secretion and is arousing. Table 38-2 outlines some of the key aspects of good sleep hygiene to improve insomnia.

COGNITIVE BEHAVIORAL THERAPY (CBT)

CBT uses a combination of the techniques above plus additional methods to improve insomnia. A trained therapist may use cognitive psychology techniques to reduce excessive worrying about sleep and to reframe faulty beliefs about the insomnia and its daytime consequences. The therapist may also teach the patient relaxation techniques, such as progressive muscle relaxation or meditation, to reduce autonomic arousal, intrusive thoughts, and anxiety.

TABLE 38-2 METHODS TO IMPROVE SLEEP HYGIENE IN INSOMNIA PATIENTS

Helpful Behaviors	Behaviors to Avoid
Use the bed only for sleep and sex • If you cannot sleep within 20 min, get out of bed and read or do other relaxing activities in dim light before returning to bed	Avoid behaviors that interfere with sleep physiology, including: • Napping, especially after 3:00 PM • Attempting to sleep too early • Caffeine after lunchtime
Make quality sleep a priority • Go to bed and get up at the same time each day • Ensure a restful environment (comfortable bed, bedroom quiet and dark)	In the 2–3 h before bedtime, avoid: • Heavy eating • Smoking or alcohol • Vigorous exercise
Develop a consistent bedtime routine. For example: • Prepare for sleep with 20–30 min of relaxation (e.g., soft music, meditation, yoga, pleasant reading) • Take a warm bath	When trying to fall asleep, avoid: • Solving problems • Thinking about life issues • Reviewing events of the day

MEDICATIONS FOR INSOMNIA

If insomnia persists after treatment of these contributing factors, pharmacotherapy is often used on a nightly or intermittent basis. A variety of sedatives can improve sleep.

Antihistamines, such as diphenhydramine, are the primary active ingredient in most over-the-counter sleep aids. These may be of benefit when used intermittently, but often produce rapid tolerance and can produce anticholinergic side effects such as dry mouth and constipation, which limit their use, particularly in the elderly.

Benzodiazepine receptor agonists (BzRAs) are an effective and well-tolerated class of medications for insomnia. BzRAs bind to the $GABA_A$ receptor and potentiate the postsynaptic response to GABA. $GABA_A$ receptors are found throughout the brain, and BzRAs may globally reduce neural activity and may enhance the activity of specific sleep-promoting GABAergic pathways. Classic BzRAs include lorazepam, triazolam, and clonazepam, whereas newer agents such as zolpidem and zaleplon have more selective affinity for the α_1 subunit of the $GABA_A$ receptor.

Specific BzRAs are often chosen based on the desired duration of action. The most commonly prescribed agents in this family are zaleplon (5–20 mg), with a half-life of 1–2 h; zolpidem (5–10 mg) and triazolam (0.125–0.25 mg), with half-lives of 2–4 h; eszopiclone (1–3 mg), with a half-life of 5–8 h; and temazepam (15–30 mg), with a half-life of 8–20 h. Generally, side effects are minimal when the dose is kept low and the serum concentration is minimized during the waking hours (by using the shortest-acting effective agent). For chronic insomnia, intermittent use is recommended, unless the consequences of untreated insomnia outweigh concerns regarding chronic use.

The heterocyclic *antidepressants* (trazodone, amitriptyline,[2] and doxepin) are the most commonly prescribed alternatives to BzRAs due to their lack of abuse potential and lower cost. Trazodone (25–100 mg) is used more commonly than the tricyclic antidepressants, because it has a much shorter half-life (5–9 h) and less anticholinergic activity.

Medications for insomnia are now among the most commonly prescribed medications, but they should be used cautiously. All sedatives increase the risk of injurious falls and confusion in the elderly, and therefore if needed, these medications should be used at the lowest effective dose. Morning sedation can interfere with driving and judgment, and when selecting a medication, one should

[2]Trazodone and amitriptyline have not been approved by the FDA for treating insomnia.

consider the duration of action. Benzodiazepines carry a risk of addiction and abuse, especially in patients with a history of alcohol or sedative abuse. Like alcohol, some sleep-promoting medications can worsen sleep apnea. Sedatives can also produce complex behaviors during sleep, such as sleep walking and sleep eating, although this seems more likely at higher doses.

RESTLESS LEGS SYNDROME

Patients with restless legs syndrome (RLS) report an irresistible urge to move the legs. Many patients report a creepy-crawly or unpleasant deep ache within the thighs or calves, and those with more severe RLS may have discomfort in the arms as well. For most patients with RLS, these dysesthesias and restlessness are much worse in the evening and first half of the night. The symptoms appear with inactivity and can make sitting still in an airplane or when watching a movie a miserable experience. The sensations are temporarily relieved by movement, stretching, or massage. This nocturnal discomfort usually interferes with sleep, and patients may report daytime sleepiness as a consequence. RLS is very common, affecting 5–10% of adults and is more common in women and older adults.

A variety of factors can cause RLS. Iron deficiency is the most common treatable cause, and iron replacement should be considered if the ferritin level is less than 50 ng/mL. RLS can also occur with peripheral neuropathies and uremia and can be worsened by pregnancy, caffeine, alcohol, antidepressants, lithium, neuroleptics, and antihistamines. Genetic factors contribute to RLS, and polymorphisms in a variety of genes (*BTBD9, MEIS1, MAP2K5/LBXCOR,* and *PTPRD*) have been linked to RLS, although as yet, the mechanism through which they cause RLS remains unknown. Roughly one-third of patients (particularly those with an early age of onset) have multiple affected family members.

RLS is treated by addressing the underlying cause such as iron deficiency if present. Otherwise, treatment is symptomatic, and dopamine agonists are used most frequently. Agonists of dopamine $D_{2/3}$ receptors such as pramipexole (0.25–0.5 mg q7PM) or ropinirole (0.5–4 mg q7PM) are considered first-line agents. Augmentation is a worsening of RLS such that symptoms begin earlier in the day and can spread to other body regions, and it can occur in about 25% of patients taking dopamine agonists. Other possible side effects of dopamine agonists include nausea, morning sedation, and increases in rewarding behavior such as gambling and sex. Opioids, benzodiazepines, pregabalin, and gabapentin may also be of therapeutic value. Most patients with restless legs also experience periodic limb movement disorder, although the reverse is not the case.

PERIODIC LIMB MOVEMENT DISORDER

Periodic limb movement disorder (PLMD) involves rhythmic twitches of the legs that disrupt sleep. The movements resemble a triple flexion reflex with extensions of the great toe and dorsiflexion of the foot for 0.5 to 5.0 s, which recur every 20–40 s during NREM sleep, in episodes lasting from minutes to hours. PLMD is diagnosed by a polysomnogram that includes recordings of the anterior tibialis and sometimes other muscles. The EEG shows that the movements of PLMD frequently cause brief arousals that disrupt sleep and can cause insomnia and daytime sleepiness. PLMD can be caused by the same factors that cause RLS (see above), and the frequency of leg movements improves with the same medications as used for RLS, including dopamine agonists. Recent genetic studies identified polymorphisms associated with RLS/PLMD, suggesting that they may have a common pathophysiology.

PARASOMNIAS

Parasomnias are abnormal behaviors or experiences that arise from or occur during sleep. A variety of parasomnias can occur during NREM sleep, from brief confusional arousals to sleepwalking and night terrors. The presenting complaint is usually related to the behavior itself, but the parasomnias can disturb sleep continuity or lead to mild impairments in daytime alertness. Two main parasomnias occur in REM sleep: REM sleep behavior disorder (RBD) and nightmares.

Sleepwalking (Somnambulism) Patients affected by this disorder carry out automatic motor activities that range from simple to complex. Individuals may walk, urinate inappropriately, eat, exit the house, or drive a car with minimal awareness. Full arousal may be difficult, and occasional individuals may respond to attempted awakening with agitation or violence. Sleepwalking arises from NREM stage N3 sleep, usually in the first few hours of the night, and the EEG usually shows the slow cortical activity of deep NREM sleep even when the patient is moving about. Sleepwalking is most common in children and adolescents, when these sleep stages are most robust. About 15% of children have occasional sleepwalking, and it persists in about 1% of adults. Episodes are usually isolated but may be recurrent in 1–6% of patients. The cause is unknown, although it has a familial basis in roughly one-third of cases. Sleepwalking can be worsened by insufficient sleep, which subsequently causes an increase in deep NREM sleep; alcohol; and stress. These should be addressed if present. Small studies have shown some efficacy of antidepressants and benzodiazepines; relaxation techniques and hypnosis can also be helpful. Patients and their families should improve home safety (e.g., replace glass doors, remove low tables to avoid tripping) to minimize the chance of injury if sleepwalking occurs.

Sleep Terrors This disorder occurs primarily in young children during the first few hours of sleep during NREM stage N3 sleep. The child often sits up during sleep and screams, exhibiting autonomic arousal with sweating, tachycardia, large pupils, and hyperventilation. The individual may be difficult to arouse and rarely recalls the episode on awakening in the morning. Treatment usually consists of reassuring the parents that the condition is self-limited and benign, and like sleepwalking, it may improve by avoiding insufficient sleep.

Sleep Bruxism Bruxism is an involuntary, forceful grinding of teeth during sleep that affects 10–20% of the population. The patient is usually unaware of the problem. The typical age of onset is 17–20 years, and spontaneous remission usually occurs by age 40. Sex distribution appears to be equal. In many cases, the diagnosis is made during dental examination, damage is minor, and no treatment is indicated. In more severe cases, treatment with a tooth guard is necessary to prevent tooth injury. Stress management or, in some cases, biofeedback can be useful when bruxism is a manifestation of psychological stress. There are anecdotal reports of benefit with benzodiazepines.

Sleep Enuresis Bedwetting, like sleepwalking and night terrors, is another parasomnia that occurs during sleep in the young. Before age 5 or 6 years, nocturnal enuresis should be considered a normal feature of development. The condition usually improves spontaneously by puberty, has a prevalence in late adolescence of 1–3%, and is rare in adulthood. Treatment consists of bladder training exercises and behavioral therapy. Symptomatic pharmacotherapy is usually accomplished in adults with desmopressin (0.2 mg qhs), oxybutynin chloride (5 mg qhs), or imipramine (10–25 mg qhs). Important causes of nocturnal enuresis in patients who were previously continent for 6–12 months include urinary tract infections or malformations, cauda equina lesions, emotional disturbances, epilepsy, sleep apnea, and certain medications.

REM Sleep Behavior Disorder (RBD) RBD (Video 38-2) is distinct from other parasomnias in that it occurs during REM sleep. The patient or the bed partner usually reports agitated or violent behavior during sleep, and upon awakening, the patient can often report a dream that accompanied the movements. During normal REM sleep, nearly all skeletal muscles are paralyzed, but in patients with RBD, the polysomnogram often shows limb movements during REM sleep, lasting for seconds to minutes. The movements can be dramatic, and it is not uncommon for the patient or the bed partner to be injured.

RBD primarily afflicts older men, and most either have or will develop a neurodegenerative disorder. In longitudinal studies of RBD, half of the patients developed a synucleinopathy such as Parkinson's disease (Chap. 449) or dementia with Lewy bodies (Chap. 448), or occasionally multiple system atrophy (Chap. 454), within 12 years, and over 80% developed a synucleinopathy by 20 years. RBD can occur in patients taking antidepressants, and in some, these medications may unmask this early indicator of neurodegeneration. Synucleinopathies probably cause neuronal loss in brainstem regions that regulate muscle atonia during REM sleep, and loss of these neurons permits movements to break through during REM sleep. RBD also occurs in about 30% of patients with narcolepsy, but the underlying cause is probably different, as they seem to be at no increased risk of a neurodegenerative disorder.

Many patients with RBD have sustained improvement with clonazepam (0.5–2.0 mg qhs).[3] Melatonin at doses up to 9 mg nightly may also prevent attacks.

CIRCADIAN RHYTHM SLEEP DISORDERS

A subset of patients presenting with either insomnia or hypersomnia may have a disorder of sleep *timing* rather than sleep *generation*. Disorders of sleep timing can be either organic (i.e., due to an abnormality of circadian pacemaker[s]) or environmental/behavioral (i.e., due to a disruption of environmental synchronizers). Effective therapies aim to entrain the circadian rhythm of sleep propensity to an appropriate phase.

Delayed Sleep-Wake Phase Disorder Delayed sleep-wake phase disorder (DSWPD) is characterized by: (1) reported sleep onset and wake times intractably later than desired; (2) actual sleep times at nearly the same clock hours daily; and (3) if conducted at the habitual delayed sleep time, essentially normal sleep on polysomnography (except for delayed sleep onset). Patients with DSWPD exhibit an abnormally delayed endogenous circadian phase, which can be assessed by measuring, in a dimly lit environment, the onset of secretion of the endogenous circadian rhythm of pineal melatonin in either the blood or saliva, as light suppresses melatonin secretion. Dim-light melatonin onset (DLMO) in DSWPD patients typically occurs later in the evening than normal, which is about 8:00–9:00 PM (i.e., about 1–2 h before habitual bedtime). Patients tend to be young adults. The delayed circadian phase could be due to: (1) an abnormally long, genetically determined intrinsic period of the endogenous circadian pacemaker; (2) reduced phase-advancing capacity of the pacemaker; (3) slower rate of buildup of homeostatic sleep drive during wakefulness; or (4) an irregular prior sleep-wake schedule, characterized by frequent nights when the patient chooses to remain awake while exposed to artificial light well past midnight (for personal, social, school, or work reasons). In most cases, it is difficult to distinguish among these factors, as patients with either a behaviorally induced or biologically driven circadian phase delay may both exhibit a similar circadian phase delay in DLMO, making it difficult for both to fall asleep at the desired hour. DSWPD is a self-perpetuating condition that can persist for years and may not respond to attempts to reestablish normal bedtime hours. Treatment methods involving phototherapy with blue-enriched light during the morning hours and/or melatonin administration in the evening hours show promise in these patients, although the relapse rate is high. Patients with this circadian rhythm sleep disorder can be distinguished from those who have sleep-onset insomnia because DSWPD patients show late onset of dim-light melatonin secretion.

Advanced Sleep-Wake Phase Disorder Advanced sleep-wake phase disorder (ASWPD) is the converse of DSWPD. Most commonly, this syndrome occurs in older people, 15% of whom report that they cannot sleep past 5:00 AM, with twice that number complaining that they wake up too early at least several times per week. Patients with ASWPD are sleepy during the evening hours, even in social settings. Sleep-wake timing in ASWPD patients can interfere with a normal social life. Patients with this circadian rhythm sleep disorder can be distinguished from those who have early wakening due to insomnia because ASWPD patients show early onset of dim-light melatonin secretion.

In addition to age-related ASWPD, an early-onset familial variant of this condition has also been reported. In two families in which ASWPD was inherited in an autosomal dominant pattern, the syndrome was due to missense mutations in a circadian clock component (in the casein kinase binding domain of *PER2* in one family, and in casein kinase I delta in the other) that altered the circadian period. Patients with ASWPD may benefit from bright-light and/or blue enriched phototherapy during the evening hours to reset the circadian pacemaker to a later hour.

Non-24-h Sleep-Wake Rhythm Disorder Non-24-h sleep-wake rhythm disorder (N24SWRD) can occur when the primary synchronizing input (i.e., the light-dark cycle) from the environment to the circadian pacemaker is compromised (as occurs in many blind people with no light perception) or when the maximal phase-advancing capacity of the circadian pacemaker cannot accommodate the difference between the 24-h geophysical day and the intrinsic period of the patient's circadian pacemaker, resulting in loss of entrainment to the 24-h day. Rarely, self-selected exposure to artificial light may, in some sighted patients, inadvertently entrain the circadian pacemaker to a >24-h schedule. Affected patients with N24SWRD have difficulty maintaining a stable phase relationship between the output of the pacemaker and the 24-h day. Such patients typically present with an incremental pattern of successive delays in sleep propensity, progressing in and out of phase with local time. When the N24SWRD patient's endogenous circadian rhythms are out of phase with the local environment, nighttime insomnia coexists with excessive daytime sleepiness. Conversely, when the endogenous circadian rhythms are in phase with the local environment, symptoms remit. The interval between symptomatic phases may last several weeks to several months in N24SWRD, depending on the period of the underlying nonentrained rhythm and the 24-h day. Nightly low-dose (0.5 mg) melatonin administration may improve sleep and, in some cases, induce synchronization of the circadian pacemaker.

Shift-Work Disorder More than 7 million workers in the United States regularly work at night, either on a permanent or rotating schedule. Many more begin the commute to work or school between 4:00 AM and 7:00 AM, requiring them to commute and then work during the time of day that they would otherwise be asleep. In addition, each week, millions of "day" workers and students elect to remain awake at night or awaken very early in the morning to work or study to meet work or school deadlines, drive long distances, compete in sporting events, or participate in recreational activities. Such schedules can result in both sleep loss and misalignment of circadian rhythms with respect to the sleep-wake cycle.

The circadian timing system usually fails to adapt successfully to the inverted schedules required by overnight work or the phase advance required by early morning (4:00 AM to 7:00 AM) start times. This leads to a misalignment between the desired work-rest schedule and the output of the pacemaker and to disturbed daytime sleep in most individuals. Excessive work hours (per day or per week), insufficient time off between consecutive days of work or school, and transmeridian travel may be contributing factors. Sleep deficiency, increased length of time awake prior to work, and misalignment of circadian phase produce decreased alertness and performance, increased reaction time, and increased risk of performance lapses, thereby resulting in greater safety hazards among night workers and other sleep-deprived individuals. Sleep disturbance nearly doubles the risk of a fatal work accident. Long-term night shift workers have higher rates of breast, colorectal, and prostate cancer and of cardiac, gastrointestinal, and reproductive disorders. The World Health Organization has added night-shift work to its list of probable carcinogens.

Sleep onset begins in local brain regions before gradually sweeping over the entire brain as sensory thresholds rise and consciousness is lost. A sleepy individual struggling to remain awake may attempt to continue performing routine and familiar motor tasks during the transition state between wakefulness and stage N1 sleep, while unable to adequately process sensory input from the environment. Motor vehicle operators who fail to heed the warning signs of sleepiness are especially vulnerable to sleep-related accidents, as sleep processes can intrude involuntarily upon the waking brain, causing catastrophic consequences. Such sleep-related attentional failures typically last only seconds but are known on occasion to persist for longer durations.

[3]No medications have been approved by the FDA for the treatment of RBD.

There is a significant increase in the risk of sleep-related, fatal-to-the-driver highway crashes in the early morning and late afternoon hours, coincident with bimodal peaks in the daily rhythm of sleep tendency.

Resident physicians constitute another group of workers at greater risk for accidents and other adverse consequences of lack of sleep and misalignment of the circadian rhythm. Recurrent scheduling of resident physicians to work shifts of ≥24 consecutive hours impairs psychomotor performance to a degree that is comparable to alcohol intoxication, doubles the risk of attentional failures among intensive care unit resident physicians working at night, and significantly increases the risk of serious medical errors in intensive care units, including a fivefold increase in the risk of serious diagnostic mistakes. Some 20% of hospital resident physicians report making a fatigue-related mistake that injured a patient, and 5% admit making a fatigue-related mistake that resulted in the death of a patient. Moreover, working for >24 consecutive hours increases the risk of percutaneous injuries and more than doubles the risk of motor vehicle crashes on the commute home. For these reasons, in 2008, the Institute of Medicine concluded that the practice of scheduling resident physicians to work for more than 16 consecutive hours without sleep is hazardous for both resident physicians and their patients.

From 5 to 15% of individuals scheduled to work at night or in the early morning hours have much greater-than-average difficulties remaining awake during night work and sleeping during the day; these individuals are diagnosed with chronic and severe shift-work disorder (SWD). Patients with this disorder have a level of excessive sleepiness during work at night or in the early morning and insomnia during day sleep that the physician judges to be clinically significant; the condition is associated with an increased risk of sleep-related accidents and with some of the illnesses associated with night-shift work. Patients with chronic and severe SWD are profoundly sleepy at work. In fact, their sleep latencies during night work average just 2 min, comparable to mean daytime sleep latency durations of patients with narcolepsy or severe sleep apnea.

TREATMENT SHIFT-WORK DISORDER

Caffeine is frequently used by night workers to promote wakefulness. However, it cannot forestall sleep indefinitely, and it does not shield users from sleep-related performance lapses. Postural changes, exercise, and strategic placement of nap opportunities can sometimes temporarily reduce the risk of fatigue-related performance lapses. Properly timed exposure to blue-enriched light or bright white light can directly enhance alertness and facilitate more rapid adaptation to night-shift work.

Modafinil (200 mg) or armodafinil (150 mg) 30–60 min before the start of each night shift is an effective treatment for the excessive sleepiness during night work in patients with SWD. Although treatment with modafinil or armodafinil significantly improves performance and reduces sleep propensity and the risk of lapses of attention during night work, affected patients remain excessively sleepy.

Fatigue risk management programs for night shift workers should promote education about sleep, increase awareness of the hazards associated with sleep deficiency and night work, and screen for common sleep disorders. Work schedules should be designed to minimize: (1) exposure to night work; (2) the frequency of shift rotations; (3) the number of consecutive night shifts; and (4) the duration of night shifts.

Jet Lag Disorder Each year, more than 60 million people fly from one time zone to another, often resulting in excessive daytime sleepiness, sleep-onset insomnia, and frequent arousals from sleep, particularly in the latter half of the night. The syndrome is transient, typically lasting 2–14 d depending on the number of time zones crossed, the direction of travel, and the traveler's age and phase-shifting capacity. Travelers who spend more time outdoors at their destination reportedly adapt more quickly than those who remain in hotel rooms, presumably due to brighter (outdoor) light exposure. Avoidance of antecedent sleep loss and obtaining naps on the afternoon prior to overnight travel can reduce the difficulties associated with extended wakefulness. Laboratory studies suggest that low doses of melatonin can enhance sleep efficiency, but only if taken when endogenous melatonin concentrations are low (i.e., during the biologic daytime).

In addition to jet lag associated with travel across time zones, many patients report a behavioral pattern that has been termed *social jet lag*, in which bedtimes and wake times on weekends or days off occur 4–8 h later than during the week. Such recurrent displacement of the timing of the sleep-wake cycle is common in adolescents and young adults and is associated with sleep-onset insomnia, poorer academic performance, increased risk of depressive symptoms, and excessive daytime sleepiness.

MEDICAL IMPLICATIONS OF CIRCADIAN RHYTHMICITY

Prominent circadian variations have been reported in the incidence of acute myocardial infarction, sudden cardiac death, and stroke, the leading causes of death in the United States. Platelet aggregability is increased in the early morning hours, coincident with the peak incidence of these cardiovascular events. Recurrent circadian disruption combined with chronic sleep deficiency, such as occurs during night-shift work, is associated with increased plasma glucose concentrations after a meal due to inadequate pancreatic insulin secretion. Night shift workers with elevated fasting glucose have an increased risk of progressing to diabetes. Blood pressure of night workers with sleep apnea is higher than that of day workers. A better understanding of the possible role of circadian rhythmicity in the acute destabilization of a chronic condition such as atherosclerotic disease could improve the understanding of its pathophysiology.

Diagnostic and therapeutic procedures may also be affected by the time of day at which data are collected. Examples include blood pressure, body temperature, the dexamethasone suppression test, and plasma cortisol levels. The timing of chemotherapy administration has been reported to have an effect on the outcome of treatment. In addition, both the toxicity and effectiveness of drugs can vary with time of day. For example, more than a fivefold difference has been observed in mortality rates following administration of toxic agents to experimental animals at different times of day. Anesthetic agents are particularly sensitive to time-of-day effects. Finally, the physician must be aware of the public health risks associated with the ever-increasing demands made by the 24/7 schedules in our round-the-clock society.

ACKNOWLEDGMENT

John W. Winkelman, MD, PhD and Gary S. Richardson, MD contributed to this chapter in the prior edition and some material from that chapter has been retained here.

VIDEO 38-1 A typical episode of severe cataplexy. The patient is joking and then falls to the ground with an abrupt loss of muscle tone. The electromyogram recordings (four lower traces on the right) show reductions in muscle activity during the period of paralysis. The electroencephalogram (top two traces) shows wakefulness throughout the episode. *(Video courtesy of Giuseppe Plazzi, University of Bologna.)*

VIDEO 38-2 Typical aggressive movements in rapid eye movement (REM) sleep behavior disorder. *(Video courtesy of Dr. Carlos Schenck, University of Minnesota Medical School.)*

SECTION 4 DISORDERS OF EYES, EARS, NOSE, AND THROAT

39 Disorders of the Eye

Jonathan C. Horton

THE HUMAN VISUAL SYSTEM

The visual system provides a supremely efficient means for the rapid assimilation of information from the environment to aid in the guidance of behavior. The act of seeing begins with the capture of images focused by the cornea and lens on a light-sensitive membrane in the back of the eye called the *retina*. The retina is actually part of the brain, banished to the periphery to serve as a transducer for the conversion of patterns of light energy into neuronal signals. Light is absorbed by pigment in two types of photoreceptors: rods and cones. In the human retina there are 100 million rods and 5 million cones. The rods operate in dim (scotopic) illumination. The cones function under daylight (photopic) conditions. The cone system is specialized for color perception and high spatial resolution. The majority of cones are within the macula, the portion of the retina that serves the central 10° of vision. In the middle of the macula a small pit termed the *fovea*, packed exclusively with cones, provides the best visual acuity.

Photoreceptors hyperpolarize in response to light, activating bipolar, amacrine, and horizontal cells in the inner nuclear layer. After processing of photoreceptor responses by this complex retinal circuit, the flow of sensory information ultimately converges on a final common pathway: the ganglion cells. These cells translate the visual image impinging on the retina into a continuously varying barrage of action potentials that propagates along the primary optic pathway to visual centers within the brain. There are a million ganglion cells in each retina and hence a million fibers in each optic nerve.

Ganglion cell axons sweep along the inner surface of the retina in the nerve fiber layer, exit the eye at the optic disc, and travel through the optic nerve, optic chiasm, and optic tract to reach targets in the brain. The majority of fibers synapse on cells in the lateral geniculate body, a thalamic relay station. Cells in the lateral geniculate body project in turn to the primary visual cortex. This afferent retinogeniculocortical sensory pathway provides the neural substrate for visual perception. Although the lateral geniculate body is the main target of the retina, separate classes of ganglion cells project to other subcortical visual nuclei involved in different functions. Ganglion cells that mediate pupillary constriction and circadian rhythms are light sensitive owing to a novel visual pigment, melanopsin. Pupil responses are mediated by input to the pretectal olivary nuclei in the midbrain. The pretectal nuclei send their output to the Edinger-Westphal nuclei, which in turn provide parasympathetic innervation to the iris sphincter via an interneuron in the ciliary ganglion. Circadian rhythms are timed by a retinal projection to the suprachiasmatic nucleus. Visual orientation and eye movements are served by retinal input to the superior colliculus. Gaze stabilization and optokinetic reflexes are governed by a group of small retinal targets known collectively as the *brainstem accessory optic system*.

The eyes must be rotated constantly within their orbits to place and maintain targets of visual interest on the fovea. This activity, called *foveation*, or looking, is governed by an elaborate efferent motor system. Each eye is moved by six extraocular muscles that are supplied by cranial nerves from the oculomotor (III), trochlear (IV), and abducens (VI) nuclei. Activity in these ocular motor nuclei is coordinated by pontine and midbrain mechanisms for smooth pursuit, saccades, and gaze stabilization during head and body movements. Large regions of the frontal and parietooccipital cortex control these brainstem eye movement centers by providing descending supranuclear input.

CLINICAL ASSESSMENT OF VISUAL FUNCTION

REFRACTIVE STATE

In approaching a patient with reduced vision, the first step is to decide whether refractive error is responsible. In *emmetropia*, parallel rays from infinity are focused perfectly on the retina. Sadly, this condition is enjoyed by only a minority of the population. In *myopia*, the globe is too long, and light rays come to a focal point in front of the retina. Near objects can be seen clearly, but distant objects require a diverging lens in front of the eye. In *hyperopia*, the globe is too short, and hence a converging lens is used to supplement the refractive power of the eye. In *astigmatism*, the corneal surface is not perfectly spherical, necessitating a cylindrical corrective lens. As an alternative to eyeglasses or contact lenses, refractive error can be corrected by performing laser in situ keratomileusis (LASIK) or photorefractive keratectomy (PRK) to alter the curvature of the cornea.

With the onset of middle age, *presbyopia* develops as the lens within the eye becomes unable to increase its refractive power to accommodate on near objects. To compensate for presbyopia an emmetropic patient must use reading glasses. A patient already wearing glasses for distance correction usually switches to bifocals. The only exception is a myopic patient, who may achieve clear vision at near simply by removing glasses containing the distance prescription.

Refractive errors usually develop slowly and remain stable after adolescence, except in unusual circumstances. For example, the acute onset of diabetes mellitus can produce sudden myopia because of lens edema induced by hyperglycemia. Testing vision through a pinhole aperture is a useful way to screen quickly for refractive error. If visual acuity is better through a pinhole than it is with the unaided eye, the patient needs refraction to obtain best corrected visual acuity.

VISUAL ACUITY

The Snellen chart is used to test acuity at a distance of 6 m (20 ft). For convenience, a scale version of the Snellen chart called the Rosenbaum card is held at 36 cm (14 in.) from the patient (Fig. 39-1). All subjects should be able to read the 6/6 m (20/20 ft) line with each eye using their refractive correction, if any. Patients who need reading glasses because of presbyopia must wear them for accurate testing with the Rosenbaum card. If 6/6 (20/20) acuity is not present in each eye, the deficiency in vision must be explained. If it is worse than 6/240 (20/800), acuity should be recorded in terms of counting fingers, hand motions, light perception, or no light perception. Legal blindness is defined by the Internal Revenue Service as a best corrected acuity of 6/60 (20/200) or less in the better eye or a binocular visual field subtending 20° or less. For driving the laws vary by state, but most states require a corrected acuity of 6/12 (20/40) in at least one eye for unrestricted privileges. Patients with a homonymous hemianopia should not drive.

PUPILS

The pupils should be tested individually in dim light with the patient fixating on a distant target. There is no need to check the near response if the pupils respond briskly to light, because isolated loss of constriction (miosis) to accommodation does not occur. For this reason, the ubiquitous abbreviation PERRLA (pupils equal, round, and reactive to light and accommodation) implies a wasted effort with the last step. However, it is important to test the near response if the light response is poor or absent. Light-near dissociation occurs with neurosyphilis (Argyll Robertson pupil), with lesions of the dorsal midbrain (*Parinaud's syndrome*), and after aberrant regeneration (oculomotor nerve palsy, Adie's tonic pupil).

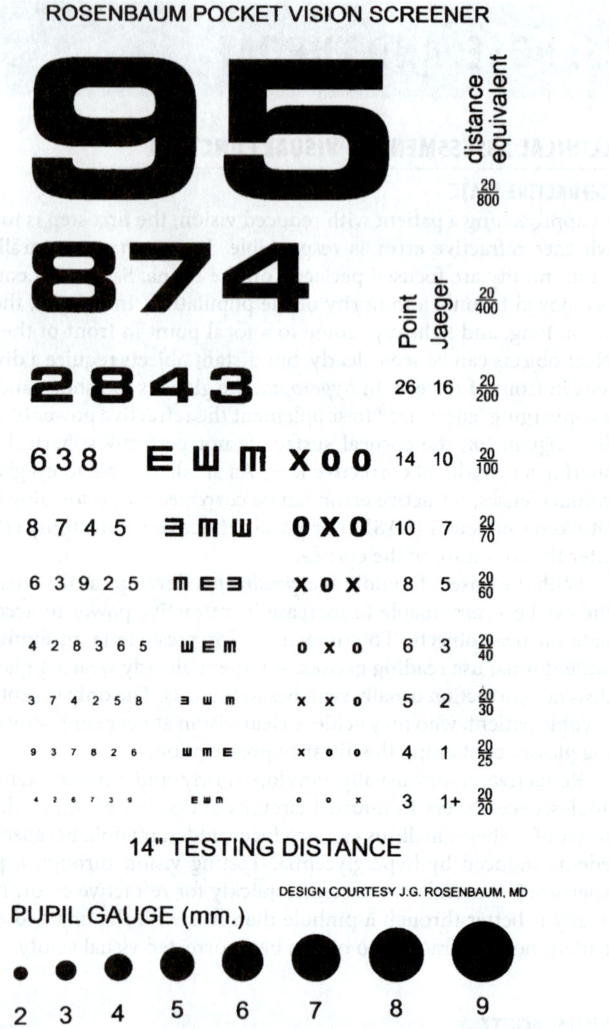

FIGURE 39-1 The Rosenbaum card is a miniature, scale version of the Snellen chart for testing visual acuity at near. When the visual acuity is recorded, the Snellen distance equivalent should bear a notation indicating that vision was tested at near, not at 6 m (20 ft), or else the Jaeger number system should be used to report the acuity.

An eye with no light perception has no pupillary response to direct light stimulation. If the retina or optic nerve is only partially injured, the direct pupillary response will be weaker than the consensual pupillary response evoked by shining a light into the healthy fellow eye. A *relative afferent pupillary defect* (Marcus Gunn pupil) can be elicited with the swinging flashlight test (Fig. 39-2). It is an extremely useful sign in retrobulbar optic neuritis and other optic nerve diseases, in which it may be the sole objective evidence for disease. In bilateral optic neuropathy, no afferent pupil defect is present if the optic nerves are affected equally.

Subtle inequality in pupil size, up to 0.5 mm, is a fairly common finding in normal persons. The diagnosis of essential or physiologic anisocoria is secure as long as the relative pupil asymmetry remains constant as ambient lighting varies. Anisocoria that increases in dim light indicates a sympathetic paresis of the iris dilator muscle. The triad of miosis with ipsilateral ptosis and anhidrosis constitutes *Horner's syndrome*, although anhidrosis is an inconstant feature. Brainstem stroke, carotid dissection, and neoplasm impinging on the sympathetic chain occasionally are identified as the cause of Horner's syndrome, but most cases are idiopathic.

Anisocoria that increases in bright light suggests a parasympathetic palsy. The first concern is an oculomotor nerve paresis. This possibility is excluded if the eye movements are full and the patient has no ptosis or diplopia. Acute pupillary dilation (mydriasis) can result from damage to the ciliary ganglion in the orbit. Common mechanisms are infection (herpes zoster, influenza), trauma (blunt, penetrating, surgical), and ischemia (diabetes, temporal arteritis). After denervation of the iris sphincter the pupil does not respond well to light, but the response to near is often relatively intact. When the near stimulus is removed, the pupil redilates very slowly compared with the normal pupil, hence the term *tonic pupil*. In *Adie's syndrome* a tonic pupil is present, sometimes in conjunction with weak or absent tendon reflexes in the lower extremities. This benign disorder, which occurs predominantly in healthy young women, is assumed to represent a mild dysautonomia. Tonic pupils are also associated with Shy-Drager syndrome, segmental hypohidrosis, diabetes, and amyloidosis. Occasionally, a tonic pupil is discovered incidentally in an otherwise completely

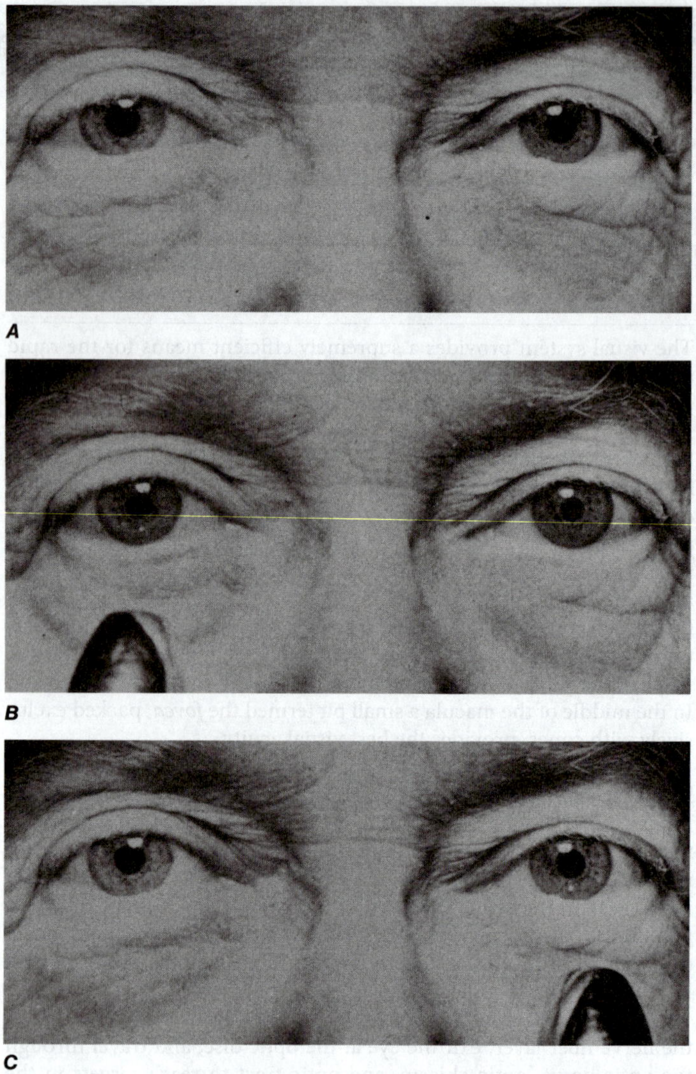

FIGURE 39-2 Demonstration of a relative afferent pupil defect (Marcus Gunn pupil) in the left eye, done with the patient fixating on a distant target. ***A.*** With dim background lighting, the pupils are equal and relatively large. ***B.*** Shining a flashlight into the right eye evokes equal, strong constriction of both pupils. ***C.*** Swinging the flashlight over to the damaged left eye causes dilation of both pupils, although they remain smaller than in ***A***. Swinging the flashlight back over to the healthy right eye would result in symmetric constriction back to the appearance shown in ***B***. Note that the pupils always remain equal; the damage to the left retina/optic nerve is revealed by weaker bilateral pupil constriction to a flashlight in the left eye compared with the right eye. *(From P Levatin: Arch Ophthalmol 62:768, 1959. Copyright © 1959 American Medical Association. All rights reserved.)*

normal, asymptomatic individual. The diagnosis is confirmed by placing a drop of dilute (0.125%) pilocarpine into each eye. Denervation hypersensitivity produces pupillary constriction in a tonic pupil, whereas the normal pupil shows no response. Pharmacologic dilatation from accidental or deliberate instillation of anticholinergic agents (atropine, scopolamine drops) into the eye also can produce pupillary mydriasis. In this situation, normal strength (1%) pilocarpine causes no constriction.

Both pupils are affected equally by systemic medications. They are small with narcotic use (morphine, heroin) and large with anticholinergics (scopolamine). Parasympathetic agents (pilocarpine, demecarium bromide) used to treat glaucoma produce miosis. In any patient with an unexplained pupillary abnormality, a slit-lamp examination is helpful to exclude surgical trauma to the iris, an occult foreign body, perforating injury, intraocular inflammation, adhesions (synechia), angle-closure glaucoma, and iris sphincter rupture from blunt trauma.

EYE MOVEMENTS AND ALIGNMENT

Eye movements are tested by asking the patient, with both eyes open, to pursue a small target such as a penlight into the cardinal fields of gaze. Normal ocular versions are smooth, symmetric, full, and maintained in all directions without nystagmus. Saccades, or quick refixation eye movements, are assessed by having the patient look back and forth between two stationary targets. The eyes should move rapidly and accurately in a single jump to their target. Ocular alignment can be judged by holding a penlight directly in front of the patient at about 1 m. If the eyes are straight, the corneal light reflex will be centered in the middle of each pupil. To test eye alignment more precisely, the cover test is useful. The patient is instructed to look at a small fixation target in the distance. One eye is covered suddenly while the second eye is observed. If the second eye shifts to fixate on the target, it was misaligned. If it does not move, the first eye is uncovered and the test is repeated on the second eye. If neither eye moves the eyes are aligned orthotropically. If the eyes are orthotropic in primary gaze but the patient complains of diplopia, the cover test should be performed with the head tilted or turned in whatever direction elicits diplopia. With practice, the examiner can detect an ocular deviation (heterotropia) as small as 1–2° with the cover test. In a patient with vertical diplopia, a small deviation can be difficult to detect and easy to dismiss. The magnitude of the deviation can be measured by placing a prism in front of the misaligned eye to determine the power required to neutralize the fixation shift evoked by covering the other eye. Temporary press-on plastic Fresnel prisms, prism eyeglasses, or eye muscle surgery can be used to restore binocular alignment.

STEREOPSIS

Stereoacuity is determined by presenting targets with retinal disparity separately to each eye by using polarized images. The most popular office tests measure a range of thresholds from 800–40 seconds of arc. Normal stereoacuity is 40 seconds of arc. If a patient achieves this level of stereoacuity, one is assured that the eyes are aligned orthotropically and that vision is intact in each eye. Random dot stereograms have no monocular depth cues and provide an excellent screening test for strabismus and amblyopia in children.

COLOR VISION

The retina contains three classes of cones, with visual pigments of differing peak spectral sensitivity: red (560 nm), green (530 nm), and blue (430 nm). The red and green cone pigments are encoded on the X chromosome, and the blue cone pigment on chromosome 7. Mutations of the blue cone pigment are exceedingly rare. Mutations of the red and green pigments cause congenital X-linked color blindness in 8% of males. Affected individuals are not truly color blind; rather, they differ from normal subjects in the way they perceive color and how they combine primary monochromatic lights to match a particular color. Anomalous trichromats have three cone types, but a mutation in one cone pigment (usually red or green) causes a shift in peak spectral sensitivity, altering the proportion of primary colors required to achieve a color match. Dichromats have only two cone types and therefore will accept a color match based on only two primary colors. Anomalous trichromats and dichromats have 6/6 (20/20) visual acuity, but their hue discrimination is impaired. Ishihara color plates can be used to detect red-green color blindness. The test plates contain a hidden number that is visible only to subjects with color confusion from red-green color blindness. Because color blindness is almost exclusively X-linked, it is worth screening only male children.

The Ishihara plates often are used to detect acquired defects in color vision, although they are intended as a screening test for congenital color blindness. Acquired defects in color vision frequently result from disease of the macula or optic nerve. For example, patients with a history of optic neuritis often complain of color desaturation long after their visual acuity has returned to normal. Color blindness also can result from bilateral strokes involving the ventral portion of the occipital lobe (cerebral achromatopsia). Such patients can perceive only shades of gray and also may have difficulty recognizing faces (prosopagnosia). Infarcts of the dominant occipital lobe sometimes give rise to color anomia. Affected patients can discriminate colors but cannot name them.

VISUAL FIELDS

Vision can be impaired by damage to the visual system anywhere from the eyes to the occipital lobes. One can localize the site of the lesion with considerable accuracy by mapping the visual field deficit by finger confrontation and then correlating it with the topographic anatomy of the visual pathway (Fig. 39-3). Quantitative visual field mapping is performed by computer-driven perimeters that present a target of variable intensity at fixed positions in the visual field (Fig. 39-3*A*). By generating an automated printout of light thresholds, these static perimeters provide a sensitive means of detecting scotomas in the visual field. They are exceedingly useful for serial assessment of visual function in chronic diseases such as glaucoma and pseudotumor cerebri.

The crux of visual field analysis is to decide whether a lesion is before, at, or behind the optic chiasm. If a scotoma is confined to one eye, it must be due to a lesion anterior to the chiasm, involving either the optic nerve or the retina. Retinal lesions produce scotomas that correspond optically to their location in the fundus. For example, a superior-nasal retinal detachment results in an inferior-temporal field cut. Damage to the macula causes a central scotoma (Fig. 39-3*B*).

Optic nerve disease produces characteristic patterns of visual field loss. Glaucoma selectively destroys axons that enter the superotemporal or inferotemporal poles of the optic disc, resulting in arcuate scotomas shaped like a Turkish scimitar, which emanate from the blind spot and curve around fixation to end flat against the horizontal meridian (Fig. 39-3*C*). This type of field defect mirrors the arrangement of the nerve fiber layer in the temporal retina. Arcuate or nerve fiber layer scotomas also result from optic neuritis, ischemic optic neuropathy, optic disc drusen, and branch retinal artery or vein occlusion.

Damage to the entire upper or lower pole of the optic disc causes an altitudinal field cut that follows the horizontal meridian (Fig. 39-3*D*). This pattern of visual field loss is typical of ischemic optic neuropathy but also results from retinal vascular occlusion, advanced glaucoma, and optic neuritis.

About half the fibers in the optic nerve originate from ganglion cells serving the macula. Damage to papillomacular fibers causes a cecocentral scotoma that encompasses the blind spot and macula (Fig. 39-3*E*). If the damage is irreversible, pallor eventually appears in the temporal portion of the optic disc. Temporal pallor from a cecocentral scotoma may develop in optic neuritis, nutritional optic neuropathy, toxic optic neuropathy, Leber's hereditary optic neuropathy, Kjer's dominant optic atrophy, and compressive optic neuropathy. It is worth mentioning that the temporal side of the optic disc is slightly paler than the nasal side in most normal individuals. Therefore, it sometimes can be difficult to decide whether the temporal pallor visible on fundus examination represents a pathologic change. Pallor of the nasal rim of the optic disc is a less equivocal sign of optic atrophy.

At the optic chiasm, fibers from nasal ganglion cells decussate into the contralateral optic tract. Crossed fibers are damaged more by

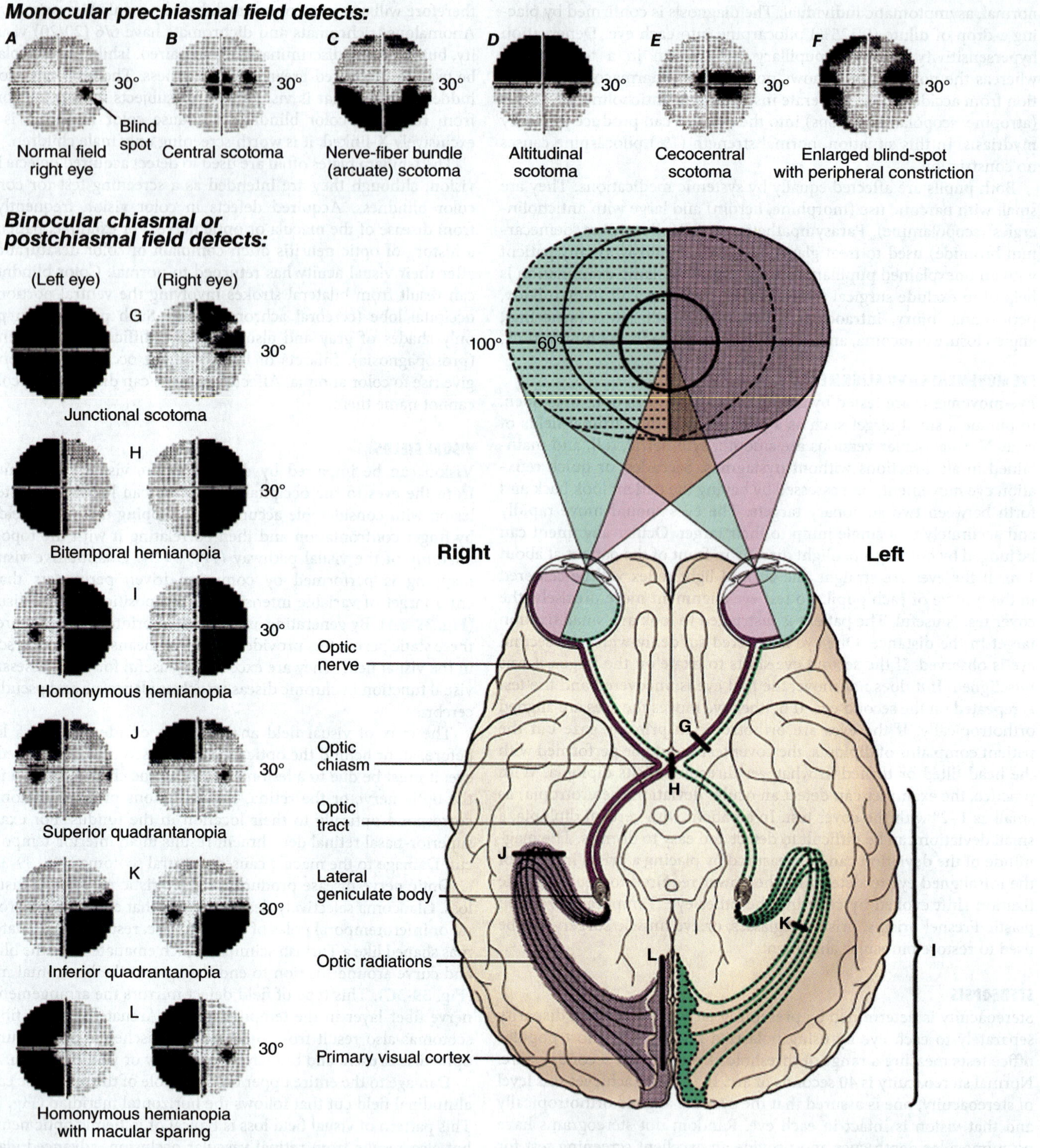

FIGURE 39-3 Ventral view of the brain, correlating patterns of visual field loss with the sites of lesions in the visual pathway. The visual fields overlap partially, creating 120° of central binocular field flanked by a 40° monocular crescent on either side. The visual field maps in this figure were done with a computer-driven perimeter (Humphrey Instruments, Carl Zeiss, Inc.). It plots the retinal sensitivity to light in the central 30° by using a gray scale format. Areas of visual field loss are shown in black. The examples of common monocular, prechiasmal field defects are all shown for the right eye. By convention, the visual fields are always recorded with the left eye's field on the left and the right eye's field on the right, just as the patient sees the world.

compression than are uncrossed fibers. As a result, mass lesions of the sellar region cause a temporal hemianopia in each eye. Tumors anterior to the optic chiasm, such as meningiomas of the tuberculum sella, produce a junctional scotoma characterized by an optic neuropathy in one eye and a superior-temporal field cut in the other eye (Fig. 39-3G). More symmetric compression of the optic chiasm by a pituitary adenoma (see Fig. 403-1), meningioma, craniopharyngioma, glioma, or aneurysm results in a bitemporal hemianopia (Fig. 39-3H). The insidious development of a bitemporal hemianopia often goes unnoticed by the patient and will escape detection by the physician unless each eye is tested separately.

It is difficult to localize a postchiasmal lesion accurately, because injury anywhere in the optic tract, lateral geniculate body, optic radiations, or visual cortex can produce a homonymous hemianopia (i.e., a temporal hemifield defect in the contralateral eye and a matching nasal hemifield defect in the ipsilateral eye) (Fig. 39-3I). A unilateral postchiasmal lesion leaves the visual acuity in each eye unaffected, although the patient may read the letters on only the left or right half of the eye chart. Lesions of the optic radiations tend to cause poorly matched or incongruous field defects in each eye. Damage to the optic radiations in the temporal lobe (Meyer's loop) produces a superior quadrantic homonymous hemianopia (Fig. 39-3*J*), whereas injury to the optic radiations in the parietal lobe results in an inferior quadrantic homonymous hemianopia (Fig. 39-3*K*). Lesions of the primary visual cortex give rise to dense, congruous hemianopic field defects. Occlusion of the posterior cerebral artery supplying the occipital lobe is a common cause of total homonymous hemianopia. Some patients with hemianopia after occipital stroke have macular sparing, because the macular representation at the tip of the occipital lobe is supplied by collaterals from the middle cerebral artery (Fig. 39-3*L*). Destruction of both occipital lobes produces cortical blindness. This condition can be distinguished from bilateral prechiasmal visual loss by noting that the pupil responses and optic fundi remain normal.

DISORDERS

RED OR PAINFUL EYE

Corneal Abrasions Corneal abrasions are seen best by placing a drop of fluorescein in the eye and looking with the slit lamp, using a cobalt-blue light. A penlight with a blue filter will suffice if a slit lamp is not available. Damage to the corneal epithelium is revealed by yellow fluorescence of the exposed basement membrane underlying the epithelium. It is important to check for foreign bodies. To search the conjunctival fornices, the lower lid should be pulled down and the upper lid everted. A foreign body can be removed with a moistened cotton-tipped applicator after a drop of a topical anesthetic such as proparacaine has been placed in the eye. Alternatively, it may be possible to flush the foreign body from the eye by irrigating copiously with saline or artificial tears. If the corneal epithelium has been abraded, antibiotic ointment and a patch should be applied to the eye. A drop of an intermediate-acting cycloplegic such as cyclopentolate hydrochloride 1% helps reduce pain by relaxing the ciliary body. The eye should be reexamined the next day. Minor abrasions may not require patching, antibiotics, or cycloplegia.

Subconjunctival Hemorrhage This results from rupture of small vessels bridging the potential space between the episclera and the conjunctiva. Blood dissecting into this space can produce a spectacular red eye, but vision is not affected and the hemorrhage resolves without treatment. Subconjunctival hemorrhage is usually spontaneous but can result from blunt trauma, eye rubbing, or vigorous coughing. Occasionally it is a clue to an underlying bleeding disorder.

Pinguecula Pinguecula is a small, raised conjunctival nodule at the temporal or nasal limbus. In adults such lesions are extremely common and have little significance unless they become inflamed (pingueculitis). They are more apt to occur in workers with frequent outdoor exposure. A *pterygium* resembles a pinguecula but has crossed the limbus to encroach on the corneal surface. Removal is justified when symptoms of irritation or blurring develop, but recurrence is a common problem.

Blepharitis This refers to inflammation of the eyelids. The most common form occurs in association with acne rosacea or seborrheic dermatitis. The eyelid margins usually are colonized heavily by staphylococci. Upon close inspection, they appear greasy, ulcerated, and crusted with scaling debris that clings to the lashes. Treatment consists of strict eyelid hygiene, using warm compresses and eyelash scrubs with baby shampoo. An external *hordeolum* (sty) is caused by staphylococcal infection of the superficial accessory glands of Zeis or Moll located in the eyelid margins. An internal hordeolum occurs after suppurative infection of the oil-secreting meibomian glands within the tarsal plate of the eyelid. Topical antibiotics such as bacitracin/polymyxin B ophthalmic ointment can be applied. Systemic antibiotics, usually tetracyclines or azithromycin, sometimes are necessary for treatment of meibomian gland inflammation (meibomitis) or chronic, severe blepharitis. A *chalazion* is a painless, chronic granulomatous inflammation of a meibomian gland that produces a pealike nodule within the eyelid. It can be incised and drained or injected with glucocorticoids. Basal cell, squamous cell, or meibomian gland carcinoma should be suspected with any nonhealing ulcerative lesion of the eyelids.

Dacryocystitis An inflammation of the lacrimal drainage system, dacryocystitis can produce epiphora (tearing) and ocular injection. Gentle pressure over the lacrimal sac evokes pain and reflux of mucus or pus from the tear puncta. Dacryocystitis usually occurs after obstruction of the lacrimal system. It is treated with topical and systemic antibiotics, followed by probing, silicone stent intubation, or surgery to reestablish patency. *Entropion* (inversion of the eyelid) or *ectropion* (sagging or eversion of the eyelid) can also lead to epiphora and ocular irritation.

Conjunctivitis Conjunctivitis is the most common cause of a red, irritated eye. Pain is minimal, and visual acuity is reduced only slightly. The most common viral etiology is adenovirus infection. It causes a watery discharge, a mild foreign-body sensation, and photophobia. Bacterial infection tends to produce a more mucopurulent exudate. Mild cases of infectious conjunctivitis usually are treated empirically with broad-spectrum topical ocular antibiotics such as sulfacetamide 10%, polymyxin-bacitracin, or a trimethoprim-polymyxin combination. Smears and cultures usually are reserved for severe, resistant, or recurrent cases of conjunctivitis. To prevent contagion, patients should be admonished to wash their hands frequently, not to touch their eyes, and to avoid direct contact with others.

Allergic Conjunctivitis This condition is extremely common and often is mistaken for infectious conjunctivitis. Itching, redness, and epiphora are typical. The palpebral conjunctiva may become hypertropic with giant excrescences called cobblestone papillae. Irritation from contact lenses or any chronic foreign body also can induce formation of cobblestone papillae. *Atopic conjunctivitis* occurs in subjects with atopic dermatitis or asthma. Symptoms caused by allergic conjunctivitis can be alleviated with cold compresses, topical vasoconstrictors, antihistamines, and mast cell stabilizers such as cromolyn sodium. Topical glucocorticoid solutions provide dramatic relief of immune-mediated forms of conjunctivitis, but their long-term use is ill advised because of the complications of glaucoma, cataract, and secondary infection. Topical nonsteroidal anti-inflammatory drugs (NSAIDs) (e.g., ketorolac tromethamine) are better alternatives.

Keratoconjunctivitis Sicca Also known as dry eye, this produces a burning foreign-body sensation, injection, and photophobia. In mild cases the eye appears surprisingly normal, but tear production measured by wetting of a filter paper (Schirmer strip) is deficient. A variety of systemic drugs, including antihistaminic, anticholinergic, and psychotropic medications, result in dry eye by reducing lacrimal secretion. Disorders that involve the lacrimal gland directly, such as sarcoidosis and Sjögren's syndrome, also cause dry eye. Patients may develop dry eye after radiation therapy if the treatment field includes the orbits. Problems with ocular drying are also common after lesions affecting cranial nerve V or VII. Corneal anesthesia is particularly dangerous, because the absence of a normal blink reflex exposes the cornea to injury without pain to warn the patient. Dry eye is managed by frequent and liberal application of artificial tears and ocular lubricants. In severe cases the tear puncta can be plugged or cauterized to reduce lacrimal outflow.

Keratitis Keratitis is a threat to vision because of the risk of corneal clouding, scarring, and perforation. Worldwide, the two leading causes of blindness from keratitis are trachoma from chlamydial infection and vitamin A deficiency related to malnutrition. In the United States, contact lenses play a major role in corneal infection and ulceration. They should not be worn by anyone with an active eye infection. In evaluating the cornea, it is important to differentiate between a superficial infection (*keratoconjunctivitis*) and a deeper, more serious ulcerative process. The latter is accompanied by greater visual loss, pain, photophobia, redness, and discharge. Slit-lamp examination shows disruption of the corneal epithelium, a cloudy infiltrate or abscess in the stroma, and an inflammatory cellular reaction in the anterior chamber. In severe cases, pus settles at the bottom of the anterior chamber, giving rise to a hypopyon. Immediate empirical antibiotic therapy should be initiated after corneal scrapings are obtained for Gram's stain, Giemsa stain, and cultures. Fortified topical antibiotics are most effective, supplemented with subconjunctival antibiotics as required. A fungal etiology should always be considered in a patient with keratitis. Fungal infection is common in warm humid climates, especially after penetration of the cornea by plant or vegetable material.

Herpes Simplex The *herpesviruses* are a major cause of blindness from keratitis. Most adults in the United States have serum antibodies to herpes simplex, indicating prior viral infection (Chap. 216). Primary ocular infection generally is caused by herpes simplex type 1 rather than type 2. It manifests as a unilateral follicular blepharoconjunctivitis that is easily confused with adenoviral conjunctivitis unless telltale vesicles appear on the periocular skin or conjunctiva. A dendritic pattern of corneal epithelial ulceration revealed by fluorescein staining is pathognomonic for herpes infection but is seen in only a minority of primary infections. Recurrent ocular infection arises from reactivation of the latent herpesvirus. Viral eruption in the corneal epithelium may result in the characteristic herpes dendrite. Involvement of the corneal stroma produces edema, vascularization, and iridocyclitis. Herpes keratitis is treated with topical antiviral agents, cycloplegics, and oral acyclovir. Topical glucocorticoids are effective in mitigating corneal scarring but must be used with extreme caution because of the danger of corneal melting and perforation. Topical glucocorticoids also carry the risk of prolonging infection and inducing glaucoma.

Herpes Zoster Herpes zoster from reactivation of latent varicella (chickenpox) virus causes a dermatomal pattern of painful vesicular dermatitis. Ocular symptoms can occur after zoster eruption in any branch of the trigeminal nerve but are particularly common when vesicles form on the nose, reflecting nasociliary (V1) nerve involvement (Hutchinson's sign). Herpes zoster ophthalmicus produces corneal dendrites, which can be difficult to distinguish from those seen in herpes simplex. Stromal keratitis, anterior uveitis, raised intraocular pressure, ocular motor nerve palsies, acute retinal necrosis, and postherpetic scarring and neuralgia are other common sequelae. Herpes zoster ophthalmicus is treated with antiviral agents and cycloplegics. In severe cases, glucocorticoids may be added to prevent permanent visual loss from corneal scarring.

Episcleritis This is an inflammation of the episclera, a thin layer of connective tissue between the conjunctiva and the sclera. Episcleritis resembles conjunctivitis, but it is a more localized process and discharge is absent. Most cases of episcleritis are idiopathic, but some occur in the setting of an autoimmune disease. *Scleritis* refers to a deeper, more severe inflammatory process that frequently is associated with a connective tissue disease such as rheumatoid arthritis, lupus erythematosus, polyarteritis nodosa, granulomatosis with polyangiitis (Wegener's), or relapsing polychondritis. The inflammation and thickening of the sclera can be diffuse or nodular. In anterior forms of scleritis, the globe assumes a violet hue and the patient complains of severe ocular tenderness and pain. With posterior scleritis, the pain and redness may be less marked, but there is often proptosis, choroidal effusion, reduced motility, and visual loss. Episcleritis and scleritis should be treated with NSAIDs. If these agents fail, topical or even systemic glucocorticoid therapy may be necessary, especially if an underlying autoimmune process is active.

Uveitis Involving the anterior structures of the eye, uveitis also is called *iritis* or *iridocyclitis*. The diagnosis requires slit-lamp examination to identify inflammatory cells floating in the aqueous humor or deposited on the corneal endothelium (keratic precipitates). Anterior uveitis develops in sarcoidosis, ankylosing spondylitis, juvenile rheumatoid arthritis, inflammatory bowel disease, psoriasis, reactive arthritis, and Behçet's disease. It also is associated with herpes infections, syphilis, Lyme disease, onchocerciasis, tuberculosis, and leprosy. Although anterior uveitis can occur in conjunction with many diseases, no cause is found to explain the majority of cases. For this reason, laboratory evaluation usually is reserved for patients with recurrent or severe anterior uveitis. Treatment is aimed at reducing inflammation and scarring by judicious use of topical glucocorticoids. Dilatation of the pupil reduces pain and prevents the formation of synechiae.

Posterior Uveitis This is diagnosed by observing inflammation of the vitreous, retina, or choroid on fundus examination. It is more likely than anterior uveitis to be associated with an identifiable systemic disease. Some patients have panuveitis, or inflammation of both the anterior and posterior segments of the eye. Posterior uveitis is a manifestation of autoimmune diseases such as sarcoidosis, Behçet's disease, Vogt-Koyanagi-Harada syndrome, and inflammatory bowel disease. It also accompanies diseases such as toxoplasmosis, onchocerciasis, cysticercosis, coccidioidomycosis, toxocariasis, and histoplasmosis; infections caused by organisms such as *Candida*, *Pneumocystis carinii*, *Cryptococcus*, *Aspergillus*, herpes, and cytomegalovirus (see Fig. 219-1); and other diseases, such as syphilis, Lyme disease, tuberculosis, cat-scratch disease, Whipple's disease, and brucellosis. In multiple sclerosis, chronic inflammatory changes can develop in the extreme periphery of the retina (pars planitis or intermediate uveitis).

Acute Angle-Closure Glaucoma This is an unusual but frequently misdiagnosed cause of a red, painful eye. Asian populations have a particularly high risk of angle-closure glaucoma. Susceptible eyes have a shallow anterior chamber because the eye has either a short axial length (hyperopia) or a lens enlarged by the gradual development of cataract. When the pupil becomes mid-dilated, the peripheral iris blocks aqueous outflow via the anterior chamber angle and the intraocular pressure rises abruptly, producing pain, injection, corneal edema, obscurations, and blurred vision. In some patients, ocular symptoms are overshadowed by nausea, vomiting, or headache, prompting a fruitless workup for abdominal or neurologic disease. The diagnosis is made by measuring the intraocular pressure during an acute attack or by performing gonioscopy, a procedure that allows one to observe a narrow chamber angle with a mirrored contact lens. Acute angle closure is treated with acetazolamide (PO or IV), topical beta blockers, prostaglandin analogues, α_2-adrenergic agonists, and pilocarpine to induce miosis. If these measures fail, a laser can be used to create a hole in the peripheral iris to relieve pupillary block. Many physicians are reluctant to dilate patients routinely for fundus examination because they fear precipitating an angle-closure glaucoma. The risk is actually remote and more than outweighed by the potential benefit to patients of discovering a hidden fundus lesion visible only through a fully dilated pupil. Moreover, a single attack of angle closure after pharmacologic dilatation rarely causes any permanent damage to the eye and serves as an inadvertent provocative test to identify patients with narrow angles who would benefit from prophylactic laser iridectomy.

Endophthalmitis This results from bacterial, viral, fungal, or parasitic infection of the internal structures of the eye. It usually is acquired by hematogenous seeding from a remote site. Chronically ill, diabetic, or immunosuppressed patients, especially those with a history of indwelling IV catheters or positive blood cultures, are at greatest risk for endogenous endophthalmitis. Although most patients have ocular pain and injection, visual loss is sometimes the only symptom. Septic emboli from a diseased heart valve or a dental abscess that lodge in the retinal circulation can give rise to endophthalmitis. White-centered retinal hemorrhages known as Roth's spots (Fig. 39-4) are considered pathognomonic for subacute bacterial endocarditis, but they also appear in leukemia, diabetes, and many other conditions. Endophthalmitis also occurs as a complication of ocular surgery, especially glaucoma filtering, occasionally months or even years after the operation. An occult penetrating foreign body or unrecognized trauma to the globe should be considered in any patient with unexplained intraocular infection or inflammation.

TRANSIENT OR SUDDEN VISUAL LOSS

Amaurosis Fugax This term refers to a transient ischemic attack of the retina (Chap. 446). Because neural tissue has a high rate of metabolism, interruption of blood flow to the retina for more than a few seconds

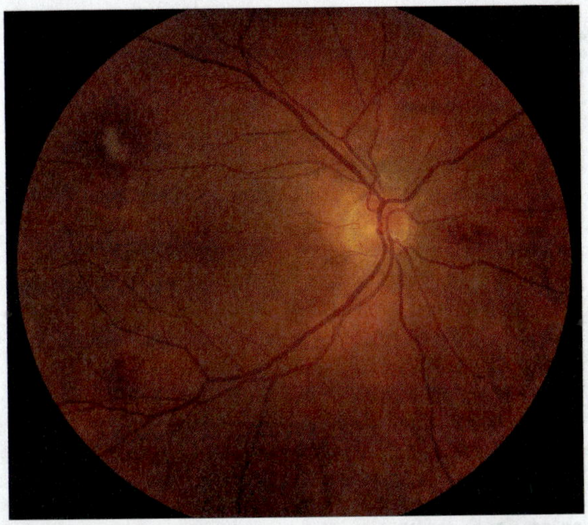

FIGURE 39-4 Roth's spot, cotton-wool spot, and retinal hemorrhages in a 48-year-old liver transplant patient with candidemia from immunosuppression.

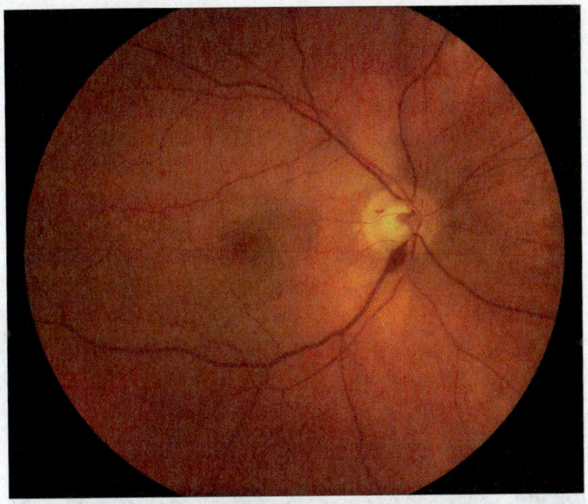

FIGURE 39-6 Central retinal artery occlusion in a 78-year-old man reducing acuity to counting fingers in the right eye. Note the splinter hemorrhage on the optic disc and the slightly milky appearance to the macula with a cherry-red fovea.

results in *transient monocular blindness*, a term used interchangeably with amaurosis fugax. Patients describe a rapid fading of vision like a curtain descending, sometimes affecting only a portion of the visual field. Amaurosis fugax usually results from an embolus that becomes stuck within a retinal arteriole (Fig. 39-5). If the embolus breaks up or passes, flow is restored and vision returns quickly to normal without permanent damage. With prolonged interruption of blood flow, the inner retina suffers infarction. Ophthalmoscopy reveals zones of whitened, edematous retina following the distribution of branch retinal arterioles. Complete occlusion of the central retinal artery produces arrest of blood flow and a milky retina with a cherry-red fovea (Fig. 39-6). Emboli are composed of cholesterol (Hollenhorst plaque), calcium, or platelet-fibrin debris. The most common source is an atherosclerotic plaque in the carotid artery or aorta, although emboli also can arise from the heart, especially in patients with diseased valves, atrial fibrillation, or wall motion abnormalities.

In rare instances, amaurosis fugax results from low central retinal artery perfusion pressure in a patient with a critical stenosis of the ipsilateral carotid artery and poor collateral flow via the circle of Willis. In this situation, amaurosis fugax develops when there is a dip in systemic blood pressure or a slight worsening of the carotid stenosis. Sometimes there is contralateral motor or sensory loss, indicating concomitant hemispheric cerebral ischemia.

Retinal arterial occlusion also occurs rarely in association with retinal migraine, lupus erythematosus, anticardiolipin antibodies, anticoagulant deficiency states (protein S, protein C, and antithrombin deficiency), pregnancy, IV drug abuse, blood dyscrasias, dysproteinemias, and temporal arteritis.

Marked *systemic hypertension* causes sclerosis of retinal arterioles, splinter hemorrhages, focal infarcts of the nerve fiber layer (cotton-wool spots), and leakage of lipid and fluid (hard exudate) into the macula (Fig. 39-7). In hypertensive crisis, sudden visual loss can result from vasospasm of retinal arterioles and retinal ischemia. In addition, acute hypertension may produce visual loss from ischemic swelling of the optic disc. Patients with acute hypertensive retinopathy should be treated by lowering the blood pressure. However, the blood pressure should not be reduced precipitously, because there is a danger of optic disc infarction from sudden hypoperfusion.

Impending *branch* or *central retinal vein occlusion* can produce prolonged visual obscurations that resemble those described by patients with amaurosis fugax. The veins appear engorged and phlebitic, with numerous retinal hemorrhages (Fig. 39-8). In some patients, venous blood flow recovers spontaneously, whereas others evolve a frank obstruction with extensive retinal bleeding ("blood and thunder" appearance), infarction, and visual loss. Venous occlusion of the retina is often idiopathic, but hypertension, diabetes, and glaucoma

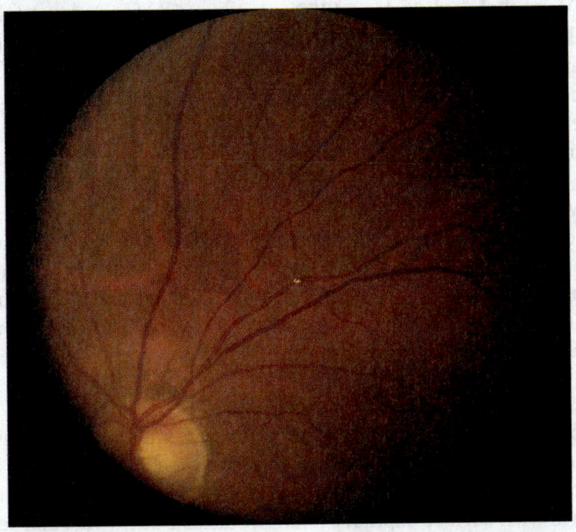

FIGURE 39-5 Hollenhorst plaque lodged at the bifurcation of a retinal arteriole proves that a patient is shedding emboli from the carotid artery, great vessels, or heart.

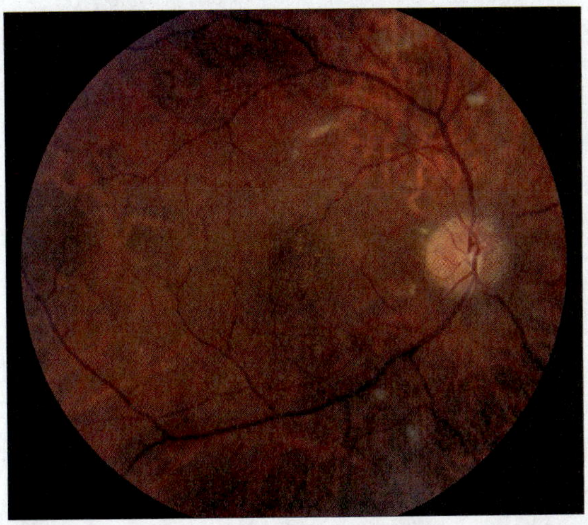

FIGURE 39-7 Hypertensive retinopathy with blurred optic disc, scattered hemorrhages, cotton-wool spots (nerve fiber layer infarcts), and foveal exudate in a 62-year-old man with chronic renal failure and a systolic blood pressure of 220.

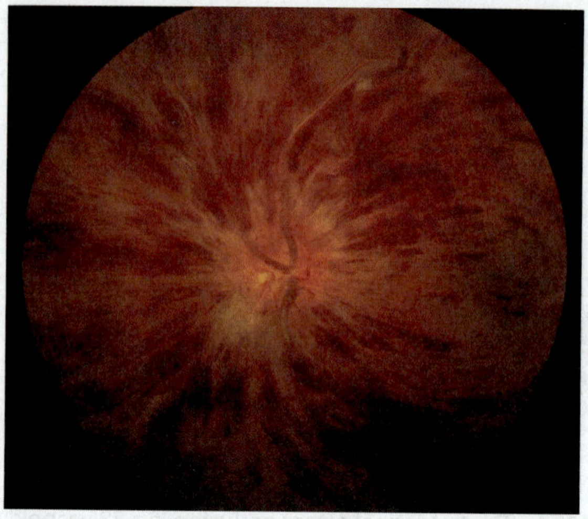

FIGURE 39-8 Central retinal vein occlusion can produce massive retinal hemorrhage ("blood and thunder"), ischemia, and vision loss.

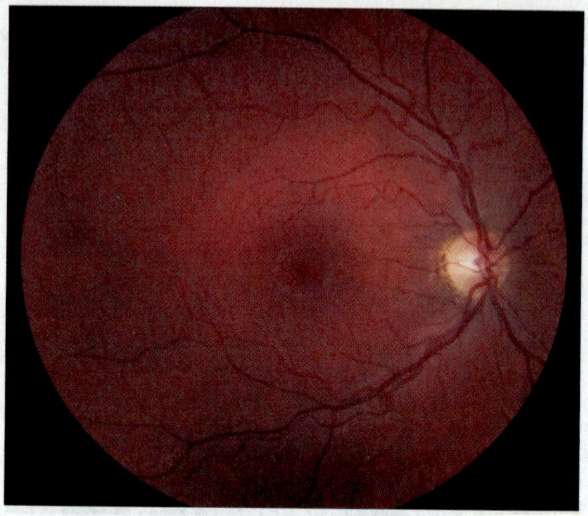

FIGURE 39-10 Retrobulbar optic neuritis is characterized by a normal fundus examination initially, hence the rubric "the doctor sees nothing, and the patient sees nothing." Optic atrophy develops after severe or repeated attacks.

are prominent risk factors. Polycythemia, thrombocythemia, or other factors leading to an underlying hypercoagulable state should be corrected; aspirin treatment may be beneficial.

Anterior Ischemic Optic Neuropathy (AION) This is caused by insufficient blood flow through the posterior ciliary arteries that supply the optic disc. It produces painless monocular visual loss that is sudden in onset, followed sometimes by stuttering progression. The optic disc appears swollen and surrounded by nerve fiber layer splinter hemorrhages (Fig. 39-9). AION is divided into two forms: arteritic and nonarteritic. The nonarteritic form is most common. No specific cause can be identified, although diabetes and hypertension are common risk factors. A crowded disc architecture and small optic cup predispose to the development of nonarteritic AION. No treatment is available. About 5% of patients, especially those age >60, develop the arteritic form of AION in conjunction with giant-cell (temporal) arteritis (Chap. 385). It is urgent to recognize arteritic AION so that high doses of glucocorticoids can be instituted immediately to prevent blindness in the second eye. Symptoms of polymyalgia rheumatica may be present; the sedimentation rate and C-reactive protein level are usually elevated. In a patient with visual loss from suspected arteritic AION, temporal artery biopsy is mandatory to confirm the diagnosis. Glucocorticoids should be started immediately, without waiting for the biopsy to be completed. The diagnosis of arteritic AION is difficult to sustain in the face of a negative temporal artery biopsy, but such cases do occur

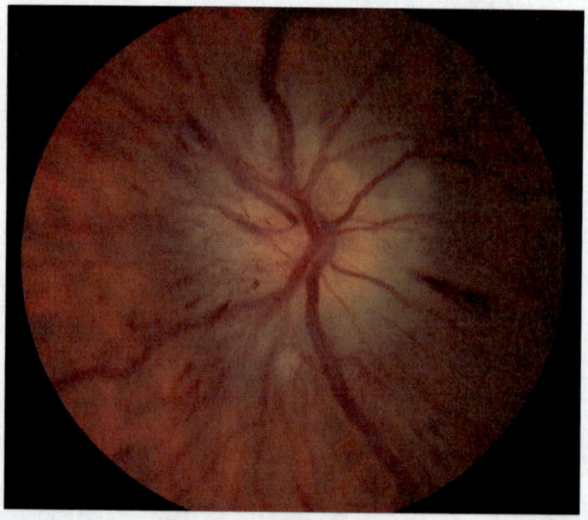

FIGURE 39-9 Anterior ischemic optic neuropathy from temporal arteritis in a 67-year-old woman with acute disc swelling, splinter hemorrhages, visual loss, and an erythrocyte sedimentation rate of 70 mm/h.

rarely. It is important to biopsy an arterial segment of at least 3 cm and to examine a sufficient number of tissue sections prepared from the specimen.

Posterior Ischemic Optic Neuropathy This is an uncommon cause of acute visual loss, induced by the combination of severe anemia and hypotension. Cases have been reported after major blood loss during surgery (especially in patients undergoing cardiac or lumbar spine operations), exsanguinating trauma, gastrointestinal bleeding, and renal dialysis. The fundus usually appears normal, although optic disc swelling develops if the process extends anteriorly far enough to reach the globe. Vision can be salvaged in some patients by prompt blood transfusion and reversal of hypotension.

Optic Neuritis This is a common inflammatory disease of the optic nerve. In the Optic Neuritis Treatment Trial (ONTT), the mean age of patients was 32 years, 77% were female, 92% had ocular pain (especially with eye movements), and 35% had optic disc swelling. In most patients, the demyelinating event was retrobulbar and the ocular fundus appeared normal on initial examination (Fig. 39-10), although optic disc pallor slowly developed over subsequent months.

Virtually all patients experience a gradual recovery of vision after a single episode of optic neuritis, even without treatment. This rule is so reliable that failure of vision to improve after a first attack of optic neuritis casts doubt on the original diagnosis. Treatment with high-dose IV methylprednisolone (250 mg every 6 h for 3 days) followed by oral prednisone (1 mg/kg per day for 11 days) makes no difference in ultimate acuity 6 months after the attack, but the recovery of visual function occurs more rapidly. Therefore, when visual loss is severe (worse than 20/100), IV followed by PO glucocorticoids are often recommended.

For some patients, optic neuritis remains an isolated event. However, the ONTT showed that the 15-year cumulative probability of developing clinically definite multiple sclerosis after optic neuritis is 50%. A brain magnetic resonance (MR) scan is advisable in every patient with a first attack of optic neuritis. If two or more plaques are present on initial imaging, treatment should be considered to prevent the development of additional demyelinating lesions (Chap. 458).

LEBER'S HEREDITARY OPTIC NEUROPATHY

This disease usually affects young men, causing gradual, painless, severe central visual loss in one eye, followed weeks to years later by the same process in the other eye. Acutely, the optic disc appears mildly plethoric with surface capillary telangiectasias but no vascular leakage on fluorescein angiography. Eventually optic atrophy ensues. Leber's optic neuropathy is caused by a point mutation at codon 11778 in the mitochondrial gene encoding nicotinamide adenine dinucleotide

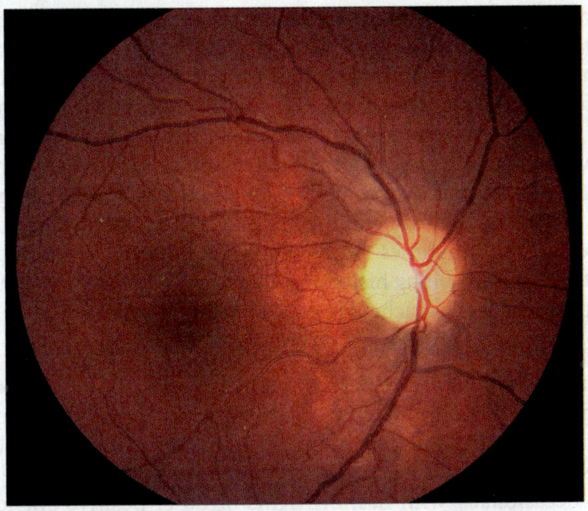

FIGURE 39-11 Optic atrophy is not a specific diagnosis but refers to the combination of optic disc pallor, arteriolar narrowing, and nerve fiber layer destruction produced by a host of eye diseases, especially optic neuropathies.

dehydrogenase (NADH) subunit 4. Additional mutations responsible for the disease have been identified, most in mitochondrial genes that encode proteins involved in electron transport. Mitochondrial mutations that cause Leber's neuropathy are inherited from the mother by all her children, but usually only sons develop symptoms.

Toxic Optic Neuropathy This can result in acute visual loss with bilateral optic disc swelling and central or cecocentral scotomas. Such cases have been reported to result from exposure to ethambutol, methyl alcohol (moonshine), ethylene glycol (antifreeze), or carbon monoxide. In toxic optic neuropathy, visual loss also can develop gradually and produce optic atrophy (Fig. 39-11) without a phase of acute optic disc edema. Many agents have been implicated as a cause of toxic optic neuropathy, but the evidence supporting the association for many is weak. The following is a partial list of potential offending drugs or toxins: disulfiram, ethchlorvynol, chloramphenicol, amiodarone, monoclonal anti-CD3 antibody, ciprofloxacin, digitalis, streptomycin, lead, arsenic, thallium, D-penicillamine, isoniazid, emetine, sildenafil, tadalafil, vardenafil, and sulfonamides. Deficiency states induced by starvation, malabsorption, or alcoholism can lead to insidious visual loss. Thiamine, vitamin B_{12}, and folate levels should be checked in any patient with unexplained bilateral central scotomas and optic pallor.

Papilledema This connotes bilateral optic disc swelling from raised intracranial pressure (Fig. 39-12). Headache is a common but not invariable accompaniment. All other forms of optic disc swelling (e.g., from optic neuritis or ischemic optic neuropathy) should be called "optic disc edema". This convention is arbitrary but serves to avoid confusion. Often it is difficult to differentiate papilledema from other forms of optic disc edema by fundus examination alone. Transient visual obscurations are a classic symptom of papilledema. They can occur in only one eye or simultaneously in both eyes. They usually last seconds but can persist longer. Obscurations follow abrupt shifts in posture or happen spontaneously. When obscurations are prolonged or spontaneous, the papilledema is more threatening. Visual acuity is not affected by papilledema unless the papilledema is severe, long-standing, or accompanied by macular edema and hemorrhage. Visual field testing shows enlarged blind spots and peripheral constriction (Fig. 39-3*F*). With unremitting papilledema, peripheral visual field loss progresses in an insidious fashion while the optic nerve develops atrophy. In this setting, reduction of optic disc swelling is an ominous sign of a dying nerve rather than an encouraging indication of resolving papilledema.

Evaluation of papilledema requires neuroimaging to exclude an intracranial lesion. MR angiography is appropriate in selected cases to search for a dural venous sinus occlusion or an arteriovenous shunt. If neuroradiologic studies are negative, the subarachnoid opening pressure should be measured by lumbar puncture. An elevated pressure, with normal cerebrospinal fluid, points by exclusion to the diagnosis of *pseudotumor cerebri* (idiopathic intracranial hypertension). The majority of patients are young, female, and obese. Treatment with a carbonic anhydrase inhibitor such as acetazolamide lowers intracranial pressure by reducing the production of cerebrospinal fluid. Weight reduction is vital: bariatric surgery should be considered in patients who cannot lose weight by diet control. If vision loss is severe or progressive, a shunt should be performed without delay to prevent blindness. Occasionally, emergency surgery is required for sudden blindness caused by fulminant papilledema.

Optic Disc Drusen These are refractile deposits within the substance of the optic nerve head (Fig. 39-13). They are unrelated to drusen of the retina, which occur in age-related macular degeneration. Optic disc drusen are most common in people of northern European descent. Their diagnosis is obvious when they are visible as glittering particles on the surface of the optic disc. However, in many patients they are hidden beneath the surface, producing pseudopapilledema. It is important to recognize optic disc drusen to avoid an unnecessary evaluation for papilledema. Ultrasound or computed tomography (CT) scanning is sensitive for detection of buried optic disc drusen because they contain calcium. In most patients, optic disc drusen are an incidental, innocuous finding, but they can produce visual obscurations. On perimetry they give rise to enlarged blind spots and arcuate

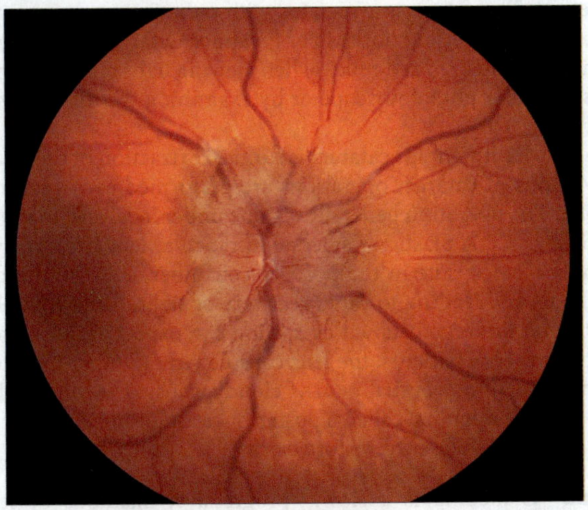

FIGURE 39-12 Papilledema means optic disc edema from raised intracranial pressure. This young woman developed acute papilledema, with hemorrhages and cotton-wool spots, as a rare side effect of treatment with tetracycline for acne.

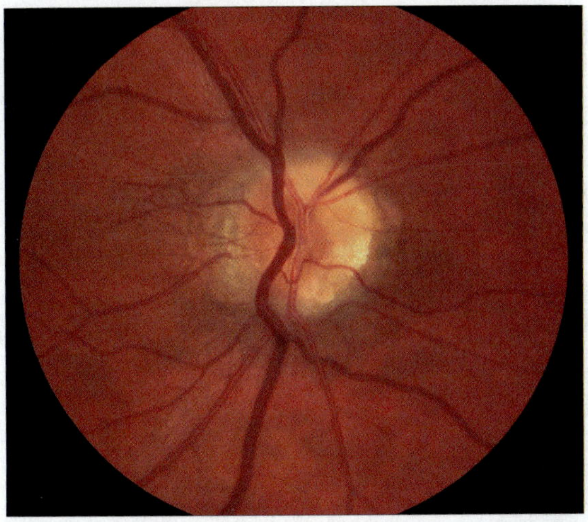

FIGURE 39-13 Optic disc drusen are calcified, mulberry-like deposits of unknown etiology within the optic disc, giving rise to "pseudopapilledema."

scotomas from damage to the optic disc. With increasing age, drusen tend to become more exposed on the disc surface as optic atrophy develops. Hemorrhage, choroidal neovascular membrane, and AION are more likely to occur in patients with optic disc drusen. No treatment is available.

Vitreous Degeneration This occurs in all individuals with advancing age, leading to visual symptoms. Opacities develop in the vitreous, casting annoying shadows on the retina. As the eye moves, these distracting "floaters" move synchronously, with a slight lag caused by inertia of the vitreous gel. Vitreous traction on the retina causes mechanical stimulation, resulting in perception of flashing lights. This photopsia is brief and is confined to one eye, in contrast to the bilateral, prolonged scintillations of cortical migraine. Contraction of the vitreous can result in sudden separation from the retina, heralded by an alarming shower of floaters and photopsia. This process, known as *vitreous detachment*, is a common involutional event in the elderly. It is not harmful unless it damages the retina. A careful examination of the dilated fundus is important in any patient complaining of floaters or photopsia to search for peripheral tears or holes. If such a lesion is found, laser application can forestall a retinal detachment. Occasionally a tear ruptures a retinal blood vessel, causing vitreous hemorrhage and sudden loss of vision. On attempted ophthalmoscopy the fundus is hidden by a dark haze of blood. Ultrasound is required to examine the interior of the eye for a retinal tear or detachment. If the hemorrhage does not resolve spontaneously, the vitreous can be removed surgically. Vitreous hemorrhage also results from the fragile neovascular vessels that proliferate on the surface of the retina in diabetes, sickle cell anemia, and other ischemic ocular diseases.

Retinal Detachment This produces symptoms of floaters, flashing lights, and a scotoma in the peripheral visual field corresponding to the detachment (Fig. 39-14). If the detachment includes the fovea, there is an afferent pupil defect and the visual acuity is reduced. In most eyes, retinal detachment starts with a hole, flap, or tear in the peripheral retina (rhegmatogenous retinal detachment). Patients with peripheral retinal thinning (lattice degeneration) are particularly vulnerable to this process. Once a break has developed in the retina, liquefied vitreous is free to enter the subretinal space, separating the retina from the pigment epithelium. The combination of vitreous traction on the retinal surface and passage of fluid behind the retina leads inexorably to detachment. Patients with a history of myopia, trauma, or prior cataract extraction are at greatest risk for retinal detachment. The diagnosis is confirmed by ophthalmoscopic examination of the dilated eye.

Classic Migraine (See also Chap. 447) This usually occurs with a visual aura lasting about 20 min. In a typical attack, a small central disturbance in the field of vision marches toward the periphery, leaving a transient scotoma in its wake. The expanding border of migraine scotoma has a scintillating, dancing, or zigzag edge, resembling the bastions of a fortified city, hence the term *fortification spectra*. Patients' descriptions of fortification spectra vary widely and can be confused with amaurosis fugax. Migraine patterns usually last longer and are perceived in both eyes, whereas amaurosis fugax is briefer and occurs in only one eye. Migraine phenomena also remain visible in the dark or with the eyes closed. Generally they are confined to either the right or the left visual hemifield, but sometimes both fields are involved simultaneously. Patients often have a long history of stereotypic attacks. After the visual symptoms recede, headache develops in most patients.

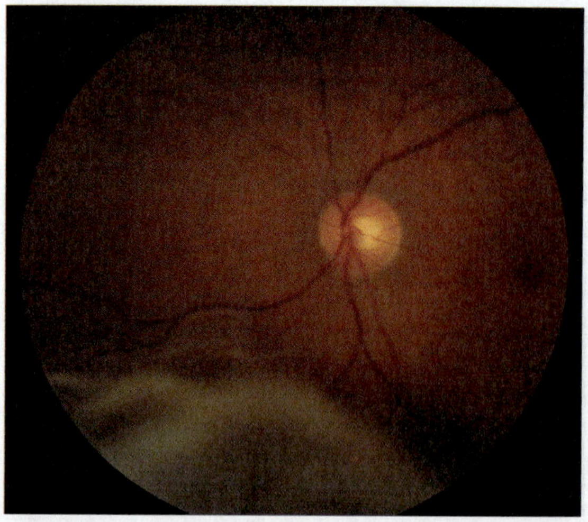

FIGURE 39-14 **Retinal detachment** appears as an elevated sheet of retinal tissue with folds. In this patient, the fovea was spared, so acuity was normal, but an inferior detachment produced a superior scotoma.

Transient Ischemic Attacks Vertebrobasilar insufficiency may result in acute homonymous visual symptoms. Many patients mistakenly describe symptoms in the left or right eye when in fact the symptoms are occurring in the left or right hemifield of both eyes. Interruption of blood supply to the visual cortex causes a sudden fogging or graying of vision, occasionally with flashing lights or other positive phenomena that mimic migraine. Cortical ischemic attacks are briefer in duration than migraine, occur in older patients, and are not followed by headache. There may be associated signs of brainstem ischemia, such as diplopia, vertigo, numbness, weakness, and dysarthria.

Stroke Stroke occurs when interruption of blood supply from the posterior cerebral artery to the visual cortex is prolonged. The only finding on examination is a homonymous visual field defect that stops abruptly at the vertical meridian. Occipital lobe stroke usually is due to thrombotic occlusion of the vertebrobasilar system, embolus, or dissection. Lobar hemorrhage, tumor, abscess, and arteriovenous malformation are other common causes of hemianopic cortical visual loss.

Factitious (Functional, Nonorganic) Visual Loss This is claimed by hysterics or malingerers. The latter account for the vast majority, seeking sympathy, special treatment, or financial gain by feigning loss of sight. The diagnosis is suspected when the history is atypical, physical findings are lacking or contradictory, inconsistencies emerge on testing, and a secondary motive can be identified. In our litigious society, the fraudulent pursuit of recompense has spawned an epidemic of factitious visual loss.

CHRONIC VISUAL LOSS

Cataract Cataract is a clouding of the lens sufficient to reduce vision. Most cataracts develop slowly as a result of aging, leading to gradual impairment of vision. The formation of cataract occurs more rapidly in patients with a history of ocular trauma, uveitis, or diabetes mellitus. Cataracts are acquired in a variety of genetic diseases, such as myotonic dystrophy, neurofibromatosis type 2, and galactosemia. Radiation therapy and glucocorticoid treatment can induce cataract as a side effect. The cataracts associated with radiation or glucocorticoids have a typical posterior subcapsular location. Cataract can be detected by noting an impaired red reflex when viewing light reflected from the fundus with an ophthalmoscope or by examining the dilated eye with the slit lamp.

The only treatment for cataract is surgical extraction of the opacified lens. Millions of cataract operations are performed each year around the globe. The operation generally is done under local anesthesia on an outpatient basis. A plastic or silicone intraocular lens is placed within the empty lens capsule in the posterior chamber, substituting for the natural lens and leading to rapid recovery of sight. More than 95% of patients who undergo cataract extraction can expect an improvement in vision. In some patients, the lens capsule remaining in the eye after cataract extraction eventually turns cloudy, causing secondary loss of vision. A small opening, called a posterior capsulotomy, is made in the lens capsule with a laser to restore clarity.

Glaucoma Glaucoma is a slowly progressive, insidious optic neuropathy that usually is associated with chronic elevation of intraocular pressure. After cataract, it is the most common cause of blindness in the world. It is especially prevalent in people of African descent. The mechanism by which raised intraocular pressure injures the optic

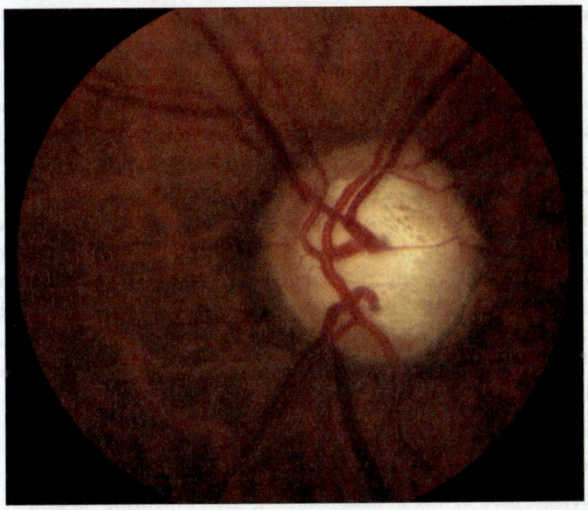

FIGURE 39-15 Glaucoma results in "cupping" as the neural rim is destroyed and the central cup becomes enlarged and excavated. The cup-to-disc ratio is about 0.8 in this patient.

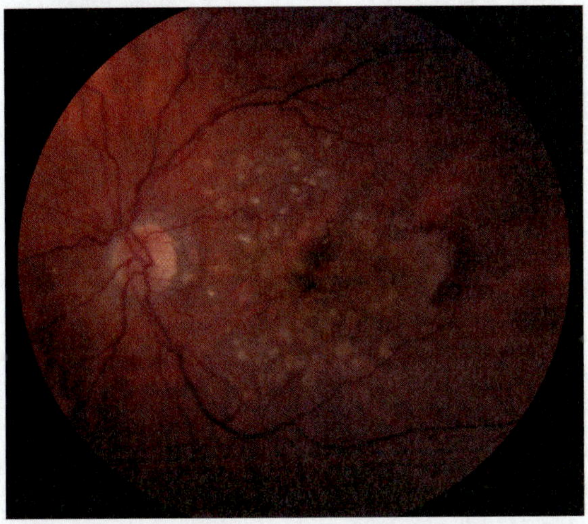

FIGURE 39-16 Age-related macular degeneration consisting of scattered yellow drusen in the macula (dry form) and a crescent of fresh hemorrhage temporal to the fovea from a subretinal neovascular membrane (wet form).

nerve is not understood. Axons entering the inferotemporal and superotemporal aspects of the optic disc are damaged first, producing typical nerve fiber bundle or arcuate scotomas on perimetric testing. As fibers are destroyed, the neural rim of the optic disc shrinks and the physiologic cup within the optic disc enlarges (Fig. 39-15). This process is referred to as pathologic "cupping." The cup-to-disc diameter is expressed as a fraction (e.g., 0.2). The cup-to-disc ratio ranges widely in normal individuals, making it difficult to diagnose glaucoma reliably simply by observing an unusually large or deep optic cup. Careful documentation of serial examinations is helpful. In a patient with physiologic cupping the large cup remains stable, whereas in a patient with glaucoma it expands relentlessly over the years. Observation of progressive cupping and detection of an arcuate scotoma or a nasal step on computerized visual field testing is sufficient to establish the diagnosis of glaucoma. Optical coherence tomography reveals corresponding loss of fibers along the arcuate pathways in the nerve fiber layer.

About 95% of patients with glaucoma have open anterior chamber angles. In most affected individuals the intraocular pressure is elevated. The cause of elevated intraocular pressure is unknown, but it is associated with gene mutations in the heritable forms. Surprisingly, a third of patients with open-angle glaucoma have an intraocular pressure within the normal range of 10–20 mmHg. For this so-called normal or low-tension form of glaucoma, high myopia is a risk factor.

Chronic angle-closure glaucoma and chronic open-angle glaucoma are usually asymptomatic. Only acute angle-closure glaucoma causes a red or painful eye, from abrupt elevation of intraocular pressure. In all forms of glaucoma, foveal acuity is spared until end-stage disease is reached. For these reasons, severe and irreversible damage can occur before either the patient or the physician recognizes the diagnosis. Screening of patients for glaucoma by noting the cup-to-disc ratio on ophthalmoscopy and by measuring intraocular pressure is vital. Glaucoma is treated with topical adrenergic agonists, cholinergic agonists, beta blockers, and prostaglandin analogues. Occasionally, systemic absorption of beta blocker from eyedrops can be sufficient to cause side effects of bradycardia, hypotension, heart block, bronchospasm, or depression. Topical or oral carbonic anhydrase inhibitors are used to lower intraocular pressure by reducing aqueous production. Laser treatment of the trabecular meshwork in the anterior chamber angle improves aqueous outflow from the eye. If medical or laser treatments fail to halt optic nerve damage from glaucoma, a filter must be constructed surgically (trabeculectomy) or a drainage device placed to release aqueous from the eye in a controlled fashion.

Macular Degeneration This is a major cause of gradual, painless, bilateral central visual loss in the elderly. It occurs in a nonexudative (dry) form and an exudative (wet) form. Inflammation may be important in both forms of macular degeneration; susceptibility is associated with variants in the gene for complement factor H, an inhibitor of the alternative complement pathway. The nonexudative process begins with the accumulation of extracellular deposits called drusen underneath the retinal pigment epithelium. On ophthalmoscopy, they are pleomorphic but generally appear as small discrete yellow lesions clustered in the macula (Fig. 39-16). With time they become larger, more numerous, and confluent. The retinal pigment epithelium becomes focally detached and atrophic, causing visual loss by interfering with photoreceptor function. Treatment with vitamins C and E, beta-carotene, and zinc may retard dry macular degeneration.

Exudative macular degeneration, which develops in only a minority of patients, occurs when neovascular vessels from the choroid grow through defects in Bruch's membrane and proliferate underneath the retinal pigment epithelium or the retina. Leakage from these vessels produces elevation of the retina, with distortion (metamorphopsia) and blurring of vision. Although the onset of these symptoms is usually gradual, bleeding from a subretinal choroidal neovascular membrane sometimes causes acute visual loss. Neovascular membranes can be difficult to see on fundus examination because they are located beneath the retina. Fluorescein angiography and optical coherence tomography, a technique for acquiring images of the retina in cross-section, are extremely useful for their detection. Major or repeated hemorrhage under the retina from neovascular membranes results in fibrosis, development of a round (disciform) macular scar, and permanent loss of central vision.

A major therapeutic advance has occurred with the discovery that exudative macular degeneration can be treated with intraocular injection of antagonists to vascular endothelial growth factor. Bevacizumab, ranibizumab, or aflibercept is administered by direct injection into the vitreous cavity, beginning on a monthly basis. These antibodies cause the regression of neovascular membranes by blocking the action of vascular endothelial growth factor, thereby improving visual acuity.

Central Serous Chorioretinopathy This primarily affects males between the ages of 20 and 50 years. Leakage of serous fluid from the choroid causes small, localized detachment of the retinal pigment epithelium and the neurosensory retina. These detachments produce acute or chronic symptoms of metamorphopsia and blurred vision when the macula is involved. They are difficult to visualize with a direct ophthalmoscope because the detached retina is transparent and only slightly elevated. Optical coherence tomography shows fluid beneath the retina, and fluorescein angiography shows dye streaming into the subretinal space. The cause of central serous chorioretinopathy is unknown. Symptoms may resolve spontaneously if the retina reattaches, but recurrent detachment is common. Laser photocoagulation has benefited some patients with this condition.

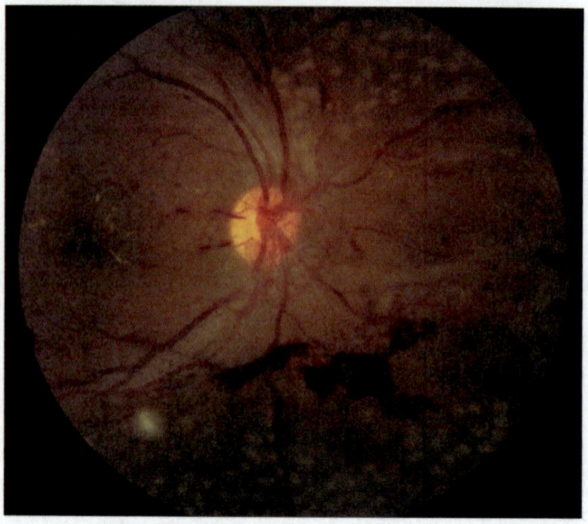

FIGURE 39-17 Proliferative diabetic retinopathy in a 25-year-old man with an 18-year history of diabetes, showing neovascular vessels emanating from the optic disc, retinal and vitreous hemorrhage, cotton-wool spots, and macular exudate. Round spots in the periphery represent recently applied panretinal photocoagulation.

Diabetic Retinopathy A rare disease until 1921, when the discovery of insulin resulted in a dramatic improvement in life expectancy for patients with diabetes mellitus, diabetic retinopathy is now a leading cause of blindness in the United States. The retinopathy takes years to develop but eventually appears in nearly all cases. Regular surveillance of the dilated fundus is crucial for any patient with diabetes. In advanced diabetic retinopathy, the proliferation of neovascular vessels leads to blindness from vitreous hemorrhage, retinal detachment, and glaucoma (Fig. 39-17). These complications can be avoided in most patients by administration of panretinal laser photocoagulation at the appropriate point in the evolution of the disease. **For further discussion of the manifestations and management of diabetic retinopathy, see Chaps. 417–419.**

Retinitis Pigmentosa This is a general term for a disparate group of rod-cone dystrophies characterized by progressive night blindness, visual field constriction with a ring scotoma, loss of acuity, and an abnormal electroretinogram (ERG). It occurs sporadically or in an autosomal recessive, dominant, or X-linked pattern. Irregular black deposits of clumped pigment in the peripheral retina, called *bone spicules* because of their vague resemblance to the spicules of cancellous bone, give the disease its name (Fig. 39-18). The name is actually a misnomer because retinitis pigmentosa is not an inflammatory process. Most cases are due to a mutation in the gene for rhodopsin, the rod photopigment, or in the gene for peripherin, a glycoprotein located in photoreceptor outer segments. Vitamin A (15,000 IU/d) slightly retards the deterioration of the ERG in patients with retinitis pigmentosa but has no beneficial effect on visual acuity or fields.

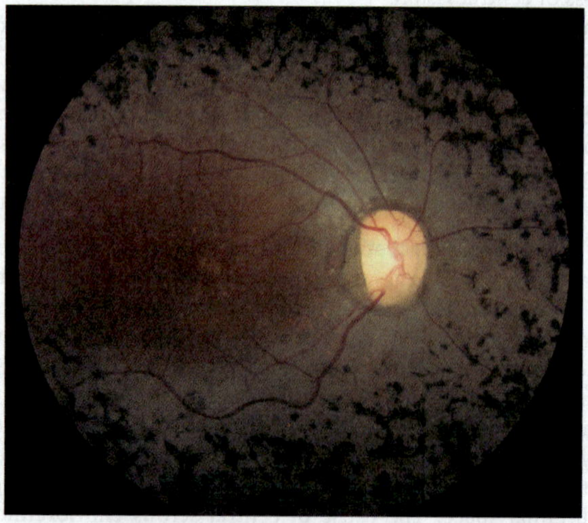

FIGURE 39-18 Retinitis pigmentosa with black clumps of pigment known as "bone spicules." The patient had peripheral visual field loss with sparing of central (macular) vision.

Leber's congenital amaurosis, a rare cone dystrophy, has been treated by replacement of the missing RPE65 protein through gene therapy, resulting in modest improvement in visual function. Some forms of retinitis pigmentosa occur in association with rare, hereditary systemic diseases (olivopontocerebellar degeneration, Bassen-Kornzweig disease, Kearns-Sayre syndrome, Refsum's disease). Chronic treatment with chloroquine, hydroxychloroquine, and phenothiazines (especially thioridazine) can produce visual loss from a toxic retinopathy that resembles retinitis pigmentosa.

Epiretinal Membrane This is a fibrocellular tissue that grows across the inner surface of the retina, causing metamorphopsia and reduced visual acuity from distortion of the macula. A crinkled, cellophane-like membrane is visible on the retinal examination. Epiretinal membrane is most common in patients over 50 years of age and is usually unilateral. Most cases are idiopathic, but some occur as a result of hypertensive retinopathy, diabetes, retinal detachment, or trauma. When visual acuity is reduced to the level of about 6/24 (20/80), vitrectomy and surgical peeling of the membrane to relieve macular puckering are recommended. Contraction of an epiretinal membrane sometimes gives rise to a *macular hole*. Most macular holes, however, are caused by local vitreous traction within the fovea. Vitrectomy can improve acuity in selected cases.

Melanoma and Other Tumors Melanoma is the most common primary tumor of the eye (Fig. 39-19). It causes photopsia, an enlarging scotoma, and loss of vision. A small melanoma is often difficult to differentiate from a benign choroidal nevus. Serial examinations are required to document a malignant pattern of growth. Treatment of melanoma is controversial. Options include enucleation, local resection, and irradiation. *Metastatic tumors* to the eye outnumber primary tumors. Breast and lung carcinomas have a special propensity to spread to the choroid or iris. Leukemia and lymphoma also commonly invade ocular tissues. Sometimes their only sign on eye examination is cellular debris in the vitreous, which can masquerade as a chronic posterior uveitis. *Retrobulbar tumor* of the optic nerve (meningioma, glioma) or *chiasmal tumor* (pituitary adenoma, meningioma) produces

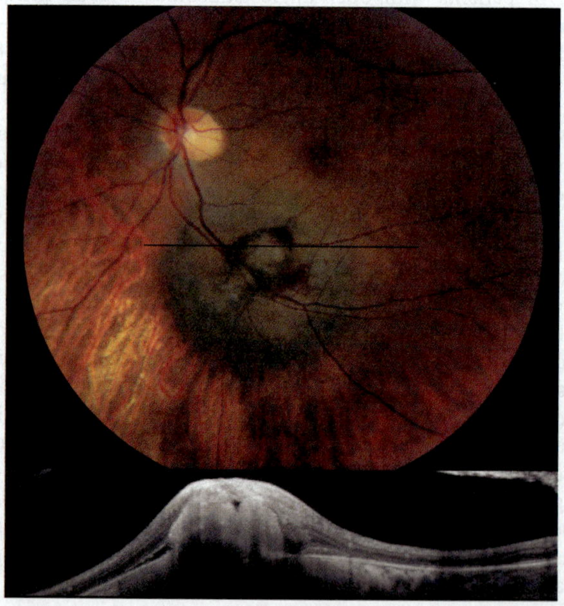

FIGURE 39-19 Melanoma of the choroid, appearing as an elevated dark mass in the inferior fundus, with overlying hemorrhage. The black line denotes the plane of the optical coherence tomography scan (*below*) showing the subretinal tumor.

gradual visual loss with few objective findings except for optic disc pallor. Rarely, sudden expansion of a pituitary adenoma from infarction and bleeding (*pituitary apoplexy*) causes acute retrobulbar visual loss, with headache, nausea, and ocular motor nerve palsies. In any patient with visual field loss or optic atrophy, CT or MR scanning should be considered if the cause remains unknown after careful review of the history and thorough examination of the eye.

PROPTOSIS

When the globes appear asymmetric, the clinician must first decide which eye is abnormal. Is one eye recessed within the orbit (*enophthalmos*), or is the other eye protuberant (*exophthalmos*, or *proptosis*)? A small globe or a Horner's syndrome can give the appearance of enophthalmos. True enophthalmos occurs commonly after trauma, from atrophy of retrobulbar fat, or from fracture of the orbital floor. The position of the eyes within the orbits is measured by using a Hertel exophthalmometer, a handheld instrument that records the position of the anterior corneal surface relative to the lateral orbital rim. If this instrument is not available, relative eye position can be judged by bending the patient's head forward and looking down upon the orbits. A proptosis of only 2 mm in one eye is detectable from this perspective. The development of proptosis implies a space-occupying lesion in the orbit and usually warrants CT or MR imaging.

Graves' Ophthalmopathy This is the leading cause of proptosis in adults (Chap. 405). The proptosis is often asymmetric and can even appear to be unilateral. Orbital inflammation and engorgement of the extraocular muscles, particularly the medial rectus and the inferior rectus, account for the protrusion of the globe. Corneal exposure, lid retraction, conjunctival injection, restriction of gaze, diplopia, and visual loss from optic nerve compression are cardinal symptoms. Graves' eye disease is a clinical diagnosis, but laboratory testing can be useful. The serum level of thyroid-stimulating immunoglobulins is often elevated. Orbital imaging usually reveals enlarged extraocular eye muscles, but not always. Graves' ophthalmopathy can be treated with oral prednisone (60 mg/d) for 1 month, followed by a taper over several months. Worsening of symptoms upon glucocorticoid withdrawal is common. Topical lubricants, taping the eyelids closed at night, moisture chambers, and eyelid surgery are helpful to limit exposure of ocular tissues. Radiation therapy is not effective. Orbital decompression should be performed for severe, symptomatic exophthalmos or if visual function is reduced by optic nerve compression. In patients with diplopia, prisms or eye muscle surgery can be used to restore ocular alignment in primary gaze.

Orbital Pseudotumor This is an idiopathic, inflammatory orbital syndrome that is distinguished from Graves' ophthalmopathy by the prominent complaint of pain. Other symptoms include diplopia, ptosis, proptosis, and orbital congestion. Evaluation for sarcoidosis, granulomatosis with polyangiitis, and other types of orbital vasculitis or collagen-vascular disease is negative. Imaging often shows swollen eye muscles (orbital myositis) with enlarged tendons. By contrast, in Graves' ophthalmopathy, the tendons of the eye muscles usually are spared. The Tolosa-Hunt syndrome (Chap. 455) may be regarded as an extension of orbital pseudotumor through the superior orbital fissure into the cavernous sinus. The diagnosis of orbital pseudotumor is difficult. Biopsy of the orbit frequently yields nonspecific evidence of fat infiltration by lymphocytes, plasma cells, and eosinophils. A dramatic response to a therapeutic trial of systemic glucocorticoids indirectly provides the best confirmation of the diagnosis.

Orbital Cellulitis This causes pain, lid erythema, proptosis, conjunctival chemosis, restricted motility, decreased acuity, afferent pupillary defect, fever, and leukocytosis. It often arises from the paranasal sinuses, especially by contiguous spread of infection from the ethmoid sinus through the lamina papyracea of the medial orbit. A history of recent upper respiratory tract infection, chronic sinusitis, thick mucus secretions, or dental disease is significant in any patient with suspected orbital cellulitis. Blood cultures should be obtained, but they are usually negative. Most patients respond to empirical therapy with broad-spectrum IV antibiotics. Occasionally, orbital cellulitis follows an overwhelming course, with massive proptosis, blindness, septic cavernous sinus thrombosis, and meningitis. To avert this disaster, orbital cellulitis should be managed aggressively in the early stages, with immediate imaging of the orbits and antibiotic therapy that includes coverage of methicillin-resistant *Staphylococcus aureus* (MRSA). Prompt surgical drainage of an orbital abscess or paranasal sinusitis is indicated if optic nerve function deteriorates despite antibiotics.

Tumors Tumors of the orbit cause painless, progressive proptosis. The most common primary tumors are cavernous hemangioma, lymphangioma, neurofibroma, schwannoma, dermoid cyst, adenoid cystic carcinoma, optic nerve glioma, optic nerve meningioma, and benign mixed tumor of the lacrimal gland. Metastatic tumor to the orbit occurs frequently in breast carcinoma, lung carcinoma, and lymphoma. Diagnosis by fine-needle aspiration followed by urgent radiation therapy sometimes can preserve vision.

Carotid Cavernous Fistulas With anterior drainage through the orbit, these fistulas produce proptosis, diplopia, glaucoma, and corkscrew, arterialized conjunctival vessels. Direct fistulas usually result from trauma. They are easily diagnosed because of the prominent signs produced by high-flow, high-pressure shunting. Indirect fistulas, or dural arteriovenous malformations, are more likely to occur spontaneously, especially in older women. The signs are more subtle, and the diagnosis frequently is missed. The combination of slight proptosis, diplopia, enlarged muscles, and an injected eye often is mistaken for thyroid ophthalmopathy. A bruit heard upon auscultation of the head or reported by the patient is a valuable diagnostic clue. Imaging shows an enlarged superior ophthalmic vein in the orbits. Carotid cavernous shunts can be eliminated by intravascular embolization.

PTOSIS

Blepharoptosis This is an abnormal drooping of the eyelid. Unilateral or bilateral ptosis can be congenital, from dysgenesis of the levator palpebrae superioris, or from abnormal insertion of its aponeurosis into the eyelid. Acquired ptosis can develop so gradually that the patient is unaware of the problem. Inspection of old photographs is helpful in dating the onset. A history of prior trauma, eye surgery, contact lens use, diplopia, systemic symptoms (e.g., dysphagia or peripheral muscle weakness), or a family history of ptosis should be sought. Fluctuating ptosis that worsens late in the day is typical of myasthenia gravis. Examination should focus on evidence for proptosis, eyelid masses or deformities, inflammation, pupil inequality, or limitation of motility. The width of the palpebral fissures is measured in primary gaze to determine the degree of ptosis. The ptosis will be underestimated if the patient compensates by lifting the brow with the frontalis muscle.

Mechanical Ptosis This occurs in many elderly patients from stretching and redundancy of eyelid skin and subcutaneous fat (dermatochalasis). The extra weight of these sagging tissues causes the lid to droop. Enlargement or deformation of the eyelid from infection, tumor, trauma, or inflammation also results in ptosis on a purely mechanical basis.

Aponeurotic Ptosis This is an acquired dehiscence or stretching of the aponeurotic tendon, which connects the levator muscle to the tarsal plate of the eyelid. It occurs commonly in older patients, presumably from loss of connective tissue elasticity. Aponeurotic ptosis is also a common sequela of eyelid swelling from infection or blunt trauma to the orbit, cataract surgery, or contact lens use.

Myogenic Ptosis The causes of *myogenic ptosis* include myasthenia gravis (Chap. 461) and a number of rare myopathies that manifest with ptosis. The term *chronic progressive external ophthalmoplegia* refers to a spectrum of systemic diseases caused by mutations of mitochondrial DNA. As the name implies, the most prominent findings are symmetric, slowly progressive ptosis and limitation of eye movements. In general, diplopia is a late symptom because all eye movements are reduced equally. In the *Kearns-Sayre* variant, retinal pigmentary changes and abnormalities of cardiac conduction develop.

Peripheral muscle biopsy shows characteristic "ragged-red fibers." *Oculopharyngeal dystrophy* is a distinct autosomal dominant disease with onset in middle age, characterized by ptosis, limited eye movements, and trouble swallowing. *Myotonic dystrophy*, another autosomal dominant disorder, causes ptosis, ophthalmoparesis, cataract, and pigmentary retinopathy. Patients have muscle wasting, myotonia, frontal balding, and cardiac abnormalities.

Neurogenic Ptosis This results from a lesion affecting the innervation to either of the two muscles that open the eyelid: Müller's muscle or the levator palpebrae superioris. Examination of the pupil helps distinguish between these two possibilities. In Horner's syndrome, the eye with ptosis has a smaller pupil and the eye movements are full. In an oculomotor nerve palsy, the eye with the ptosis has a larger or a normal pupil. If the pupil is normal but there is limitation of adduction, elevation, and depression, a pupil-sparing oculomotor nerve palsy is likely (see next section). Rarely, a lesion affecting the small, central subnucleus of the oculomotor complex will cause bilateral ptosis with normal eye movements and pupils.

DOUBLE VISION (DIPLOPIA)

The first point to clarify is whether diplopia persists in either eye after the opposite eye is covered. If it does, the diagnosis is monocular diplopia. The cause is usually intrinsic to the eye and therefore has no dire implications for the patient. Corneal aberrations (e.g., keratoconus, pterygium), uncorrected refractive error, cataract, or foveal traction may give rise to monocular diplopia. Occasionally it is a symptom of malingering or psychiatric disease. Diplopia alleviated by covering one eye is binocular diplopia and is caused by disruption of ocular alignment. Inquiry should be made into the nature of the double vision (purely side-by-side versus partial vertical displacement of images), mode of onset, duration, intermittency, diurnal variation, and associated neurologic or systemic symptoms. If the patient has diplopia while being examined, motility testing should reveal a deficiency corresponding to the patient's symptoms. However, subtle limitation of ocular excursions is often difficult to detect. For example, a patient with a slight left abducens nerve paresis may appear to have full eye movements despite a complaint of horizontal diplopia upon looking to the left. In this situation, the cover test provides a more sensitive method for demonstrating the ocular misalignment. It should be conducted in primary gaze and then with the head turned and tilted in each direction. In the above example, a cover test with the head turned to the right will maximize the fixation shift evoked by the cover test.

Occasionally, a cover test performed in an asymptomatic patient during a routine examination will reveal an ocular deviation. If the eye movements are full and the ocular misalignment is equal in all directions of gaze (concomitant deviation), the diagnosis is strabismus. In this condition, which affects about 1% of the population, fusion is disrupted in infancy or early childhood. To avoid diplopia, vision is suppressed from the nonfixating eye. In some children, this leads to impaired vision (amblyopia, or "lazy" eye) in the deviated eye.

Binocular diplopia results from a wide range of processes: infectious, neoplastic, metabolic, degenerative, inflammatory, and vascular. One must decide whether the diplopia is neurogenic in origin or is due to restriction of globe rotation by local disease in the orbit. Orbital pseudotumor, myositis, infection, tumor, thyroid disease, and muscle entrapment (e.g., from a blowout fracture) cause restrictive diplopia. The diagnosis of restriction is usually made by recognizing other associated signs and symptoms of local orbital disease. Omission of high-resolution orbital imaging is a common mistake in the evaluation of diplopia.

Myasthenia Gravis (See also Chap. 461) This is a major cause of diplopia. The diplopia is often intermittent, variable, and not confined to any single ocular motor nerve distribution. The pupils are always normal. Fluctuating ptosis may be present. Many patients have a purely ocular form of the disease, with no evidence of systemic muscular weakness. The diagnosis can be confirmed by an IV edrophonium injection, which produces a transient reversal of eyelid or eye muscle weakness. Blood tests for antibodies against the acetylcholine receptor or the MuSK protein can establish the diagnosis but are frequently negative in the purely ocular form of myasthenia gravis. *Botulism* from food or wound poisoning can mimic ocular myasthenia.

After restrictive orbital disease and myasthenia gravis are excluded, a lesion of a cranial nerve supplying innervation to the extraocular muscles is the most likely cause of binocular diplopia.

Oculomotor Nerve The third cranial nerve innervates the medial, inferior, and superior recti; inferior oblique; levator palpebrae superioris; and the iris sphincter. Total palsy of the oculomotor nerve causes ptosis, a dilated pupil, and leaves the eye "down and out" because of the unopposed action of the lateral rectus and superior oblique. This combination of findings is obvious. More challenging is the diagnosis of early or partial oculomotor nerve palsy. In this setting any combination of ptosis, pupil dilation, and weakness of the eye muscles supplied by the oculomotor nerve may be encountered. Frequent serial examinations during the evolving phase of the palsy help ensure that the diagnosis is not missed. The advent of an oculomotor nerve palsy with a pupil involvement, especially when accompanied by pain, suggests a compressive lesion, such as a tumor or circle of Willis aneurysm. Neuroimaging should be obtained, along with a CT or MR angiogram. Occasionally, a catheter arteriogram must be done to exclude an aneurysm.

A lesion of the oculomotor nucleus in the rostral midbrain produces signs that differ from those caused by a lesion of the nerve itself. There is bilateral ptosis because the levator muscle is innervated by a single central subnucleus. There is also weakness of the contralateral superior rectus, because it is supplied by the oculomotor nucleus on the other side. Occasionally both superior recti are weak. Isolated nuclear oculomotor palsy is rare. Usually neurologic examination reveals additional signs that suggest brainstem damage from infarction, hemorrhage, tumor, or infection.

Injury to structures surrounding fascicles of the oculomotor nerve descending through the midbrain has given rise to a number of classic eponymic designations. In *Nothnagel's syndrome*, injury to the superior cerebellar peduncle causes ipsilateral oculomotor palsy and contralateral cerebellar ataxia. In *Benedikt's syndrome*, injury to the red nucleus results in ipsilateral oculomotor palsy and contralateral tremor, chorea, and athetosis. *Claude's syndrome* incorporates features of both of these syndromes, by injury to both the red nucleus and the superior cerebellar peduncle. Finally, in *Weber's syndrome*, injury to the cerebral peduncle causes ipsilateral oculomotor palsy with contralateral hemiparesis.

In the subarachnoid space the oculomotor nerve is vulnerable to aneurysm, meningitis, tumor, infarction, and compression. In cerebral herniation, the nerve becomes trapped between the edge of the tentorium and the uncus of the temporal lobe. Oculomotor palsy also can result from midbrain torsion and hemorrhages during herniation. In the cavernous sinus, oculomotor palsy arises from carotid aneurysm, carotid cavernous fistula, cavernous sinus thrombosis, tumor (pituitary adenoma, meningioma, metastasis), herpes zoster infection, and the Tolosa-Hunt syndrome.

The etiology of an isolated, pupil-sparing oculomotor palsy often remains an enigma even after neuroimaging and extensive laboratory testing. Most cases are thought to result from microvascular infarction of the nerve somewhere along its course from the brainstem to the orbit. Usually the patient complains of pain. Diabetes, hypertension, and vascular disease are major risk factors. Spontaneous recovery over a period of months is the rule. If this fails to occur or if new findings develop, the diagnosis of microvascular oculomotor nerve palsy should be reconsidered. Aberrant regeneration is common when the oculomotor nerve is injured by trauma or compression (tumor, aneurysm). Miswiring of sprouting fibers to the levator muscle and the rectus muscles results in elevation of the eyelid upon downgaze or adduction. The pupil also constricts upon attempted adduction, elevation, or depression of the globe. Aberrant regeneration is not seen after oculomotor palsy from microvascular infarct and hence vitiates that diagnosis.

Trochlear Nerve The fourth cranial nerve originates in the midbrain, just caudal to the oculomotor nerve complex. Fibers exit the brainstem dorsally and cross to innervate the contralateral superior oblique. The principal actions of this muscle are to depress and intort the globe. A palsy therefore results in hypertropia and excyclotorsion. The cyclotorsion seldom is noticed by patients. Instead, they complain of vertical diplopia, especially upon reading or looking down. The vertical diplopia also is exacerbated by tilting the head toward the side with the muscle palsy and alleviated by tilting it away. This "head tilt test" is a cardinal diagnostic feature.

Isolated trochlear nerve palsy results from all the causes listed above for the oculomotor nerve except aneurysm. The trochlear nerve is particularly apt to suffer injury after closed head trauma. The free edge of the tentorium is thought to impinge on the nerve during a concussive blow. Most isolated trochlear nerve palsies are idiopathic and hence are diagnosed by exclusion as "microvascular." Spontaneous improvement occurs over a period of months in most patients. A base-down prism (conveniently applied to the patient's glasses as a stick-on Fresnel lens) may serve as a temporary measure to alleviate diplopia. If the palsy does not resolve, the eyes can be realigned by weakening the inferior oblique muscle.

Abducens Nerve The sixth cranial nerve innervates the lateral rectus muscle. A palsy produces horizontal diplopia, worse on gaze to the side of the lesion. A nuclear lesion has different consequences, because the abducens nucleus contains interneurons that project via the medial longitudinal fasciculus to the medial rectus subnucleus of the contralateral oculomotor complex. Therefore, an abducens nuclear lesion produces a complete lateral gaze palsy from weakness of both the ipsilateral lateral rectus and the contralateral medial rectus. *Foville's syndrome* after dorsal pontine injury includes lateral gaze palsy, ipsilateral facial palsy, and contralateral hemiparesis incurred by damage to descending corticospinal fibers. *Millard-Gubler syndrome* from ventral pontine injury is similar except for the eye findings. There is lateral rectus weakness only, instead of gaze palsy, because the abducens fascicle is injured rather than the nucleus. Infarct, tumor, hemorrhage, vascular malformation, and multiple sclerosis are the most common etiologies of brainstem abducens palsy.

After leaving the ventral pons, the abducens nerve runs forward along the clivus to pierce the dura at the petrous apex, where it enters the cavernous sinus. Along its subarachnoid course it is susceptible to meningitis, tumor (meningioma, chordoma, carcinomatous meningitis), subarachnoid hemorrhage, trauma, and compression by aneurysm or dolichoectatic vessels. At the petrous apex, mastoiditis can produce deafness, pain, and ipsilateral abducens palsy (*Gradenigo's syndrome*). In the cavernous sinus, the nerve can be affected by carotid aneurysm, carotid cavernous fistula, tumor (pituitary adenoma, meningioma, nasopharyngeal carcinoma), herpes infection, and Tolosa-Hunt syndrome.

Unilateral or bilateral abducens palsy is a classic sign of raised intracranial pressure. The diagnosis can be confirmed if papilledema is observed on fundus examination. The mechanism is still debated but probably is related to rostral-caudal displacement of the brainstem. The same phenomenon accounts for abducens palsy from Chiari malformation or low intracranial pressure (e.g., after lumbar puncture, spinal anesthesia, or spontaneous dural cerebrospinal fluid leak).

Treatment of abducens palsy is aimed at prompt correction of the underlying cause. However, the cause remains obscure in many instances despite diligent evaluation. As was mentioned above for isolated trochlear or oculomotor palsy, most cases are assumed to represent microvascular infarcts because they often occur in the setting of diabetes or other vascular risk factors. Some cases may develop as a postinfectious mononeuritis (e.g., after a viral flu). Patching one eye, occluding one eyeglass lens with tape, or applying a temporary prism will provide relief of diplopia until the palsy resolves. If recovery is incomplete, eye muscle surgery nearly always can realign the eyes, at least in primary position. A patient with an abducens palsy that fails to improve should be reevaluated for an occult etiology (e.g., chordoma, carcinomatous meningitis, carotid cavernous fistula, myasthenia gravis). Skull base tumors are easily missed even on contrast-enhanced neuroimaging studies.

Multiple Ocular Motor Nerve Palsies These should not be attributed to spontaneous microvascular events affecting more than one cranial nerve at a time. This remarkable coincidence does occur, especially in diabetic patients, but the diagnosis is made only in retrospect after all other diagnostic alternatives have been exhausted. Neuroimaging should focus on the cavernous sinus, superior orbital fissure, and orbital apex, where all three ocular motor nerves are in close proximity. In a diabetic or immunocompromised host, fungal infection (*Aspergillus*, Mucorales, *Cryptococcus*) is a common cause of multiple nerve palsies. In a patient with systemic malignancy, carcinomatous meningitis is a likely diagnosis. Cytologic examination may be negative despite repeated sampling of the cerebrospinal fluid. The cancer-associated Lambert-Eaton myasthenic syndrome also can produce ophthalmoplegia. Giant cell (temporal) arteritis occasionally manifests as diplopia from ischemic palsies of extraocular muscles. Fisher's syndrome, an ocular variant of Guillain-Barré, produces ophthalmoplegia with areflexia and ataxia. Often the ataxia is mild, and the reflexes are normal. Antiganglioside antibodies (GQ1b) can be detected in about 50% of cases.

Supranuclear Disorders of Gaze These are often mistaken for multiple ocular motor nerve palsies. For example, Wernicke's encephalopathy can produce nystagmus and a partial deficit of horizontal and vertical gaze that mimics a combined abducens and oculomotor nerve palsy. The disorder occurs in malnourished or alcoholic patients and can be reversed by thiamine. Infarct, hemorrhage, tumor, multiple sclerosis, encephalitis, vasculitis, and Whipple's disease are other important causes of supranuclear gaze palsy. Disorders of vertical gaze, especially downward saccades, are an early feature of progressive supranuclear palsy. Smooth pursuit is affected later in the course of the disease. Parkinson's disease, Huntington's disease, and olivopontocerebellar degeneration also can affect vertical gaze.

The *frontal eye field* of the cerebral cortex is involved in generation of saccades to the contralateral side. After hemispheric stroke, the eyes usually deviate toward the lesioned side because of the unopposed action of the frontal eye field in the normal hemisphere. With time, this deficit resolves. Seizures generally have the opposite effect: the eyes deviate conjugately away from the irritative focus. *Parietal lesions* disrupt smooth pursuit of targets moving toward the side of the lesion. Bilateral parietal lesions produce *Bálint's syndrome*, which is characterized by impaired eye-hand coordination (optic ataxia), difficulty initiating voluntary eye movements (ocular apraxia), and visuospatial disorientation (simultanagnosia).

Horizontal Gaze Descending cortical inputs mediating horizontal gaze ultimately converge at the level of the pons. Neurons in the paramedian pontine reticular formation are responsible for controlling conjugate gaze toward the same side. They project directly to the ipsilateral abducens nucleus. A lesion of either the paramedian pontine reticular formation or the abducens nucleus causes an ipsilateral conjugate gaze palsy. Lesions at either locus produce nearly identical clinical syndromes, with the following exception: vestibular stimulation (oculocephalic maneuver or caloric irrigation) will succeed in driving the eyes conjugately to the side in a patient with a lesion of the paramedian pontine reticular formation but not in a patient with a lesion of the abducens nucleus.

INTERNUCLEAR OPHTHALMOPLEGIA This results from damage to the medial longitudinal fasciculus ascending from the abducens nucleus in the pons to the oculomotor nucleus in the midbrain (hence, "internuclear"). Damage to fibers carrying the conjugate signal from abducens interneurons to the contralateral medial rectus motoneurons results in a failure of adduction on attempted lateral gaze. For example, a patient with a left internuclear ophthalmoplegia (INO) will have slowed or absent adducting movements of the left eye (Fig. 39-20). A patient

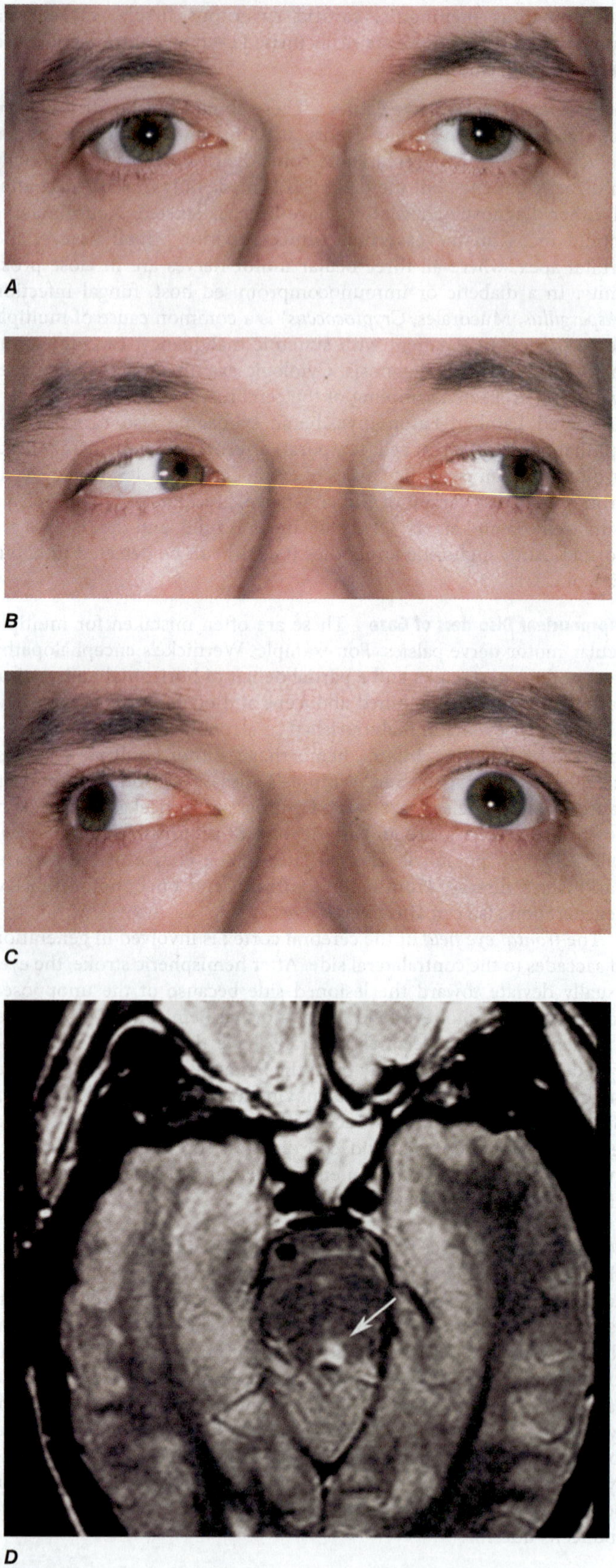

FIGURE 39-20 Left internuclear ophthalmoplegia (INO). ***A.*** In primary position of gaze, the eyes appear normal. ***B.*** Horizontal gaze to the left is intact. ***C.*** On attempted horizontal gaze to the right, the left eye fails to adduct. In mildly affected patients, the eye may adduct partially or more slowly than normal. Nystagmus is usually present in the abducted eye. ***D.*** T2-weighted axial magnetic resonance image through the pons showing a demyelinating plaque in the left medial longitudinal fasciculus (*arrow*).

with bilateral injury to the medial longitudinal fasciculus will have bilateral INO. Multiple sclerosis is the most common cause, although tumor, stroke, trauma, or any brainstem process may be responsible. *One-and-a-half syndrome* is due to a combined lesion of the medial longitudinal fasciculus and the abducens nucleus on the same side. The patient's only horizontal eye movement is abduction of the eye on the other side.

Vertical Gaze This is controlled at the level of the midbrain. The neuronal circuits affected in disorders of vertical gaze are not fully elucidated, but lesions of the rostral interstitial nucleus of the medial longitudinal fasciculus and the interstitial nucleus of Cajal cause supranuclear paresis of upgaze, downgaze, or all vertical eye movements. Distal basilar artery ischemia is the most common etiology. *Skew deviation* refers to a vertical misalignment of the eyes, usually constant in all positions of gaze. The finding has poor localizing value because skew deviation has been reported after lesions in widespread regions of the brainstem and cerebellum.

PARINAUD'S SYNDROME Also known as dorsal midbrain syndrome, this is a distinct supranuclear vertical gaze disorder caused by damage to the posterior commissure. It is a classic sign of hydrocephalus from aqueductal stenosis. Pineal region or midbrain tumors, cysticercosis, and stroke also cause Parinaud's syndrome. Features include loss of upgaze (and sometimes downgaze), convergence-retraction nystagmus on attempted upgaze, downward ocular deviation ("setting sun" sign), lid retraction (Collier's sign), skew deviation, pseudoabducens palsy, and light-near dissociation of the pupils.

Nystagmus This is a rhythmic oscillation of the eyes, occurring physiologically from vestibular and optokinetic stimulation or pathologically in a wide variety of diseases (Chap. 28). Abnormalities of the eyes or optic nerves, present at birth or acquired in childhood, can produce a complex, searching nystagmus with irregular pendular (sinusoidal) and jerk features. Examples are albinism, Leber's congenital amaurosis, and bilateral cataract. This nystagmus is commonly referred to as *congenital sensory nystagmus*. This is a poor term because even in children with congenital lesions, the nystagmus does not appear until weeks after birth. *Congenital motor nystagmus*, which looks similar to congenital sensory nystagmus, develops in the absence of any abnormality of the sensory visual system. Visual acuity also is reduced in congenital motor nystagmus, probably by the nystagmus itself, but seldom below a level of 20/200.

JERK NYSTAGMUS This is characterized by a slow drift off the target, followed by a fast corrective saccade. By convention, the nystagmus is named after the quick phase. Jerk nystagmus can be downbeat, upbeat, horizontal (left or right), and torsional. The pattern of nystagmus may vary with gaze position. Some patients will be oblivious to their nystagmus. Others will complain of blurred vision or a subjective to-and-fro movement of the environment (oscillopsia) corresponding to the nystagmus. Fine nystagmus may be difficult to see on gross examination of the eyes. Observation of nystagmoid movements of the optic disc on ophthalmoscopy is a sensitive way to detect subtle nystagmus.

GAZE-EVOKED NYSTAGMUS This is the most common form of jerk nystagmus. When the eyes are held eccentrically in the orbits, they have a natural tendency to drift back to primary position. The subject compensates by making a corrective saccade to maintain the deviated eye position. Many normal patients have mild gaze-evoked nystagmus. Exaggerated gaze-evoked nystagmus can be induced by drugs (sedatives, anticonvulsants, alcohol); muscle paresis; myasthenia gravis; demyelinating disease; and cerebellopontine angle, brainstem, and cerebellar lesions.

VESTIBULAR NYSTAGMUS *Vestibular nystagmus* results from dysfunction of the labyrinth (Ménière's disease), vestibular nerve, or vestibular nucleus in the brainstem. Peripheral vestibular nystagmus often occurs in discrete attacks, with symptoms of nausea and vertigo. There may be associated tinnitus and hearing loss. Sudden shifts in head position may provoke or exacerbate symptoms.

DOWNBEAT NYSTAGMUS *Downbeat nystagmus* results from lesions near the craniocervical junction (Chiari malformation, basilar invagination). It also has been reported in brainstem or cerebellar stroke, lithium or anticonvulsant intoxication, alcoholism, and multiple sclerosis. *Upbeat nystagmus* is associated with damage to the pontine tegmentum from stroke, demyelination, or tumor.

Opsoclonus This rare, dramatic disorder of eye movements consists of bursts of consecutive saccades (saccadomania). When the saccades are confined to the horizontal plane, the term *ocular flutter* is preferred. It can result from viral encephalitis, trauma, or a paraneoplastic effect of neuroblastoma, breast carcinoma, and other malignancies. It has also been reported as a benign, transient phenomenon in otherwise healthy patients.

40e Use of the Hand-Held Ophthalmoscope

Homayoun Tabandeh, Morton F. Goldberg

This is a digital-only chapter. It is available on the DVD that accompanies this book, as well as on Access Medicine/Harrison's Online, and the eBook and edition of HPIM 19e.

Examination of the living human retina provides a unique opportunity for the direct study of nervous, vascular, and connective tissues. Many systemic disorders have retinal manifestations that are valuable for screening, diagnosis, and management of these conditions. Furthermore, retinal involvement in systemic disorders, such as diabetes mellitus, is a major cause of morbidity. Early recognition by ophthalmoscopic screening is a key factor in effective treatment. Ophthalmoscopy has the potential to be one of the most "high-yield" elements of the physical examination. Effective ophthalmoscopy requires a basic understanding of ocular structures and ophthalmoscopic techniques and recognition of abnormal findings.

41e Video Library of Neuro-Ophthalmology

Shirley H. Wray

This is a digital-only chapter. It is available on the DVD that accompanies this book, as well as on Access Medicine/Harrison's Online, and the eBook edition of HPIM 19e.

The proper control of eye movements requires the coordinated activity of many different anatomic structures in the peripheral and central nervous system, and in turn, manifestations of a diverse array of neurologic and medical disorders are revealed as disorders of eye movement. In this remarkable video collection, an introduction to distinctive eye movement disorders encountered in the context of neuromuscular, paraneoplastic, demyelinating, neurovascular, and neurodegenerative disorders is presented.

42 Disorders of Smell and Taste

Richard L. Doty, Steven M. Bromley

All environmental chemicals necessary for life enter the body by the nose and mouth. The senses of smell (olfaction) and taste (gustation) monitor such chemicals, determine the flavor and palatability of foods and beverages, and warn of dangerous environmental conditions, including fire, air pollution, leaking natural gas, and bacteria-laden foodstuffs. These senses contribute significantly to quality of life and, when dysfunctional, can have untoward physical and psychological consequences. A basic understanding of these senses in health and disease is critical for the physician, because thousands of patients present to doctors' offices each year with complaints of chemosensory dysfunction. Among the more important recent developments in neurology is the discovery that decreased smell function is among the first signs, if not the first sign, of such neurodegenerative diseases as Parkinson's disease (PD) and Alzheimer's disease (AD), signifying their "presymptomatic" phase.

ANATOMY AND PHYSIOLOGY

Olfactory System Odorous chemicals enter the front of nose during inhalation and active sniffing, as well as the back of the nose (nasopharynx) during deglutition. After reaching the highest recesses of the nasal cavity, they dissolve in the olfactory mucus and diffuse or are actively transported by specialized proteins to receptors located on the cilia of olfactory receptor cells. The cilia, dendrites, cell bodies, and proximal axonal segments of these bipolar cells are located within a unique neuroepithelium covering the cribriform plate, the superior nasal septum, superior turbinate, and sectors of the middle turbinate (Fig. 42-1). Each of the ~6 million bipolar receptor cells expresses only one of ~450 receptor protein types, most of which respond to more than a single chemical. When damaged, the receptor cells can be replaced by stem cells near the basement membrane. Unfortunately, such replacement is often incomplete.

After coalescing into bundles surrounded by glia-like ensheathing cells (termed fila), the receptor cell axons pass through the cribriform plate to the olfactory bulbs, where they synapse with dendrites of other cell types within the glomeruli (Fig. 42-2). These spherical structures, which make up a distinct layer of the olfactory bulb, are a site of convergence of information, because many more fibers enter than leave them. Receptor cells that express the same type of receptor project to the same glomeruli, effectively making each glomerulus a functional unit. The major projection neurons of the olfactory system—the mitral and tufted cells—send primary dendrites into the glomeruli, connecting not only with the incoming receptor cell axons, but with dendrites of periglomerular cells. The activity of the mitral/tufted cells is modulated by the periglomerular cells, secondary dendrites from other mitral/tufted cells, and granule cells, the most numerous cells of the bulb. The latter cells, which are largely GABAergic, receive inputs from central brain structures and modulate the output of the mitral/tufted cells. Interestingly, like the olfactory receptor cells, some cells within the bulb undergo replacement. Thus, neuroblasts formed within the anterior subventricular zone of the brain migrate along the rostral migratory stream, ultimately becoming granule and periglomerular cells.

The axons of the mitral and tufted cells synapse within the primary olfactory cortex (POC) (Fig. 42-3). The POC is defined as those cortical structures that receive direct projections from the olfactory bulb, most notably the piriform and entorhinal cortices. Although olfaction is unique in that its initial afferent projections bypass the thalamus, persons with damage to the thalamus can exhibit olfactory deficits, particularly ones of odor identification. Such deficits likely reflect the involvement of thalamic connections between the primary olfactory cortex and the orbitofrontal cortex (OFC), where odor identification occurs. The close anatomic ties between the olfactory system and the

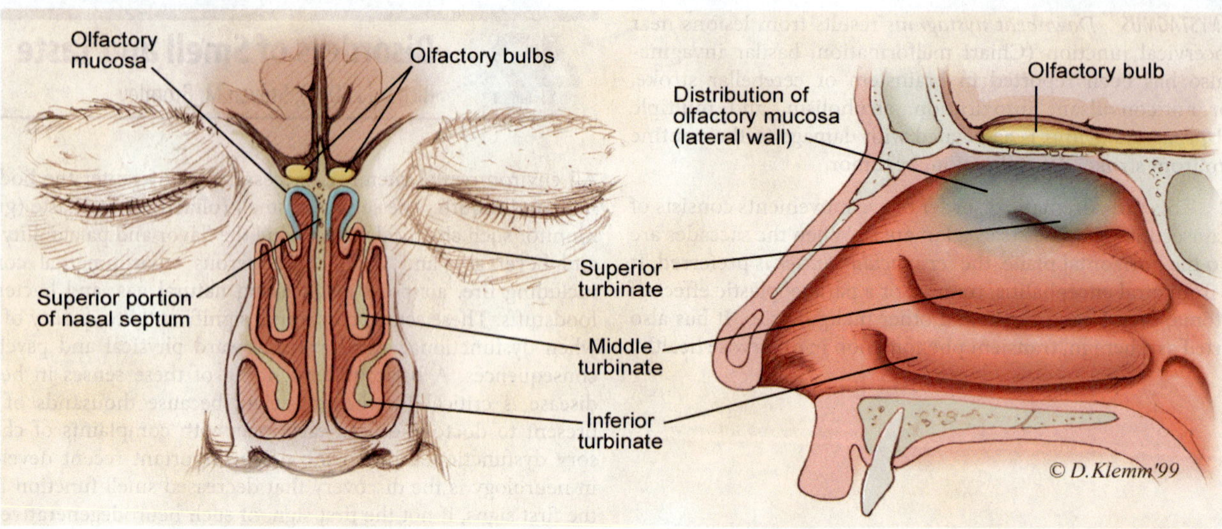

FIGURE 42-1 Anatomy of the olfactory neural pathways, showing the distribution of olfactory receptors in the roof of the nasal cavity. *(Copyright David Klemm, Faculty and Curriculum Support [FACS], Georgetown University Medical Center; used with permission.)*

amygdala, hippocampus, and hypothalamus help to explain the intimate associations between odor perception and cognitive functions such as memory, motivation, arousal, autonomic activity, digestion, and sex.

Taste System Tastants are sensed by specialized receptor cells present within taste buds—small grapefruit-like segmented structures located on the lateral margins and dorsum of the tongue, roof of the mouth, pharynx, larynx, and superior esophagus (Fig. 42-4). Lingual taste buds are imbedded in well-defined protuberances, termed fungiform, foliate, and circumvallate papillae. After dissolving in a liquid, tastants enter the opening of the taste bud—the taste pore—and bind to receptors on microvilli, small extensions of receptor cells within each taste bud. Such binding changes the electrical potential across the taste cell, resulting in neurotransmitter release onto the first-order taste neurons. Although humans have ~7500 taste buds, not all harbor taste-sensitive cells; some contain only one class of receptor (e.g., cells responsive only to sugars), whereas others contain cells sensitive to more than one class. The number of taste receptor cells per taste bud ranges from zero to well over 100. A small family of three G-protein-coupled receptors (GPCRs), namely T1R1, T1R2, and T1R3, mediate sweet and umami taste sensations. Bitter sensations, on the other hand, depend on T2R receptors, a family of ~30 GPCRs expressed on cells different from those that express the sweet and umami receptors. T2Rs sense a wide range of bitter substances but do not distinguish among them. Sour tastants are sensed by the PKD2L1 receptor, a member of the transient receptor potential protein (TRP) family. Perception of salty sensations, such as induced by sodium chloride, arises from the entry of Na^+ ions into the cells via specialized membrane channels, such as the amiloride-sensitive Na^+ channel.

Recent studies have found that both bitter and sweet taste-related receptors are also present elsewhere in the body, most notably in the

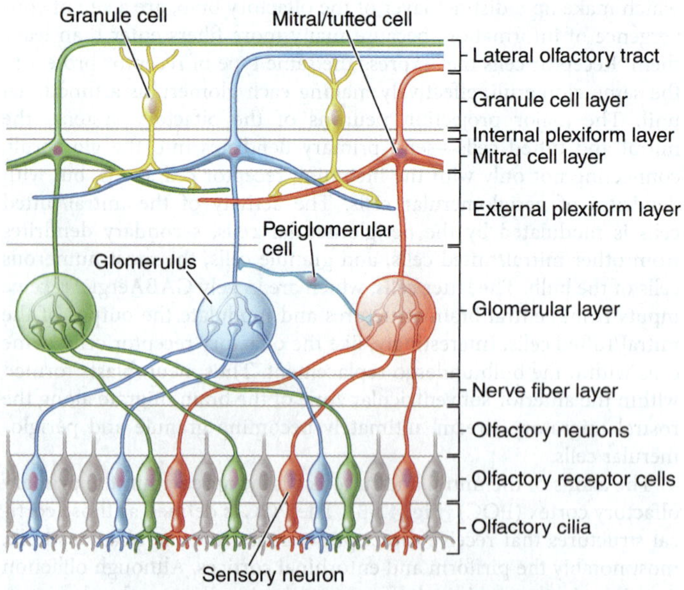

FIGURE 42-2 Schematic of the layers and wiring of the olfactory bulb. Each receptor type (red, green, blue) projects to a common glomerulus. The neural activity within each glomerulus is modulated by periglomerular cells. The activity of the primary projection cells, the mitral and tufted cells, is modulated by granule cells, periglomerular cells, and secondary dendrites from adjacent mitral and tufted cells. *(From www.med.yale.edu/neurosurg/treloar/index.html.)*

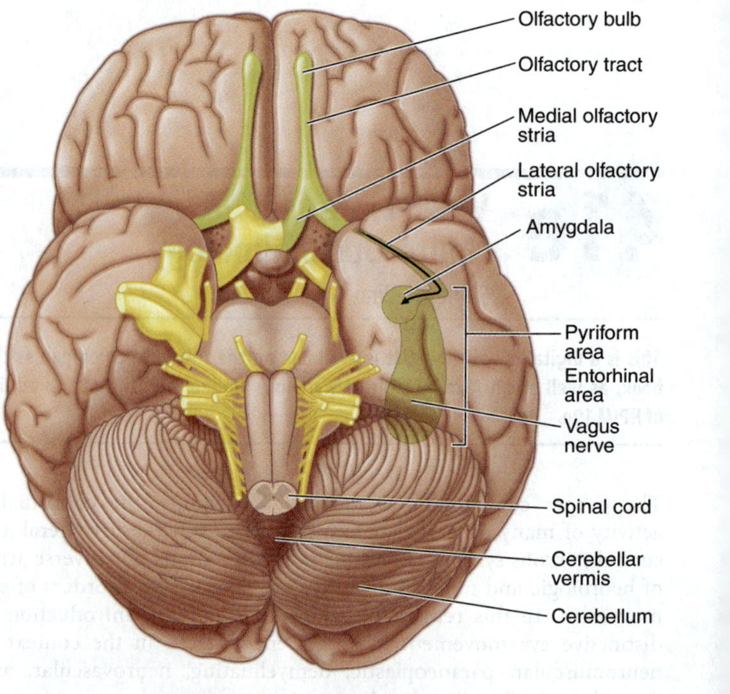

FIGURE 42-3 Anatomy of the base of the brain showing the primary olfactory cortex.

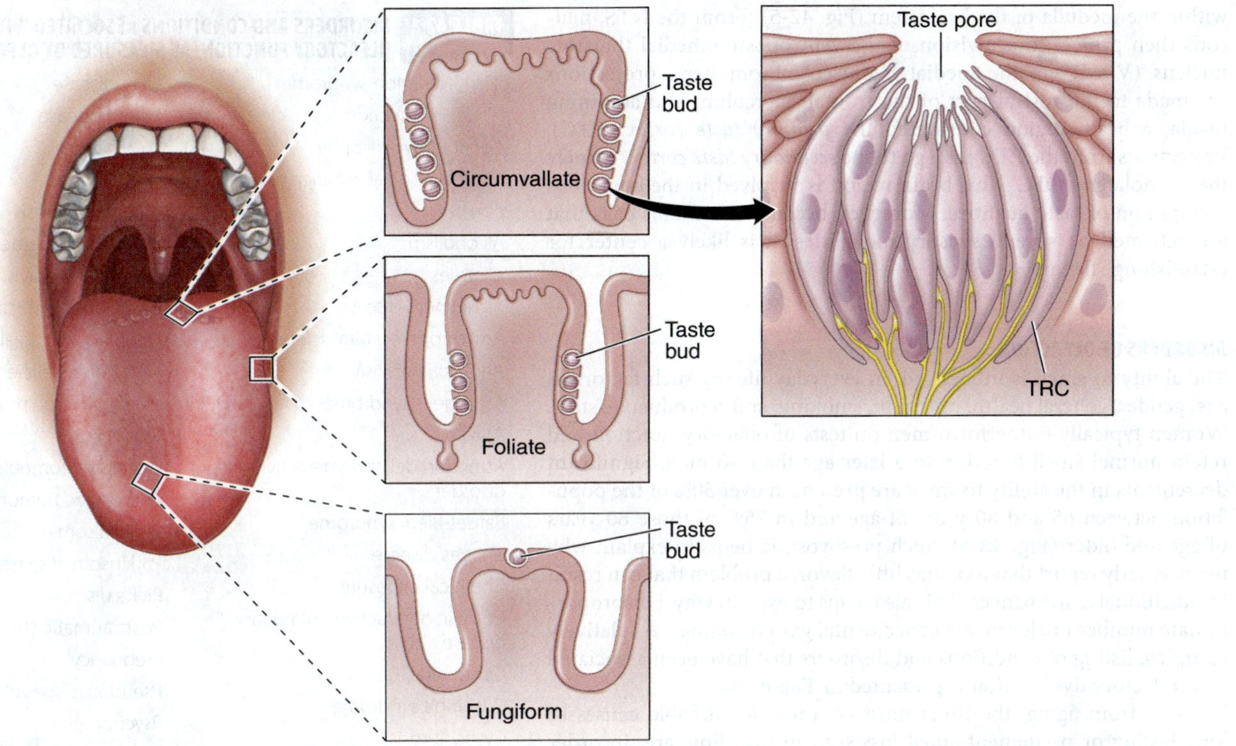

FIGURE 42-4 Schematic of the taste bud and its opening (pore), as well as the location of buds on the three major types of papillae: fungiform (anterior), foliate (lateral), and circumvallate (posterior).

alimentary and respiratory tracts. This important discovery generalizes the concept of taste-related chemoreception to areas of the body beyond the mouth and throat, with α-gustducin, the taste-specific G-protein α-subunit, expressed in so-called brush cells found specifically within the human trachea, lung, pancreas, and gallbladder. These brush cells are rich in nitric oxide (NO) synthase, known to defend against xenobiotic organisms, protect the mucosa from acid-induced lesions, and, in the case of the gastrointestinal tract, stimulate vagal and splanchnic afferent neurons. NO further acts on nearby cells, including enteroendocrine cells, absorptive or secretory epithelial cells, mucosal blood vessels, and cells of the immune system. Members of the T2R family of bitter receptors and the sweet receptors of the T1R family have been identified within the gastrointestinal tract and in enteroendocrine cell lines. In some cases, these receptors are important for metabolism, with the T1R3 receptors and gustducin playing decisive roles in the sensing and transport of dietary sugars from the intestinal lumen into absorptive enterocytes via a sodium-dependent glucose transporter and in regulation of hormone release from gut enteroendocrine cells. In other cases, these receptors may be important for airway protection, with a number of T2R bitter receptors in the motile cilia of the human airway that responded to bitter compounds by increasing their beat frequency. One specific T2R38 taste receptor is expressed in human upper respiratory epithelia and responds to acyl-monoserine lactone quorum-sensing molecules secreted by *Pseudomonas aeruginosa* and other gram-negative bacteria. Differences in T2R38 functionality, as related to TAS2R38 genotype, correlate with susceptibility to upper respiratory infections in humans.

Taste information is sent to the brain via three cranial nerves (CNs): CN VII (the *facial nerve*, which involves the intermediate nerve with its branches, the greater petrosal and chorda tympani nerves), CN IX (the *glossopharyngeal nerve*), and CN X (the *vagus nerve*) (Fig. 42-5). CN VII innervates the anterior tongue and all of the soft palate, CN IX innervates the posterior tongue, and CN X innervates the laryngeal surface of the epiglottis, larynx, and proximal portion of the esophagus. The mandibular branch of CN V (V_3) conveys somatosensory information (e.g., touch, burning, cooling, irritation) to the brain. Although not technically a gustatory nerve, CN V shares primary nerve routes with many of the gustatory nerve fibers and adds temperature, texture, pungency, and spiciness to the taste experience. The chorda tympani nerve is famous for taking a recurrent course through the facial canal in the petrosal portion of the temporal bone, passing through the middle ear, and then exiting the skull via the petrotympanic fissure, where it joins the lingual nerve (a division of CN V) near the tongue. This nerve also carries parasympathetic fibers to the submandibular and sublingual glands, whereas the greater petrosal nerve supplies the palatine glands, thereby influencing saliva production.

The axons of the projection cells, which synapse with taste buds, enter the rostral portion of the nucleus of the solitary tract (NTS)

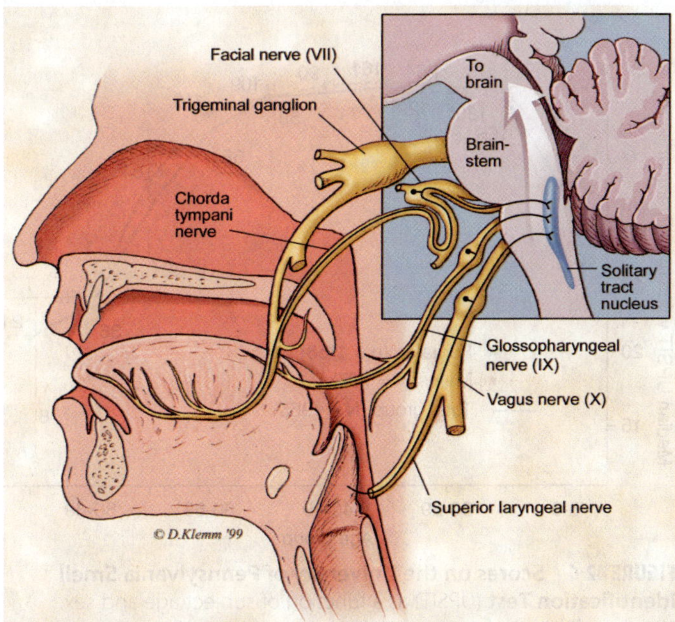

FIGURE 42-5 Schematic of the cranial nerves (CNs) that mediate taste function, including the chorda tympani nerve (CN VII), the glossopharyngeal nerve (CN IX), and the vagus nerve (CN X).

within the medulla of the brainstem (Fig. 42-5). From the NTS, neurons then project to a division of the ventroposteromedial thalamic nucleus (VPM) via the medial lemniscus. From here, projections are made to the rostral part of the frontal operculum and adjoining insula, a brain region considered the *primary taste cortex* (PTC). Projections from the PTC then go to the *secondary taste cortex*, namely the caudolateral OFC. This brain region is involved in the conscious recognition of taste qualities. Moreover, because it contains cells that are activated by several sensory modalities, it is likely a center for establishing "flavor."

DISORDERS OF OLFACTION

The ability to smell is influenced, in everyday life, by such factors as age, gender, general health, nutrition, smoking, and reproductive state. Women typically outperform men on tests of olfactory function and retain normal smell function to a later age than do men. Significant decrements in the ability to smell are present in over 50% of the population between 65 and 80 years of age and in 75% of those 80 years of age and older (Fig. 42-6). Such presbyosmia helps to explain why many elderly report that food has little flavor, a problem that can result in nutritional disturbances. This also helps to explain why a disproportionate number of elderly die in accidental gas poisonings. A relatively complete listing of conditions and disorders that have been associated with olfactory dysfunction is presented in Table 42-1.

Aside from aging, the three most common identifiable causes of long-lasting or permanent smell loss seen in the clinic are, in order of frequency, severe upper respiratory infections, head trauma, and chronic rhinosinusitis. The physiologic basis for most head trauma–related losses is the shearing and subsequent scarring of the olfactory fila as they pass from the nasal cavity into the brain cavity. The cribriform plate does not have to be fractured or show pathology for smell loss to be present. Severity of trauma, as indexed by a poor Glasgow Coma Scale score on presentation and the length of posttraumatic amnesia, is associated with higher risk of olfactory impairment. Less than 10% of posttraumatic anosmic patients will recover age-related normal function over time. This increases to nearly 25% of those with less-than-total loss. Upper respiratory infections, such as those associated with the common cold, influenza, pneumonia, or HIV, can directly and permanently harm the olfactory epithelium by decreasing receptor cell number, damaging cilia on remaining receptor cells, and inducing the replacement of sensory epithelium with respiratory epithelium. The smell loss associated with chronic rhinosinusitis is related to disease severity, with most loss occurring in cases where rhinosinusitis and polyposis are both present. Although systemic glucocorticoid therapy can usually induce short-term functional improvement, it does not, on average, return smell test scores to normal, implying that chronic permanent neural loss is present and/or that short-term administration of systemic glucocorticoids does not completely mitigate the inflammation. It is well established that microinflammation in an otherwise seemingly normal epithelium can influence smell function.

A number of neurodegenerative diseases are accompanied by olfactory impairment, including PD, AD, Huntington's disease, Down's syndrome, parkinsonism-dementia complex of Guam, dementia with Lewy bodies (DLB), multiple system atrophy, corticobasal degeneration, and frontotemporal dementia; smell loss can also occur in multiple sclerosis (MS) and idiopathic rapid eye movement (REM) behavioral sleep disorder (iRBD). Olfactory impairment in PD often predates the clinical diagnosis by at least 4 years. In staged cases, studies of the sequence of formation of abnormal α-synuclein aggregates and Lewy bodies suggest that the olfactory bulbs may be, along with the dorsomotor nucleus of the vagus, the first site of neural damage

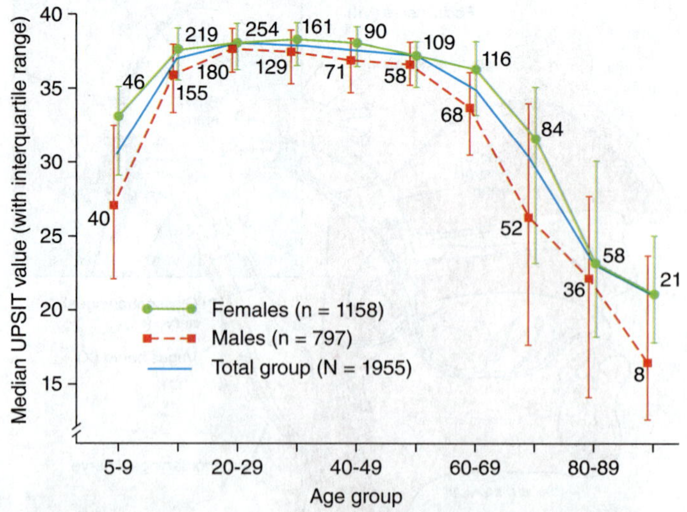

FIGURE 42-6 Scores on the University of Pennsylvania Smell Identification Test (UPSIT) as a function of subject age and sex. Numbers by each data point indicate sample sizes. Note that women identify odorants better than men at all ages. *(From RL Doty et al: Science 226:1421, 1984. Copyright © 1984 American Association for the Advancement of Science.)*

TABLE 42-1 DISORDERS AND CONDITIONS ASSOCIATED WITH COMPROMISED OLFACTORY FUNCTION, AS MEASURED BY OLFACTORY TESTING

22q11 deletion syndrome	Liver disease
AIDS/HIV infection	Lubag disease
Adenoid hypertrophy	Medications
Adrenal cortical insufficiency	Migraine
Age	Multiple sclerosis
Alcoholism	Multi-infarct dementia
Allergies	Myasthenia gravis
Alzheimer's disease	Narcolepsy with cataplexy
Amyotrophic lateral sclerosis (ALS)	Neoplasms, cranial/nasal
Anorexia nervosa	Nutritional deficiencies
Asperger's syndrome	Obstructive pulmonary disease
Ataxias	Obesity
Attention deficit/hyperactivity disorder	Obsessive compulsive disorder
Bardet-Biedl syndrome	Orthostatic tremor
Chagas' disease	Panic disorder
Chemical exposure	Parkinson's disease (PD)
Chronic obstructive pulmonary disease	Pick's disease
Congenital	Posttraumatic stress disorder
Cushing's syndrome	Pregnancy
Cystic fibrosis	Pseudohypoparathyroidism
Degenerative ataxias	Psychopathy
Diabetes	Radiation (therapeutic, cranial)
Down's syndrome	REM behavior disorder
Epilepsy	Refsum's disease
Facial paralysis	Renal failure/end-stage kidney disease
Frontotemporal lobe degeneration	Restless leg syndrome
Gonadal dysgenesis (Turner's syndrome)	Rhinosinusitis/polyposis
Guamanian ALS/PD/dementia syndrome	Schizophrenia
Head trauma	Seasonal affective disorder
Herpes simplex encephalitis	Sjögren's syndrome
Hypothyroidism	Stroke
Huntington's disease	Tobacco smoking
Iatrogenesis	Toxic chemical exposure
Kallmann's syndrome	Upper respiratory infections
Korsakoff's psychosis	Usher syndrome
Leprosy	Vitamin B_{12} deficiency

in PD. In postmortem studies of patients with very mild "presymptomatic" signs of AD, poorer smell function has been associated with higher levels of AD-related pathology. Smell loss is more marked in patients with early clinical manifestations of DLB than in those with mild AD. Interestingly, smell loss is minimal or nonexistent in progressive supranuclear palsy and 1-methyl-4-phenyl-1,2,3,6-tetrahydropyridine (MPTP)-induced parkinsonism. In MS, the olfactory disturbance varies as a function of the plaque activity within the frontal and temporal lobes.

The smell loss seen in iRBD is of the same magnitude as that found in PD. This is of particular interest because patients with iRBD frequently develop PD and hyposmia. There is some evidence that iRBD may actually represent an early associated condition of PD. REM behavior disorder is not only seen in its idiopathic form, but can also be associated with narcolepsy. This led to a recent study of narcoleptic patients with and without REM behavior disorder, which demonstrated that narcolepsy, independent of REM behavior disorder, was associated with impairments in olfactory function. Orexin A, also known as hypocretin-1, is dramatically diminished or undetectable in the cerebrospinal fluid of patients with narcolepsy and cataplexy (Chap. 38). The orexin-containing neurons in the hypothalamus project throughout the entire olfactory system (from the olfactory epithelium to the olfactory cortex), and damage to these orexin-containing projections may be one underlying mechanism for impaired olfactory performance in narcoleptic patients. The administration of intranasal orexin A (hypocretin-1) appears to result in improved olfactory function, supporting the notion that mild olfactory impairment is not only a primary feature of narcolepsy with cataplexy, but that central nervous system orexin deficiency may be a fundamental part of the mechanism for this loss.

DISORDERS OF TASTE

The majority of patients who present with taste dysfunction exhibit olfactory, not taste, loss. This is because most flavors attributed to taste actually depend on retronasal stimulation of the olfactory receptors during deglutition. As noted earlier, taste buds only mediate basic tastes such as sweet, sour, bitter, salty, and umami. Significant impairment of whole-mouth gustatory function is rare outside of generalized metabolic disturbances or systemic use of some medications, because taste bud regeneration occurs and peripheral damage alone would require the involvement of multiple cranial nerve pathways. Nonetheless, taste can be influenced by (1) the release of foul-tasting materials from the oral cavity from oral medical conditions or appliances (e.g., gingivitis, purulent sialadenitis), (2) transport problems of tastants to the taste buds (e.g., drying of the orolingual mucosa, infections, inflammatory conditions), (3) damage to the taste buds themselves (e.g., local trauma, invasive carcinomas), (4) damage to the neural pathways innervating the taste buds (e.g., middle ear infections), (5) damage to central structures (e.g., multiple sclerosis, tumor, epilepsy, stroke), and (6) systemic disturbances of metabolism (e.g., diabetes, thyroid disease, medications). Unlike CN VII, CN IX is relatively protected along its path, although iatrogenic interventions such as tonsillectomy, bronchoscopy, laryngoscopy, endotracheal intubation, and radiation therapy can result in selective injury. CN VII damage commonly results from mastoidectomy, tympanoplasty, and stapedectomy, in some cases inducing persistent metallic sensations. Bell's palsy (Chap. 455) is one of the most common causes of CN VII injury that results in taste disturbance. On rare occasions, migraines (Chap. 447) are associated with a gustatory prodrome or aura, and in some cases, tastants can trigger a migraine attack. Interestingly, dysgeusia occurs in some cases of burning mouth syndrome (BMS; also termed *glossodynia* or *glossalgia*), as do dry mouth and thirst. BMS is likely associated with dysfunction of the trigeminal nerve (CN V). Some of the etiologies suggested for this poorly understood syndrome are amenable to treatment, including (1) nutritional deficiencies (e.g., iron, folic acid, B vitamins, zinc), (2) diabetes mellitus (possibly predisposing to oral candidiasis), (3) denture allergy, (4) mechanical irritation from dentures or oral devices, (5) repetitive movements of the mouth (e.g., tongue thrusting, teeth grinding, jaw clenching), (6) tongue ischemia as a result of temporal arteritis, (7) periodontal disease, (8) reflux esophagitis, and (9) geographic tongue.

Although both taste and smell can be adversely influenced by pharmacologic agents, drug-related taste alterations are more common. Indeed, over 250 medications have been reported to alter the ability to taste. Major offenders include antineoplastic agents, antirheumatic drugs, antibiotics, and blood pressure medications. Terbinafine, a commonly used antifungal, has been linked to taste disturbance lasting up to 3 years. In a recent controlled trial, nearly two-thirds of individuals taking eszopiclone (Lunesta) experienced a bitter dysgeusia that was stronger in women, systematically related to the time since drug administration, and positively correlated with both blood and saliva levels of the drug. Intranasal use of nasal gels and sprays containing zinc, which are common over-the-counter prophylactics for upper respiratory viral infections, has been implicated in loss of smell function. Whether their efficacy in preventing such infections, which are the most common cause of anosmia and hyposmia, outweighs their potential detriment to smell function requires study. Dysgeusia occurs commonly in the context of drugs used to treat or minimize symptoms of cancer, with a weighted prevalence from 56–76% depending on the type of cancer treatment. Attempts to prevent taste problems from such drugs using prophylactic zinc sulfate or amifostine have proven to be minimally beneficial. Although antiepileptic medications are occasionally used to treat smell or taste disturbances, the use of topiramate has been reported to result in a reversible loss of an ability to detect and recognize tastes and odors during treatment.

As with olfaction, a number of systemic disorders can affect taste. These include chronic renal failure, end-stage liver disease, vitamin and mineral deficiencies, diabetes mellitus, and hypothyroidism (to name a few). In diabetes, there appears to be a progressive loss of taste beginning with glucose and then extending to other sweeteners, salty stimuli, and then all stimuli. Psychiatric conditions can be associated with chemosensory alterations (e.g., depression, schizophrenia, bulimia). A recent review of tactile, gustatory, and olfactory hallucinations demonstrated that no one type of hallucinatory experience is pathognomonic to any given diagnosis.

Pregnancy proves to be a unique condition with regard to taste function. There appears to be an increase in dislike and intensity of bitter tastes during the first trimester that may help to ensure that pregnant women avoid poisons during a critical phase of fetal development. Similarly, a relative increase in the preference for salt and bitter in the second and third trimesters may support the ingestion of much needed electrolytes to expand fluid volume and support a varied diet.

CLINICAL EVALUATION

In most cases, a careful clinical history will establish the probable etiology of a chemosensory problem, including questions about its nature, onset, duration, and pattern of fluctuations. *Sudden loss* suggests the possibility of head trauma, ischemia, infection, or a psychiatric condition. *Gradual loss* can reflect the development of a progressive obstructive lesion. *Intermittent loss* suggests the likelihood of an inflammatory process. The patient should be asked about potential precipitating events, such as cold or flu infections prior to symptom onset, because these often go underappreciated. Information regarding head trauma, smoking habits, drug and alcohol abuse (e.g., intranasal cocaine, chronic alcoholism in the context of Wernicke's and Korsakoff's syndromes), exposures to pesticides and other toxic agents, and medical interventions is also informative. A determination of all the medications that the patient was taking before and at the time of symptom onset is important, because many can cause chemosensory disturbances. Comorbid medical conditions associated with smell impairment, such as renal failure, liver disease, hypothyroidism, diabetes, or dementia, should be assessed. Delayed puberty in association with anosmia (with or without midline craniofacial abnormalities, deafness, and renal anomalies) suggests the possibility of Kallmann's syndrome. Recollection of epistaxis, discharge (clear, purulent, or bloody), nasal obstruction, allergies, and somatic symptoms, including headache or irritation, may have localizing value. Questions related to memory, parkinsonian signs, and seizure activity (e.g., automatisms, blackouts, auras, déjà vu) should be posed. Pending litigation and the possibility of malingering should be considered. Modern forced-choice olfactory tests can detect malingering from improbable responses.

Neurologic and otorhinolaryngologic (ORL) examinations, along with appropriate brain and nasosinus imaging, aid in the evaluation of patients with olfactory or gustatory complaints. The neural evaluation should focus on cranial nerve function, with particular attention to possible skull base and intracranial lesions. Visual acuity, field, and optic disc examinations aid in the detection of intracranial mass lesions that induce intracranial pressure (papilledema) and optic atrophy, especially when considering Foster Kennedy syndrome. The ORL examination should thoroughly assess the intranasal architecture and mucosal surfaces. Polyps, masses, and adhesions of the turbinates to the septum may compromise the flow of air to the olfactory receptors, because less than a fifth of the inspired air traverses the olfactory cleft in the unobstructed state. Blood tests may be helpful to identify such conditions as diabetes, infection, heavy metal exposure, nutritional deficiency (e.g., vitamin B_6 or B_{12}), allergy, and thyroid, liver, and kidney disease.

As with other sensory disorders, quantitative sensory testing is advised. Self-reports of patients can be misleading, and a number of patients who complain of chemosensory dysfunction have normal function for their age and gender. Quantitative smell and taste testing provides valid information for worker's compensation and other legal claims, as well as a way to accurately assess treatment interventions. A number of standardized olfactory and taste tests are commercially available. Most evaluate the ability of patients to detect and identify odors or tastes. For example, the most widely used of these tests, the 40-item University of Pennsylvania Smell Identification Test (UPSIT), uses norms based on nearly 4000 normal subjects. A determination is made of both absolute dysfunction (i.e., mild loss, moderate loss, severe loss, total loss, probable malingering) and relative dysfunction (percentile rank for age and gender). Although electrophysiologic testing is available at some smell and taste centers (e.g., odor event-related potentials), they require complex stimulus presentation and recording equipment and rarely provide additional diagnostic information. With the exception of electrogustometers, commercially available taste tests have only recently become available. Most use filter paper strips impregnated with tastants, so no stimulus preparation is required.

TREATMENT AND MANAGEMENT

Given the various mechanisms by which olfactory and gustatory disturbance can occur, management of patients tends to be condition specific. For example, patients with hypothyroidism, diabetes, or infections often benefit from specific treatments to correct the underlying disease process that is adversely influencing chemoreception. For most patients who present primarily with obstructive/transport loss affecting the nasal and paranasal regions (e.g., allergic rhinitis, polyposis, intranasal neoplasms, nasal deviations), medical and/or surgical intervention is often beneficial. Antifungal and antibiotic treatments may reverse taste problems secondary to candidiasis or other oral infections. Chlorhexidine mouthwash mitigates some salty or bitter dysgeusias, conceivably as a result of its strong positive charge. Excessive dryness of the oral mucosa is a problem with many medications and conditions, and artificial saliva (e.g., Xerolube) or oral pilocarpine treatments may prove beneficial. Other methods to improve salivary flow include the use of mints, lozenges, or sugarless gum. Flavor enhancers may make food more palatable (e.g., monosodium glutamate), but caution is advised to avoid overusing ingredients containing sodium or sugar, particularly in circumstances when a patient also has underlying hypertension or diabetes. Medications that induce distortions of taste can often be discontinued and replaced with other types of medications or modes of therapy. As mentioned earlier, pharmacologic agents result in taste disturbances much more frequently than smell disturbances, and over 250 medications have been reported to alter the sense of taste. It is important to note, however, that many drug-related effects are long lasting and not reversed by short-term drug discontinuance.

A recent study of endoscopic sinus surgery in patients with chronic rhinosinusitis and hyposmia revealed that patients with severe olfactory dysfunction prior to the surgery had a more dramatic and sustained improvement over time compared to patients with more mild olfactory dysfunction prior to intervention. In the case of intranasal and sinus-related inflammatory conditions, such as seen with allergy, viruses, and traumas, the use of intranasal or systemic glucocorticoids may also be helpful. One common approach is to use a tapering course of oral prednisone. The utility of restoring olfaction with either topical or systemic glucocorticoids has been studied. Topical intranasal administration was found to be less effective in general than systemic administration; however, the effects of different nasal administration techniques were not analyzed; for example, intranasal glucocorticoids are more effective if administered in the Moffett's position (head in the inverted position such as over the edge of the bed with the bridge of the nose perpendicular to the floor). After head trauma, an initial trial of glucocorticoids may help to reduce local edema and the potential deleterious deposition of scar tissue around olfactory fila at the level of the cribriform plate.

Treatments are limited for patients with chemosensory loss or primary injury to neural pathways. Nonetheless, spontaneous recovery can occur. In a follow-up study of 542 patients presenting to our center with smell loss from a variety of causes, modest improvement occurred over an average time period of 4 years in about half of the participants. However, only 11% of the anosmic and 23% of the hyposmic patients regained normal age-related function. Interestingly, the amount of dysfunction present at the time of presentation, not etiology, was the best predictor of prognosis. Other predictors were age and the duration of dysfunction prior to initial testing.

A nonblinded study has reported that patients with hyposmia may benefit from smelling strong odors (e.g., eucalyptol, citronella, eugenol, and phyenyl ethyl alcohol) before going to bed and immediately upon awakening each day over the course of several months. The rationale for such an approach comes from animal studies demonstrating that prolonged exposure to odorants can induce increased neural activity within the olfactory bulb. In an uncontrolled study, α-lipoic acid (400 mg/d), an essential cofactor for many enzyme complexes with possible antioxidant effects, was reported to be beneficial in mitigating smell loss following viral infection of the upper respiratory tract; controlled studies are needed to confirm this observation. This agent has also been suggested to be useful in some cases of hypogeusia and BMS.

The use of zinc and vitamin A in treating olfactory disturbances is controversial, and there does not appear to be much benefit beyond replenishing established deficiencies. However, zinc has been shown to improve taste function secondary to hepatic deficiencies, and retinoids (bioactive vitamin A derivatives) are known to play an essential role in the survival of olfactory neurons. One protocol in which zinc was infused with chemotherapy treatments suggested a possible protective effect against developing taste impairment. Diseases of the alimentary tract can not only influence chemoreceptive function, but also occasionally influence vitamin B_{12} absorption. This can result in a relative deficiency of vitamin B_{12}, theoretically contributing to olfactory nerve disturbance. Vitamin B_2 (riboflavin) and magnesium supplements are reported in the alternative literature to aid in the management of migraine that, in turn, may be associated with smell dysfunction. Because vitamin D deficiency is a cofactor of chemotherapy-induced mucocutaneous toxicity and dysgeusia, adding vitamin D_3, 1000–2000 units per day, may benefit some patients with smell and taste complaints during or following chemotherapy.

A number of medications have reportedly been used with success in ameliorating olfactory symptoms, although strong scientific evidence for efficacy is generally lacking. A report that theophylline improved smell function was uncontrolled and failed to account for the fact that some meaningful improvement occurs without treatment; indeed, the percentage of responders was about the same (~50%) as that noted by others to show spontaneous improvement over a similar time period. Antiepileptics and some antidepressants (e.g., amitriptyline) have been used to treat dysosmias and smell distortions, particularly following head trauma. Ironically, amitriptyline is also frequently on the list of medications that can ultimately distort smell and taste function, possibly from its anticholinergic effects. A recent study suggests that the use of the centrally acting acetylcholinesterase inhibitor donepezil in AD resulted in improvements on smell identification measures that correlated with overall clinician-based impressions of change in dementia severity scores.

Alternative therapies, such as acupuncture, meditation, cognitive-behavioral therapy, and yoga, can help patients manage uncomfortable experiences associated with chemosensory disturbance and oral pain syndromes and to cope with the psychosocial stressors surrounding the impairment. Additionally, modification of diet and eating habits is also important. By accentuating the other sensory experiences of a meal, such as food texture, aroma, temperature, and color, one can optimize the overall eating experience for a patient. In some cases, a flavor enhancer like monosodium glutamate (MSG) can be added to foods to increase palatability and encourage intake.

Proper oral and nasal hygiene and routine dental care are extremely important ways for patients to protect themselves from disorders of the mouth and nose that can ultimately result in chemosensory disturbance. Patients should be warned not to overcompensate for their taste loss by adding excessive amounts of sugar or salt. Smoking cessation and the discontinuance of oral tobacco use are essential in the management of any patient with smell and/or taste disturbance and should be repeatedly emphasized.

A major and often overlooked element of therapy comes from chemosensory testing itself. Confirmation or lack of conformation of loss is beneficial to patients who come to believe, in light of unsupportive family members and medical providers, that they may be "crazy." In cases where the loss is minor, patients can be informed of the likelihood of a more positive prognosis. Importantly, quantitative testing places the patient's problem into overall perspective. Thus, it is often therapeutic for an older person to know that, while his or her smell function is not what it used to be, it still falls above the average of his or her peer group. Without testing, many such patients are simply told they are getting old and nothing can be done for them, leading in some cases to depression and decreased self-esteem.

43 Disorders of Hearing

Anil K. Lalwani

Hearing loss is one of the most common sensory disorders in humans and can present at any age. Nearly 10% of the adult population has some hearing loss, and one-third of individuals age >65 years have a hearing loss of sufficient magnitude to require a hearing aid.

PHYSIOLOGY OF HEARING

The function of the external and middle ear is to amplify sound to facilitate conversion of the mechanical energy of the sound wave into an electrical signal by the inner ear hair cells, a process called mechanotransduction (Fig. 43-1). Sound waves enter the external auditory canal and set the tympanic membrane (eardrum) in motion, which in turn moves the malleus, incus, and stapes of the middle ear. Movement of the footplate of the stapes causes pressure changes in the fluid-filled inner ear, eliciting a traveling wave in the basilar membrane of the cochlea. The tympanic membrane and the ossicular chain in the middle ear serve as an impedance-matching mechanism, improving the efficiency of energy transfer from air to the fluid-filled inner ear.

Stereocilia of the hair cells of the organ of Corti, which rests on the basilar membrane, are in contact with the tectorial membrane and are deformed by the traveling wave. A point of maximal displacement of the basilar membrane is determined by the frequency of the stimulating tone. High-frequency tones cause maximal displacement of the basilar membrane near the base of the cochlea, whereas for low-frequency sounds, the point of maximal displacement is toward the apex of the cochlea.

The inner and outer hair cells of the organ of Corti have different innervation patterns, but both are mechanoreceptors. The afferent innervation relates principally to the inner hair cells, and the efferent innervation relates principally to outer hair cells. The motility of the outer hair cells alters the micromechanics of the inner hair cells, creating a cochlear amplifier, which explains the exquisite sensitivity and frequency selectivity of the cochlea.

Beginning in the cochlea, the frequency specificity is maintained at each point of the central auditory pathway: dorsal and ventral cochlear nuclei, trapezoid body, superior olivary complex, lateral lemniscus, inferior colliculus, medial geniculate body, and auditory cortex. At low frequencies, individual auditory nerve fibers can respond more or less synchronously with the stimulating tone. At higher frequencies, phase-locking occurs so that neurons alternate in response to particular phases of the cycle of the sound wave. Intensity is encoded by the amount of neural activity in individual neurons, the number of neurons that are active, and the specific neurons that are activated.

There is evidence that the right and left ears as well as the central nervous system may process speech asymmetrically. Generally, a sound is processed symmetrically from the peripheral to the central auditory system. However, a "right ear advantage" exists for dichotic listening tasks, in which subjects are asked to report on competing sounds presented to each ear. In most individuals, a perceptual right ear advantage for consonant-vowel syllables, stop consonants, and words also exists. Similarly, whereas central auditory processing for sounds is symmetric with minimal lateral specialization for the most part, speech processing is lateralized. There is specialization of the left auditory cortex for speech recognition and production, and of the right hemisphere for emotional and tonal aspects of speech. Left hemisphere dominance for speech is found in 95–98% of right-handed persons and 70–80% of left-handed persons.

DISORDERS OF THE SENSE OF HEARING

Hearing loss can result from disorders of the auricle, external auditory canal, middle ear, inner ear, or central auditory pathways (Fig. 43-2). *In general, lesions in the auricle, external auditory canal, or middle ear that impede the transmission of sound from the external environment to the inner ear cause conductive hearing loss, whereas lesions that impair mechanotransduction in the inner ear or transmission of the electrical signal along the eighth nerve to the brain cause sensorineural hearing loss.*

Conductive Hearing Loss The external ear, the external auditory canal, and the middle ear apparatus is designed to collect and amplify sound and efficiently transfer the mechanical energy of the sound wave to the fluid-filled cochlea. Factors that obstruct the transmission of sound or serve to dampen the acoustical energy result in conductive hearing loss. Conductive hearing loss can occur from obstruction of the external auditory canal by cerumen, debris, and foreign bodies; swelling of the lining of the canal; atresia or neoplasms of the canal; perforations of the tympanic membrane; disruption of the ossicular chain, as occurs with necrosis of the long process of the incus in trauma or infection; otosclerosis; or fluid, scarring, or neoplasms in the middle ear. Rarely, inner ear malformations or pathologies, such as superior semicircular canal dehiscence, lateral semicircular canal dysplasia, incomplete partition of the inner ear, and large vestibular aqueduct, may also be associated with conductive hearing loss.

Eustachian tube dysfunction is extremely common in adults and may predispose to acute otitis media (AOM) or serous otitis media (SOM). Trauma, AOM, and chronic otitis media are the usual factors responsible for tympanic membrane perforation. While small perforations often heal spontaneously, larger defects usually require surgical intervention. Tympanoplasty is highly effective (>90%) in the repair of tympanic membrane perforations. Otoscopy is usually sufficient to diagnose AOM, SOM, chronic otitis media, cerumen impaction, tympanic membrane perforation, and eustachian tube dysfunction; tympanometry can be useful to confirm the clinical suspicion of these conditions.

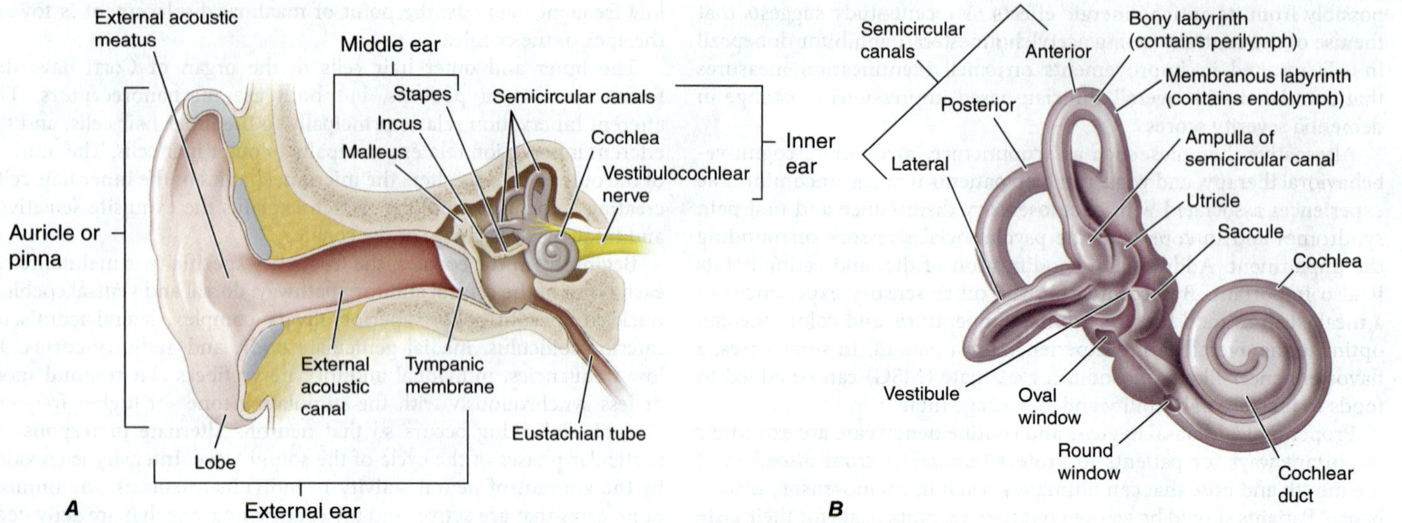

FIGURE 43-1 **Ear anatomy.** ***A.*** Drawing of modified coronal section through external ear and temporal bone, with structures of the middle and inner ear demonstrated. ***B.*** High-resolution view of inner ear.

Cholesteatoma, a benign tumor composed of stratified squamous epithelium in the middle ear or mastoid, occurs frequently in adults. This is a slowly growing lesion that destroys bone and normal ear tissue. Theories of pathogenesis include traumatic immigration and invasion of squamous epithelium through a retraction pocket, implantation of squamous epithelia in the middle ear through a perforation or surgery, and metaplasia following chronic infection and irritation. On examination, there is often a perforation of the tympanic membrane filled with cheesy white squamous debris. The presence of an aural polyp obscuring the tympanic membrane is highly suggestive of an underlying cholesteatoma. A chronically draining ear that fails to respond to appropriate antibiotic therapy should raise suspicion of a cholesteatoma. Conductive hearing loss secondary to ossicular erosion is common. Surgery is required to remove this destructive process.

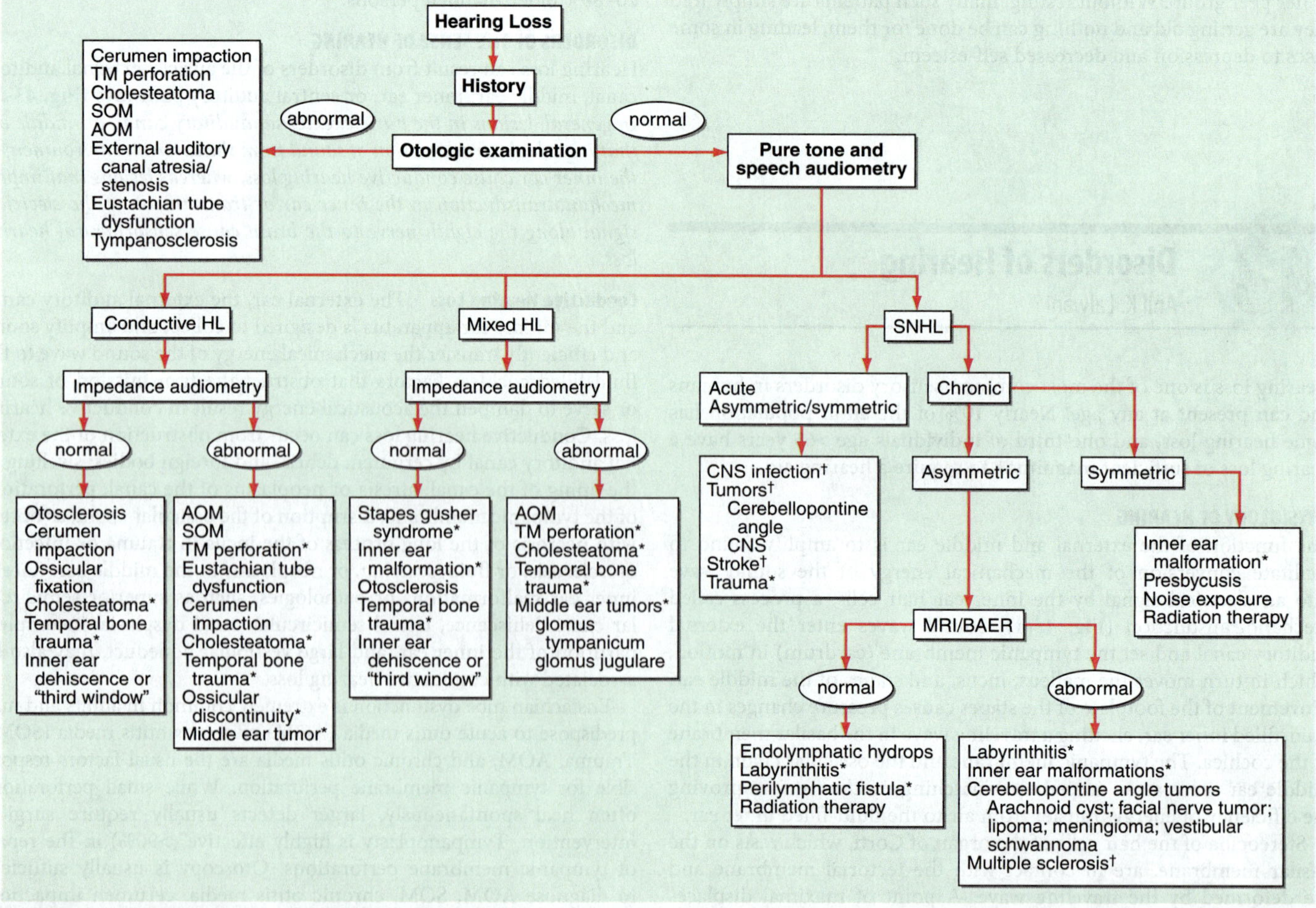

FIGURE 43-2 **An algorithm for the approach to hearing loss.** AOM, acute otitis media; BAER, brainstem auditory evoked response; CNS, central nervous system; HL, hearing loss; SNHL, sensorineural hearing loss; SOM, serous otitis media; TM, tympanic membrane. *Computed tomography scan of temporal bone. †Magnetic resonance imaging (MRI) scan.

Conductive hearing loss with a normal ear canal and intact tympanic membrane suggests either ossicular pathology or the presence of "third window" in the inner ear (see below). Fixation of the stapes from *otosclerosis* is a common cause of low-frequency conductive hearing loss. It occurs equally in men and women and is inherited as an autosomal dominant trait with incomplete penetrance; in some cases, it may be a manifestation of osteogenesis imperfecta. Hearing impairment usually presents between the late teens and the forties. In women, the otosclerotic process is accelerated during pregnancy, and the hearing loss is often first noticeable at this time. A hearing aid or a simple outpatient surgical procedure (stapedectomy) can provide adequate auditory rehabilitation. Extension of otosclerosis beyond the stapes footplate to involve the cochlea (cochlear otosclerosis) can lead to mixed or sensorineural hearing loss. Fluoride therapy to prevent hearing loss from cochlear otosclerosis is of uncertain value.

Disorders that lead to the formation of a pathologic "third window" in the inner ear can be associated with conductive hearing loss. There are normally two major openings, or windows, that connect the inner ear with the middle ear and serve as conduits for transmission of sound; these are, respectively, the oval and round windows. A third window is formed where the normally hard otic bone surrounding the inner ear is eroded; dissipation of the acoustic energy at the third window is responsible for the "inner ear conductive hearing loss." The superior semicircular canal dehiscence syndrome resulting from erosion of the otic bone over the superior circular canal can present with conductive hearing loss that mimics otosclerosis. A common symptom is vertigo evoked by loud sounds (Tullio phenomenon), by Valsalva maneuvers that change middle ear pressure, or by applying positive pressure on the tragus (the cartilage anterior to the external opening of the ear canal). Patients with this syndrome also complain of being able to hear the movement of their eyes and neck. A large jugular bulb or jugular bulb diverticulum can create a "third window" by eroding into the vestibular aqueduct or posterior semicircular canal; the symptoms are similar to those of the superior semicircular canal dehiscence syndrome.

Sensorineural Hearing Loss Sensorineural hearing loss results from either damage to the mechanotransduction apparatus of the cochlea or disruption of the electrical conduction pathway from the inner ear to the brain. Thus, injury to hair cells, supporting cells, auditory neurons, or the central auditory pathway can cause sensorineural hearing loss. Damage to the hair cells of the organ of Corti may be caused by intense noise, viral infections, ototoxic drugs (e.g., salicylates, quinine and its synthetic analogues, aminoglycoside antibiotics, loop diuretics such as furosemide and ethacrynic acid, and cancer chemotherapeutic agents such as cisplatin), fractures of the temporal bone, meningitis, cochlear otosclerosis (see above), Ménière's disease, and aging. Congenital malformations of the inner ear may be the cause of hearing loss in some adults. Genetic predisposition alone or in concert with environmental exposures may also be responsible (see below).

Presbycusis (age-associated hearing loss) is the most common cause of sensorineural hearing loss in adults. In the early stages, it is characterized by symmetric, gentle to sharply sloping high-frequency hearing loss (Fig. 43-3). With progression, the hearing loss involves all frequencies. More importantly, the hearing impairment is associated with significant loss in clarity. There is a loss of discrimination for phonemes, recruitment (abnormal growth of loudness), and particular difficulty in understanding speech in noisy environments such as at restaurants and social events. Hearing aids are helpful in enhancing the signal-to-noise ratio by amplifying sounds that are close to the listener. *Although hearing aids are able to amplify sounds, they cannot restore the clarity of hearing.* Thus, amplification with hearing aids may provide only limited rehabilitation once the word recognition score deteriorates below 50%. Cochlear implants are the treatment of choice when hearing aids prove inadequate, even when hearing loss is incomplete (see below).

Ménière's disease is characterized by episodic vertigo, fluctuating sensorineural hearing loss, tinnitus, and aural fullness. Tinnitus and/or deafness may be absent during the initial attacks of vertigo, but it

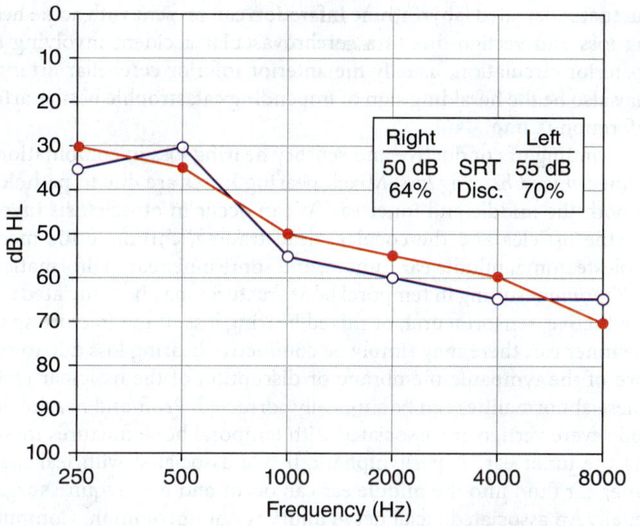

FIGURE 43-3 Presbyacusis or age-related hearing loss. The audiogram shows a moderate to severe downsloping sensorineural hearing loss typical of presbyacusis. The loss of high-frequency hearing is associated with a decreased speech discrimination score; consequently, patients complain of lack of clarity of hearing, especially in a noisy background. HL, hearing threshold level; SRT, speech reception threshold.

invariably appears as the disease progresses and increases in severity during acute attacks. The annual incidence of Ménière's disease is 0.5–7.5 per 1000; onset is most frequently in the fifth decade of life but may also occur in young adults or the elderly. Histologically, there is distention of the endolymphatic system (endolymphatic hydrops) leading to degeneration of vestibular and cochlear hair cells. This may result from endolymphatic sac dysfunction secondary to infection, trauma, autoimmune disease, inflammatory causes, or tumor; an idiopathic etiology constitutes the largest category and is most accurately referred to as Ménière's disease. Although any pattern of hearing loss can be observed, typically, low-frequency, unilateral sensorineural hearing impairment is present. Magnetic resonance imaging (MRI) should be obtained to exclude retrocochlear pathology such as a cerebellopontine angle tumor or demyelinating disorder. Therapy is directed toward the control of vertigo. A 2-g/d low-salt diet is the mainstay of treatment for control of rotatory vertigo. Diuretics, a short course of glucocorticoids, and intratympanic gentamicin may also be useful adjuncts in recalcitrant cases. Surgical therapy of vertigo is reserved for unresponsive cases and includes endolymphatic sac decompression, labyrinthectomy, and vestibular nerve section. Both labyrinthectomy and vestibular nerve section abolish rotatory vertigo in >90% of cases. Unfortunately, there is no effective therapy for hearing loss, tinnitus, or aural fullness from Ménière's disease.

Sensorineural hearing loss may also result from any neoplastic, vascular, demyelinating, infectious, or degenerative disease or trauma affecting the central auditory pathways. HIV leads to both peripheral and central auditory system pathology and is associated with sensorineural hearing impairment.

Primary diseases of the central nervous system can also present with hearing impairment. Characteristically, a reduction in clarity of hearing and speech comprehension is much greater than the loss of the ability to hear pure tone. Auditory testing is consistent with an auditory neuropathy; normal otoacoustic emissions (OAE) and an abnormal auditory brainstem response (ABR) is typical (see below). Hearing loss can accompany hereditary sensorimotor neuropathies and inherited disorders of myelin. Tumors of the cerebellopontine angle such as vestibular schwannoma and meningioma usually present with asymmetric sensorineural hearing loss with greater deterioration of speech understanding than pure tone hearing. Multiple sclerosis may present with acute unilateral or bilateral hearing loss; typically, pure tone testing remains relatively stable while speech understanding fluctuates. Isolated labyrinthine infarction can present with acute hearing loss and vertigo due to a cerebrovascular accident involving the posterior circulation, usually the anterior inferior cerebellar artery; it may also be the heralding sign of impending catastrophic basilar artery infarction (Chap. 446).

A finding of conductive and sensory hearing loss in combination is termed *mixed hearing loss*. Mixed hearing losses are due to pathology of both the middle and inner ear, as can occur in otosclerosis involving the ossicles and the cochlea, head trauma, chronic otitis media, cholesteatoma, middle ear tumors, and some inner ear malformations.

Trauma resulting in temporal bone fractures may be associated with conductive, sensorineural, or mixed hearing loss. If the fracture spares the inner ear, there may simply be conductive hearing loss due to rupture of the tympanic membrane or disruption of the ossicular chain. These abnormalities can be surgically corrected. Profound hearing loss and severe vertigo are associated with temporal bone fractures involving the inner ear. A perilymphatic fistula associated with leakage of inner ear fluid into the middle ear can occur and may require surgical repair. An associated facial nerve injury is not uncommon. Computed tomography (CT) is best suited to assess fracture of the traumatized temporal bone, evaluate the ear canal, and determine the integrity of the ossicular chain and the involvement of the inner ear. Cerebrospinal fluid leaks that accompany temporal bone fractures are usually self-limited; the value of prophylactic antibiotics is uncertain.

Tinnitus is defined as the perception of a sound when there is no sound in the environment. It may have a buzzing, roaring, or ringing quality and may be pulsatile (synchronous with the heartbeat). Tinnitus is often associated with either a conductive or sensorineural hearing loss. The pathophysiology of tinnitus is not well understood. The cause of the tinnitus can usually be determined by finding the cause of the associated hearing loss. Tinnitus may be the first symptom of a serious condition such as a vestibular schwannoma. Pulsatile tinnitus requires evaluation of the vascular system of the head to exclude vascular tumors such as glomus jugulare tumors, aneurysms, dural arteriovenous fistulas, and stenotic arterial lesions; it may also occur with SOM. It is most commonly associated with some abnormality of the jugular bulb such as a large jugular bulb or jugular bulb diverticulum.

GENETIC CAUSES OF HEARING LOSS

More than half of childhood hearing impairment is thought to be hereditary; hereditary hearing impairment (HHI) can also manifest later in life. HHI may be classified as either nonsyndromic, when hearing loss is the only clinical abnormality, or syndromic, when hearing loss is associated with anomalies in other organ systems. Nearly two-thirds of HHIs are nonsyndromic, and the remaining one-third are syndromic. Between 70 and 80% of nonsyndromic HHI is inherited in an autosomal recessive manner and designated DFNB; another 15–20% is autosomal dominant (DFNA). Less than 5% is X-linked (DFNX) or maternally inherited via the mitochondria.

More than 150 loci harboring genes for nonsyndromic HHI have been mapped, with recessive loci outnumbering dominant; numerous genes have now been identified (Table 43-1). The hearing genes fall into the categories of structural proteins (*MYH9, MYO7A, MYO15, TECTA, DIAPH1*), transcription factors (*POU3F4, POU4F3*), ion channels (*KCNQ4, SLC26A4*), and gap junction proteins (*GJB2, GJB3, GJB6*). Several of these genes, including *GJB2*, *TECTA*, and *TMC1*, cause both autosomal dominant and recessive forms of nonsyndromic HHI. In general, the hearing loss associated with dominant genes has its onset in adolescence or adulthood, varies in severity, and progresses with age, whereas the hearing loss associated with recessive inheritance is congenital and profound. Connexin 26, product of the *GJB2* gene, is particularly important because it is responsible for nearly 20% of all cases of childhood deafness; half of genetic deafness in children is *GJB2*-related. Two frameshift mutations, 35delG and 167delT, account for >50% of the cases; however, screening for these two mutations alone is insufficient, and sequencing of the entire gene is required to diagnose *GJB2*-related recessive deafness. The 167delT mutation is highly prevalent in Ashkenazi Jews; ~1 in 1765 individuals in this population are homozygous and affected. The hearing loss can also vary among the members of the same family, suggesting that other genes or factors influence the auditory phenotype.

In addition to *GJB2*, several other nonsyndromic genes are associated with hearing loss that progresses with age. The contribution of genetics to presbycusis is also becoming better understood. Sensitivity to aminoglycoside ototoxicity can be maternally transmitted through a mitochondrial mutation. Susceptibility to noise-induced hearing loss may also be genetically determined.

There are >400 syndromic forms of hearing loss. These include Usher's syndrome (retinitis pigmentosa and hearing loss), Waardenburg's syndrome (pigmentary abnormality and hearing loss), Pendred's syndrome (thyroid organification defect and hearing loss), Alport's syndrome (renal disease and hearing loss), Jervell and Lange-Nielsen syndrome (prolonged QT interval and hearing loss), neurofibromatosis type 2 (bilateral acoustic schwannoma), and mitochondrial disorders (mitochondrial encephalopathy, lactic acidosis, and stroke-like episodes [MELAS]; myoclonic epilepsy and ragged red fibers [MERRF]; progressive external ophthalmoplegia [PEO]) (Table 43-2).

APPROACH TO THE PATIENT: **Disorders of the Sense of Hearing**

The goal in the evaluation of a patient with auditory complaints is to determine (1) the nature of the hearing impairment (conductive vs sensorineural vs mixed), (2) the severity of the impairment (mild, moderate, severe, or profound), (3) the anatomy of the impairment (external ear, middle ear, inner ear, or central auditory pathway), and (4) the etiology. The history should elicit characteristics of the hearing loss, including the duration of deafness, unilateral versus bilateral involvement, nature of onset (sudden vs insidious), and rate of progression (rapid vs slow). Symptoms of tinnitus, vertigo, imbalance, aural fullness, otorrhea, headache, facial nerve dysfunction, and head and neck paresthesias should be noted. Information regarding head trauma, exposure to ototoxins, occupational or recreational noise exposure, and family history of hearing impairment may also be important. A sudden onset of unilateral hearing loss, with or without tinnitus, may represent a viral infection of the inner ear, vestibular schwannoma, or a stroke. Patients with unilateral hearing loss (sensory or conductive) usually complain of reduced hearing, poor sound localization, and difficulty hearing clearly with background noise. Gradual progression of a hearing deficit is common with otosclerosis, noise-induced hearing loss, vestibular schwannoma, or Ménière's disease. Small vestibular schwannomas typically present with asymmetric hearing impairment, tinnitus, and imbalance (rarely vertigo); cranial neuropathy, in particular of the trigeminal or facial nerve, may accompany larger tumors. In addition to hearing loss, Ménière's disease may be associated with episodic vertigo, tinnitus, and aural fullness. Hearing loss with otorrhea is most likely due to chronic otitis media or cholesteatoma.

Examination should include the auricle, external ear canal, and tympanic membrane. The external ear canal of the elderly is often dry and fragile; it is preferable to clean cerumen with wall-mounted suction or cerumen loops and to avoid irrigation. In examining the eardrum, the topography of the tympanic membrane is more important than the presence or absence of the light reflex. In addition to the pars tensa (the lower two-thirds of the tympanic membrane), the pars flaccida (upper one-third of the tympanic membrane) above the short process of the malleus should also be examined for retraction pockets that may be evidence of chronic eustachian tube dysfunction or cholesteatoma. Insufflation of the ear canal is necessary to assess tympanic membrane mobility and compliance. Careful inspection of the nose, nasopharynx, and upper respiratory tract is indicated. Unilateral serous effusion should prompt a fiberoptic examination of the nasopharynx to exclude neoplasms. Cranial nerves should be evaluated with special attention to facial and trigeminal nerves, which are commonly affected with tumors involving the cerebellopontine angle.

TABLE 43-1 HEREDITARY HEARING IMPAIRMENT GENES

Designation	Gene	Function
Autosomal Dominant		
	CRYM	Thyroid hormone–binding protein
DFNA1	*DIAPH1*	Cytoskeletal protein
DFNA2A	*KCNQ4*	Potassium channel
DFNA2B	*GJB3 (Cx31)*	Gap junction
DFNA3A	*GJB2 (Cx26)*	Gap junction
DFNA3B	*GJB6 (Cx30)*	Gap junction
DFNA4	*MYH14*	Class II nonmuscle myosin
	CEACAM16	Cell adhesion molecule
DFNA5	*DFNA5*	Unknown
DFNA6/14/38	*WFS1*	Transmembrane protein
DFNA8/12	*TECTA*	Tectorial membrane protein
DFNA9	*COCH*	Unknown
DFNA10	*EYA4*	Developmental gene
DFNA11	*MYO7A*	Cytoskeletal protein
DFNA13	*COL11A2*	Cytoskeletal protein
DFNA15	*POU4F3*	Transcription factor
DFNA17	*MYH9*	Cytoskeletal protein
DFNA20/26	*ACTG1*	Cytoskeletal protein
DFNA22	*MYO6*	Unconventional myosin
DFNA23	*SIX1*	Developmental gene
DFNA25	*SLC17AB*	Vesicular glutamate transporter
DFNA28	*TFCP2L3*	Transcription factor
DFNA36	*TMC1*	Transmembrane protein
DFNA41	*P2RX2*	Purinergic receptor
DFNA44	*CCDC50*	Effector of epidermal growth factor–mediated signaling
DFNA48	*MYO1A*	Unconventional myosin
DFNA50	*MIRN96*	MicroRNA
DFNA51	*TJP2*	Tight junction protein
DFNA56	*TNC*	Extracellular matrix protein
DFNA64	*SMAC/DIABLO*	Mitochondrial proapoptotic protein
Autosomal Recessive		
DFNB1A	*GJB2 (CX26)*	Gap junction
DFNB1B	*GJB6 (CX30)*	Gap junction
DFNB2	*MYO7A*	Cytoskeletal protein
DFNB3	*MYO15*	Cytoskeletal protein
DFNB4	*PDS (SLC26A4)*	Chloride/iodide transporter
DFNB6	*TMIE*	Transmembrane protein
DFNB7/B11	*TMC1*	Transmembrane protein
DFNB9	*OTOF*	Trafficking of membrane vesicles
DFNB8/10	*TMPRSS3*	Transmembrane serine protease
DFNB12	*CDH23*	Intercellular adherence protein
DFNB15/72/95	*GIPC3*	PDZ domain containing protein
DFNB16	*STRC*	Stereocilia protein
DFNB18	*USH1C*	Unknown
DFNB21	*TECTA*	Tectorial membrane protein
DFNB22	*OTOA*	Gel attachment to nonsensory cell
DFNB23	*PCDH15*	Morphogenesis and cohesion
DFNB24	*RDX*	Cytoskeletal protein
DFNB25	*GRXCR1*	Reversible S-glutathionylation of proteins
DFNB28	*TRIOBP*	Cytoskeletal-organizing protein
DFNB29	*CLDN14*	Tight junctions
DFNB30	*MYO3A*	Hybrid motor-signaling myosin
DFNB31	*WHRN*	PDZ domain–containing protein
DFNB35	*ESRRB*	Estrogen-related receptor beta protein
DFNB36	*ESPN*	Ca-insensitive actin-bundling protein
DFNB37	*MYO6*	Unconventional myosin
DFNB39	*HFG*	Hepatocyte growth factor
DFNB42	*ILDR1*	Ig-like domain-containing receptor
DFNB48	*CIB2*	Calcium and integrin binding protein
DFNB49	*MARVELD2*	Tight junction protein
DFNB53	*COL11A2*	Collagen protein
DFNB59	*PJVK*	Zn-binding protein
DFNB61	*SLC26A5*	Motor protein
DFNB63	*LRTOMT/COMT2*	Putative methyltransferase
DFNB66/67	*LHFPL5*	Tetraspan protein
DFNB70	*PNPT1*	Mitochondrial-RNA-import protein
DFNB74	*MSRB3*	Methionine sulfoxide reductase
DFNB77	*LOXHD1*	Stereociliary protein
DFNB79	*TPRN*	Unknown
DFNB82	*GPSM2*	G protein signaling modulator
DFNB84	*PTPRQ*	Type III receptor-like protein-tyrosine phosphatase family
DFNB86	*TBC1D24*	GTPase-activating protein
DFNB88	*ELMOD3*	GTPase-activating protein
DFNB89	*KARS*	Lysyl-tRNA synthetase
DFNB91	*GJB3*	Gap junction
DFNB93	*CABP2*	Calcium binding protein
DFNB98	*TSPEAR*	Epilepsy-associated repeats containing protein
	SERPINB6	Protease inhibitor

The Rinne and Weber tuning fork tests, with a 512-Hz tuning fork, are used to screen for hearing loss, differentiate conductive from sensorineural hearing losses, and confirm the findings of audiologic evaluation. The Rinne test compares the ability to hear by air conduction with the ability to hear by bone conduction. The tines of a vibrating tuning fork are held near the opening of the external auditory canal, and then the stem is placed on the mastoid process; for direct contact, it may be placed on teeth or dentures. The patient is asked to indicate whether the tone is louder by air conduction or bone conduction. Normally, and in the presence of sensorineural hearing loss, a tone is heard louder by air conduction than by bone conduction; however, with conductive hearing loss of ≥30 dB (see "Audiologic Assessment," below), the bone-conduction stimulus is perceived as louder than the air-conduction stimulus. For the Weber test, the stem of a vibrating tuning fork is placed on the head in the midline and the patient is asked whether the tone is heard in both ears or better in one ear than in the other. With a unilateral conductive hearing loss, the tone is perceived in the affected ear. With a unilateral sensorineural hearing loss, the tone is perceived in the unaffected ear. A 5-dB difference in hearing between the two ears is required for lateralization.

LABORATORY ASSESSMENT OF HEARING

Audiologic Assessment The minimum audiologic assessment for hearing loss should include the measurement of pure tone air-conduction and bone-conduction thresholds, speech reception threshold, word recognition score, tympanometry, acoustic reflexes, and acoustic-reflex decay. This test battery provides a screening evaluation of the entire auditory system and allows one to determine whether further

TABLE 43-2 SYNDROMIC HEREDITARY HEARING IMPAIRMENT GENES

Syndrome	Gene	Function
Alport's syndrome	*COL4A3-5*	Cytoskeletal protein
BOR syndrome	*EYA1*	Developmental gene
	SIX5	Developmental gene
	SIX1	Developmental gene
Jervell and Lange-Nielsen syndrome	*KCNQ1*	Delayed rectifier K+ channel
	KCNE1	Delayed rectifier K+ channel
Norrie's disease	*NDP*	Cell-cell interactions
Pendred's syndrome	*SLC26A4*	Chloride/iodide transporter
	FOXI1	Transcriptional activator of *SLC26A4*
	KCNJ10	Inwardly rectifying K+ channel
Treacher Collins syndrome	*TCOF1*	Nucleolar-cytoplasmic transport
	POLR1D	Subunit of RNA polymerases I and III
	POLR1C	Subunit of RNA polymerases I and III
Usher's syndrome	*MYO7A*	Cytoskeletal protein
	USH1C	Unknown
	CDH23	Intercellular adherence protein
	PCDH15	Cell adhesion molecule
	SANS	Harmonin-associated protein
	CIB2	Calcium and integrin binding protein
	USH2A	Cell adhesion molecule
	VLGR1	G protein–coupled receptor
	WHRN	PDZ domain–containing protein
	CLRN1	Cellular synapse protein?
	PDZD7	PDZ domain containing protein
WS type I, III	*PAX3*	Transcription factor
WS type II	*MITF*	Transcription factor
	SNAI2	Transcription factor
WS type IV	*EDNRB*	Endothelin B receptor
	EDN3	Endothelin B receptor ligand
	SOX10	Transcription factor

Abbreviations: BOR, branchio-oto-renal syndrome; WS, Waardenburg's syndrome.

differentiation of a sensory (cochlear) from a neural (retrocochlear) hearing loss is indicated.

Pure tone audiometry assesses hearing acuity for pure tones. The test is administered by an audiologist and is performed in a sound-attenuated chamber. The pure tone stimulus is delivered with an audiometer, an electronic device that allows the presentation of specific frequencies (generally between 250 and 8000 Hz) at specific intensities. Air- and bone-conduction thresholds are established for each ear. Air-conduction thresholds are determined by presenting the stimulus in air with the use of headphones. Bone-conduction thresholds are determined by placing the stem of a vibrating tuning fork or an oscillator of an audiometer in contact with the head. In the presence of a hearing loss, broad-spectrum noise is presented to the nontest ear for *masking* purposes so that responses are based on perception from the ear under test.

The responses are measured in decibels. An *audiogram* is a plot of intensity in decibels of hearing threshold versus frequency. A decibel (dB) is equal to 20 times the logarithm of the ratio of the sound pressure required to achieve threshold in the patient to the sound pressure required to achieve threshold in a normal-hearing person. Therefore, a change of 6 dB represents doubling of sound pressure, and a change of 20 dB represents a tenfold change in sound pressure. Loudness, which depends on the frequency, intensity, and duration of a sound, doubles with approximately each 10-dB increase in sound pressure level. Pitch, on the other hand, does not directly correlate with frequency. The perception of pitch changes slowly in the low and high frequencies. In the middle tones, which are important for human speech, pitch varies more rapidly with changes in frequency.

Pure tone audiometry establishes the presence and severity of hearing impairment, unilateral versus bilateral involvement, and the type of hearing loss. Conductive hearing losses with a large mass component, as is often seen in middle ear effusions, produce elevation of thresholds that predominate in the higher frequencies. Conductive hearing losses with a large stiffness component, as in fixation of the footplate of the stapes in early otosclerosis, produce threshold elevations in the lower frequencies. Often, the conductive hearing loss involves all frequencies, suggesting involvement of both stiffness and mass. In general, sensorineural hearing losses such as presbycusis affect higher frequencies more than lower frequencies (Fig. 43-3). An exception is Ménière's disease, which is characteristically associated with low-frequency sensorineural hearing loss. Noise-induced hearing loss has an unusual pattern of hearing impairment in which the loss at 4000 Hz is greater than at higher frequencies. Vestibular schwannomas characteristically affect the higher frequencies, but any pattern of hearing loss can be observed.

Speech recognition requires greater synchronous neural firing than is necessary for appreciation of pure tones. *Speech audiometry* tests the clarity with which one hears. The *speech reception threshold* (SRT) is defined as the intensity at which speech is recognized as a meaningful symbol and is obtained by presenting two-syllable words with an equal accent on each syllable. The intensity at which the patient can repeat 50% of the words correctly is the SRT. Once the SRT is determined, discrimination or word recognition ability is tested by presenting one-syllable words at 25–40 dB above the SRT. The words are phonetically balanced in that the phonemes (speech sounds) occur in the list of words at the same frequency that they occur in ordinary conversational English. An individual with normal hearing or conductive hearing loss can repeat 88–100% of the phonetically balanced words correctly. Patients with a sensorineural hearing loss have variable loss of discrimination. As a general rule, neural lesions produce greater deficits in discrimination than do cochlear lesions. For example, in a patient with mild asymmetric sensorineural hearing loss, a clue to the diagnosis of vestibular schwannoma is the presence of greater than expected deterioration in discrimination ability. Deterioration in discrimination ability at higher intensities above the SRT also suggests a lesion in the eighth nerve or central auditory pathways.

Tympanometry measures the impedance of the middle ear to sound and is useful in diagnosis of middle ear effusions. A *tympanogram* is the graphic representation of change in impedance or compliance as the pressure in the ear canal is changed. Normally, the middle ear is most compliant at atmospheric pressure, and the compliance decreases as the pressure is increased or decreased (type A); this pattern is seen with normal hearing or in the presence of sensorineural hearing loss. Compliance that does not change with change in pressure suggests middle ear effusion (type B). With a negative pressure in the middle ear, as with eustachian tube obstruction, the point of maximal compliance occurs with negative pressure in the ear canal (type C). A tympanogram in which no point of maximal compliance can be obtained is most commonly seen with discontinuity of the ossicular chain (type A_d). A reduction in the maximal compliance peak can be seen in otosclerosis (type A_s).

During tympanometry, an intense tone elicits contraction of the stapedius muscle. The change in compliance of the middle ear with contraction of the stapedius muscle can be detected. The presence or absence of this *acoustic reflex* is important in determining the etiology of hearing loss as well as in the anatomic localization of facial nerve paralysis. The acoustic reflex can help differentiate between conductive hearing loss due to otosclerosis and that caused by an inner ear "third window": it is absent in otosclerosis and present in inner ear conductive hearing loss. Normal or elevated acoustic reflex thresholds in an individual with sensorineural hearing impairment suggest a cochlear hearing loss. An absent acoustic reflex in the setting of sensorineural hearing loss is not helpful in localizing the site of lesion. Assessment of *acoustic reflex decay* helps differentiate sensory from neural hearing losses. In neural hearing loss, such as with vestibular schwannoma, the reflex adapts or decays with time.

OAEs generated by outer hair cells only can be measured with microphones inserted into the external auditory canal. The emissions may be spontaneous or evoked with sound stimulation. The presence of OAEs indicates that the outer hair cells of the organ of Corti are intact and can be used to assess auditory thresholds and to distinguish sensory from neural hearing losses.

Evoked Responses *Electrocochleography* measures the earliest evoked potentials generated in the cochlea and the auditory nerve. Receptor potentials recorded include the cochlear microphonic, generated by the outer hair cells of the organ of Corti, and the summating potential, generated by the inner hair cells in response to sound. The whole nerve action potential representing the composite firing of the first-order neurons can also be recorded during electrocochleography. Clinically, the test is useful in the diagnosis of Ménière's disease, where an elevation of the ratio of summating potential to action potential is seen.

Brainstem auditory evoked responses (BAERs), also known as *auditory brainstem responses* (ABRs), are useful in differentiating the site of sensorineural hearing loss. In response to sound, five distinct electrical potentials arising from different stations along the peripheral and central auditory pathway can be identified using computer averaging from scalp surface electrodes. BAERs are valuable in situations in which patients cannot or will not give reliable voluntary thresholds. They are also used to assess the integrity of the auditory nerve and brainstem in various clinical situations, including intraoperative monitoring, and in determination of brain death.

The *vestibular-evoked myogenic potential (VEMP) test* elicits a vestibulocolic reflex whose afferent limb arises from acoustically sensitive cells in the saccule, with signals conducted via the inferior vestibular nerve. VEMP is a biphasic, short-latency response recorded from the tonically contracted sternocleidomastoid muscle in response to loud auditory clicks or tones. VEMPs may be diminished or absent in patients with early and late Ménière's disease, vestibular neuritis, benign paroxysmal positional vertigo, and vestibular schwannoma. On the other hand, the threshold for VEMPs may be lower in cases of superior canal dehiscence, other inner ear dehiscence, and perilymphatic fistula.

Imaging Studies The choice of radiologic tests is largely determined by whether the goal is to evaluate the bony anatomy of the external, middle, and inner ear or to image the auditory nerve and brain. Axial and coronal CT of the temporal bone with fine 0.3- to 0.6-mm cuts is ideal for determining the caliber of the external auditory canal, integrity of the ossicular chain, and presence of middle ear or mastoid disease; it can also detect inner ear malformations. CT is also ideal for the detection of bone erosion with chronic otitis media and cholesteatoma. Pöschl reformatting in the plane of the superior semicircular canal is required for the identification of dehiscence or absence of bone over the superior semicircular canal. MRI is superior to CT for imaging of retrocochlear pathology such as vestibular schwannoma, meningioma, other lesions of the cerebellopontine angle, demyelinating lesions of the brainstem, and brain tumors. Both CT and MRI are equally capable of identifying inner ear malformations and assessing cochlear patency for preoperative evaluation of patients for cochlear implantation.

TREATMENT DISORDERS OF THE SENSE OF HEARING

In general, conductive hearing losses are amenable to surgical correction, whereas sensorineural hearing losses are usually managed medically. Atresia of the ear canal can be surgically repaired, often with significant improvement in hearing. Tympanic membrane perforations due to chronic otitis media or trauma can be repaired with an outpatient tympanoplasty. Likewise, conductive hearing loss associated with otosclerosis can be treated by stapedectomy, which is successful in >95% of cases. Tympanostomy tubes allow the prompt return of normal hearing in individuals with middle ear effusions. Hearing aids are effective and well tolerated in patients with conductive hearing losses.

Patients with mild, moderate, and severe sensorineural hearing losses are regularly rehabilitated with hearing aids of varying configuration and strength. Hearing aids have been improved to provide greater fidelity and have been miniaturized. The current generation of hearing aids can be placed entirely within the ear canal, thus reducing any stigma associated with their use. In general, the more severe the hearing impairment, the larger the hearing aid required for auditory rehabilitation. Digital hearing aids lend themselves to individual programming, and multiple and directional microphones at the ear level may be helpful in noisy surroundings. Because all hearing aids amplify noise as well as speech, the only absolute solution to the problem of noise is to place the microphone closer to the speaker than the noise source. This arrangement is not possible with a self-contained, cosmetically acceptable device. A significant limitation of rehabilitation with a hearing aid is that although it is able to enhance detection of sound with amplification, it cannot restore clarity of hearing that is lost with presbycusis.

Patients with unilateral deafness have difficulty with sound localization and reduced clarity of hearing in background noise. They may benefit from a CROS (contralateral routing of signal) hearing aid in which a microphone is placed on the hearing-impaired side and the sound is transmitted to the receiver placed on the contralateral ear. The same result may be obtained with a bone-anchored hearing aid (BAHA), in which a hearing aid clamps to a screw integrated into the skull on the hearing-impaired side. Like the CROS hearing aid, the BAHA transfers the acoustic signal to the contralateral hearing ear, but it does so by vibrating the skull. Patients with profound deafness on one side and some hearing loss in the better ear are candidates for a BICROS hearing aid; it differs from the CROS hearing aid in that the patient wears a hearing aid, and not simply a receiver, in the better ear. Unfortunately, while CROS and BAHA devices provide benefit, they do not restore hearing in the deaf ear. Only cochlear implants can restore hearing (see below). Increasingly, cochlear implants are being investigated for the treatment of patients with single-sided deafness; early reports show great promise in not only restoring hearing but also improving sound localization and performance in background noise.

In many situations, including lectures and the theater, hearing-impaired persons benefit from assistive devices that are based on the principle of having the speaker closer to the microphone than any source of noise. Assistive devices include infrared and frequency-modulated (FM) transmission as well as an electromagnetic loop around the room for transmission to the individual's hearing aid. Hearing aids with telecoils can also be used with properly equipped telephones in the same way.

In the event that the hearing aid provides inadequate rehabilitation, cochlear implants may be appropriate (Fig. 43-4). Criteria for implantation include severe to profound hearing loss with open-set sentence cognition of ≤40% under best aided conditions. Worldwide, more than 300,000 hearing-impaired individuals have received cochlear implants. Cochlear implants are neural prostheses that convert sound energy to electrical energy and can be used to stimulate the auditory division of the eighth nerve directly. In most cases of profound hearing impairment, the auditory hair cells are lost but the ganglionic cells of the auditory division of the eighth nerve are preserved. Cochlear implants consist of electrodes that are inserted into the cochlea through the round window, speech processors that extract acoustical elements of speech for conversion to electrical currents, and a means of transmitting the electrical energy through the skin. Patients with implants experience sound that helps with speech reading, allows open-set word recognition, and helps in modulating the person's own voice. Usually, within the first 3–6 months after implantation, adult patients can understand speech without visual cues. With the current generation of multichannel cochlear implants, nearly 75% of patients are able to converse on the telephone.

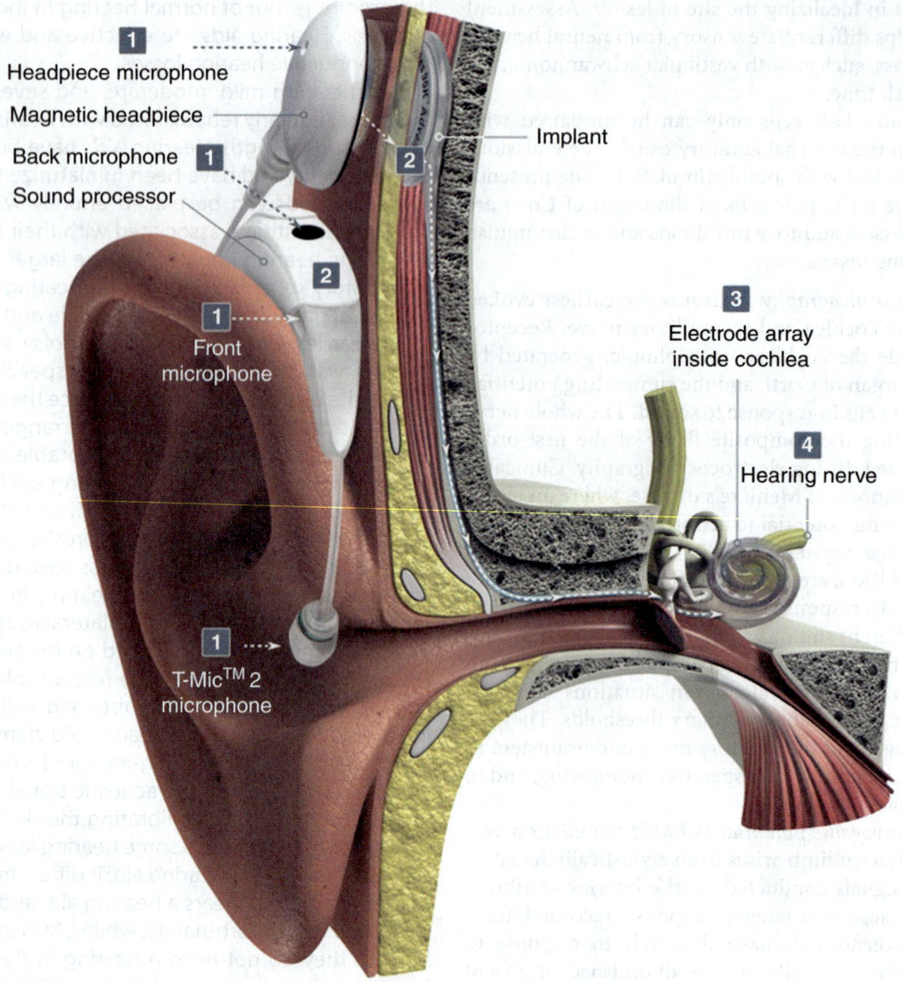

FIGURE 43-4 A cochlear implant is composed of an external microphone and speech processor worn on the ear and a receiver implanted underneath the temporalis muscle. The internal receiver is attached to an electrode that is placed surgically in the cochlea.

The U.S. Food and Drug Administration recently approved the first hybrid cochlear implant for the treatment of high-frequency hearing loss. Patients with presbyacusis typically have normal low-frequency hearing, while suffering from high-frequency hearing loss associated with loss of clarity that cannot always be adequately rehabilitated with a hearing aid. However, these patients are not candidates for conventional cochlear implants because they have too much residual hearing. The hybrid implant has been specifically designed for this patient population; it has a shorter electrode than a conventional cochlear implant and can be introduced into the cochlea atraumatically, thus preserving low-frequency hearing. Individuals with a hybrid implant use their own natural low-frequency "acoustic" hearing and rely on the implant for providing "electrical" high-frequency hearing. Patients who have received the hybrid implant perform better on speech testing in both quiet and noisy backgrounds.

For individuals who have had both eighth nerves destroyed by trauma or bilateral vestibular schwannomas (e.g., neurofibromatosis type 2), brainstem auditory implants placed near the cochlear nucleus may provide auditory rehabilitation.

Tinnitus often accompanies hearing loss. As for background noise, tinnitus can degrade speech comprehension in individuals with hearing impairment. Therapy for tinnitus is usually directed toward minimizing the appreciation of tinnitus. Relief of the tinnitus may be obtained by masking it with background music. Hearing aids are also helpful in tinnitus suppression, as are tinnitus maskers, devices that present a sound to the affected ear that is more pleasant to listen to than the tinnitus. The use of a tinnitus masker is often followed by several hours of inhibition of the tinnitus. Antidepressants have been shown to be beneficial in helping patients cope with tinnitus.

Hard-of-hearing individuals often benefit from a reduction in unnecessary noise in the environment (e.g., radio or television) to enhance the signal-to-noise ratio. Speech comprehension is aided by lip reading; therefore, the impaired listener should be seated so that the face of the speaker is well illuminated and easily seen. Although speech should be in a loud, clear voice, one should be aware that in sensorineural hearing losses in general and in hard-of-hearing elderly in particular, recruitment (abnormal perception of loud sounds) may be troublesome. Above all, optimal communication cannot take place without both parties giving it their full and undivided attention.

PREVENTION

Conductive hearing losses may be prevented by prompt antibiotic therapy of adequate duration for AOM and by ventilation of the middle ear with tympanostomy tubes in middle ear effusions lasting ≥12 weeks. Loss of vestibular function and deafness due to aminoglycoside antibiotics can largely be prevented by careful monitoring of serum peak and trough levels.

Some 10 million Americans have noise-induced hearing loss, and 20 million are exposed to hazardous noise in their employment. Noise-induced hearing loss can be prevented by avoidance of exposure to loud noise or by regular use of ear plugs or fluid-filled ear muffs to attenuate intense sound. Table 43-3 lists loudness levels for a variety of

TABLE 43-3 DECIBEL (LOUDNESS) LEVEL OF COMMON ENVIRONMENTAL NOISE

Source	Decibel (dB)
Weakest sound heard	0
Whisper	30
Normal conversation	55–65
City traffic inside car	85
OSHA monitoring requirement begins	**90**
Jackhammer	95
Subway train at 200 ft	95
Power mower	107
Power saw	110
Painful sound	**125**
Jet engine at 100 feet	140
12-gauge shotgun blast	165
Loudest sound that can occur	194

Abbreviation: OSHA, Occupational Safety and Health Administration.

environmental sounds. High-risk activities for noise-induced hearing loss include use of electrical equipment for wood and metal working and target practice or hunting with small firearms. All internal-combustion and electric engines, including snow and leaf blowers, snowmobiles, outboard motors, and chainsaws, require protection of the user with hearing protectors. Virtually all noise-induced hearing loss is preventable through education, which should begin before the teenage years. Programs for conservation of hearing in the workplace are required by the Occupational Safety and Health Administration (OSHA) whenever the exposure over an 8-h period averages 85 dB. OSHA mandates that workers in such noisy environments have hearing monitoring and protection programs that include a preemployment screen, an annual audiologic assessment, and the mandatory use of hearing protectors. Exposure to loud sounds above 85 dB in the work environment is restricted by OSHA, with halving of allowed exposure time for each increment of 5 dB above this threshold; for example, exposure to 90 dB is permitted for 8 h; 95 dB for 4 h, and 100 dB for 2 h (Table 43-4).

TABLE 43-4 OSHA DAILY PERMISSIBLE NOISE LEVEL EXPOSURE

Sound Level (dB)	Duration per Day (h)
90	8
92	6
95	4
97	3
100	2
102	1.5
105	1
110	0.5
115	≤0.25

Note: Exposure to impulsive or impact noise should not exceed 140-dB peak sound pressure level.

Source: From *https://www.osha.gov/pls/oshaweb/owadisp.show_document?p_table=standards&p_id=9735.*

44 Sore Throat, Earache, and Upper Respiratory Symptoms

Michael A. Rubin, Larry C. Ford, Ralph Gonzales

Infections of the upper respiratory tract (URIs) have a tremendous impact on public health. They are among the most common reasons for visits to primary care providers, and although the illnesses are typically mild, their high incidence and transmission rates place them among the leading causes of time lost from work or school. Even though a minority (~25%) of cases are caused by bacteria, URIs are the leading diagnoses for which antibiotics are prescribed on an outpatient basis in the United States. The enormous consumption of antibiotics for these illnesses has contributed to the rise in antibiotic resistance among common community-acquired pathogens such as *Streptococcus pneumoniae*—a trend that in itself has an enormous influence on public health.

Although most URIs are caused by viruses, distinguishing patients with primary viral infection from those with primary bacterial infection is difficult. Signs and symptoms of bacterial and viral URIs are typically indistinguishable. Until consistent, inexpensive, and rapid testing becomes available and is used widely, acute infections will be diagnosed largely on clinical grounds. The judicious use and potential for misuse of antibiotics in this setting pose definite challenges.

NONSPECIFIC INFECTIONS OF THE UPPER RESPIRATORY TRACT

Nonspecific URIs are a broadly defined group of disorders that collectively constitute the leading cause of ambulatory care visits in the United States. By definition, nonspecific URIs have no prominent localizing features. They are identified by a variety of descriptive names, including *acute infective rhinitis, acute rhinopharyngitis/nasopharyngitis, acute coryza,* and *acute nasal catarrh,* as well as by the inclusive label *common cold.*

ETIOLOGY

The large assortment of URI classifications reflects the wide variety of causative infectious agents and the varied manifestations of common pathogens. Nearly all nonspecific URIs are caused by viruses spanning multiple virus families and many antigenic types. For instance, there are at least 100 immunotypes of rhinovirus (Chap. 223), the most common cause of URI (~30–40% of cases); other causes include influenza virus (three immunotypes; Chap. 224) as well as parainfluenza virus (four immunotypes), coronavirus (at least three immunotypes), and adenovirus (47 immunotypes) (Chap. 223). Respiratory syncytial virus (RSV), a well-established pathogen in pediatric populations, is also a recognized cause of significant disease in elderly and immunocompromised individuals. A host of additional viruses, including some viruses not typically associated with URIs (e.g., enteroviruses, rubella virus, and varicella-zoster virus), account for a small percentage of cases in adults each year. Although new diagnostic modalities (e.g., nasopharyngeal swab for polymerase chain reaction [PCR]) can assign a viral etiology, there are few specific treatment options, and no pathogen is identified in a substantial proportion of cases. A specific diagnostic workup beyond a clinical diagnosis is generally unnecessary in an otherwise healthy adult.

CLINICAL MANIFESTATIONS

The signs and symptoms of nonspecific URI are similar to those of other URIs but lack a pronounced localization to one particular anatomic location, such as the sinuses, pharynx, or lower airway. Nonspecific URI commonly presents as an acute, mild, and self-limited catarrhal syndrome with a median duration of ~1 week (range, 2–10 days). Signs and symptoms are diverse and frequently variable across patients, even when caused by the same virus. The principal signs and symptoms of nonspecific URI include rhinorrhea (with or without purulence), nasal congestion, cough, and sore throat. Other manifestations, such as fever, malaise, sneezing, lymphadenopathy, and hoarseness, are more variable, with fever more common among infants and young children. This varying presentation may reflect differences in host response as well as in infecting organisms; myalgias and fatigue, for example, sometimes are seen with influenza and parainfluenza infections, whereas conjunctivitis may suggest infection with adenovirus or enterovirus. Findings on physical examination are frequently nonspecific and unimpressive. Between 0.5% and 2% of colds are complicated by secondary bacterial infections (e.g., rhinosinusitis, otitis media, and pneumonia), particularly in higher-risk populations such as infants, elderly persons, and chronically ill or immunosuppressed individuals. Secondary bacterial infections usually are associated with a prolonged course of illness, increased severity of illness, and localization of signs and symptoms, often as a rebound after initial clinical improvement (the "double-dip" sign). Purulent secretions from the nares or throat often are misinterpreted as an indication of bacterial sinusitis or pharyngitis. These secretions, however, can be seen in nonspecific URI and, in the absence of other clinical features, are poor predictors of bacterial infection.

TREATMENT NONSPECIFIC UPPER RESPIRATORY INFECTIONS

Antibiotics have no role in the treatment of uncomplicated nonspecific URI, and their misuse facilitates the emergence of antimicrobial resistance; in healthy volunteers, a single course of a commonly prescribed antibiotic like azithromycin can result in macrolide resistance in oral streptococci many months later. In the absence of clinical evidence of bacterial infection, treatment remains entirely symptom based, with use of decongestants and nonsteroidal anti-inflammatory drugs. Clinical trials of zinc, vitamin C, echinacea, and other alternative remedies have revealed no consistent benefit in the treatment of nonspecific URI.

INFECTIONS OF THE SINUS

Rhinosinusitis refers to an inflammatory condition involving the nasal sinuses. Although most cases of sinusitis involve more than one sinus, the maxillary sinus is most commonly involved; next, in order of frequency, are the ethmoid, frontal, and sphenoid sinuses. Each sinus is lined with a respiratory epithelium that produces mucus, which is transported out by ciliary action through the sinus ostium and into the nasal cavity. Normally, mucus does not accumulate in the sinuses, which remain mostly sterile despite their adjacency to the bacterium-filled nasal passages. When the sinus ostia are obstructed or when ciliary clearance is impaired or absent, the secretions can be retained, producing the typical signs and symptoms of sinusitis. As these secretions accumulate with obstruction, they become more susceptible to infection with a variety of pathogens, including viruses, bacteria, and fungi. Sinusitis affects a tremendous proportion of the population, accounts for millions of visits to primary care physicians each year, and is the fifth leading diagnosis for which antibiotics are prescribed. It typically is classified by duration of illness (acute vs. chronic); by etiology (infectious vs. noninfectious); and, when infectious, by the offending pathogen type (viral, bacterial, or fungal).

ACUTE RHINOSINUSITIS

Acute rhinosinusitis—defined as sinusitis of <4 weeks' duration—constitutes the vast majority of sinusitis cases. Most cases are diagnosed in the ambulatory care setting and occur primarily as a consequence of a preceding viral URI. Differentiating acute bacterial from viral sinusitis on clinical grounds is difficult. Therefore, it is perhaps not surprising that antibiotics are prescribed frequently (in 85–98% of all cases) for this condition.

Etiology The ostial obstruction in rhinosinusitis can arise from both infectious and noninfectious causes. Noninfectious etiologies include allergic rhinitis (with either mucosal edema or polyp obstruction), barotrauma (e.g., from deep-sea diving or air travel), and exposure to chemical irritants. Obstruction can also occur with nasal and sinus tumors (e.g., squamous cell carcinoma) or granulomatous diseases (e.g., granulomatosis with polyangiitis, rhinoscleroma), and conditions leading to altered mucus content (e.g., cystic fibrosis) can cause sinusitis through impaired mucus clearance. In ICUs, nasotracheal intubation and nasogastric tubes are major risk factors for nosocomial sinusitis.

Viral rhinosinusitis is far more common than bacterial sinusitis, although relatively few studies have sampled sinus aspirates for the presence of different viruses. In the studies that have done so, the viruses most commonly isolated—both alone and with bacteria—have been rhinovirus, parainfluenza virus, and influenza virus. Bacterial causes of sinusitis have been better described. Among community-acquired cases, *S. pneumoniae* and nontypable *Haemophilus influenzae* are the most common pathogens, accounting for 50–60% of cases. *Moraxella catarrhalis* causes disease in a significant percentage (20%) of children but a lesser percentage of adults. Other streptococcal species and *Staphylococcus aureus* cause only a small percentage of cases, although there is increasing concern about methicillin-resistant *S. aureus* (MRSA) as an emerging cause. It is difficult to assess whether a cultured bacterium represents a true infecting organism, an insufficiently deep sample (which would not be expected to be sterile), or—especially in the case of previous sinus surgeries—a colonizing organism. Anaerobes occasionally are found in association with infections of the roots of premolar teeth that spread to the adjacent maxillary sinuses. The role of atypical organisms like *Chlamydia pneumoniae* and *Mycoplasma pneumoniae* in the pathogenesis of acute sinusitis is unclear. Nosocomial cases commonly are associated with bacteria prevalent in the hospital environment, including *S. aureus*, *Pseudomonas aeruginosa*, *Serratia marcescens*, *Klebsiella pneumoniae*, and *Enterobacter* species. Often, these infections are polymicrobial and can involve organisms that are highly resistant to numerous antibiotics. Fungi also are established causes of sinusitis, although most acute cases are in immunocompromised patients and represent invasive, life-threatening infections. The best-known example is rhinocerebral mucormycosis caused by fungi of the order Mucorales, which includes *Rhizopus*, *Rhizomucor*, *Mucor*, *Lichtheimia* (formerly *Mycocladus*, formerly *Absidia*), and *Cunninghamella* (Chap. 242). These infections classically occur in diabetic patients with ketoacidosis but can also develop in transplant recipients, patients with hematologic malignancies, and patients receiving chronic glucocorticoid or deferoxamine therapy. Other hyaline molds, such as *Aspergillus* and *Fusarium* species, also are occasional causes of this disease.

Clinical Manifestations Most cases of acute sinusitis present after or in conjunction with a viral URI, and it can be difficult to discriminate the clinical features of one from the other, with timing becoming important in diagnosis (see below). A large proportion of patients with colds have sinus inflammation, although, as previously stated, true bacterial sinusitis complicates only 0.2–2% of these viral infections. Common presenting symptoms of sinusitis include nasal drainage and congestion, facial pain or pressure, and headache. Thick, purulent or discolored nasal discharge is often thought to indicate bacterial sinusitis but also occurs early in viral infections such as the common cold and is not specific to bacterial infection. Other nonspecific manifestations include cough, sneezing, and fever. Tooth pain, most often involving the upper molars, as well as halitosis are occasionally associated with bacterial sinusitis.

In acute sinusitis, sinus pain or pressure often localizes to the involved sinus (particularly the maxillary sinus) and can be worse when the patient bends over or is supine. Although rare, manifestations of advanced sphenoid or ethmoid sinus infection can be profound, including severe frontal or retroorbital pain radiating to the occiput, thrombosis of the cavernous sinus, and signs of orbital cellulitis. Acute focal sinusitis is uncommon but should be considered with severe symptoms involving the maxillary sinus and fever, regardless of illness duration. Similarly, patients with advanced frontal sinusitis can present with a condition known as *Pott's puffy tumor*, with soft tissue swelling and pitting edema over the frontal bone from a communicating subperiosteal abscess. Life-threatening complications of sinusitis include meningitis, epidural abscess, and cerebral abscess.

Patients with acute fungal rhinosinusitis (such as mucormycosis; Chap. 242) often present with symptoms related to pressure effects, particularly when the infection has spread to the orbits and cavernous sinus. Signs such as orbital swelling and cellulitis, proptosis, ptosis, and decreased extraocular movement are common, as is retro- or periorbital pain. Nasopharyngeal ulcerations, epistaxis, and headaches are also common, and involvement of cranial nerves V and VII has been described in more advanced cases. Bony erosion may be evident on examination or endoscopy. Often the patient does not appear seriously ill despite the rapidly progressive nature of these infections.

Patients with acute nosocomial sinusitis are often critically ill and thus do not manifest the typical clinical features of sinus disease. This diagnosis should be suspected, however, when hospitalized patients with appropriate risk factors (e.g., nasotracheal intubation) develop fever without another apparent cause.

Diagnosis Distinguishing viral from bacterial rhinosinusitis in the ambulatory setting is usually difficult because of the relatively low sensitivity and specificity of the common clinical features. One clinical feature that has been used to help guide diagnostic and therapeutic decision-making is illness duration. Because acute bacterial sinusitis is uncommon in patients whose symptoms have lasted <10 days, expert panels now recommend reserving this diagnosis for patients with "persistent" symptoms (i.e., symptoms lasting >10 days in adults or >10–14 days in children) accompanied by the three cardinal signs of purulent nasal discharge, nasal obstruction, and facial pain (Table 44-1). Even among patients who meet these criteria, only 40–50% have true bacterial sinusitis. The use of CT or sinus radiography is not recommended for acute disease, particularly early in the course of illness (i.e., at <10 days) in light of the high prevalence of similar findings among patients with acute viral rhinosinusitis. In the evaluation of persistent, recurrent, or chronic sinusitis, CT of the sinuses becomes the radiographic study of choice.

The clinical history and/or setting often can identify cases of acute anaerobic bacterial sinusitis, acute fungal sinusitis, or sinusitis from noninfectious causes (e.g., allergic rhinosinusitis). In the case of an immunocompromised patient with acute fungal sinus infection, immediate examination by an otolaryngologist is required. Biopsy specimens from involved areas should be examined by a pathologist for evidence of fungal hyphal elements and tissue invasion. Cases of suspected acute nosocomial sinusitis should be confirmed by sinus CT. Because therapy should target the offending organism, a sinus aspirate for culture and susceptibility testing should be obtained, whenever possible, before the initiation of antimicrobial therapy.

TABLE 44-1 GUIDELINES FOR THE DIAGNOSIS AND TREATMENT OF ACUTE SINUSITIS IN ADULTS

Diagnostic Criteria	Treatment Recommendations[a]
Moderate symptoms (e.g., nasal purulence/congestion or cough) for >10 d *or*	*Initial therapy:*
	Amoxicillin, 500 mg PO tid; *or*
	Amoxicillin/clavulanate, 500/125 mg PO tid or 875/125 mg PO bid[b]
Severe symptoms of any duration, including unilateral/focal facial swelling or tooth pain	*Penicillin allergy:*
	Doxycycline, 100 mg PO bid; *or*
	Clindamycin, 300 mg PO tid
	Exposure to antibiotics within 30 d or >30% prevalence of penicillin-resistant Streptococcus pneumoniae:
	Amoxicillin/clavulanate (extended release), 2000/125 mg PO bid; *or*
	An antipneumococcal fluoroquinolone (e.g., moxifloxacin, 400 mg PO daily)
	Recent treatment failure:
	Amoxicillin/clavulanate (extended release), 2000 mg PO bid; *or*
	An antipneumococcal fluoroquinolone (e.g., moxifloxacin, 400 mg PO daily)

[a]The duration of therapy is generally 7–10 days (with consideration of a 5-day course), with appropriate follow-up. Severe disease may warrant IV antibiotics and consideration of hospital admission. [b]Although the evidence is not as strong, amoxicillin/clavulanate may be considered for initial use, particularly if local rates of penicillin resistance or β-lactamase production are high.

TREATMENT ACUTE RHINOSINUSITIS

Most patients with a clinical diagnosis of acute rhinosinusitis improve without antibiotic therapy. The preferred initial approach in patients with mild to moderate symptoms of short duration is therapy aimed at symptom relief and facilitation of sinus drainage, such as with oral and topical decongestants, nasal saline lavage, and—at least in patients with a history of chronic sinusitis or allergies—nasal glucocorticoids. Newer studies have cast doubt on the role of antibiotics and nasal glucocorticoids in acute rhinosinusitis. In one notable double-blind, randomized, placebo-controlled trial, neither antibiotics nor topical glucocorticoids had a significant impact on cure in the study population of patients, the majority of whom had had symptoms for <7 days. Similarly, another high-profile randomized trial comparing antibiotics to placebo in patients with acute rhinosinusitis demonstrated no significant improvement in symptoms by the third day of therapy. Still, antibiotic therapy can be considered for adult patients whose condition does not improve after 10 days, and patients with more severe symptoms (regardless of duration) should be treated with antibiotics (Table 44-1). However, watchful waiting remains a viable option in many cases.

Empirical antibiotic therapy for adults with community-acquired sinusitis should consist of the narrowest-spectrum agent active against the most common bacterial pathogens, including *S. pneumoniae* and *H. influenzae*—e.g., amoxicillin or amoxicillin/clavulanate (with the decision guided by local rates of β-lactamase-producing *H. influenzae*). No clinical trials support the use of broader-spectrum agents for routine cases of bacterial sinusitis, even in the current era of drug-resistant *S. pneumoniae*. For those patients who do not respond to initial antimicrobial therapy, sinus aspiration and/or lavage by an otolaryngologist should be considered. Antibiotic prophylaxis to prevent episodes of recurrent acute bacterial sinusitis is not recommended.

Surgical intervention and IV antibiotic administration usually are reserved for patients with severe disease or those with intracranial complications such as abscess and orbital involvement. Immunocompromised patients with acute invasive fungal sinusitis usually require extensive surgical debridement and treatment with IV antifungal agents active against fungal hyphal forms, such as amphotericin B. Specific therapy should be individualized according to the fungal species and its susceptibilities as well as the individual patient's characteristics.

Treatment of nosocomial sinusitis should begin with broad-spectrum antibiotics to cover common and often resistant pathogens such as *S. aureus* and gram-negative bacilli. Therapy then should be tailored to the results of culture and susceptibility testing of sinus aspirates.

CHRONIC SINUSITIS

Chronic sinusitis is characterized by symptoms of sinus inflammation lasting >12 weeks. This illness is most commonly associated with either bacteria or fungi, and clinical cure in most cases is very difficult. Many patients have undergone treatment with repeated courses of antibacterial agents and multiple sinus surgeries, increasing their risk of colonization with antibiotic-resistant pathogens and of surgical complications. These patients often have high rates of morbidity, sometimes over many years.

In *chronic bacterial sinusitis*, infection is thought to be due to the impairment of mucociliary clearance from repeated infections rather than to persistent bacterial infection. The pathogenesis of this condition, however, is poorly understood. Although certain conditions (e.g., cystic fibrosis) can predispose patients to chronic bacterial sinusitis, most patients with chronic rhinosinusitis do not have obvious underlying conditions that result in the obstruction of sinus drainage, the impairment of ciliary action, or immune dysfunction. Patients experience constant nasal congestion and sinus pressure, with intermittent periods of greater severity, which may persist for years. CT can be helpful in determining the extent of disease, detecting an underlying anatomic defect or obstructing process (e.g., a polyp), and assessing the response to therapy. Management should involve an otolaryngologist to conduct endoscopic examinations and obtain tissue samples for histologic examination and culture. An endoscopy-derived culture not only has a higher yield but also allows direct visualization for abnormal anatomy.

Chronic fungal sinusitis is a disease of immunocompetent hosts and is usually noninvasive, although slowly progressive invasive disease is sometimes seen. Noninvasive disease, which typically is associated with hyaline molds such as *Aspergillus* species and dematiaceous molds such as *Curvularia* or *Bipolaris* species, can present as a number of different scenarios. In mild, indolent disease, which usually occurs in the setting of repeated failures of antibacterial therapy, only nonspecific mucosal changes may be seen on sinus CT. Although there is some controversy on this point, endoscopic surgery is usually curative in these cases, with no need for antifungal therapy. Another form of disease presents as long-standing, often unilateral symptoms and opacification of a single sinus on imaging studies as a result of a mycetoma (fungus ball) within the sinus. Treatment for this condition also is surgical, although systemic antifungal therapy may be warranted in the rare case in which bony erosion occurs. A third form of disease, known as *allergic fungal sinusitis*, is seen in patients with a history of nasal polyposis and asthma, who often have had multiple sinus surgeries. Patients with this condition produce a thick, eosinophil-laden mucus with the consistency of peanut butter that contains sparse fungal hyphae on histologic examination. These patients often present with pansinusitis.

TREATMENT CHRONIC SINUSITIS

Treatment of chronic bacterial sinusitis can be challenging and consists primarily of repeated culture-guided courses of antibiotics, sometimes for 3–4 weeks or longer at a time; administration of intranasal glucocorticoids; and mechanical irrigation of the sinus with sterile saline solution. When this management approach fails, sinus surgery may be indicated and sometimes provides significant, albeit short-term, alleviation. Treatment of chronic fungal sinusitis consists of surgical removal of impacted mucus. Recurrence, unfortunately, is common.

INFECTIONS OF THE EAR AND MASTOID

Infections of the ear and associated structures can involve both the middle and the external ear, including the skin, cartilage, periosteum, ear canal, and tympanic and mastoid cavities. Both viruses and bacteria are known causes of these infections, some of which result in significant morbidity if not treated appropriately.

INFECTIONS OF EXTERNAL EAR STRUCTURES

Infections involving the structures of the external ear are often difficult to differentiate from noninfectious inflammatory conditions with similar clinical manifestations. Clinicians should consider inflammatory disorders as possible causes of external ear irritation, particularly in the absence of local or regional adenopathy. Aside from the more salient causes of inflammation, such as trauma, insect bite, and overexposure to sunlight or extreme cold, the differential diagnosis should include less common conditions such as autoimmune disorders (e.g., lupus or relapsing polychondritis) and vasculitides (e.g., granulomatosis with polyangiitis).

Auricular Cellulitis Auricular cellulitis is an infection of the skin overlying the external ear and typically follows minor local trauma. It presents as the typical signs and symptoms of cellulitis, with tenderness, erythema, swelling, and warmth of the external ear (particularly the lobule) but without apparent involvement of the ear canal or inner structures. Treatment consists of warm compresses and oral antibiotics such as cephalexin or dicloxacillin that are active against typical skin and soft tissue pathogens (specifically, *S. aureus* and streptococci). IV antibiotics such as a first-generation cephalosporin (e.g., cefazolin) or a penicillinase-resistant penicillin (e.g., nafcillin) occasionally are needed for more severe cases, with consideration of MRSA if either risk factors or failure of therapy point to this organism.

Perichondritis Perichondritis, an infection of the perichondrium of the auricular cartilage, typically follows local trauma (e.g., piercings, burns, or lacerations). Occasionally, when the infection spreads down to the cartilage of the pinna itself, patients may develop chondritis. The infection may closely resemble auricular cellulitis, with erythema, swelling, and extreme tenderness of the pinna, although the lobule is less often involved in perichondritis. The most common pathogens are *P. aeruginosa* and *S. aureus*, although other gram-negative and gram-positive organisms occasionally are involved. Treatment consists of systemic antibiotics active against both *P. aeruginosa* and *S. aureus*. An antipseudomonal penicillin (e.g., piperacillin) or a combination of a penicillinase-resistant penicillin and an antipseudomonal quinolone (e.g., nafcillin plus ciprofloxacin) is typically used. Incision and drainage may be helpful for culture and for resolution of infection, which often takes weeks. When perichondritis fails to respond to adequate antimicrobial therapy, clinicians should consider a noninfectious inflammatory etiology such as relapsing polychondritis.

Otitis Externa The term *otitis externa* refers to a collection of diseases involving primarily the auditory meatus. Otitis externa usually results from a combination of heat and retained moisture, with desquamation and maceration of the epithelium of the outer ear canal. The disease exists in several forms: localized, diffuse, chronic, and invasive. All forms are predominantly bacterial in origin, with *P. aeruginosa* and *S. aureus* the most common pathogens.

Acute localized otitis externa (*furunculosis*) can develop in the outer third of the ear canal, where skin overlies cartilage and hair follicles are numerous. As in furunculosis elsewhere on the body, *S. aureus* is the usual pathogen, and treatment typically consists of an oral antistaphylococcal penicillin (e.g., dicloxacillin or cephalexin), with incision and drainage in cases of abscess formation.

Acute diffuse otitis externa is also known as *swimmer's ear*, although it can develop in patients who have not recently been swimming. Heat, humidity, and the loss of protective cerumen lead to excessive moisture and elevation of the pH in the ear canal, which in turn lead to skin maceration and irritation. Infection may then follow; the predominant pathogen is *P. aeruginosa*, although other gram-negative and gram-positive organisms—and rarely yeasts—have been recovered from patients with this condition. The illness often starts with itching and progresses to severe pain, which is usually elicited by manipulation of the pinna or tragus. The onset of pain is generally accompanied by the development of an erythematous, swollen ear canal, often with scant white, clumpy discharge. Treatment consists of cleansing the canal to remove debris and enhance the activity of topical therapeutic agents—usually hypertonic saline or mixtures of alcohol and acetic acid. Inflammation can also be decreased by adding glucocorticoids to the treatment regimen or by using Burow's solution (aluminum acetate in water). Antibiotics are most effective when given topically. Otic mixtures provide adequate pathogen coverage; these preparations usually combine neomycin with polymyxin, with or without glucocorticoids. Systemic antimicrobial agents typically are reserved for severe disease or infections in immunocompromised hosts.

Chronic otitis externa is caused primarily by repeated local irritation, most commonly arising from persistent drainage from a chronic middle-ear infection. Other causes of repeated irritation, such as insertion of cotton swabs or other foreign objects into the ear canal, can lead to this condition, as can rare chronic infections such as syphilis, tuberculosis, and leprosy. Chronic otitis externa typically presents as erythematous, scaling dermatitis in which the predominant symptom is pruritus rather than pain; this condition must be differentiated from several others that produce a similar clinical picture, such as atopic dermatitis, seborrheic dermatitis, psoriasis, and dermatomycosis. Therapy consists of identifying and treating or removing the offending process, although successful resolution is frequently difficult.

Invasive otitis externa, also known as *malignant* or *necrotizing* otitis externa, is an aggressive and potentially life-threatening disease that occurs predominantly in elderly diabetic patients and other immunocompromised persons. The disease begins in the external canal as a soft tissue infection that progresses slowly over weeks to months and often is difficult to distinguish from a severe case of chronic otitis externa because of the presence of purulent otorrhea and an erythematous swollen ear and external canal. Severe, deep-seated otalgia, frequently out of proportion to findings on examination, is often noted and can help differentiate invasive from chronic otitis externa. The characteristic finding on examination is granulation tissue in the posteroinferior wall of the external canal, near the junction of bone and cartilage. If left unchecked, the infection can migrate to the base of the skull (resulting in skull-base osteomyelitis) and onward to the meninges and brain, with a high mortality rate. Cranial nerve involvement is seen occasionally, with the facial nerve usually affected first and most often. Thrombosis of the sigmoid sinus can occur if the infection extends to the area. CT, which can reveal osseous erosion of the temporal bone and skull base, can be used to help determine the extent of disease, as can gallium and technetium-99 scintigraphy studies. *P. aeruginosa* is by far the most common offender, although *S. aureus, Staphylococcus epidermidis, Aspergillus, Actinomyces,* and some gram-negative bacteria also have been associated with this disease. In all cases, the external ear canal should be cleansed and a biopsy specimen of the granulation tissue within the canal (or of deeper tissues) obtained for culture of the offending organism. IV antibiotic therapy should be given for a prolonged course (6–8 weeks) and directed specifically toward the recovered pathogen. For *P. aeruginosa,* the regimen typically includes an antipseudomonal penicillin or cephalosporin (e.g., piperacillin or cefepime), often with an aminoglycoside or a fluoroquinolone, the latter of which can even be administered orally given its excellent bioavailability. In addition, antibiotic drops containing an agent active against *Pseudomonas* (e.g., ciprofloxacin) are usually prescribed and are combined with glucocorticoids to reduce inflammation. Cases of invasive *Pseudomonas* otitis externa recognized in the early stages can sometimes be treated with oral and otic fluoroquinolones alone, albeit with close follow-up. Extensive surgical debridement, once an important component of the treatment approach, is now rarely indicated.

In *necrotizing otitis externa,* recurrence is documented up to 20% of the time. Aggressive glycemic control in diabetics is important not only for effective treatment but also for prevention of recurrence. The role of hyperbaric oxygen has not been clearly established.

INFECTIONS OF MIDDLE-EAR STRUCTURES

Otitis media is an inflammatory condition of the middle ear that results from dysfunction of the eustachian tube in association with a number of illnesses, including URIs and chronic rhinosinusitis. The inflammatory response in these conditions leads to the development of a sterile transudate within the middle ear and mastoid cavities. Infection may occur if bacteria or viruses from the nasopharynx contaminate this fluid, producing an acute (or sometimes chronic) illness.

Acute Otitis Media Acute otitis media results when pathogens from the nasopharynx are introduced into the inflammatory fluid collected in the middle ear (e.g., by nose blowing during a URI). Pathogenic proliferation in this space leads to the development of the typical signs and symptoms of acute middle-ear infection. The diagnosis of acute otitis media requires the demonstration of fluid in the middle ear (with tympanic membrane [TM] immobility) and the accompanying signs or symptoms of local or systemic illness (Table 44-2).

ETIOLOGY Acute otitis media typically follows a viral URI. The causative viruses (most commonly RSV, influenza virus, rhinovirus, and enterovirus) can themselves cause subsequent acute otitis media; more often, they predispose the patient to bacterial otitis media. Studies using tympanocentesis have consistently found *S. pneumoniae* to be the most important bacterial cause, isolated in up to 35% of cases. *H. influenzae* (nontypable strains) and *M. catarrhalis* also are

TABLE 44-2 GUIDELINES FOR THE DIAGNOSIS AND TREATMENT OF ACUTE OTITIS MEDIA

Illness Severity	Diagnostic Criteria	Treatment Recommendations
Mild to moderate	>2 yrs *or* 6 mo to 2 yrs without middle-ear effusion	*Observation alone* (deferring antibiotic therapy for 48–72 h and limiting management to symptom relief)
	<6 mo; *or*	*Initial therapy*[a]
	6 mo to 2 yrs with middle-ear effusion (fluid in the middle ear, evidenced by decreased TM mobility, air/fluid level behind TM, bulging TM, purulent otorrhea) *and* acute onset of signs and symptoms of middle-ear inflammation, including fever, otalgia, decreased hearing, tinnitus, vertigo, erythematous TM; *or*	Amoxicillin, 80–90 mg/kg qd (up to 2 g) PO in divided doses (bid or tid); *or* Cefdinir, 14 mg/kg qd PO in 1 dose or divided doses (bid); *or* Cefuroxime, 30 mg/kg qd PO in divided doses (bid); *or* Azithromycin, 10 mg/kg qd PO on day 1 followed by 5 mg/kg qd PO for 4 d
	>2 yrs with bilateral disease, TM perforation, high fever, immunocompromise, emesis	*Exposure to antibiotics within 30 d or recent treatment failure*[a,b]: Amoxicillin, 90 mg/kg qd (up to 2 g) PO in divided doses (bid), plus clavulanate, 6.4 mg/kg qd PO in divided doses (bid); *or* Ceftriaxone, 50 mg/kg IV/IM qd for 3 d; *or* Clindamycin, 30–40 mg/kg qd PO in divided doses (tid)
Severe	As above, with temperature ≥39.0°C (102°F); *or* Moderate to severe otalgia	*Initial therapy*[a] Amoxicillin, 90 mg/kg qd (up to 2 g) PO in divided doses (bid), plus clavulanate, 6.4 mg/kg qd PO in divided doses (bid); *or* Ceftriaxone, 50 mg/kg IV/IM qd for 3 d
		Exposure to antibiotics within 30 d or recent treatment failure[a,b] Ceftriaxone, 50 mg/kg IV/IM qd for 3 d; *or* Clindamycin, 30–40 mg/kg qd PO in divided doses (tid); *or* Consider tympanocentesis with culture

[a]Duration (unless otherwise specified): 10 days for patients <6 years old and patients with severe disease; 5–7 days (with consideration of observation only in previously healthy individuals with mild disease) for patients ≥6 years old. [b]Failure to improve and/or clinical worsening after 48–72 h of observation or treatment.

Abbreviation: TM, tympanic membrane.

Source: American Academy of Pediatrics Subcommittee on Management of Acute Otitis Media, 2004.

common bacterial causes of acute otitis media, and concern is increasing with MRSA as an emerging etiologic agent. Viruses, such as those mentioned above, have been recovered either alone or with bacteria in 17–40% of cases.

CLINICAL MANIFESTATIONS Fluid in the middle ear is typically demonstrated or confirmed with pneumatic otoscopy. In the absence of fluid, the TM moves visibly with the application of positive and negative pressure, but this movement is dampened when fluid is present. With bacterial infection, the TM can also be erythematous, bulging, or retracted and occasionally can perforate spontaneously. The signs and symptoms accompanying infection can be local or systemic, including otalgia, otorrhea, diminished hearing, and fever. Erythema of the TM is often evident but is nonspecific as it frequently is seen in association with inflammation of the upper respiratory mucosa. Other signs and symptoms occasionally reported include vertigo, nystagmus, and tinnitus.

TREATMENT ACUTE OTITIS MEDIA

There has been considerable debate on the usefulness of antibiotics for the treatment of acute otitis media. A higher proportion of treated than untreated patients are free of illness 3–5 days after diagnosis. The difficulty of predicting which patients will benefit from antibiotic therapy has led to different approaches. In the Netherlands, for instance, physicians typically manage acute otitis media with initial observation, administering anti-inflammatory agents for aggressive pain management and reserving antibiotics for high-risk patients, patients with complicated disease, or patients whose condition does not improve after 48–72 h. In contrast, many experts in the United States continue to recommend antibiotic therapy for children <6 months old in light of the higher frequency of secondary complications in this young and functionally immunocompromised population. However, observation without antimicrobial therapy is now the recommended option in the United States for acute otitis media in children >2 years of age and for mild to moderate disease without middle-ear effusion in children 6 months to 2 years of age. Treatment is typically indicated for patients <6 months old; for children 6 months to 2 years old who have middle-ear effusion and signs/symptoms of middle-ear inflammation; for all patients >2 years old who have bilateral disease, TM perforation, immunocompromise, or emesis; and for any patient who has severe symptoms, including a fever ≥39°C or moderate to severe otalgia (Table 44-2).

Because most studies of the etiologic agents of acute otitis media consistently document similar pathogen profiles, therapy is generally empirical except in those few cases in which tympanocentesis is warranted—e.g., cases refractory to therapy and cases in patients who are severely ill or immunodeficient. Despite resistance to penicillin and amoxicillin in roughly one-quarter of *S. pneumoniae* isolates, one-third of *H. influenzae* isolates, and nearly all *M. catarrhalis* isolates, outcome studies continue to find that amoxicillin is as successful as any other agent, and it remains the drug of first choice in recommendations from multiple sources (Table 44-2). Therapy for uncomplicated acute otitis media typically is administered for 5–7 days to patients ≥6 years old; longer courses (e.g., 10 days) should be reserved for patients with severe disease, in whom short-course therapy may be inadequate.

A switch in regimen is recommended if there is no clinical improvement by the third day of therapy, given the possibility of infection with a β-lactamase-producing strain of *H. influenzae* or *M. catarrhalis* or with a strain of penicillin-resistant *S. pneumoniae.* Decongestants and antihistamines are frequently used as adjunctive agents to reduce congestion and relieve obstruction of the eustachian tube, but clinical trials have yielded no significant evidence of benefit with either class of agents.

Recurrent Acute Otitis Media Recurrent acute otitis media (more than three episodes within 6 months or four episodes within 12 months) generally is due to relapse or reinfection, although data indicate that the majority of early recurrences are new infections. In general, the same pathogens responsible for acute otitis media cause recurrent disease; even so, the recommended treatment consists of antibiotics active against β-lactamase-producing organisms. Antibiotic prophylaxis (e.g., with trimethoprim-sulfamethoxazole [TMP-SMX] or amoxicillin) can reduce recurrences in patients with recurrent acute otitis media by an average of one episode per year, but this benefit is small compared with the high likelihood of colonization with antibiotic-resistant pathogens. Other approaches, including placement of tympanostomy tubes, adenoidectomy, and tonsillectomy plus adenoidectomy, are of questionable overall value in light of the relatively small benefit compared with the potential for complications.

Serous Otitis Media In serous otitis media (otitis media with effusion), fluid is present in the middle ear for an extended period in the absence of signs and symptoms of infection. In general, acute effusions are self-limited; most resolve in 2–4 weeks. In some cases, however (in particular after an episode of acute otitis media), effusions can persist for months. These chronic effusions are often associated with significant hearing loss in the affected ear. The great majority of cases of otitis media with effusion resolve spontaneously within 3 months without antibiotic therapy. Antibiotic therapy or myringotomy with insertion of tympanostomy tubes typically is reserved for patients in whom bilateral effusion (1) has persisted for at least 3 months and (2) is associated with significant bilateral hearing loss. With this conservative approach and the application of strict diagnostic criteria for acute otitis media and otitis media with effusion, it is estimated that 6–8 million courses of antibiotics could be avoided each year in the United States.

Chronic Otitis Media Chronic suppurative otitis media is characterized by persistent or recurrent purulent otorrhea in the setting of TM perforation. Usually, there is also some degree of conductive hearing loss. This condition can be categorized as active or inactive. Inactive disease is characterized by a central perforation of the TM, which allows drainage of purulent fluid from the middle ear. When the perforation is more peripheral, squamous epithelium from the auditory canal may invade the middle ear through the perforation, forming a mass of keratinaceous debris (*cholesteatoma*) at the site of invasion. This mass can enlarge and has the potential to erode bone and promote further infection, which can lead to meningitis, brain abscess, or paralysis of cranial nerve VII. Treatment of chronic active otitis media is surgical; mastoidectomy, myringoplasty, and tympanoplasty can be performed as outpatient surgical procedures, with an overall success rate of ~80%. Chronic inactive otitis media is more difficult to cure, usually requiring repeated courses of topical antibiotic drops during periods of drainage. Systemic antibiotics may offer better cure rates, but their role in the treatment of this condition remains unclear.

Mastoiditis Acute mastoiditis was relatively common among children before the introduction of antibiotics. Because the mastoid air cells connect with the middle ear, the process of fluid collection and infection is usually the same in the mastoid as in the middle ear. Early and frequent treatment of acute otitis media is most likely the reason that the incidence of acute mastoiditis has declined to only 1.2–2.0 cases per 100,000 person-years in countries with high prescribing rates for acute otitis media.

In countries such as the Netherlands, where antibiotics are used sparingly for acute otitis media, the incidence rate of acute mastoiditis is roughly twice that in countries like the United States. However, neighboring Denmark has a rate of acute mastoiditis similar to that in the Netherlands but an antibiotic-prescribing rate for acute otitis media more similar to that in the United States.

In typical acute mastoiditis, purulent exudate collects in the mastoid air cells (Fig. 44-1), producing pressure that may result in erosion of the surrounding bone and formation of abscess-like cavities that are

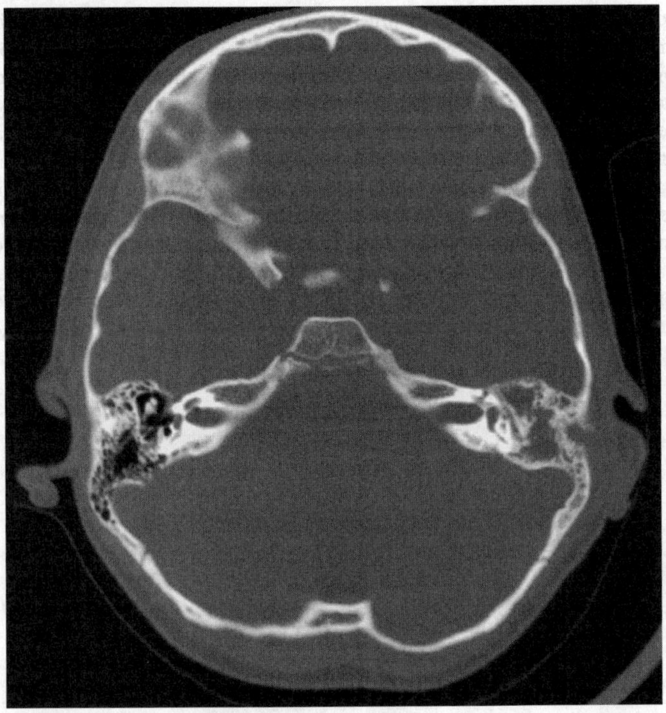

FIGURE 44-1 Acute mastoiditis. Axial CT image shows an acute fluid collection within the mastoid air cells on the left.

usually evident on CT. Patients typically present with pain, erythema, and swelling of the mastoid process along with displacement of the pinna, usually in conjunction with the typical signs and symptoms of acute middle-ear infection. Rarely, patients can develop severe complications if the infection tracks under the periosteum of the temporal bone to cause a subperiosteal abscess, erodes through the mastoid tip to cause a deep neck abscess, or extends posteriorly to cause septic thrombosis of the lateral sinus.

Purulent fluid should be cultured whenever possible to help guide antimicrobial therapy. Initial empirical therapy usually is directed against the typical organisms associated with acute otitis media, such as *S. pneumoniae*, *H. influenzae*, and *M. catarrhalis*. Patients with more severe or prolonged courses of illness should be treated for infection with *S. aureus* and gram-negative bacilli (including *Pseudomonas*). Broad empirical therapy should be narrowed once culture results become available. Most patients can be treated conservatively with IV antibiotics; surgery (cortical mastoidectomy) is reserved for complicated cases and those in which conservative treatment has failed.

INFECTIONS OF THE PHARYNX AND ORAL CAVITY

Oropharyngeal infections range from mild, self-limited viral illnesses to serious, life-threatening bacterial infections. The most common presenting symptom is sore throat—one of the most common reasons for ambulatory care visits by both adults and children. Although sore throat is a symptom in many noninfectious illnesses as well, the overwhelming majority of patients with a new sore throat have acute pharyngitis of viral or bacterial etiology.

ACUTE PHARYNGITIS

Millions of visits to primary care providers each year are for sore throat; the majority of cases of acute pharyngitis are caused by typical respiratory viruses. The most important source of concern is infection with group A β-hemolytic *Streptococcus* (*S. pyogenes*) that is associated with acute glomerulonephritis and acute rheumatic fever. The risk of rheumatic fever can be reduced by timely penicillin therapy.

Etiology A wide variety of organisms cause acute pharyngitis. The relative importance of the different pathogens can only be estimated, since a significant proportion of cases (~30%) have no identified cause. Together, respiratory viruses are the most common identifiable cause of acute pharyngitis, with rhinoviruses and coronaviruses accounting for large proportions of cases (~20% and at least 5%, respectively). Influenza virus, parainfluenza virus, and adenovirus also account for a measurable share of cases, with the former two more seasonal and the latter as part of the more clinically severe syndrome of pharyngoconjunctival fever. Other important but less common viral causes include herpes simplex virus (HSV) types 1 and 2, coxsackievirus A, cytomegalovirus (CMV), and Epstein-Barr virus (EBV). Acute HIV infection can present as acute pharyngitis and should be considered in at-risk populations.

Acute bacterial pharyngitis is typically caused by *S. pyogenes*, which accounts for ~5–15% of all cases of acute pharyngitis in adults; rates vary with the season and with utilization of the health care system. Group A streptococcal pharyngitis is primarily a disease of children 5–15 years of age; it is uncommon among children <3 years old, as is rheumatic fever. Streptococci of groups C and G account for a minority of cases, although these serogroups are nonrheumatogenic. *Fusobacterium necrophorum* has been increasingly recognized as a cause of pharyngitis in adolescents and young adults and is isolated nearly as often as group A streptococci. This organism is important because of the rare but life-threatening *Lemierre's disease*, which is generally associated with *F. necrophorum* and is usually preceded by pharyngitis (see "Oral Infections," below). The remaining bacterial causes of acute pharyngitis are seen infrequently (<1% of cases each) but should be considered in appropriate exposure groups because of the severity of illness if left untreated; these etiologic agents include *Neisseria gonorrhoeae*, *Corynebacterium diphtheriae*, *Corynebacterium ulcerans*, *Yersinia enterocolitica*, and *Treponema pallidum* (in secondary syphilis). Anaerobic bacteria also can cause acute pharyngitis (*Vincent's angina*) and can contribute to more serious polymicrobial infections, such as peritonsillar or retropharyngeal abscesses (see below). Atypical organisms such as *M. pneumoniae* and *C. pneumoniae* have been recovered from patients with acute pharyngitis; whether these agents are commensals or causes of acute infection is debatable.

Clinical Manifestations Although the signs and symptoms accompanying acute pharyngitis are not reliable predictors of the etiologic agent, the clinical presentation occasionally suggests one etiology over another. Acute pharyngitis due to respiratory viruses such as rhinovirus or coronavirus usually is not severe and typically is associated with a constellation of coryzal symptoms better characterized as nonspecific URI. Findings on physical examination are uncommon; fever is rare, and tender cervical adenopathy and pharyngeal exudates are not seen. In contrast, acute pharyngitis from influenza virus can be severe and is much more likely to be associated with fever as well as with myalgias, headache, and cough. The presentation of pharyngoconjunctival fever due to adenovirus infection is similar. Since pharyngeal exudate may be present on examination, this condition can be difficult to differentiate from streptococcal pharyngitis. However, adenoviral pharyngitis is distinguished by the presence of conjunctivitis in one-third to one-half of patients. Acute pharyngitis from primary HSV infection can also mimic streptococcal pharyngitis in some cases, with pharyngeal inflammation and exudate, but the presence of vesicles and shallow ulcers on the palate can help differentiate the two diseases. This HSV syndrome is distinct from pharyngitis caused by coxsackievirus (*herpangina*), which is associated with small vesicles that develop on the soft palate and uvula and then rupture to form shallow white ulcers. Acute exudative pharyngitis coupled with fever, fatigue, generalized lymphadenopathy, and (on occasion) splenomegaly is characteristic of infectious mononucleosis due to EBV or CMV. Acute primary infection with HIV is frequently associated with fever and acute pharyngitis as well as with myalgias, arthralgias, malaise, and occasionally a nonpruritic maculopapular rash, which may be followed by lymphadenopathy and mucosal ulcerations without exudate.

The clinical features of acute pharyngitis caused by streptococci of groups A, C, and G are similar, ranging from a relatively mild illness without many accompanying symptoms to clinically severe cases with profound pharyngeal pain, fever, chills, and abdominal pain.

A hyperemic pharyngeal membrane with tonsillar hypertrophy and exudate is usually seen, along with tender anterior cervical adenopathy. Coryzal manifestations, including cough, are typically absent; when present, they suggest a viral etiology. Strains of *S. pyogenes* that generate erythrogenic toxin can also produce scarlet fever characterized by an erythematous rash and strawberry tongue. The other types of acute bacterial pharyngitis (e.g., gonococcal, diphtherial, and yersinial) often present as exudative pharyngitis with or without other clinical features. Their etiologies are often suggested only by the clinical history.

Diagnosis The primary goal of diagnostic testing is to separate acute streptococcal pharyngitis from pharyngitis of other etiologies (particularly viral) so that antibiotics can be prescribed more efficiently for patients in whom they may be beneficial. The most appropriate standard for the diagnosis of streptococcal pharyngitis, however, has not been established definitively. Throat swab culture is generally regarded as the most appropriate but cannot distinguish between infection and colonization and requires 24–48 h to yield results that vary with technique and culture conditions. Rapid antigen-detection tests offer good specificity (>90%) but lower sensitivity when implemented in routine practice. The sensitivity has also been shown to vary across the clinical spectrum of disease (65–90%). Several clinical prediction systems (Fig. 44-2) can increase the sensitivity of rapid antigen-detection tests to >90% in controlled settings. Since the

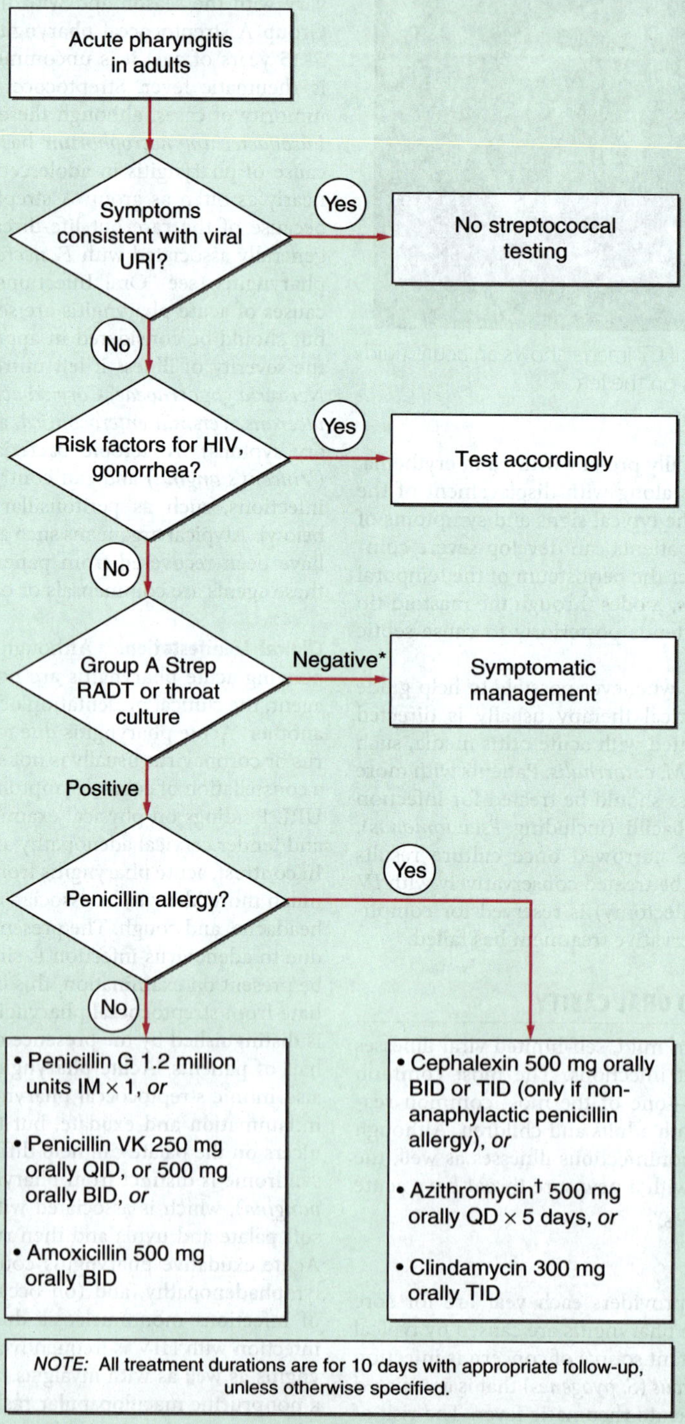

*Confirmation of a negative rapid antigen-detection test by a throat culture is not required in adults.
†Macrolides do not treat *F. necrophorum*, a cause of pharyngitis in young adults (see text).
Abbreviations: URI, upper respiratory infection; RADT, rapid antigen detection test

FIGURE 44-2 Algorithm for the diagnosis and treatment of acute pharyngitis.

sensitivities achieved in routine clinical practice are often lower, several medical and professional societies continue to recommend that all negative rapid antigen-detection tests in children be confirmed by a throat culture to limit transmission and complications of illness caused by group A streptococci. The Centers for Disease Control and Prevention, the Infectious Diseases Society of America, and the American Academy of Family Physicians do not recommend backup culture when adults have negative results from a highly sensitive rapid antigen-detection test, however, because of the lower prevalence and smaller benefit in this age group.

Cultures and rapid diagnostic tests for other causes of acute pharyngitis, such as influenza virus, adenovirus, HSV, EBV, CMV, and *M. pneumoniae*, are available in many locations and can be used when suspected. The diagnosis of acute EBV infection depends primarily on the detection of antibodies to the virus with a heterophile agglutination assay (monospot slide test) or enzyme-linked immunosorbent assay. Testing for HIV RNA or antigen (p24) should be performed when acute primary HIV infection is suspected. If other bacterial causes are suspected (particularly *N. gonorrhoeae*, *C. diphtheriae*, or *Y. enterocolitica*), specific cultures should be requested since these organisms may be missed on routine throat swab culture.

TREATMENT PHARYNGITIS

Antibiotic treatment of pharyngitis due to *S. pyogenes* confers numerous benefits, including a decrease in the risk of rheumatic fever, the primary focus of treatment. The magnitude of this benefit is fairly small, since rheumatic fever is now a rare disease, even among untreated patients. Nevertheless, when therapy is started within 48 h of illness onset, symptom duration is decreased modestly. An additional benefit of therapy is the potential to reduce the transmission of streptococcal pharyngitis, particularly in areas of overcrowding or close contact. Antibiotic therapy for acute pharyngitis is therefore recommended in cases in which *S. pyogenes* is confirmed as the etiologic agent by rapid antigen-detection test or throat swab culture. Otherwise, antibiotics should be given in routine cases only when another bacterial cause has been identified. Effective therapy for streptococcal pharyngitis consists of either a single dose of IM benzathine penicillin or a full 10-day course of oral penicillin (Fig. 44-2).

Azithromycin can be used in place of penicillin, although resistance to azithromycin among *S. pyogenes* strains in some parts of the world (particularly Europe) can prohibit the use of this drug. Newer (and more expensive) antibiotics also are active against streptococci but offer no greater efficacy than the agents mentioned above. Testing for cure is unnecessary and may reveal only chronic colonization. There is no evidence to support antibiotic treatment of group C or G streptococcal pharyngitis or pharyngitis in which mycoplasmas or chlamydiae have been recovered. Cultures can be of benefit because *F. necrophorum*, an increasingly common cause of bacterial pharyngitis in young adults, is not covered by macrolide therapy. Long-term penicillin prophylaxis (benzathine penicillin G, 1.2 million units IM every 3–4 weeks; or penicillin VK, 250 mg PO bid) is indicated for patients at risk of recurrent rheumatic fever.

Treatment of viral pharyngitis is entirely symptom based except in infection with influenza virus or HSV. For influenza, the armamentarium includes the adamantanes amantadine and rimantadine and the neuraminidase inhibitors oseltamivir and zanamivir. Administration of all these agents needs to be started within 48 h of symptom onset to reduce illness duration meaningfully. Among these agents, only oseltamivir and zanamivir are active against both influenza A and influenza B and therefore can be used when local patterns of infection and antiviral resistance are unknown. Oropharyngeal HSV infection sometimes responds to treatment with antiviral agents such as acyclovir, although these drugs are often reserved for immunosuppressed patients.

Complications Although rheumatic fever is the best-known complication of acute streptococcal pharyngitis, the risk of its following acute infection remains quite low. Other complications include acute glomerulonephritis and numerous suppurative conditions, such as peritonsillar abscess (*quinsy*), otitis media, mastoiditis, sinusitis, bacteremia, and pneumonia—all of which occur at low rates. Although antibiotic treatment of acute streptococcal pharyngitis can prevent the development of rheumatic fever, there is no evidence that it can prevent acute glomerulonephritis. Some evidence supports antibiotic use to prevent the suppurative complications of streptococcal pharyngitis, particularly peritonsillar abscess, which can also involve oral anaerobes such as *Fusobacterium*. Abscesses usually are accompanied by severe pharyngeal pain, dysphagia, fever, and dehydration; in addition, medial displacement of the tonsil and lateral displacement of the uvula are often evident on examination. Although early use of IV antibiotics (e.g., clindamycin, penicillin G with metronidazole) may obviate the need for surgical drainage in some cases, treatment typically involves needle aspiration or incision and drainage.

ORAL INFECTIONS

Aside from periodontal disease such as gingivitis, infections of the oral cavity most commonly involve HSV or *Candida* species. In addition to causing painful cold sores on the lips, HSV can infect the tongue and buccal mucosa, causing the formation of irritating vesicles. Although topical antiviral agents (e.g., acyclovir and penciclovir) can be used externally for cold sores, oral or IV acyclovir is often needed for primary infections, extensive oral infections, and infections in immunocompromised patients. Oropharyngeal candidiasis (*thrush*) is caused by a variety of *Candida* species, most often *C. albicans*. Thrush occurs predominantly in neonates, immunocompromised patients (especially those with AIDS), and recipients of prolonged antibiotic or glucocorticoid therapy. In addition to sore throat, patients often report a burning tongue, and physical examination reveals friable white or gray plaques on the gingiva, tongue, and oral mucosa. Treatment, which usually consists of an oral antifungal suspension (nystatin or clotrimazole) or oral fluconazole, is typically successful. In the uncommon cases of fluconazole-refractory thrush that are seen in some patients with HIV/AIDS, other therapeutic options include oral formulations of itraconazole or voriconazole as well as an IV echinocandin (caspofungin, micafungin, or anidulafungin) or amphotericin B deoxycholate, if needed. In these cases, therapy based on culture and susceptibility test results is ideal.

Vincent's angina, also known as *acute necrotizing ulcerative gingivitis* or *trench mouth*, is a unique and dramatic form of gingivitis characterized by painful, inflamed gingiva with ulcerations of the interdental papillae that bleed easily. Since oral anaerobes are the cause, patients typically have halitosis and frequently present with fever, malaise, and lymphadenopathy. Treatment consists of debridement and oral administration of penicillin plus metronidazole, with clindamycin or doxycycline alone as an alternative.

Ludwig's angina is a rapidly progressive, potentially fulminant form of cellulitis that involves the bilateral sublingual and submandibular spaces and that typically originates from an infected or recently extracted tooth, most commonly the lower second and third molars. Improved dental care has reduced the incidence of this disorder substantially. Infection in these areas leads to dysphagia, odynophagia, and "woody" edema in the sublingual region, forcing the tongue up and back with the potential for airway obstruction. Fever, dysarthria, and drooling also may be noted, and patients may speak in a "hot potato" voice. Intubation or tracheostomy may be necessary to secure the airway, as asphyxiation is the most common cause of death. Patients should be monitored closely and treated promptly with IV antibiotics directed against streptococci and oral anaerobes. Recommended agents include ampicillin/sulbactam, clindamycin, or high-dose penicillin plus metronidazole.

Postanginal septicemia (*Lemierre's disease*) is a rare anaerobic oropharyngeal infection caused predominantly by *F. necrophorum*. The illness typically starts as a sore throat (most commonly in adolescents and young adults), which may present as exudative tonsillitis or peritonsillar abscess. Infection of the deep pharyngeal tissue allows organisms to drain into the lateral pharyngeal space, which contains the carotid artery and internal jugular vein. Septic thrombophlebitis of the internal jugular vein can result, with associated pain, dysphagia, and neck swelling and stiffness. Sepsis usually occurs 3–10 days after the onset of sore throat and is often coupled with metastatic infection to the lung and other distant sites. Occasionally, the infection can extend along the carotid sheath and into the posterior mediastinum, resulting in mediastinitis, or it can erode into the carotid artery, with the early sign of repeated small bleeds into the mouth. The mortality rate from these invasive infections can be as high as 50%. Treatment consists of IV antibiotics (clindamycin or ampicillin/sulbactam) and surgical drainage of any purulent collections. The concomitant use of anticoagulants to prevent embolization remains controversial and is sometimes advised, with careful consideration of both the risks and the benefits.

INFECTIONS OF THE LARYNX AND EPIGLOTTIS

LARYNGITIS

Laryngitis is defined as any inflammatory process involving the larynx and can be caused by a variety of infectious and noninfectious processes. The vast majority of laryngitis cases seen in clinical practice in developed countries are acute. Acute laryngitis is a common syndrome caused predominantly by the same viruses responsible for many other URIs. In fact, most cases of acute laryngitis occur in the setting of a viral URI.

Etiology Nearly all major respiratory viruses have been implicated in acute viral laryngitis, including rhinovirus, influenza virus, parainfluenza virus, adenovirus, coxsackievirus, coronavirus, and RSV. Acute laryngitis can also be associated with acute bacterial respiratory infections such as those caused by group A *Streptococcus* or *C. diphtheriae* (although diphtheria has been virtually eliminated in the United States). Another bacterial pathogen thought to play a role (albeit unclear) in the pathogenesis of acute laryngitis is *M. catarrhalis*, which has been recovered from nasopharyngeal culture in a significant percentage of cases.

Chronic laryngitis of infectious etiology is much less common in developed than in developing countries. Laryngitis due to *Mycobacterium tuberculosis* is often difficult to distinguish from laryngeal cancer, in part because of the frequent absence of signs, symptoms, and radiographic findings typical of pulmonary disease. *Histoplasma* and *Blastomyces* may cause laryngitis, often as a complication of systemic infection. *Candida* species can cause laryngitis as well, often in association with thrush or esophagitis and particularly in immunosuppressed patients. Rare cases of chronic laryngitis are due to *Coccidioides* and *Cryptococcus*.

Clinical Manifestations Laryngitis is characterized by hoarseness and also can be associated with reduced vocal pitch or aphonia. As acute laryngitis is caused predominantly by respiratory viruses, these symptoms usually occur in association with other symptoms and signs of URI, including rhinorrhea, nasal congestion, cough, and sore throat. Direct laryngoscopy often reveals diffuse laryngeal erythema and edema, along with vascular engorgement of the vocal folds. In addition, chronic disease (e.g., tuberculous laryngitis) often includes mucosal nodules and ulcerations visible on laryngoscopy; these lesions are sometimes mistaken for laryngeal cancer.

TREATMENT LARYNGITIS

Acute laryngitis is usually treated with humidification and voice rest alone. Antibiotics are not recommended except when group A *Streptococcus* is cultured, in which case penicillin is the drug of choice. The choice of therapy for chronic laryngitis depends on the pathogen, whose identification usually requires biopsy with culture. Patients with laryngeal tuberculosis are highly contagious because of the large number of organisms that are easily aerosolized. These patients should be managed in the same way as patients with active pulmonary disease.

CROUP

The term *croup* actually denotes a group of diseases collectively referred to as "croup syndrome," all of which are acute and predominantly viral respiratory illnesses characterized by marked swelling of the subglottic region of the larynx. Croup primarily affects children <6 years old. For a detailed discussion of this entity, the reader should consult a textbook of pediatric medicine.

EPIGLOTTITIS

Acute epiglottitis (supraglottitis) is an acute, rapidly progressive form of cellulitis of the epiglottis and adjacent structures that can result in complete—and potentially fatal—airway obstruction in both children and adults. Before the widespread use of *H. influenzae* type b (Hib) vaccine, this entity was much more common among children, with a peak incidence at ~3.5 years of age. In some countries, mass vaccination against Hib has reduced the annual incidence of acute epiglottitis in children by >90%; in contrast, the annual incidence in adults has changed little since the introduction of Hib vaccine. Because of the danger of airway obstruction, acute epiglottitis constitutes a medical emergency, particularly in children, and prompt diagnosis and airway protection are of the utmost importance.

Etiology After the introduction of the Hib vaccine in the mid-1980s, disease incidence among children in the United States declined dramatically. Nevertheless, lack of vaccination or vaccine failure has meant that many pediatric cases seen today are still due to Hib. In adults and (more recently) in children, a variety of other bacterial pathogens have been associated with epiglottitis, the most common being group A *Streptococcus*. Other pathogens—seen less frequently—include *S. pneumoniae*, *Haemophilus parainfluenzae*, and *S. aureus* (including MRSA). Viruses have not been established as causes of acute epiglottitis.

Clinical Manifestations and Diagnosis Epiglottitis typically presents more acutely in young children than in adolescents or adults. On presentation, most children have had symptoms for <24 h, including high fever, severe sore throat, tachycardia, systemic toxicity, and (in many cases) drooling while sitting forward. Symptoms and signs of respiratory obstruction also may be present and may progress rapidly. The somewhat milder illness in adolescents and adults often follows 1–2 days of severe sore throat and is commonly accompanied by dyspnea, drooling, and stridor. Physical examination of patients with acute epiglottitis may reveal moderate or severe respiratory distress, with inspiratory stridor and retractions of the chest wall. These findings *diminish* as the disease progresses and the patient tires. Conversely, oropharyngeal examination reveals infection that is much less severe than would be predicted from the symptoms—a finding that should alert the clinician to a cause of symptoms and obstruction that lies beyond the tonsils. The diagnosis often is made on clinical grounds, although direct fiberoptic laryngoscopy is frequently performed in a controlled environment (e.g., an operating room) to visualize and culture the typical edematous "cherry-red" epiglottis and facilitate placement of an endotracheal tube. Direct visualization in an examination room (i.e., with a tongue blade and indirect laryngoscopy) is not recommended because of the risk of immediate laryngospasm and complete airway obstruction. Lateral neck radiographs and laboratory tests can assist in the diagnosis but may delay the critical securing of the airway and cause the patient to be moved or repositioned more than is necessary, thereby increasing the risk of further airway compromise. Neck radiographs typically reveal an enlarged edematous epiglottis (the "thumbprint sign," Fig. 44-3), usually with a dilated hypopharynx and normal subglottic structures. Laboratory tests characteristically document mild to moderate leukocytosis with a predominance of neutrophils. Blood cultures are positive in a significant proportion of cases.

TREATMENT EPIGLOTTITIS

Security of the airway is always of primary concern in acute epiglottitis, even if the diagnosis is only suspected. Mere observation for signs of impending airway obstruction is not routinely recommended,

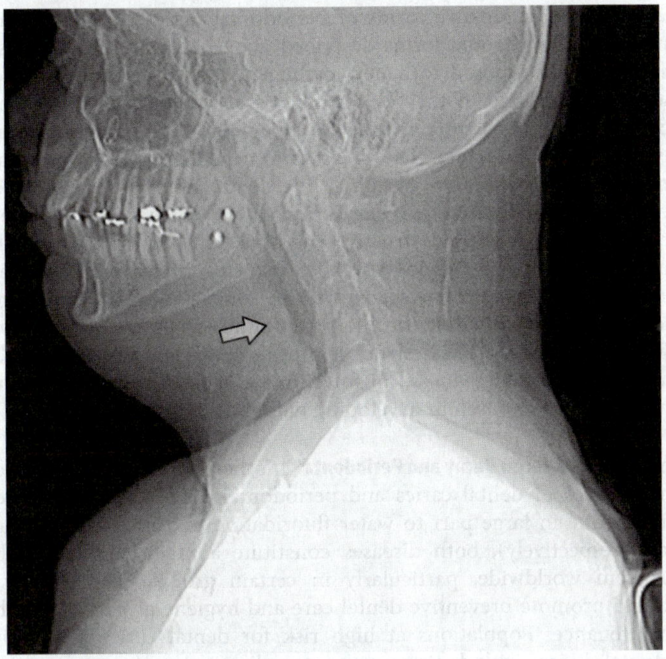

FIGURE 44-3 Acute epiglottitis. In this lateral soft tissue radiograph of the neck, the arrow indicates the enlarged edematous epiglottis (the "thumbprint sign").

particularly in children. Many adults have been managed with observation only since the illness is perceived to be milder in this age group, but some data suggest that this approach may be risky and probably should be reserved only for adult patients who have yet to develop dyspnea or stridor. Once the airway has been secured and specimens of blood and epiglottis tissue have been obtained for culture, treatment with IV antibiotics should be given to cover the most likely organisms, particularly *H. influenzae*. Because rates of ampicillin resistance in this organism have risen significantly in recent years, therapy with a β-lactam/β-lactamase inhibitor combination or a second- or third-generation cephalosporin is recommended. Typically, ampicillin/sulbactam, cefuroxime, cefotaxime, or ceftriaxone is given, with clindamycin and TMP-SMX reserved for patients allergic to β-lactams. Antibiotic therapy should be continued for 7–10 days and should be tailored to the organism recovered in culture. If the household contacts of a patient with *H. influenzae* epiglottitis include an unvaccinated child under age 4, all members of the household (including the patient) should receive prophylactic rifampin for 4 days to eradicate carriage of *H. influenzae*.

INFECTIONS OF DEEP NECK STRUCTURES

Deep neck infections are usually extensions of infection from other primary sites, most often within the pharynx or oral cavity. Many of these infections are life threatening but are difficult to detect at early stages, when they may be more easily managed. Three of the most clinically relevant spaces in the neck are the submandibular (and sublingual) space, the lateral pharyngeal (or parapharyngeal) space, and the retropharyngeal space. These spaces communicate with one another and with other important structures in the head, neck, and thorax, providing pathogens with easy access to areas that include the mediastinum, carotid sheath, skull base, and meninges. Once infection reaches these sensitive areas, mortality rates can be as high as 20–50%.

Infection of the submandibular and/or sublingual space typically originates from an infected or recently extracted lower tooth. The result is the severe, life-threatening infection referred to as Ludwig's angina (see "Oral Infections," above). Infection of the lateral pharyngeal (or parapharyngeal) space is most often a complication of common infections of the oral cavity and upper respiratory tract, including tonsillitis, peritonsillar abscess, pharyngitis, mastoiditis, and periodontal infection. This space, situated deep in the lateral wall of the pharynx, contains a number of sensitive structures, including the carotid artery, internal jugular vein, cervical sympathetic chain, and portions of cranial nerves IX through XII; at its distal end, it opens into the posterior mediastinum. Involvement of this space with infection can therefore be rapidly fatal. Examination may reveal some tonsillar displacement, trismus, and neck rigidity, but swelling of the lateral pharyngeal wall can easily be missed. The diagnosis can be confirmed by CT. Treatment consists of airway management, operative drainage of fluid collections, and at least 10 days of IV therapy with an antibiotic active against streptococci and oral anaerobes (e.g., ampicillin/sulbactam). A particularly severe form of this infection involving the components of the carotid sheath (postanginal septicemia, Lemierre's disease) is described above (see "Oral Infections"). Infection of the retropharyngeal space also can be extremely dangerous, as this space runs posterior to the pharynx from the skull base to the superior mediastinum. Infections in this space are more common among children <5 years old because of the presence of several small retropharyngeal lymph nodes that typically atrophy by age 4 years. Infection is usually a consequence of extension from another site of infection—most commonly, acute pharyngitis. Other sources include otitis media, tonsillitis, dental infections, Ludwig's angina, and anterior extension of vertebral osteomyelitis. Retropharyngeal space infection also can follow penetrating trauma to the posterior pharynx (e.g., from an endoscopic procedure). Infections are commonly polymicrobial, involving a mixture of aerobes and anaerobes; group A β-hemolytic streptococci and *S. aureus* are the most common pathogens. *M. tuberculosis* was a common cause in the past but now is rarely involved in the United States.

Patients with retropharyngeal abscess typically present with sore throat, fever, dysphagia, and neck pain and are often drooling because of difficulty and pain with swallowing. Examination may reveal tender cervical adenopathy, neck swelling, and diffuse erythema and edema of the posterior pharynx as well as a bulge in the posterior pharyngeal wall that may not be obvious on routine inspection. A soft tissue mass is usually demonstrable by lateral neck radiography or CT. Because of the risk of airway obstruction, treatment begins with securing of the airway, followed by a combination of surgical drainage and IV antibiotic administration. Initial empirical therapy should cover streptococci, oral anaerobes, and *S. aureus*; ampicillin/sulbactam, clindamycin plus ceftriaxone, or meropenem is usually effective. Complications result primarily from extension to other areas (e.g., rupture into the posterior pharynx may lead to aspiration pneumonia and empyema). Extension may also occur to the lateral pharyngeal space and mediastinum, resulting in mediastinitis and pericarditis, or into nearby major blood vessels. All these events are associated with a high mortality rate.

45 Oral Manifestations of Disease

Samuel C. Durso

As primary care physicians and consultants, internists are often asked to evaluate patients with disease of the oral soft tissues, teeth, and pharynx. Knowledge of the oral milieu and its unique structures is necessary to guide preventive services and recognize oral manifestations of local or systemic disease (Chap. 46e). Furthermore, internists frequently collaborate with dentists in the care of patients who have a variety of medical conditions that affect oral health or who undergo dental procedures that increase their risk of medical complications.

DISEASES OF THE TEETH AND PERIODONTAL STRUCTURES

Tooth formation begins during the sixth week of embryonic life and continues through 17 years of age. Teeth start to develop in utero and continue to develop until after the tooth erupts. Normally, all 20 deciduous teeth have erupted by age 3 and have been shed by age 13. Permanent teeth, eventually totaling 32, begin to erupt by age 6 and have completely erupted by age 14, though third molars ("wisdom teeth") may erupt later.

The erupted tooth consists of the visible *crown* covered with enamel and the root submerged below the gum line and covered with bonelike *cementum*. *Dentin*, a material that is denser than bone and exquisitely sensitive to pain, forms the majority of the tooth substance, surrounding a core of myxomatous *pulp* containing the vascular and nerve supply. The tooth is held firmly in the alveolar socket by the *periodontium*, supporting structures that consist of the gingivae, alveolar bone, cementum, and periodontal ligament. The periodontal ligament tenaciously binds the tooth's cementum to the alveolar bone. Above this ligament is a collar of attached gingiva just below the crown. A few millimeters of unattached or free gingiva (1–3 mm) overlap the base of the crown, forming a shallow sulcus along the gum-tooth margin.

Dental Caries, Pulpal and Periapical Disease, and Complications Dental caries usually begin asymptomatically as a destructive infectious process of the enamel. Bacteria—principally *Streptococcus mutans*—colonize the organic buffering biofilm (*plaque*) on the tooth surface. If not removed by brushing or by the natural cleansing and antibacterial action of saliva, bacterial acids can demineralize the enamel. Fissures and pits on the occlusal surfaces are the most frequent sites of early decay. Surfaces between the teeth, adjacent to tooth restorations and exposed roots, are also vulnerable, particularly as individuals age. Over time, dental caries extend to the underlying dentin, leading to cavitation of the enamel. Without management, the caries will penetrate to the tooth pulp, producing *acute pulpitis*. At this stage, when the pulp infection is limited, the tooth may become sensitive to percussion and to hot or cold, and pain resolves immediately when the irritating stimulus is removed. Should the infection spread throughout the pulp, *irreversible pulpitis* occurs, leading to *pulp necrosis*. At this later stage, pain can be severe and has a sharp or throbbing visceral quality that may be worse when the patient lies down. Once pulp necrosis is complete, pain may be constant or intermittent, but cold sensitivity is lost.

Treatment of caries involves removal of the softened and infected hard tissue and restoration of the tooth structure with silver amalgam, glass ionomer, composite resin, or gold. Once irreversible pulpitis occurs, root canal therapy becomes necessary; removal of the contents of the pulp chamber and root canals is followed by thorough cleaning and filling with an inert material. Alternatively, the tooth may be extracted.

Pulpal infection leads to *periapical abscess* formation, which can produce pain on chewing. If the infection is mild and chronic, a *periapical granuloma* or eventually a *periapical cyst* forms, either of which produces radiolucency at the root apex. When unchecked, a periapical abscess can erode into the alveolar bone, producing osteomyelitis; penetrate and drain through the gingivae, producing a parulis (gumboil); or track along deep fascial planes, producing virulent cellulitis (Ludwig's angina) involving the submandibular space and floor of the mouth (Chap. 201). Elderly patients, patients with diabetes mellitus, and patients taking glucocorticoids may experience little or no pain or fever as these complications develop.

Periodontal Disease Periodontal disease and dental caries are the primary causes of tooth loss. Like dental caries, chronic infection of the gingiva and anchoring structures of the tooth begins with formation of bacterial plaque. The process begins at the gum line. Plaque and *calculus* (calcified plaque) are preventable by appropriate daily oral hygiene, including periodic professional cleaning. Left undisturbed, chronic inflammation can ensue and produce hyperemia of the free and attached gingivae (*gingivitis*), which then typically bleed with brushing. If this issue is ignored, severe *periodontitis* can develop, leading to deepening of the physiologic sulcus and destruction of the periodontal ligament. Gingival pockets develop around the teeth. As the periodontium (including the supporting bone) is destroyed, the teeth loosen. A role for chronic inflammation due to chronic periodontal disease in promoting coronary heart disease and stroke has been proposed. Epidemiologic studies have demonstrated a moderate but significant association between chronic periodontal inflammation and atherogenesis, though a causal role remains unproven.

Acute and aggressive forms of periodontal disease are less common than the chronic forms described above. However, if the host is stressed or exposed to a new pathogen, rapidly progressive and destructive disease of the periodontal tissue can occur. A virulent example is *acute necrotizing ulcerative gingivitis*. Stress and poor oral hygiene are risk factors. The presentation includes sudden gingival inflammation, ulceration, bleeding, interdental gingival necrosis, and fetid halitosis. *Localized juvenile periodontitis*, which is seen in adolescents, is particularly destructive and appears to be associated with impaired neutrophil chemotaxis. *AIDS-related periodontitis* resembles acute necrotizing ulcerative gingivitis in some patients and a more destructive form of adult chronic periodontitis in others. It may also produce a gangrene-like destructive process of the oral soft tissues and bone that resembles *noma*, an infectious condition seen in severely malnourished children in developing nations.

Prevention of Tooth Decay and Periodontal Infection Despite the reduced prevalences of dental caries and periodontal disease in the United States (due in large part to water fluoridation and improved dental care, respectively), both diseases constitute a major public health problem worldwide, particularly in certain groups. The internist should promote preventive dental care and hygiene as part of health maintenance. Populations at high risk for dental caries and periodontal disease include those with hyposalivation and/or xerostomia, diabetics, alcoholics, tobacco users, persons with Down syndrome, and those with gingival hyperplasia. Furthermore, patients lacking access to dental care (e.g., as a result of low socioeconomic status) and patients with a reduced ability to provide self-care (e.g., individuals with disabilities, nursing home residents, and persons with dementia or upper-extremity disability) suffer at a disproportionate rate. It is important to provide counseling regarding regular dental hygiene and professional cleaning, use of fluoride-containing toothpaste, professional fluoride treatments, and (for patients with limited dexterity) use of electric toothbrushes and also to instruct persons caring for those who are not capable of self-care. Cost, fear of dental care, and differences in language and culture create barriers that prevent some people from seeking preventive dental services.

Developmental and Systemic Disease Affecting the Teeth and Periodontium In addition to posing cosmetic issues, *malocclusion*, the most common developmental oral problem, can interfere with mastication unless corrected through orthodontic and surgical techniques. Impacted third molars are common and can become infected or erupt into an insufficient space. Acquired prognathism due to *acromegaly* may also lead to malocclusion, as may deformity of the maxilla and mandible due to *Paget's disease* of the bone. Delayed tooth eruption, a receding chin, and a protruding tongue are occasional features of *cretinism* and *hypopituitarism*. Congenital syphilis produces tapering, notched (*Hutchinson's*) incisors and finely nodular (*mulberry*) molar crowns. *Enamel hypoplasia* results in crown defects ranging from pits to deep fissures of primary or permanent teeth. Intrauterine infection (syphilis, rubella), vitamin deficiency (A, C, or D), disorders of calcium metabolism (malabsorption, vitamin D–resistant rickets, hypoparathyroidism), prematurity, high fever, and rare inherited defects (*amelogenesis imperfecta*) are all causes. Tetracycline, given in sufficiently high doses during the first 8 years of life, may produce enamel hypoplasia and discoloration. Exposure to endogenous pigments can discolor developing teeth; etiologies include *erythroblastosis fetalis* (green or bluish-black), congenital liver disease (green or yellow-brown), and porphyria (red or brown that fluoresces with ultraviolet light). *Mottled enamel* occurs if excessive fluoride is ingested during development. Worn enamel is seen with age, bruxism, or excessive acid exposure (e.g., chronic gastric reflux or bulimia). Celiac disease is associated with nonspecific enamel defects in children but not in adults.

Total or partial tooth loss resulting from periodontitis is seen with cyclic neutropenia, Papillon-Lefévre syndrome, Chédiak-Higashi syndrome, and leukemia. Rapid focal tooth loosening is most often due to infection, but rarer causes include Langerhans cell histiocytosis, Ewing's sarcoma, osteosarcoma, and Burkitt's lymphoma. Early loss of primary teeth is a feature of *hypophosphatasia*, a rare congenital error of metabolism.

Pregnancy may produce gingivitis and localized *pyogenic granulomas*. Severe periodontal disease occurs in uncontrolled diabetes mellitus. *Gingival hyperplasia* may be caused by phenytoin, calcium channel blockers (e.g., nifedipine), and cyclosporine, though excellent daily oral care can prevent or reduce its occurrence. *Idiopathic familial gingival fibromatosis* and several syndrome-related disorders cause similar conditions. Discontinuation of the medication may reverse the drug-induced form, though surgery may be needed to control both of the latter entities. *Linear gingival erythema* is variably seen in patients with advanced HIV infection and probably represents immune deficiency and decreased neutrophil activity. Diffuse or focal gingival swelling may be a feature of early or late acute myelomonocytic leukemia as well as of other lymphoproliferative disorders. A rare but pathognomonic sign of granulomatosis with polyangiitis is a red-purplish, granular gingivitis (*strawberry gums*).

DISEASES OF THE ORAL MUCOSA

Infections Most oral mucosal diseases involve microorganisms (Table 45-1).

Pigmented Lesions See Table 45-2.

Dermatologic Diseases See Tables 45-1, 45-2, and 45-3 and Chaps. 70–74.

Diseases of the Tongue See Table 45-4.

HIV Disease and AIDS See Tables 45-1, 45-2, 45-3, and 45-5; Chap. 226; and Fig. 218-3.

Ulcers Ulceration is the most common oral mucosal lesion. Although there are many causes, the host and the pattern of lesions, including the presence of organ system features, narrow the differential diagnosis (Table 45-1). Most acute ulcers are painful and self-limited. Recurrent aphthous ulcers and herpes simplex account for the majority. Persistent and deep aphthous ulcers can be idiopathic or can accompany HIV/AIDS. Aphthous lesions are often the presenting symptom in *Behçet's syndrome* (Chap. 387). Similar-appearing, though less painful, lesions may occur in reactive arthritis, and aphthous ulcers are occasionally present during phases of *discoid* or *systemic lupus erythematosus* (Chap. 382). Aphthous-like ulcers are seen in *Crohn's disease* (Chap. 351), but, unlike the common aphthous variety, they may exhibit granulomatous inflammation on histologic examination. Recurrent aphthae are more prevalent in patients with *celiac disease* and have been reported to remit with elimination of gluten.

Of major concern are chronic, relatively painless ulcers and mixed red/white patches (erythroplakia and leukoplakia) of >2 weeks' duration. Squamous cell carcinoma and premalignant dysplasia should be considered early and a diagnostic biopsy performed. This awareness and this procedure are critically important because early-stage malignancy is vastly more treatable than late-stage disease. High-risk sites include the lower lip, floor of the mouth, ventral and lateral tongue, and soft palate–tonsillar pillar complex. Significant risk factors for oral cancer in Western countries include sun exposure (lower lip), tobacco and alcohol use, and human papillomavirus infection. In India and some other Asian countries, smokeless tobacco mixed with betel nut, slaked lime, and spices is a common cause of oral cancer. Rarer causes of chronic oral ulcer, such as tuberculosis, fungal infection, granulomatosis with polyangiitis, and midline granuloma may look identical to carcinoma. Making the correct diagnosis depends on recognizing other clinical features and performing a biopsy of the lesion. The syphilitic chancre is typically painless and therefore easily missed. Regional lymphadenopathy is invariably present. The syphilitic etiology is confirmed with appropriate bacterial and serologic tests.

Disorders of mucosal fragility often produce painful oral ulcers that fail to heal within 2 weeks. *Mucous membrane pemphigoid* and *pemphigus vulgaris* are the major acquired disorders. While their clinical features are often distinctive, a biopsy or immunohistochemical examination should be performed to diagnose these entities and to distinguish them from *lichen planus* and drug reactions.

Hematologic and Nutritional Disease Internists are more likely to encounter patients with acquired, rather than congenital, bleeding disorders. Bleeding should stop 15 min after minor trauma and within an hour after tooth extraction if local pressure is applied. More prolonged bleeding, if not due to continued injury or rupture of a large vessel, should lead to investigation for a clotting abnormality. In addition to bleeding, petechiae and ecchymoses are prone to occur at the vibrating line between the soft and hard palates in patients with platelet dysfunction or thrombocytopenia.

All forms of leukemia, but particularly *acute myelomonocytic leukemia*, can produce gingival bleeding, ulcers, and gingival enlargement. Oral ulcers are a feature of agranulocytosis, and ulcers and mucositis are often severe complications of chemotherapy and radiation therapy for hematologic and other malignancies. *Plummer-Vinson syndrome* (iron deficiency, angular stomatitis, glossitis, and dysphagia) raises the risk of oral squamous cell cancer and esophageal cancer at the postcricoidal tissue web. Atrophic papillae and a red, burning tongue may occur with pernicious anemia. Deficiencies in B-group vitamins produce many of these same symptoms as well as oral ulceration and cheilosis. Consequences of *scurvy* include swollen, bleeding gums; ulcers; and loosening of the teeth.

NONDENTAL CAUSES OF ORAL PAIN

Most, but not all, oral pain emanates from inflamed or injured tooth pulp or periodontal tissues. Nonodontogenic causes are often overlooked. In most instances, toothache is predictable and proportional to the stimulus applied, and an identifiable condition (e.g., caries, abscess) is found. Local anesthesia eliminates pain originating from dental or periodontal structures, but not referred pains. The most common nondental source of pain is myofascial pain referred from muscles of mastication, which become tender and ache with increased use. Many sufferers exhibit *bruxism* (grinding of the teeth) secondary to stress and anxiety. *Temporomandibular joint disorder* is closely related. It affects both sexes, with a higher prevalence among women. Features include pain, limited mandibular movement, and temporomandibular joint sounds. The etiologies are complex; malocclusion does not play the primary role once attributed to it. *Osteoarthritis* is a common cause of masticatory pain. Anti-inflammatory medication, jaw rest, soft foods, and heat provide relief. The temporomandibular joint is involved in 50% of patients with *rheumatoid arthritis*, and its involvement is usually a late feature of severe disease. Bilateral preauricular pain, particularly in the morning, limits range of motion.

Migrainous neuralgia may be localized to the mouth. Episodes of pain and remission without an identifiable cause and a lack of relief with local anesthesia are important clues. *Trigeminal neuralgia* (*tic douloureux*) can involve the entire branch or part of the mandibular or maxillary branch of the fifth cranial nerve and can produce pain in one or a few teeth. Pain may occur spontaneously or may be triggered by touching the lip or gingiva, brushing the teeth, or chewing. *Glossopharyngeal neuralgia* produces similar acute neuropathic symptoms in the distribution of the ninth cranial nerve. Swallowing, sneezing, coughing, or pressure on the tragus of the ear triggers pain that is felt in the base of the tongue, pharynx, and soft palate and may be referred to the temporomandibular joint. *Neuritis* involving the maxillary and mandibular divisions of the trigeminal nerve (e.g., maxillary sinusitis, neuroma, and leukemic infiltrate) is distinguished from ordinary toothache by the neuropathic quality of the pain. Occasionally, *phantom pain* follows tooth extraction. Pain and hyperalgesia behind the ear and on the side of the face in the day or so before facial weakness develops often constitute the earliest symptom of *Bell's palsy*. Likewise, similar symptoms may precede visible lesions of herpes zoster infecting the seventh nerve (*Ramsey-Hunt syndrome*) or trigeminal nerve. *Postherpetic neuralgia* may follow either condition. *Coronary ischemia* may produce pain exclusively in the face and jaw; as in typical angina pectoris, this pain is usually reproducible with increased myocardial demand. Aching in several upper molar or

TABLE 45-1 VESICULAR, BULLOUS, OR ULCERATIVE LESIONS OF THE ORAL MUCOSA

Condition	Usual Location	Clinical Features	Course
Viral Diseases			
Primary acute herpetic gingivostomatitis (HSV type 1; rarely type 2)	Lip and oral mucosa (buccal, gingival, lingual mucosa)	Labial vesicles that rupture and crust, and intraoral vesicles that quickly ulcerate; extremely painful; acute gingivitis, fever, malaise, foul odor, and cervical lymphadenopathy; occurs primarily in infants, children, and young adults	Heals spontaneously in 10–14 days; unless secondarily infected, lesions lasting >3 weeks are not due to primary HSV infection
Recurrent herpes labialis	Mucocutaneous junction of lip, perioral skin	Eruption of groups of vesicles that may coalesce, then rupture and crust; painful to pressure or spicy foods	Lasts ~1 week, but condition may be prolonged if secondarily infected; if severe, topical or oral antiviral treatment may reduce healing time
Recurrent intraoral herpes simplex	Palate and gingiva	Small vesicles on keratinized epithelium that rupture and coalesce; painful	Heals spontaneously in ~1 week; if severe, topical or oral antiviral treatment may reduce healing time
Chickenpox (VZV)	Gingiva and oral mucosa	Skin lesions may be accompanied by small vesicles on oral mucosa that rupture to form shallow ulcers; may coalesce to form large bullous lesions that ulcerate; mucosa may have generalized erythema	Lesions heal spontaneously within 2 weeks
Herpes zoster (VZV reactivation)	Cheek, tongue, gingiva, or palate	Unilateral vesicular eruptions and ulceration in linear pattern following sensory distribution of trigeminal nerve or one of its branches	Gradual healing without scarring unless secondarily infected; postherpetic neuralgia is common; oral acyclovir, famciclovir, or valacyclovir reduces healing time and postherpetic neuralgia
Infectious mononucleosis (Epstein-Barr virus)	Oral mucosa	Fatigue, sore throat, malaise, fever, and cervical lymphadenopathy; numerous small ulcers usually appear several days before lymphadenopathy; gingival bleeding and multiple petechiae at junction of hard and soft palates	Oral lesions disappear during convalescence; no treatment is given, though glucocorticoids are indicated if tonsillar swelling compromises the airway
Herpangina (coxsackievirus A; also possibly coxsackievirus B and echovirus)	Oral mucosa, pharynx, tongue	Sudden onset of fever, sore throat, and oropharyngeal vesicles, usually in children <4 years old, during summer months; diffuse pharyngeal congestion and vesicles (1–2 mm), grayish-white surrounded by red areola; vesicles enlarge and ulcerate	Incubation period of 2–9 days; fever for 1–4 days; recovery uneventful
Hand-foot-and-mouth disease (most commonly coxsackievirus A16)	Oral mucosa, pharynx, palms, and soles	Fever, malaise, headache with oropharyngeal vesicles that become painful, shallow ulcers; highly infectious; usually affects children under age 10	Incubation period 2–18 days; lesions heal spontaneously in 2–4 weeks
Primary HIV infection	Gingiva, palate, and pharynx	Acute gingivitis and oropharyngeal ulceration, associated with febrile illness resembling mononucleosis and including lymphadenopathy	Followed by HIV seroconversion, asymptomatic HIV infection, and usually ultimately by HIV disease
Bacterial or Fungal Diseases			
Acute necrotizing ulcerative gingivitis ("trench mouth")	Gingiva	Painful, bleeding gingiva characterized by necrosis and ulceration of gingival papillae and margins plus lymphadenopathy and foul breath	Debridement and diluted (1:3) peroxide lavage provide relief within 24 h; antibiotics in acutely ill patients; relapse may occur
Prenatal (congenital) syphilis	Palate, jaws, tongue, and teeth	Gummatous involvement of palate, jaws, and facial bones; Hutchinson's incisors, mulberry molars, glossitis, mucous patches, and fissures at corner of mouth	Tooth deformities in permanent dentition irreversible
Primary syphilis (chancre)	Lesion appearing where organism enters body; may occur on lips, tongue, or tonsillar area	Small papule developing rapidly into a large, painless ulcer with indurated border; unilateral lymphadenopathy; chancre and lymph nodes containing spirochetes; serologic tests positive by third to fourth weeks	Healing of chancre in 1–2 months, followed by secondary syphilis in 6–8 weeks
Secondary syphilis	Oral mucosa frequently involved with mucous patches, which occur primarily on palate and also at commissures of mouth	Maculopapular lesions of oral mucosa, 5–10 mm in diameter with central ulceration covered by grayish membrane; eruptions occurring on various mucosal surfaces and skin, accompanied by fever, malaise, and sore throat	Lesions may persist from several weeks to a year
Tertiary syphilis	Palate and tongue	Gummatous infiltration of palate or tongue followed by ulceration and fibrosis; atrophy of tongue papillae produces characteristic bald tongue and glossitis	Gumma may destroy palate, causing complete perforation
Gonorrhea	Lesions may occur in mouth at site of inoculation or secondarily by hematogenous spread from a primary focus	Most pharyngeal infection is asymptomatic; may produce burning or itching sensation; oropharynx and tonsils may be ulcerated and erythematous; saliva viscous and fetid	More difficult to eradicate than urogenital infection, though pharyngitis usually resolves with appropriate antimicrobial treatment
Tuberculosis	Tongue, tonsillar area, soft palate	Painless, solitary, 1- to 5-cm, irregular ulcer covered with persistent exudate; ulcer has firm undermined border	Autoinoculation from pulmonary infection is usual; lesions resolve with appropriate antimicrobial therapy

(Continued)

TABLE 45-1 VESICULAR, BULLOUS, OR ULCERATIVE LESIONS OF THE ORAL MUCOSA (*CONTINUED*)

Condition	Usual Location	Clinical Features	Course
Cervicofacial actinomycosis	Swellings in region of face, neck, and floor of mouth	Infection may be associated with extraction, jaw fracture, or eruption of molar tooth; in acute form, resembles acute pyogenic abscess, but contains yellow "sulfur granules" (gram-positive mycelia and their hyphae)	Typically, swelling is hard and grows painlessly; multiple abscesses with draining tracts develop; penicillin first choice; surgery usually necessary
Histoplasmosis	Any area of the mouth, particularly tongue, gingiva, or palate	Nodular, verrucous, or granulomatous lesions; ulcers are indurated and painful; usual source hematogenous or pulmonary, but may be primary	Systemic antifungal therapy necessary
Candidiasis[a]			
Dermatologic Diseases			
Mucous membrane pemphigoid	Typically produces marked gingival erythema and ulceration; other areas of oral cavity, esophagus, and vagina may be affected	Painful, grayish-white collapsed vesicles or bullae of full-thickness epithelium with peripheral erythematous zone; gingival lesions desquamate, leaving ulcerated area	Protracted course with remissions and exacerbations; involvement of different sites develops slowly; glucocorticoids may temporarily reduce symptoms but do not control disease
EM minor and EM major (Stevens-Johnson syndrome)	Primarily oral mucosa and skin of hands and feet	Intraoral ruptured bullae surrounded by inflammatory area; lips may show hemorrhagic crusts; "iris" or "target" lesion on skin is pathognomonic; patient may have severe signs of toxicity	Onset very rapid; usually idiopathic, but may be associated with trigger such as drug reaction; condition may last 3–6 weeks; mortality rate for untreated EM major is 5–15%
Pemphigus vulgaris	Oral mucosa and skin; sites of mechanical trauma (soft/hard palate, frenulum, lips, buccal mucosa)	Usually (>70%) presents with oral lesions; fragile, ruptured bullae and ulcerated oral areas; mostly in older adults	With repeated occurrence of bullae, toxicity may lead to cachexia, infection, and death within 2 years; often controllable with oral glucocorticoids
Lichen planus	Oral mucosa and skin	White striae in mouth; purplish nodules on skin at sites of friction; occasionally causes oral mucosal ulcers and erosive gingivitis	White striae alone usually asymptomatic; erosive lesions often difficult to treat, but may respond to glucocorticoids
Other Conditions			
Recurrent aphthous ulcers	Usually on nonkeratinized oral mucosa (buccal and labial mucosa, floor of mouth, soft palate, lateral and ventral tongue)	Single or clustered painful ulcers with surrounding erythematous border; lesions may be 1–2 mm in diameter in crops (herpetiform), 1–5 mm (minor), or 5–15 mm (major)	Lesions heal in 1–2 weeks but may recur monthly or several times a year; protective barrier with benzocaine and topical glucocorticoids relieve symptoms; systemic glucocorticoids may be needed in severe cases
Behçet's syndrome	Oral mucosa, eyes, genitalia, gut, and CNS	Multiple aphthous ulcers in mouth; inflammatory ocular changes, ulcerative lesions on genitalia; inflammatory bowel disease and CNS disease	Oral lesions often first manifestation; persist several weeks and heal without scarring
Traumatic ulcers	Anywhere on oral mucosa; dentures frequently responsible for ulcers in vestibule	Localized, discrete ulcerated lesions with red border; produced by accidental biting of mucosa, penetration by foreign object, or chronic irritation by dentures	Lesions usually heal in 7–10 days when irritant is removed, unless secondarily infected
Squamous cell carcinoma	Any area of mouth, most commonly on lower lip, lateral borders of tongue, and floor of mouth	Red, white, or red and white ulcer with elevated or indurated border; failure to heal; pain not prominent in early lesions	Invades and destroys underlying tissues; frequently metastasizes to regional lymph nodes
Acute myeloid leukemia (usually monocytic)	Gingiva	Gingival swelling and superficial ulceration followed by hyperplasia of gingiva with extensive necrosis and hemorrhage; deep ulcers may occur elsewhere on mucosa, complicated by secondary infection	Usually responds to systemic treatment of leukemia; occasionally requires local irradiation
Lymphoma	Gingiva, tongue, palate, and tonsillar area	Elevated, ulcerated area that may proliferate rapidly, giving appearance of traumatic inflammation	Fatal if untreated; may indicate underlying HIV infection
Chemical or thermal burns	Any area in mouth	White slough due to contact with corrosive agents (e.g., aspirin, hot cheese) applied locally; removal of slough leaves raw, painful surface	Lesion heals in several weeks if not secondarily infected

[a]See Table 45-3.

Abbreviations: CNS, central nervous system; EM, erythema multiforme; HSV, herpes simplex virus; VZV, varicella-zoster virus.

premolar teeth that is unrelieved by anesthetizing the teeth may point to *maxillary sinusitis*.

Giant cell arteritis is notorious for producing headache, but it may also produce facial pain or sore throat without headache. Jaw and tongue claudication with chewing or talking is relatively common. Tongue infarction is rare. Patients with subacute thyroiditis often experience pain referred to the face or jaw before the tenderness of the thyroid gland and transient hyperthyroidism are appreciated.

"Burning mouth syndrome" (*glossodynia*) occurs in the absence of an identifiable cause (e.g., vitamin B_{12} deficiency, iron deficiency, diabetes mellitus, low-grade *Candida* infection, food sensitivity, or subtle xerostomia) and predominantly affects postmenopausal women. The etiology may be neuropathic. Clonazepam, α-lipoic acid, and cognitive behavioral therapy have benefited some patients. Some cases associated with an angiotensin-converting enzyme inhibitor have remitted when treatment with the drug was discontinued.

DISEASES OF THE SALIVARY GLANDS

Saliva is essential to oral health. Its absence leads to dental caries, periodontal disease, and difficulties in wearing dental prostheses, masticating, and speaking. Its major components, water and mucin, serve as a cleansing solvent and lubricating fluid. In addition, saliva contains antimicrobial factors (e.g., lysozyme, lactoperoxidase, secretory IgA), epidermal growth factor, minerals, and buffering systems. The

TABLE 45-2 PIGMENTED LESIONS OF THE ORAL MUCOSA

Condition	Usual Location	Clinical Features	Course
Oral melanotic macule	Any area of mouth	Discrete or diffuse, localized, brown to black macule	Remains indefinitely; no growth
Diffuse melanin pigmentation	Any area of mouth	Diffuse pale to dark-brown pigmentation; may be physiologic ("racial") or due to smoking	Remains indefinitely
Nevi	Any area of mouth	Discrete, localized, brown to black pigmentation	Remains indefinitely
Malignant melanoma	Any area of mouth	Can be flat and diffuse, painless, brown to black; or can be raised and nodular	Expands and invades early; metastasis leads to death
Addison's disease	Any area of mouth, but mostly buccal mucosa	Blotches or spots of bluish-black to dark-brown pigmentation occurring early in disease, accompanied by diffuse pigmentation of skin; other symptoms of adrenal insufficiency	Condition controlled by adrenal steroid replacement
Peutz-Jeghers syndrome	Any area of mouth	Dark-brown spots on lips, buccal mucosa, with characteristic distribution of pigment around lips, nose, and eyes and on hands; concomitant intestinal polyposis	Oral pigmented lesions remain indefinitely; gastrointestinal polyps may become malignant
Drug ingestion (neuroleptics, oral contraceptives, minocycline, zidovudine, quinine derivatives)	Any area of mouth	Brown, black, or gray areas of pigmentation	Gradually disappears following cessation of drug intake
Amalgam tattoo	Gingiva and alveolar mucosa	Small blue-black pigmented areas associated with embedded amalgam particles in soft tissues; may show up on radiographs as radiopaque particles in some cases	Remains indefinitely
Heavy metal pigmentation (bismuth, mercury, lead)	Gingival margin	Thin blue-black pigmented line along gingival margin; rarely seen except in children exposed to lead-based paint	Indicative of systemic absorption; no significance for oral health
Black hairy tongue	Dorsum of tongue	Elongation of filiform papillae of tongue, which become stained by coffee, tea, tobacco, or pigmented bacteria	Improves within 1–2 weeks with gentle brushing of tongue or (if due to bacterial overgrowth) discontinuation of antibiotic
Fordyce spots	Buccal and labial mucosa	Numerous small yellowish spots just beneath mucosal surface; no symptoms; due to hyperplasia of sebaceous glands	Benign; remains without apparent change
Kaposi's sarcoma	Palate most common, but may occur at any other site	Red or blue plaques of variable size and shape; often enlarge, become nodular, and may ulcerate	Usually indicative of HIV infection or non-Hodgkin's lymphoma; rarely fatal, but may require treatment for comfort or cosmesis
Mucous retention cysts	Buccal and labial mucosa	Bluish, clear fluid–filled cyst due to extravasated mucus from injured minor salivary gland	Benign; painless unless traumatized; may be removed surgically

TABLE 45-3 WHITE LESIONS OF ORAL MUCOSA

Condition	Usual Location	Clinical Features	Course
Lichen planus	Buccal mucosa, tongue, gingiva, and lips; skin	Striae, white plaques, red areas, ulcers in mouth; purplish papules on skin; may be asymptomatic, sore, or painful; lichenoid drug reactions may look similar	Protracted; responds to topical glucocorticoids
White sponge nevus	Oral mucosa, vagina, anal mucosa	Painless white thickening of epithelium; adolescence/early adulthood onset; familial	Benign and permanent
Smoker's leukoplakia and smokeless tobacco lesions	Any area of oral mucosa, sometimes related to location of habit	White patch that may become firm, rough, or red-fissured and ulcerated; may become sore and painful but is usually painless	May or may not resolve with cessation of habit; 2% of patients develop squamous cell carcinoma; early biopsy essential
Erythroplakia with or without white patches	Floor of mouth commonly affected in men; tongue and buccal mucosa in women	Velvety, reddish plaque; occasionally mixed with white patches or smooth red areas	High risk of squamous cell cancer; early biopsy essential
Candidiasis	Any area in mouth	*Pseudomembranous type* ("thrush"): creamy white curdlike patches that reveal a raw, bleeding surface when scraped; found in sick infants, debilitated elderly patients receiving high-dose glucocorticoids or broad-spectrum antibiotics, and patients with AIDS	Responds favorably to antifungal therapy and correction of predisposing causes where possible
		Erythematous type: flat, red, sometimes sore areas in same groups of patients	Course same as for pseudomembranous type
		Candidal leukoplakia: nonremovable white thickening of epithelium due to *Candida*	Responds to prolonged antifungal therapy
		Angular cheilitis: sore fissures at corner of mouth	Responds to topical antifungal therapy
Hairy leukoplakia	Usually on lateral tongue, rarely elsewhere on oral mucosa	White areas ranging from small and flat to extensive accentuation of vertical folds; found in HIV carriers (all risk groups for AIDS)	Due to Epstein-Barr virus; responds to high-dose acyclovir but recurs; rarely causes discomfort unless secondarily infected with *Candida*
Warts (human papillomavirus)	Anywhere on skin and oral mucosa	Single or multiple papillary lesions with thick, white, keratinized surfaces containing many pointed projections; cauliflower lesions covered with normal-colored mucosa or multiple pink or pale bumps (focal epithelial hyperplasia)	Lesions grow rapidly and spread; squamous cell carcinoma must be ruled out with biopsy; excision or laser therapy; may regress in HIV-infected patients receiving antiretroviral therapy

TABLE 45-4 ALTERATIONS OF THE TONGUE

Type of Change	Clinical Features
Size or Morphology	
Macroglossia	Enlarged tongue that may be part of a syndrome found in developmental conditions such as Down syndrome, Simpson-Golabi-Behmel syndrome, or Beckwith-Wiedemann syndrome; may be due to tumor (hemangioma or lymphangioma), metabolic disease (e.g., primary amyloidosis), or endocrine disturbance (e.g., acromegaly or cretinism); may occur when all teeth are removed
Fissured ("scrotal") tongue	Dorsal surface and sides of tongue covered by painless shallow or deep fissures that may collect debris and become irritated
Median rhomboid glossitis	Congenital abnormality with ovoid, denuded area in median posterior portion of tongue; may be associated with candidiasis and may respond to antifungal treatment
Color	
"Geographic" tongue (benign migratory glossitis)	Asymptomatic inflammatory condition of tongue, with rapid loss and regrowth of filiform papillae leading to appearance of denuded red patches "wandering" across surface
Hairy tongue	Elongation of filiform papillae of medial dorsal surface area due to failure of keratin layer of papillae to desquamate normally; brownish-black coloration may be due to staining by tobacco, food, or chromogenic organisms
"Strawberry" and "raspberry" tongue	Appearance of tongue during scarlet fever due to hypertrophy of fungiform papillae as well as changes in filiform papillae
"Bald" tongue	Atrophy may be associated with xerostomia, pernicious anemia, iron-deficiency anemia, pellagra, or syphilis; may be accompanied by painful burning sensation; may be an expression of erythematous candidiasis and respond to antifungal treatment

TABLE 45-5 ORAL LESIONS ASSOCIATED WITH HIV INFECTION

Lesion Morphology	Etiologies
Papules, nodules, plaques	Candidiasis (hyperplastic and pseudomembranous)[a]
	Condyloma acuminatum (human papillomavirus infection)
	Squamous cell carcinoma (preinvasive and invasive)
	Non-Hodgkin's lymphoma[a]
	Hairy leukoplakia[a]
Ulcers	Recurrent aphthous ulcers[a]
	Angular cheilitis
	Squamous cell carcinoma
	Acute necrotizing ulcerative gingivitis[a]
	Necrotizing ulcerative periodontitis[a]
	Necrotizing ulcerative stomatitis
	Non-Hodgkin's lymphoma[a]
	Viral infection (herpes simplex, herpes zoster, cytomegalovirus infection)
	Infection caused by *Mycobacterium tuberculosis* or *Mycobacterium avium-intracellulare*
	Fungal infection (histoplasmosis, cryptococcosis, candidiasis, geotrichosis, aspergillosis)
	Bacterial infection (*Escherichia coli, Enterobacter cloacae, Klebsiella pneumoniae, Pseudomonas aeruginosa*)
	Drug reactions (single or multiple ulcers)
Pigmented lesions	Kaposi's sarcoma[a]
	Bacillary angiomatosis (skin and visceral lesions more common than oral)
	Zidovudine pigmentation (skin, nails, and occasionally oral mucosa)
	Addison's disease
Miscellaneous	Linear gingival erythema[a]

[a]Strongly associated with HIV infection.

major salivary glands secrete intermittently in response to autonomic stimulation, which is high during a meal but low otherwise. Hundreds of minor glands in the lips and cheeks secrete mucus continuously throughout the day and night. Consequently, oral function becomes impaired when salivary function is reduced. The sensation of a dry mouth (*xerostomia*) is perceived when salivary flow is reduced by 50%. The most common etiology is medication, especially drugs with anticholinergic properties but also alpha and beta blockers, calcium channel blockers, and diuretics. Other causes include Sjögren's syndrome, chronic parotitis, salivary duct obstruction, diabetes mellitus, HIV/AIDS, and radiation therapy that includes the salivary glands in the field (e.g., for Hodgkin's disease and for head and neck cancer). Management involves the elimination or limitation of drying medications, preventive dental care, and supplementation with oral liquid or salivary substitutes. Sugarless mints or chewing gum may stimulate salivary secretion if dysfunction is mild. When sufficient exocrine tissue remains, pilocarpine or cevimeline has been shown to increase secretions. Commercial saliva substitutes or gels relieve dryness. Fluoride supplementation is critical to prevent caries.

Sialolithiasis presents most often as painful swelling but in some instances as only swelling or only pain. Conservative therapy consists of local heat, massage, and hydration. Promotion of salivary secretion with mints or lemon drops may flush out small stones. Antibiotic treatment is necessary when bacterial infection in suspected. In adults, *acute bacterial parotitis* is typically unilateral and most commonly affects postoperative, dehydrated, and debilitated patients. *Staphylococcus aureus* (including methicillin-resistant strains) and anaerobic bacteria are the most common pathogens. Chronic bacterial *sialadenitis* results from lowered salivary secretion and recurrent bacterial infection. When suspected bacterial infection is not responsive to therapy, the differential diagnosis should be expanded to include benign and malignant neoplasms, lymphoproliferative disorders, Sjögren's syndrome, sarcoidosis, tuberculosis, lymphadenitis, actinomycosis, and granulomatosis with polyangiitis. Bilateral nontender parotid enlargement occurs with diabetes mellitus, cirrhosis, bulimia, HIV/AIDS, and drugs (e.g., iodide, propylthiouracil).

Pleomorphic adenoma comprises two-thirds of all salivary neoplasms. The parotid is the principal salivary gland affected, and the tumor presents as a firm, slow-growing mass. Although this tumor is benign, its recurrence is common if resection is incomplete. Malignant tumors such as mucoepidermoid carcinoma, adenoid cystic carcinoma, and adenocarcinoma tend to grow relatively fast, depending upon grade. They may ulcerate and invade nerves, producing numbness and facial paralysis. Surgical resection is the primary treatment. Radiation therapy (particularly neutron-beam therapy) is used when surgery is not feasible and as post-resection for certain histologic types with a high risk of recurrence. Malignant salivary gland tumors have a 5-year survival rate of ~68%.

DENTAL CARE FOR MEDICALLY COMPLEX PATIENTS

Routine dental care (e.g., uncomplicated extraction, scaling and cleaning, tooth restoration, and root canal) is remarkably safe. The most common concerns regarding care of dental patients with medical disease are excessive bleeding for patients taking anticoagulants, infection of the heart valves and prosthetic devices from hematogenous seeding by the oral flora, and cardiovascular complications resulting from vasopressors used with local anesthetics during dental treatment. Experience confirms that the risk of any of these complications is very low.

Patients undergoing tooth extraction or alveolar and gingival surgery rarely experience uncontrolled bleeding when warfarin anticoagulation is maintained within the therapeutic range currently recommended for prevention of venous thrombosis, atrial fibrillation, or mechanical heart valve. Embolic complications and death, however, have been reported during subtherapeutic anticoagulation. Therapeutic anticoagulation should be confirmed before and continued through the procedure. Likewise, low-dose aspirin (e.g., 81–325 mg) can safely be continued. For patients taking aspirin and another antiplatelet medication (e.g., clopidogrel), the decision to continue the second antiplatelet medication should be based on individual consideration of the risks of thrombosis and bleeding.

Patients at risk for bacterial endocarditis (Chap. 155) should maintain optimal oral hygiene, including flossing, and have regular professional cleanings. Currently, guidelines recommend that prophylactic antibiotics be restricted to those patients at high risk for bacterial endocarditis who undergo dental and oral procedures involving significant manipulation of gingival or periapical tissue or penetration of the oral mucosa. If unexpected bleeding occurs, antibiotics given within 2 h after the procedure provide effective prophylaxis.

Hematogenous bacterial seeding from oral infection can undoubtedly produce late prosthetic-joint infection and therefore requires removal of the infected tissue (e.g., drainage, extraction, root canal) and appropriate antibiotic therapy. However, evidence that late prosthetic-joint infection follows routine dental procedures is lacking. For this reason, antibiotic prophylaxis is not recommended before dental surgery for patients with orthopedic pins, screws, and plates. Antibiotic prophylaxis is recommended for patients within the first 2 years after joint replacement who have inflammatory arthropathies, immunosuppression, type 1 diabetes mellitus, previous prosthetic-joint infection, hemophilia, or malnourishment.

Concern often arises regarding the use of vasoconstrictors to treat patients with hypertension and heart disease. Vasoconstrictors enhance the depth and duration of local anesthesia, thus reducing the anesthetic dose and potential toxicity. If intravascular injection is avoided, 2% lidocaine with 1:100,000 epinephrine (limited to a total of 0.036 mg of epinephrine) can be used safely in patients with controlled hypertension and stable coronary heart disease, arrhythmia, or congestive heart failure. Precautions should be taken with patients taking tricyclic antidepressants and nonselective beta blockers because these drugs may potentiate the effect of epinephrine.

Elective dental treatments should be postponed for at least 1 month and preferably for 6 months after myocardial infarction, after which the risk of reinfarction is low provided the patient is medically stable (e.g., stable rhythm, stable angina, and no heart failure). Patients who have suffered a stroke should have elective dental care deferred for 6 months. In both situations, effective stress reduction requires good pain control, including the use of the minimal amount of vasoconstrictor necessary to provide good hemostasis and local anesthesia.

Bisphosphonate therapy is associated with *osteonecrosis* of the jaw. However, the risk with oral bisphosphonate therapy is very low. Most patients affected have received high-dose aminobisphosphonate therapy for multiple myeloma or metastatic breast cancer and have undergone tooth extraction or dental surgery. Intraoral lesions, of which two-thirds are painful, appear as exposed yellow-white hard bone involving the mandible or maxilla. Screening tests for determining risk of osteonecrosis are unreliable. Patients slated for aminobisphosphonate therapy should receive preventive dental care that reduces the risk of infection and the need for future dentoalveolar surgery.

HALITOSIS

Halitosis typically emanates from the oral cavity or nasal passages. Volatile sulfur compounds resulting from bacterial decay of food and cellular debris account for the malodor. Periodontal disease, caries, acute forms of gingivitis, poorly fitting dentures, oral abscess, and tongue coating are common causes. Treatment includes correcting poor hygiene, treating infection, and tongue brushing. Hyposalivation can produce and exacerbate halitosis. Pockets of decay in the tonsillar crypts, esophageal diverticulum, esophageal stasis (e.g., achalasia, stricture), sinusitis, and lung abscess account for some instances. A few systemic diseases produce distinctive odors: renal failure (ammoniacal), hepatic (fishy), and ketoacidosis (fruity). *Helicobacter pylori* gastritis can also produce ammoniacal breath. If a patient presents because of concern about halitosis but no odor is detectable, then pseudohalitosis or halitophobia must be considered.

AGING AND ORAL HEALTH

While tooth loss and dental disease are not normal consequences of aging, a complex array of structural and functional changes that occur with age can affect oral health. Subtle changes in tooth structure (e.g., diminished pulp space and volume, sclerosis of dentinal tubules, and altered proportions of nerve and vascular pulp content) result in the elimination or diminution of pain sensitivity and a reduction in the reparative capacity of the teeth. In addition, age-associated fatty replacement of salivary acini may reduce physiologic reserve, thus increasing the risk of hyposalivation. In healthy older adults, there is minimal, if any, reduction in salivary flow.

Poor oral hygiene often results when general health fails or when patients lose manual dexterity and upper-extremity flexibility. This situation is particularly common among frail older adults and nursing home residents and must be emphasized because regular oral cleaning and dental care reduce the incidence of pneumonia and oral disease as well as the mortality risk in this population. Other risks for dental decay include limited lifetime fluoride exposure. Without assiduous care, decay can become quite advanced yet remain asymptomatic. Consequently, much of a tooth—or the entire tooth—can be destroyed before the patient is aware of the process.

Periodontal disease, a leading cause of tooth loss, is indicated by loss of alveolar bone height. More than 90% of the U.S. population has some degree of periodontal disease by age 50. Healthy adults who have not had significant alveolar bone loss by the sixth decade of life do not typically experience significant worsening with advancing age.

Complete edentulousness with advanced age, though less common than in previous decades, still affects ~50% of the U.S. population ≥85 years of age. Speech, mastication, and facial contours are dramatically affected. Edentulousness may also exacerbate obstructive sleep apnea, particularly in asymptomatic individuals who wear dentures. Dentures can improve verbal articulation and restore diminished facial contours. Mastication can also be restored; however, patients expecting dentures to facilitate oral intake are often disappointed. Accommodation to dentures requires a period of adjustment. Pain can result from friction or traumatic lesions produced by loose dentures. Poor fit and poor oral hygiene may permit the development of candidiasis. This fungal infection may be either asymptomatic or painful and is suggested by erythematous smooth or granular tissue conforming to an area covered by the appliance. Individuals with dentures and no natural teeth need regular (annual) professional oral examinations.

46e Atlas of Oral Manifestations of Disease

Samuel C. Durso, Janet A. Yellowitz

This is a digital-only chapter. It is available on the DVD that accompanies this book, as well as on Access Medicine/Harrison's Online, and the eBook and "app" editions of HPIM 19e.

The health status of the oral cavity is linked to cardiovascular disease, diabetes, and other systemic illnesses. Thus, examining the oral cavity for signs of disease is a key part of the physical exam. This chapter presents numerous outstanding clinical photographs illustrating many of the conditions discussed in Chap. 45, Oral Manifestations of Disease. Conditions affecting the teeth, periodontal tissues, and oral mucosa are all represented.

47e Dyspnea

Richard M. Schwartzstein

This is a digital-only chapter. It is available on the DVD that accompanies this book, as well as on Access Medicine/Harrison's Online, and the eBook and "app" editions of HPIM 19e.

DYSPNEA

The American Thoracic Society defines *dyspnea* as a "subjective experience of breathing discomfort that consists of qualitatively distinct sensations that vary in intensity. The experience derives from interactions among multiple physiological, psychological, social, and environmental factors and may induce secondary physiological and behavioral responses." Dyspnea, a symptom, can be perceived only by the person experiencing it and must be distinguished from the signs of increased work of breathing.

48 Cough and Hemoptysis

Patricia A. Kritek, Christopher H. Fanta

COUGH

Cough performs an essential protective function for human airways and lungs. Without an effective cough reflex, we are at risk for retained airway secretions and aspirated material predisposing to infection, atelectasis, and respiratory compromise. At the other extreme, excessive coughing can be exhausting; can be complicated by emesis, syncope, muscular pain, or rib fractures; and can aggravate abdominal or inguinal hernias and urinary incontinence. Cough is often a clue to the presence of respiratory disease. In many instances, cough is an expected and accepted manifestation of disease, as in acute respiratory tract infection. However, persistent cough in the absence of other respiratory symptoms commonly causes patients to seek medical attention.

COUGH MECHANISM

Spontaneous cough is triggered by stimulation of sensory nerve endings that are thought to be primarily rapidly adapting receptors and C fibers. Both chemical (e.g., capsaicin) and mechanical (e.g., particulates in air pollution) stimuli may initiate the cough reflex. A cationic ion channel—the type 1 vanilloid receptor—found on rapidly adapting receptors and C fibers is the receptor for capsaicin, and its expression is increased in patients with chronic cough. Afferent nerve endings richly innervate the pharynx, larynx, and airways to the level of the terminal bronchioles and extend into the lung parenchyma. They may also be located in the external auditory meatus (the auricular branch of the vagus nerve, or the Arnold nerve) and in the esophagus. Sensory signals travel via the vagus and superior laryngeal nerves to a region of the brainstem in the nucleus tractus solitarius vaguely identified as the "cough center." The cough reflex involves a highly orchestrated series of involuntary muscular actions, with the potential for input from cortical pathways as well. The vocal cords adduct, leading to transient upper-airway occlusion. Expiratory muscles contract, generating positive intrathoracic pressures as high as 300 mmHg. With sudden release of the laryngeal contraction, rapid expiratory flows are generated,

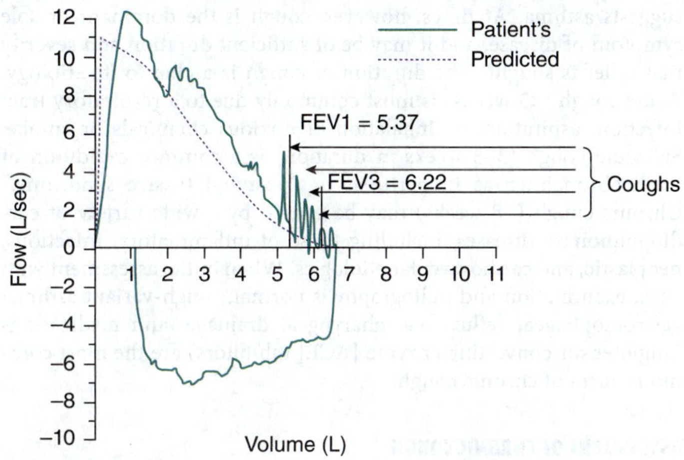

FIGURE 48-1 Flow-volume curve shows spikes of high expiratory flow achieved with cough. FEV_1, forced expiratory volume in 1 s.

exceeding the normal "envelope" of maximal expiratory flow seen on the flow-volume curve (Fig. 48-1). Bronchial smooth-muscle contraction together with dynamic compression of airways narrows airway lumens and maximizes the velocity of exhalation. The kinetic energy available to dislodge mucus from the inside of airway walls is directly proportional to the square of the velocity of expiratory airflow. A deep breath preceding a cough optimizes the function of the expiratory muscles; a series of repetitive coughs at successively lower lung volumes sweeps the point of maximal expiratory velocity progressively further into the lung periphery.

IMPAIRED COUGH

Weak or ineffective cough compromises the ability to clear lower respiratory tract infections, predisposing to more serious infections and their sequelae. Weakness, paralysis, or pain of the expiratory (abdominal and intercostal) muscles is foremost on the list of causes of impaired cough (Table 48-1). Cough strength is generally assessed qualitatively; peak expiratory flow or maximal expiratory pressure at the mouth can be used as a surrogate marker for cough strength. A variety of assistive devices and techniques have been developed to improve cough strength, running the gamut from simple (splinting of the abdominal muscles with a tightly-held pillow to reduce postoperative pain while coughing) to complex (a mechanical cough-assist device supplied via face mask or tracheal tube that applies a cycle of positive pressure followed rapidly by negative pressure). Cough may fail to clear secretions despite a preserved ability to generate normal expiratory velocities; such failure may be due to either abnormal airway secretions (e.g., bronchiectasis due to cystic fibrosis) or structural abnormalities of the airways (e.g., tracheomalacia with expiratory collapse during cough).

SYMPTOMATIC COUGH

The cough of chronic bronchitis in long-term cigarette smokers rarely leads the patient to seek medical advice. It lasts for only seconds to a

TABLE 48-1 CAUSES OF IMPAIRED COUGH

Decreased expiratory-muscle strength
Decreased inspiratory-muscle strength
Chest wall deformity
Impaired glottic closure or tracheostomy
Tracheomalacia
Abnormal airway secretions
Central respiratory depression (e.g., anesthesia, sedation, or coma)

few minutes, is productive of benign-appearing mucoid sputum, and generally does not cause discomfort. Cough may occur in the context of other respiratory symptoms that together point to a diagnosis; for example, cough accompanied by wheezing, shortness of breath, and chest tightness after exposure to a cat or other sources of allergens suggests asthma. At times, however, cough is the dominant or sole symptom of disease, and it may be of sufficient duration and severity that relief is sought. The duration of cough is a clue to its etiology. Acute cough (<3 weeks) is most commonly due to a respiratory tract infection, aspiration, or inhalation of noxious chemicals or smoke. Subacute cough (3–8 weeks in duration) is a common residuum of tracheobronchitis, as in pertussis or "postviral tussive syndrome." Chronic cough (>8 weeks) may be caused by a wide variety of cardiopulmonary diseases, including those of inflammatory, infectious, neoplastic, and cardiovascular etiologies. When initial assessment with chest examination and radiography is normal, cough-variant asthma, gastroesophageal reflux, nasopharyngeal drainage, and medications (angiotensin-converting enzyme [ACE] inhibitors) are the most common causes of chronic cough.

ASSESSMENT OF CHRONIC COUGH

Details as to the sound, the time of occurrence during the day, and the pattern of coughing infrequently provide useful etiologic clues. Regardless of cause, cough often worsens upon first lying down at night, with talking, or with the hyperpnea of exercise; it frequently improves with sleep. An exception may involve the cough that occurs only with certain allergic exposures or exercise in cold air, as in asthma. Useful historical questions include what circumstances surround the onset of cough, what makes the cough better or worse, and whether or not the cough produces sputum.

The physical examination seeks clues suggesting the presence of cardiopulmonary disease, including findings such as wheezing or crackles on chest examination. Examination of the auditory canals and tympanic membranes (for irritation of the latter resulting in stimulation of Arnold's nerve), the nasal passageways (for rhinitis or polyps), and the nails (for clubbing) may also provide etiologic clues. Because cough can be a manifestation of a systemic disease such as sarcoidosis or vasculitis, a thorough general examination is equally important.

In virtually all instances, evaluation of chronic cough merits a chest radiograph. The list of diseases that can cause persistent cough without other symptoms and without detectable abnormalities on physical examination is long. It includes serious illnesses such as sarcoidosis or Hodgkin's disease in young adults, lung cancer in older patients, and (worldwide) pulmonary tuberculosis. An abnormal chest film prompts an evaluation aimed at explaining the cough. In a patient with chronic productive cough, examination of expectorated sputum is warranted. Purulent-appearing sputum should be sent for routine bacterial culture and, in certain circumstances, mycobacterial culture as well. Cytologic examination of mucoid sputum may be useful to assess for malignancy and to distinguish neutrophilic from eosinophilic bronchitis. Expectoration of blood—whether streaks of blood, blood mixed with airway secretions, or pure blood—deserves a special approach to assessment and management (see "Hemoptysis," below).

CHRONIC COUGH WITH A NORMAL CHEST RADIOGRAPH

It is commonly held that (alone or in combination) the use of an ACE inhibitor; postnasal drainage; gastroesophageal reflux; and asthma account for more than 90% of cases of chronic cough with a normal or noncontributory chest radiograph. However, clinical experience does not support this contention, and strict adherence to this concept discourages the search for alternative explanations by both clinicians and researchers. ACE inhibitor–induced cough occurs in 5–30% of patients taking these agents and is not dose dependent. ACE metabolizes bradykinin and other tachykinins, such as substance P. The mechanism of ACE inhibitor–associated cough may involve sensitization of sensory nerve endings due to accumulation of bradykinin. In support of this hypothesis, polymorphisms in the neurokinin-2 receptor gene are associated with ACE inhibitor–induced cough. Any patient with chronic unexplained cough who is taking an ACE inhibitor should have a trial period off the medication, regardless of the timing of the onset of cough relative to the initiation of ACE inhibitor therapy. In most instances, a safe alternative is available; angiotensin-receptor blockers do not cause cough. Failure to observe a decrease in cough after 1 month off medication argues strongly against this etiology. Postnasal drainage of any etiology can cause cough as a response to stimulation of sensory receptors of the cough-reflex pathway in the hypopharynx or aspiration of draining secretions into the trachea. Clues suggesting this etiology include postnasal drip, frequent throat clearing, and sneezing and rhinorrhea. On speculum examination of the nose, excess mucoid or purulent secretions, inflamed and edematous nasal mucosa, and/or polyps may be seen; in addition, secretions or a cobblestoned appearance of the mucosa along the posterior pharyngeal wall may be noted. Unfortunately, there is no means by which to quantitate postnasal drainage. In many instances, this diagnosis must rely on subjective information provided by the patient. This assessment must also be counterbalanced by the fact that many people who have chronic postnasal drainage do not experience cough.

Linking gastroesophageal reflux to chronic cough poses similar challenges. It is thought that reflux of gastric contents into the lower esophagus may trigger cough via reflex pathways initiated in the esophageal mucosa. Reflux to the level of the pharynx (laryngopharyngeal reflux), with consequent aspiration of gastric contents, causes a chemical bronchitis and possibly pneumonitis that can elicit cough for days afterward. Retrosternal burning after meals or on recumbency, frequent eructation, hoarseness, and throat pain may be indicative of gastroesophageal reflux. Nevertheless, reflux may also elicit minimal or no symptoms. Glottic inflammation detected on laryngoscopy may be a manifestation of recurrent reflux to the level of the throat, but it is a nonspecific finding. Quantification of the frequency and level of reflux requires a somewhat invasive procedure to measure esophageal pH directly (either nasopharyngeal placement of a catheter with a pH probe into the esophagus for 24 h or endoscopic placement of a radiotransmitter capsule into the esophagus). The precise interpretation of test results that permits an etiologic linking of reflux events and cough remains debated. Again, assigning the cause of cough to gastroesophageal reflux must be weighed against the observation that many people with symptomatic reflux do not experience chronic cough.

Cough alone as a manifestation of asthma is common among children but not among adults. Cough due to asthma in the absence of wheezing, shortness of breath, and chest tightness is referred to as "cough-variant asthma." A history suggestive of cough-variant asthma ties the onset of cough to exposure to typical triggers for asthma and the resolution of cough to discontinuation of exposure. Objective testing can establish the diagnosis of asthma (airflow obstruction on spirometry that varies over time or reverses in response to a bronchodilator) or exclude it with certainty (a negative response to a bronchoprovocation challenge—e.g., with methacholine). In a patient capable of taking reliable measurements, home expiratory peak flow monitoring can be a cost-effective method to support or discount a diagnosis of asthma.

Chronic eosinophilic bronchitis causes chronic cough with a normal chest radiograph. This condition is characterized by sputum eosinophilia in excess of 3% without airflow obstruction or bronchial hyperresponsiveness and is successfully treated with inhaled glucocorticoids.

Treatment of chronic cough in a patient with a normal chest radiograph is often empirical and is targeted at the most likely cause(s) of cough as determined by history, physical examination, and possibly pulmonary-function testing. Therapy for postnasal drainage depends on the presumed etiology (infection, allergy, or vasomotor rhinitis) and may include systemic antihistamines; antibiotics; nasal saline irrigation; and nasal pump sprays with glucocorticoids, antihistamines, or anticholinergics. Antacids, histamine type 2 (H2) receptor antagonists, and proton-pump inhibitors are used to neutralize or decrease the production of gastric acid in gastroesophageal reflux disease; dietary changes, elevation of the head and torso during sleep, and medications to improve gastric emptying are additional therapeutic measures.

Cough-variant asthma typically responds well to inhaled glucocorticoids and intermittent use of inhaled β-agonist bronchodilators.

Patients who fail to respond to treatment targeting the common causes of chronic cough or who have had these causes excluded by appropriate diagnostic testing should undergo chest CT. Diseases causing cough that may be missed on chest x-ray include tumors, early interstitial lung disease, bronchiectasis, and atypical mycobacterial pulmonary infection. On the other hand, patients with chronic cough who have normal findings on chest examination, lung function testing, oxygenation assessment, and chest CT can be reassured as to the absence of serious pulmonary pathology.

SYMPTOM-BASED TREATMENT OF COUGH

Chronic idiopathic cough, also called *cough hypersensitivity syndrome*, is distressingly common. It is often experienced as a tickle or sensitivity in the throat, occurs more often in women, and is typically "dry" or at most productive of scant amounts of mucoid sputum. It can be exhausting, interfere with work, and cause social embarrassment. Once serious underlying cardiopulmonary pathology has been excluded, an attempt at cough suppression is appropriate. Most effective are narcotic cough suppressants, such as codeine or hydrocodone, which are thought to act in the "cough center" in the brainstem. The tendency of narcotic cough suppressants to cause drowsiness and constipation and their potential for addictive dependence limit their appeal for long-term use. *Dextromethorphan* is an over-the-counter, centrally acting cough suppressant with fewer side effects and less efficacy than the narcotic cough suppressants. Dextromethorphan is thought to have a different site of action than narcotic cough suppressants and can be used in combination with them if necessary. *Benzonatate* is thought to inhibit neural activity of sensory nerves in the cough-reflex pathway. It is generally free of side effects; however, its effectiveness in suppressing cough is variable and unpredictable. Case series have reported benefit from off-label use of *gabapentin* or *amitriptyline* for chronic idiopathic cough. Novel cough suppressants without the limitations of currently available agents are greatly needed. Approaches that are being explored include the development of neurokinin receptor antagonists, type 1 vanilloid receptor antagonists, and novel opioid and opioid-like receptor agonists.

HEMOPTYSIS

Hemoptysis, the expectoration of blood from the respiratory tract, can arise at any location from the alveoli to the glottis. It is important to distinguish hemoptysis from *epistaxis* (bleeding from the nasopharynx) and *hematemesis* (bleeding from the upper gastrointestinal tract). Hemoptysis can range from the expectoration of blood-tinged sputum to that of life-threatening large volumes of bright red blood. For most patients, any degree of hemoptysis can cause anxiety and often prompts medical evaluation.

While precise epidemiologic data are lacking, the most common etiology of hemoptysis is infection of the medium-sized airways. In the United States, the cause is usually viral or bacterial bronchitis. Hemoptysis can arise in the setting of acute bronchitis or during an exacerbation of chronic bronchitis. Worldwide, the most common cause of hemoptysis is infection with *Mycobacterium tuberculosis*, presumably because of the high prevalence of tuberculosis and its predilection for cavity formation. While these are the most common causes, the differential diagnosis for hemoptysis is extensive, and a step-wise approach to evaluation is appropriate.

ETIOLOGY

One way to approach the source of hemoptysis is to search systematically for potential sites of bleeding from the alveolus to the mouth. Diffuse bleeding in the alveolar space, often referred to as *diffuse alveolar hemorrhage* (DAH), may present as hemoptysis. Causes of DAH can be inflammatory or noninflammatory. Inflammatory DAH is due to small-vessel vasculitis/capillaritis from a variety of diseases, including granulomatosis with polyangiitis and microscopic polyangiitis. Similarly, systemic autoimmune diseases such as systemic lupus erythematosus can manifest as pulmonary capillaritis. Antibodies to the alveolar basement membrane, as are seen in Goodpasture's disease, can also result in alveolar hemorrhage. In the early period after bone marrow transplantation, patients can develop a form of inflammatory DAH that can be catastrophic and life-threatening. The exact pathophysiology of this process is not well understood, but DAH should be suspected in patients with sudden-onset dyspnea and hypoxemia in the first 100 days after bone marrow transplantation.

Alveoli can also bleed due to direct inhalational injury, including thermal injury from fires, inhalation of illicit substances (e.g., cocaine), and inhalation of toxic chemicals. If alveoli are irritated from any process, patients with thrombocytopenia, coagulopathy, or antiplatelet or anticoagulant use will be at increased risk of hemoptysis.

Bleeding in hemoptysis most commonly arises from the small- to medium-sized airways. Irritation and injury of the bronchial mucosa can lead to small-volume bleeding. More significant hemoptysis can result from the proximity of the bronchial artery and vein to the airway, with these vessels and the bronchus running together in what is often referred to as the *bronchovascular bundle*. In the smaller airways, these blood vessels are close to the airspace, and lesser degrees of inflammation or injury can therefore result in their rupture into the airways. While alveolar hemorrhage arises from capillaries that are part of the low-pressure pulmonary circulation, bronchial bleeding generally originates from bronchial arteries, which are under systemic pressure and thus are predisposed to larger-volume bleeding.

Any infection of the airways can result in hemoptysis, although acute bronchitis is most commonly caused by viral infection. In patients with a history of chronic bronchitis, bacterial superinfection with organisms such as *Streptococcus pneumoniae*, *Haemophilus influenzae*, or *Moraxella catarrhalis* can also result in hemoptysis. Patients with bronchiectasis (a permanent dilation of the airways with loss of mucosal integrity) are particularly prone to hemoptysis due to chronic inflammation and anatomic abnormalities that bring the bronchial arteries closer to the mucosal surface. One common presentation of patients with advanced cystic fibrosis—the prototypical bronchiectatic lung disease—is hemoptysis, which can be life-threatening.

Pneumonias of any sort can cause hemoptysis. Tuberculous infection, which can lead to bronchiectasis or cavitary pneumonia, is a very common cause of hemoptysis worldwide. Patients may present with a chronic cough productive of blood-streaked sputum or with larger-volume bleeding. *Rasmussen's aneurysm* (the dilation of a pulmonary artery in a cavity formed by previous tuberculous infection) remains a source of massive, life-threatening hemoptysis in the developing world. Community-acquired pneumonia and lung abscess can also result in bleeding. Once again, if the infection results in cavitation, there is a greater likelihood of bleeding due to erosion into blood vessels. Infections with *Staphylococcus aureus* and gram-negative rods (e.g., *Klebsiella pneumoniae*) are especially likely to cause necrotizing lung infections and thus to be associated with hemoptysis.

While not common in North America, pulmonary paragonimiasis (i.e., infection with the lung fluke *Paragonimus westermani*) often presents as fever, cough, and hemoptysis. This infection is a public health issue in Southeast Asia and China and is frequently confused with active tuberculosis, in which the clinical picture can be similar. Paragonimiasis should be considered in recent immigrants from endemic areas who have new or recurrent hemoptysis. In addition, pulmonary paragonimiasis has been reported secondary to ingestion of crayfish or small crabs in the United States.

Other causes of airway irritation resulting in hemoptysis include inhalation of toxic chemicals, thermal injury, and direct trauma from suctioning of the airways (particularly in intubated patients). All of these etiologies should be considered in light of the individual patient's history and exposures.

Perhaps the most feared cause of hemoptysis is bronchogenic lung cancer, although hemoptysis is a presenting symptom in only ~10% of patients. Cancers arising in the proximal airways are much more likely to cause hemoptysis, but any malignancy in the chest can do so. Because both squamous cell carcinomas and small-cell carcinomas are more commonly in or adjacent to the proximal airways, and large at presentation, they are more often a cause of hemoptysis. These cancers can present with large-volume and life-threatening hemoptysis because of erosion into the hilar vessels. Carcinoid tumors, which are found almost exclusively as endobronchial lesions with friable mucosa, can also present with hemoptysis.

In addition to cancers arising in the lung, metastatic disease in the pulmonary parenchyma can bleed. Malignancies that commonly metastasize to the lungs include renal cell, breast, colon, testicular, and thyroid cancers as well as melanoma. While hemoptysis is not a common manifestation of pulmonary metastases, the combination of multiple pulmonary nodules and hemoptysis should raise suspicion of this etiology. Finally, disease of the pulmonary vasculature can cause hemoptysis. Perhaps most frequently, congestive heart failure with transmission of elevated left atrial pressures can lead to rupture of small alveolar capillaries. These patients rarely present with bright red blood but more commonly have pink, frothy sputum or blood-tinged secretions. Patients with a focal jet of mitral regurgitation can present with an upper-lobe opacity on chest radiography together with hemoptysis. This finding is thought to be due to focal increases in pulmonary capillary pressure due to the regurgitant jet. Pulmonary arteriovenous malformations are prone to bleeding. Pulmonary embolism can also lead to the development of hemoptysis, which is generally associated with pulmonary infarction. Pulmonary arterial hypertension from other causes rarely results in hemoptysis.

EVALUATION

As with most signs of possible illness, the initial step in the evaluation of hemoptysis is a thorough history and physical examination (Fig. 48-2). As already mentioned, initial questioning should focus on ascertaining whether the bleeding is truly from the respiratory tract and not the nasopharynx or gastrointestinal tract; bleeding from the latter sources requires different approaches to evaluation and treatment.

History and Physical Examination The specific characteristics of hemoptysis may be helpful in determining an etiology, such as whether the expectorated material consists of blood-tinged, purulent secretions; pink, frothy sputum; or pure blood. Information on specific triggers of the bleeding (e.g., recent inhalation exposures) as well as any previous episodes of hemoptysis should be elicited during history-taking. Monthly hemoptysis in a woman suggests catamenial hemoptysis from pulmonary endometriosis. Moreover, the volume of blood expectorated is important not only in determining the cause but also in gauging the urgency for further diagnostic and therapeutic maneuvers. Patients rarely exsanguinate from hemoptysis but can effectively "drown" in aspirated blood. Large-volume hemoptysis, referred to as *massive hemoptysis*, is variably defined as hemoptysis of >200–600 mL in 24 h. Massive hemoptysis should be considered a medical emergency. All patients should be asked about current or former cigarette smoking; this behavior predisposes to chronic bronchitis and increases the likelihood of bronchogenic cancer. Practitioners should inquire about symptoms and signs suggestive of respiratory tract infection (including fever, chills, and dyspnea), recent inhalation exposures, recent use of illicit substances, and risk factors for venous thromboembolism.

A medical history of malignancy or treatment thereof, rheumatologic disease, vascular disease, or underlying lung disease (e.g., bronchiectasis) may be relevant to the cause of hemoptysis. Because many causes of DAH can be part of a pulmonary-renal syndrome, specific inquiry into a history of renal insufficiency is important.

The physical examination begins with an assessment of vital signs and oxygen saturation to gauge whether there is evidence of life-threatening bleeding. Tachycardia, hypotension, and decreased oxygen saturation mandate a more expedited evaluation of hemoptysis. A specific focus on respiratory and cardiac examinations is important; these examinations should include inspection of the nares, auscultation of the lungs and heart, assessment of the lower extremities for symmetric or asymmetric edema, and evaluation for jugular venous distention. Clubbing of the digits may suggest underlying lung diseases such as bronchogenic carcinoma or bronchiectasis, which predispose to hemoptysis. Similarly, mucocutaneous telangiectasias should raise the specter of pulmonary arterial-venous malformations.

Diagnostic Evaluation For most patients, the next step in evaluation of hemoptysis should be a standard chest radiograph. If a source of bleeding is not identified on plain film, CT of the chest should be performed. CT allows better delineation of bronchiectasis, alveolar filling, cavitary

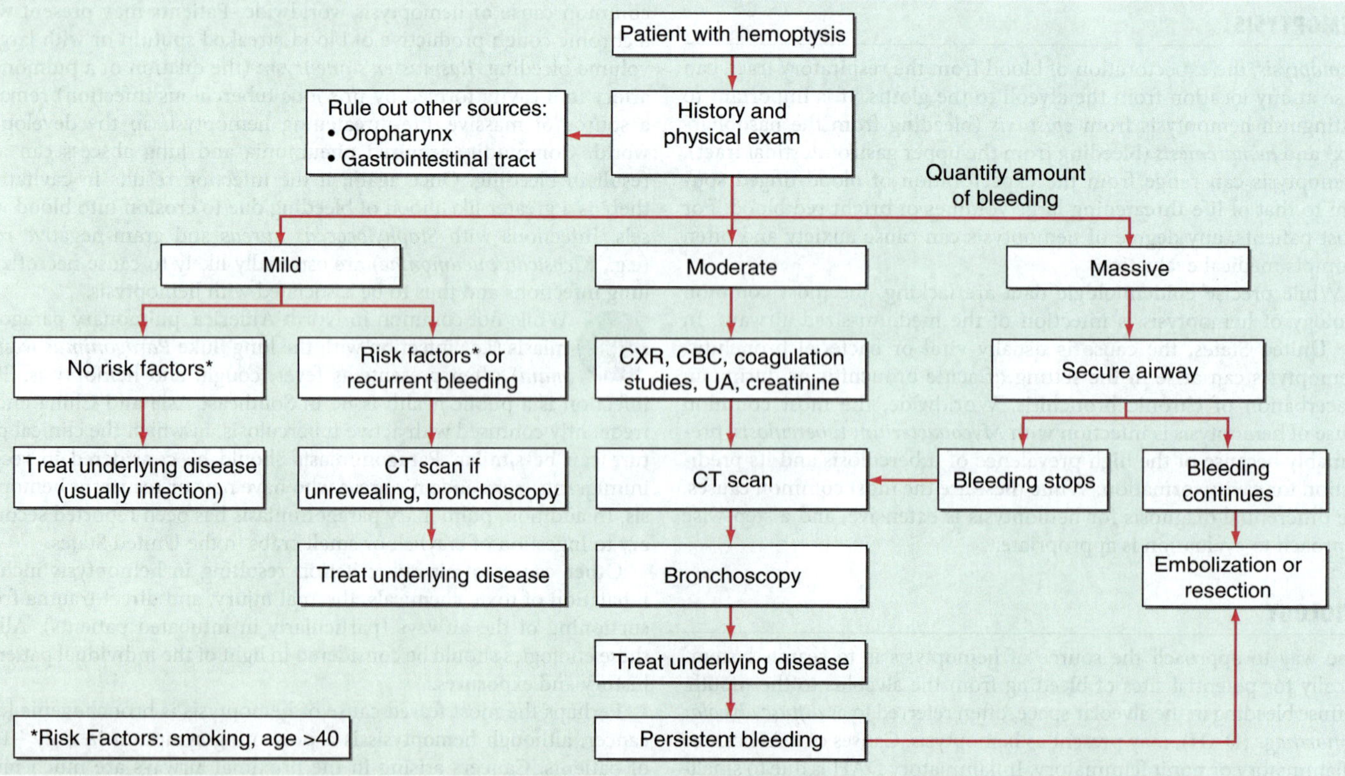

FIGURE 48-2 **Decision tree for evaluation of hemoptysis.** CBC, complete blood count; CT, computed tomography; CXR, chest x-ray; UA, urinalysis.

infiltrates, and masses than does chest radiograph. The practitioner should consider a CT protocol to assess for pulmonary embolism if the history or examination suggests venous thromboembolism as a cause of bleeding.

Laboratory studies should include a complete blood count to assess both the hematocrit and the platelet count as well as coagulation studies. Renal function should be evaluated and urinalysis conducted because of the possibility of pulmonary-renal syndromes presenting with hemoptysis. The documentation of acute renal insufficiency or the detection of red blood cells or their casts on urinalysis should elevate suspicion of small-vessel vasculitis, and studies such as antineutrophil cytoplasmic antibody, antiglomerular basement membrane antibody, and antinuclear antibody should be considered. If a patient is producing sputum, Gram's and acid-fast staining as well as culture should be undertaken.

If all of these studies are unrevealing, bronchoscopy should be considered. In any patient with a history of cigarette smoking, airway inspection should be part of the evaluation of new-onset hemoptysis as endobronchial lesions are not reliably visualized on CT.

TREATMENT HEMOPTYSIS

For the most part, the treatment of hemoptysis varies with its etiology. However, large-volume, life-threatening hemoptysis generally requires immediate intervention regardless of the cause. The first step is to establish a patent airway, usually by endotracheal intubation and subsequent mechanical ventilation. As large-volume hemoptysis usually arises from an airway lesion, it is ideal to identify the site of bleeding by either chest imaging or bronchoscopy (more commonly rigid rather than flexible). The goals are then to isolate the bleeding to one lung and not to allow the preserved airspaces in the other lung to be filled with blood so that gas exchange is further impaired. Patients should be placed with the bleeding lung in a dependent position (i.e., bleeding-side down), and, if possible, dual-lumen endotracheal tubes or an airway blocker should be placed in the proximal airway of the bleeding lung. These interventions generally require the assistance of anesthesiologists, interventional pulmonologists, or thoracic surgeons.

If the bleeding does not stop with treatment of the underlying cause and the passage of time, severe hemoptysis from bronchial arteries can be treated with angiographic embolization of the responsible bronchial artery. This intervention should be entertained only in the most severe and life-threatening cases of hemoptysis because of the risk of unintentional spinal-artery embolization and consequent paraplegia. Endobronchial lesions can be treated with a variety of bronchoscopically directed interventions, including cauterization and laser therapy. In extreme circumstances, surgical resection of the affected region of the lung is considered. Most cases of hemoptysis resolve with treatment of the infection or inflammatory process or with removal of the offending stimulus.

49 Hypoxia and Cyanosis

Joseph Loscalzo

HYPOXIA

The fundamental purpose of the cardiorespiratory system is to deliver O_2 and nutrients to cells and to remove CO_2 and other metabolic products from them. Proper maintenance of this function depends not only on intact cardiovascular and respiratory systems, but also on an adequate number of red blood cells and hemoglobin and a supply of inspired gas containing adequate O_2.

RESPONSES TO HYPOXIA

Decreased O_2 availability to cells results in an inhibition of oxidative phosphorylation and increased anaerobic glycolysis. This switch from aerobic to anaerobic metabolism, the Pasteur effect, maintains some, albeit reduced, adenosine 5′-triphosphate (ATP) production. In severe hypoxia, when ATP production is inadequate to meet the energy requirements of ionic and osmotic equilibrium, cell membrane depolarization leads to uncontrolled Ca^{2+} influx and activation of Ca^{2+}-dependent phospholipases and proteases. These events, in turn, cause cell swelling, activation of apoptotic pathways, and, ultimately, cell death.

The adaptations to hypoxia are mediated, in part, by the upregulation of genes encoding a variety of proteins, including glycolytic enzymes, such as phosphoglycerate kinase and phosphofructokinase, as well as the glucose transporters Glut-1 and Glut-2; and by growth factors, such as vascular endothelial growth factor (VEGF) and erythropoietin, which enhance erythrocyte production. The hypoxia-induced increase in expression of these key proteins is governed by the hypoxia-sensitive transcription factor, hypoxia-inducible factor-1 (HIF-1).

During hypoxia, systemic arterioles dilate, at least in part, by opening of K_{ATP} channels in vascular smooth-muscle cells due to the hypoxia-induced reduction in ATP concentration. By contrast, in pulmonary vascular smooth-muscle cells, inhibition of K^+ channels causes depolarization which, in turn, activates voltage-gated Ca^{2+} channels raising the cytosolic $[Ca^{2+}]$ and causing smooth-muscle cell contraction. Hypoxia-induced pulmonary arterial constriction shunts blood away from poorly ventilated portions toward better ventilated portions of the lung; however, it also increases pulmonary vascular resistance and right ventricular afterload.

Effects on the Central Nervous System Changes in the central nervous system (CNS), particularly the higher centers, are especially important consequences of hypoxia. Acute hypoxia causes impaired judgment, motor incoordination, and a clinical picture resembling acute alcohol intoxication. High-altitude illness is characterized by headache secondary to cerebral vasodilation, gastrointestinal symptoms, dizziness, insomnia, fatigue, or somnolence. Pulmonary arterial and sometimes venous constriction causes capillary leakage and high-altitude pulmonary edema (HAPE) (Chap. 47e), which intensifies hypoxia, further promoting vasoconstriction. Rarely, high-altitude cerebral edema (HACE) develops, which is manifest by severe headache and papilledema and can cause coma. As hypoxia becomes more severe, the regulatory centers of the brainstem are affected, and death usually results from respiratory failure.

Effects on the Cardiovascular System Acute hypoxia stimulates the chemoreceptor reflex arc to induce venoconstriction and systemic arterial vasodilation. These acute changes are accompanied by transiently increased myocardial contractility, which is followed by depressed myocardial contractility with prolonged hypoxia.

CAUSES OF HYPOXIA

Respiratory Hypoxia When hypoxia occurs from respiratory failure, Pa_{O_2} declines, and when respiratory failure is persistent, the hemoglobin-oxygen (Hb-O_2) dissociation curve (see Fig. 127-2) is displaced to the right, with greater quantities of O_2 released at any level of tissue P_{O_2}. Arterial hypoxemia, i.e., a reduction of O_2 saturation of arterial blood (Sa_{O_2}), and consequent cyanosis are likely to be more marked when such depression of Pa_{O_2} results from pulmonary disease than when the depression occurs as the result of a decline in the fraction of oxygen in inspired air (FI_{O_2}). In this latter situation, Pa_{CO_2} falls secondary to anoxia-induced hyperventilation and the Hb-O_2 dissociation curve is displaced to the left, limiting the decline in Sa_{O_2} at any level of Pa_{O_2}.

The most common cause of respiratory hypoxia is *ventilation-perfusion mismatch* resulting from perfusion of poorly ventilated alveoli. Respiratory hypoxemia may also be caused by *hypoventilation*, in which case it is associated with an elevation of Pa_{CO_2} (Chap. 306e). These two forms of respiratory hypoxia are usually correctable by inspiring 100% O_2 for several minutes. A third cause of respiratory hypoxia is shunting of blood across the lung from the pulmonary arterial to the venous bed (*intrapulmonary right-to-left shunting*) by perfusion of nonventilated portions of the lung, as in pulmonary atelectasis or through pulmonary arteriovenous connections. The low Pa_{O_2} in this situation is only partially corrected by an F_{IO_2} of 100%.

Hypoxia Secondary to High Altitude As one ascends rapidly to 3000 m (~10,000 ft), the reduction of the O_2 content of inspired air (F_{IO_2}) leads to a decrease in alveolar P_{O_2} to approximately 60 mmHg, and a condition termed *high-altitude illness* develops (see above). At higher altitudes, arterial saturation declines rapidly and symptoms become more serious; and at 5000 m, unacclimated individuals usually cease to be able to function normally owing to the changes in CNS function described above.

Hypoxia Secondary to Right-to-Left Extrapulmonary Shunting From a physiologic viewpoint, this cause of hypoxia resembles intrapulmonary right-to-left shunting but is caused by congenital cardiac malformations, such as tetralogy of Fallot, transposition of the great arteries, and Eisenmenger's syndrome (Chap. 282). As in pulmonary right-to-left shunting, the Pa_{O_2} cannot be restored to normal with inspiration of 100% O_2.

Anemic Hypoxia A reduction in hemoglobin concentration of the blood is accompanied by a corresponding decline in the O_2-carrying capacity of the blood. Although the Pa_{O_2} is normal in anemic hypoxia, the absolute quantity of O_2 transported per unit volume of blood is diminished. As the anemic blood passes through the capillaries and the usual quantity of O_2 is removed from it, the P_{O_2} and saturation in the venous blood decline to a greater extent than normal.

Carbon Monoxide (CO) Intoxication (See also Chap. 472e) Hemoglobin that binds with CO (carboxy-hemoglobin, COHb) is unavailable for O_2 transport. In addition, the presence of COHb shifts the Hb-O_2 dissociation curve to the left (see Fig. 127-2) so that O_2 is unloaded only at lower tensions, further contributing to tissue hypoxia.

Circulatory Hypoxia As in anemic hypoxia, the Pa_{O_2} is usually normal, but venous and tissue P_{O_2} values are reduced as a consequence of reduced tissue perfusion and greater tissue O_2 extraction. This pathophysiology leads to an increased arterial-mixed venous O_2 difference (a-v-O_2 difference), or gradient. Generalized circulatory hypoxia occurs in heart failure (Chap. 279) and in most forms of shock (Chap. 324).

Specific Organ Hypoxia Localized circulatory hypoxia may occur as a result of decreased perfusion secondary to arterial obstruction, as in localized atherosclerosis in any vascular bed, or as a consequence of vasoconstriction, as observed in Raynaud's phenomenon (Chap. 302). Localized hypoxia may also result from venous obstruction and the resultant expansion of interstitial fluid causing arteriolar compression and, thereby, reduction of arterial inflow. Edema, which increases the distance through which O_2 must diffuse before it reaches cells, can also cause localized hypoxia. In an attempt to maintain adequate perfusion to more vital organs in patients with reduced cardiac output secondary to heart failure or hypovolemic shock, vasoconstriction may reduce perfusion in the limbs and skin, causing hypoxia of these regions.

Increased O_2 Requirements If the O_2 consumption of tissues is elevated without a corresponding increase in perfusion, tissue hypoxia ensues and the P_{O_2} in venous blood declines. Ordinarily, the clinical picture of patients with hypoxia due to an elevated metabolic rate, as in fever or thyrotoxicosis, is quite different from that in other types of hypoxia: the skin is warm and flushed owing to increased cutaneous blood flow that dissipates the excessive heat produced, and cyanosis is usually absent.

Exercise is a classic example of increased tissue O_2 requirements. These increased demands are normally met by several mechanisms operating simultaneously: (1) increase in the cardiac output and ventilation and, thus, O_2 delivery to the tissues; (2) a preferential shift in blood flow to the exercising muscles by changing vascular resistances in the circulatory beds of exercising tissues, directly and/or reflexly; (3) an increase in O_2 extraction from the delivered blood and a widening of the arteriovenous O_2 difference; and (4) a reduction in the pH of the tissues and capillary blood, shifting the Hb-O_2 curve to the right (see Fig. 127-2), and unloading more O_2 from hemoglobin. If the capacity of these mechanisms is exceeded, then hypoxia, especially of the exercising muscles, will result.

Improper Oxygen Utilization Cyanide (Chap. 473e) and several other similarly acting poisons cause cellular hypoxia. The tissues are unable to use O_2, and, as a consequence, the venous blood tends to have a high O_2 tension. This condition has been termed *histotoxic hypoxia*.

ADAPTATION TO HYPOXIA

An important component of the respiratory response to hypoxia originates in special chemosensitive cells in the carotid and aortic bodies and in the respiratory center in the brainstem. The stimulation of these cells by hypoxia increases ventilation, with a loss of CO_2, and can lead to respiratory alkalosis. When combined with the metabolic acidosis resulting from the production of lactic acid, the serum bicarbonate level declines (Chap. 66).

With the reduction of Pa_{O_2}, cerebrovascular resistance decreases and cerebral blood flow increases in an attempt to maintain O_2 delivery to the brain. However, when the reduction of Pa_{O_2} is accompanied by hyperventilation and a reduction of Pa_{CO_2}, cerebrovascular resistance rises, cerebral blood flow falls, and tissue hypoxia intensifies.

The diffuse, systemic vasodilation that occurs in generalized hypoxia increases the cardiac output. In patients with underlying heart disease, the requirements of peripheral tissues for an increase of cardiac output with hypoxia may precipitate congestive heart failure. In patients with ischemic heart disease, a reduced Pa_{O_2} may intensify myocardial ischemia and further impair left ventricular function.

One of the important compensatory mechanisms for chronic hypoxia is an increase in the hemoglobin concentration and in the number of red blood cells in the circulating blood, i.e., the development of polycythemia secondary to erythropoietin production (Chap. 131). In persons with chronic hypoxemia secondary to prolonged residence at a high altitude (>13,000 ft, 4200 m), a condition termed *chronic mountain sickness* develops. This disorder is characterized by a blunted respiratory drive, reduced ventilation, erythrocytosis, cyanosis, weakness, right ventricular enlargement secondary to pulmonary hypertension, and even stupor.

CYANOSIS

Cyanosis refers to a bluish color of the skin and mucous membranes resulting from an increased quantity of reduced hemoglobin (i.e., deoxygenated hemoglobin) or of hemoglobin derivatives (e.g., methemoglobin or sulfhemoglobin) in the small blood vessels of those tissues. It is usually most marked in the lips, nail beds, ears, and malar eminences. Cyanosis, especially if developed recently, is more commonly detected by a family member than the patient. The florid skin characteristic of polycythemia vera (Chap. 131) must be distinguished from the true cyanosis discussed here. A cherry-colored flush, rather than cyanosis, is caused by COHb (Chap. 473e).

The degree of cyanosis is modified by the color of the cutaneous pigment and the thickness of the skin, as well as by the state of the cutaneous capillaries. The accurate clinical detection of the presence and degree of cyanosis is difficult, as proved by oximetric studies. In some instances, central cyanosis can be detected reliably when the Sa_{O_2} has fallen to 85%; in others, particularly in dark-skinned persons, it may not be detected until it has declined to 75%. In the latter case, examination of the mucous membranes in the oral cavity and the conjunctivae rather than examination of the skin is more helpful in the detection of cyanosis.

The increase in the quantity of reduced hemoglobin in the mucocutaneous vessels that produces cyanosis may be brought about either by an increase in the quantity of venous blood as a result of dilation of the venules (including precapillary venules) or by a reduction in the Sa_{O_2} in the capillary blood. In general, cyanosis becomes apparent when the concentration of reduced hemoglobin in capillary blood exceeds 40 g/L (4 g/dL).

It is the *absolute*, rather than the *relative*, quantity of reduced hemoglobin that is important in producing cyanosis. Thus, in a patient with severe anemia, the *relative* quantity of reduced hemoglobin in the venous blood may be very large when considered in relation to the total quantity of hemoglobin in the blood. However, since the concentration of the latter is markedly reduced, the *absolute* quantity of reduced hemoglobin may still be low, and, therefore, patients with severe anemia and even *marked* arterial desaturation may not display cyanosis. Conversely, the higher the total hemoglobin content, the greater the tendency toward cyanosis; thus, patients with marked polycythemia tend to be cyanotic at higher levels of Sao_2 than patients with normal hematocrit values. Likewise, local passive congestion, which causes an increase in the total quantity of reduced hemoglobin in the vessels in a given area, may cause cyanosis. Cyanosis is also observed when nonfunctional hemoglobin, such as methemoglobin (consequential or acquired) or sulfhemoglobin (Chap. 127), is present in blood.

Cyanosis may be subdivided into central and peripheral types. In *central* cyanosis, the Sao_2 is reduced or an abnormal hemoglobin derivative is present, and the mucous membranes and skin are both affected. *Peripheral* cyanosis is due to a slowing of blood flow and abnormally great extraction of O_2 from normally saturated arterial blood; it results from vasoconstriction and diminished peripheral blood flow, such as occurs in cold exposure, shock, congestive failure, and peripheral vascular disease. Often in these conditions, the mucous membranes of the oral cavity or those beneath the tongue may be spared. Clinical differentiation between central and peripheral cyanosis may not always be simple, and in conditions such as cardiogenic shock with pulmonary edema, there may be a mixture of both types.

DIFFERENTIAL DIAGNOSIS

Central Cyanosis (Table 49-1) Decreased Sao_2 results from a marked reduction in the Pao_2. This reduction may be brought about by a decline in the Fio_2 without sufficient compensatory alveolar hyperventilation to maintain alveolar Po_2. Cyanosis usually becomes manifest in an ascent to an altitude of 4000 m (13,000 ft).

Seriously *impaired pulmonary function*, through perfusion of unventilated or poorly ventilated areas of the lung or alveolar hypoventilation, is a common cause of central cyanosis (Chap. 306e).

TABLE 49-1 CAUSES OF CYANOSIS

Central Cyanosis
Decreased arterial oxygen saturation
Decreased atmospheric pressure—high altitude
Impaired pulmonary function
Alveolar hypoventilation
Inhomogeneity in pulmonary ventilation and perfusion (perfusion of hypoventilated alveoli)
Impaired oxygen diffusion
Anatomic shunts
Certain types of congenital heart disease
Pulmonary arteriovenous fistulas
Multiple small intrapulmonary shunts
Hemoglobin with low affinity for oxygen
Hemoglobin abnormalities
Methemoglobinemia—hereditary, acquired
Sulfhemoglobinemia—acquired
Carboxyhemoglobinemia (not true cyanosis)
Peripheral Cyanosis
Reduced cardiac output
Cold exposure
Redistribution of blood flow from extremities
Arterial obstruction
Venous obstruction

This condition may occur acutely, as in extensive pneumonia or pulmonary edema, or chronically, with chronic pulmonary diseases (e.g., emphysema). In the latter situation, secondary polycythemia is generally present and clubbing of the fingers (see below) may occur. Another cause of reduced Sao_2 is *shunting of systemic venous blood into the arterial circuit*. Certain forms of congenital heart disease are associated with cyanosis on this basis (see above and Chap. 282).

Pulmonary arteriovenous fistulae may be congenital or acquired, solitary or multiple, microscopic or massive. The severity of cyanosis produced by these fistulae depends on their size and number. They occur with some frequency in hereditary hemorrhagic telangiectasia. Sao_2 reduction and cyanosis may also occur in some patients with cirrhosis, presumably as a consequence of pulmonary arteriovenous fistulae or portal vein–pulmonary vein anastomoses.

In patients with cardiac or pulmonary right-to-left shunts, the presence and severity of cyanosis depend on the size of the shunt relative to the systemic flow as well as on the Hb-O_2 saturation of the venous blood. With increased extraction of O_2 from the blood by the exercising muscles, the venous blood returning to the right side of the heart is more unsaturated than at rest, and shunting of this blood intensifies the cyanosis. Secondary polycythemia occurs frequently in patients in this setting and contributes to the cyanosis.

Cyanosis can be caused by small quantities of circulating methemoglobin (Hb Fe^{3+}) and by even smaller quantities of sulfhemoglobin (Chap. 127); both of these hemoglobin derivatives impair oxygen delivery to the tissues. Although they are uncommon causes of cyanosis, these abnormal hemoglobin species should be sought by spectroscopy when cyanosis is not readily explained by malfunction of the circulatory or respiratory systems. Generally, digital clubbing does not occur with them.

Peripheral Cyanosis Probably the most common cause of peripheral cyanosis is the normal vasoconstriction resulting from exposure to cold air or water. When cardiac output is reduced, cutaneous vasoconstriction occurs as a compensatory mechanism so that blood is diverted from the skin to more vital areas such as the CNS and heart, and cyanosis of the extremities may result even though the arterial blood is normally saturated.

Arterial obstruction to an extremity, as with an embolus, or arteriolar constriction, as in cold-induced vasospasm (Raynaud's phenomenon) (Chap. 302), generally results in pallor and coldness, and there may be associated cyanosis. Venous obstruction, as in thrombophlebitis or deep venous thrombosis, dilates the subpapillary venous plexuses and thereby intensifies cyanosis.

APPROACH TO THE PATIENT: Cyanosis

Certain features are important in arriving at the cause of cyanosis:

1. It is important to ascertain the time of onset of cyanosis. Cyanosis present since birth or infancy is usually due to congenital heart disease.
2. Central and peripheral cyanosis must be differentiated. Evidence of disorders of the respiratory or cardiovascular systems is helpful. Massage or gentle warming of a cyanotic extremity will increase peripheral blood flow and abolish peripheral, but not central, cyanosis.
3. The presence or absence of clubbing of the digits (see below) should be ascertained. The combination of cyanosis and clubbing is frequent in patients with congenital heart disease and right-to-left shunting and is seen occasionally in patients with pulmonary disease, such as lung abscess or pulmonary arteriovenous fistulae. In contrast, peripheral cyanosis or acutely developing central cyanosis is *not* associated with clubbed digits.
4. Pao_2 and Sao_2 should be determined, and, in patients with cyanosis in whom the mechanism is obscure, spectroscopic examination of the blood should be performed to look for abnormal types of hemoglobin (critical in the differential diagnosis of cyanosis).

CLUBBING

The selective bulbous enlargement of the distal segments of the fingers and toes due to proliferation of connective tissue, particularly on the dorsal surface, is termed *clubbing*; there is also increased sponginess of the soft tissue at the base of the clubbed nail. Clubbing may be hereditary, idiopathic, or acquired and associated with a variety of disorders, including cyanotic congenital heart disease (see above), infective endocarditis, and a variety of pulmonary conditions (among them primary and metastatic lung cancer, bronchiectasis, asbestosis, sarcoidosis, lung abscess, cystic fibrosis, tuberculosis, and mesothelioma), as well as with some gastrointestinal diseases (including inflammatory bowel disease and hepatic cirrhosis). In some instances, it is occupational, e.g., in jackhammer operators.

Clubbing in patients with primary and metastatic lung cancer, mesothelioma, bronchiectasis, or hepatic cirrhosis may be associated with *hypertrophic osteoarthropathy*. In this condition, the subperiosteal formation of new bone in the distal diaphyses of the long bones of the extremities causes pain and symmetric arthritis-like changes in the shoulders, knees, ankles, wrists, and elbows. The diagnosis of hypertrophic osteoarthropathy may be confirmed by bone radiograph or magnetic resonance imaging (MRI). Although the mechanism of clubbing is unclear, it appears to be secondary to humoral substances that cause dilation of the vessels of the distal digits as well as growth factors released from platelet precursors in the digital circulation. In certain circumstances, clubbing is reversible, such as following lung transplantation for cystic fibrosis.

50 Edema

Eugene Braunwald, Joseph Loscalzo

STARLING FORCES AND FLUID EXCHANGE

About one-third of total-body water is confined to the extracellular space. Approximately 75% of the latter is interstitial fluid, and the remainder is the plasma. The forces that regulate the disposition of fluid between these two components of the extracellular compartment frequently are referred to as the *Starling forces*. The hydrostatic pressure within the capillaries and the colloid oncotic pressure in the interstitial fluid tend to promote movement of fluid from the vascular to the extravascular space. By contrast, the colloid oncotic pressure contributed by plasma proteins and the hydrostatic pressure within the interstitial fluid promote the movement of fluid into the vascular compartment. As a consequence, there is movement of water and diffusible solutes from the vascular space at the arteriolar end of the capillaries. Fluid is returned from the interstitial space into the vascular system at the venous end of the capillaries and by way of the lymphatics. These movements are usually balanced so that there is a steady state in the sizes of the intravascular and interstitial compartments, yet a large exchange between them occurs. However, if either the capillary hydrostatic pressure is increased and/or the oncotic pressure is reduced, a further net movement of fluid from intravascular to the interstitial spaces will take place.

Edema is defined as a clinically apparent increase in the interstitial fluid volume, which develops when Starling forces are altered so that there is increased flow of fluid from the vascular system into the interstitium. Edema due to an increase in capillary pressure may result from an elevation of venous pressure caused by obstruction to venous and/or lymphatic drainage. An increase in capillary pressure may be generalized, as occurs in heart failure, or it may be localized to one extremity when venous pressure is elevated due to unilateral thrombophlebitis (see below). The Starling forces also may be imbalanced when the colloid oncotic pressure of the plasma is reduced owing to any factor that may induce hypoalbuminemia, as when large quantities of protein are lost in the urine such as in the nephrotic syndrome (see below), or when synthesis is reduced in a severe catabolic state.

CAPILLARY DAMAGE

Edema may also result from damage to the capillary endothelium, which increases its permeability and permits the transfer of proteins into the interstitial compartment. Injury to the capillary wall can result from drugs (see below), viral or bacterial agents, and thermal or mechanical trauma. Increased capillary permeability also may be a consequence of a hypersensitivity reaction and of immune injury. Damage to the capillary endothelium is presumably responsible for inflammatory edema, which is usually nonpitting, localized, and accompanied by other signs of inflammation—i.e., erythema, heat, and tenderness.

REDUCTION OF EFFECTIVE ARTERIAL VOLUME

In many forms of edema, despite the increase in extracellular fluid volume, the effective arterial blood volume, a parameter that represents the filling of the arterial tree and that effectively perfuses the tissues, is reduced. Underfilling of the arterial tree may be caused by a reduction of cardiac output and/or systemic vascular resistance, by pooling of blood in the splanchnic veins (as in cirrhosis), and by hypoalbuminemia (Fig. 50-1*A*). As a consequence of underfilling, a series of physiologic responses designed to restore the effective arterial volume to normal are set into motion. A key element of these responses is the renal retention of sodium and, therefore, water, thereby restoring effective arterial volume, but sometimes also leading to or intensifying edema.

RENAL FACTORS AND THE RENIN-ANGIOTENSIN-ALDOSTERONE SYSTEM

The diminished renal blood flow characteristic of states in which the effective arterial blood volume is reduced is translated by the renal juxtaglomerular cells (specialized myoepithelial cells surrounding the afferent arteriole) into a signal for increased renin release. Renin is an enzyme with a molecular mass of about 40,000 Da that acts on its substrate, angiotensinogen, an α_2-globulin synthesized by the liver, to release angiotensin I, a decapeptide, which in turn is converted to angiotensin II (AII), an octapeptide. AII has generalized vasoconstrictor properties, particularly on the renal efferent arterioles. This action reduces the hydrostatic pressure in the peritubular capillaries, whereas the increased filtration fraction raises the colloid osmotic pressure in these vessels, thereby enhancing salt and water reabsorption in the proximal tubule as well as in the ascending limb of the loop of Henle.

The renin-angiotensin-aldosterone system (RAAS) operates as both a hormonal and paracrine system. Its activation causes sodium and water retention and thereby contributes to edema formation. Blockade of the conversion of angiotensin I to AII and blockade of the AII receptor enhance sodium and water excretion and reduce many forms of edema. AII that enters the systemic circulation stimulates the production of aldosterone by the zona glomerulosa of the adrenal cortex. Aldosterone in turn enhances sodium reabsorption (and potassium excretion) by the collecting tubule, further favoring edema formation. In patients with heart failure, not only is aldosterone secretion elevated but the biologic half-life of the hormone is prolonged secondary to the depression of hepatic blood flow, which reduces its hepatic catabolism and increases further the plasma level of the hormone. Blockade of the action of aldosterone by spironolactone or eplerenone (aldosterone antagonists) or by amiloride (a blocker of epithelial sodium channels) often induces a moderate diuresis in edematous states.

ARGININE VASOPRESSIN

(See also Chap. 404) The secretion of arginine vasopressin (AVP) occurs in response to increased intracellular osmolar concentration, and, by stimulating V_2 receptors, AVP increases the reabsorption of free water in the distal tubules and collecting ducts of the kidneys, thereby increasing total-body water. Circulating AVP is elevated in many patients with heart failure secondary to a nonosmotic stimulus associated with decreased effective arterial volume and reduced compliance of the left atrium. Such patients fail to show the normal reduction of AVP with a reduction of osmolality, contributing to edema formation and hyponatremia.

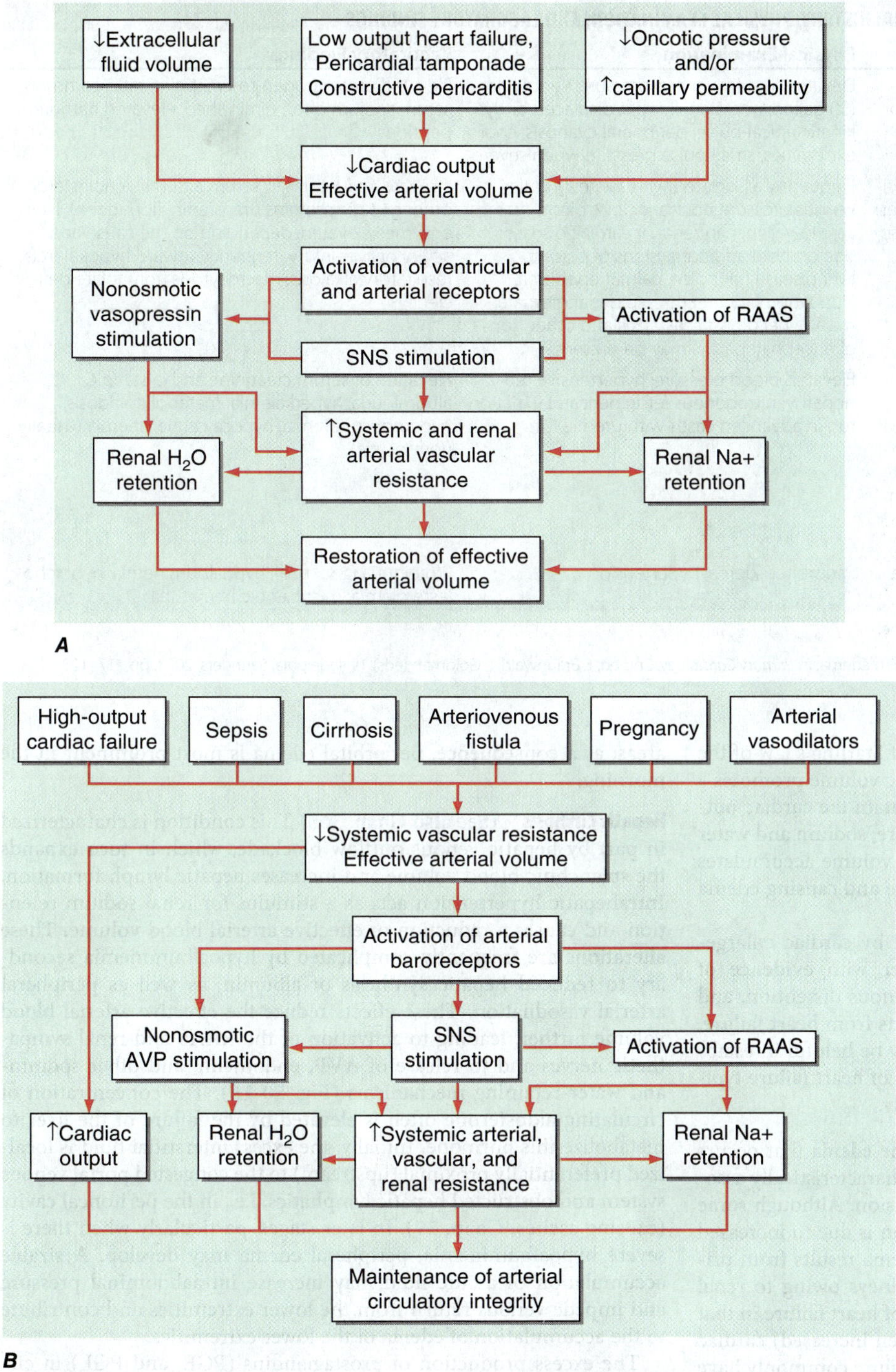

FIGURE 50-1 Clinical conditions in which a decrease in cardiac output (*A*) and systemic vascular resistance (*B*) cause arterial underfilling with resulting neurohumoral activation and renal sodium and water retention. In addition to activating the neurohumoral axis, adrenergic stimulation causes renal vasoconstriction and enhances sodium and fluid transport by the proximal tubule epithelium. RAAS, renin-angiotensin aldosterone system; SNS, sympathetic nervous system. *(Modified from RW Schrier: Ann Intern Med 113:155, 1990.)*

ENDOTHELIN-1

This potent peptide vasoconstrictor is released by endothelial cells. Its concentration in the plasma is elevated in patients with severe heart failure and contributes to renal vasoconstriction, sodium retention, and edema.

NATRIURETIC PEPTIDES

Atrial distention causes release into the circulation of atrial natriuretic peptide (ANP), a polypeptide; a high-molecular-weight precursor of ANP is stored in secretory granules within atrial myocytes. The closely related brain natriuretic peptide (pre-prohormone BNP) is stored primarily in ventricular myocytes and is released when ventricular diastolic pressure rises. Released ANP and BNP (which is derived from its precursor) bind to the natriuretic receptor-A, which causes: (1) excretion of sodium and water by augmenting glomerular filtration rate, inhibiting sodium reabsorption in the proximal tubule, and inhibiting release of renin and aldosterone; and (2) dilation of arterioles and venules by antagonizing the vasoconstrictor actions of AII, AVP, and sympathetic stimulation. Thus, elevated levels of natriuretic peptides have the capacity to oppose sodium retention in hypervolemic and edematous states.

Although circulating levels of ANP and BNP are elevated in heart failure and in cirrhosis with ascites, the natriuretic peptides are not sufficiently potent to prevent edema formation. Indeed, in edematous states, resistance to the actions of natriuretic peptides may be increased, further reducing their effectiveness.

Further discussion of the control of sodium and water balance is found in Chap. 64e.

CLINICAL CAUSES OF EDEMA

A weight gain of several kilograms usually precedes overt manifestations of generalized edema, and a similar weight loss from diuresis can be induced in a slightly edematous patient before "dry weight" is achieved. *Anasarca* refers to gross, generalized edema. *Ascites* (Chap. 59) and *hydrothorax* refer to accumulation of excess fluid in the peritoneal and pleural cavities, respectively, and are considered special forms of edema.

Edema is recognized by the persistence of an indentation of the skin after pressure; this is known as "pitting" edema. In its more subtle form, edema may be detected by noting that after the stethoscope is removed from the chest wall, the rim of the bell leaves an indentation on the skin of the chest for a few minutes. Edema may be present when the ring on a finger fits more snugly than in the past or when a patient complains of difficulty putting on shoes, particularly in the evening. Edema may also be recognized by puffiness of the face, which is most readily apparent in the periorbital areas.

GENERALIZED EDEMA

The differences among the major causes of generalized edema are shown in Table 50-1. Cardiac, renal, hepatic, or nutritional disorders are responsible for a majority of patients with generalized edema. Consequently, the differential diagnosis of generalized edema should be directed toward identifying or excluding these several conditions.

Heart Failure (See also Chap. 279) In heart failure, the impaired systolic emptying of the ventricle(s) and/or the impairment of ventricular relaxation promotes an accumulation of blood in the venous circulation at the expense of the effective arterial volume. In addition, the heightened tone of the sympathetic nervous system causes renal vasoconstriction and reduction of glomerular filtration. In mild heart failure, a small increment of total blood volume may repair the deficit of

TABLE 50-1 PRINCIPAL CAUSES OF GENERALIZED EDEMA: HISTORY, PHYSICAL EXAMINATION, AND LABORATORY FINDINGS

Organ System	History	Physical Examination	Laboratory Findings
Cardiac	Dyspnea with exertion prominent—often associated with orthopnea—or paroxysmal nocturnal dyspnea	Elevated jugular venous pressure, ventricular (S_3) gallop; occasionally with displaced or dyskinetic apical pulse; peripheral cyanosis, cool extremities, small pulse pressure when severe	Elevated urea nitrogen-to-creatinine ratio common; serum sodium often diminished; elevated natriuretic peptides
Hepatic	Dyspnea uncommon, except if associated with significant degree of ascites; most often a history of ethanol abuse	Frequently associated with ascites; jugular venous pressure normal or low; blood pressure lower than in renal or cardiac disease; one or more additional signs of chronic liver disease (jaundice, palmar erythema, Dupuytren's contracture, spider angiomata, male gynecomastia; asterixis and other signs of encephalopathy) may be present	If severe, reductions in serum albumin, cholesterol, other hepatic proteins (transferrin, fibrinogen); liver enzymes elevated, depending on the cause and acuity of liver injury; tendency toward hypokalemia, respiratory alkalosis; macrocytosis from folate deficiency
Renal (CRF)	Usually chronic: may be associated with uremic signs and symptoms, including decreased appetite, altered (metallic or fishy) taste, altered sleep pattern, difficulty concentrating, restless legs, or myoclonus; dyspnea can be present, but generally less prominent than in heart failure	Elevated blood pressure; hypertensive retinopathy; nitrogenous fetor; pericardial friction rub in advanced cases with uremia	Elevation of serum creatinine and cystatin C; albuminuria; hyperkalemia, metabolic acidosis, hyperphosphatemia, hypocalcemia, anemia (usually normocytic)
Renal (NS)	Childhood diabetes mellitus; plasma cell dyscrasias	Periorbital edema; hypertension	Proteinuria (≥3.5 g/d); hypoalbuminemia; hypercholesterolemia; microscopic hematuria

Abbreviations: CRF, chronic renal failure; NS, nephrotic syndrome.

Source: Modified from GM Chertow: Approach to the patient with edema, in *Primary Cardiology*, 2nd ed, E Braunwald, L Goldman (eds). Philadelphia, Saunders, 2003, pp 117–128.

effective arterial volume through the operation of Starling's law of the heart, in which an increase in ventricular diastolic volume promotes a more forceful contraction and may thereby maintain the cardiac output. However, if the cardiac disorder is more severe, sodium and water retention continue, and the increment in blood volume accumulates in the venous circulation, raising venous pressure and causing edema (Fig. 50-1).

The presence of heart disease, as manifested by cardiac enlargement and/or ventricular hypertrophy, together with evidence of cardiac failure, such as dyspnea, basilar rales, venous distention, and hepatomegaly, usually indicates that edema results from heart failure. Noninvasive tests such as echocardiography may be helpful in establishing the diagnosis of heart disease. The edema of heart failure typically occurs in the dependent portions of the body.

Edema of Renal Disease (See also Chap. 338) The edema that occurs during the acute phase of glomerulonephritis is characteristically associated with hematuria, proteinuria, and hypertension. Although some evidence supports the view that the fluid retention is due to increased capillary permeability, in most instances, the edema results from primary retention of sodium and water by the kidneys owing to renal insufficiency. This state differs from most forms of heart failure in that it is characterized by a normal (or sometimes even increased) cardiac output. Patients with edema due to acute renal failure commonly have arterial hypertension as well as pulmonary congestion on chest roentgenogram, often without considerable cardiac enlargement, but they may not develop orthopnea. Patients with *chronic* renal failure may also develop edema due to primary renal retention of sodium and water.

Nephrotic Syndrome and other Hypoalbuminemic States The primary alteration in the nephrotic syndrome is a diminished colloid oncotic pressure due to losses of large quantities (≥3.5 g/d) of protein into the urine. With severe hypoalbuminemia (<35 g/L) and the consequent reduced colloid osmotic pressure, the sodium and water that are retained cannot be restrained within the vascular compartment, and total and effective arterial blood volumes decline. This process initiates the edema-forming sequence of events described above, including activation of the RAAS. The nephrotic syndrome may occur during the course of a variety of kidney diseases, which include glomerulonephritis, diabetic glomerulosclerosis, and hypersensitivity reactions. The edema is diffuse, symmetric, and most prominent in the dependent areas; as a consequence, periorbital edema is most prominent in the morning.

Hepatic Cirrhosis (See also Chap. 365) This condition is characterized in part by hepatic venous outflow blockade, which in turn expands the splanchnic blood volume and increases hepatic lymph formation. Intrahepatic hypertension acts as a stimulus for renal sodium retention and causes a reduction of effective arterial blood volume. These alterations are frequently complicated by hypoalbuminemia secondary to reduced hepatic synthesis of albumin, as well as peripheral arterial vasodilation. These effects reduce the effective arterial blood volume further, leading to activation of the RAAS and renal sympathetic nerves and to release of AVP, endothelin, and other sodium- and water-retaining mechanisms (Fig. 50-1*B*). The concentration of circulating aldosterone often is elevated by the failure of the liver to metabolize this hormone. Initially, the excess interstitial fluid is localized preferentially proximal (upstream) to the congested portal venous system and obstructed hepatic lymphatics, i.e., in the peritoneal cavity (causing ascites, Chap. 59). In later stages, particularly when there is severe hypoalbuminemia, peripheral edema may develop. A sizable accumulation of ascitic fluid may increase intraabdominal pressure and impede venous return from the lower extremities and contribute to the accumulation of edema of the lower extremities.

The excess production of prostaglandins (PGE_2 and PGI_2) in cirrhosis attenuates renal sodium retention. When the synthesis of these substances is inhibited by nonsteroidal anti-inflammatory drugs (NSAIDs), renal function may deteriorate, and this may increase sodium retention further.

Drug-Induced Edema A large number of widely used drugs can cause edema (Table 50-2). Mechanisms include renal vasoconstriction (NSAIDs and cyclosporine), arteriolar dilation (vasodilators), augmented renal sodium reabsorption (steroid hormones), and capillary damage.

Edema of Nutritional Origin A diet grossly deficient in protein over a prolonged period may produce hypoproteinemia and edema. The latter may be intensified by the development of beriberi heart disease, which also is of nutritional origin, in which multiple peripheral arteriovenous fistulae result in reduced effective systemic perfusion and effective arterial blood volume, thereby enhancing edema formation (Chap. 96e) (Fig. 50-1*B*). Edema may actually become intensified

TABLE 50-2 DRUGS ASSOCIATED WITH EDEMA FORMATION

Nonsteroidal anti-inflammatory drugs
Antihypertensive agents
Direct arterial/arteriolar vasodilators
Hydralazine
Clonidine
Methyldopa
Guanethidine
Minoxidil
Calcium channel antagonists
α-Adrenergic antagonists
Thiazolidinediones
Steroid hormones
Glucocorticoids
Anabolic steroids
Estrogens
Progestins
Cyclosporine
Growth hormone
Immunotherapies
Interleukin 2
OKT3 monoclonal antibody

Source: Modified from Chertow GM: Approach to the patient with edema, in *Primary Cardiology*, 2nd ed, E Braunwald, L Goldman (eds). Philadelphia, Saunders, 2003, pp 117–128.

when famished subjects are first provided with an adequate diet. The ingestion of more food may increase the quantity of sodium ingested, which is then retained along with water. So-called refeeding edema also may be linked to increased release of insulin, which directly increases tubular sodium reabsorption. In addition to hypoalbuminemia, hypokalemia and caloric deficits may be involved in the edema of starvation.

LOCALIZED EDEMA

In this condition, the hydrostatic pressure in the capillary bed upstream (proximal) of the obstruction increases so that an abnormal quantity of fluid is transferred from the vascular to the interstitial space. Since the alternative route (i.e., the lymphatic channels) also may be obstructed or maximally filled, an increased volume of interstitial fluid in the limb develops (i.e., there is trapping of fluid in the interstitium of the extremity). The displacement of large quantities of fluid into a limb may occur at the expense of the blood volume in the remainder of the body, thereby reducing effective arterial blood volume and leading to the retention of NaCl and H_2O until the deficit in plasma volume has been corrected.

Localized edema due to venous or lymphatic obstruction may be caused by thrombophlebitis, chronic lymphangitis, resection of regional lymph nodes, and filariasis, among other causes. Lymphedema is particularly intractable because restriction of lymphatic flow results in increased protein concentration in the interstitial fluid, a circumstance that aggravates fluid retention.

Other Causes of Edema These causes include hypothyroidism (myxedema) and hyperthyroidism (pretibial myxedema secondary to Graves' disease), the edema in which is typically nonpitting and due to deposition of hyaluronic acid and, in Graves' disease, lymphocytic infiltration and inflammation; exogenous hyperadrenocortism; pregnancy; and administration of estrogens and vasodilators, particularly dihydropyridines such as nifedipine.

DISTRIBUTION OF EDEMA

The distribution of edema is an important guide to its cause. Edema associated with heart failure tends to be more extensive in the legs and to be accentuated in the evening, a feature also determined largely by posture. When patients with heart failure are confined to bed, edema may be most prominent in the presacral region. Severe heart failure may cause ascites that may be distinguished from the ascites caused by hepatic cirrhosis by the jugular venous pressure, which is usually elevated in heart failure and normal in cirrhosis.

Edema resulting from hypoproteinemia, as occurs in the nephrotic syndrome, characteristically is generalized, but it is especially evident in the very soft tissues of the eyelids and face and tends to be most pronounced in the morning owing to the recumbent posture assumed during the night. Less common causes of facial edema include trichinosis, allergic reactions, and myxedema. Edema limited to one leg or to one or both arms is usually the result of venous and/or lymphatic obstruction. Unilateral paralysis reduces lymphatic and venous drainage on the affected side and may also be responsible for unilateral edema. In patients with obstruction of the superior vena cava, edema is confined to the face, neck, and upper extremities in which the venous pressure is elevated compared with that in the lower extremities.

APPROACH TO THE PATIENT: Edema

An important first question is whether the edema is localized or generalized. If it is localized, the local phenomena that may be responsible should be considered. If the edema is generalized, one should first determine if there is serious hypoalbuminemia, e.g., serum albumin <25 g/L. If so, the history, physical examination, urinalysis, and other laboratory data will help evaluate the question of cirrhosis, severe malnutrition, or the nephrotic syndrome as the underlying disorder. If hypoalbuminemia is not present, it should be determined if there is evidence of heart failure severe enough to promote generalized edema. Finally, it should be ascertained as to whether or not the patient has an adequate urine output or if there is significant oliguria or anuria. These abnormalities are discussed in Chaps. 61, 334, and 335.

51e Approach to the Patient with a Heart Murmur

Patrick T. O'Gara, Joseph Loscalzo

This is a digital-only chapter. It is available on the DVD that accompanies this book, as well as on Access Medicine/Harrison's Online, and the eBook and "app" editions of HPIM 19e.

The differential diagnosis of a heart murmur begins with a careful assessment of its major attributes and response to bedside maneuvers. The history, clinical context, and associated physical examination findings provide additional clues by which the significance of a heart murmur can be established. Accurate bedside identification of a heart murmur can inform decisions regarding the indications for noninvasive testing and the need for referral to a cardiovascular specialist. Preliminary discussions can be held with the patient regarding antibiotic or rheumatic fever prophylaxis, the need to restrict various forms of physical activity, and the potential role for family screening.

52 Palpitations

Joseph Loscalzo

Palpitations are extremely common among patients who present to their internists and can best be defined as an intermittent "thumping," "pounding," or "fluttering" sensation in the chest. This sensation can be either intermittent or sustained and either regular or irregular. Most patients interpret palpitations as an unusual awareness of the heartbeat and become especially concerned when they sense that they have had "skipped" or "missing" heartbeats. Palpitations are often noted when the patient is quietly resting, during which time other stimuli are minimal. Palpitations that are positional generally reflect a structural process within (e.g., atrial myxoma) or adjacent to (e.g., mediastinal mass) the heart.

Palpitations are brought about by cardiac (43%), psychiatric (31%), miscellaneous (10%), and unknown (16%) causes, according to one large series. Among the cardiovascular causes are premature atrial and ventricular contractions, supraventricular and ventricular arrhythmias, mitral valve prolapse (with or without associated arrhythmias), aortic insufficiency, atrial myxoma, and pulmonary embolism. Intermittent palpitations are commonly caused by premature atrial or ventricular contractions: the post-extrasystolic beat is sensed by the patient owing to the increase in ventricular end-diastolic dimension following the pause in the cardiac cycle and the increased strength of contraction (post-extrasystolic potentiation) of that beat. Regular, sustained palpitations can be caused by regular supraventricular and ventricular tachycardias. Irregular, sustained palpitations can be caused by atrial fibrillation. It is important to note that most arrhythmias are not associated with palpitations. In those that are, it is often useful either to ask the patient to "tap out" the rhythm of the palpitations or to take his/her pulse during palpitations. In general, hyperdynamic cardiovascular states caused by catecholaminergic stimulation from exercise, stress, or pheochromocytoma can lead to palpitations. Palpitations are common among athletes, especially older endurance athletes. In addition, the enlarged ventricle of aortic regurgitation and accompanying hyperdynamic precordium frequently lead to the sensation of palpitations. Other factors that enhance the strength of myocardial contraction, including tobacco, caffeine, aminophylline, atropine, thyroxine, cocaine, and amphetamines, can cause palpitations.

Psychiatric causes of palpitations include panic attacks or disorders, anxiety states, and somatization, alone or in combination. Patients with psychiatric causes for palpitations more commonly report a longer duration of the sensation (>15 min) and other accompanying symptoms than do patients with other causes. Among the miscellaneous causes of palpitations are thyrotoxicosis, drugs (see above) and ethanol, spontaneous skeletal muscle contractions of the chest wall, pheochromocytoma, and systemic mastocytosis.

APPROACH TO THE PATIENT: Palpitations

The principal goal in assessing patients with palpitations is to determine whether the symptom is caused by a life-threatening arrhythmia. Patients with preexisting coronary artery disease (CAD) or risk factors for CAD are at greatest risk for ventricular arrhythmias (Chap. 276) as a cause for palpitations. In addition, the association of palpitations with other symptoms suggesting hemodynamic compromise, including syncope or lightheadedness, supports this diagnosis. Palpitations caused by sustained tachyarrhythmias in patients with CAD can be accompanied by angina pectoris or dyspnea, and, in patients with ventricular dysfunction (systolic or diastolic), aortic stenosis, hypertrophic cardiomyopathy, or mitral stenosis (with or without CAD), can be accompanied by dyspnea from increased left atrial and pulmonary venous pressure.

Key features of the physical examination that will help confirm or refute the presence of an arrhythmia as a cause for palpitations (as well as its adverse hemodynamic consequences) include measurement of the vital signs, assessment of the jugular venous pressure and pulse, and auscultation of the chest and precordium. A resting electrocardiogram can be used to document the arrhythmia. If exertion is known to induce the arrhythmia and accompanying palpitations, exercise electrocardiography can be used to make the diagnosis. If the arrhythmia is sufficiently infrequent, other methods must be used, including continuous electrocardiographic (Holter) monitoring; telephonic monitoring, through which the patient can transmit an electrocardiographic tracing during a sensed episode; loop recordings (external or implantable), which can capture the electrocardiographic event for later review; and mobile cardiac outpatient telemetry. Data suggest that Holter monitoring is of limited clinical utility, while the implantable loop recorder and mobile cardiac outpatient telemetry are safe and possibly more cost-effective in the assessment of patients with (infrequent) recurrent, unexplained palpitations.

Most patients with palpitations do not have serious arrhythmias or underlying structural heart disease. If sufficiently troubling to the patient, occasional benign atrial or ventricular premature contractions can often be managed with beta-blocker therapy. Palpitations incited by alcohol, tobacco, or illicit drugs need to be managed by abstention, while those caused by pharmacologic agents should be addressed by considering alternative therapies when appropriate or possible. Psychiatric causes of palpitations may benefit from cognitive therapy or pharmacotherapy. The physician should note that palpitations are at the very least bothersome and, on occasion, frightening to the patient. Once serious causes for the symptom have been excluded, the patient should be reassured that the palpitations will not adversely affect prognosis.

SECTION 6 ALTERATIONS IN GASTROINTESTINAL FUNCTION

53 Dysphagia

Ikuo Hirano, Peter J. Kahrilas

Dysphagia—difficulty with swallowing—refers to problems with the transit of food or liquid from the mouth to the hypopharynx or through the esophagus. Severe dysphagia can compromise nutrition, cause aspiration, and reduce quality of life. Additional terminology pertaining to swallowing dysfunction is as follows. *Aphagia* (inability to swallow) typically denotes complete esophageal obstruction, most commonly encountered in the acute setting of a food bolus or foreign body impaction. *Odynophagia* refers to painful swallowing, typically resulting from mucosal ulceration within the oropharynx or esophagus. It commonly is accompanied by dysphagia, but the converse is not true. *Globus pharyngeus* is a foreign body sensation localized in the neck that does not interfere with swallowing and sometimes is relieved by swallowing. *Transfer dysphagia* frequently results in nasal regurgitation and pulmonary aspiration during swallowing and is characteristic of oropharyngeal dysphagia. *Phagophobia* (fear of swallowing) and *refusal to swallow* may be psychogenic or related to anticipatory anxiety about food bolus obstruction, odynophagia, or aspiration.

PHYSIOLOGY OF SWALLOWING

Swallowing begins with a voluntary (oral) phase that includes preparation during which food is masticated and mixed with saliva. This is followed by a transfer phase during which the bolus is pushed into the pharynx by the tongue. Bolus entry into the hypopharynx initiates the pharyngeal swallow response, which is centrally mediated and involves a complex series of actions, the net result of which is to propel food through the pharynx into the esophagus while preventing its entry into the airway. To accomplish this, the larynx is elevated and pulled forward, actions that also facilitate upper esophageal sphincter (UES) opening. Tongue pulsion then propels the bolus through the UES, followed by a peristaltic contraction that clears residue from the pharynx and through the esophagus. The lower esophageal sphincter (LES) relaxes as the food enters the esophagus and remains relaxed until the peristaltic contraction has delivered the bolus into the stomach. Peristaltic contractions elicited in response to a swallow are called *primary peristalsis* and involve sequenced inhibition followed by contraction of the musculature along the entire length of the esophagus. The inhibition that precedes the peristaltic contraction is called *deglutitive inhibition*. Local distention of the esophagus anywhere along its length, as may occur with gastroesophageal reflux, activates *secondary peristalsis* that begins at the point of distention and proceeds distally. Tertiary esophageal contractions are nonperistaltic, disordered esophageal contractions that may be observed to occur spontaneously during fluoroscopic observation.

The musculature of the oral cavity, pharynx, UES, and cervical esophagus is striated and directly innervated by lower motor neurons carried in cranial nerves (Fig. 53-1). Oral cavity muscles are innervated by the fifth (trigeminal) and seventh (facial) cranial nerves; the tongue, by the twelfth (hypoglossal) cranial nerve. Pharyngeal muscles are innervated by the ninth (glossopharyngeal) and tenth (vagus) cranial nerves.

Physiologically, the UES consists of the cricopharyngeus muscle, the adjacent inferior pharyngeal constrictor, and the proximal portion of the cervical esophagus. UES innervation is derived from the vagus nerve, whereas the innervation to the musculature acting on the UES to facilitate its opening during swallowing comes from the fifth, seventh, and twelfth cranial nerves. The UES remains closed at rest owing to both its inherent elastic properties and neurogenically mediated contraction of the cricopharyngeus muscle. UES opening during swallowing involves both cessation of vagal excitation to the cricopharyngeus and simultaneous contraction of the suprahyoid and geniohyoid muscles that pull open the UES in conjunction with the upward and forward displacement of the larynx.

The neuromuscular apparatus for peristalsis is distinct in proximal and distal parts of the esophagus. The cervical esophagus, like the pharyngeal musculature, consists of striated muscle and is directly innervated by lower motor neurons of the vagus nerve. Peristalsis in the proximal esophagus is governed by the sequential activation of the vagal motor neurons in the nucleus ambiguus. In contrast, the distal esophagus and LES are composed of smooth muscle and are controlled by excitatory and inhibitory neurons within the esophageal myenteric plexus. Medullary preganglionic neurons from the dorsal motor nucleus of the vagus trigger peristalsis via these ganglionic neurons during primary peristalsis. Neurotransmitters of the excitatory ganglionic neurons are acetylcholine and substance P; those of the inhibitory neurons are vasoactive intestinal peptide and nitric oxide. Peristalsis results from the patterned activation of inhibitory followed by excitatory ganglionic neurons, with progressive dominance of the inhibitory neurons distally. Similarly, LES relaxation occurs with the onset of deglutitive inhibition and persists until the peristaltic sequence is complete. At rest, the LES is contracted because of excitatory ganglionic stimulation and its intrinsic myogenic tone, a property that distinguishes it from the adjacent esophagus. The function of the LES is supplemented by the surrounding muscle of the right diaphragmatic crus, which acts as an external sphincter during inspiration, cough, or abdominal straining.

PATHOPHYSIOLOGY OF DYSPHAGIA

Dysphagia can be subclassified both by location and by the circumstances in which it occurs. With respect to location, distinct considerations apply to oral, pharyngeal, or esophageal dysphagia. Normal transport of an ingested bolus depends on the consistency and size of the bolus, the caliber of the lumen, the integrity of peristaltic contraction, and deglutitive inhibition of both the UES and the LES. Dysphagia caused by an oversized bolus or a narrow lumen is called *structural dysphagia*, whereas dysphagia due to abnormalities of peristalsis or impaired sphincter relaxation after swallowing is called *propulsive* or

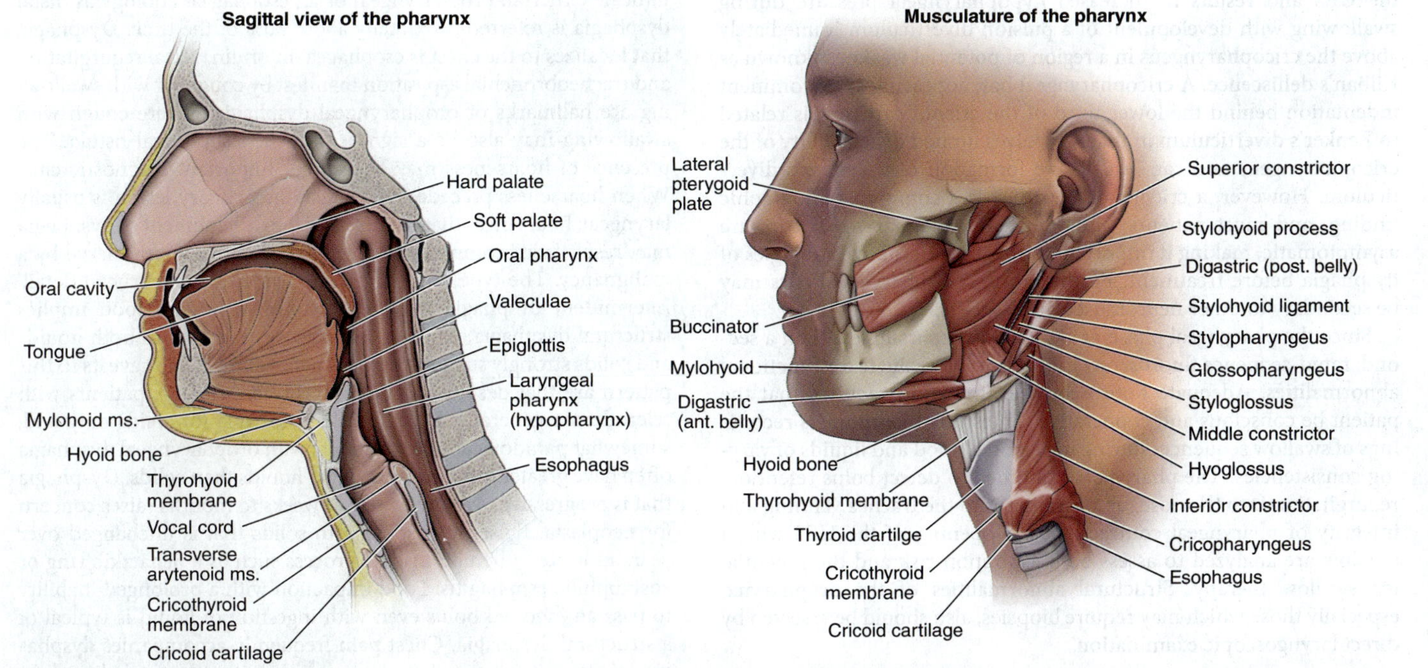

FIGURE 53-1 Sagittal and diagrammatic views of the musculature involved in enacting oropharyngeal swallowing. Note the dominance of the tongue in the sagittal view and the intimate relationship between the entrance to the larynx (airway) and the esophagus. In the resting configuration illustrated, the esophageal inlet is closed. This is transiently reconfigured such that the esophageal inlet is open and the laryngeal inlet closed during swallowing. *(Adapted from PJ Kahrilas, in DW Gelfand and JE Richter [eds]: Dysphagia: Diagnosis and Treatment. New York: Igaku-Shoin Medical Publishers, 1989, pp. 11–28.)*

motor dysphagia. More than one mechanism may be operative in a patient with dysphagia. Scleroderma commonly presents with absent peristalsis as well as a weakened LES that predisposes patients to peptic stricture formation. Likewise, radiation therapy for head and neck cancer may compound the functional deficits in the oropharyngeal swallow attributable to the tumor and cause cervical esophageal stenosis.

Oral and Pharyngeal (Oropharyngeal) Dysphagia Oral-phase dysphagia is associated with poor bolus formation and control so that food has prolonged retention within the oral cavity and may seep out of the mouth. Drooling and difficulty in initiating swallowing are other characteristic signs. Poor bolus control also may lead to premature spillage of food into the hypopharynx with resultant aspiration into the trachea or regurgitation into the nasal cavity. Pharyngeal-phase dysphagia is associated with retention of food in the pharynx due to poor tongue or pharyngeal propulsion or obstruction at the UES. Signs and symptoms of concomitant hoarseness or cranial nerve dysfunction may be associated with oropharyngeal dysphagia.

Oropharyngeal dysphagia may be due to neurologic, muscular, structural, iatrogenic, infectious, and metabolic causes. Iatrogenic, neurologic, and structural pathologies are most common. Iatrogenic causes include surgery and radiation, often in the setting of head and neck cancer. Neurogenic dysphagia resulting from cerebrovascular accidents, Parkinson's disease, and amyotrophic lateral sclerosis is a major source of morbidity related to aspiration and malnutrition. Medullary nuclei directly innervate the oropharynx. Lateralization of pharyngeal dysphagia implies either a structural pharyngeal lesion or a neurologic process that selectively targeted the ipsilateral brainstem nuclei or cranial nerve. Advances in functional brain imaging have elucidated an important role of the cerebral cortex in swallow function and dysphagia. Asymmetry in the cortical representation of the pharynx provides an explanation for the dysphagia that occurs as a consequence of unilateral cortical cerebrovascular accidents.

Oropharyngeal structural lesions causing dysphagia include Zenker's diverticulum, cricopharyngeal bar, and neoplasia. Zenker's diverticulum typically is encountered in elderly patients, with an estimated prevalence between 1:1000 and 1:10,000. In addition to dysphagia, patients may present with regurgitation of particulate food debris, aspiration, and halitosis. The pathogenesis is related to stenosis of the cricopharyngeus that causes diminished opening of the UES and results in increased hypopharyngeal pressure during swallowing with development of a pulsion diverticulum immediately above the cricopharyngeus in a region of potential weakness known as Killian's dehiscence. A cricopharyngeal bar, appearing as a prominent indentation behind the lower third of the cricoid cartilage, is related to Zenker's diverticulum in that it involves limited distensibility of the cricopharyngeus and can lead to the formation of a Zenker's diverticulum. However, a cricopharyngeal bar is a common radiographic finding, and most patients with transient cricopharyngeal bars are asymptomatic, making it important to rule out alternative etiologies of dysphagia before treatment. Furthermore, cricopharyngeal bars may be secondary to other neuromuscular disorders.

Since the pharyngeal phase of swallowing occurs in less than a second, rapid-sequence fluoroscopy is necessary to evaluate for functional abnormalities. Adequate fluoroscopic examination requires that the patient be conscious and cooperative. The study incorporates recordings of swallow sequences during ingestion of food and liquids of varying consistencies. The pharynx is examined to detect bolus retention, regurgitation into the nose, or aspiration into the trachea. Timing and integrity of pharyngeal contraction and opening of the UES with a swallow are analyzed to assess both aspiration risk and the potential for swallow therapy. Structural abnormalities of the oropharynx, especially those which may require biopsies, also should be assessed by direct laryngoscopic examination.

Esophageal Dysphagia The adult esophagus measures 18–26 cm in length and is anatomically divided into the cervical esophagus, extending from the pharyngoesophageal junction to the suprasternal notch, and the thoracic esophagus, which continues to the diaphragmatic hiatus. When distended, the esophageal lumen has internal dimensions of about 2 cm in the anteroposterior plane and 3 cm in the lateral plane. Solid food dysphagia becomes common when the lumen is narrowed to <13 mm but also can occur with larger diameters in the setting of poorly masticated food or motor dysfunction. Circumferential lesions are more likely to cause dysphagia than are lesions that involve only a partial circumference of the esophageal wall. The most common structural causes of dysphagia are Schatzki's rings, eosinophilic esophagitis, and peptic strictures. Dysphagia also occurs in the setting of gastroesophageal reflux disease without a stricture, perhaps on the basis of altered esophageal sensation, distensibility, or motor function.

Propulsive disorders leading to esophageal dysphagia result from abnormalities of peristalsis and/or deglutitive inhibition, potentially affecting the cervical or thoracic esophagus. Since striated muscle pathology usually involves both the oropharynx and the cervical esophagus, the clinical manifestations usually are dominated by oropharyngeal dysphagia. Diseases affecting smooth muscle involve both the thoracic esophagus and the LES. A dominant manifestation of this, absent peristalsis, refers to either the complete absence of swallow-induced contraction or the presence of nonperistaltic, disordered contractions. Absent peristalsis and failure of deglutitive LES relaxation are the defining features of achalasia. In diffuse esophageal spasm (DES), LES function is normal, with the disordered motility restricted to the esophageal body. Absent peristalsis combined with severe weakness of the LES is a nonspecific pattern commonly found in patients with scleroderma.

APPROACH TO THE PATIENT: Dysphagia

Figure 53-2 shows an algorithm for the approach to a patient with dysphagia.

HISTORY

The patient history is extremely valuable in making a presumptive diagnosis or at least substantially restricting the differential diagnoses in most patients. Key elements of the history are the localization of dysphagia, the circumstances in which dysphagia is experienced, other symptoms associated with dysphagia, and progression. Dysphagia that localizes to the suprasternal notch may indicate either an oropharyngeal or an esophageal etiology as distal dysphagia is referred proximally about 30% of the time. Dysphagia that localizes to the chest is esophageal in origin. Nasal regurgitation and tracheobronchial aspiration manifest by coughing with swallowing are hallmarks of oropharyngeal dysphagia. Severe cough with swallowing may also be a sign of a tracheoesophageal fistula. The presence of hoarseness may be another important diagnostic clue. When hoarseness precedes dysphagia, the primary lesion is usually laryngeal; hoarseness that occurs after the development of dysphagia may result from compromise of the recurrent laryngeal nerve by a malignancy. The type of food causing dysphagia is a crucial detail. Intermittent dysphagia that occurs only with solid food implies structural dysphagia, whereas constant dysphagia with both liquids and solids strongly suggests a motor abnormality. Two caveats to this pattern are that despite having a motor abnormality, patients with scleroderma generally develop mild dysphagia for solids only and, somewhat paradoxically, that patients with oropharyngeal dysphagia often have greater difficulty managing liquids than solids. Dysphagia that is progressive over the course of weeks to months raises concern for neoplasia. Episodic dysphagia to solids that is unchanged over years indicates a benign disease process such as a Schatzki's ring or eosinophilic esophagitis. Food impaction with a prolonged inability to pass an ingested bolus even with ingestion of liquid is typical of a structural dysphagia. Chest pain frequently accompanies dysphagia whether it is related to motor disorders, structural disorders, or reflux disease. A prolonged history of heartburn preceding the onset of dysphagia is suggestive of peptic stricture and, infrequently, esophageal adenocarcinoma. A history of prolonged nasogastric intubation, esophageal or head and neck surgery, ingestion of caustic

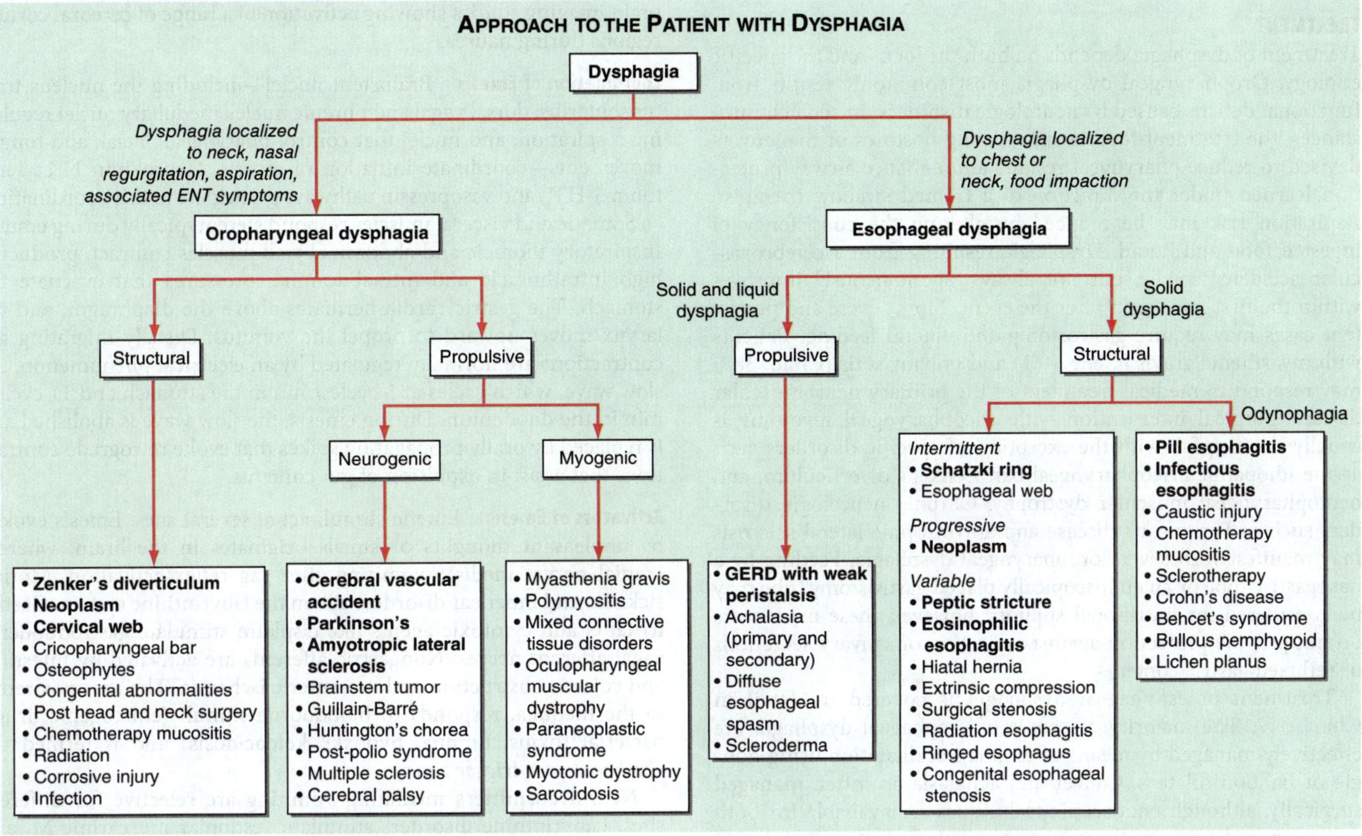

FIGURE 53-2 Approach to the patient with dysphagia. Etiologies in bold print are the most common. ENT, ear, nose, and throat; GERD, gastroesophageal reflux disease.

agents or pills, previous radiation or chemotherapy, or associated mucocutaneous diseases may help isolate the cause of dysphagia. With accompanying odynophagia, which usually is indicative of ulceration, infectious or pill-induced esophagitis should be suspected. In patients with AIDS or other immunocompromised states, esophagitis due to opportunistic infections such as *Candida*, herpes simplex virus, or cytomegalovirus and to tumors such as Kaposi's sarcoma and lymphoma should be considered. A strong history of atopy increases concerns for eosinophilic esophagitis.

PHYSICAL EXAMINATION

Physical examination is important in the evaluation of oral and pharyngeal dysphagia because dysphagia is usually only one of many manifestations of a more global disease process. Signs of bulbar or pseudobulbar palsy, including dysarthria, dysphonia, ptosis, tongue atrophy, and hyperactive jaw jerk, in addition to evidence of generalized neuromuscular disease, should be elicited. The neck should be examined for thyromegaly. A careful inspection of the mouth and pharynx should disclose lesions that may interfere with passage of food. Missing dentition can interfere with mastication and exacerbate an existing cause of dysphagia. Physical examination is less helpful in the evaluation of esophageal dysphagia as most relevant pathology is restricted to the esophagus. The notable exception is skin disease. Changes in the skin may suggest a diagnosis of scleroderma or mucocutaneous diseases such as pemphigoid, lichen planus and epidermolysis bullosa, all of which can involve the esophagus.

DIAGNOSTIC PROCEDURES

Although most instances of dysphagia are attributable to benign disease processes, dysphagia is also a cardinal symptom of several malignancies, making it an important symptom to evaluate. Cancer may result in dysphagia due to intraluminal obstruction (esophageal or proximal gastric cancer, metastatic deposits), extrinsic compression (lymphoma, lung cancer), or paraneoplastic syndromes. Even when not attributable to malignancy, dysphagia is usually a manifestation of an identifiable and treatable disease entity, making its evaluation beneficial to the patient and gratifying to the practitioner. The specific diagnostic algorithm to pursue is guided by the details of the history (Fig. 53-2). If oral or pharyngeal dysphagia is suspected, a fluoroscopic swallow study, usually done by a swallow therapist, is the procedure of choice. Otolaryngoscopic and neurologic evaluation also can be important, depending on the circumstances. For suspected esophageal dysphagia, upper endoscopy is the single most useful test. Endoscopy allows better visualization of mucosal lesions than does barium radiography and also allows one to obtain mucosal biopsies. Endoscopic or histologic abnormalities are evident in the leading causes of esophageal dysphagia: Schatzki ring, gastroesophageal reflux disease and eosinophilic esophagitis. Furthermore, therapeutic intervention with esophageal dilation can be done as part of the procedure if it is deemed necessary. The emergence of eosinophilic esophagitis as a leading cause of dysphagia in both children and adults has led to the recommendation that esophageal mucosal biopsies be obtained routinely in the evaluation of unexplained dysphagia even if endoscopically identified esophageal mucosal lesions are absent. For cases of suspected esophageal motility disorders, endoscopy is still the appropriate initial evaluation as neoplastic and inflammatory conditions can secondarily produce patterns of either achalasia or esophageal spasm. Esophageal manometry is done if dysphagia is not adequately explained by endoscopy or to confirm the diagnosis of a suspected esophageal motor disorder. Barium radiography can provide useful adjunctive information in cases of subtle or complex esophageal strictures, prior esophageal surgery, esophageal diverticula, or paraesophageal herniation. In specific cases, computed tomography (CT) examination and endoscopic ultrasonography may be useful.

TREATMENT

Treatment of dysphagia depends on both the locus and the specific etiology. Oropharyngeal dysphagia most commonly results from functional deficits caused by neurologic disorders. In such circumstances, the treatment focuses on utilizing postures or maneuvers devised to reduce pharyngeal residue and enhance airway protection learned under the direction of a trained swallow therapist. Aspiration risk may be reduced by altering the consistency of ingested food and liquid. Dysphagia resulting from a cerebrovascular accident usually, but not always, spontaneously improves within the first few weeks after the event. More severe and persistent cases may require gastrostomy and enteral feeding. Patients with myasthenia gravis (Chap. 461) and polymyositis (Chap. 388) may respond to medical treatment of the primary neuromuscular disease. Surgical intervention with cricopharyngeal myotomy is usually not helpful, with the exception of specific disorders such as the idiopathic cricopharyngeal bar, Zenker's diverticulum, and oculopharyngeal muscular dystrophy. Chronic neurologic disorders such as Parkinson's disease and amyotrophic lateral sclerosis may manifest with severe oropharyngeal dysphagia. Feeding by a nasogastric tube or an endoscopically placed gastrostomy tube may be considered for nutritional support; however, these maneuvers do not provide protection against aspiration of salivary secretions or refluxed gastric contents.

Treatment of esophageal dysphagia is covered in detail in Chap. 347. The majority of causes of esophageal dysphagia are effectively managed by means of esophageal dilatation using bougie or balloon dilators. Cancer and achalasia are often managed surgically, although endoscopic techniques are available for both palliation and primary therapy, respectively. Infectious etiologies respond to antimicrobial medications or treatment of the underlying immunosuppressive state. Finally, eosinophilic esophagitis has emerged as an important cause of dysphagia that is amenable to treatment by elimination of dietary allergens or administration of swallowed, topically acting glucocorticoids.

54 Nausea, Vomiting, and Indigestion

William L. Hasler

Nausea is the subjective feeling of a need to vomit. *Vomiting* (emesis) is the oral expulsion of gastrointestinal contents due to contractions of gut and thoracoabdominal wall musculature. Vomiting is contrasted with *regurgitation,* the effortless passage of gastric contents into the mouth. *Rumination* is the repeated regurgitation of food residue, which may be rechewed and reswallowed. In contrast to emesis, these phenomena may exhibit volitional control. *Indigestion* is a term encompassing a range of complaints including nausea, vomiting, heartburn, regurgitation, and dyspepsia (the presence of symptoms thought to originate in the gastroduodenal region). Some individuals with dyspepsia report predominantly epigastric burning, gnawing, or pain. Others experience postprandial fullness, early satiety (an inability to complete a meal due to premature fullness), bloating, eructation (belching), and anorexia.

NAUSEA AND VOMITING

MECHANISMS

Vomiting is coordinated by the brainstem and is effected by responses in the gut, pharynx, and somatic musculature. Mechanisms underlying nausea are poorly understood but likely involve the cerebral cortex, as nausea requires conscious perception. This is supported by functional brain imaging studies showing activation of a range of cerebral cortical regions during nausea.

Coordination of Emesis Brainstem nuclei—including the nucleus tractus solitarius; dorsal vagal and phrenic nuclei; medullary nuclei regulating respiration; and nuclei that control pharyngeal, facial, and tongue movements—coordinate initiation of emesis. Neurokinin NK_1, serotonin 5-HT_3, and vasopressin pathways participate in this coordination.

Somatic and visceral muscles respond stereotypically during emesis. Inspiratory thoracic and abdominal wall muscles contract, producing high intrathoracic and intraabdominal pressures that evacuate the stomach. The gastric cardia herniates above the diaphragm, and the larynx moves upward to propel the vomitus. Distally migrating gut contractions are normally regulated by an electrical phenomenon, the slow wave, which cycles at 3 cycles/min in the stomach and 11 cycles/min in the duodenum. During emesis, the slow wave is abolished and is replaced by orally propagating spikes that evoke retrograde contractions that assist in expulsion of gut contents.

Activators of Emesis Emetic stimuli act at several sites. Emesis evoked by unpleasant thoughts or smells originates in the brain, whereas cranial nerves mediate vomiting after gag reflex activation. Motion sickness and inner ear disorders act on the labyrinthine system. Gastric irritants and cytotoxic agents like cisplatin stimulate gastroduodenal vagal afferent nerves. Nongastric afferents are activated by intestinal and colonic obstruction and mesenteric ischemia. The area postrema, in the medulla, responds to bloodborne stimuli (emetogenic drugs, bacterial toxins, uremia, hypoxia, ketoacidosis) and is termed the *chemoreceptor trigger zone.*

Neurotransmitters mediating vomiting are selective for different sites. Labyrinthine disorders stimulate vestibular muscarinic M_1 and histaminergic H_1 receptors. Vagal afferent stimuli activate serotonin 5-HT_3 receptors. The area postrema is served by nerves acting on 5-HT_3, M_1, H_1, and dopamine D_2 subtypes. Cannabinoid CB_1 pathways may participate in the cerebral cortex. Optimal pharmacologic therapy of vomiting requires understanding of these pathways.

DIFFERENTIAL DIAGNOSIS

Nausea and vomiting are caused by conditions within and outside the gut as well as by drugs and circulating toxins (Table 54-1).

Intraperitoneal Disorders Visceral obstruction and inflammation of hollow and solid viscera may elicit vomiting. Gastric obstruction results from ulcers and malignancy, whereas small-bowel and colon blockage occur because of adhesions, benign or malignant tumors, volvulus, intussusception, or inflammatory diseases like Crohn's disease. The superior mesenteric artery syndrome, occurring after weight loss or prolonged bed rest, results when the duodenum is compressed by the overlying superior mesenteric artery. Abdominal irradiation impairs intestinal motor function and induces strictures. Biliary colic causes nausea by acting on local afferent nerves. Vomiting with pancreatitis, cholecystitis, and appendicitis is due to visceral irritation and induction of ileus. Enteric infections with viruses like norovirus or rotavirus or bacteria such as *Staphylococcus aureus* and *Bacillus cereus* often cause vomiting, especially in children. Opportunistic infections like cytomegalovirus or herpes simplex virus induce emesis in immunocompromised individuals.

Gut sensorimotor dysfunction often causes nausea and vomiting. *Gastroparesis* presents with symptoms of gastric retention with evidence of delayed gastric emptying and occurs after vagotomy or with pancreatic carcinoma, mesenteric vascular insufficiency, or organic diseases like diabetes, scleroderma, and amyloidosis. Idiopathic gastroparesis is the most common etiology. It occurs in the absence of systemic illness and may follow a viral illness, suggesting an infectious trigger. *Intestinal pseudoobstruction* is characterized by disrupted intestinal and colonic motor activity with retention of food residue and secretions; bacterial overgrowth; nutrient malabsorption; and symptoms of nausea, vomiting, bloating, pain, and altered defecation. Intestinal pseudoobstruction may be idiopathic, inherited as a familial visceral myopathy or neuropathy, result from systemic disease, or

TABLE 54-1 CAUSES OF NAUSEA AND VOMITING

Intraperitoneal	Extraperitoneal	Medications/ Metabolic Disorders
Obstructing disorders	Cardiopulmonary disease	Drugs
Pyloric obstruction	Cardiomyopathy	Cancer chemotherapy
Small-bowel obstruction	Myocardial infarction	Antibiotics
Colonic obstruction	Labyrinthine disease	Cardiac antiarrhythmics
Superior mesenteric artery syndrome	Motion sickness	Digoxin
Enteric infections	Labyrinthitis	Oral hypoglycemics
Viral	Malignancy	Oral contraceptives
Bacterial	Intracerebral disorders	Endocrine/metabolic disease
Inflammatory diseases	Malignancy	Pregnancy
Cholecystitis	Hemorrhage	Uremia
Pancreatitis	Abscess	Ketoacidosis
Appendicitis	Hydrocephalus	Thyroid and parathyroid disease
Hepatitis	Psychiatric illness	Adrenal insufficiency
Altered sensorimotor function	Anorexia and bulimia nervosa	Toxins
Gastroparesis	Depression	Liver failure
Intestinal pseudoobstruction	Postoperative vomiting	Ethanol
Gastroesophageal reflux		
Chronic idiopathic nausea		
Functional vomiting		
Cyclic vomiting syndrome		
Cannabinoid hyperemesis syndrome		
Rumination syndrome		
Biliary colic		
Abdominal irradiation		

occur as a paraneoplastic consequence of malignancy (e.g., small-cell lung carcinoma). Patients with gastroesophageal reflux may report nausea and vomiting, as do some with irritable bowel syndrome (IBS) or chronic constipation.

Other functional gastroduodenal disorders without organic abnormalities have been characterized in adults. *Chronic idiopathic nausea* is defined as nausea without vomiting occurring several times a week. *Functional vomiting* is defined as one or more vomiting episodes weekly in the absence of an eating disorder or psychiatric disease. *Cyclic vomiting syndrome* presents with periodic discrete episodes of relentless nausea and vomiting in children and adults and shows an association with migraine headaches, suggesting that some cases may be migraine variants. Some adult cases have been described in association with rapid gastric emptying. A related condition, *cannabinoid hyperemesis syndrome*, presents with cyclical vomiting with intervening well periods in individuals (mostly men) who use large quantities of cannabis over many years and resolves with its discontinuation. Pathologic behaviors such as taking prolonged hot baths or showers are associated with the syndrome. *Rumination syndrome*, characterized by repetitive regurgitation of recently ingested food, is often misdiagnosed as refractory vomiting.

Extraperitoneal Disorders Myocardial infarction and congestive heart failure may cause nausea and vomiting. Postoperative emesis occurs after 25% of surgeries, most commonly laparotomy and orthopedic surgery. Increased intracranial pressure from tumors, bleeding, abscess, or blockage of cerebrospinal fluid outflow produces vomiting with or without nausea. Patients with psychiatric illnesses including anorexia nervosa, bulimia nervosa, anxiety, and depression often report significant nausea that may be associated with delayed gastric emptying.

Medications and Metabolic Disorders Drugs evoke vomiting by action on the stomach (analgesics, erythromycin) or area postrema (opiates, anti-parkinsonian drugs). Other emetogenic agents include antibiotics, cardiac antiarrhythmics, antihypertensives, oral hypoglycemics, antidepressants (selective serotonin and serotonin norepinephrine reuptake inhibitors), smoking cessation drugs (varenicline, nicotine), and contraceptives. Cancer chemotherapy causes vomiting that is acute (within hours of administration), delayed (after 1 or more days), or anticipatory. Acute emesis from highly emetogenic agents (e.g., cisplatin) is mediated by 5-HT_3 pathways, whereas delayed emesis is less dependent on 5-HT_3 mechanisms. Anticipatory nausea may respond to anxiolytic therapy rather than antiemetics.

Metabolic disorders elicit nausea and vomiting. Pregnancy is the most prevalent endocrinologic cause, and nausea affects 70% of women in the first trimester. Hyperemesis gravidarum is a severe form of nausea of pregnancy that produces significant fluid loss and electrolyte disturbances. Uremia, ketoacidosis, adrenal insufficiency, and parathyroid and thyroid disease are other metabolic etiologies.

Circulating toxins evoke emesis via effects on the area postrema. Endogenous toxins are generated in fulminant liver failure, whereas exogenous enterotoxins may be produced by enteric bacterial infection. Ethanol intoxication is a common toxic etiology of nausea and vomiting.

APPROACH TO THE PATIENT: Nausea and Vomiting

HISTORY AND PHYSICAL EXAMINATION

The history helps define the etiology of nausea and vomiting. Drugs, toxins, and infections often cause acute symptoms, whereas established illnesses evoke chronic complaints. Gastroparesis and pyloric obstruction elicit vomiting within an hour of eating. Emesis from intestinal blockage occurs later. Vomiting occurring within minutes of meal consumption prompts consideration of rumination syndrome. With severe gastric emptying delays, the vomitus may contain food residue ingested hours or days before. Hematemesis raises suspicion of an ulcer, malignancy, or Mallory-Weiss tear. Feculent emesis is noted with distal intestinal or colonic obstruction. Bilious vomiting excludes gastric obstruction, whereas emesis of undigested food is consistent with a Zenker's diverticulum or achalasia. Vomiting can relieve abdominal pain from a bowel obstruction, but has no effect in pancreatitis or cholecystitis. Profound weight loss raises concern about malignancy or obstruction. Fevers suggest inflammation. An intracranial source is considered if there are headaches or visual field changes. Vertigo or tinnitus indicates labyrinthine disease.

The physical examination complements the history. Orthostatic hypotension and reduced skin turgor indicate intravascular fluid loss. Pulmonary abnormalities raise concern for aspiration of vomitus. Abdominal auscultation may reveal absent bowel sounds with ileus. High-pitched rushes suggest bowel obstruction, whereas a succussion splash upon abrupt lateral movement of the patient is found with gastroparesis or pyloric obstruction. Tenderness or involuntary guarding raises suspicion of inflammation, whereas fecal blood suggests mucosal injury from ulcer, ischemia, or tumor. Neurologic disease presents with papilledema, visual field loss, or focal neural abnormalities. Neoplasm is suggested by palpation of masses or adenopathy.

DIAGNOSTIC TESTING

For intractable symptoms or an elusive diagnosis, selected screening tests can direct clinical care. Electrolyte replacement is indicated for hypokalemia or metabolic alkalosis. Iron-deficiency anemia mandates a search for mucosal injury. Pancreaticobiliary disease is indicated by abnormal pancreatic or liver biochemistries, whereas endocrinologic, rheumatologic, or paraneoplastic etiologies are suggested by hormone or serologic abnormalities. If bowel obstruction is suspected, supine and upright abdominal radiographs may show intestinal air-fluid levels with reduced colonic air. Ileus is characterized by diffusely dilated air-filled bowel loops.

Anatomic studies may be indicated if initial testing is nondiagnostic. Upper endoscopy detects ulcers, malignancy, and retained gastric food residue in gastroparesis. Small-bowel barium radiography or computed tomography (CT) diagnoses partial bowel obstruction. Colonoscopy or contrast enema radiography detects colonic obstruction. Ultrasound or CT defines intraperitoneal inflammation; CT and magnetic resonance imaging (MRI) enterography provide superior definition of inflammation in Crohn's disease. CT or MRI of the head can delineate intracranial disease. Mesenteric angiography, CT, or MRI is useful for suspected ischemia.

Gastrointestinal motility testing may detect an underlying motor disorder when anatomic abnormalities are absent. Gastroparesis commonly is diagnosed by gastric scintigraphy, by which emptying of a radiolabeled meal is measured. Isotopic breath tests and wireless motility capsule methods are alternatives tests to define gastroparesis in different regions of the world. Intestinal pseudoobstruction often is suggested by abnormal barium transit and luminal dilation on small-bowel contrast radiography. Delayed small-bowel transit also may be detected by wireless capsule techniques. Small-intestinal manometry can confirm the diagnosis and further characterize the motor abnormality as neuropathic or myopathic based on contractile patterns. Such investigation can obviate the need for surgical intestinal biopsy to evaluate for smooth muscle or neuronal degeneration. Combined ambulatory esophageal pH/impedance testing and high-resolution manometry can facilitate diagnosis of rumination syndrome.

TREATMENT NAUSEA AND VOMITING

GENERAL PRINCIPLES

Therapy of vomiting is tailored to correcting remediable abnormalities if possible. Hospitalization is considered for severe dehydration, especially if oral fluid replenishment cannot be sustained. Once oral intake is tolerated, nutrients are restarted with low-fat liquids, because lipids delay gastric emptying. Foods high in indigestible residue are avoided because these prolong gastric retention. Controlling blood glucose in poorly controlled diabetics can reduce hospitalizations in gastroparesis.

ANTIEMETIC MEDICATIONS

The most commonly used antiemetic agents act on central nervous system sites (Table 54-2). Antihistamines like dimenhydrinate and meclizine and anticholinergics like scopolamine act on labyrinthine pathways to treat motion sickness and inner ear disorders. Dopamine D_2 antagonists treat emesis evoked by area postrema stimuli and are used for medication, toxic, and metabolic etiologies. Dopamine antagonists cross the blood-brain barrier and cause anxiety, movement disorders, and hyperprolactinemic effects (galactorrhea, sexual dysfunction).

Other classes exhibit antiemetic properties. 5-HT_3 antagonists such as ondansetron and granisetron can prevent postoperative vomiting, radiation therapy–induced symptoms, and cancer chemotherapy–induced emesis, but also are used for other causes of emesis with limited evidence for efficacy. Tricyclic antidepressant agents provide symptomatic benefit in patients with chronic idiopathic nausea and functional vomiting as well as in long-standing diabetic patients with nausea and vomiting. Other antidepressants such as mirtazapine and olanzapine also may exhibit antiemetic effects.

GASTROINTESTINAL MOTOR STIMULANTS

Drugs that stimulate gastric emptying are used for gastroparesis (Table 54-2). Metoclopramide, a combined 5-HT_4 agonist and D_2 antagonist, is effective in gastroparesis, but antidopaminergic side effects, such as dystonias and mood and sleep disturbances, limit use in ~25% of cases. Erythromycin increases gastroduodenal motility by action on receptors for motilin, an endogenous stimulant of fasting motor activity. Intravenous erythromycin is useful for inpatients with refractory gastroparesis, but oral forms have some utility. Domperidone, a D_2 antagonist not available in the United States, exhibits prokinetic and antiemetic effects but does not cross into most brain regions; thus, anxiety and dystonic reactions are rare. The main side effects of domperidone relate to induction of

TABLE 54-2 TREATMENT OF NAUSEA AND VOMITING

Treatment	Mechanism	Examples	Clinical Indications
Antiemetic agents	Antihistaminergic	Dimenhydrinate, meclizine	Motion sickness, inner ear disease
	Anticholinergic	Scopolamine	Motion sickness, inner ear disease
	Antidopaminergic	Prochlorperazine, thiethylperazine	Medication-, toxin-, or metabolic-induced emesis
	5-HT_3 antagonist	Ondansetron, granisetron	Chemotherapy- and radiation-induced emesis, postoperative emesis
	NK_1 antagonist	Aprepitant	Chemotherapy-induced nausea and vomiting
	Tricyclic antidepressant	Amitriptyline, nortriptyline	Functional vomiting, chronic idiopathic nausea, cyclic vomiting syndrome, ?gastroparesis
	Other antidepressant	Mirtazapine, olanzapine	?Functional vomiting, ?chronic idiopathic nausea, ?gastroparesis
Prokinetic agents	5-HT_4 agonist and antidopaminergic	Metoclopramide	Gastroparesis
	Motilin agonist	Erythromycin	Gastroparesis, ?intestinal pseudoobstruction
	Peripheral antidopaminergic	Domperidone	Gastroparesis
	Somatostatin analogue	Octreotide	Intestinal pseudoobstruction
	Acetylcholinesterase inhibitor	Pyridostigmine	?Small-intestinal dysmotility/pseudoobstruction
Special settings	Benzodiazepines	Lorazepam	Anticipatory nausea and vomiting with chemotherapy
	Glucocorticoids	Methylprednisolone, dexamethasone	Chemotherapy-induced emesis
	Cannabinoids	Tetrahydrocannabinol	Chemotherapy-induced emesis

Note: ?, indication is uncertain.

hyperprolactinemia via effects on pituitary regions served by a porous blood-brain barrier.

Refractory motility disorders pose significant challenges. Intestinal pseudoobstruction may respond to the somatostatin analogue octreotide, which induces propagative small-intestinal motor complexes. Acetylcholinesterase inhibitors such as pyridostigmine are also observed to benefit some patients with small-bowel dysmotility. Pyloric injections of botulinum toxin are reported in uncontrolled studies to reduce gastroparesis symptoms, but small controlled trials observe benefits no greater than sham treatments. Surgical pyloroplasty has improved symptoms in case series. Placing a feeding jejunostomy reduces hospitalizations and improves overall health in some patients with drug-refractory gastroparesis. Postvagotomy gastroparesis may improve with near-total gastric resection; similar operations are now being tried for other gastroparesis etiologies. Implanted gastric electrical stimulators may reduce symptoms, enhance nutrition, improve quality of life, and decrease health care expenditures in medication-refractory gastroparesis, but small controlled trials do not report convincing benefits.

SAFETY CONSIDERATIONS

Safety concerns about selected antiemetics have been emphasized. Centrally acting antidopaminergics, especially metoclopramide, can cause irreversible movement disorders such as tardive dyskinesia, particularly in older patients. This complication should be carefully explained and documented in the medical record. Some agents with antiemetic properties including domperidone, erythromycin, tricyclics, and 5-HT_3 antagonists can induce dangerous cardiac rhythm disturbances, especially in those with QTc interval prolongation on electrocardiography (ECG). Surveillance ECG testing has been advocated for some of these agents.

SELECTED CLINICAL SETTINGS

Some cancer chemotherapies are intensely emetogenic (Chap. 103e). Combining a 5-HT_3 antagonist, an NK_1 antagonist, and a glucocorticoid provides significant control of both acute and delayed vomiting after highly emetogenic chemotherapy. Unlike other drugs in the same class, the 5-HT_3 antagonist palonosetron exhibits efficacy at preventing delayed chemotherapy-induced vomiting. Benzodiazepines such as lorazepam can reduce anticipatory nausea and vomiting. Miscellaneous therapies with benefit in chemotherapy-induced emesis include cannabinoids, olanzapine, and alternative therapies like ginger. Most antiemetic regimens produce greater reductions in vomiting than in nausea.

Clinicians should exercise caution in managing pregnant patients with nausea. Studies of the teratogenic effects of antiemetic agents provide conflicting results. Few controlled trials have been performed in nausea of pregnancy. Antihistamines such as meclizine and doxylamine, antidopaminergics such as prochlorperazine, and antiserotonergics such as ondansetron demonstrate limited efficacy. Some obstetricians offer alternative therapies such as pyridoxine, acupressure, or ginger.

Managing cyclic vomiting syndrome is a challenge. Prophylaxis with tricyclic antidepressants, cyproheptadine, or β-adrenoceptor antagonists can reduce the severity and frequency of attacks. Intravenous 5-HT_3 antagonists combined with the sedating effects of a benzodiazepine like lorazepam are a mainstay of treatment of acute flares. Small studies report benefits with antimigraine agents, including the 5-HT_1 agonist sumatriptan, as well as selected anticonvulsants such as zonisamide and levetiracetam.

INDIGESTION

MECHANISMS

The most common causes of indigestion are gastroesophageal reflux and functional dyspepsia. Other cases are a consequence of organic illness.

Gastroesophageal Reflux Gastroesophageal reflux results from many physiologic defects. Reduced lower esophageal sphincter (LES) tone contributes to reflux in scleroderma and pregnancy and may be a factor in some patients without systemic illness. Others exhibit frequent transient LES relaxations (TLESRs) that cause bathing of the esophagus by acid or nonacidic fluid. Overeating and aerophagia override the barrier function of the LES, whereas reductions in esophageal body motility or salivary secretion prolong fluid exposure. Increased intragastric pressure promotes gastroesophageal reflux in obesity. The role of hiatal hernias is controversial—most reflux patients have hiatal hernias, but most with hiatal hernias do not have excess heartburn.

Gastric Motor Dysfunction Disturbed gastric motility may contribute to gastroesophageal reflux in up to one-third of cases. Delayed gastric emptying is also found in ~30% of functional dyspeptics. Conversely, some dyspeptics exhibit rapid gastric emptying. The relation of these defects to symptom induction is uncertain; studies show poor correlation between symptom severity and degrees of motor dysfunction. Impaired gastric fundus relaxation after eating (i.e., accommodation) may underlie selected dyspeptic symptoms like bloating, nausea, and early satiety in ~40% of patients.

Visceral Afferent Hypersensitivity Disturbed gastric sensation is another pathogenic factor in functional dyspepsia. Visceral hypersensitivity was first reported in IBS with demonstration of heightened perception of rectal balloon inflation without changes in compliance. Similarly, ~35% of dyspeptic patients note discomfort with fundic distention to lower pressures than healthy controls. Others with dyspepsia exhibit hypersensitivity to chemical stimulation with capsaicin or with acid or lipid exposure in the duodenum. Some individuals with functional heartburn without increased acid or nonacid reflux are believed to have heightened perception of normal esophageal pH and volume.

Other Factors *Helicobacter pylori* has a clear etiologic role in peptic ulcer disease, but ulcers cause a minority of dyspepsia cases. *H. pylori* is a minor factor in the genesis of functional dyspepsia. Functional dyspepsia is associated with chronic fatigue, produces reduced physical and mental well-being, and is exacerbated by stress. Anxiety, depression, and somatization may have contributing roles in some cases. Functional MRI studies show increased activation of several brain regions, emphasizing contributions from central nervous system factors. Analgesics cause dyspepsia, whereas nitrates, calcium channel blockers, theophylline, and progesterone promote gastroesophageal reflux. Other stimuli that induce reflux include ethanol, tobacco, and caffeine via LES relaxation. Genetic factors may promote development of reflux and dyspepsia.

DIFFERENTIAL DIAGNOSIS

Gastroesophageal Reflux Disease Gastroesophageal reflux disease (GERD) is prevalent. Heartburn is reported once monthly by 40% of Americans and daily by 7–10%. Most cases of heartburn occur because of excess acid reflux, but reflux of nonacidic fluid produces similar symptoms. Alkaline reflux esophagitis produces GERD-like symptoms most often in patients who have had surgery for peptic ulcer disease. Ten percent of patients with heartburn exhibit normal esophageal acid exposure and no increase in nonacidic reflux (functional heartburn).

Functional Dyspepsia Nearly 25% of the populace has dyspepsia at least six times yearly, but only 10–20% present to clinicians. Functional dyspepsia, the cause of symptoms in >60% of dyspeptic patients, is defined as ≥3 months of bothersome postprandial fullness, early satiety, or epigastric pain or burning with symptom onset at least 6 months before diagnosis in the absence of organic cause. Functional dyspepsia is subdivided into postprandial distress syndrome, characterized by meal-induced fullness, early satiety, and discomfort, and epigastric pain syndrome, which presents with epigastric burning pain unrelated to meals. Most cases follow a benign course, but some with *H. pylori* infection or on nonsteroidal anti-inflammatory drugs

(NSAIDs) develop ulcers. As with idiopathic gastroparesis, some cases of functional dyspepsia result from prior infection.

Ulcer Disease In most GERD patients, there is no destruction of the esophagus. However, 5% develop esophageal ulcers, and some form strictures. Symptoms cannot distinguish nonerosive from erosive or ulcerative esophagitis. A minority of cases of dyspepsia stem from gastric or duodenal ulcers. The most common causes of ulcer disease are *H. pylori* infection and use of NSAIDs. Other rare causes of gastroduodenal ulcers include Crohn's disease (Chap. 351) and Zollinger-Ellison syndrome (Chap. 348), resulting from gastrin overproduction by an endocrine tumor.

Malignancy Dyspeptic patients often seek care because of fear of cancer, but few cases result from malignancy. Esophageal squamous cell carcinoma occurs most often with long-standing tobacco or ethanol intake. Other risks include prior caustic ingestion, achalasia, and the hereditary disorder tylosis. Esophageal adenocarcinoma usually complicates prolonged acid reflux. Eight to 20% of GERD patients exhibit esophageal intestinal metaplasia, termed *Barrett's metaplasia,* a condition that predisposes to esophageal adenocarcinoma (Chap. 109). Gastric malignancies include adenocarcinoma, which is prevalent in certain Asian societies, and lymphoma.

Other Causes Opportunistic fungal or viral esophageal infections may produce heartburn but more often cause odynophagia. Other causes of esophageal inflammation include eosinophilic esophagitis and pill esophagitis. Biliary colic is in the differential diagnosis of unexplained upper abdominal pain, but most patients with biliary colic report discrete acute episodes of right upper quadrant or epigastric pain rather than the chronic burning, discomfort, and fullness of dyspepsia. Twenty percent of patients with gastroparesis report a predominance of pain or discomfort rather than nausea and vomiting. Intestinal lactase deficiency as a cause of gas, bloating, and discomfort occurs in 15–25% of whites of northern European descent but is more common in blacks and Asians. Intolerance of other carbohydrates (e.g., fructose, sorbitol) produces similar symptoms. Small-intestinal bacterial overgrowth may cause dyspepsia, often associated with bowel dysfunction, distention, and malabsorption. Eosinophilic infiltration of the duodenal mucosa is described in some dyspeptics, particularly with postprandial distress syndrome. Celiac disease, pancreatic disease (chronic pancreatitis, malignancy), hepatocellular carcinoma, Ménétrier's disease, infiltrative diseases (sarcoidosis, eosinophilic gastroenteritis), mesenteric ischemia, thyroid and parathyroid disease, and abdominal wall strain cause dyspepsia. Gluten sensitivity in the absence of celiac disease is reported to evoke unexplained upper abdominal symptoms. Extraperitoneal etiologies of indigestion include congestive heart failure and tuberculosis.

APPROACH TO THE PATIENT: Indigestion

HISTORY AND PHYSICAL EXAMINATION

Care of the indigestion patient requires a thorough interview. GERD classically produces heartburn, a substernal warmth that moves toward the neck. Heartburn often is exacerbated by meals and may awaken the patient. Associated symptoms include regurgitation of acid or nonacidic fluid and water brash, the reflex release of salty salivary secretions into the mouth. Atypical symptoms include pharyngitis, asthma, cough, bronchitis, hoarseness, and chest pain that mimics angina. Some patients with acid reflux on esophageal pH testing do not report heartburn, but note abdominal pain or other symptoms.

Dyspeptic patients typically report symptoms referable to the upper abdomen that may be meal-related, as with postprandial distress syndrome, or independent of food ingestion, as in epigastric pain syndrome. Functional dyspepsia overlaps with other disorders including GERD, IBS, and idiopathic gastroparesis.

TABLE 54-3 ALARM SYMPTOMS IN GASTROESOPHAGEAL REFLUX DISEASE

Odynophagia
Unexplained weight loss
Recurrent vomiting
Occult or gross gastrointestinal bleeding
Jaundice
Palpable mass or adenopathy
Family history of gastrointestinal malignancy

The physical exam with GERD and functional dyspepsia usually is normal. In atypical GERD, pharyngeal erythema and wheezing may be noted. Recurrent acid regurgitation may cause poor dentition. Dyspeptics may exhibit epigastric tenderness or distention.

Discriminating functional and organic causes of indigestion mandates excluding certain historic and exam features. Odynophagia suggests esophageal infection. Dysphagia is concerning for a benign or malignant esophageal blockage. Other alarm features include unexplained weight loss, recurrent vomiting, occult or gross bleeding, jaundice, palpable mass or adenopathy, and a family history of gastrointestinal neoplasm.

DIAGNOSTIC TESTING

Because indigestion is prevalent and most cases result from GERD or functional dyspepsia, a general principle is to perform only limited and directed diagnostic testing of selected individuals.

Once alarm factors are excluded (Table 54-3), patients with typical GERD do not need further evaluation and are treated empirically. Upper endoscopy is indicated to exclude mucosal injury in cases with atypical symptoms, symptoms unresponsive to acid suppression, or alarm factors. For heartburn >5 years in duration, especially in patients >50 years old, endoscopy is advocated to screen for Barrett's metaplasia. The benefits and cost-effectiveness of this approach have not been validated in controlled studies. Ambulatory esophageal pH testing using a catheter method or a wireless capsule endoscopically attached to the esophageal wall is considered for drug-refractory symptoms and atypical symptoms like unexplained chest pain. High-resolution esophageal manometry is ordered when surgical treatment of GERD is considered. A low LES pressure predicts failure of drug therapy and provides a rationale to proceed to surgery. Poor esophageal body peristalsis raises concern about postoperative dysphagia and directs the choice of surgical technique. Nonacidic reflux may be detected by combined esophageal impedance-pH testing in medication-unresponsive patients.

Upper endoscopy is recommended as the initial test in patients with unexplained dyspepsia who are >55 years old or who have alarm factors because of the purported elevated risks of malignancy and ulcer in these groups. However, endoscopic findings in unexplained dyspepsia include erosive esophagitis in 13%, peptic ulcer in 8%, and gastric or esophageal malignancy in only 0.3%. Management of patients <55 years old without alarm factors depends on the local prevalence of *H. pylori* infection. In regions with low *H. pylori* prevalence (<10%), a 4-week trial of an acid-suppressing medication such as a proton pump inhibitor (PPI) is recommended. If this fails, a "test and treat" approach is most commonly applied. *H. pylori* status is determined with urea breath testing, stool antigen measurement, or blood serology testing. Those who are *H. pylori* positive are given therapy to eradicate the infection. If symptoms resolve on either regimen, no further intervention is required. For patients in areas with high *H. pylori* prevalence (>10%), an initial test and treat approach is advocated, with a subsequent trial of an acid-suppressing regimen offered for those in whom *H. pylori* treatment fails or for those who are negative for the infection. In each of these patient subsets, upper endoscopy is reserved for those whose symptoms fail to respond to therapy.

Further testing is indicated in some settings. If bleeding is noted, a blood count can exclude anemia. Thyroid chemistries or calcium levels screen for metabolic disease, whereas specific serologies may suggest celiac disease. Pancreatic and liver chemistries are obtained for possible pancreaticobiliary causes. Ultrasound, CT, or MRI is performed if abnormalities are found. Gastric emptying testing is considered to exclude gastroparesis for dyspeptic symptoms that resemble postprandial distress when drug therapy fails and in some GERD patients, especially if surgical intervention is an option. Breath testing after carbohydrate ingestion detects lactase deficiency, intolerance to other carbohydrates, or small-intestinal bacterial overgrowth.

TREATMENT INDIGESTION

GENERAL PRINCIPLES

For mild indigestion, reassurance that a careful evaluation revealed no serious organic disease may be the only intervention needed. Drugs that cause gastroesophageal reflux or dyspepsia should be stopped, if possible. Patients with GERD should limit ethanol, caffeine, chocolate, and tobacco use due to their effects on the LES. Other measures in GERD include ingesting a low-fat diet, avoiding snacks before bedtime, and elevating the head of the bed. Patients with functional dyspepsia also may be advised to reduce intake of fat, spicy foods, caffeine, and alcohol.

Specific therapies for organic disease should be offered when possible. Surgery is appropriate for biliary colic, whereas diet changes are indicated for lactase deficiency or celiac disease. Peptic ulcers may be cured by specific medical regimens. However, because most indigestion is caused by GERD or functional dyspepsia, medications that reduce gastric acid, modulate motility, or blunt gastric sensitivity are used.

ACID-SUPPRESSING OR -NEUTRALIZING MEDICATIONS

Drugs that reduce or neutralize gastric acid are often prescribed for GERD. Histamine H_2 antagonists like cimetidine, ranitidine, famotidine, and nizatidine are useful in mild to moderate GERD. For severe symptoms or for many cases of erosive or ulcerative esophagitis, PPIs such as omeprazole, lansoprazole, rabeprazole, pantoprazole, esomeprazole, or dexlansoprazole are needed. These drugs inhibit gastric H^+, K^+-ATPase and are more potent than H_2 antagonists. Up to one-third of GERD patients do not respond to standard PPI doses; one-third of these patients have nonacidic reflux, whereas 10% have persistent acid-related disease. Furthermore, heartburn typically responds better to PPI therapy than regurgitation or atypical GERD symptoms. Some individuals respond to doubling of the PPI dose or adding an H_2 antagonist at bedtime. Infrequent complications of long-term PPI therapy include infection, diarrhea (from *Clostridium difficile* infection or microscopic colitis), small-intestinal bacterial overgrowth, nutrient deficiency (vitamin B_{12}, iron, calcium), hypomagnesemia, bone demineralization, interstitial nephritis, and impaired medication absorption (e.g., clopidogrel). Many patients started on a PPI can be stepped down to an H_2 antagonist or be switched to an on-demand schedule.

Acid-suppressing drugs are also effective in selected patients with functional dyspepsia. A meta-analysis of eight controlled trials calculated a risk ratio of 0.86, with a 95% confidence interval of 0.78–0.95, favoring PPI therapy over placebo. H_2 antagonists also reportedly improve symptoms in functional dyspepsia; however, findings of trials of this drug class likely are influenced by inclusion of large numbers of GERD patients.

Antacids are useful for short-term control of mild GERD but have less benefit in severe cases unless given at high doses that cause side effects (diarrhea and constipation with magnesium- and aluminum-containing agents, respectively). Alginic acid combined with antacids forms a floating barrier to reflux in patients with upright symptoms. Sucralfate, a salt of aluminum hydroxide and sucrose octasulfate that buffers acid and binds pepsin and bile salts, shows efficacy in GERD similar to H_2 antagonists.

HELICOBACTER PYLORI ERADICATION

H. pylori eradication is definitively indicated only for peptic ulcer and mucosa-associated lymphoid tissue gastric lymphoma. The utility of eradication therapy in functional dyspepsia is limited, although some cases (particularly with the epigastric pain syndrome subtype) relate to this infection. A meta-analysis of 18 controlled trials calculated a relative risk reduction of 10%, with a 95% confidence interval of 6–14%, favoring *H. pylori* eradication over placebo. Most drug combinations (Chaps. 188 and 348) include 10–14 days of a PPI or bismuth subsalicylate in concert with two antibiotics. *H. pylori* infection is associated with reduced prevalence of GERD, especially in the elderly. However, eradication of the infection does not worsen GERD symptoms. No consensus recommendations regarding *H. pylori* eradication in GERD patients have been offered.

AGENTS THAT MODIFY GASTROINTESTINAL MOTOR ACTIVITY

Prokinetics like metoclopramide, erythromycin, and domperidone have limited utility in GERD. The γ-aminobutyric acid B (GABA-B) agonist baclofen reduces esophageal exposure to acid and nonacidic fluids by reducing TLESRs by 40%; this drug is proposed for refractory acid and nonacid reflux. Several studies have promoted the efficacy of motor-stimulating drugs in functional dyspepsia, but publication bias and small sample sizes raise questions about reported benefits of these agents. Some clinicians suggest that patients with the postprandial distress subtype may respond preferentially to prokinetic drugs. The 5-HT_1 agonist buspirone may improve some functional dyspepsia symptoms by enhancing meal-induced gastric accommodation. Acotiamide promotes gastric emptying and augments accommodation by enhancing gastric acetylcholine release via muscarinic receptor antagonism and acetylcholinesterase inhibition. This agent is approved for functional dyspepsia in Japan and is in testing elsewhere.

OTHER OPTIONS

Antireflux surgery (fundoplication) to increase LES pressure may be offered to GERD patients who are young and require lifelong therapy, have typical heartburn and regurgitation, are responsive to PPIs, and show evidence of acid reflux on pH monitoring. Surgery also is effective for some cases of nonacidic reflux. Individuals who respond less well to fundoplication include those with atypical symptoms or who have esophageal body motor disturbances. Dysphagia, gas-bloat syndrome, and gastroparesis are long-term complications of these procedures; ~60% develop recurrent GERD symptoms over time. The utility and safety of endoscopic therapies (radiofrequency ablation, transoral incisionless fundoplication) to enhance gastroesophageal barrier function have unproved durable benefits for refractory GERD.

Some patients with functional heartburn and functional dyspepsia refractory to standard therapies may respond to antidepressants in tricyclic and selective serotonin reuptake inhibitor classes, although studies are limited. Their mechanism of action may involve blunting of visceral pain processing in the brain. Gas and bloating are among the most troubling symptoms in some patients with indigestion and can be difficult to treat. Dietary exclusion of gas-producing foods such as legumes and use of simethicone or activated charcoal provide benefits in some cases. Low FODMAP (fermentable oligosaccharide, disaccharide, monosaccharide, and polyol) diets and therapies to modify gut flora (nonabsorbable antibiotics, probiotics) reduce gaseous symptoms in some IBS patients. The utility of low-FODMAP diets, antibiotics, and probiotics in functional dyspepsia is unproven. Herbal remedies such as STW 5 (Iberogast, a mixture of nine herbal agents) are useful in some dyspeptic patients. Psychological treatments (e.g., behavioral therapy, psychotherapy, hypnotherapy) may be offered for refractory functional dyspepsia, but no convincing data confirm their efficacy.

55 Diarrhea and Constipation

Michael Camilleri, Joseph A. Murray

Diarrhea and constipation are exceedingly common and, together, exact an enormous toll in terms of mortality, morbidity, social inconvenience, loss of work productivity, and consumption of medical resources. Worldwide, >1 billion individuals suffer one or more episodes of acute diarrhea each year. Among the 100 million persons affected annually by acute diarrhea in the United States, nearly half must restrict activities, 10% consult physicians, ~250,000 require hospitalization, and ~5000 die (primarily the elderly). The annual economic burden to society may exceed $20 billion. Acute infectious diarrhea remains one of the most common causes of mortality in developing countries, particularly among impoverished infants, accounting for 1.8 million deaths per year. Recurrent, acute diarrhea in children in tropical countries results in environmental enteropathy with long-term impacts on physical and intellectual development.

Constipation, by contrast, is rarely associated with mortality and is exceedingly common in developed countries, leading to frequent self-medication and, in a third of those, to medical consultation. Population statistics on chronic diarrhea and constipation are more uncertain, perhaps due to variable definitions and reporting, but the frequency of these conditions is also high. United States population surveys put prevalence rates for chronic diarrhea at 2–7% and for chronic constipation at 12–19%, with women being affected twice as often as men. Diarrhea and constipation are among the most common patient complaints presenting to internists and primary care physicians, and they account for nearly 50% of referrals to gastroenterologists.

Although diarrhea and constipation may present as mere nuisance symptoms at one extreme, they can be severe or life-threatening at the other. Even mild symptoms may signal a serious underlying gastrointestinal lesion, such as colorectal cancer, or systemic disorder, such as thyroid disease. Given the heterogeneous causes and potential severity of these common complaints, it is imperative for clinicians to appreciate the pathophysiology, etiologic classification, diagnostic strategies, and principles of management of diarrhea and constipation, so that rational and cost-effective care can be delivered.

NORMAL PHYSIOLOGY

While the primary function of the small intestine is the digestion and assimilation of nutrients from food, the small intestine and colon together perform important functions that regulate the secretion and absorption of water and electrolytes, the storage and subsequent transport of intraluminal contents aborally, and the salvage of some nutrients that are not absorbed in the small intestine after bacterial metabolism of carbohydrate allows salvage of short-chain fatty acids. The main motor functions are summarized in Table 55-1. Alterations in fluid and electrolyte handling contribute significantly to diarrhea. Alterations in motor and sensory functions of the colon result in highly prevalent syndromes such as irritable bowel syndrome (IBS), chronic diarrhea, and chronic constipation.

TABLE 55-1 NORMAL GASTROINTESTINAL MOTILITY: FUNCTIONS AT DIFFERENT ANATOMIC LEVELS

Stomach and Small Bowel
Synchronized MMC in fasting
Accommodation, trituration, mixing, transit
Stomach ~3 h
Small bowel ~3 h
Ileal reservoir empties boluses
Colon: Irregular Mixing, Fermentation, Absorption, Transit
Ascending, transverse: reservoirs
Descending: conduit
Sigmoid/rectum: volitional reservoir

Abbreviation: MMC, migrating motor complex.

NEURAL CONTROL

The small intestine and colon have intrinsic and extrinsic innervation. The *intrinsic innervation*, also called the enteric nervous system, comprises myenteric, submucosal, and mucosal neuronal layers. The function of these layers is modulated by interneurons through the actions of neurotransmitter amines or peptides, including acetylcholine, vasoactive intestinal peptide (VIP), opioids, norepinephrine, serotonin, adenosine triphosphate (ATP), and nitric oxide (NO). The myenteric plexus regulates smooth-muscle function through intermediary pacemaker-like cells called the interstitial cells of Cajal, and the submucosal plexus affects secretion, absorption, and mucosal blood flow. The enteric nervous system receives input from the extrinsic nerves, but it is capable of independent control of these functions.

The *extrinsic innervations* of the small intestine and colon are part of the autonomic nervous system and also modulate motor and secretory functions. The parasympathetic nerves convey visceral sensory pathways from and excitatory pathways to the small intestine and colon. Parasympathetic fibers via the vagus nerve reach the small intestine and proximal colon along the branches of the superior mesenteric artery. The distal colon is supplied by sacral parasympathetic nerves (S_{2-4}) via the pelvic plexus; these fibers course through the wall of the colon as ascending intracolonic fibers as far as, and in some instances including, the proximal colon. The chief excitatory neurotransmitters controlling motor function are acetylcholine and the tachykinins, such as substance P. The sympathetic nerve supply modulates motor functions and reaches the small intestine and colon alongside their arterial vessels. Sympathetic input to the gut is generally excitatory to sphincters and inhibitory to non-sphincteric muscle. Visceral afferents convey sensation from the gut to the central nervous system (CNS); initially, they course along sympathetic fibers, but as they approach the spinal cord they separate, have cell bodies in the dorsal root ganglion, and enter the dorsal horn of the spinal cord. Afferent signals are conveyed to the brain along the lateral spinothalamic tract and the nociceptive dorsal column pathway and are then projected beyond the thalamus and brainstem to the insula and cerebral cortex to be perceived. Other afferent fibers synapse in the prevertebral ganglia and reflexly modulate intestinal motility, blood flow, and secretion.

INTESTINAL FLUID ABSORPTION AND SECRETION

On an average day, 9 L of fluid enter the gastrointestinal (GI) tract, ~1 L of residual fluid reaches the colon, and the stool excretion of fluid constitutes about 0.2 L/d. The colon has a large capacitance and functional reserve and may recover up to four times its usual volume of 0.8 L/d, provided the rate of flow permits reabsorption to occur. Thus, the colon can partially compensate for excess fluid delivery to the colon that may result from intestinal absorptive or secretory disorders.

In the small intestine and colon, sodium absorption is predominantly electrogenic (i.e., it can be measured as an ionic current across the membrane because there is not an equivalent loss of a cation from the cell), and uptake takes place at the apical membrane; it is compensated for by the export functions of the basolateral sodium pump. There are several active transport proteins at the apical membrane, especially in the small intestine, whereby sodium ion entry is coupled to monosaccharides (e.g., glucose through the transporter SGLT1, or fructose through GLUT-5). Glucose then exits the basal membrane through a specific transport protein, GLUT-5, creating a glucose concentration gradient between the lumen and the intercellular space, drawing water and electrolytes passively from the lumen. A variety of neural and nonneural mediators regulate colonic fluid and electrolyte balance, including cholinergic, adrenergic, and serotonergic mediators. Angiotensin and aldosterone also influence colonic absorption, reflecting the common embryologic development of the distal colonic epithelium and the renal tubules.

SMALL-INTESTINAL MOTILITY

During the fasting period, the motility of the small intestine is characterized by a cyclical event called the migrating motor complex (MMC), which serves to clear nondigestible residue from the small intestine (the intestinal "housekeeper"). This organized, propagated series of contractions lasts, on average, 4 min, occurs every 60–90 min, and usually involves the entire small intestine. After food ingestion, the small intestine produces irregular, mixing contractions of relatively low amplitude, except in the distal ileum where more powerful contractions occur intermittently and empty the ileum by bolus transfers.

ILEOCOLONIC STORAGE AND SALVAGE

The distal ileum acts as a reservoir, emptying intermittently by bolus movements. This action allows time for salvage of fluids, electrolytes, and nutrients. Segmentation by haustra compartmentalizes the colon and facilitates mixing, retention of residue, and formation of solid stools. There is increased appreciation of the intimate interaction between the colonic function and the luminal ecology. The resident microorganisms, predominantly anaerobic bacteria, in the colon are necessary for the digestion of unabsorbed carbohydrates that reach the colon even in health, thereby providing a vital source of nutrients to the mucosa. Normal colonic flora also keeps pathogens at bay by a variety of mechanisms. In health, the ascending and transverse regions of colon function as reservoirs (average transit time, 15 h), and the descending colon acts as a conduit (average transit time, 3 h). The colon is efficient at conserving sodium and water, a function that is particularly important in sodium-depleted patients in whom the small intestine alone is unable to maintain sodium balance. Diarrhea or constipation may result from alteration in the reservoir function of the proximal colon or the propulsive function of the left colon. Constipation may also result from disturbances of the rectal or sigmoid reservoir, typically as a result of dysfunction of the pelvic floor, the anal sphincters, the coordination of defecation, or dehydration.

COLONIC MOTILITY AND TONE

The small intestinal MMC only rarely continues into the colon. However, short duration or phasic contractions mix colonic contents, and high-amplitude (>75 mmHg) propagated contractions (HAPCs) are sometimes associated with mass movements through the colon and normally occur approximately five times per day, usually on awakening in the morning and postprandially. Increased frequency of HAPCs may result in diarrhea or urgency. The predominant phasic contractions in the colon are irregular and non-propagated and serve a "mixing" function.

Colonic tone refers to the background contractility upon which phasic contractile activity (typically contractions lasting <15 s) is superimposed. It is an important cofactor in the colon's capacitance (volume accommodation) and sensation.

COLONIC MOTILITY AFTER MEAL INGESTION

After meal ingestion, colonic phasic and tonic contractility increase for a period of ~2 h. The initial phase (~10 min) is mediated by the vagus nerve in response to mechanical distention of the stomach. The subsequent response of the colon requires caloric stimulation (e.g., intake of at least 500 kcal) and is mediated, at least in part, by hormones (e.g., gastrin and serotonin).

DEFECATION

Tonic contraction of the puborectalis muscle, which forms a sling around the rectoanal junction, is important to maintain continence; during defecation, sacral parasympathetic nerves relax this muscle, facilitating the straightening of the rectoanal angle (Fig. 55-1). Distention of the rectum results in transient relaxation of the internal anal sphincter via intrinsic and reflex sympathetic innervation. As sigmoid and rectal contractions, as well as straining (Valsalva maneuver), which increases intraabdominal pressure, increase the pressure within the rectum, the rectosigmoid angle opens by >15°. Voluntary relaxation of the external anal sphincter (striated muscle innervated by the pudendal nerve) in response to the sensation produced by distention permits the evacuation of feces. Defecation can also be delayed voluntarily by contraction of the external anal sphincter.

DIARRHEA

DEFINITION

Diarrhea is loosely defined as passage of abnormally liquid or unformed stools at an increased frequency. For adults on a typical Western diet, stool weight >200 g/d can generally be considered diarrheal. Diarrhea may be further defined as *acute* if <2 weeks, *persistent* if 2–4 weeks, and *chronic* if >4 weeks in duration.

Two common conditions, usually associated with the passage of stool totaling <200 g/d, must be distinguished from diarrhea, because diagnostic and therapeutic algorithms differ. *Pseudodiarrhea*, or the frequent passage of small volumes of stool, is often associated with rectal urgency, tenesmus, or a feeling of incomplete evacuation, and accompanies IBS or proctitis. *Fecal incontinence* is the involuntary discharge of rectal contents and is most often caused by neuromuscular disorders or structural anorectal problems. Diarrhea and urgency, especially if severe, may aggravate or cause incontinence. Pseudodiarrhea and fecal incontinence occur at prevalence rates comparable to or higher than that of chronic diarrhea and should always be considered in patients complaining of "diarrhea." Overflow diarrhea may occur in nursing home patients due to fecal impaction that is readily detectable by rectal examination. A careful history and physical examination generally allow these conditions to be discriminated from true diarrhea.

ACUTE DIARRHEA

More than 90% of cases of acute diarrhea are caused by infectious agents; these cases are often accompanied by vomiting, fever, and abdominal pain. The remaining 10% or so are caused by medications, toxic ingestions, ischemia, food indiscretions, and other conditions.

Infectious Agents Most infectious diarrheas are acquired by fecal-oral transmission or, more commonly, via ingestion of food or water contaminated with pathogens from human or animal feces. In the immunocompetent person, the resident fecal microflora, containing >500 taxonomically distinct species, are rarely the source of diarrhea

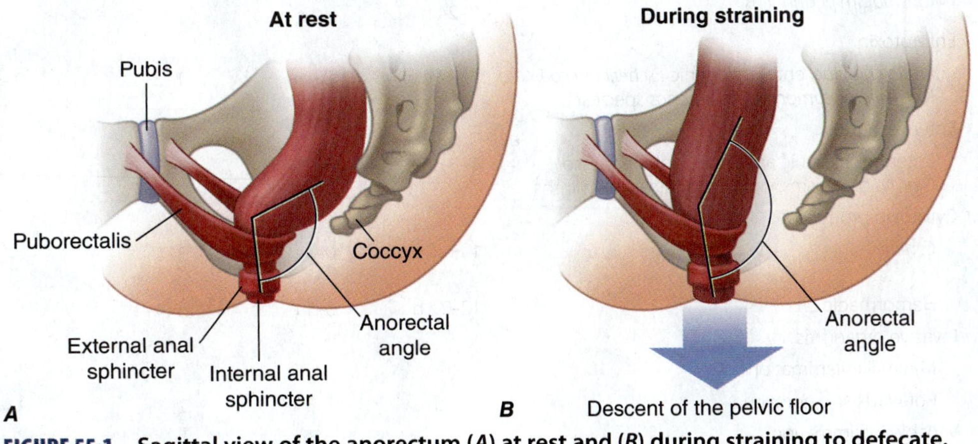

FIGURE 55-1 Sagittal view of the anorectum (*A*) at rest and (*B*) during straining to defecate. Continence is maintained by normal rectal sensation and tonic contraction of the internal anal sphincter and the puborectalis muscle, which wraps around the anorectum, maintaining an anorectal angle between 80° and 110°. During defecation, the pelvic floor muscles (including the puborectalis) relax, allowing the anorectal angle to straighten by at least 15°, and the perineum descends by 1–3.5 cm. The external anal sphincter also relaxes and reduces pressure on the anal canal. *(Reproduced with permission from A Lembo, M Camilleri: N Engl J Med 349:1360, 2003.)*

and may actually play a role in suppressing the growth of ingested pathogens. Disturbances of flora by antibiotics can lead to diarrhea by reducing the digestive function or by allowing the overgrowth of pathogens, such as *Clostridium difficile* (Chap. 161). Acute infection or injury occurs when the ingested agent overwhelms or bypasses the host's mucosal immune and nonimmune (gastric acid, digestive enzymes, mucus secretion, peristalsis, and suppressive resident flora) defenses. Established clinical associations with specific enteropathogens may offer diagnostic clues.

In the United States, five high-risk groups are recognized:

1. *Travelers.* Nearly 40% of tourists to endemic regions of Latin America, Africa, and Asia develop so-called traveler's diarrhea, most commonly due to enterotoxigenic or enteroaggregative *Escherichia coli* as well as to *Campylobacter*, *Shigella*, *Aeromonas*, norovirus, *Coronavirus*, and *Salmonella*. Visitors to Russia (especially St. Petersburg) may have increased risk of *Giardia*-associated diarrhea; visitors to Nepal may acquire *Cyclospora*. Campers, backpackers, and swimmers in wilderness areas may become infected with *Giardia*. Cruise ships may be affected by outbreaks of gastroenteritis caused by agents such as norovirus.
2. *Consumers of certain foods.* Diarrhea closely following food consumption at a picnic, banquet, or restaurant may suggest infection with *Salmonella*, *Campylobacter*, or *Shigella* from chicken; enterohemorrhagic *E. coli* (O157:H7) from undercooked hamburger; *Bacillus cereus* from fried rice or other reheated food; *Staphylococcus aureus* or *Salmonella* from mayonnaise or creams; *Salmonella* from eggs; *Listeria* from uncooked foods or soft cheeses; and *Vibrio* species, *Salmonella*, or acute hepatitis A from seafood, especially if raw. State departments of public health issue communications regarding food-related illnesses, which may have originated domestically or been imported, but ultimately cause epidemics in the United States (e.g., the *Cyclospora* epidemic of 2013 in midwestern states that resulted from bagged salads).
3. *Immunodeficient persons.* Individuals at risk for diarrhea include those with either primary immunodeficiency (e.g., IgA deficiency, common variable hypogammaglobulinemia, chronic granulomatous disease) or the much more common secondary immunodeficiency states (e.g., AIDS, senescence, pharmacologic suppression). Common enteric pathogens often cause a more severe and protracted diarrheal illness, and, particularly in persons with AIDS, opportunistic infections, such as by *Mycobacterium* species, certain viruses (cytomegalovirus, adenovirus, and herpes simplex), and protozoa (*Cryptosporidium*, *Isospora belli*, Microsporida, and *Blastocystis hominis*) may also play a role (Chap. 226). In patients with AIDS, agents transmitted venereally per rectum (e.g., *Neisseria gonorrhoeae*, *Treponema pallidum*, *Chlamydia*) may contribute to proctocolitis. Persons with hemochromatosis are especially prone to invasive, even fatal, enteric infections with *Vibrio* species and *Yersinia* infections and should avoid raw fish.
4. *Daycare attendees and their family members.* Infections with *Shigella*, *Giardia*, *Cryptosporidium*, rotavirus, and other agents are very common and should be considered.
5. *Institutionalized persons.* Infectious diarrhea is one of the most frequent categories of nosocomial infections in many hospitals and long-term care facilities; the causes are a variety of microorganisms but most commonly *C. difficile*. *C. difficile* can affect those with no history of antibiotic use and may be acquired in the community.

The pathophysiology underlying acute diarrhea by infectious agents produces specific clinical features that may also be helpful in diagnosis (Table 55-2). Profuse, watery diarrhea secondary to small-bowel hypersecretion occurs with ingestion of preformed bacterial toxins, enterotoxin-producing bacteria, and enteroadherent pathogens. Diarrhea associated with marked vomiting and minimal or no fever may occur abruptly within a few hours after ingestion of the former two types; vomiting is usually less, abdominal cramping or bloating is greater, and fever is higher with the latter. Cytotoxin-producing and invasive microorganisms all cause high fever and abdominal pain. Invasive bacteria and *Entamoeba histolytica* often cause bloody diarrhea (referred to as *dysentery*). *Yersinia* invades the terminal ileal and proximal colon mucosa and may cause especially severe abdominal pain with tenderness mimicking acute appendicitis.

Finally, infectious diarrhea may be associated with systemic manifestations. Reactive arthritis (formerly known as Reiter's syndrome), arthritis, urethritis, and conjunctivitis may accompany or follow

TABLE 55-2 ASSOCIATION BETWEEN PATHOBIOLOGY OF CAUSATIVE AGENTS AND CLINICAL FEATURES IN ACUTE INFECTIOUS DIARRHEA

Pathobiology/Agents	Incubation Period	Vomiting	Abdominal Pain	Fever	Diarrhea
Toxin producers					
Preformed toxin					
Bacillus cereus, Staphylococcus aureus, Clostridium perfringens	1–8 h 8–24 h	3–4+	1–2+	0–1+	3–4+, watery
Enterotoxin					
Vibrio cholerae, enterotoxigenic *Escherichia coli*, *Klebsiella pneumoniae*, *Aeromonas* species	8–72 h	2–4+	1–2+	0–1+	3–4+, watery
Enteroadherent					
Enteropathogenic and enteroadherent *E. coli*, *Giardia* organisms, cryptosporidiosis, helminths	1–8 d	0–1+	1–3+	0–2+	1–2+, watery, mushy
Cytotoxin producers					
C. difficile	1–3 d	0–1+	3–4+	1–2+	1–3+, usually watery, occasionally bloody
Hemorrhagic *E. coli*	12–72 h	0–1+	3–4+	1–2+	1–3+, initially watery, quickly bloody
Invasive organisms					
Minimal inflammation					
Rotavirus and norovirus	1–3 d	1–3+	2–3+	3–4+	1–3+, watery
Variable inflammation					
Salmonella, *Campylobacter*, and *Aeromonas* species, *Vibrio parahaemolyticus*, *Yersinia*	12 h–11 d	0–3+	2–4+	3–4+	1–4+, watery or bloody
Severe inflammation					
Shigella species, enteroinvasive *E. coli*, *Entamoeba histolytica*	12 h–8 d	0–1+	3–4+	3–4+	1–2+, bloody

Source: Adapted from DW Powell, in T Yamada (ed): *Textbook of Gastroenterology and Hepatology*, 4th ed. Philadelphia, Lippincott Williams & Wilkins, 2003.

infections by *Salmonella*, *Campylobacter*, *Shigella*, and *Yersinia*. Yersiniosis may also lead to an autoimmune-type thyroiditis, pericarditis, and glomerulonephritis. Both enterohemorrhagic *E. coli* (O157:H7) and *Shigella* can lead to the *hemolytic-uremic syndrome* with an attendant high mortality rate. The syndrome of postinfectious IBS has now been recognized as a complication of infectious diarrhea. Similarly, acute gastroenteritis may precede the diagnosis of celiac disease or Crohn's disease. Acute diarrhea can also be a major symptom of several systemic infections including *viral hepatitis*, *listeriosis*, *legionellosis*, and *toxic shock syndrome*.

Other Causes Side effects from medications are probably the most common noninfectious causes of acute diarrhea, and etiology may be suggested by a temporal association between use and symptom onset. Although innumerable medications may produce diarrhea, some of the more frequently incriminated include antibiotics, cardiac antidysrhythmics, antihypertensives, nonsteroidal anti-inflammatory drugs (NSAIDs), certain antidepressants, chemotherapeutic agents, bronchodilators, antacids, and laxatives. Occlusive or nonocclusive *ischemic colitis* typically occurs in persons >50 years; often presents as acute lower abdominal pain preceding watery, then bloody diarrhea; and generally results in acute inflammatory changes in the sigmoid or left colon while sparing the rectum. Acute diarrhea may accompany colonic *diverticulitis* and *graft-versus-host disease*. Acute diarrhea, often associated with systemic compromise, can follow ingestion of toxins including organophosphate insecticides; amanita and other mushrooms; arsenic; and preformed environmental toxins in seafood, such as ciguatera and scombroid. Acute anaphylaxis to food ingestion can have a similar presentation. Conditions causing chronic diarrhea can also be confused with acute diarrhea early in their course. This confusion may occur with inflammatory bowel disease (IBD) and some of the other inflammatory chronic diarrheas that may have an abrupt rather than insidious onset and exhibit features that mimic infection.

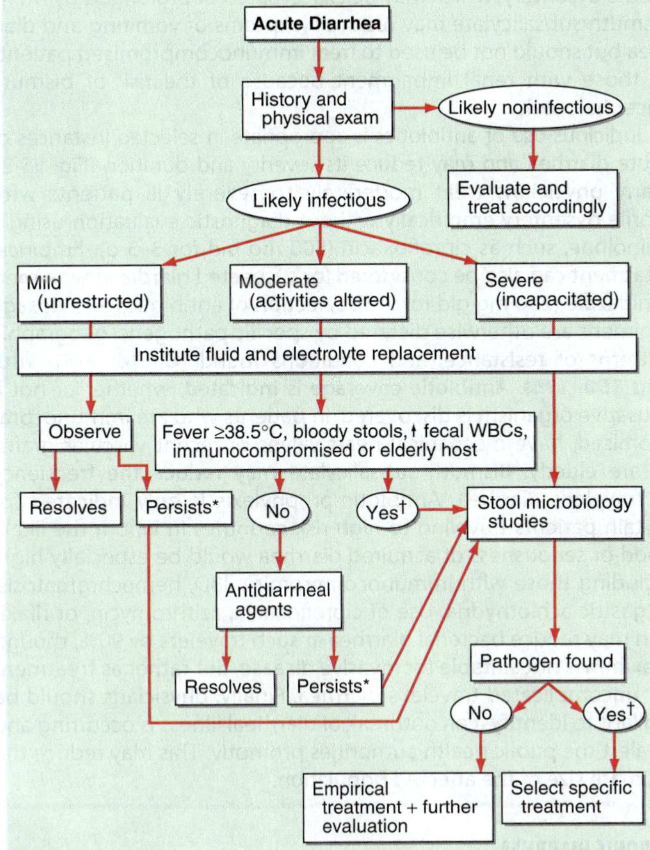

FIGURE 55-2 Algorithm for the management of acute diarrhea. Consider empirical treatment before evaluation with (*) metronidazole and with (†) quinolone. WBCs, white blood cells.

APPROACH TO THE PATIENT: Acute Diarrhea

The decision to evaluate acute diarrhea depends on its severity and duration and on various host factors (Fig. 55-2). Most episodes of acute diarrhea are mild and self-limited and do not justify the cost and potential morbidity rate of diagnostic or pharmacologic interventions. Indications for evaluation include profuse diarrhea with dehydration, grossly bloody stools, fever ≥38.5°C (≥101°F), duration >48 h without improvement, recent antibiotic use, new community outbreaks, associated severe abdominal pain in patients >50 years, and elderly (≥70 years) or immunocompromised patients. In some cases of moderately severe febrile diarrhea associated with fecal leukocytes (or increased fecal levels of the leukocyte proteins, such as calprotectin) or with gross blood, a diagnostic evaluation might be avoided in favor of an empirical antibiotic trial (see below).

The cornerstone of diagnosis in those suspected of severe acute infectious diarrhea is microbiologic analysis of the stool. Workup includes cultures for bacterial and viral pathogens, direct inspection for ova and parasites, and immunoassays for certain bacterial toxins (*C. difficile*), viral antigens (rotavirus), and protozoal antigens (*Giardia*, *E. histolytica*). The aforementioned clinical and epidemiologic associations may assist in focusing the evaluation. If a particular pathogen or set of possible pathogens is so implicated, then either the whole panel of routine studies may not be necessary or, in some instances, special cultures may be appropriate as for enterohemorrhagic and other types of *E. coli*, *Vibrio* species, and *Yersinia*. Molecular diagnosis of pathogens in stool can be made by identification of unique DNA sequences; and evolving microarray technologies have led to more rapid, sensitive, specific, and cost-effective diagnosis.

Persistent diarrhea is commonly due to *Giardia* (Chap. 247), but additional causative organisms that should be considered include *C. difficile* (especially if antibiotics had been administered), *E. histolytica*, *Cryptosporidium*, *Campylobacter*, and others. If stool studies are unrevealing, flexible sigmoidoscopy with biopsies and upper endoscopy with duodenal aspirates and biopsies may be indicated. Brainerd diarrhea is an increasingly recognized entity characterized by an abrupt-onset diarrhea that persists for at least 4 weeks, but may last 1–3 years, and is thought to be of infectious origin. It may be associated with subtle inflammation of the distal small intestine or proximal colon.

Structural examination by sigmoidoscopy, colonoscopy, or abdominal computed tomography (CT) scanning (or other imaging approaches) may be appropriate in patients with uncharacterized persistent diarrhea to exclude IBD or as an initial approach in patients with suspected noninfectious acute diarrhea such as might be caused by ischemic colitis, diverticulitis, or partial bowel obstruction.

TREATMENT ACUTE DIARRHEA

Fluid and electrolyte replacement are of central importance to all forms of acute diarrhea. Fluid replacement alone may suffice for mild cases. Oral sugar-electrolyte solutions (iso-osmolar sport drinks or designed formulations) should be instituted promptly with severe diarrhea to limit dehydration, which is the major cause of death. Profoundly dehydrated patients, especially infants and the elderly, require IV rehydration.

In moderately severe nonfebrile and nonbloody diarrhea, antimotility and antisecretory agents such as loperamide can be useful adjuncts to control symptoms. Such agents should be avoided with febrile dysentery, which may be exacerbated or prolonged by them. Bismuth subsalicylate may reduce symptoms of vomiting and diarrhea but should not be used to treat immunocompromised patients or those with renal impairment because of the risk of bismuth encephalopathy.

Judicious use of antibiotics is appropriate in selected instances of acute diarrhea and may reduce its severity and duration (Fig. 55-2). Many physicians treat moderately to severely ill patients with febrile dysentery empirically without diagnostic evaluation using a quinolone, such as ciprofloxacin (500 mg bid for 3–5 d). Empirical treatment can also be considered for suspected giardiasis with metronidazole (250 mg qid for 7 d). Selection of antibiotics and dosage regimens are otherwise dictated by specific pathogens, geographic patterns of resistance, and conditions found **(Chaps. 160, 186, and 190–196)**. Antibiotic coverage is indicated, whether or not a causative organism is discovered, in patients who are immunocompromised, have mechanical heart valves or recent vascular grafts, or are elderly. Bismuth subsalicylate may reduce the frequency of traveler's diarrhea. Antibiotic prophylaxis is only indicated for certain patients traveling to high-risk countries in whom the likelihood or seriousness of acquired diarrhea would be especially high, including those with immunocompromise, IBD, hemochromatosis, or gastric achlorhydria. Use of ciprofloxacin, azithromycin, or rifaximin may reduce bacterial diarrhea in such travelers by 90%, though rifaximin is not suitable for invasive disease, but rather as treatment for uncomplicated traveler's diarrhea. Finally, physicians should be vigilant to identify if an outbreak of diarrheal illness is occurring and to alert the public health authorities promptly. This may reduce the ultimate size of the affected population.

CHRONIC DIARRHEA

Diarrhea lasting >4 weeks warrants evaluation to exclude serious underlying pathology. In contrast to acute diarrhea, most of the causes of chronic diarrhea are noninfectious. The classification of chronic diarrhea by pathophysiologic mechanism facilitates a rational approach to management, although many diseases cause diarrhea by more than one mechanism (Table 55-3).

Secretory Causes Secretory diarrheas are due to derangements in fluid and electrolyte transport across the enterocolonic mucosa. They are characterized clinically by watery, large-volume fecal outputs that are typically painless and persist with fasting. Because there is no malabsorbed solute, stool osmolality is accounted for by normal endogenous electrolytes with no fecal osmotic gap.

MEDICATIONS Side effects from regular ingestion of drugs and toxins are the most common secretory causes of chronic diarrhea. Hundreds of prescription and over-the-counter medications (see earlier section, "Acute Diarrhea, Other Causes") may produce diarrhea. Surreptitious or habitual use of stimulant laxatives (e.g., senna, cascara, bisacodyl, ricinoleic acid [castor oil]) must also be considered. Chronic ethanol consumption may cause a secretory-type diarrhea due to enterocyte injury with impaired sodium and water absorption as well as rapid transit and other alterations. Inadvertent ingestion of certain environmental toxins (e.g., arsenic) may lead to chronic rather than acute forms of diarrhea. Certain bacterial infections may occasionally persist and be associated with a secretory-type diarrhea.

BOWEL RESECTION, MUCOSAL DISEASE, OR ENTEROCOLIC FISTULA These conditions may result in a secretory-type diarrhea because of inadequate surface for reabsorption of secreted fluids and electrolytes. Unlike other secretory diarrheas, this subset of conditions tends to worsen with eating. With disease (e.g., Crohn's ileitis) or resection of <100 cm of terminal ileum, dihydroxy bile acids may escape absorption and stimulate colonic secretion (cholerheic diarrhea). This mechanism may contribute to so-called *idiopathic secretory diarrhea or bile acid diarrhea (BAD)*, in which bile acids are functionally malabsorbed from a normal-appearing terminal ileum. This *idiopathic bile acid malabsorption (BAM)* may account for an average of 40% of unexplained chronic diarrhea. Reduced negative feedback regulation of bile acid synthesis in hepatocytes by fibroblast growth factor 19 (FGF-19) produced by ileal enterocytes results in a degree of bile-acid synthesis that exceeds the normal capacity for ileal reabsorption, producing BAD. An alternative cause of BAD is a genetic variation in the receptor proteins (β-klotho and fibroblast growth factor 4) on the hepatocyte that normally mediate the effect of FGF-19. Dysfunction of these proteins prevents FGF-19 inhibition of hepatocyte bile acid synthesis.

TABLE 55-3 MAJOR CAUSES OF CHRONIC DIARRHEA ACCORDING TO PREDOMINANT PATHOPHYSIOLOGIC MECHANISM

Secretory Causes
Exogenous stimulant laxatives
Chronic ethanol ingestion
Other drugs and toxins
Endogenous laxatives (dihydroxy bile acids)
Idiopathic secretory diarrhea or bile acid diarrhea
Certain bacterial infections
Bowel resection, disease, or fistula (↓ absorption)
Partial bowel obstruction or fecal impaction
Hormone-producing tumors (carcinoid, VIPoma, medullary cancer of thyroid, mastocytosis, gastrinoma, colorectal villous adenoma)
Addison's disease
Congenital electrolyte absorption defects
Osmotic Causes
Osmotic laxatives (Mg^{2+}, PO_4^{-3}, SO_4^{-2})
Lactase and other disaccharide deficiencies
Nonabsorbable carbohydrates (sorbitol, lactulose, polyethylene glycol)
Gluten and FODMAP intolerance
Steatorrheal Causes
Intraluminal maldigestion (pancreatic exocrine insufficiency, bacterial overgrowth, bariatric surgery, liver disease)
Mucosal malabsorption (celiac sprue, Whipple's disease, infections, abetalipoproteinemia, ischemia, drug-induced enteropathy)
Postmucosal obstruction (1° or 2° lymphatic obstruction)
Inflammatory Causes
Idiopathic inflammatory bowel disease (Crohn's, chronic ulcerative colitis)
Lymphocytic and collagenous colitis
Immune-related mucosal disease (1° or 2° immunodeficiencies, food allergy, eosinophilic gastroenteritis, graft-versus-host disease)
Infections (invasive bacteria, viruses, and parasites, Brainerd diarrhea)
Radiation injury
Gastrointestinal malignancies
Dysmotile Causes
Irritable bowel syndrome (including postinfectious IBS)
Visceral neuromyopathies
Hyperthyroidism
Drugs (prokinetic agents)
Postvagotomy
Factitial Causes
Munchausen
Eating disorders
Iatrogenic Causes
Cholecystectomy
Ileal resection
Bariatric surgery
Vagotomy, fundoplication

Abbreviation: FODMAP, fermentable oligosaccharides, disaccharides, monosaccharides, and polyols.

Partial bowel obstruction, ostomy stricture, or fecal impaction may paradoxically lead to increased fecal output due to fluid hypersecretion.

HORMONES Although uncommon, the classic examples of secretory diarrhea are those mediated by hormones. *Metastatic gastrointestinal* *carcinoid tumors* or, rarely, *primary bronchial carcinoids* may produce watery diarrhea alone or as part of the carcinoid syndrome that comprises episodic flushing, wheezing, dyspnea, and right-sided valvular heart disease. Diarrhea is due to the release into the circulation of potent intestinal secretagogues including serotonin, histamine, prostaglandins, and various kinins. Pellagra-like skin lesions may rarely occur as the result of serotonin overproduction with niacin depletion. *Gastrinoma*, one of the most common neuroendocrine tumors, most typically presents with refractory peptic ulcers, but diarrhea occurs in up to one-third of cases and may be the only clinical manifestation in 10%. While other secretagogues released with gastrin may play a role, the diarrhea most often results from fat maldigestion owing to pancreatic enzyme inactivation by low intraduodenal pH. The watery diarrhea hypokalemia achlorhydria syndrome, also called *pancreatic cholera*, is due to a non-β cell pancreatic adenoma, referred to as a *VIPoma*, that secretes VIP and a host of other peptide hormones including pancreatic polypeptide, secretin, gastrin, gastrin-inhibitory polypeptide (also called glucose-dependent insulinotropic peptide), neurotensin, calcitonin, and prostaglandins. The secretory diarrhea is often massive with stool volumes >3 L/d; daily volumes as high as 20 L have been reported. Life-threatening dehydration; neuromuscular dysfunction from associated hypokalemia, hypomagnesemia, or hypercalcemia; flushing; and hyperglycemia may accompany a VIPoma. *Medullary carcinoma of the thyroid* may present with watery diarrhea caused by calcitonin, other secretory peptides, or prostaglandins. Prominent diarrhea is often associated with metastatic disease and poor prognosis. *Systemic mastocytosis*, which may be associated with the skin lesion urticaria pigmentosa, may cause diarrhea that is either secretory and mediated by histamine or inflammatory due to intestinal infiltration by mast cells. Large *colorectal villous adenomas* may rarely be associated with a secretory diarrhea that may cause hypokalemia, can be inhibited by NSAIDs, and are apparently mediated by prostaglandins.

CONGENITAL DEFECTS IN ION ABSORPTION Rarely, defects in specific carriers associated with ion absorption cause watery diarrhea from birth. These disorders include defective Cl^-/HCO_3^- exchange (*congenital chloridorrhea*) with alkalosis (which results from a mutated *DRA* [down-regulated in adenoma] gene) and defective Na^+/H^+ exchange (*congenital sodium diarrhea)*, which results from a mutation in the *NHE3* (sodium-hydrogen exchanger) gene and results in acidosis.

Some hormone deficiencies may be associated with watery diarrhea, such as occurs with adrenocortical insufficiency (Addison's disease) that may be accompanied by skin hyperpigmentation.

Osmotic Causes Osmotic diarrhea occurs when ingested, poorly absorbable, osmotically active solutes draw enough fluid into the lumen to exceed the reabsorptive capacity of the colon. Fecal water output increases in proportion to such a solute load. Osmotic diarrhea characteristically ceases with fasting or with discontinuation of the causative agent.

OSMOTIC LAXATIVES Ingestion of magnesium-containing antacids, health supplements, or laxatives may induce osmotic diarrhea typified by a stool osmotic gap (>50 mosmol/L): serum osmolarity (typically 290 mosmol/kg) − (2 × [fecal sodium + potassium concentration]). Measurement of fecal osmolarity is no longer recommended because, even when measured immediately after evacuation, it may be erroneous because carbohydrates are metabolized by colonic bacteria, causing an increase in osmolarity.

CARBOHYDRATE MALABSORPTION Carbohydrate malabsorption due to acquired or congenital defects in brush-border disaccharidases and other enzymes leads to osmotic diarrhea with a low pH. One of the most common causes of chronic diarrhea in adults is *lactase deficiency*, which affects three-fourths of nonwhites worldwide and 5–30% of persons in the United States; the total lactose load at any one time influences the symptoms experienced. Most patients learn to avoid milk products without requiring treatment with enzyme supplements. Some sugars, such as sorbitol, lactulose, or fructose, are frequently malabsorbed, and diarrhea ensues with ingestion of medications, gum, or candies sweetened with these poorly or incompletely absorbed sugars.

WHEAT AND FODMAP INTOLERANCE Chronic diarrhea, bloating, and abdominal pain are recognized as symptoms of nonceliac gluten intolerance (which is associated with impaired intestinal or colonic barrier function) and intolerance of fermentable oligosaccharides, disaccharides, monosaccharides, and polyols (FODMAPs). The latter's effects represent the interaction between the GI microbiome and the nutrients.

Steatorrheal Causes Fat malabsorption may lead to greasy, foul-smelling, difficult-to-flush diarrhea often associated with weight loss and nutritional deficiencies due to concomitant malabsorption of amino acids and vitamins. Increased fecal output is caused by the osmotic effects of fatty acids, especially after bacterial hydroxylation, and, to a lesser extent, by the neutral fat. Quantitatively, steatorrhea is defined as stool fat exceeding the normal 7 g/d; rapid-transit diarrhea may result in fecal fat up to 14 g/d; daily fecal fat averages 15–25 g with small-intestinal diseases and is often >32 g with pancreatic exocrine insufficiency. Intraluminal maldigestion, mucosal malabsorption, or lymphatic obstruction may produce steatorrhea.

INTRALUMINAL MALDIGESTION This condition most commonly results from pancreatic exocrine insufficiency, which occurs when >90% of pancreatic secretory function is lost. *Chronic pancreatitis*, usually a sequel of ethanol abuse, most frequently causes pancreatic insufficiency. Other causes include *cystic fibrosis*; *pancreatic duct obstruction*; and, rarely, *somatostatinoma*. Bacterial overgrowth in the small intestine may deconjugate bile acids and alter micelle formation, impairing fat digestion; it occurs with stasis from a blind-loop, small-bowel diverticulum or dysmotility and is especially likely in the elderly. Finally, cirrhosis or biliary obstruction may lead to mild steatorrhea due to deficient intraluminal bile acid concentration.

MUCOSAL MALABSORPTION Mucosal malabsorption occurs from a variety of enteropathies, but it most commonly occurs from *celiac disease*. This gluten-sensitive enteropathy affects all ages and is characterized by villous atrophy and crypt hyperplasia in the proximal small bowel and can present with fatty diarrhea associated with multiple nutritional deficiencies of varying severity. Celiac disease is much more frequent than previously thought; it affects ~1% of the population, frequently presents without steatorrhea, can mimic IBS, and has many other GI and extraintestinal manifestations. *Tropical sprue* may produce a similar histologic and clinical syndrome but occurs in residents of or travelers to tropical climates; abrupt onset and response to antibiotics suggest an infectious etiology. *Whipple's disease*, due to the bacillus *Tropheryma whipplei* and histiocytic infiltration of the small-bowel mucosa, is a less common cause of steatorrhea that most typically occurs in young or middle-aged men; it is frequently associated with arthralgias, fever, lymphadenopathy, and extreme fatigue, and it may affect the CNS and endocardium. A similar clinical and histologic picture results from *Mycobacterium avium-intracellulare* infection in patients with AIDS. *Abetalipoproteinemia* is a rare defect of chylomicron formation and fat malabsorption in children, associated with acanthocytic erythrocytes, ataxia, and retinitis pigmentosa. Several other conditions may cause mucosal malabsorption including infections, especially with protozoa such as *Giardia*; numerous medications (e.g., olmesartan, mycophenolate mofetil, colchicine, cholestyramine, neomycin); amyloidosis; and chronic ischemia.

POSTMUCOSAL LYMPHATIC OBSTRUCTION The pathophysiology of this condition, which is due to the rare *congenital intestinal lymphangiectasia* or to *acquired lymphatic obstruction* secondary to trauma, tumor, cardiac disease or infection, leads to the unique constellation of fat malabsorption with enteric losses of protein (often causing edema) and lymphocytopenia. Carbohydrate and amino acid absorption are preserved.

Inflammatory Causes Inflammatory diarrheas are generally accompanied by pain, fever, bleeding, or other manifestations of inflammation. The mechanism of diarrhea may not only be exudation but, depending on lesion site, may include fat malabsorption, disrupted fluid/electrolyte absorption, and hypersecretion or hypermotility from release of cytokines and other inflammatory mediators. The unifying feature on stool analysis is the presence of leukocytes or leukocyte-derived proteins such as calprotectin. With severe inflammation, exudative protein loss can lead to anasarca (generalized edema). Any middle-aged or older person with chronic inflammatory-type diarrhea, especially with blood, should be carefully evaluated to exclude a colorectal tumor.

IDIOPATHIC INFLAMMATORY BOWEL DISEASE The illnesses in this category, which include *Crohn's disease* and *chronic ulcerative colitis*, are among the most common organic causes of chronic diarrhea in adults and range in severity from mild to fulminant and life-threatening. They may be associated with uveitis, polyarthralgias, cholestatic liver disease (primary sclerosing cholangitis), and skin lesions (erythema nodosum, pyoderma gangrenosum). *Microscopic colitis*, including both lymphocytic and *collagenous colitis*, is an increasingly recognized cause of chronic watery diarrhea, especially in middle-aged women and those on NSAIDs, statins, proton pump inhibitors (PPIs), and selective serotonin reuptake inhibitors (SSRIs); biopsy of a normal-appearing colon is required for histologic diagnosis. It may coexist with symptoms suggesting IBS or with celiac sprue or drug-induced enteropathy. It typically responds well to anti-inflammatory drugs (e.g., bismuth), to the opioid agonist loperamide, or to budesonide.

PRIMARY OR SECONDARY FORMS OF IMMUNODEFICIENCY Immunodeficiency may lead to prolonged infectious diarrhea. With selective IgA deficiency or common variable *hypogammaglobulinemia*, diarrhea is particularly prevalent and often the result of giardiasis, bacterial overgrowth, or sprue.

EOSINOPHILIC GASTROENTERITIS Eosinophil infiltration of the mucosa, muscularis, or serosa at any level of the GI tract may cause diarrhea, pain, vomiting, or ascites. Affected patients often have an atopic history, Charcot-Leyden crystals due to extruded eosinophil contents may be seen on microscopic inspection of stool, and peripheral eosinophilia is present in 50–75% of patients. While hypersensitivity to certain foods occurs in adults, true food allergy causing chronic diarrhea is rare.

OTHER CAUSES Chronic inflammatory diarrhea may be caused by *radiation enterocolitis, chronic graft-versus-host disease, Behçet's syndrome*, and *Cronkhite-Canada syndrome*, among others.

Dysmotility Causes Rapid transit may accompany many diarrheas as a secondary or contributing phenomenon, but primary dysmotility is an unusual etiology of true diarrhea. Stool features often suggest a secretory diarrhea, but mild steatorrhea of up to 14 g of fat per day can be produced by maldigestion from rapid transit alone. *Hyperthyroidism, carcinoid syndrome*, and certain drugs (e.g., prostaglandins, prokinetic agents) may produce hypermotility with resultant diarrhea. Primary visceral neuromyopathies or idiopathic acquired intestinal pseudoobstruction may lead to stasis with secondary bacterial overgrowth causing diarrhea. *Diabetic diarrhea*, often accompanied by peripheral and generalized autonomic neuropathies, may occur in part because of intestinal dysmotility.

The exceedingly common IBS (10% point prevalence, 1–2% per year incidence) is characterized by disturbed intestinal and colonic motor and sensory responses to various stimuli. Symptoms of stool frequency typically cease at night, alternate with periods of constipation, are accompanied by abdominal pain relieved with defecation, and rarely result in weight loss.

Factitial Causes Factitial diarrhea accounts for up to 15% of unexplained diarrheas referred to tertiary care centers. Either as a form of *Munchausen syndrome* (deception or self-injury for secondary gain) or *eating disorders*, some patients covertly self-administer laxatives alone or in combination with other medications (e.g., diuretics) or surreptitiously add water or urine to stool sent for analysis. Such patients are typically women, often with histories of psychiatric illness, and disproportionately from careers in health care. Hypotension and hypokalemia are common co-presenting features. The evaluation of such patients may be difficult: contamination of the stool with water or urine is suggested by very low or high stool osmolarity, respectively. Such patients often deny this possibility when confronted, but they do benefit from psychiatric counseling when they acknowledge their behavior.

APPROACH TO THE PATIENT: Chronic Diarrhea

The laboratory tools available to evaluate the very common problem of chronic diarrhea are extensive, and many are costly and invasive. As such, the diagnostic evaluation must be rationally directed by a careful history, including medications, and physical examination (Fig. 55-3*A*). When this strategy is unrevealing, simple triage tests are often warranted to direct the choice of more complex investigations (Fig. 55-3*B*). The history, physical examination (Table 55-4), and routine blood studies should attempt to characterize the mechanism of diarrhea, identify diagnostically helpful associations, and assess the patient's fluid/electrolyte and nutritional status. Patients should be questioned about the onset, duration, pattern, aggravating (especially diet) and relieving factors, and stool characteristics of their diarrhea. The presence or absence of fecal incontinence, fever, weight loss, pain, certain exposures (travel, medications, contacts with diarrhea), and common extraintestinal manifestations (skin changes, arthralgias, oral aphthous ulcers) should be noted. A family history of IBD or sprue may indicate those possibilities. Physical findings may offer clues such as a thyroid mass, wheezing, heart murmurs, edema, hepatomegaly, abdominal masses, lymphadenopathy, mucocutaneous abnormalities, perianal fistulas, or anal sphincter laxity. Peripheral blood leukocytosis, elevated sedimentation rate, or C-reactive protein suggests inflammation; anemia reflects blood loss or nutritional deficiencies; or eosinophilia may occur with parasitoses, neoplasia, collagen-vascular disease, allergy, or eosinophilic gastroenteritis. Blood chemistries may demonstrate electrolyte, hepatic, or other metabolic disturbances. Measuring IgA tissue transglutaminase antibodies may help detect celiac disease. Bile acid diarrhea is confirmed by a scintigraphic radiolabeled bile acid retention test; however, this is not available in many countries. Alternative approaches are a screening blood test (serum C4 or FGF-19), measurement of fecal bile acids, or a therapeutic trial with a bile acid sequestrant (e.g., cholestyramine or colesevelam).

A therapeutic trial is often appropriate, definitive, and highly cost-effective when a specific diagnosis is suggested on the initial physician encounter. For example, chronic watery diarrhea, which ceases with fasting in an otherwise healthy young adult, may justify a trial of a lactose-restricted diet; bloating and diarrhea persisting since a mountain backpacking trip may warrant a trial of metronidazole for likely giardiasis; and postprandial diarrhea persisting following resection of terminal ileum might be due to bile acid malabsorption and be treated with cholestyramine or colesevelam before further evaluation. Persistent symptoms require additional investigation.

Certain diagnoses may be suggested on the initial encounter (e.g., idiopathic IBD); however, additional focused evaluations may be necessary to confirm the diagnosis and characterize the severity or extent of disease so that treatment can be best guided. Patients suspected of having IBS should be initially evaluated with flexible sigmoidoscopy with colorectal biopsies to exclude IBD, or particularly microscopic colitis, which is clinically indistinguishable from IBS with diarrhea; those with normal findings might be reassured and, as indicated, treated empirically with antispasmodics, antidiarrheals, or antidepressants (e.g., tricyclic agents). Any patient who presents with chronic diarrhea and hematochezia should be evaluated with stool microbiologic studies and colonoscopy.

In an estimated two-thirds of cases, the cause for chronic diarrhea remains unclear after the initial encounter, and further testing is required. Quantitative stool collection and analyses can yield

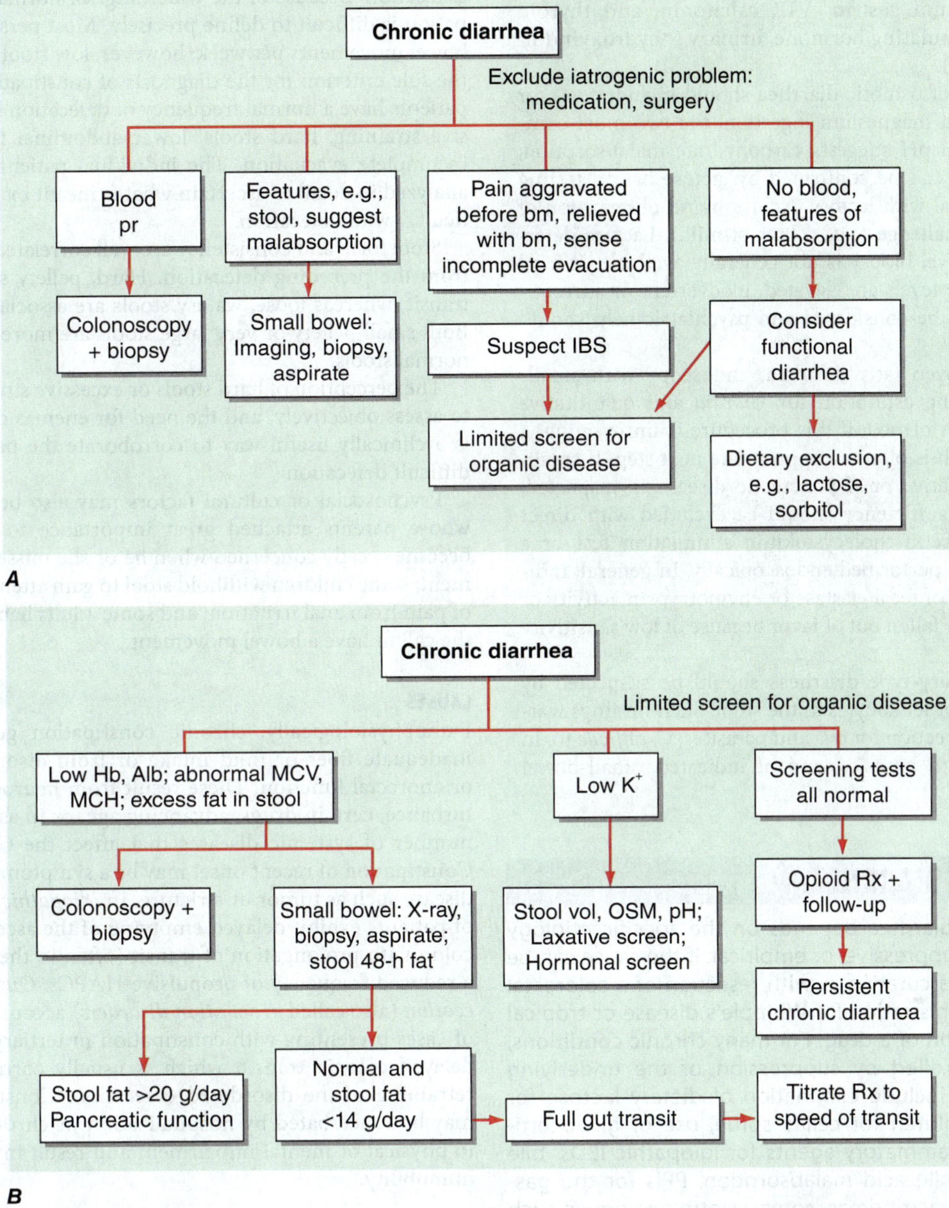

FIGURE 55-3 **Chronic diarrhea.** ***A.*** Initial management based on accompanying symptoms or features. ***B.*** Evaluation based on findings from a limited age-appropriate screen for organic disease. Alb, albumin; bm, bowel movement; Hb, hemoglobin; IBS, irritable bowel syndrome; MCH, mean corpuscular hemoglobin; MCV, mean corpuscular volume; OSM, osmolality; pr, per rectum. *(Reprinted from M Camilleri: Clin Gastroenterol Hepatol. 2:198, 2004.)*

important objective data that may establish a diagnosis or characterize the type of diarrhea as a triage for focused additional studies (Fig. 55-3*B*). If stool weight is >200 g/d, additional stool analyses should be performed that might include electrolyte concentration, pH, occult blood testing, leukocyte inspection (or leukocyte protein assay), fat quantitation, and laxative screens.

For secretory diarrheas (watery, normal osmotic gap), possible medication-related side effects or surreptitious laxative use should be reconsidered. Microbiologic studies should be done including fecal bacterial cultures (including media for *Aeromonas* and *Plesiomonas*), inspection for ova and parasites, and *Giardia* antigen assay (the most sensitive test for giardiasis). Small-bowel bacterial overgrowth can be excluded by intestinal aspirates with quantitative cultures or with glucose or lactulose breath tests involving measurement of breath hydrogen, methane, or other metabolite. However, interpretation of these breath tests may be confounded by disturbances of intestinal transit. Upper endoscopy and colonoscopy with biopsies and small-bowel x-rays (formerly barium, but increasingly CT with enterography or magnetic resonance with enteroclysis) are helpful to rule out structural or occult inflammatory disease. When suggested by history or other findings, screens for peptide hormones should

TABLE 55-4 PHYSICAL EXAMINATION IN PATIENTS WITH CHRONIC DIARRHEA

1. Are there general features to suggest malabsorption or inflammatory bowel disease (IBD) such as anemia, dermatitis herpetiformis, edema, or clubbing?
2. Are there features to suggest underlying autonomic neuropathy or collagen-vascular disease in the pupils, orthostasis, skin, hands, or joints?
3. Is there an abdominal mass or tenderness?
4. Are there any abnormalities of rectal mucosa, rectal defects, or altered anal sphincter functions?
5. Are there any mucocutaneous manifestations of systemic disease such as dermatitis herpetiformis (celiac disease), erythema nodosum (ulcerative colitis), flushing (carcinoid), or oral ulcers for IBD or celiac disease?

be pursued (e.g., serum gastrin, VIP, calcitonin, and thyroid hormone/thyroid-stimulating hormone, urinary 5-hydroxyindolacetic acid, histamine).

Further evaluation of osmotic diarrhea should include tests for lactose intolerance and magnesium ingestion, the two most common causes. Low fecal pH suggests carbohydrate malabsorption; lactose malabsorption can be confirmed by lactose breath testing or by a therapeutic trial with lactose exclusion and observation of the effect of lactose challenge (e.g., a liter of milk). Lactase determination on small-bowel biopsy is not generally available. If fecal magnesium or laxative levels are elevated, inadvertent or surreptitious ingestion should be considered and psychiatric help should be sought.

For those with proven fatty diarrhea, endoscopy with small-bowel biopsy (including aspiration for *Giardia* and quantitative cultures) should be performed; if this procedure is unrevealing, a small-bowel radiograph is often an appropriate next step. If small-bowel studies are negative or if pancreatic disease is suspected, pancreatic exocrine insufficiency should be excluded with direct tests, such as the secretin-cholecystokinin stimulation test or a variation that could be performed endoscopically. In general, indirect tests such as assay of fecal elastase or chymotrypsin activity or a bentiromide test have fallen out of favor because of low sensitivity and specificity.

Chronic inflammatory-type diarrheas should be suspected by the presence of blood or leukocytes in the stool. Such findings warrant stool cultures; inspection for ova and parasites; *C. difficile* toxin assay; colonoscopy with biopsies; and, if indicated, small-bowel contrast studies.

TREATMENT CHRONIC DIARRHEA

Treatment of chronic diarrhea depends on the specific etiology and may be curative, suppressive, or empirical. If the cause can be eradicated, treatment is curative as with resection of a colorectal cancer, antibiotic administration for Whipple's disease or tropical sprue, or discontinuation of a drug. For many chronic conditions, diarrhea can be controlled by suppression of the underlying mechanism. Examples include elimination of dietary lactose for lactase deficiency or gluten for celiac sprue, use of glucocorticoids or other anti-inflammatory agents for idiopathic IBDs, bile acid sequestrants for bile acid malabsorption, PPIs for the gastric hypersecretion of gastrinomas, somatostatin analogues such as octreotide for malignant carcinoid syndrome, prostaglandin inhibitors such as indomethacin for medullary carcinoma of the thyroid, and pancreatic enzyme replacement for pancreatic insufficiency. When the specific cause or mechanism of chronic diarrhea evades diagnosis, empirical therapy may be beneficial. Mild opiates, such as diphenoxylate or loperamide, are often helpful in mild or moderate watery diarrhea. For those with more severe diarrhea, codeine or tincture of opium may be beneficial. Such antimotility agents should be avoided with severe IBD, because toxic megacolon may be precipitated. Clonidine, an α_2-adrenergic agonist, may allow control of diabetic diarrhea, although the medication may be poorly tolerated because it causes postural hypotension. The 5-HT_3 receptor antagonists (e.g., alosetron) may relieve diarrhea and urgency in patients with IBS diarrhea. For all patients with chronic diarrhea, fluid and electrolyte repletion is an important component of management (see "Acute Diarrhea," earlier). Replacement of fat-soluble vitamins may also be necessary in patients with chronic steatorrhea.

CONSTIPATION

DEFINITION

Constipation is a common complaint in clinical practice and usually refers to persistent, difficult, infrequent, or seemingly incomplete defecation. Because of the wide range of normal bowel habits, constipation is difficult to define precisely. Most persons have at least three bowel movements per week; however, low stool frequency alone is not the sole criterion for the diagnosis of constipation. Many constipated patients have a normal frequency of defecation but complain of excessive straining, hard stools, lower abdominal fullness, or a sense of incomplete evacuation. The individual patient's symptoms must be analyzed in detail to ascertain what is meant by "constipation" or "difficulty" with defecation.

Stool form and consistency are well correlated with the time elapsed from the preceding defecation. Hard, pellety stools occur with slow transit, whereas loose, watery stools are associated with rapid transit. Both small pellety or very large stools are more difficult to expel than normal stools.

The perception of hard stools or excessive straining is more difficult to assess objectively, and the need for enemas or digital disimpaction is a clinically useful way to corroborate the patient's perceptions of difficult defecation.

Psychosocial or cultural factors may also be important. A person whose parents attached great importance to daily defecation will become greatly concerned when he or she misses a daily bowel movement; some children withhold stool to gain attention or because of fear of pain from anal irritation; and some adults habitually ignore or delay the call to have a bowel movement.

CAUSES

Pathophysiologically, chronic constipation generally results from inadequate fiber or fluid intake or from disordered colonic transit or anorectal function. These result from neurogastroenterologic disturbance, certain drugs, advancing age, or in association with a large number of systemic diseases that affect the GI tract (Table 55-5). Constipation of recent onset may be a symptom of significant organic disease such as tumor or stricture. In *idiopathic constipation*, a subset of patients exhibit delayed emptying of the ascending and transverse colon with prolongation of transit (often in the proximal colon) and a reduced frequency of propulsive HAPCs. *Outlet obstruction to defecation* (also called *evacuation disorders*) accounts for about a quarter of cases presenting with constipation in tertiary care and may cause delayed colonic transit, which is usually corrected by biofeedback retraining of the disordered defecation. Constipation of any cause may be exacerbated by hospitalization or chronic illnesses that lead to physical or mental impairment and result in inactivity or physical immobility.

TABLE 55-5 CAUSES OF CONSTIPATION IN ADULTS

Types of Constipation and Causes	Examples
Recent Onset	
Colonic obstruction	Neoplasm; stricture: ischemic, diverticular, inflammatory
Anal sphincter spasm	Anal fissure, painful hemorrhoids
Medications	
Chronic	
Irritable bowel syndrome	Constipation-predominant, alternating
Medications	Ca^{2+} blockers, antidepressants
Colonic pseudoobstruction	Slow-transit constipation, megacolon (rare Hirschsprung's, Chagas' diseases)
Disorders of rectal evacuation	Pelvic floor dysfunction; anismus; descending perineum syndrome; rectal mucosal prolapse; rectocele
Endocrinopathies	Hypothyroidism, hypercalcemia, pregnancy
Psychiatric disorders	Depression, eating disorders, drugs
Neurologic disease	Parkinsonism, multiple sclerosis, spinal cord injury
Generalized muscle disease	Progressive systemic sclerosis

APPROACH TO THE PATIENT: Constipation

A careful history should explore the patient's symptoms and confirm whether he or she is indeed constipated based on frequency (e.g., fewer than three bowel movements per week), consistency (lumpy/hard), excessive straining, prolonged defecation time, or need to support the perineum or digitate the anorectum to facilitate stool evacuation. In the vast majority of cases (probably >90%), there is no underlying cause (e.g., cancer, depression, or hypothyroidism), and constipation responds to ample hydration, exercise, and supplementation of dietary fiber (15–25 g/d). A good diet and medication history and attention to psychosocial issues are key. Physical examination and, particularly, a rectal examination should exclude fecal impaction and most of the important diseases that present with constipation and possibly indicate features suggesting an evacuation disorder (e.g., high anal sphincter tone, failure of perineal descent, or paradoxical puborectalis contraction during straining to simulate stool evacuation).

The presence of weight loss, rectal bleeding, or anemia with constipation mandates either flexible sigmoidoscopy plus barium enema or colonoscopy alone, particularly in patients >40 years, to exclude structural diseases such as cancer or strictures. Colonoscopy alone is most cost-effective in this setting because it provides an opportunity to biopsy mucosal lesions, perform polypectomy, or dilate strictures. Barium enema has advantages over colonoscopy in the patient with isolated constipation because it is less costly and identifies colonic dilation and all significant mucosal lesions or strictures that are likely to present with constipation. Melanosis coli, or pigmentation of the colon mucosa, indicates the use of anthraquinone laxatives such as cascara or senna; however, this is usually apparent from a careful history. An unexpected disorder such as megacolon or cathartic colon may also be detected by colonic radiographs. Measurement of serum calcium, potassium, and thyroid-stimulating hormone levels will identify rare patients with metabolic disorders.

Patients with more troublesome constipation may not respond to fiber alone and may be helped by a bowel-training regimen, which involves taking an osmotic laxative (e.g., magnesium salts, lactulose, sorbitol, polyethylene glycol) and evacuating with enema or suppository (e.g., glycerine or bisacodyl) as needed. After breakfast, a distraction-free 15–20 min on the toilet without straining is encouraged. Excessive straining may lead to development of hemorrhoids, and, if there is weakness of the pelvic floor or injury to the pudendal nerve, may result in obstructed defecation from descending perineum syndrome several years later. Those few who do not benefit from the simple measures delineated above or require long-term treatment or fail to respond to potent laxatives should undergo further investigation (Fig. 55-4). Novel agents that induce secretion (e.g., lubiprostone, a chloride channel activator, or linaclotide, a guanylate cyclase C agonist that activates chloride secretion) are also available.

INVESTIGATION OF SEVERE CONSTIPATION

A small minority (probably <5%) of patients have severe or "intractable" constipation; about 25% have evacuation disorders. These are the patients most likely to require evaluation by gastroenterologists or in referral centers. Further observation of the patient may occasionally reveal a previously unrecognized cause, such as an evacuation disorder, laxative abuse, malingering, or psychological disorder. In these patients, evaluations of the physiologic function of the colon and pelvic floor and of psychological status aid in the rational choice of treatment. Even among these highly selected patients with severe constipation, a cause can be identified in only about one-third of tertiary referral patients, with the others being diagnosed with normal transit constipation.

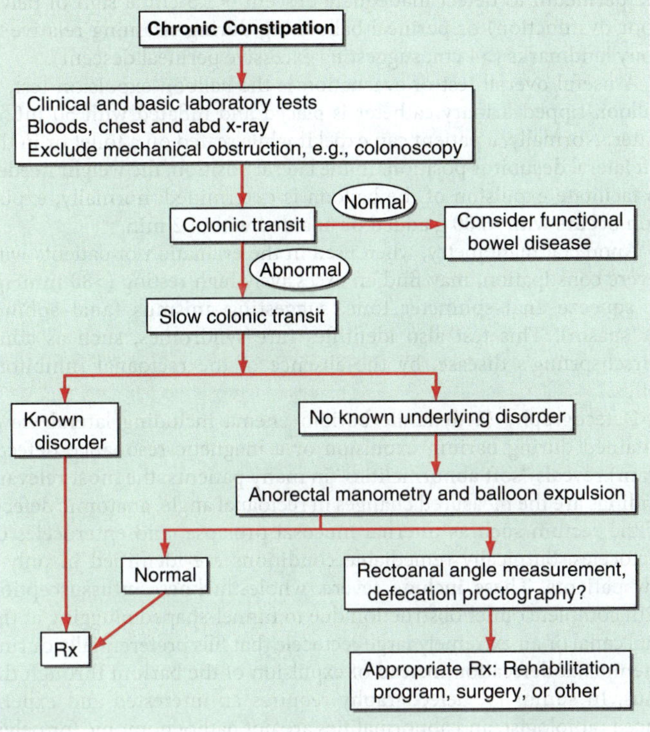

FIGURE 55-4 Algorithm for the management of constipation. abd, abdominal.

Measurement of Colonic Transit Radiopaque marker transit tests are easy, repeatable, generally safe, inexpensive, reliable, and highly applicable in evaluating constipated patients in clinical practice. Several validated methods are very simple. For example, radiopaque markers are ingested; an abdominal flat film taken 5 days later should indicate passage of 80% of the markers out of the colon without the use of laxatives or enemas. This test does not provide useful information about the transit profile of the stomach and small bowel.

Radioscintigraphy with a delayed-release capsule containing radiolabeled particles has been used to noninvasively characterize normal, accelerated, or delayed colonic function over 24–48 h with low radiation exposure. This approach simultaneously assesses gastric, small bowel (which may be important in ~20% of patients with delayed colonic transit because they reflect a more generalized GI motility disorder), and colonic transit. The disadvantages are the greater cost and the need for specific materials prepared in a nuclear medicine laboratory.

Anorectal and Pelvic Floor Tests Pelvic floor dysfunction is suggested by the inability to evacuate the rectum, a feeling of persistent rectal fullness, rectal pain, the need to extract stool from the rectum digitally, application of pressure on the posterior wall of the vagina, support of the perineum during straining, and excessive straining. These significant symptoms should be contrasted with the simple sense of incomplete rectal evacuation, which is common in IBS.

Formal psychological evaluation may identify eating disorders, "control issues," depression, or post-traumatic stress disorders that may respond to cognitive or other intervention and may be important in restoring quality of life to patients who might present with chronic constipation.

A simple clinical test in the office to document a non-relaxing puborectalis muscle is to have the patient strain to expel the index finger during a digital rectal examination. Motion of the puborectalis posteriorly during straining indicates proper coordination of the pelvic floor muscles. Motion anteriorly with paradoxical contraction during simulated evacuation indicates pelvic floor dysfunction.

Measurement of perineal descent is relatively easy to gauge clinically by placing the patient in the left decubitus position and watching the perineum to detect inadequate descent (<1.5 cm, a sign of pelvic floor dysfunction) or perineal ballooning during straining relative to bony landmarks (>4 cm, suggesting excessive perineal descent).

A useful overall test of evacuation is the balloon expulsion test. A balloon-tipped urinary catheter is placed and inflated with 50 mL of water. Normally, a patient can expel it while seated on a toilet or in the left lateral decubitus position. In the lateral position, the weight needed to facilitate expulsion of the balloon is determined; normally, expulsion occurs with <200 g added or unaided within 2 min.

Anorectal manometry, when used in the evaluation of patients with severe constipation, may find an excessively high resting (>80 mmHg) or squeeze anal sphincter tone, suggesting anismus (anal sphincter spasm). This test also identifies rare syndromes, such as adult Hirschsprung's disease, by the absence of the rectoanal inhibitory reflex.

Defecography (a dynamic barium enema including lateral views obtained during barium expulsion or a magnetic resonance defecogram) reveals "soft abnormalities" in many patients; the most relevant findings are the measured changes in rectoanal angle, anatomic defects of the rectum such as internal mucosal prolapse, and enteroceles or rectoceles. Surgically remediable conditions are identified in only a few patients. These include severe, whole-thickness intussusception with complete outlet obstruction due to funnel-shaped plugging at the anal canal or an extremely large rectocele that fills preferentially during attempts at defecation instead of expulsion of the barium through the anus. In summary, defecography requires an interested and experienced radiologist, and abnormalities are not pathognomonic for pelvic floor dysfunction. The most common cause of outlet obstruction is failure of the puborectalis muscle to relax; this is not identified by barium defecography, but can be demonstrated by magnetic resonance defecography, which provides more information about the structure and function of the pelvic floor, distal colorectum, and anal sphincters.

Neurologic testing (electromyography) is more helpful in the evaluation of patients with incontinence than of those with symptoms suggesting obstructed defecation. The absence of neurologic signs in the lower extremities suggests that any documented denervation of the puborectalis results from pelvic (e.g., obstetric) injury or from stretching of the pudendal nerve by chronic, long-standing straining. Constipation is common among patients with spinal cord injuries, neurologic diseases such as Parkinson's disease, multiple sclerosis, and diabetic neuropathy.

Spinal-evoked responses during electrical rectal stimulation or stimulation of external anal sphincter contraction by applying magnetic stimulation over the lumbosacral cord identify patients with limited sacral neuropathies with sufficient residual nerve conduction to attempt biofeedback training.

In summary, a balloon expulsion test is an important screening test for anorectal dysfunction. Rarely, an anatomic evaluation of the rectum or anal sphincters and an assessment of pelvic floor relaxation are the tools for evaluating patients in whom obstructed defecation is suspected and is associated with symptoms of rectal mucosal prolapse, pressure of the posterior wall of the vagina to facilitate defecation (suggestive of anterior rectocele), or prior pelvic surgery that may be complicated by enterocele.

TREATMENT CONSTIPATION

After the cause of constipation is characterized, a treatment decision can be made. Slow-transit constipation requires aggressive medical or surgical treatment; anismus or pelvic floor dysfunction usually responds to biofeedback management (Fig. 40-4). The remaining ~60% of patients with constipation has normal colonic transit and can be treated symptomatically. Patients with spinal cord injuries or other neurologic disorders require a dedicated bowel regimen that often includes rectal stimulation, enema therapy, and carefully timed laxative therapy.

Patients with constipation are treated with bulk, osmotic, prokinetic, secretory, and stimulant laxatives including fiber, psyllium, milk of magnesia, lactulose, polyethylene glycol (colonic lavage solution), lubiprostone, linaclotide, and bisacodyl, or, in some countries, prucalopride, a 5-HT_4 agonist. If a 3-to 6-month trial of medical therapy fails, unassociated with obstructed defecation, the patients should be considered for laparoscopic colectomy with ileorectostomy; however, this should not be undertaken if there is continued evidence of an evacuation disorder or a generalized GI dysmotility. Referral to a specialized center for further tests of colonic motor function is warranted. The decision to resort to surgery is facilitated in the presence of megacolon and megarectum. The complications after surgery include small-bowel obstruction (11%) and fecal soiling, particularly at night during the first postoperative year. Frequency of defecation is 3–8 per day during the first year, dropping to 1–3 per day from the second year after surgery.

Patients who have a combined (evacuation and transit/motility) disorder should pursue pelvic floor retraining (biofeedback and muscle relaxation), psychological counseling, and dietetic advice first. If symptoms are intractable despite biofeedback and optimized medical therapy, colectomy and ileorectostomy could be considered as long as the evacuation disorder is resolved and optimized medical therapy is unsuccessful. In patients with pelvic floor dysfunction alone, biofeedback training has a 70–80% success rate, measured by the acquisition of comfortable stool habits. Attempts to manage pelvic floor dysfunction with operations (internal anal sphincter or puborectalis muscle division) or injections with botulinum toxin have achieved only mediocre success and have been largely abandoned.

56 Involuntary Weight Loss

Russell G. Robertson, J. Larry Jameson

Involuntary weight loss (IWL) is frequently insidious and can have important implications, often serving as a harbinger of serious underlying disease. Clinically important weight loss is defined as the loss of 10 pounds (4.5 kg) or >5% of one's body weight over a period of 6–12 months. IWL is encountered in up to 8% of all adult outpatients and 27% of frail persons age 65 years and older. There is no identifiable cause in up to one-quarter of patients despite extensive investigation. Conversely, up to half of people who claim to have lost weight have no documented evidence of weight loss. People with no known cause of weight loss generally have a better prognosis than do those with known causes, particularly when the source is neoplastic. Weight loss in older persons is associated with a variety of deleterious effects, including hip fracture, pressure ulcers, impaired immune function, and decreased functional status. Not surprisingly, significant weight loss is associated with increased mortality, which can range from 9% to as high as 38% within 1 to 2.5 years in the absence of clinical awareness and attention.

PHYSIOLOGY OF WEIGHT REGULATION WITH AGING

(See also Chaps. 94e and 415e) Among healthy aging people, total body weight peaks in the sixth decade of life and generally remains stable until the ninth decade, after which it gradually falls. In contrast, lean body mass (fat-free mass) begins to decline at a rate of 0.3 kg per year in the third decade, and the rate of decline increases further beginning at age 60 in men and age 65 in women. These changes in lean body mass largely reflect the age-dependent decline in growth hormone secretion and, consequently, circulating levels of insulin-like growth factor type I (IGF-I) that occur with normal aging. Loss of sex steroids, at menopause in women and more gradually with aging in men, also contributes to these changes in body composition. In the healthy elderly, an increase in fat tissue balances the loss in lean body mass until very old age, when loss of both fat and skeletal muscle occurs. Age-dependent changes also occur at the cellular level. Telomeres shorten, and body cell mass—the fat-free portion of cells—declines steadily with aging.

Between ages 20 and 80, mean energy intake is reduced by up to 1200 kcal/d in men and 800 kcal/d in women. Decreased hunger is a reflection of reduced physical activity and loss of lean body mass, producing lower demand for calories and food intake. Several important age-associated physiologic changes also predispose elderly persons to weight loss, such as declining chemosensory function (smell and taste), reduced efficiency of chewing, slowed gastric emptying, and alterations in the neuroendocrine axis, including changes in levels of leptin, cholecystokinin, neuropeptide Y, and other hormones and peptides. These changes are associated with early satiety and a decline in both appetite and the hedonistic appreciation of food. Collectively, they contribute to the "anorexia of aging."

CAUSES OF INVOLUNTARY WEIGHT LOSS

Most causes of IWL belong to one of four categories: (1) malignant neoplasms, (2) chronic inflammatory or infectious diseases, (3) metabolic disorders (e.g., hyperthyroidism and diabetes), or (4) psychiatric disorders (Table 56-1). Not infrequently, more than one of these causes can be responsible for IWL. In most series, IWL is caused by malignant disease in a quarter of patients and by organic disease in one-third, with the remainder due to psychiatric disease, medications, or uncertain causes.

The most common malignant causes of IWL are gastrointestinal, hepatobiliary, hematologic, lung, breast, genitourinary, ovarian, and prostate. Half of all patients with cancer lose some body weight; one-third lose more than 5% of their original body weight, and up to 20% of all cancer deaths are caused directly by cachexia (through immobility and/or cardiac/respiratory failure). The greatest incidence of weight loss is seen among patients with solid tumors. Malignancy that reveals itself through significant weight loss usually has a very poor prognosis.

In addition to malignancies, gastrointestinal causes are among the most prominent causes of IWL. Peptic ulcer disease, inflammatory bowel disease, dysmotility syndromes, chronic pancreatitis, celiac disease, constipation, and atrophic gastritis are some of the more common entities. Oral and dental problems are easily overlooked and may manifest with halitosis, poor oral hygiene, xerostomia, inability to chew, reduced masticatory force, nonocclusion, temporomandibular joint syndrome, edentulousness, and pain due to caries or abscesses.

Tuberculosis, fungal diseases, parasites, subacute bacterial endocarditis, and HIV are well-documented causes of IWL. Cardiovascular and pulmonary diseases cause unintentional weight loss through increased metabolic demand and decreased appetite and caloric intake. Uremia produces nausea, anorexia, and vomiting. Connective tissue diseases may increase metabolic demand and disrupt nutritional balance. As the incidence of diabetes mellitus increases with aging, the associated glucosuria can contribute to weight loss. Hyperthyroidism in the elderly may have less prominent sympathomimetic features and may present as "apathetic hyperthyroidism" or T_3 toxicosis (Chap. 405).

Neurologic injuries such as stroke, quadriplegia, and multiple sclerosis may lead to visceral and autonomic dysfunction that can impair caloric intake. Dysphagia from these neurologic insults is a common mechanism. Functional disability that compromises activities of daily living (ADLs) is a common cause of undernutrition in the elderly. Visual impairment from ophthalmic or central nervous system disorders such as a tremor can limit the ability of people to prepare and eat meals. IWL may be one of the earliest manifestations of Alzheimer's dementia.

Isolation and depression are significant causes of IWL that may manifest as an inability to care for oneself, including nutritional needs. A cytokine-mediated inflammatory metabolic cascade can be both a cause of and a manifestation of depression. Bereavement can be a cause of IWL and, when present, is more pronounced in men. More intense forms of mental illness such as paranoid disorders may lead to delusions about food and cause weight loss. Alcoholism can be a significant source of weight loss and malnutrition.

Elderly persons living in poverty may have to choose whether to purchase food or use the money for other expenses, including medications. Institutionalization is an independent risk factor, as up to 30–50% of nursing home patients have inadequate food intake.

Medications can cause anorexia, nausea, vomiting, gastrointestinal distress, diarrhea, dry mouth, and changes in taste. This is particularly an issue in the elderly, many of whom take five or more medications.

ASSESSMENT

The four major manifestations of IWL are (1) anorexia (loss of appetite), (2) sarcopenia (loss of muscle mass), (3) cachexia (a syndrome that combines weight loss, loss of muscle and adipose tissue, anorexia, and weakness), and (4) dehydration. The current obesity epidemic adds complexity, as excess adipose tissue can mask the development of sarcopenia and delay awareness of the development of cachexia. If it is not possible to measure weight directly, a change in clothing size, corroboration of weight loss by a relative or friend, and a numeric estimate of weight loss provided by the patient are suggestive of true weight loss.

Initial assessment includes a comprehensive history and physical, a complete blood count, tests of liver enzyme levels, C-reactive protein, erythrocyte sedimentation rate, renal function studies, thyroid function tests, chest radiography, and an abdominal ultrasound (Table 56-2). Age, sex, and risk factor–specific cancer screening tests, such as mammography and colonoscopy, should be performed (Chap. 100). Patients at risk should have HIV testing. All elderly patients with weight loss should undergo screening for dementia and depression by using instruments such as the

TABLE 56-1 CAUSES OF INVOLUNTARY WEIGHT LOSS

Cancer	**Medications**
Colon	Sedatives
Hepatobiliary	Antibiotics
Hematologic	Nonsteroidal anti-inflammatory drugs
Lung	Serotonin reuptake inhibitors
Breast	Metformin
Genitourinary	Levodopa
Ovarian	Angiotensin-converting enzyme inhibitors
Prostate	Other drugs
Gastrointestinal disorders	**Disorders of the mouth and teeth**
Malabsorption	Caries
Peptic ulcer	Dysgeusia
Inflammatory bowel disease	**Age-related factors**
Pancreatitis	Physiologic changes
Obstruction/constipation	Visual impairment
Pernicious anemia	Decreased taste and smell
Endocrine and metabolic	Functional disabilities
Hyperthyroidism	**Neurologic**
Diabetes mellitus	Stroke
Pheochromocytoma	Parkinson's disease
Adrenal insufficiency	Neuromuscular disorders
Cardiac disorders	Dementia
Chronic ischemia	**Social**
Chronic congestive heart failure	Isolation
Respiratory disorders	Economic hardship
Emphysema	**Psychiatric and behavioral**
Chronic obstructive pulmonary disease	Depression
Renal insufficiency	Anxiety
Rheumatologic disease	Paranoia
Infections	Bereavement
HIV	Alcoholism
Tuberculosis	Eating disorders
Parasitic infection	Increased activity or exercise
Subacute bacterial endocarditis	**Idiopathic**

TABLE 56-2 ASSESSMENT AND TESTING FOR INVOLUNTARY WEIGHT LOSS

Indications	Laboratory
5% weight loss in 30 d	Complete blood count
10% weight loss in 180 d	Comprehensive electrolyte and metabolic panel, including liver and renal function tests
Body mass index <21	Thyroid function tests
25% of food left uneaten after 7 d	Erythrocyte sedimentation rate
Change in fit of clothing	C-reactive protein
Change in appetite, smell, or taste	Ferritin
Abdominal pain, nausea, vomiting, diarrhea, constipation, dysphagia	HIV testing, if indicated
Assessment	**Radiology**
Complete physical exam, including dental evaluation	Chest x-ray
Medication review	Abdominal ultrasound
Recommended cancer screening	
Mini-Mental State Examination[a]	
Mini-Nutritional Assessment[a]	
Nutrition Screening Initiative[a]	
Simplified Nutritional Assessment Questionnaire[a]	
Observation of eating[a]	
Activities of daily living[a]	
Instrumental activities of daily living[a]	

[a]May be more specific to assess weight loss in the elderly.

Mini-Mental State Examination and the Geriatric Depression Scale, respectively (Chap. 11). The Mini Nutritional Assessment (*www.mna-elderly.com*) and the Nutrition Screening Initiative (*http://www.ncbi.nlm.nih.gov/pmc/articles/PMC1694757/*) are also available for the nutritional assessment of elderly patients. Almost all patients with a malignancy and >90% of those with other organic diseases have at least one laboratory abnormality. In patients presenting with substantial IWL, major organic and malignant diseases are unlikely when a baseline evaluation is completely normal. Careful follow-up rather than undirected testing is advised since the prognosis of weight loss of undetermined cause is generally favorable.

TREATMENT UNINTENTIONAL WEIGHT LOSS

The first priority in managing weight loss is to identify and treat the underlying causes systematically. Treatment of underlying metabolic, psychiatric, infectious, or other systemic disorders may be sufficient to restore weight and functional status gradually. Medications that cause nausea or anorexia should be withdrawn or changed, if possible. For those with unexplained IWL, oral nutritional supplements such as high-energy drinks sometimes reverse weight loss. Advising patients to consume supplements between meals rather than with a meal may help minimize appetite suppression and facilitate increased overall intake. Orexigenic, anabolic, and anticytokine agents are under investigation. In selected patients, the antidepressant mirtazapine results in a significant increase in body weight, body fat mass, and leptin concentration. Patients with wasting conditions who can comply with an appropriate exercise program gain muscle protein mass, strength, and endurance and may be more capable of performing ADLs.

57 Gastrointestinal Bleeding

Loren Laine

Gastrointestinal bleeding (GIB) accounts for ~150 hospitalizations per 100,000 population annually in the United States, with upper GIB (UGIB) ~1.5–2 times more common than lower GIB (LGIB) The incidence of GIB has decreased in recent decades, primarily due to a reduction in UGIB, and the mortality has also decreased to <5%. Patients today rarely die from exsanguination, but rather die due to decompensation of other underlying illnesses.

GIB presents as either overt or occult bleeding. *Overt GIB* is manifested by *hematemesis*, vomitus of red blood or "coffee-grounds" material; *melena*, black, tarry, foul-smelling stool; and/or *hematochezia*, passage of bright red or maroon blood from the rectum. *Occult GIB* may be identified in the absence of overt bleeding when patients present with *symptoms of blood loss or anemia* such as lightheadedness, syncope, angina, or dyspnea; or when routine diagnostic evaluation reveals iron deficiency anemia or a positive fecal occult blood test. GIB is also categorized by the site of bleeding as UGIB, LGIB, or obscure GIB if the source is unclear.

SOURCES OF GASTROINTESTINAL BLEEDING

Upper Gastrointestinal Sources of Bleeding (Table 57-1) Peptic ulcers are the most common cause of UGIB, accounting for ~50% of cases. Mallory-Weiss tears account for ~5–10% of cases. The proportion of patients bleeding from varices varies widely from ~5–40%, depending on the population. Hemorrhagic or erosive gastropathy (e.g., due to nonsteroidal anti-inflammatory drugs [NSAIDs] or alcohol) and erosive esophagitis often cause mild UGIB, but major bleeding is rare.

PEPTIC ULCERS Characteristics of an ulcer at endoscopy provide important prognostic information. One-third of patients with active bleeding or a nonbleeding visible vessel have further bleeding that requires urgent surgery if they are treated conservatively. These patients benefit from endoscopic therapy with bipolar electrocoagulation, heater probe, injection therapy (e.g., absolute alcohol, 1:10,000 epinephrine), and/or clips with reductions in bleeding, hospital stay, mortality, and costs. In contrast, patients with clean-based ulcers have rates of recurrent bleeding approaching zero. If stable with no other reason for hospitalization, such patients may be discharged home after endoscopy. Patients without clean-based ulcers usually remain in the hospital for 3 days because most episodes of recurrent bleeding occur within 3 days.

Randomized controlled trials document that high-dose, constant-infusion IV proton pump inhibitor (PPI) (80-mg bolus and 8-mg/h infusion), designed to sustain intragastric pH >6 and enhance clot stability, decreases further bleeding and mortality in patients with high-risk ulcers (active bleeding, nonbleeding visible vessel, adherent clot) when given after endoscopic therapy. Patients with lower-risk findings (flat pigmented spot or clean base) do not require endoscopic

TABLE 57-1 SOURCES OF BLEEDING IN PATIENTS HOSPITALIZED FOR UPPER GASTROINTESTINAL BLEEDING

Sources of Bleeding	Proportion of Patients, %
Ulcers	31–67
Varices	6–39
Mallory-Weiss tears	2–8
Gastroduodenal erosions	2–18
Erosive esophagitis	1–13
Neoplasm	2–8
Vascular ectasias	0–6
No source identified	5–14

Source: Data on hospitalizations from year 2000 onward from Am J Gastroenterol 98:1494, 2003; Gastrointest Endosc 57:AB147, 2003; 60;875, 2004; Eur J Gastroenterol Hepatol 16:177, 2004; 17:641, 2005; J Clin Gastroenterol 42:128, 2008; World J Gastroenterol 14:5046, 2008; Dig Dis Sci 54:333, 2009; Gut 60:1327, 2011; Endoscopy 44:998, 2012; J Clin Gastroenterol 48:113, 2014.

therapy and receive standard doses of oral PPI. Approximately one-third of patients with bleeding ulcers will rebleed within the next 1–2 years if no preventive strategies are employed. Prevention of recurrent bleeding focuses on the three main factors in ulcer pathogenesis, *Helicobacter pylori*, NSAIDs, and acid. Eradication of *H. pylori* in patients with bleeding ulcers decreases rates of rebleeding to <5%. If a bleeding ulcer develops in a patient taking NSAIDs, the NSAIDs should be discontinued. If NSAIDs must be given, a cyclooxygenase 2 (COX-2) selective inhibitor (coxib) plus a PPI should be used. PPI co-therapy alone or a coxib alone is associated with an annual rebleeding rate of ~10% in patients with a recent bleeding ulcer, whereas the combination of a coxib and PPI provides a further significant decrease in recurrent ulcer bleeding. Patients with established cardiovascular disease who develop bleeding ulcers while taking low-dose aspirin should restart aspirin as soon as possible after their bleeding episode (1–7 days). A randomized trial showed that failure to restart aspirin was associated with no significant difference in rebleeding (5% vs. 10% at 30 days) but a significant increase in mortality at 30 days (9% vs. 1%) and 8 weeks (13% vs. 1%) compared with immediate reinstitution of aspirin. Patients with bleeding ulcers unrelated to *H. pylori* or NSAIDs should remain on PPI therapy indefinitely. Peptic ulcers are discussed in Chap. 348.

MALLORY-WEISS TEARS The classic history is vomiting, retching, or coughing preceding hematemesis, especially in an alcoholic patient. Bleeding from these tears, which are usually on the gastric side of the gastroesophageal junction, stops spontaneously in 80–90% of patients and recurs in only 0–10%. Endoscopic therapy is indicated for actively bleeding Mallory-Weiss tears. Angiographic therapy with embolization and operative therapy with oversewing of the tear are rarely required. Mallory-Weiss tears are discussed in Chap. 347.

ESOPHAGEAL VARICES Patients with variceal hemorrhage have poorer outcomes than patients with other sources of UGIB. Urgent endoscopy within 12 h is recommended in cirrhotics with UGIB, and if esophageal varices are present, endoscopic ligation is performed and an IV vasoactive medication (e.g., octreotide 50 μg bolus and 50 μg/h infusion) is given for 2–5 days. Combination endoscopic and medical therapy appears to be superior to either therapy alone in decreasing rebleeding. In patients with advanced liver disease (e.g., Child-Pugh class C with score 10–13), a transjugular intrahepatic portosystemic shunt (TIPS) should be strongly considered within the first 1–2 days of hospitalization because randomized trials show significant decreases in rebleeding and mortality compared with standard endoscopic and medical therapy. Over the long term, treatment with nonselective beta blockers plus endoscopic ligation is recommended because the combination of endoscopic and medical therapy is more effective than either alone in reduction of recurrent esophageal variceal bleeding.

In patients who have persistent or recurrent bleeding despite endoscopic and medical therapy, TIPS is recommended. Decompressive surgery (e.g., distal splenorenal shunt) may be considered instead of TIPS in patients with well-compensated cirrhosis.

Portal hypertension is also responsible for bleeding from gastric varices, varices in the small and large intestine, and portal hypertensive gastropathy and enterocolopathy. Bleeding gastric varices due to cirrhosis are treated with endoscopic injection of tissue adhesive (e.g., *n*-butyl cyanoacrylate), if available; if not, TIPS is performed.

HEMORRHAGIC AND EROSIVE GASTROPATHY ("GASTRITIS") Hemorrhagic and erosive gastropathy, often labeled gastritis, refers to endoscopically visualized subepithelial hemorrhages and erosions. These are mucosal lesions and do not cause major bleeding due to the absence of arteries and veins in the mucosa. Erosions develop in various clinical settings, the most important of which are NSAID use, alcohol intake, and stress. Half of patients who chronically ingest NSAIDs have erosions, whereas up to 20% of actively drinking alcoholic patients with symptoms of UGIB have evidence of subepithelial hemorrhages or erosions.

Stress-related gastric mucosal injury occurs only in extremely sick patients, such as those who have experienced serious trauma, major surgery, burns covering more than one-third of the body surface area, major intracranial disease, or severe medical illness (i.e., ventilator dependence, coagulopathy). Severe bleeding should not develop unless ulceration occurs. The mortality rate in these patients is quite high because of their serious underlying illnesses.

The incidence of bleeding from stress-related gastric mucosal injury has decreased dramatically in recent years, most likely due to better care of critically ill patients. Pharmacologic prophylaxis for bleeding may be considered in the high-risk patients mentioned above. Meta-analyses of randomized trials indicate that PPIs are more effective than H_2 receptor antagonists in reduction of overt and clinically important UGIB without differences in mortality or nosocomial pneumonia.

OTHER CAUSES Other less frequent causes of UGIB include erosive duodenitis, neoplasms, aortoenteric fistulas, vascular lesions (including hereditary hemorrhagic telangiectasias [Osler-Weber-Rendu] and gastric antral vascular ectasia ["watermelon stomach"]), Dieulafoy's lesion (in which an aberrant vessel in the mucosa bleeds from a pinpoint mucosal defect), prolapse gastropathy (prolapse of proximal stomach into esophagus with retching, especially in alcoholics), and hemobilia or hemosuccus pancreaticus (bleeding from the bile duct or pancreatic duct).

Small-Intestinal Sources of Bleeding Small-intestinal sources of bleeding (bleeding from sites beyond the reach of the standard upper endoscope) are often difficult to diagnose and are responsible for the majority of cases of obscure GIB. Fortunately, small-intestinal bleeding is uncommon. The most common causes in adults are vascular ectasias, tumors (e.g., GI stromal tumor, carcinoid, adenocarcinoma, lymphoma, metastases), and NSAID-induced erosions and ulcers. Other less common causes in adults include Crohn's disease, infection, ischemia, vasculitis, small-bowel varices, diverticula, Meckel's diverticulum, duplication cysts, and intussusception.

Meckel's diverticulum is the most common cause of significant LGIB in children, decreasing in frequency as a cause of bleeding with age. In adults <40–50 years, small-bowel tumors often account for obscure GIB; in patients >50–60 years, vascular ectasias and NSAID-induced lesions are more commonly responsible.

Vascular ectasias should be treated with endoscopic therapy if possible. Although estrogen/progesterone compounds have been used for vascular ectasias, a large double-blind trial found no benefit in prevention of recurrent bleeding. Octreotide is also used, based on case series but no randomized trials. A randomized trial reported significant benefit of thalidomide and awaits further confirmation. Other isolated lesions, such as tumors, are generally treated with surgical resection.

Colonic Sources of Bleeding Hemorrhoids are probably the most common cause of LGIB; anal fissures also cause minor bleeding and pain. If these local anal processes, which rarely require hospitalization, are excluded, the most common causes of LGIB in adults are diverticula, vascular ectasias (especially in the proximal colon of patients >70 years), neoplasms (primarily adenocarcinoma), colitis (ischemic, infectious, idiopathic inflammatory bowel disease), and postpolypectomy bleeding. Less common causes include NSAID-induced ulcers or colitis, radiation proctopathy, solitary rectal ulcer syndrome, trauma, varices (most commonly rectal), lymphoid nodular hyperplasia, vasculitis, and aortocolic fistulas. In children and adolescents, the most common colonic causes of significant GIB are inflammatory bowel disease and juvenile polyps.

Diverticular bleeding is abrupt in onset, usually painless, sometimes massive, and often from the right colon; chronic or occult bleeding is not characteristic. Clinical reports suggest that bleeding colonic diverticula stop bleeding spontaneously in ~80% of patients and, on long-term follow-up, rebleed in ~15–25% of patients. Case series suggest endoscopic therapy may decrease recurrent bleeding in the uncommon case when colonoscopy identifies the specific bleeding diverticulum. When diverticular bleeding is found at angiography, transcatheter arterial embolization by superselective technique stops bleeding in a majority of patients. If bleeding persists or recurs, segmental surgical resection is indicated.

Bleeding from right colonic vascular ectasias in the elderly may be overt or occult; it tends to be chronic and only occasionally is hemodynamically significant. Endoscopic hemostatic therapy may be useful in the treatment of vascular ectasias, as well as discrete bleeding ulcers and postpolypectomy bleeding. Surgical therapy is generally required for major, persistent, or recurrent bleeding from the wide variety of colonic sources of GIB that cannot be treated medically, angiographically, or endoscopically.

APPROACH TO THE PATIENT: **Gastrointestinal Bleeding**

INITIAL ASSESSMENT

Measurement of the heart rate and blood pressure is the best way to initially assess a patient with GIB. Clinically significant bleeding leads to postural changes in heart rate or blood pressure, tachycardia, and, finally, recumbent hypotension. In contrast, the hemoglobin does not fall immediately with acute GIB, due to proportionate reductions in plasma and red cell volumes (i.e., "people bleed whole blood"). Thus, hemoglobin may be normal or only minimally decreased at the initial presentation of a severe bleeding episode. As extravascular fluid enters the vascular space to restore volume, the hemoglobin falls, but this process may take up to 72 h. Transfusion is recommended when the hemoglobin drops below 7 g/dL, based on a large randomized trial showing this restrictive transfusion strategy decreases rebleeding and death in acute UGIB compared with a transfusion threshold of 9 g/dL. Patients with slow, chronic GIB may have very low hemoglobin values despite normal blood pressure and heart rate. With the development of iron-deficiency anemia, the mean corpuscular volume will be low and red blood cell distribution width will increase.

DIFFERENTIATION OF UGIB FROM LGIB

Hematemesis indicates an upper GI source of bleeding (above the ligament of Treitz). Melena indicates blood has been present in the GI tract for at least 14 h, and as long as 3–5 days. The more proximal the bleeding site, the more likely melena will occur. Hematochezia usually represents a lower GI source of bleeding, although an upper GI lesion may bleed so briskly that blood transits the bowel before melena develops. When hematochezia is the presenting symptom of UGIB, it is associated with hemodynamic instability and dropping hemoglobin. Bleeding lesions of the small bowel may present as melena or hematochezia. Other clues to UGIB include hyperactive bowel sounds and an elevated blood urea nitrogen (due to volume depletion and blood proteins absorbed in the small intestine).

A nonbloody nasogastric aspirate may be seen in up to ~18% of patients with UGIB, usually from a duodenal source. Even a bile-stained appearance does not exclude a bleeding postpyloric lesion because reports of bile in the aspirate are incorrect in ~50% of cases. Testing of aspirates that are not grossly bloody for occult blood is not useful.

EVALUATION AND MANAGEMENT OF UGIB (FIG. 57-1)

At presentation, patients are generally stratified as higher or lower risk for further bleeding and death. Baseline characteristics predictive of rebleeding and death include hemodynamic compromise (tachycardia or hypotension), increasing age, and comorbidities. PPI infusion may be considered at presentation: it decreases high-risk ulcer stigmata (e.g., active bleeding) and need for endoscopic therapy but does not improve clinical outcomes such as further bleeding, surgery, or death. Treatment to improve endoscopic visualization with the promotility agent erythromycin, 250 mg intravenously ~30 min before endoscopy, also may be considered: it provides a small but significant increase in diagnostic yield and decrease in second endoscopies but is not documented to decrease further bleeding or death. Cirrhotic patients presenting with UGIB should be placed on antibiotics (e.g., quinolone, ceftriaxone) and started on a vasoactive medication (octreotide, terlipressin, somatostatin, vapreotide) upon presentation, even before endoscopy. Antibiotics decrease bacterial infections, rebleeding, and mortality in this population, and vasoactive medications appear to improve control of bleeding in the first 12 h after presentation.

Upper endoscopy should be performed within 24 h in most patients with UGIB. Patients at higher risk (e.g., hemodynamic instability, cirrhosis) may benefit from more urgent endoscopy within 12 h. Early endoscopy is also beneficial in low-risk patients for management decisions. Patients with major bleeding and high-risk endoscopic findings (e.g., varices, ulcers with active bleeding or a visible vessel) benefit from endoscopic hemostatic therapy, whereas patients with low-risk lesions (e.g., clean-based ulcers, nonbleeding Mallory-Weiss tears, erosive or hemorrhagic gastropathy) who have stable vital signs and hemoglobin and no other medical problems can be discharged home.

EVALUATION AND MANAGEMENT OF LGIB (FIG. 57-2)

Patients with hematochezia and hemodynamic instability should have upper endoscopy to rule out an upper GI source before evaluation of the lower GI tract.

Colonoscopy after an oral lavage solution is the procedure of choice in most patients admitted with LGIB unless bleeding is too massive,

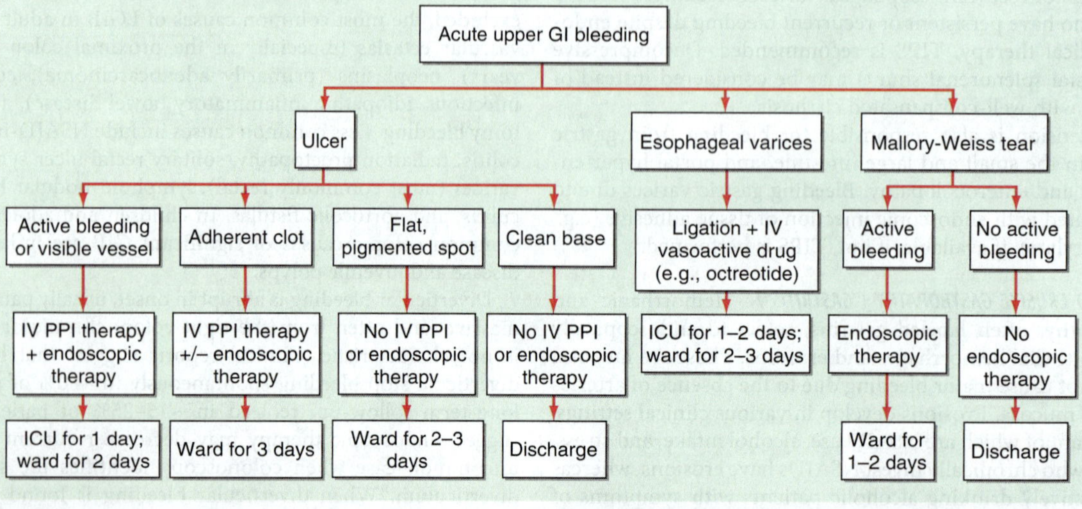

FIGURE 57-1 Suggested algorithm for patients with acute upper gastrointestinal (GI) bleeding. Recommendations on level of care and time of discharge assume patient is stabilized without further bleeding or other concomitant medical problems. ICU, intensive care unit; PPI, proton pump inhibitor.

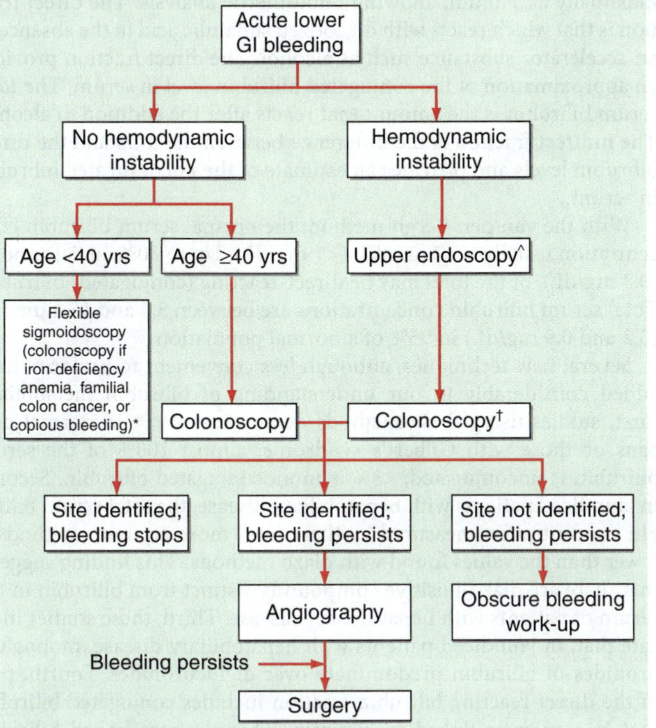

FIGURE 57-2 Suggested algorithm for patients with acute lower gastrointestinal (GI) bleeding. *Some suggest colonoscopy for any degree of rectal bleeding in patients <40 years as well. ^If upper GI endoscopy reveals definite source, no further evaluation is needed. †If massive bleeding does not allow time for colonic lavage, proceed to angiography.

in which case angiography is recommended. Sigmoidoscopy is used primarily in patients <40 years old with minor bleeding. In patients with no source identified on colonoscopy, imaging studies may be employed. ^{99m}Tc-labeled red cell scan allows repeated imaging for up to 24 h and may identify the general location of bleeding. However, radionuclide scans should be interpreted with caution because results, especially from later images, are highly variable. Multidector computed tomography (CT) "angiography" is an increasingly used technique that is likely superior to nuclear scintigraphy. In active LGIB, angiography can detect the site of bleeding (extravasation of contrast into the gut) and permits treatment with embolization. Even after bleeding has stopped, angiography may identify lesions with abnormal vasculature, such as vascular ectasias or tumors.

EVALUATION AND MANAGEMENT OF OBSCURE GIB

Obscure GIB is defined as persistent or recurrent bleeding for which no source has been identified by routine endoscopic and contrast x-ray studies; it may be overt (melena, hematochezia) or occult (iron-deficiency anemia). Current guidelines suggest angiography as the initial test for massive obscure bleeding, and video capsule endoscopy, which allows examination of the entire small intestine, for all others. Push enteroscopy, usually performed with a pediatric colonoscope, to inspect the entire duodenum and proximal jejunum also may be considered as an initial evaluation. A systematic review of 14 trials comparing push enteroscopy to capsule revealed "clinically significant findings" in 26% and 56% of patients, respectively. However, in contrast to enteroscopy, lack of control of the capsule prevents its manipulation and full visualization of the intestine; in addition, tissue cannot be sampled and therapy cannot be applied.

If capsule endoscopy is positive, management is dictated by the finding. If capsule endoscopy is negative, current recommendations suggest patients may either be observed or, if their clinical course mandates (e.g., recurrent bleeding, need for transfusions or hospitalization), undergo further testing. "Deep" enteroscopy (e.g., double-balloon, single-balloon, and spiral enteroscopy) is commonly the next test undertaken in patients with clinically important obscure GIB because it allows the endoscopist to examine, obtain specimens from, and provide therapy to much or all of the small intestine. CT and magnetic resonance enterography also are used to examine the small intestine. Other imaging techniques sometimes used in evaluation of obscure GIB include ^{99m}Tc-labeled red blood cell scintigraphy, multidetector CT "angiography," angiography, and ^{99m}Tc-pertechnetate scintigraphy for Meckel's diverticulum (especially in young patients). If all tests are unrevealing, intraoperative endoscopy is indicated in patients with severe recurrent or persistent bleeding requiring repeated transfusions.

POSITIVE FECAL OCCULT BLOOD TEST

Fecal occult blood testing is recommended only for colorectal cancer screening and may be used beginning at age 50 in average-risk adults and beginning at age 40 in adults with a first-degree relative with colorectal neoplasm at ≥60 years or two second-degree relatives with colorectal cancer. A positive test necessitates colonoscopy. If evaluation of the colon is negative, further workup is not recommended unless iron-deficiency anemia or GI symptoms are present.

58 Jaundice

Savio John, Daniel S. Pratt

Jaundice, or icterus, is a yellowish discoloration of tissue resulting from the deposition of bilirubin. Tissue deposition of bilirubin occurs only in the presence of serum hyperbilirubinemia and is a sign of either liver disease or, less often, a hemolytic disorder. The degree of serum bilirubin elevation can be estimated by physical examination. Slight increases in serum bilirubin level are best detected by examining the sclerae, which have a particular affinity for bilirubin due to their high elastin content. The presence of scleral icterus indicates a serum bilirubin level of at least 51 μmol/L (3 mg/dL). The ability to detect scleral icterus is made more difficult if the examining room has fluorescent lighting. If the examiner suspects scleral icterus, a second site to examine is underneath the tongue. As serum bilirubin levels rise, the skin will eventually become yellow in light-skinned patients and even green if the process is long-standing; the green color is produced by oxidation of bilirubin to biliverdin.

The differential diagnosis for yellowing of the skin is limited. In addition to jaundice, it includes carotenoderma, the use of the drug quinacrine, and excessive exposure to phenols. Carotenoderma is the yellow color imparted to the skin of healthy individuals who ingest excessive amounts of vegetables and fruits that contain carotene, such as carrots, leafy vegetables, squash, peaches, and oranges. In jaundice the yellow coloration of the skin is uniformly distributed over the body, whereas in carotenoderma the pigment is concentrated on the palms, soles, forehead, and nasolabial folds. Carotenoderma can be distinguished from jaundice by the sparing of the sclerae. Quinacrine causes a yellow discoloration of the skin in 4–37% of patients treated with it.

Another sensitive indicator of increased serum bilirubin is darkening of the urine, which is due to the renal excretion of conjugated bilirubin. Patients often describe their urine as tea- or cola-colored. Bilirubinuria indicates an elevation of the direct serum bilirubin fraction and, therefore, the presence of liver disease.

Serum bilirubin levels increase when an imbalance exists between bilirubin production and clearance. A logical evaluation of the patient who is jaundiced requires an understanding of bilirubin production and metabolism.

PRODUCTION AND METABOLISM OF BILIRUBIN

(See also Chap. 359) Bilirubin, a tetrapyrrole pigment, is a breakdown product of heme (ferroprotoporphyrin IX). About 70–80% of the 250–300 mg of bilirubin produced each day is derived from the breakdown of hemoglobin in senescent red blood cells. The remainder comes from prematurely destroyed erythroid cells in bone marrow and from the turnover of hemoproteins such as myoglobin and cytochromes found in tissues throughout the body.

The formation of bilirubin occurs in reticuloendothelial cells, primarily in the spleen and liver. The first reaction, catalyzed by the microsomal enzyme heme oxygenase, oxidatively cleaves the α bridge of the porphyrin group and opens the heme ring. The end products of this reaction are biliverdin, carbon monoxide, and iron. The second reaction, catalyzed by the cytosolic enzyme biliverdin reductase, reduces the central methylene bridge of biliverdin and converts it to bilirubin. Bilirubin formed in the reticuloendothelial cells is virtually insoluble in water due to tight internal hydrogen bonding between the water-soluble moieties of bilirubin—i.e., the bonding of the proprionic acid carboxyl groups of one dipyrrolic half of the molecule with the imino and lactam groups of the opposite half. This configuration blocks solvent access to the polar residues of bilirubin and places the hydrophobic residues on the outside. To be transported in blood, bilirubin must be solubilized. Solubilization is accomplished by the reversible, noncovalent binding of bilirubin to albumin. Unconjugated bilirubin bound to albumin is transported to the liver. There, the bilirubin—but not the albumin—is taken up by hepatocytes via a process that at least partly involves carrier-mediated membrane transport. No specific bilirubin transporter has yet been identified (Chap. 359, Fig. 359-1).

After entering the hepatocyte, unconjugated bilirubin is bound in the cytosol to a number of proteins including proteins in the glutathione-S-transferase superfamily. These proteins serve both to reduce efflux of bilirubin back into the serum and to present the bilirubin for conjugation. In the endoplasmic reticulum, bilirubin is solubilized by conjugation to glucuronic acid, a process that disrupts the internal hydrogen bonds and yields bilirubin monoglucuronide and diglucuronide. The conjugation of glucuronic acid to bilirubin is catalyzed by bilirubin uridine diphosphate-glucuronosyl transferase (UDPGT). The now-hydrophilic bilirubin conjugates diffuse from the endoplasmic reticulum to the canalicular membrane, where bilirubin monoglucuronide and diglucuronide are actively transported into canalicular bile by an energy-dependent mechanism involving the multidrug resistance–associated protein 2 (MRP2).

The conjugated bilirubin excreted into bile drains into the duodenum and passes unchanged through the proximal small bowel. Conjugated bilirubin is not taken up by the intestinal mucosa. When the conjugated bilirubin reaches the distal ileum and colon, it is hydrolyzed to unconjugated bilirubin by bacterial β-glucuronidases. The unconjugated bilirubin is reduced by normal gut bacteria to form a group of colorless tetrapyrroles called *urobilinogens*. About 80–90% of these products are excreted in feces, either unchanged or oxidized to orange derivatives called *urobilins*. The remaining 10–20% of the urobilinogens are passively absorbed, enter the portal venous blood, and are re-excreted by the liver. A small fraction (usually <3 mg/dL) escapes hepatic uptake, filters across the renal glomerulus, and is excreted in urine.

MEASUREMENT OF SERUM BILIRUBIN

The terms *direct* and *indirect* bilirubin—i.e., conjugated and unconjugated bilirubin, respectively—are based on the original van den Bergh reaction. This assay, or a variation of it, is still used in most clinical chemistry laboratories to determine the serum bilirubin level. In this assay, bilirubin is exposed to diazotized sulfanilic acid and splits into two relatively stable dipyrrylmethene azopigments that absorb maximally at 540 nm, allowing photometric analysis. The direct fraction is that which reacts with diazotized sulfanilic acid in the absence of an accelerator substance such as alcohol. The direct fraction provides an approximation of the conjugated bilirubin level in serum. The *total* serum bilirubin is the amount that reacts after the addition of alcohol. The indirect fraction is the difference between the total and the direct bilirubin levels and provides an estimate of the unconjugated bilirubin in serum.

With the van den Bergh method, the normal serum bilirubin concentration usually is 17 μmol/L (<1 mg/dL). Up to 30%, or 5.1 μmol/L (0.3 mg/dL), of the total may be direct-reacting (conjugated) bilirubin. Total serum bilirubin concentrations are between 3.4 and 15.4 μmol/L (0.2 and 0.9 mg/dL) in 95% of a normal population.

Several new techniques, although less convenient to perform, have added considerably to our understanding of bilirubin metabolism. First, studies using these methods demonstrate that, in normal persons or those with Gilbert's syndrome, almost 100% of the serum bilirubin is unconjugated; <3% is monoconjugated bilirubin. Second, in jaundiced patients with hepatobiliary disease, the total serum bilirubin concentration measured by these new, more accurate methods is lower than the values found with diazo methods. This finding suggests that there are diazo-positive compounds distinct from bilirubin in the serum of patients with hepatobiliary disease. Third, these studies indicate that, in jaundiced patients with hepatobiliary disease, monoglucuronides of bilirubin predominate over diglucuronides. Fourth, part of the direct-reacting bilirubin fraction includes conjugated bilirubin that is covalently linked to albumin. This albumin-linked bilirubin fraction (*delta fraction*, or *biliprotein*) represents an important fraction of total serum bilirubin in patients with cholestasis and hepatobiliary disorders. The delta fraction (delta bilirubin) is formed in serum when hepatic excretion of bilirubin glucuronides is impaired and the glucuronides accumulate in serum. By virtue of its tight binding to albumin, the clearance rate of delta bilirubin from serum approximates the half-life of albumin (12–14 days) rather than the short half-life of bilirubin (about 4 h).

The prolonged half-life of albumin-bound conjugated bilirubin accounts for two previously unexplained enigmas in jaundiced patients with liver disease: (1) that some patients with conjugated hyperbilirubinemia do not exhibit bilirubinuria during the recovery phase of their disease because the bilirubin is covalently bound to albumin and therefore not filtered by the renal glomeruli, and (2) that the elevated serum bilirubin level declines more slowly than expected in some patients who otherwise appear to be recovering satisfactorily. Late in the recovery phase of hepatobiliary disorders, all the conjugated bilirubin may be in the albumin-linked form.

MEASUREMENT OF URINE BILIRUBIN

Unconjugated bilirubin is always bound to albumin in the serum, is not filtered by the kidney, and is not found in the urine. Conjugated bilirubin is filtered at the glomerulus, and the majority is reabsorbed by the proximal tubules; a small fraction is excreted in the urine. Any bilirubin found in the urine is conjugated bilirubin. The presence of bilirubinuria implies the presence of liver disease. A urine dipstick test (Ictotest) gives the same information as fractionation of the serum bilirubin and is very accurate. A false-negative result is possible in patients with prolonged cholestasis due to the predominance of delta bilirubin, which is covalently bound to albumin and therefore not filtered by the renal glomeruli.

APPROACH TO THE PATIENT: Jaundice

The goal of this chapter is not to provide an encyclopedic review of all of the conditions that can cause jaundice. Rather, the chapter is intended to offer a framework that helps a physician to evaluate the patient with jaundice in a logical way (Fig. 58-1).

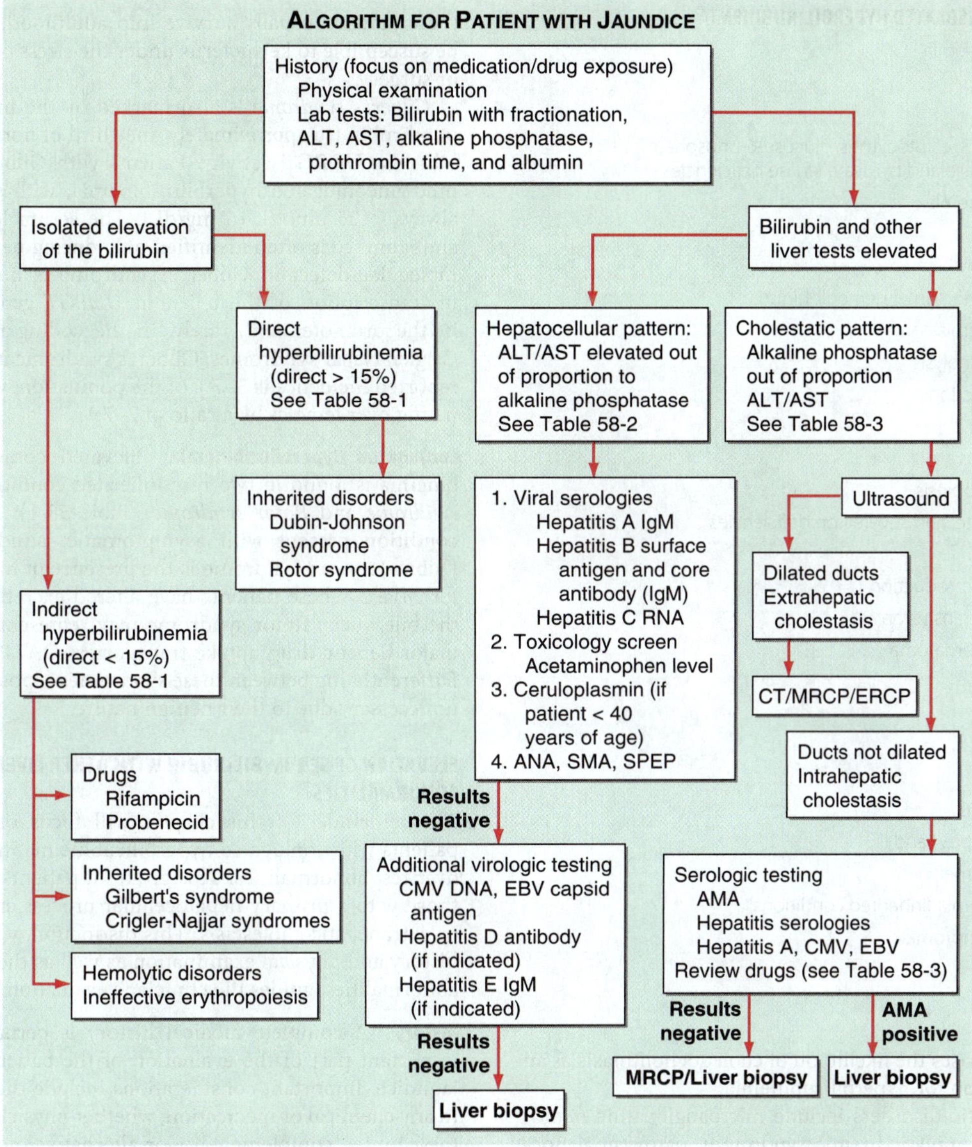

FIGURE 58-1 Evaluation of the patient with jaundice. ALT, alanine aminotransferase; AMA, antimitochondrial antibody; ANA, antinuclear antibody; AST, aspartate aminotransferase; CMV, cytomegalovirus; EBV, Epstein-Barr virus; LKM, liver-kidney microsomal antibody; MRCP, magnetic resonance cholangiopancreatography; SMA, smooth-muscle antibody; SPEP, serum protein electrophoresis.

Simply stated, the initial step is to perform appropriate blood tests in order to determine whether the patient has an isolated elevation of serum bilirubin. If so, is the bilirubin elevation due to an increased unconjugated or conjugated fraction? If the hyperbilirubinemia is accompanied by other liver test abnormalities, is the disorder hepatocellular or cholestatic? If cholestatic, is it intra- or extrahepatic? All of these questions can be answered with a thoughtful history, physical examination, and interpretation of laboratory and radiologic tests and procedures.

The bilirubin present in serum represents a balance between input from the production of bilirubin and hepatic/biliary removal of the pigment. Hyperbilirubinemia may result from (1) overproduction of bilirubin; (2) impaired uptake, conjugation, or excretion of bilirubin; or (3) regurgitation of unconjugated or conjugated bilirubin from damaged hepatocytes or bile ducts. An increase in unconjugated bilirubin in serum results from overproduction, impaired uptake, or conjugation of bilirubin. An increase in conjugated bilirubin is due to decreased excretion into the bile ductules or backward leakage of the pigment. The initial steps in evaluating the patient with jaundice are to determine (1) whether the hyperbilirubinemia is predominantly conjugated or unconjugated in nature and (2) whether other biochemical liver tests are abnormal. The thoughtful interpretation of limited data permits a rational evaluation of the patient (Fig. 58-1). The following discussion will focus solely on the evaluation of the adult patient with jaundice.

ISOLATED ELEVATION OF SERUM BILIRUBIN

Unconjugated Hyperbilirubinemia The differential diagnosis of isolated unconjugated hyperbilirubinemia is limited (Table 58-1). The critical determination is whether the patient is suffering from a hemolytic process resulting in an overproduction of bilirubin (hemolytic disorders and ineffective erythropoiesis) or from impaired hepatic uptake/conjugation of bilirubin (drug effect or genetic disorders).

Hemolytic disorders that cause excessive heme production may be either inherited or acquired. Inherited disorders include spherocytosis, sickle cell anemia, thalassemia, and deficiency of red cell enzymes such as pyruvate kinase and glucose-6-phosphate dehydrogenase. In these conditions, the serum bilirubin level rarely exceeds 86 μmol/L (5 mg/dL). Higher levels may occur when there is coexistent renal or hepatocellular dysfunction or in acute hemolysis, such as a sickle cell crisis. In evaluating jaundice in patients with chronic hemolysis, it is important to remember the high incidence of pigmented (calcium bilirubinate) gallstones found in these

TABLE 58-1 CAUSES OF ISOLATED HYPERBILIRUBINEMIA

I. Indirect hyperbilirubinemia
  A. Hemolytic disorders
    1. Inherited
      a. Spherocytosis, elliptocytosis, glucose-6-phosphate dehydrogenase and pyruvate kinase deficiencies
      b. Sickle cell anemia
    2. Acquired
      a. Microangiopathic hemolytic anemias
      b. Paroxysmal nocturnal hemoglobinuria
      c. Spur cell anemia
      d. Immune hemolysis
      e. Parasitic infections
        (1) Malaria
        (2) Babesiosis
  B. Ineffective erythropoiesis
    1. Cobalamin, folate, and severe iron deficiencies
    2. Thalassemia
  C. Increased bilirubin production
    1. Massive blood transfusion
    2. Resorption of hematoma
  D. Drugs
    1. Rifampin
    2. Probenecid
    3. Ribavirin
  E. Inherited conditions
    1. Crigler-Najjar types I and II
    2. Gilbert's syndrome
II. Direct hyperbilirubinemia (inherited conditions)
  A. Dubin-Johnson syndrome
  B. Rotor syndrome

patients, which increases the likelihood of choledocholithiasis as an alternative explanation for hyperbilirubinemia.

Acquired hemolytic disorders include microangiopathic hemolytic anemia (e.g., hemolytic-uremic syndrome), paroxysmal nocturnal hemoglobinuria, spur cell anemia, immune hemolysis, and parasitic infections (e.g., malaria and babesiosis). Ineffective erythropoiesis occurs in cobalamin, folate, and iron deficiencies. Resorption of hematomas and massive blood transfusions both can result in increased hemoglobin release and overproduction of bilirubin.

In the absence of hemolysis, the physician should consider a problem with the hepatic uptake or conjugation of bilirubin. Certain drugs, including rifampin and probenecid, may cause unconjugated hyperbilirubinemia by diminishing hepatic uptake of bilirubin. Impaired bilirubin conjugation occurs in three genetic conditions: Crigler-Najjar syndrome types I and II and Gilbert's syndrome. *Crigler-Najjar type I* is an exceptionally rare condition found in neonates and characterized by severe jaundice (bilirubin >342 μmol/L [>20 mg/dL]) and neurologic impairment due to kernicterus, frequently leading to death in infancy or childhood. These patients have a complete absence of bilirubin UDPGT activity, usually due to mutations in the critical 3′ domain of the *UDPGT* gene; are totally unable to conjugate bilirubin; and hence cannot excrete it.

Crigler-Najjar type II is somewhat more common than type I. Patients live into adulthood with serum bilirubin levels of 103–428 μmol/L (6–25 mg/dL). In these patients, mutations in the bilirubin *UDPGT* gene cause the reduction—but not the complete eradication—of the enzyme's activity. Bilirubin UDPGT activity can be induced by the administration of phenobarbital, which can reduce serum bilirubin levels in these patients. Despite marked jaundice, these patients usually survive into adulthood, although they may be susceptible to kernicterus under the stress of intercurrent illness or surgery.

Gilbert's syndrome is also marked by the impaired conjugation of bilirubin (to approximately one-third of normal) due to reduced bilirubin UDPGT activity. Patients with Gilbert's syndrome have mild unconjugated hyperbilirubinemia, with serum levels almost always <103 μmol/L (6 mg/dL). The serum levels may fluctuate, and jaundice is often identified only during periods of fasting. The molecular defect in Gilbert's syndrome is linked to a reduction in transcription of the bilirubin *UDPGT* gene due to mutations in the promoter and, rarely, in the coding region. Unlike both Crigler-Najjar syndromes, Gilbert's syndrome is very common. The reported incidence is 3–7% of the population, with males predominating over females by a ratio of 2–7:1.

Conjugated Hyperbilirubinemia Elevated conjugated hyperbilirubinemia is found in two rare inherited conditions: *Dubin-Johnson syndrome* and *Rotor syndrome* (Table 58-1). Patients with either condition present with asymptomatic jaundice. The defect in Dubin-Johnson syndrome is the presence of mutations in the gene for MRP2. These patients have altered excretion of bilirubin into the bile ducts. Rotor syndrome may represent a deficiency of the major hepatic drug uptake transporters OATP1B1 and OATP1B3. Differentiating between these syndromes is possible but is clinically unnecessary due to their benign nature.

ELEVATION OF SERUM BILIRUBIN WITH OTHER LIVER TEST ABNORMALITIES

The remainder of this chapter will focus on the evaluation of patients with conjugated hyperbilirubinemia in the setting of other liver test abnormalities. This group of patients can be divided into those with a primary hepatocellular process and those with intra- or extrahepatic cholestasis. This distinction, which is based on the history and physical examination as well as the pattern of liver test abnormalities, guides the clinician's evaluation (Fig. 58-1).

History A complete medical history is perhaps the single most important part of the evaluation of the patient with unexplained jaundice. Important considerations include the use of or exposure to any chemical or medication, whether physician-prescribed, over-the-counter, complementary, or alternative medicines (e.g., herbal and vitamin preparations) or other drugs such as anabolic steroids. The patient should be carefully questioned about possible parenteral exposures, including transfusions, intravenous and intranasal drug use, tattooing, and sexual activity. Other important points include recent travel history; exposure to people with jaundice; exposure to possibly contaminated foods; occupational exposure to hepatotoxins; alcohol consumption; the duration of jaundice; and the presence of any accompanying signs and symptoms, such as arthralgias, myalgias, rash, anorexia, weight loss, abdominal pain, fever, pruritus, and changes in the urine and stool. While none of the latter manifestations is specific for any one condition, any of them can suggest a particular diagnosis. A history of arthralgias and myalgias predating jaundice suggests hepatitis, either viral or drug-related. Jaundice associated with the sudden onset of severe right-upper-quadrant pain and shaking chills suggests choledocholithiasis and ascending cholangitis.

Physical Examination The general assessment should include evaluation of the patient's nutritional status. Temporal and proximal muscle wasting suggests long-standing disease such as pancreatic cancer or cirrhosis. Stigmata of chronic liver disease, including spider nevi, palmar erythema, gynecomastia, caput medusae, Dupuytren's contractures, parotid gland enlargement, and testicular atrophy, are commonly seen in advanced alcoholic (Laennec's) cirrhosis and occasionally in other types of cirrhosis. An enlarged left supraclavicular node (Virchow's node) or a periumbilical nodule (Sister Mary Joseph's nodule) suggests an abdominal malignancy.

Jugular venous distention, a sign of right-sided heart failure, suggests hepatic congestion. Right pleural effusion in the absence of clinically apparent ascites may be seen in advanced cirrhosis.

The abdominal examination should focus on the size and consistency of the liver, on whether the spleen is palpable and hence enlarged, and on whether ascites is present. Patients with cirrhosis may have an enlarged left lobe of the liver, which is felt below the xiphoid, and an enlarged spleen. A grossly enlarged nodular liver or an obvious abdominal mass suggests malignancy. An enlarged tender liver could signify viral or alcoholic hepatitis; an infiltrative process such as amyloidosis; or, less often, an acutely congested liver secondary to right-sided heart failure. Severe right-upper-quadrant tenderness with respiratory arrest on inspiration (Murphy's sign) suggests cholecystitis. Ascites in the presence of jaundice suggests either cirrhosis or malignancy with peritoneal spread.

Laboratory Tests A battery of tests are helpful in the initial evaluation of a patient with unexplained jaundice. These include total and direct serum bilirubin measurement with fractionation; determination of serum aminotransferase, alkaline phosphatase, and albumin concentrations; and prothrombin time tests. Enzyme tests (alanine aminotransferase [ALT], aspartate aminotransferase [AST], and alkaline phosphatase [ALP]) are helpful in differentiating between a hepatocellular process and a cholestatic process (Table 358-1; Fig. 58-1)—a critical step in determining what additional workup is indicated. Patients with a hepatocellular process generally have a rise in the aminotransferases that is disproportionate to that in ALP, whereas patients with a cholestatic process have a rise in ALP that is disproportionate to that of the aminotransferases. The serum bilirubin can be prominently elevated in both hepatocellular and cholestatic conditions and therefore is not necessarily helpful in differentiating between the two.

In addition to enzyme tests, all jaundiced patients should have additional blood tests—specifically, an albumin level and a prothrombin time—to assess liver function. A low albumin level suggests a chronic process such as cirrhosis or cancer. A normal albumin level is suggestive of a more acute process such as viral hepatitis or choledocholithiasis. An elevated prothrombin time indicates either vitamin K deficiency due to prolonged jaundice and malabsorption of vitamin K or significant hepatocellular dysfunction. The failure of the prothrombin time to correct with parenteral administration of vitamin K indicates severe hepatocellular injury.

The results of the bilirubin, enzyme, albumin, and prothrombin time tests will usually indicate whether a jaundiced patient has a hepatocellular or a cholestatic disease and offer some indication of the duration and severity of the disease. The causes and evaluations of hepatocellular and cholestatic diseases are quite different.

Hepatocellular Conditions Hepatocellular diseases that can cause jaundice include viral hepatitis, drug or environmental toxicity, alcohol, and end-stage cirrhosis from any cause (Table 58-2). Wilson's disease occurs primarily in young adults. Autoimmune hepatitis is typically seen in young to middle-aged women but may affect men and women of any age. Alcoholic hepatitis can be differentiated from viral and toxin-related hepatitis by the pattern of the aminotransferases: patients with alcoholic hepatitis typically have an AST-to-ALT ratio of at least 2:1, and the AST level rarely exceeds 300 U/L. Patients with acute viral hepatitis and toxin-related injury severe enough to produce jaundice typically have aminotransferase levels >500 U/L, with the ALT greater than or equal to the AST. While ALT and AST values <8 times normal may be seen in either hepatocellular or cholestatic liver disease, values 25 times normal or higher are seen primarily in acute hepatocellular diseases. Patients with jaundice from cirrhosis can have normal or only slightly elevated aminotransferase levels.

When the clinician determines that a patient has a hepatocellular disease, appropriate testing for acute viral hepatitis includes a hepatitis A IgM antibody assay, a hepatitis B surface antigen and core IgM antibody assay, a hepatitis C viral RNA test, and, depending on the circumstances, a hepatitis E IgM antibody assay. Because it can take many weeks for hepatitis C antibody to become detectable, its assay is an unreliable test if acute hepatitis C is suspected. Studies for hepatitis D and E viruses, Epstein-Barr virus (EBV), and cytomegalovirus (CMV) may also be indicated. Ceruloplasmin is the initial screening test for Wilson's disease. Testing for autoimmune hepatitis usually includes an antinuclear antibody assay and measurement of specific immunoglobulins.

TABLE 58-2 HEPATOCELLULAR CONDITIONS THAT MAY PRODUCE JAUNDICE

Viral hepatitis
Hepatitis A, B, C, D, and E
Epstein-Barr virus
Cytomegalovirus
Herpes simplex virus
Alcoholic hepatitis
Drug toxicity
Predictable, dose-dependent (e.g., acetaminophen)
Unpredictable, idiosyncratic (e.g., isoniazid)
Environmental toxins
Vinyl chloride
Jamaica bush tea—pyrrolizidine alkaloids
Kava Kava
Wild mushrooms—*Amanita phalloides, A. verna*
Wilson's disease
Autoimmune hepatitis

Drug-induced hepatocellular injury can be classified as either predictable or unpredictable. Predictable drug reactions are dose-dependent and affect all patients who ingest a toxic dose of the drug in question. The classic example is acetaminophen hepatotoxicity. Unpredictable or idiosyncratic drug reactions are not dose-dependent and occur in a minority of patients. A great number of drugs can cause idiosyncratic hepatic injury. Environmental toxins are also an important cause of hepatocellular injury. Examples include industrial chemicals such as vinyl chloride, herbal preparations containing pyrrolizidine alkaloids (Jamaica bush tea) or Kava Kava, and the mushrooms *Amanita phalloides* and *A. verna*, which contain highly hepatotoxic amatoxins.

Cholestatic Conditions When the pattern of the liver tests suggests a cholestatic disorder, the next step is to determine whether it is intra- or extrahepatic cholestasis (Fig. 58-1). Distinguishing intrahepatic from extrahepatic cholestasis may be difficult. History, physical examination, and laboratory tests often are not helpful. The next appropriate test is an ultrasound. The ultrasound is inexpensive, does not expose the patient to ionizing radiation, and can detect dilation of the intra- and extrahepatic biliary tree with a high degree of sensitivity and specificity. The absence of biliary dilation suggests intrahepatic cholestasis, while its presence indicates extrahepatic cholestasis. False-negative results occur in patients with partial obstruction of the common bile duct or in patients with cirrhosis or primary sclerosing cholangitis (PSC), in which scarring prevents the intrahepatic ducts from dilating.

Although ultrasonography may indicate extrahepatic cholestasis, it rarely identifies the site or cause of obstruction. The distal common bile duct is a particularly difficult area to visualize by ultrasound because of overlying bowel gas. Appropriate next tests include CT, magnetic resonance cholangiopancreatography (MRCP), endoscopic retrograde cholangiopancreatography (ERCP), and endoscopic ultrasound (EUS). CT scanning and MRCP are better than ultrasonography for assessing the head of the pancreas and for identifying choledocholithiasis in the distal common bile duct, particularly when the ducts are not dilated. ERCP is the "gold standard" for identifying choledocholithiasis. Beyond its diagnostic capabilities, ERCP allows therapeutic interventions, including the removal of common bile duct stones and the placement of stents. MRCP has replaced ERCP as the initial diagnostic test in cases where the need for intervention is thought to be small. EUS displays sensitivity and specificity comparable to that of MRCP in the detection of bile duct obstruction. EUS also allows biopsy of suspected malignant lesions, but is invasive and requires sedation.

In patients with apparent *intrahepatic cholestasis*, the diagnosis is often made by serologic testing in combination with percutaneous liver biopsy. The list of possible causes of intrahepatic cholestasis is long and varied (Table 58-3). A number of conditions that typically cause a hepatocellular pattern of injury can also present as a cholestatic variant. Both hepatitis B and C viruses can cause cholestatic hepatitis (fibrosing cholestatic hepatitis). This disease variant has been reported in patients who have undergone solid organ transplantation. Hepatitis A and E, alcoholic hepatitis, and EBV or CMV infections may also present as cholestatic liver disease.

Drugs may cause intrahepatic cholestasis that is usually reversible after discontinuation of the offending agent, although it may take many months for cholestasis to resolve. Drugs most commonly associated with cholestasis are the anabolic and contraceptive steroids. Cholestatic hepatitis has been reported with chlorpromazine, imipramine, tolbutamide, sulindac, cimetidine, and erythromycin estolate. It also occurs in patients taking trimethoprim; sulfamethoxazole; and penicillin-based antibiotics such as ampicillin, dicloxacillin, and clavulanic acid. Rarely, cholestasis may be chronic and associated with progressive fibrosis despite early discontinuation of the offending drug. Chronic cholestasis has been associated with chlorpromazine and prochlorperazine.

Primary biliary cirrhosis is an autoimmune disease predominantly affecting middle-aged women and characterized by progressive destruction of interlobular bile ducts. The diagnosis is made by the detection of antimitochondrial antibody, which is found in 95% of patients. *Primary sclerosing cholangitis* is characterized by the destruction and fibrosis of larger bile ducts. The diagnosis of PSC is made with cholangiography (either MRCP or ERCP), which demonstrates the pathognomonic segmental strictures. Approximately 75% of patients with PSC have inflammatory bowel disease.

The *vanishing bile duct syndrome* and *adult bile ductopenia* are rare conditions in which a decreased number of bile ducts are seen in liver biopsy specimens. The histologic picture is similar to that in primary biliary cirrhosis. This picture is seen in patients who develop chronic rejection after liver transplantation and in those who develop graft-versus-host disease after bone marrow transplantation. Vanishing bile duct syndrome also occurs in rare cases of sarcoidosis, in patients taking certain drugs (including chlorpromazine), and idiopathically.

There are also familial forms of intrahepatic cholestasis. The familial intrahepatic cholestatic syndromes include *progressive familial intrahepatic cholestasis* (PFIC) *types 1–3* and *benign recurrent cholestasis* (BRC). PFIC1 and BRC are autosomal recessive diseases that result from mutations in the *ATP8B1* gene that encodes a protein belonging to the subfamily of P-type ATPases; the exact function of this protein remains poorly defined. While PFIC1 is a progressive condition that manifests in childhood, BRC presents later and is marked by recurrent episodes of jaundice and pruritus; the episodes are self-limited but can be debilitating. PFIC2 is caused by mutations in the *ABCB11* gene, which encodes the bile salt export pump, and PFIC3 is caused by mutations in the multidrug-resistant P-glycoprotein 3. *Cholestasis of pregnancy* occurs in the second and third trimesters and resolves after delivery. Its cause is unknown, but the condition is probably inherited, and cholestasis can be triggered by estrogen administration.

TABLE 58-3 CHOLESTATIC CONDITIONS THAT MAY PRODUCE JAUNDICE

- I. Intrahepatic
  - A. Viral hepatitis
    - 1. Fibrosing cholestatic hepatitis—hepatitis B and C
    - 2. Hepatitis A, Epstein-Barr virus infection, cytomegalovirus infection
  - B. Alcoholic hepatitis
  - C. Drug toxicity
    - 1. Pure cholestasis—anabolic and contraceptive steroids
    - 2. Cholestatic hepatitis—chlorpromazine, erythromycin estolate
    - 3. Chronic cholestasis—chlorpromazine and prochlorperazine
  - D. Primary biliary cirrhosis
  - E. Primary sclerosing cholangitis
  - F. Vanishing bile duct syndrome
    - 1. Chronic rejection of liver transplants
    - 2. Sarcoidosis
    - 3. Drugs
  - G. Congestive hepatopathy and ischemic hepatitis
  - H. Inherited conditions
    - 1. Progressive familial intrahepatic cholestasis
    - 2. Benign recurrent cholestasis
  - I. Cholestasis of pregnancy
  - J. Total parenteral nutrition
  - K. Nonhepatobiliary sepsis
  - L. Benign postoperative cholestasis
  - M. Paraneoplastic syndrome
  - N. Veno-occlusive disease
  - O. Graft-versus-host disease
  - P. Infiltrative disease
    - 1. Tuberculosis
    - 2. Lymphoma
    - 3. Amyloidosis
  - Q. Infections
    - 1. Malaria
    - 2. Leptospirosis
- II. Extrahepatic
  - A. Malignant
    - 1. Cholangiocarcinoma
    - 2. Pancreatic cancer
    - 3. Gallbladder cancer
    - 4. Ampullary cancer
    - 5. Malignant involvement of the porta hepatis lymph nodes
  - B. Benign
    - 1. Choledocholithiasis
    - 2. Postoperative biliary strictures
    - 3. Primary sclerosing cholangitis
    - 4. Chronic pancreatitis
    - 5. AIDS cholangiopathy
    - 6. Mirizzi's syndrome
    - 7. Parasitic disease (ascariasis)

Other causes of intrahepatic cholestasis include total parenteral nutrition (TPN); nonhepatobiliary sepsis; benign postoperative cholestasis; and a paraneoplastic syndrome associated with a number of different malignancies, including Hodgkin's disease, medullary thyroid cancer, renal cell cancer, renal sarcoma, T cell lymphoma, prostate cancer, and several gastrointestinal malignancies. The term *Stauffer's syndrome* has been used for intrahepatic cholestasis specifically associated with renal cell cancer. In patients developing cholestasis in the intensive care unit, the major considerations should be sepsis, ischemic hepatitis ("shock liver"), and TPN jaundice. Jaundice occurring after bone marrow transplantation is most likely due to veno-occlusive disease or graft-versus-host disease. In addition to hemolysis, sickle cell disease may cause intrahepatic and extrahepatic cholestasis. Jaundice is a late finding in heart failure caused by hepatic congestion and hepatocellular hypoxia. Ischemic hepatitis is a distinct entity of acute hypoperfusion characterized by an acute and dramatic elevation in the serum aminotransferases followed by a gradual peak in serum bilirubin.

Jaundice with associated liver dysfunction can be seen in severe cases of *Plasmodium falciparum* malaria. The jaundice in these cases is due to a combination of indirect hyperbilirubinemia from hemolysis and both cholestatic and hepatocellular jaundice. Weil's disease, a severe presentation of leptospirosis, is marked by jaundice with renal failure, fever, headache, and muscle pain.

Causes of *extrahepatic cholestasis* can be split into malignant and benign (Table 58-3). Malignant causes include pancreatic, gallbladder, and ampullary cancers as well as cholangiocarcinoma. This last malignancy is most commonly associated with PSC and is exceptionally difficult to diagnose because its appearance is often identical to that of PSC. Pancreatic and gallbladder tumors as well as cholangiocarcinoma are rarely resectable and have poor prognoses. Ampullary carcinoma has the highest surgical cure rate of all the tumors that present as painless jaundice. Hilar lymphadenopathy due to metastases from other cancers may cause obstruction of the extrahepatic biliary tree.

Choledocholithiasis is the most common cause of extrahepatic cholestasis. The clinical presentation can range from mild right-upper-quadrant discomfort with only minimal elevations of enzyme test values to ascending cholangitis with jaundice, sepsis, and circulatory collapse. PSC may occur with clinically important strictures limited to the extrahepatic biliary tree. IgG4-associated cholangitis is marked by stricturing of the biliary tree. It is critical that the clinician differentiate this condition from PSC as it is responsive to glucocorticoid therapy. In rare instances, chronic pancreatitis causes strictures of the distal common bile duct, where it passes through the head of the pancreas. AIDS cholangiopathy is a condition that is usually due to infection of the bile duct epithelium with CMV or cryptosporidia and has a cholangiographic appearance similar to that of PSC. The affected patients usually present with greatly elevated serum alkaline phosphatase levels (mean, 800 IU/L), but the bilirubin level is often near normal. These patients do not typically present with jaundice.

GLOBAL CONSIDERATIONS

While extrahepatic biliary obstruction and drugs are common causes of new-onset jaundice in developed countries, infections remain the leading cause in developing countries. Liver involvement and jaundice are observed with numerous infections, particularly malaria, babesiosis, severe leptospirosis, infections due to *Mycobacterium tuberculosis* and the *Mycobacterium avium* complex, typhoid fever, viral hepatitis secondary to infection with hepatitis viruses A–E, EBV and CMV infections, late phases of yellow fever, dengue hemorrhagic fever, schistosomiasis, fascioliasis, clonorchiasis, opisthorchiasis, ascariasis, echinococcosis, hepatosplenic candidiasis, disseminated histoplasmosis, cryptococcosis, coccidioimycosis, ehrlichiosis, chronic Q fever, yersiniosis, brucellosis, syphilis, and leprosy. Bacterial infections that do not necessarily involve the liver and bile ducts may also lead to jaundice, as in cholestasis of sepsis.

Acknowledgment

This chapter is a revised version of chapters that have appeared in prior editions of Harrison's in which Marshall M. Kaplan was a co-author together with Daniel Pratt.

59 Abdominal Swelling and Ascites

Kathleen E. Corey, Lawrence S. Friedman

ABDOMINAL SWELLING

Abdominal swelling is a manifestation of numerous diseases. Patients may complain of bloating or abdominal fullness and may note increasing abdominal girth on the basis of increased clothing or belt size. Abdominal discomfort is often reported, but pain is less frequent. When abdominal pain does accompany swelling, it is frequently the result of an intraabdominal infection, peritonitis, or pancreatitis. Patients with abdominal distention from *ascites* (fluid in the abdomen) may report the new onset of an inguinal or umbilical hernia. Dyspnea may result from pressure against the diaphragm and the inability to expand the lungs fully.

CAUSES

The causes of abdominal swelling can be remembered conveniently as the *six Fs*: flatus, fat, fluid, fetus, feces, or a "fatal growth" (often a neoplasm).

Flatus Abdominal swelling may be the result of increased intestinal gas. The normal small intestine contains approximately 200 mL of gas made up of nitrogen, oxygen, carbon dioxide, hydrogen, and methane. Nitrogen and oxygen are consumed (swallowed), whereas carbon dioxide, hydrogen, and methane are produced intraluminally by bacterial fermentation. Increased intestinal gas can occur in a number of conditions. *Aerophagia*, the swallowing of air, can result in increased amounts of oxygen and nitrogen in the small intestine and lead to abdominal swelling. Aerophagia typically results from gulping food; chewing gum; smoking; or as a response to anxiety, which can lead to repetitive belching. In some cases, increased intestinal gas is the consequence of bacterial metabolism of excess fermentable substances such as lactose and other oligosaccharides, which can lead to production of hydrogen, carbon dioxide, or methane. In many cases, the precise cause of abdominal distention cannot be determined. In some persons, particularly those with irritable bowel syndrome and bloating, the subjective sense of abdominal pressure is attributable to impaired intestinal transit of gas rather than increased gas volume. Abdominal distention—an objective increase in girth—is the result of a lack of coordination between diaphragmatic contraction and anterior abdominal wall relaxation, a response in some cases to an increase in intraabdominal volume loads. Occasionally, increased lumbar lordosis accounts for apparent abdominal distention.

Fat Weight gain with an increase in abdominal fat can result in an increase in abdominal girth and can be perceived as abdominal swelling. Abdominal fat may be caused by an imbalance between caloric intake and energy expenditure associated with a poor diet and sedentary lifestyle; it also can be a manifestation of certain diseases, such as Cushing's syndrome. Excess abdominal fat has been associated with an increased risk of insulin resistance and cardiovascular disease.

Fluid The accumulation of fluid within the abdominal cavity (ascites) often results in abdominal distention and is discussed in detail below.

Fetus Pregnancy results in increased abdominal girth. Typically, an increase in abdominal size is first noted at 12–14 weeks of gestation, when the uterus moves from the pelvis into the abdomen. Abdominal distention may be seen before this point as a result of fluid retention and relaxation of the abdominal muscles.

Feces In the setting of severe constipation or intestinal obstruction, increased stool in the colon leads to increased abdominal girth. These conditions are often accompanied by abdominal discomfort or pain, nausea, and vomiting and can be diagnosed by imaging studies.

Fatal Growth An abdominal mass can result in abdominal swelling. Enlargement of the intraabdominal organs, specifically the liver (hepatomegaly) or spleen (splenomegaly), or an abdominal aortic aneurysm can result in abdominal distention. Bladder distention also may result in abdominal swelling. In addition, malignancies, abscesses, or cysts can grow to sizes that lead to increased abdominal girth.

APPROACH TO THE PATIENT: **Abdominal Swelling**

HISTORY

Determining the etiology of abdominal swelling begins with history-taking and a physical examination. Patients should be questioned regarding symptoms suggestive of malignancy, including weight loss, night sweats, and anorexia. Inability to pass stool or flatus together with nausea or vomiting suggests bowel obstruction, severe constipation, or an ileus (lack of peristalsis). Increased eructation and flatus may point toward aerophagia or increased intestinal production of gas. Patients should be questioned about risk factors for or symptoms of chronic liver disease, including excessive alcohol use and jaundice, which suggest ascites. Patients should also be asked about other symptoms of medical conditions, including heart failure and tuberculosis, which may cause ascites.

PHYSICAL EXAMINATION

Physical examination should include an assessment for signs of systemic disease. The presence of lymphadenopathy, especially supraclavicular lymphadenopathy (*Virchow's node*), suggests metastatic abdominal malignancy. Care should be taken during the cardiac examination to evaluate for elevation of jugular venous pressure (JVP); *Kussmaul's sign* (elevation of the JVP during inspiration); a pericardial knock, which may be seen in heart failure or constrictive pericarditis; or a murmur of tricuspid regurgitation. Spider angiomas, palmar erythema, dilated superficial veins around the umbilicus (*caput medusae*), and gynecomastia suggest chronic liver disease.

The abdominal examination should begin with inspection for the presence of uneven distention or an obvious mass. Auscultation should follow. The absence of bowel sounds or the presence of high-pitched localized bowel sounds points toward an ileus or intestinal obstruction. An umbilical venous hum may suggest the presence of portal hypertension, and a harsh bruit over the liver is heard rarely in patients with hepatocellular carcinoma or alcoholic hepatitis. Abdominal swelling caused by intestinal gas can be differentiated from swelling caused by fluid or a solid mass by percussion; an abdomen filled with gas is tympanic, whereas an abdomen containing a mass or fluid is dull to percussion. The absence of abdominal dullness, however, does not exclude ascites, because a minimum of 1500 mL of ascitic fluid is required for detection on physical examination. Finally, the abdomen should be palpated to assess for tenderness, a mass, enlargement of the spleen or liver, or presence of a nodular liver suggesting cirrhosis or tumor. Light palpation of the liver may detect pulsations suggesting retrograde vascular flow from the heart in patients with right-sided heart failure, particularly tricuspid regurgitation.

IMAGING AND LABORATORY EVALUATION

Abdominal x-rays can be used to detect dilated loops of bowel suggesting intestinal obstruction or ileus. Abdominal ultrasonography can detect as little as 100 mL of ascitic fluid, hepatosplenomegaly, a nodular liver, or a mass. Ultrasonography is often inadequate to detect retroperitoneal lymphadenopathy or a pancreatic lesion because of overlying bowel gas. If malignancy or pancreatic disease is suspected, CT can be performed. CT may also detect changes associated with advanced cirrhosis and portal hypertension (Fig. 59-1).

Laboratory evaluation should include liver biochemical testing, serum albumin level measurement, and prothrombin time determination (international normalized ratio) to assess hepatic function as well as a complete blood count to evaluate for the presence of cytopenias that may result from portal hypertension or of leukocytosis, anemia, and thrombocytosis that may result from systemic infection. Serum amylase and lipase levels should be checked to evaluate the patient for acute pancreatitis. Urinary protein quantitation is indicated when nephrotic syndrome, which may cause ascites, is suspected.

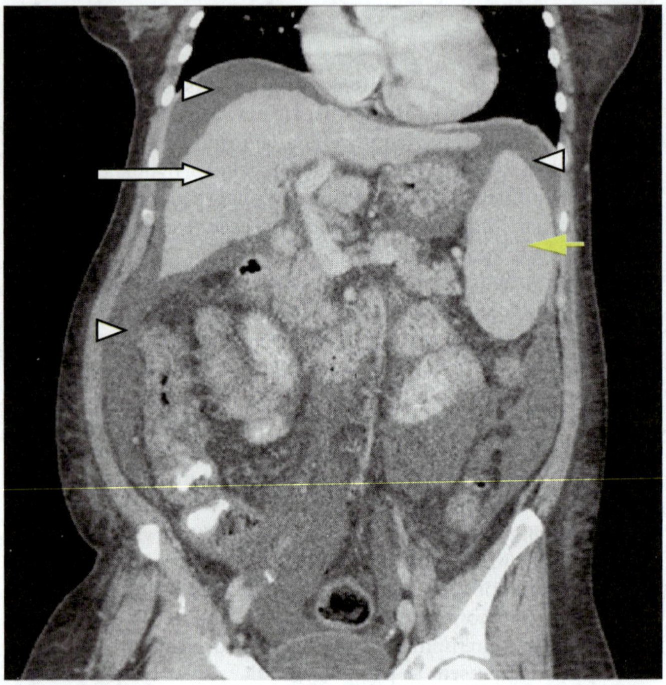

FIGURE 59-1 CT of a patient with a cirrhotic, nodular liver (white arrow), splenomegaly (yellow arrow), and ascites (arrowheads).

In selected cases, the hepatic venous pressure gradient (pressure across the liver between the portal and hepatic veins) can be measured via cannulation of the hepatic vein to confirm that ascites is caused by cirrhosis (Chap. 365). In some cases, a liver biopsy may be necessary to confirm cirrhosis.

ASCITES

PATHOGENESIS IN THE PRESENCE OF CIRRHOSIS

Ascites in patients with cirrhosis is the result of portal hypertension and renal salt and water retention. Similar mechanisms contribute to ascites formation in heart failure. Portal hypertension signifies elevation of the pressure within the portal vein. According to Ohm's law, pressure is the product of resistance and flow. Increased hepatic resistance occurs by several mechanisms. First, the development of hepatic fibrosis, which defines cirrhosis, disrupts the normal architecture of the hepatic sinusoids and impedes normal blood flow through the liver. Second, activation of hepatic stellate cells, which mediate fibrogenesis, leads to smooth-muscle contraction and fibrosis. Finally, cirrhosis is associated with a decrease in endothelial nitric oxide synthetase (eNOS) production, which results in decreased nitric oxide production and increased intrahepatic vasoconstriction.

The development of cirrhosis is also associated with increased systemic circulating levels of nitric oxide (contrary to the decrease seen intrahepatically) as well as increased levels of vascular endothelial growth factor and tumor necrosis factor that result in splanchnic arterial vasodilation. Vasodilation of the splanchnic circulation results in pooling of blood and a decrease in the effective circulating volume, which is perceived by the kidneys as hypovolemia. Compensatory vasoconstriction via release of antidiuretic hormone ensues; the consequences are free water retention and activation of the sympathetic nervous system and the renin angiotensin aldosterone system, which lead in turn to renal sodium and water retention.

PATHOGENESIS IN THE ABSENCE OF CIRRHOSIS

Ascites in the absence of cirrhosis generally results from peritoneal carcinomatosis, peritoneal infection, or pancreatic disease. Peritoneal carcinomatosis can result from primary peritoneal malignancies such as mesothelioma or sarcoma, abdominal malignancies such as gastric or colonic adenocarcinoma, or metastatic disease from breast or lung

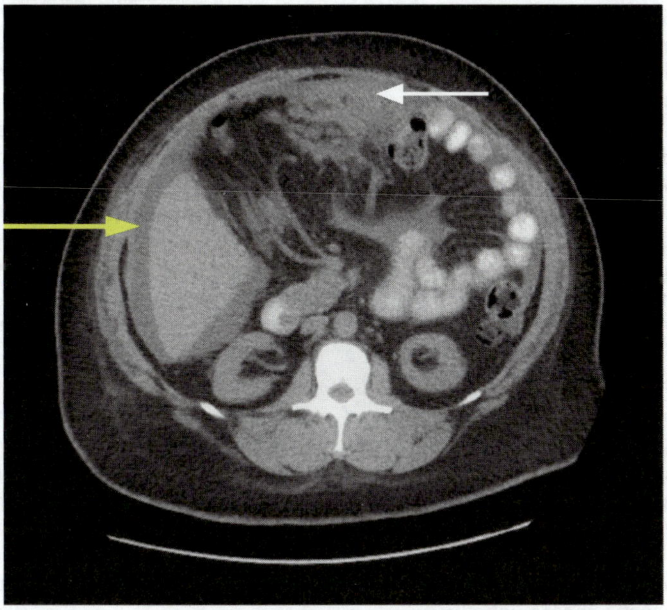

FIGURE 59-2 CT of a patient with peritoneal carcinomatosis (white arrow) and ascites (yellow arrow).

carcinoma or melanoma (Fig. 59-2). The tumor cells lining the peritoneum produce a protein-rich fluid that contributes to the development of ascites. Fluid from the extracellular space is drawn into the peritoneum, further contributing to the development of ascites. Tuberculous peritonitis causes ascites via a similar mechanism; tubercles deposited on the peritoneum exude a proteinaceous fluid. Pancreatic ascites results from leakage of pancreatic enzymes into the peritoneum.

CAUSES

Cirrhosis accounts for 84% of cases of ascites. Cardiac ascites, peritoneal carcinomatosis, and "mixed" ascites resulting from cirrhosis and a second disease account for 10–15% of cases. Less common causes of ascites include massive hepatic metastasis, infection (tuberculosis, *Chlamydia* infection), pancreatitis, and renal disease (nephrotic syndrome). Rare causes of ascites include hypothyroidism and familial Mediterranean fever.

EVALUATION

Once the presence of ascites has been confirmed, the etiology of the ascites is best determined by *paracentesis*, a bedside procedure in which a needle or small catheter is passed transcutaneously to extract ascitic fluid from the peritoneum. The lower quadrants are the most frequent sites for paracentesis. The left lower quadrant is preferred because of the greater depth of ascites and the thinner abdominal wall. Paracentesis is a safe procedure even in patients with coagulopathy; complications, including abdominal wall hematomas, hypotension, hepatorenal syndrome, and infection, are infrequent.

Once ascitic fluid has been extracted, its gross appearance should be examined. Turbid fluid can result from the presence of infection or tumor cells. White, milky fluid indicates a triglyceride level >200 mg/dL (and often >1000 mg/dL), which is the hallmark of *chylous ascites*. Chylous ascites results from lymphatic disruption that may occur with trauma, cirrhosis, tumor, tuberculosis, or certain congenital abnormalities. Dark brown fluid can reflect a high bilirubin concentration and indicates biliary tract perforation. Black fluid may indicate the presence of pancreatic necrosis or metastatic melanoma.

The ascitic fluid should be sent for measurement of albumin and total protein levels, cell and differential counts, and, if infection is suspected, Gram's stain and culture, with inoculation into blood culture bottles at the patient's bedside to maximize the yield. A serum albumin level should be measured simultaneously to permit calculation of the *serum-ascites albumin gradient* (SAAG).

The SAAG is useful for distinguishing ascites caused by portal hypertension from nonportal hypertensive ascites (Fig. 59-3). The SAAG reflects the pressure within the hepatic sinusoids and correlates with the hepatic venous pressure gradient. The SAAG is calculated by subtracting the ascitic albumin concentration from the serum albumin level and does not change with diuresis. A SAAG ≥1.1 g/dL reflects the presence of portal hypertension and indicates that the ascites is due to increased pressure in the hepatic sinusoids. According to Starling's law, a high SAAG reflects the oncotic pressure that counterbalances the portal pressure. Possible causes include cirrhosis, cardiac ascites, hepatic vein thrombosis (Budd-Chiari syndrome), sinusoidal obstruction syndrome (veno-occlusive disease), or massive liver metastases. A SAAG <1.1 g/dL indicates that the ascites is not related to portal hypertension, as in tuberculous peritonitis, peritoneal carcinomatosis, or pancreatic ascites.

For high-SAAG (≥1.1) ascites, the ascitic protein level can provide further clues to the etiology (Fig. 59-3). An ascitic protein level of ≥2.5 g/dL indicates that the hepatic sinusoids are normal and are allowing passage of protein into the ascites, as occurs in cardiac ascites, early Budd-Chiari syndrome, or sinusoidal obstruction syndrome. An ascitic protein level <2.5 g/dL indicates that the hepatic sinusoids have been damaged and scarred and no longer allow passage of protein, as occurs with cirrhosis, late Budd-Chiari syndrome, or massive liver metastases. Pro-brain-type natriuretic peptide (BNP) is a natriuretic hormone released by the heart as a result of increased volume and ventricular wall stretch. High levels of BNP in serum occur in heart failure and may be useful in identifying heart failure as the cause of high-SAAG ascites.

Further tests are indicated only in specific clinical circumstances. When secondary peritonitis resulting from a perforated hollow viscus is suspected, ascitic glucose and lactate dehydrogenase (LDH) levels can

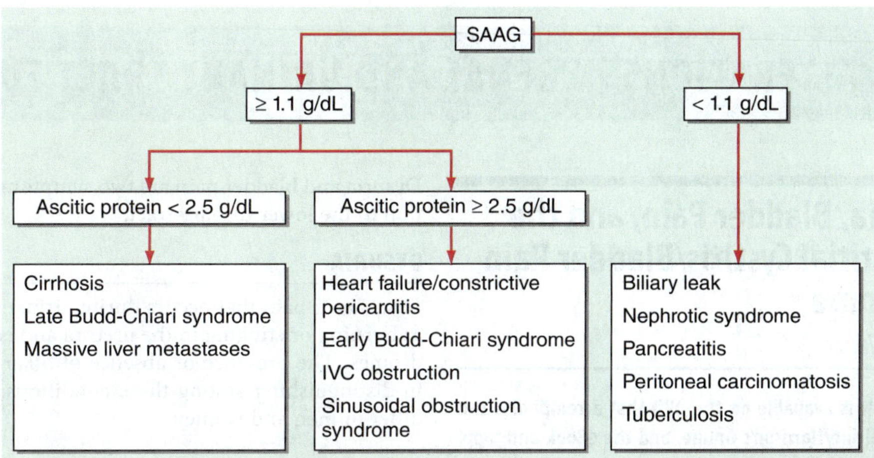

FIGURE 59-3 Algorithm for the diagnosis of ascites according to the serum-ascites albumin gradient (SAAG). IVC, inferior vena cava.

be measured. In contrast to "spontaneous" bacterial peritonitis, which may complicate cirrhotic ascites (see "Complications," below), secondary peritonitis is suggested by an ascitic glucose level <50 mg/dL, an ascitic LDH level higher than the serum LDH level, and the detection of multiple pathogens on ascitic fluid culture. When pancreatic ascites is suspected, the ascitic amylase level should be measured and is typically >1000 mg/dL. Cytology can be useful in the diagnosis of peritoneal carcinomatosis. At least 50 mL of fluid should be obtained and sent for immediate processing. Tuberculous peritonitis is typically associated with ascitic fluid lymphocytosis but can be difficult to diagnose by paracentesis. A smear for acid-fast bacilli has a diagnostic sensitivity of only 0 to 3%; a culture increases the sensitivity to 35–50%. In patients without cirrhosis, an elevated ascitic adenosine deaminase level has a sensitivity of >90% when a cut-off value of 30–45 U/L is used. When the cause of ascites remains uncertain, laparotomy or laparoscopy with peritoneal biopsies for histology and culture remains the gold standard.

TREATMENT ASCITES

The initial treatment for cirrhotic ascites is restriction of sodium intake to 2 g/d. When sodium restriction alone is inadequate to control ascites, oral diuretics—typically the combination of spironolactone and furosemide—are used. Spironolactone is an aldosterone antagonist that inhibits sodium resorption in the distal convoluted tubule of the kidney. Use of spironolactone may be limited by hyponatremia, hyperkalemia, and painful gynecomastia. If the gynecomastia is distressing, amiloride (5–40 mg/d) may be substituted for spironolactone. Furosemide is a loop diuretic that is generally combined with spironolactone in a ratio of 40:100; maximal daily doses of spironolactone and furosemide are 400 mg and 160 mg, respectively.

Refractory cirrhotic ascites is defined by the persistence of ascites despite sodium restriction and maximal (or maximally tolerated) diuretic use. Pharmacologic therapy for refractory ascites includes the addition of midodrine, an α_1-adrenergic antagonist, or clonidine, an α_2-adrenergic antagonist, to diuretic therapy. These agents act as vasoconstrictors, counteracting splanchnic vasodilation. Midodrine alone or in combination with clonidine improves systemic hemodynamics and control of ascites over that obtained with diuretics alone. Although β-adrenergic blocking agents (beta blockers) are often prescribed to prevent variceal hemorrhage in patients with cirrhosis, the use of beta blockers in patients with refractory ascites is associated with decreased survival rates.

When medical therapy alone is insufficient, refractory ascites can be managed by repeated large-volume paracentesis (LVP) or a transjugular intrahepatic peritoneal shunt (TIPS)—a radiologically placed portosystemic shunt that decompresses the hepatic sinusoids. Intravenous infusion of albumin accompanying LVP decreases the risk of "post-paracentesis circulatory dysfunction" and death. Patients undergoing LVP should receive IV albumin infusions of 6–8 g/L of ascitic fluid removed. TIPS placement is superior to LVP in reducing the reaccumulation of ascites but is associated with an increased frequency of hepatic encephalopathy, with no difference in mortality rates.

Malignant ascites does not respond to sodium restriction or diuretics. Patients must undergo serial LVPs, transcutaneous drainage catheter placement, or, rarely, creation of a peritoneovenous shunt (a shunt from the abdominal cavity to the vena cava).

Ascites caused by tuberculous peritonitis is treated with standard antituberculosis therapy. Noncirrhotic ascites of other causes is treated by correction of the precipitating condition.

COMPLICATIONS

Spontaneous bacterial peritonitis (SBP; Chap. 159) is a common and potentially lethal complication of cirrhotic ascites. Occasionally, SBP also complicates ascites caused by nephrotic syndrome, heart failure, acute hepatitis, and acute liver failure but is rare in malignant ascites. Patients with SBP generally note an increase in abdominal girth; however, abdominal tenderness is found in only 40% of patients, and rebound tenderness is uncommon. Patients may present with fever, nausea, vomiting, or the new onset of or exacerbation of preexisting hepatic encephalopathy.

SBP is defined by a polymorphonuclear neutrophil (PMN) count of ≥250/μL in the ascitic fluid. Cultures of ascitic fluid typically reveal one bacterial pathogen. The presence of multiple pathogens in the setting of an elevated ascitic PMN count suggests *secondary peritonitis* from a ruptured viscus or abscess (Chap. 159). The presence of multiple pathogens without an elevated PMN count suggests bowel perforation from the paracentesis needle. SBP is generally the result of enteric bacteria that have translocated across an edematous bowel wall. The most common pathogens are gram-negative rods, including *Escherichia coli* and *Klebsiella*, as well as streptococci and enterococci.

Treatment of SBP with an antibiotic such as IV cefotaxime is effective against gram-negative and gram-positive aerobes. A 5-day course of treatment is sufficient if the patient improves clinically. Nosocomial or health care–acquired SBP is frequently caused by multidrug-resistant bacteria, and initial antibiotic therapy should be guided by the local bacterial epidemiology.

Cirrhotic patients with a history of SBP, an ascitic fluid total protein concentration <1 g/dL, or active gastrointestinal bleeding should receive prophylactic antibiotics to prevent SBP; oral daily norfloxacin is commonly used. Diuresis increases the activity of ascitic fluid protein opsonins and may decrease the risk of SBP.

Hepatic hydrothorax occurs when ascites, often caused by cirrhosis, migrates via fenestrae in the diaphragm into the pleural space. This condition can result in shortness of breath, hypoxia, and infection. Treatment is similar to that for cirrhotic ascites and includes sodium restriction, diuretics, and, if needed, thoracentesis or TIPS placement. Chest tube placement should be avoided.

SECTION 7 ALTERATIONS IN RENAL AND URINARY TRACT FUNCTION

60e Dysuria, Bladder Pain, and the Interstitial Cystitis/Bladder Pain Syndrome

John W. Warren

This is a digital-only chapter. It is available on the DVD that accompanies this book, as well as on Access Medicine/Harrison's Online, and the eBook and "app" editions of HPIM 19e.

Dysuria and bladder pain are two symptoms that commonly call attention to the lower urinary tract.

DYSURIA

Dysuria, or pain that occurs during urination, is commonly perceived as burning or stinging in the urethra and is a symptom of several syndromes. The presence or absence of *other* symptoms is often helpful in distinguishing among these conditions. Some of these syndromes differ in men and women.

61 Azotemia and Urinary Abnormalities

Julie Lin, Bradley M. Denker

Normal kidney functions occur through numerous cellular processes to maintain body homeostasis. Disturbances in any of these functions can lead to abnormalities that may be detrimental to survival. Clinical manifestations of these disorders depend on the pathophysiology of renal injury and often are identified as a complex of symptoms, abnormal physical findings, and laboratory changes that constitute specific syndromes. These renal syndromes (Table 61-1) may arise from systemic illness or as primary renal disease. Nephrologic syndromes usually consist of several elements that reflect the underlying pathologic processes, typically including one or more of the following: (1) reduction in glomerular filtration rate (GFR) (azotemia), (2) abnormalities of urine sediment (red blood cells [RBCs], white blood cells [WBCs], casts, and crystals), (3) abnormal excretion of serum proteins (proteinuria), (4) disturbances in urine volume (oliguria, anuria, polyuria), (5) presence of hypertension and/or expanded total body fluid volume (edema), (6) electrolyte abnormalities, and (7) in some syndromes, fever/pain. The specific combination of these findings should permit identification of one of the major nephrologic syndromes (Table 61-1) and allow differential diagnoses to be narrowed so that the appropriate diagnostic and therapeutic course can be determined. All these syndromes and their associated diseases are discussed in more detail in subsequent chapters. This chapter focuses on several aspects of renal abnormalities that are critically important for distinguishing among those processes: (1) reduction in GFR leading to azotemia, (2) alterations of the urinary sediment and/or protein excretion, and (3) abnormalities of urinary volume.

TABLE 61-1 INITIAL CLINICAL AND LABORATORY DATA BASE FOR DEFINING MAJOR SYNDROMES IN NEPHROLOGY

Syndrome	Important Clues to Diagnosis	Common Findings	Chap(s). Discussing Disease-Causing Syndrome
Acute or rapidly progressive renal failure	Anuria	Hypertension, hematuria	334, 338, 340, 343
	Oliguria	Proteinuria, pyuria	
	Documented recent decline in GFR	Casts, edema	
Acute nephritis	Hematuria, RBC casts	Proteinuria	338
	Azotemia, oliguria	Pyuria	
	Edema, hypertension	Circulatory congestion	
Chronic renal failure	Azotemia for >3 months	Proteinuria	333e, 335
	Prolonged symptoms or signs of uremia	Casts	
	Symptoms or signs of renal osteodystrophy	Polyuria, nocturia	
	Kidneys reduced in size bilaterally	Edema, hypertension	
	Broad casts in urinary sediment	Electrolyte disorders	
Nephrotic syndrome	Proteinuria, with >3.5 g/24 h per 1.73 m^2	Casts	338
	Hypoalbuminemia	Lipiduria	
	Edema	Hypercoagulable state	
	Hyperlipidemia		
Asymptomatic urinary abnormalities	Hematuria		338
	Proteinuria (below nephrotic range)		
	Sterile pyuria, casts		
Urinary tract infection/pyelonephritis	Bacteriuria, with >10^5 cfu/mL	Hematuria	162
	Other infectious agent documented in urine	Mild azotemia	
	Pyuria, leukocyte casts	Mild proteinuria	
	Frequency, urgency	Fever	
	Bladder tenderness, flank tenderness		
Renal tubule defects	Electrolyte disorders	Hematuria	339, 340
	Polyuria, nocturia	"Tubular" proteinuria (<1 g/24 h)	
	Renal calcification	Enuresis	
	Large kidneys		
	Renal transport defects		
Hypertension	Systolic/diastolic hypertension	Proteinuria	298, 341
		Casts	
		Azotemia	
Nephrolithiasis	Previous history of stone passage or removal	Hematuria	342
	Previous history of stone seen by x-ray	Pyuria	
	Renal colic	Frequency, urgency	
Urinary tract obstruction	Azotemia, oliguria, anuria	Hematuria	343
	Polyuria, nocturia, urinary retention	Pyuria	
	Slowing of urinary stream	Enuresis, dysuria	
	Large prostate, large kidneys		
	Flank tenderness, full bladder after voiding		

Abbreviations: cfu, colony-forming units; GFR; glomerular filtration rate; RBC, red blood cell.

ASSESSMENT OF GFR

Monitoring the GFR is important in both hospital and outpatient settings, and several different methodologies are available. GFR is the primary metric for kidney "function," and its direct measurement involves administration of a radioactive isotope (such as inulin or iothalamate) that is filtered at the glomerulus into the urinary space but is neither reabsorbed nor secreted throughout the tubule. GFR—i.e., the clearance of inulin or iothalamate in milliliters per minute—is calculated from the rate of appearance of the isotope in the urine over several hours. In most clinical circumstances, direct GFR measurement is not feasible, and the plasma creatinine level is used as a surrogate to estimate GFR. Plasma creatinine (P_{Cr}) is the most widely used marker for GFR, which is related directly to urine creatinine (U_{Cr}) excretion and inversely to P_{Cr}. On the basis of this relationship (with some important caveats, as discussed below), GFR will fall in roughly inverse proportion to the rise in P_{Cr}. Failure to account for GFR reductions in drug dosing can lead to significant morbidity and death from drug toxicities (e.g., digoxin, aminoglycosides). In the outpatient setting, P_{Cr} serves as an estimate for GFR (although much less accurate; see below). In patients with chronic progressive renal disease, there is an approximately linear relationship between $1/P_{Cr}$ (*y* axis) and time (*x* axis). The slope of that line will remain constant for an individual; when values deviate, an investigation for a superimposed acute process (e.g., volume depletion, drug reaction) should be initiated. Signs and symptoms of uremia develop at significantly different levels of P_{Cr}, depending on the patient (size, age, and sex), underlying renal disease, existence of concurrent diseases, and true GFR. Generally, patients do not develop symptomatic uremia until renal insufficiency is severe (GFR <15 mL/min).

A significantly reduced GFR (either acute or chronic) is usually reflected in a rise in P_{Cr}, leading to retention of nitrogenous waste products (defined as azotemia) such as urea. Azotemia may result from reduced renal perfusion, intrinsic renal disease, or postrenal processes (ureteral obstruction; see below and Fig. 61-1). Precise determination of GFR is problematic, as both commonly measured indices (urea and creatinine) have characteristics that affect their accuracy as markers of clearance. Urea clearance may underestimate GFR significantly because of urea reabsorption by the tubule. In contrast, creatinine is derived from muscle metabolism of creatine, and its generation varies little from day to day.

Creatinine clearance (CrCl), an approximation of GFR, is measured from plasma and urinary creatinine excretion rates for a defined period (usually 24 h) and is expressed in milliliters per minute: $CrCl = (U_{vol} \times U_{Cr})/(P_{Cr} \times T_{min})$. Creatinine is useful for estimating GFR because it is a small, freely filtered solute that is not reabsorbed by the tubules. P_{Cr} levels can increase acutely from

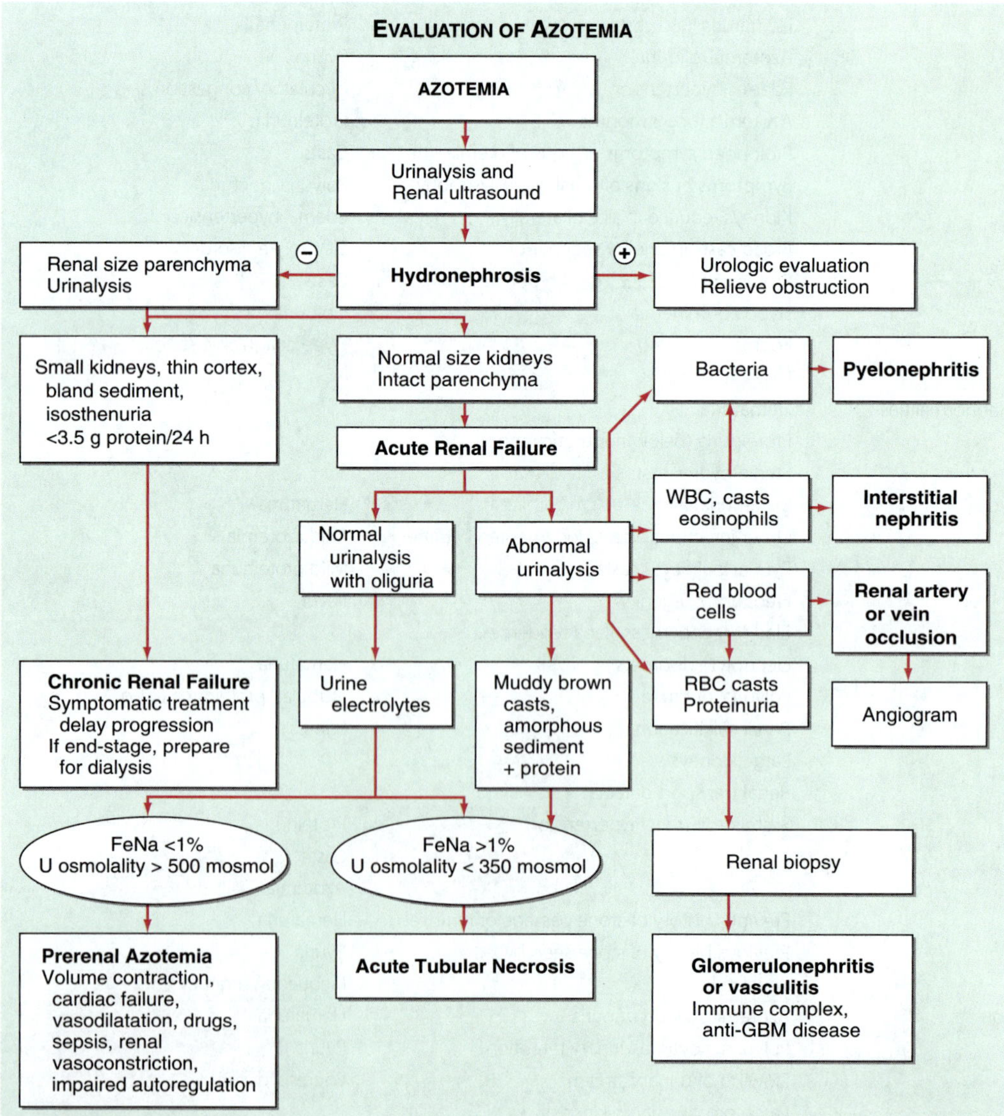

FIGURE 61-1 Approach to the patient with azotemia. FeNa, fractional excretion of sodium; GBM, glomerular basement membrane; RBC, red blood cell; WBC, white blood cell.

dietary ingestion of cooked meat, however, and creatinine can be secreted into the proximal tubule through an organic cation pathway (especially in advanced progressive chronic kidney disease), leading to overestimation of GFR. When a timed collection for CrCl is not available, decisions about drug dosing must be based on P_{Cr} alone. Two formulas are used widely to estimate kidney function from P_{Cr}: (1) Cockcroft-Gault and (2) four-variable MDRD (Modification of Diet in Renal Disease).

$$\text{Cockcroft-Gault: CrCl (mL/min)} = (140 - \text{age (years)} \times \text{weight (kg)} \times [0.85 \text{ if female}])/(72 \times P_{Cr} \text{ (mg/dL)}.$$

$$\text{MDRD: eGFR (mL/min per 1.73 m}^2) = 186.3 \times P_{Cr}\ (e^{-1.154}) \times \text{age}\ (e^{-0.203}) \times (0.742 \text{ if female}) \times (1.21 \text{ if black}).$$

Numerous websites are available to assist with these calculations (*www.kidney.org/professionals/kdoqi/gfr_calculator.cfm*). A newer CKD-EPI eGFR, which was developed by pooling several cohorts with and without kidney disease who had data on directly measured GFR, appears to be more accurate:

$$\text{CKD-EPI: eGFR} = 141 \times \min (P_{Cr}/k, 1)^a \times \max (P_{Cr}/k, 1)^{-1.209} \times 0.993^{Age} \times 1.018 \text{ [if female]} \times 1.159 \text{ [if black]},$$

where P_{Cr} is plasma creatinine, k is 0.7 for females and 0.9 for males, a is −0.329 for females and −0.411 for males, *min* indicates the minimum of P_{Cr}/k or 1, and *max* indicates the maximum of P_{Cr}/k or 1 (*http://www.qxmd.com/renal/Calculate-CKD-EPI-GFR.php*).

There are limitations to all creatinine-based estimates of GFR. Each equation, along with 24-h urine collection for measurement of creatinine clearance, is based on the assumption that the patient is in *steady state*, without daily increases or decreases in P_{Cr} as a result of rapidly changing GFR. The MDRD equation is better correlated with true GFR when the GFR is <60 mL/min per 1.73 m². The gradual loss of muscle from chronic illness, chronic use of glucocorticoids, or malnutrition can mask significant changes in GFR with small or imperceptible changes in P_{Cr}. Cystatin C, a member of the cystatin superfamily of cysteine protease inhibitors, is produced at a relatively constant rate from all nucleated cells. Serum cystatin C has been proposed to be a more sensitive marker of early GFR decline than is P_{Cr}; however, like serum creatinine, cystatin C is influenced by the patient's age, race, and sex and also is associated with diabetes, smoking, and markers of inflammation.

APPROACH TO THE PATIENT: Azotemia

Once GFR reduction has been established, the physician must decide if it represents acute or chronic renal injury. The clinical situation, history, and laboratory data often make this an easy distinction. However, the laboratory abnormalities characteristic of chronic renal failure, including anemia, hypocalcemia, and hyperphosphatemia, often are present as well in patients presenting with acute renal failure. Radiographic evidence of renal osteodystrophy (Chap. 335) can be seen only in chronic renal failure but is a very late finding, and these patients are usually undergoing dialysis. The urinalysis and renal ultrasound can facilitate distinguishing acute from chronic renal failure. An approach to the evaluation of azotemic patients is shown in Fig. 61-1. Patients with advanced chronic renal insufficiency often have some proteinuria, nonconcentrated urine (isosthenuria; isosmotic with plasma), and small kidneys on ultrasound, characterized by increased echogenicity and cortical thinning. Treatment should be directed toward slowing the progression of renal disease and providing symptomatic relief for edema, acidosis, anemia, and hyperphosphatemia, as discussed in Chap. 335. Acute renal failure (Chap. 334) can result from processes that affect renal blood flow (prerenal azotemia), intrinsic renal diseases (affecting small vessels, glomeruli, or tubules), or postrenal processes (obstruction of urine flow in ureters, bladder, or urethra) (Chap. 343).

PRERENAL FAILURE

Decreased renal perfusion accounts for 40–80% of cases of acute renal failure and, if appropriately treated, is readily reversible. The etiologies of prerenal azotemia include any cause of decreased circulating blood volume (gastrointestinal hemorrhage, burns, diarrhea, diuretics), volume sequestration (pancreatitis, peritonitis, rhabdomyolysis), or decreased effective arterial volume (cardiogenic shock, sepsis). Renal perfusion also can be affected by reductions in cardiac output from peripheral vasodilation (sepsis, drugs) or profound renal vasoconstriction (severe heart failure, hepatorenal syndrome, agents such as nonsteroidal anti-inflammatory drugs [NSAIDs]). True or "effective" arterial hypovolemia leads to a fall in mean arterial pressure, which in turn triggers a series of neural and humoral responses, including activation of the sympathetic nervous and renin-angiotensin-aldosterone systems and antidiuretic hormone (ADH) release. GFR is maintained by prostaglandin-mediated relaxation of afferent arterioles and angiotensin II–mediated constriction of efferent arterioles. Once the mean arterial pressure falls below 80 mmHg, GFR declines steeply.

Blockade of prostaglandin production by NSAIDs can result in severe vasoconstriction and acute renal failure. Blocking angiotensin action with angiotensin-converting enzyme (ACE) inhibitors or angiotensin receptor blockers (ARBs) decreases efferent arteriolar tone and in turn decreases glomerular capillary perfusion pressure. Patients taking NSAIDs and/or ACE inhibitors/ARBs are most susceptible to hemodynamically mediated acute renal failure when blood volume is reduced for any reason. Patients with bilateral renal artery stenosis (or stenosis in a solitary kidney) are dependent on efferent arteriolar vasoconstriction for maintenance of glomerular filtration pressure and are particularly susceptible to a precipitous decline in GFR when given ACE inhibitors or ARBs.

Prolonged renal hypoperfusion may lead to acute tubular necrosis (ATN), an intrinsic renal disease that is discussed below. The urinalysis and urinary electrolyte measurements can be useful in distinguishing prerenal azotemia from ATN (Table 61-2). The urine Na and osmolality of patients with prerenal azotemia can be predicted from the stimulatory actions of norepinephrine, angiotensin II, ADH, and low tubule fluid flow rate. In prerenal conditions, the tubules are intact, leading to a concentrated urine (>500 mosmol), avid Na retention (urine Na concentration, <20 mmol/L; fractional excretion of Na, <1%), and U_{Cr}/P_{Cr} >40 (Table 61-2). The prerenal urine sediment is usually normal or has hyaline and granular casts, whereas the sediment of ATN usually is filled with cellular debris, tubular epithelial casts, and dark (muddy brown) granular casts.

POSTRENAL AZOTEMIA

Urinary tract obstruction accounts for <5% of cases of acute renal failure but is usually reversible and must be ruled out early in the evaluation (Fig. 61-1). Since a single kidney is capable of adequate

TABLE 61-2 LABORATORY FINDINGS IN ACUTE RENAL FAILURE

Index	Prerenal Azotemia	Oliguric Acute Renal Failure
BUN/P_{Cr} ratio	>20:1	10–15:1
Urine sodium U_{Na}, meq/L	<20	>40
Urine osmolality, mosmol/L H_2O	>500	<350
Fractional excretion of sodium[a]	<1%	>2%
Urine/plasma creatinine U_{Cr}/P_{Cr}	>40	<20
Urinalysis (casts)	None or hyaline/granular	Muddy brown

[a] $FE_{Na} = \dfrac{U_{Na} \times P_{Cr} \times 100}{P_{Na} \times U_{Cr}}$.

Abbreviations: BUN, blood urea nitrogen; P_{Cr}, plasma creatinine concentration; P_{Na}, plasma sodium concentration; U_{Cr}, urine creatinine concentration; U_{Na}, urine sodium concentration.

clearance, obstructive acute renal failure requires obstruction at the urethra or bladder outlet, bilateral ureteral obstruction, or unilateral obstruction in a patient with a single functioning kidney. Obstruction is usually diagnosed by the presence of ureteral and renal pelvic dilation on renal ultrasound. However, early in the course of obstruction or if the ureters are unable to dilate (e.g., encasement by pelvic or periureteral tumors), the ultrasound examination may be negative. **The specific urologic conditions that cause obstruction are discussed in Chap. 343.**

INTRINSIC RENAL DISEASE

When prerenal and postrenal azotemia have been excluded as etiologies of renal failure, an intrinsic parenchymal renal disease is present. Intrinsic renal disease can arise from processes involving large renal vessels, intrarenal microvasculature and glomeruli, or the tubulointerstitium. Ischemic and toxic ATN account for ~90% of cases of acute intrinsic renal failure. As outlined in Fig. 61-1, the clinical setting and urinalysis are helpful in separating the possible etiologies. Prerenal azotemia and ATN are part of a spectrum of renal hypoperfusion; evidence of structural tubule injury is present in ATN, whereas prompt reversibility occurs with prerenal azotemia upon restoration of adequate renal perfusion. Thus, ATN often can be distinguished from prerenal azotemia by urinalysis and urine electrolyte composition (Table 61-2 and Fig. 61-1). Ischemic ATN is observed most frequently in patients who have undergone major surgery, trauma, severe hypovolemia, overwhelming sepsis, or extensive burns. Nephrotoxic ATN complicates the administration of many common medications, usually by inducing a combination of intrarenal vasoconstriction, direct tubule toxicity, and/or tubule obstruction. The kidney is vulnerable to toxic injury by virtue of its rich blood supply (25% of cardiac output) and its ability to concentrate and metabolize toxins. A diligent search for hypotension and nephrotoxins usually uncovers the specific etiology of ATN. Discontinuation of nephrotoxins and stabilization of blood pressure often suffice without the need for dialysis while the tubules recover. **An extensive list of potential drugs and toxins implicated in ATN is found in Chap. 334.**

Processes involving the tubules and interstitium can lead to acute kidney injury (AKI), a subtype of acute renal failure. These processes include drug-induced interstitial nephritis (especially by antibiotics, NSAIDs, and diuretics), severe infections (both bacterial and viral), systemic diseases (e.g., systemic lupus erythematosus), and infiltrative disorders (e.g., sarcoidosis, lymphoma, or leukemia). A list of drugs associated with allergic interstitial nephritis is found in Chap. 340. Urinalysis usually shows mild to moderate proteinuria, hematuria, and pyuria (~75% of cases) and occasionally WBC casts. The finding of RBC casts in interstitial nephritis has been reported but should prompt a search for glomerular diseases (Fig. 61-1). Occasionally, renal biopsy will be needed to distinguish among these possibilities. The finding of eosinophils in the urine is suggestive of allergic interstitial nephritis or atheroembolic renal disease and is optimally observed with Hansel staining. The absence of eosinophiluria, however, does not exclude these etiologies.

Occlusion of large renal vessels, including arteries and veins, is an uncommon cause of acute renal failure. A significant reduction in GFR by this mechanism suggests bilateral processes or, in a patient with a single functioning kidney, a unilateral process. Renal arteries can be occluded with atheroemboli, thromboemboli, in situ thrombosis, aortic dissection, or vasculitis. Atheroembolic renal failure can occur spontaneously but most often is associated with recent aortic instrumentation. The emboli are cholesterol-rich and lodge in medium and small renal arteries, with a consequent eosinophil-rich inflammatory reaction. Patients with atheroembolic acute renal failure often have a normal urinalysis, but the urine may contain eosinophils and casts. The diagnosis can be confirmed by renal biopsy, but this procedure is often unnecessary when other stigmata of atheroemboli are present (livedo reticularis, distal peripheral infarcts, eosinophilia). Renal artery thrombosis may lead to mild proteinuria and hematuria, whereas renal vein thrombosis typically induces heavy proteinuria and hematuria. **These vascular complications often require angiography for confirmation and are discussed in Chap. 341.**

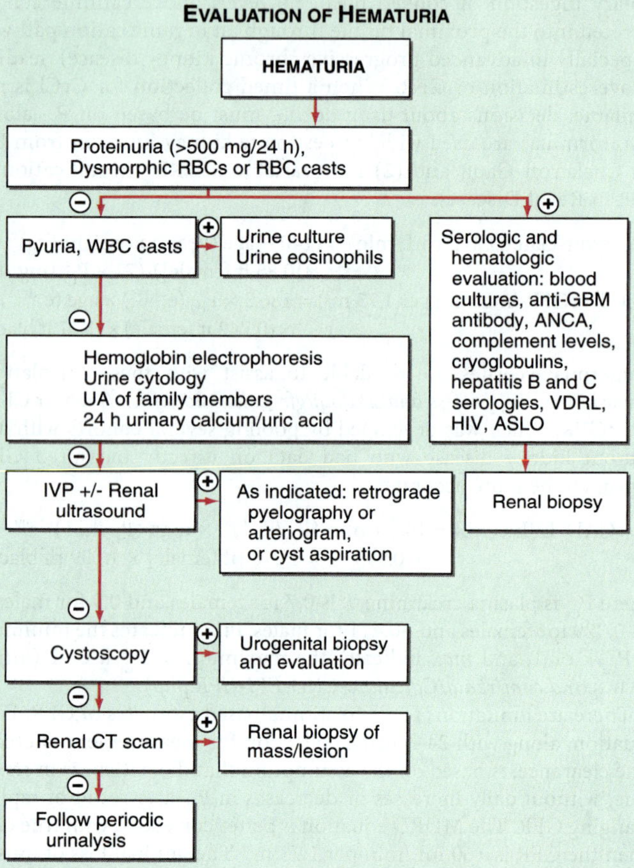

FIGURE 61-2 Approach to the patient with hematuria. ANCA, antineutrophil cytoplasmic antibody; ASLO, antistreptolysin O; CT, computed tomography; GBM, glomerular basement membrane; IVP, intravenous pyelography; RBC, red blood cell; UA, urinalysis; VDRL, Venereal Disease Research Laboratory; WBC, white blood cell.

Diseases of the glomeruli (glomerulonephritis and vasculitis) and the renal microvasculature (hemolytic-uremic syndromes, thrombotic thrombocytopenic purpura, and malignant hypertension) usually present with various combinations of glomerular injury: proteinuria, hematuria, reduced GFR, and alterations of sodium excretion that lead to hypertension, edema, and circulatory congestion (acute nephritic syndrome). These findings may occur as primary renal diseases or as renal manifestations of systemic diseases. The clinical setting and other laboratory data help distinguish primary renal diseases from systemic diseases. The finding of RBC casts in the urine is an indication for early renal biopsy (Fig. 61-1), as the pathologic pattern has important implications for diagnosis, prognosis, and treatment. Hematuria without RBC casts can also be an indication of glomerular disease; this evaluation is summarized in Fig. 61-2. **A detailed discussion of glomerulonephritis and diseases of the microvasculature is found in Chap. 340.**

OLIGURIA AND ANURIA

Oliguria refers to a 24-h urine output <400 mL, and *anuria* is the complete absence of urine formation (<100 mL). Anuria can be caused by total urinary tract obstruction, total renal artery or vein occlusion, and shock (manifested by severe hypotension and intense renal vasoconstriction). Cortical necrosis, ATN, and rapidly progressive glomerulonephritis occasionally cause anuria. Oliguria can accompany acute renal failure of any etiology and carries a more serious prognosis for renal recovery in all conditions except prerenal azotemia. *Nonoliguria* refers to urine output >400 mL/d in patients with acute or chronic azotemia. With nonoliguric ATN, disturbances of potassium and hydrogen balance are less severe than in oliguric patients, and recovery to normal renal function is usually more rapid.

ABNORMALITIES OF THE URINE

PROTEINURIA

The evaluation of proteinuria is shown schematically in Fig. 61-3 and typically is initiated after detection of proteinuria by dipstick examination. The dipstick measurement detects only albumin and gives false-positive results at pH >7.0 or when the urine is very concentrated or contaminated with blood. Because the dipstick relies on urinary albumin concentration, a very dilute urine may obscure significant proteinuria on dipstick examination. Quantification of urinary albumin on a spot urine sample (ideally from a first morning void) by measurement of an albumin-to-creatinine ratio (ACR) is helpful in approximating a 24-h albumin excretion rate (AER), where ACR (mg/g) ≈AER (mg/24 h). Furthermore, proteinuria that is not predominantly due to albumin will be missed by dipstick screening. This information is particularly important for the detection of Bence-Jones proteins in the urine of patients with multiple myeloma. Tests to measure total urine protein concentration accurately rely on precipitation with sulfosalicylic or trichloracetic acid (Fig. 61-3).

The magnitude of proteinuria and its composition in the urine depend on the mechanism of renal injury that leads to protein losses. Both charge and size selectivity normally prevent virtually all plasma albumin, globulins, and other high-molecular-weight proteins from crossing the glomerular wall; however, if this barrier is disrupted, plasma proteins may leak into the urine (glomerular proteinuria; Fig. 61-3). Smaller proteins (<20 kDa) are freely filtered but are readily reabsorbed by the proximal tubule. Traditionally, healthy individuals excrete <150 mg/d of total protein and <30 mg/d of albumin. However, even at albuminuria levels <30 mg/d, risk for progression to overt nephropathy or subsequent cardiovascular disease is increased. The remainder of the protein in the urine is secreted by the tubules (Tamm-Horsfall, IgA, and urokinase) or represents small amounts of filtered β_2-microglobulin, apoproteins, enzymes, and peptide hormones. Another mechanism of proteinuria entails excessive production of an abnormal protein that exceeds the capacity of the tubule for reabsorption. This situation most commonly occurs with plasma cell dyscrasias, such as multiple myeloma, amyloidosis, and lymphomas, that are associated with monoclonal production of immunoglobulin light chains.

The normal glomerular endothelial cell forms a barrier composed of pores of ~100 nm that retain blood cells but offer little impediment to passage of most proteins. The glomerular basement membrane traps most large proteins (>100 kDa), and the foot processes of epithelial cells (podocytes) cover the urinary side of the glomerular basement membrane and produce a series of narrow channels (slit diaphragms) to allow molecular passage of small solutes and water but not proteins. Some glomerular diseases, such as minimal change disease, cause fusion of glomerular epithelial cell foot processes, resulting in predominantly "selective" (Fig. 61-3) loss of albumin. Other glomerular diseases can present with disruption of the basement membrane and slit diaphragms (e.g., by immune complex deposition), resulting in losses of albumin and other plasma proteins. The fusion of foot processes causes increased pressure across the capillary basement membrane, resulting in areas with larger pore sizes (and more severe "nonselective" proteinuria (Fig. 61-3).

When the total daily urinary excretion of protein is >3.5 g, hypoalbuminemia, hyperlipidemia, and edema (nephrotic syndrome; Fig. 61-3) are often present as well. However, total daily urinary protein excretion >3.5 g can occur without the other features of the nephrotic syndrome in a variety of other renal diseases, including diabetes (Fig. 61-3). Plasma cell dyscrasias (multiple myeloma) can be associated with large amounts of excreted light chains in the urine, which may not be detected by dipstick. The light chains are filtered by the glomerulus and overwhelm the reabsorptive capacity of the proximal tubule. Renal failure from these disorders occurs through a variety of mechanisms, including proximal tubule injury, tubule obstruction (cast nephropathy), and light chain deposition (Chap. 340). However, not all excreted light chains are nephrotoxic.

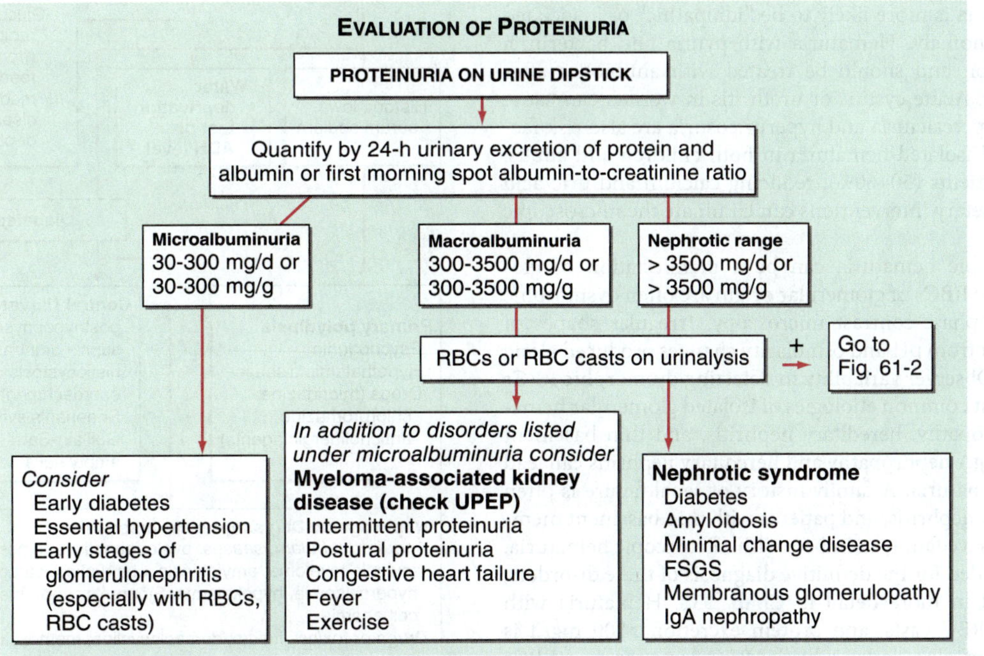

FIGURE 61-3 Approach to the patient with proteinuria. Investigation of proteinuria is often initiated by a positive dipstick on routine urinalysis. Conventional dipsticks detect predominantly albumin and provide a semiquantitative assessment (trace, 1+, 2+, or 3+), which is influenced by urinary concentration as reflected by urine specific gravity (minimum, <1.005; maximum, 1.030). However, more exact determination of proteinuria should employ a spot morning protein/creatinine ratio (mg/g) or a 24-h urine collection (mg/24 h). FSGS, focal segmental glomerulosclerosis; RBC, red blood cell; UPEP, urine protein electrophoresis.

Hypoalbuminemia in nephrotic syndrome occurs through excessive urinary losses and increased proximal tubule catabolism of filtered albumin. Edema forms from renal sodium retention and reduced plasma oncotic pressure, which favors fluid movement from capillaries to interstitium. To compensate for the perceived decrease in effective intravascular volume, activation of the renin-angiotensin system, stimulation of ADH, and activation of the sympathetic nervous system take place, promoting continued renal salt and water reabsorption and progressive edema. Despite these changes, hypertension is uncommon in primary kidney diseases resulting in the nephrotic syndrome (Fig. 61-3 and Chap. 338). The urinary loss of regulatory proteins and changes in hepatic synthesis contribute to the other manifestations of the nephrotic syndrome. A hypercoagulable state may arise from urinary losses of antithrombin III, reduced serum levels of proteins S and C, hyperfibrinogenemia, and enhanced platelet aggregation. Hypercholesterolemia may be severe and results from increased hepatic lipoprotein synthesis. Loss of immunoglobulins contributes to an increased risk of infection. Many diseases (some listed in Fig. 61-3) and drugs can cause the nephrotic syndrome; a complete list is found in Chap. 338.

HEMATURIA, PYURIA, AND CASTS

Isolated hematuria without proteinuria, other cells, or casts is often indicative of bleeding from the urinary tract. Hematuria is defined as two to five RBCs per high-power field (HPF) and can be detected by dipstick. A false-positive dipstick for hematuria (where no RBCs are seen on urine microscopy) may occur when myoglobinuria is present, often in the setting of rhabdomyolysis. Common causes of isolated hematuria include stones, neoplasms, tuberculosis, trauma, and prostatitis. Gross hematuria with blood clots usually is not an intrinsic renal process; rather, it suggests a postrenal source in the urinary collecting system. Evaluation of patients presenting with microscopic hematuria is outlined in Fig. 61-2. A single urinalysis with hematuria is common and can result from menstruation, viral illness, allergy, exercise, or mild trauma. Persistent or significant hematuria (>3 RBCs/HPF on three urinalyses, a single urinalysis with >100 RBCs, or gross hematuria) is associated with significant renal or urologic lesions in 9.1% of cases. The level of suspicion for urogenital neoplasms in patients with isolated painless hematuria and nondysmorphic RBCs increases with age. Neoplasms are rare in the pediatric population, and isolated hematuria is more likely to be "idiopathic" or associated with a congenital anomaly. Hematuria with pyuria and bacteriuria is typical of infection and should be treated with antibiotics after appropriate cultures. Acute cystitis or urethritis in women can cause gross hematuria. Hypercalciuria and hyperuricosuria are also risk factors for unexplained isolated hematuria in both children and adults. In some of these patients (50–60%), reducing calcium and uric acid excretion through dietary interventions can eliminate the microscopic hematuria.

Isolated microscopic hematuria can be a manifestation of glomerular diseases. The RBCs of glomerular origin are often dysmorphic when examined by phase-contrast microscopy. Irregular shapes of RBCs may also result from pH and osmolarity changes produced along the distal nephron. Observer variability in detecting dysmorphic RBCs is common. The most common etiologies of isolated glomerular hematuria are IgA nephropathy, hereditary nephritis, and thin basement membrane disease. IgA nephropathy and hereditary nephritis can lead to episodic gross hematuria. A family history of renal failure is often present in hereditary nephritis, and patients with thin basement membrane disease often have family members with microscopic hematuria. A renal biopsy is needed for the definitive diagnosis of these disorders, which are discussed in more detail in Chap. 338. Hematuria with dysmorphic RBCs, RBC casts, and protein excretion >500 mg/d is virtually diagnostic of glomerulonephritis. RBC casts form as RBCs that enter the tubule fluid and become trapped in a cylindrical mold of gelled Tamm-Horsfall protein. Even in the absence of azotemia, these patients should undergo serologic evaluation and renal biopsy as outlined in Fig. 61-2.

Isolated pyuria is unusual since inflammatory reactions in the kidney or collecting system also are associated with hematuria. The presence of bacteria suggests infection, and WBC casts with bacteria are indicative of pyelonephritis. WBCs and/or WBC casts also may be seen in acute glomerulonephritis as well as in tubulointerstitial processes such as interstitial nephritis and transplant rejection.

Casts can be seen in chronic renal diseases. Degenerated cellular casts called *waxy casts* or *broad casts* (arising in the dilated tubules that have undergone compensatory hypertrophy in response to reduced renal mass) may be seen in the urine.

ABNORMALITIES OF URINE VOLUME

POLYURIA

By history, it is often difficult for patients to distinguish urinary frequency (often of small volumes) from true polyuria (>3 L/d), and a quantification of volume by 24-h urine collection may be needed (Fig. 61-4). Polyuria results from two potential mechanisms: (1) excretion of nonabsorbable solutes (such as glucose) or (2) excretion of water (usually from a defect in ADH production or renal responsiveness). To distinguish a solute diuresis from a water diuresis and to determine whether the diuresis is appropriate for the clinical circumstances, urine osmolality is measured. The average person excretes between 600 and 800 mosmol of solutes per day, primarily as urea and electrolytes. If the urine output is >3 L/d and the urine is dilute (<250 mosmol/L), total mosmol excretion is normal and a water diuresis is present. This circumstance could arise from polydipsia, inadequate secretion of vasopressin (*central diabetes insipidus*), or failure of renal tubules to respond to vasopressin (*nephrogenic diabetes insipidus*). If the urine volume is >3 L/d and urine

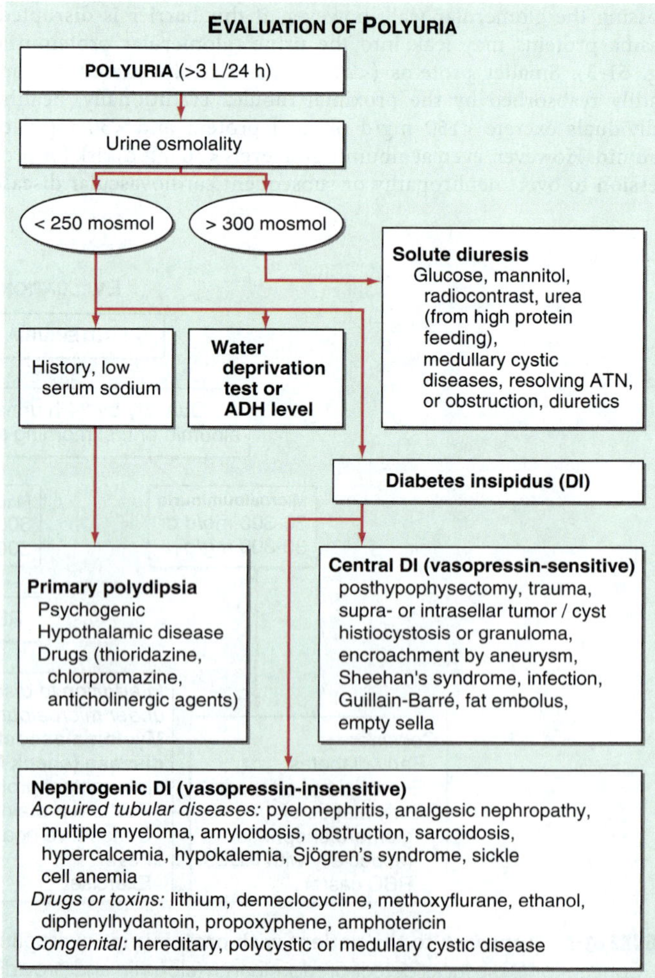

FIGURE 61-4 Approach to the patient with polyuria. ADH, antidiuretic hormone; ATN, acute tubular necrosis.

osmolality is >300 mosmol/L, a solute diuresis is clearly present and a search for the responsible solute(s) is mandatory.

Excessive filtration of a poorly reabsorbed solute such as glucose or mannitol can depress reabsorption of NaCl and water in the proximal tubule and lead to enhanced excretion in the urine. Poorly controlled diabetes mellitus with glucosuria is the most common cause of a solute diuresis, leading to volume depletion and serum hypertonicity. Since the urine sodium concentration is less than that of blood, more water than sodium is lost, causing hypernatremia and hypertonicity. Common iatrogenic solute diuresis occurs in association with mannitol administration, radiocontrast media, and high-protein feedings (enteral or parenteral), leading to increased urea production and excretion. Less commonly, excessive sodium loss may result from cystic renal diseases or Bartter's syndrome or may develop during a tubulointerstitial process (such as resolving ATN). In these so-called salt-wasting disorders, the tubule damage results in direct impairment of sodium reabsorption and indirectly reduces the responsiveness of the tubule to aldosterone. Usually, the sodium losses are mild, and the obligatory urine output is <2 L/d; resolving ATN and postobstructive diuresis are exceptions and may be associated with significant natriuresis and polyuria.

Formation of large volumes of dilute urine is usually due to polydipsic states or diabetes insipidus. Primary polydipsia can result from habit, psychiatric disorders, neurologic lesions, or medications. During deliberate polydipsia, extracellular fluid volume is normal or expanded and plasma vasopressin levels are reduced because serum osmolality tends to be near the lower limits of normal. Urine osmolality is also maximally dilute at 50 mosmol/L.

Central diabetes insipidus may be idiopathic in origin or secondary to a variety of conditions, including hypophysectomy, trauma, neoplastic, inflammatory, vascular, or infectious hypothalamic diseases. Idiopathic central diabetes insipidus is associated with selective destruction of the vasopressin-secreting neurons in the supraoptic and paraventricular nuclei and can either be inherited as an autosomal dominant trait or occur spontaneously. Nephrogenic diabetes insipidus can occur in a variety of clinical situations, as summarized in Fig. 61-4.

A plasma vasopressin level is recommended as the best method for distinguishing between central and nephrogenic diabetes insipidus. Alternatively, a water deprivation test plus exogenous vasopressin may distinguish primary polydipsia from central and nephrogenic diabetes insipidus. For a detailed discussion, see Chap. 404.

62e Atlas of Urinary Sediments and Renal Biopsies

Agnes B. Fogo, Eric G. Neilson

This is a digital-only chapter. It is available on the DVD that accompanies this book, as well as on Access Medicine/Harrison's Online, and the eBook and "app" editions of HPIM 19e.

Key diagnostic features of selected diseases in renal biopsy are illustrated, with light, immunofluorescence, and electron microscopic images. Common urinalysis findings are also documented.

63 Fluid and Electrolyte Disturbances

David B. Mount

SODIUM AND WATER

COMPOSITION OF BODY FLUIDS

Water is the most abundant constituent in the body, comprising approximately 50% of body weight in women and 60% in men. Total-body water is distributed in two major compartments: 55–75% is intracellular (intracellular fluid [ICF]), and 25–45% is extracellular (extracellular fluid [ECF]). The ECF is further subdivided into intravascular (plasma water) and extravascular (interstitial) spaces in a ratio of 1:3. Fluid movement between the intravascular and interstitial spaces occurs across the capillary wall and is determined by Starling forces, i.e., capillary hydraulic pressure and colloid osmotic pressure. The transcapillary hydraulic pressure gradient exceeds the corresponding oncotic pressure gradient, thereby favoring the movement of plasma ultrafiltrate into the extravascular space. The return of fluid into the intravascular compartment occurs via lymphatic flow.

The solute or particle concentration of a fluid is known as its osmolality, expressed as milliosmoles per kilogram of water (mOsm/kg). Water easily diffuses across most cell membranes to achieve osmotic equilibrium (ECF osmolality = ICF osmolality). Notably, the extracellular and intracellular solute compositions differ considerably owing to the activity of various transporters, channels, and ATP-driven membrane pumps. The major ECF particles are Na^+ and its accompanying anions Cl^- and HCO_3^-, whereas K^+ and organic phosphate esters (ATP, creatine phosphate, and phospholipids) are the predominant ICF osmoles. Solutes that are restricted to the ECF or the ICF determine the "tonicity" or effective osmolality of that compartment. Certain solutes, particularly urea, do not contribute to water shifts across most membranes and are thus known as *ineffective osmoles.*

Water Balance Vasopressin secretion, water ingestion, and renal water transport collaborate to maintain human body fluid osmolality between 280 and 295 mOsm/kg. Vasopressin (AVP) is synthesized in magnocellular neurons within the hypothalamus; the distal axons of these neurons project to the posterior pituitary or neurohypophysis, from which AVP is released into the circulation. A network of central "osmoreceptor" neurons, which includes the AVP-expressing magnocellular neurons themselves, sense circulating osmolality via nonselective, stretch-activated cation channels. These osmoreceptor neurons are activated or inhibited by modest increases and decreases in circulating osmolality, respectively; activation leads to AVP release and thirst.

AVP secretion is stimulated as systemic osmolality increases above a threshold level of ~285 mOsm/kg, above which there is a linear relationship between osmolality and circulating AVP (Fig. 63-1). Thirst and thus water ingestion are also activated at ~285 mOsm/kg, beyond which there is an equivalent linear increase in the perceived intensity of thirst as a function of circulating osmolality. Changes in blood volume and blood pressure are also direct stimuli for AVP release and thirst, albeit with a less sensitive response profile. Of perhaps greater clinical relevance to the pathophysiology of water homeostasis, ECF volume strongly modulates the relationship between circulating osmolality and AVP release, such that hypovolemia reduces the osmotic threshold and increases the slope of the response curve to osmolality; *hypervolemia* has an opposite effect, increasing the osmotic threshold and reducing the slope of the response curve (Fig. 63-1). Notably, AVP has a half-life in the circulation of only 10–20 minutes; thus, changes in ECF volume and/or circulating osmolality can rapidly affect water homeostasis. In addition to volume status, a number of other "nonosmotic" stimuli have potent activating effects on osmosensitive neurons and AVP release, including nausea, intracerebral angiotensin II, serotonin, and multiple drugs.

The excretion or retention of electrolyte-free water by the kidney is modulated by circulating AVP. AVP acts on renal, V_2-type receptors in

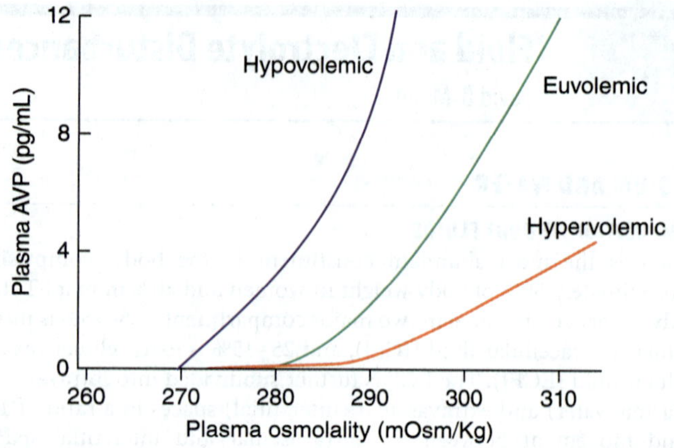

FIGURE 63-1 Circulating levels of vasopressin (AVP) in response to changes in osmolality. Plasma AVP becomes detectable in euvolemic, healthy individuals at a threshold of ~285 mOsm/kg, above which there is a linear relationship between osmolality and circulating AVP. The vasopressin response to osmolality is modulated strongly by volume status. The osmotic threshold is thus slightly lower in hypovolemia, with a steeper response curve; hypervolemia reduces the sensitivity of circulating AVP levels to osmolality.

the thick ascending limb of Henle and principal cells of the collecting duct (CD), increasing intracellular levels of cyclic AMP and activating protein kinase A (PKA)–dependent phosphorylation of multiple transport proteins. The AVP- and PKA-dependent activation of Na^+-Cl^- and K^+ transport by the thick ascending limb of the loop of Henle (TALH) is a key participant in the countercurrent mechanism (Fig. 63-2). The countercurrent mechanism ultimately increases the interstitial osmolality in the inner medulla of the kidney, driving water absorption across the renal CD. However, water, salt, and solute transport by both proximal and distal nephron segments participates in the renal concentrating mechanism (Fig. 63-2). Water transport across apical and basolateral aquaporin-1 water channels in the descending thin limb of the loop of Henle is thus involved, as is passive absorption of Na^+-Cl^- by the thin ascending limb, via apical and basolateral CLC-K1 chloride channels and paracellular Na^+ transport. Renal urea transport in turn plays important roles in the generation of the medullary osmotic gradient and the ability to excrete solute-free water under conditions of both high and low protein intake (Fig. 63-2).

AVP-induced, PKA-dependent phosphorylation of the aquaporin-2 water channel in principal cells stimulates the insertion of active water channels into the lumen of the CD, resulting in transepithelial water absorption down the medullary osmotic gradient (Fig. 63-3). Under "antidiuretic" conditions, with increased circulating AVP, the kidney reabsorbs water filtered by the glomerulus, equilibrating the osmolality across the CD epithelium to excrete a hypertonic, "concentrated" urine (osmolality of up to 1200 mOsm/kg). In the absence of circulating AVP, insertion of aquaporin-2 channels and water absorption across the CD is essentially abolished, resulting in secretion of a hypotonic, dilute urine (osmolality as low as 30–50 mOsm/kg). Abnormalities in this "final common pathway" are involved in most disorders of water homeostasis, e.g., a reduced or absent insertion of active aquaporin-2 water channels into the membrane of principal cells in diabetes insipidus.

Maintenance of Arterial Circulatory Integrity Sodium is actively pumped out of cells by the Na^+/K^+-ATPase membrane pump. In consequence, 85–90% of body Na^+ is extracellular, and the ECF volume (ECFV) is a function of total-body Na^+ content. Arterial perfusion and circulatory integrity are, in turn, determined by renal Na^+ retention or excretion, in addition to the modulation of systemic arterial resistance. Within the kidney, Na^+ is filtered by the glomeruli and then sequentially reabsorbed by the renal tubules. The Na^+ cation is typically reabsorbed with the chloride anion (Cl^-), and, thus, chloride homeostasis also affects the ECFV. On a quantitative level, at a glomerular filtration rate (GFR) of 180 L/d and serum Na^+ of ~140 m*M*, the kidney filters some 25,200 mmol/d of Na^+. This is equivalent to ~1.5 kg of salt, which would occupy roughly 10 times the extracellular space; 99.6% of filtered Na^+-Cl^- must be reabsorbed to excrete 100 m*M* per day. Minute changes in renal Na^+-Cl^- excretion will thus have significant effects on the ECFV, leading to edema syndromes or hypovolemia.

Approximately two-thirds of filtered Na^+-Cl^- is reabsorbed by the renal proximal tubule, via both paracellular and transcellular mechanisms. The TALH subsequently reabsorbs another 25–30% of filtered Na^+-Cl^- via the apical, furosemide-sensitive Na^+-K^+-$2Cl^-$ cotransporter. The adjacent aldosterone-sensitive distal nephron, comprising the distal convoluted tubule (DCT), connecting tubule (CNT), and CD, accomplishes the "fine-tuning" of renal Na^+-Cl^- excretion. The thiazide-sensitive apical Na^+-Cl^- cotransporter (NCC) reabsorbs 5–10% of filtered Na^+-Cl^- in the DCT. Principal cells in the CNT and CD reabsorb Na^+ via electrogenic, amiloride-sensitive epithelial Na^+ channels (ENaC); Cl^- ions are primarily reabsorbed by adjacent intercalated cells, via apical Cl^- exchange (Cl^--OH^- and Cl^--HCO_3^- exchange, mediated by the SLC26A4 anion exchanger) (Fig. 63-4).

Renal tubular reabsorption of filtered Na^+-Cl^- is regulated by multiple circulating and paracrine hormones, in addition to the activity of renal nerves. Angiotensin II activates proximal Na^+-Cl^- reabsorption, as do adrenergic receptors under the influence of renal sympathetic innervation; locally generated dopamine, in contrast, has a *natriuretic* effect. Aldosterone primarily activates Na^+-Cl^- reabsorption within the aldosterone-sensitive distal nephron. In particular, aldosterone activates the ENaC channel in principal cells, inducing Na^+ absorption and promoting K^+ excretion (Fig. 63-4).

Circulatory integrity is critical for the perfusion and function of vital organs. "Underfilling" of the arterial circulation is sensed by ventricular and vascular pressure receptors, resulting in a neurohumoral activation (increased sympathetic tone, activation of the

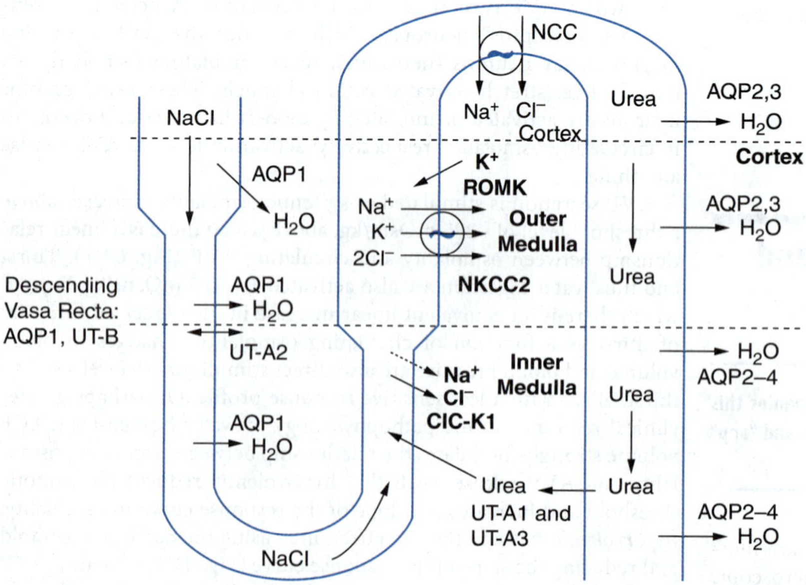

FIGURE 63-2 The renal concentrating mechanism. Water, salt, and solute transport by both proximal and distal nephron segments participates in the renal concentrating mechanism (see text for details). Diagram showing the location of the major transport proteins involved; a loop of Henle is depicted on the *left*, collecting duct on the *right*. AQP, aquaporin; CLC-K1, chloride channel; NKCC2, Na-K-2Cl cotransporter; ROMK, renal outer medullary K^+ channel; UT, urea transporter. *(Used with permission from JM Sands: Molecular approaches to urea transporters. J Am Soc Nephrol 13:2795, 2002.)*

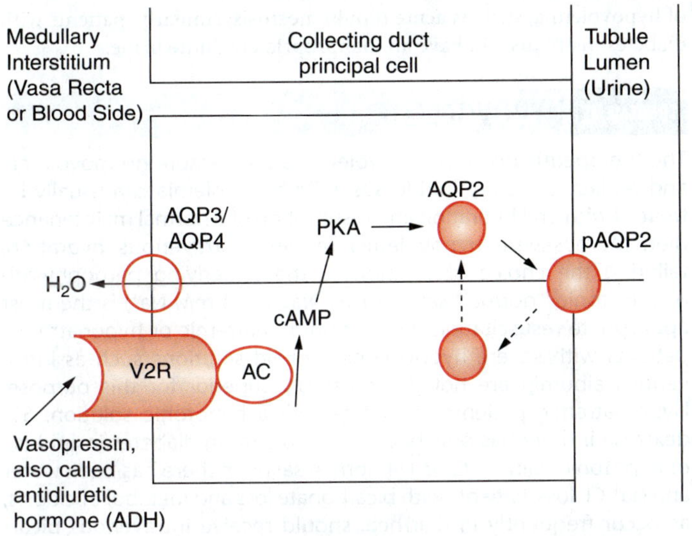

FIGURE 63-3 Vasopressin and the regulation of water permeability in the renal collecting duct. Vasopressin binds to the type 2 vasopressin receptor (V2R) on the basolateral membrane of principal cells, activates adenylyl cyclase (AC), increases intracellular cyclic adenosine monophosphatase (cAMP), and stimulates protein kinase A (PKA) activity. Cytoplasmic vesicles carrying aquaporin-2 (AQP) water channel proteins are inserted into the luminal membrane in response to vasopressin, thereby increasing the water permeability of this membrane. When vasopressin stimulation ends, water channels are retrieved by an endocytic process and water permeability returns to its low basal rate. The AQP3 and AQP4 water channels are expressed on the basolateral membrane and complete the transcellular pathway for water reabsorption. pAQP2, phosphorylated aquaporin-2. *(From JM Sands, DG Bichet: Nephrogenic diabetes insipidus. Ann Intern Med 144:186, 2006, with permission.)*

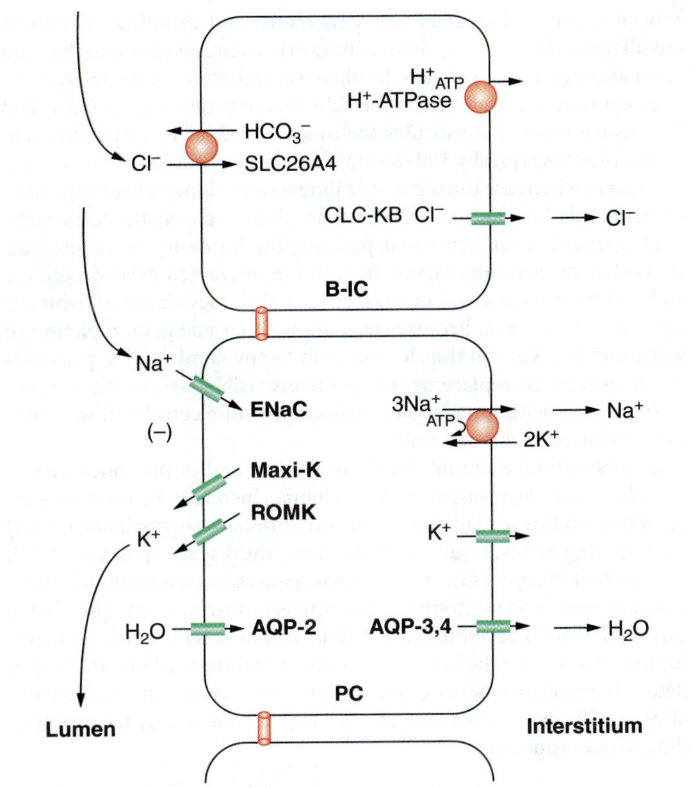

FIGURE 63-4 Sodium, water, and potassium transport in principal cells (PC) and adjacent β-intercalated cells (B-IC). The absorption of Na^+ via the amiloride-sensitive epithelial sodium channel (ENaC) generates a lumen-negative potential difference, which drives K^+ excretion through the apical secretory K^+ channel ROMK (renal outer medullary K^+ channel) and/or the flow-dependent BK channel. Transepithelial Cl^- transport occurs in adjacent β-intercalated cells, via apical Cl^--HCO_3^- and Cl^--OH^- exchange (SLC26A4 anion exchanger, also known as pendrin) basolateral CLC chloride channels. Water is absorbed down the osmotic gradient by principal cells, through the apical aquaporin-2 (AQP-2) and basolateral aquaporin-3 and aquaporin-4 (Fig. 63-3).

renin-angiotensin-aldosterone axis, and increased circulating AVP) that synergistically increases renal Na^+-Cl^- reabsorption, vascular resistance, and renal water reabsorption. This occurs in the context of decreased cardiac output, as occurs in hypovolemic states, low-output cardiac failure, decreased oncotic pressure, and/or increased capillary permeability. Alternatively, excessive arterial vasodilation results in *relative* arterial underfilling, leading to neurohumoral activation in the defense of tissue perfusion. These physiologic responses play important roles in many of the disorders discussed in this chapter. In particular, it is important to appreciate that AVP functions in the defense of circulatory integrity, inducing vasoconstriction, increasing sympathetic nervous system tone, increasing renal retention of both water and Na^+-Cl^-, and modulating the arterial baroreceptor reflex. Most of these responses involve activation of systemic V_{1A} AVP receptors, but concomitant activation of V_2 receptors in the kidney can result in renal water retention and hyponatremia.

HYPOVOLEMIA

Etiology True volume depletion, or hypovolemia, generally refers to a state of combined salt and water loss, leading to contraction of the ECFV. The loss of salt and water may be renal or nonrenal in origin.

RENAL CAUSES Excessive urinary Na^+-Cl^- and water loss is a feature of several conditions. A high filtered load of endogenous solutes, such as glucose and urea, can impair tubular reabsorption of Na^+-Cl^- and water, leading to an osmotic diuresis. Exogenous mannitol, often used to decrease intracerebral pressure, is filtered by glomeruli but not reabsorbed by the proximal tubule, thus causing an osmotic diuresis. Pharmacologic diuretics selectively impair Na^+-Cl^- reabsorption at specific sites along the nephron, leading to increased urinary Na^+-Cl^- excretion. Other drugs can induce natriuresis as a side effect. For example, acetazolamide can inhibit proximal tubular Na^+-Cl^- absorption via its inhibition of carbonic anhydrase; other drugs, such as the antibiotics trimethoprim and pentamidine, inhibit distal tubular Na^+ reabsorption through the amiloride-sensitive ENaC channel, leading to urinary Na^+-Cl^- loss. Hereditary defects in renal transport proteins are also associated with reduced reabsorption of filtered Na^+-Cl^- and/or water. Alternatively, mineralocorticoid deficiency, mineralocorticoid resistance, or inhibition of the mineralocorticoid receptor (MLR) can reduce Na^+-Cl^- reabsorption by the aldosterone-sensitive distal nephron. Finally, tubulointerstitial injury, as occurs in interstitial nephritis, acute tubular injury, or obstructive uropathy, can reduce distal tubular Na^+-Cl^- and/or water absorption.

Excessive excretion of free water, i.e., water without electrolytes, can also lead to hypovolemia. However, the effect on ECFV is usually less marked, given that two-thirds of the water volume is lost from the ICF. Excessive renal water excretion occurs in the setting of decreased circulating AVP or renal resistance to AVP (central and nephrogenic diabetes insipidus, respectively).

EXTRARENAL CAUSES Nonrenal causes of hypovolemia include fluid loss from the gastrointestinal tract, skin, and respiratory system. Accumulations of fluid within specific tissue compartments, typically the interstitium, peritoneum, or gastrointestinal tract, can also cause hypovolemia.

Approximately 9 L of fluid enter the gastrointestinal tract daily, 2 L by ingestion and 7 L by secretion; almost 98% of this volume is absorbed, such that daily fecal fluid loss is only 100–200 mL. Impaired gastrointestinal reabsorption or enhanced secretion of fluid can cause hypovolemia. Because gastric secretions have a low pH (high H^+

concentration), whereas biliary, pancreatic, and intestinal secretions are alkaline (high HCO_3^- concentration), vomiting and diarrhea are often accompanied by metabolic alkalosis and acidosis, respectively.

Evaporation of water from the skin and respiratory tract (so-called "insensible losses") constitutes the major route for loss of solute-free water, which is typically 500–650 mL/d in healthy adults. This evaporative loss can increase during febrile illness or prolonged heat exposure. Hyperventilation can also increase insensible losses via the respiratory tract, particularly in ventilated patients; the humidity of inspired air is another determining factor. In addition, increased exertion and/or ambient temperature will increase insensible losses via sweat, which is hypotonic to plasma. Profuse sweating without adequate repletion of water and Na^+-Cl^- can thus lead to both hypovolemia and hypertonicity. Alternatively, replacement of these insensible losses with a surfeit of free water, without adequate replacement of electrolytes, may lead to hypovolemic hyponatremia.

Excessive fluid accumulation in interstitial and/or peritoneal spaces can also cause intravascular hypovolemia. Increases in vascular permeability and/or a reduction in oncotic pressure (hypoalbuminemia) alter Starling forces, resulting in excessive "third spacing" of the ECFV. This occurs in sepsis syndrome, burns, pancreatitis, nutritional hypoalbuminemia, and peritonitis. Alternatively, distributive hypovolemia can occur due to accumulation of fluid within specific compartments, for example within the bowel lumen in gastrointestinal obstruction or ileus. Hypovolemia can also occur after extracorporeal hemorrhage or after significant hemorrhage into an expandable space, for example, the retroperitoneum.

Diagnostic Evaluation A careful history will usually determine the etiologic cause of hypovolemia. Symptoms of hypovolemia are nonspecific and include fatigue, weakness, thirst, and postural dizziness; more severe symptoms and signs include oliguria, cyanosis, abdominal and chest pain, and confusion or obtundation. Associated electrolyte disorders may cause additional symptoms, for example, muscle weakness in patients with hypokalemia. On examination, diminished skin turgor and dry oral mucous membranes are less than ideal markers of a decreased ECFV in adult patients; more reliable signs of hypovolemia include a decreased jugular venous pressure (JVP), orthostatic tachycardia (an increase of >15–20 beats/min upon standing), and orthostatic hypotension (a >10–20 mmHg drop in blood pressure on standing). More severe fluid loss leads to hypovolemic shock, with hypotension, tachycardia, peripheral vasoconstriction, and peripheral hypoperfusion; these patients may exhibit peripheral cyanosis, cold extremities, oliguria, and altered mental status.

Routine chemistries may reveal an increase in blood urea nitrogen (BUN) and creatinine, reflective of a decrease in GFR. Creatinine is the more dependable measure of GFR, because BUN levels may be influenced by an increase in tubular reabsorption ("prerenal azotemia"), an increase in urea generation in catabolic states, hyperalimentation, or gastrointestinal bleeding, and/or a decreased urea generation in decreased protein intake. In hypovolemic shock, liver function tests and cardiac biomarkers may show evidence of hepatic and cardiac ischemia, respectively. Routine chemistries and/or blood gases may reveal evidence of acid-base disorders. For example, bicarbonate loss due to diarrheal illness is a very common cause of metabolic acidosis; alternatively, patients with severe hypovolemic shock may develop lactic acidosis with an elevated anion gap.

The neurohumoral response to hypovolemia stimulates an increase in renal tubular Na^+ and water reabsorption. Therefore, the urine Na^+ concentration is typically <20 m*M* in nonrenal causes of hypovolemia, with a urine osmolality of >450 mOsm/kg. The reduction in both GFR and distal tubular Na^+ delivery may cause a defect in renal potassium excretion, with an increase in plasma K^+ concentration. Of note, patients with hypovolemia and a hypochloremic alkalosis due to vomiting, diarrhea, or diuretics will typically have a urine Na^+ concentration >20 m*M* and urine pH of >7.0, due to the increase in filtered HCO_3^-; the urine Cl^- concentration in this setting is a more accurate indicator of volume status, with a level <25 m*M* suggestive of hypovolemia. The urine Na^+ concentration is often >20 m*M* in patients with *renal* causes of hypovolemia, such as acute tubular necrosis; similarly, patients with diabetes insipidus will have an inappropriately dilute urine.

TREATMENT HYPOVOLEMIA

The therapeutic goals in hypovolemia are to restore normovolemia and replace ongoing fluid losses. Mild hypovolemia can usually be treated with oral hydration and resumption of a normal maintenance diet. More severe hypovolemia requires intravenous hydration, tailoring the choice of solution to the underlying pathophysiology. Isotonic, "normal" saline (0.9% NaCl, 154 m*M* Na^+) is the most appropriate resuscitation fluid for normonatremic or hyponatremic patients with severe hypovolemia; colloid solutions such as intravenous albumin are not demonstrably superior for this purpose. Hypernatremic patients should receive a hypotonic solution, 5% dextrose if there has only been water loss (as in diabetes insipidus), or hypotonic saline (1/2 or 1/4 normal saline) if there has been water and Na^+-Cl^- loss. Patients with bicarbonate loss and metabolic acidosis, as occur frequently in diarrhea, should receive intravenous bicarbonate, either an isotonic solution (150 meq of Na^+-HCO_3^- in 5% dextrose) or a more hypotonic bicarbonate solution in dextrose or dilute saline. Patients with severe hemorrhage or anemia should receive red cell transfusions, without increasing the hematocrit beyond 35%.

SODIUM DISORDERS

Disorders of serum Na^+ concentration are caused by abnormalities in water homeostasis, leading to changes in the relative ratio of Na^+ to body water. Water intake and circulating AVP constitute the two key effectors in the defense of serum osmolality; defects in one or both of these two defense mechanisms cause most cases of hyponatremia and hypernatremia. In contrast, abnormalities in sodium homeostasis per se lead to a deficit or surplus of whole-body Na^+-Cl^- content, a key determinant of the ECFV and circulatory integrity. Notably, volume status also modulates the release of AVP by the posterior pituitary, such that hypovolemia is associated with higher circulating levels of the hormone at each level of serum osmolality. Similarly, in "hypervolemic" causes of arterial underfilling, e.g., heart failure and cirrhosis, the associated neurohumoral activation is associated with an increase in circulating AVP, leading to water retention and hyponatremia. Therefore, a key concept in sodium disorders is that the absolute plasma Na^+ concentration tells one nothing about the volume status of a given patient, which furthermore must be taken into account in the diagnostic and therapeutic approach.

HYPONATREMIA

Hyponatremia, which is defined as a plasma Na^+ concentration <135 m*M*, is a very common disorder, occurring in up to 22% of hospitalized patients. This disorder is almost always the result of an increase in circulating AVP and/or increased renal sensitivity to AVP, combined with an intake of free water; a notable exception is hyponatremia due to low solute intake (see below). The underlying pathophysiology for the exaggerated or "inappropriate" AVP response differs in patients with hyponatremia as a function of their ECFV. Hyponatremia is thus subdivided diagnostically into three groups, depending on clinical history and volume status, i.e., "hypovolemic," "euvolemic," and "hypervolemic" (Fig. 63-5).

Hypovolemic Hyponatremia Hypovolemia causes a marked neurohumoral activation, increasing circulating levels of AVP. The increase in circulating AVP helps preserve blood pressure via vascular and baroreceptor V_{1A} receptors and increases water reabsorption via renal V_2 receptors; activation of V_2 receptors can lead to hyponatremia in the setting of increased free water intake. Nonrenal causes of hypovolemic hyponatremia include GI loss (e.g., vomiting, diarrhea, tube drainage) and insensible loss (sweating, burns) of Na^+-Cl^- and water, in the absence of adequate oral replacement; urine Na^+ concentration is typically <20 m*M*. Notably, these patients may be clinically classified as euvolemic, with only the reduced urinary Na^+ concentration to

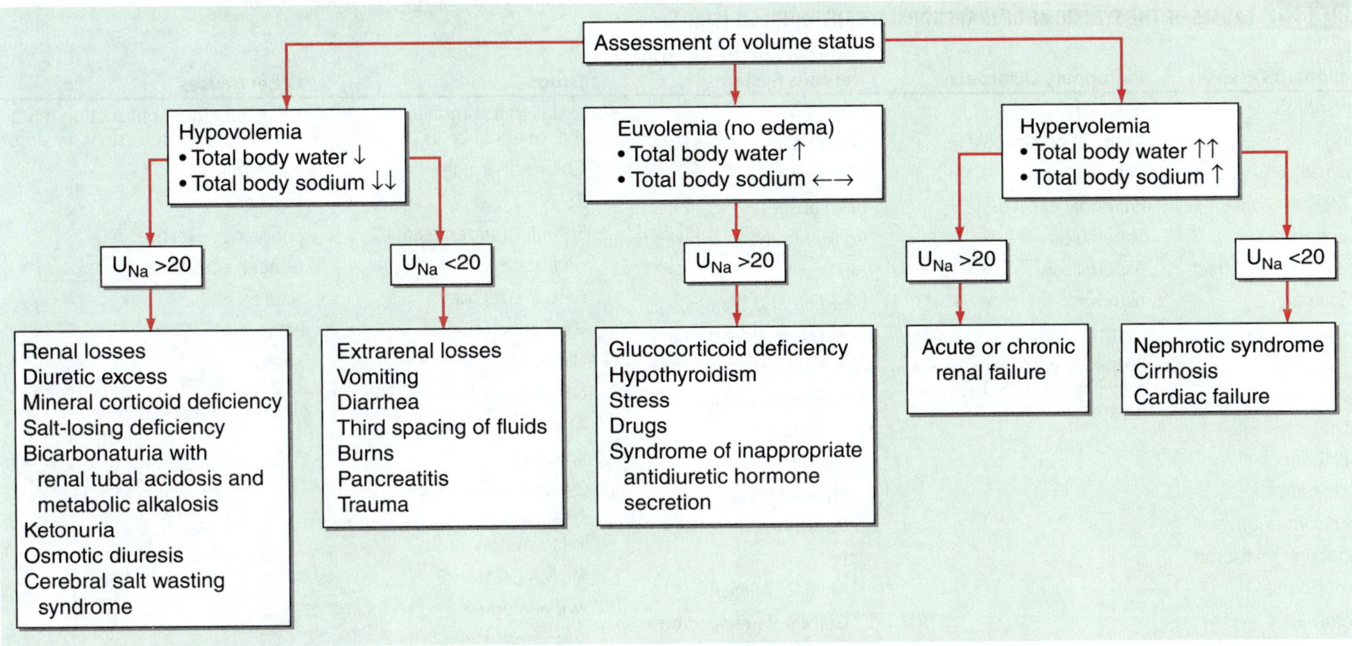

FIGURE 63-5 The diagnostic approach to hyponatremia. *(From S Kumar, T Berl: Diseases of water metabolism, in Atlas of Diseases of the Kidney, RW Schrier [ed]. Philadelphia, Current Medicine, Inc, 1999; with permission.)*

indicate the cause of their hyponatremia. Indeed, a urine Na^+ concentration <20 m*M*, in the absence of a cause of hypervolemic hyponatremia, predicts a rapid increase in plasma Na^+ concentration in response to intravenous normal saline; saline therapy thus induces a water diuresis in this setting, as circulating AVP levels plummet.

The *renal* causes of hypovolemic hyponatremia share an inappropriate loss of Na^+-Cl^- in the urine, leading to volume depletion and an increase in circulating AVP; urine Na^+ concentration is typically >20 m*M* (Fig. 63-5). A deficiency in circulating aldosterone and/or its renal effects can lead to hyponatremia in primary adrenal insufficiency and other causes of hypoaldosteronism; hyperkalemia and hyponatremia in a hypotensive and/or hypovolemic patient with high urine Na^+ concentration (much greater than 20 m*M*) should strongly suggest this diagnosis. Salt-losing nephropathies may lead to hyponatremia when sodium intake is reduced, due to impaired renal tubular function; typical causes include reflux nephropathy, interstitial nephropathies, postobstructive uropathy, medullary cystic disease, and the recovery phase of acute tubular necrosis. Thiazide diuretics cause hyponatremia via a number of mechanisms, including polydipsia and diuretic-induced volume depletion. Notably, thiazides do not inhibit the renal concentrating mechanism, such that circulating AVP retains a full effect on renal water retention. In contrast, loop diuretics, which are less frequently associated with hyponatremia, inhibit Na^+-Cl^- and K^+ absorption by the TALH, blunting the countercurrent mechanism and reducing the ability to concentrate the urine. Increased excretion of an osmotically active nonreabsorbable or poorly reabsorbable solute can also lead to volume depletion and hyponatremia; important causes include glycosuria, ketonuria (e.g., in starvation or in diabetic or alcoholic ketoacidosis), and bicarbonaturia (e.g., in renal tubular acidosis or metabolic alkalosis, where the associated bicarbonaturia leads to loss of Na^+).

Finally, the syndrome of "cerebral salt wasting" is a rare cause of hypovolemic hyponatremia, encompassing hyponatremia with clinical hypovolemia and inappropriate natriuresis in association with intracranial disease; associated disorders include subarachnoid hemorrhage, traumatic brain injury, craniotomy, encephalitis, and meningitis. Distinction from the more common syndrome of inappropriate antidiuresis is critical because cerebral salt wasting will typically respond to aggressive Na^+-Cl^- repletion.

Hypervolemic Hyponatremia Patients with hypervolemic hyponatremia develop an increase in total-body Na^+-Cl^- that is accompanied by a proportionately *greater* increase in total-body water, leading to a reduced plasma Na^+ concentration. As in hypovolemic hyponatremia, the causative disorders can be separated by the effect on urine Na^+ concentration, with acute or chronic renal failure uniquely associated with an increase in urine Na^+ concentration (Fig. 63-5). The pathophysiology of hyponatremia in the sodium-avid edematous disorders (congestive heart failure [CHF], cirrhosis, and nephrotic syndrome) is similar to that in hypovolemic hyponatremia, except that arterial filling and circulatory integrity is decreased due to the specific etiologic factors (e.g., cardiac dysfunction in CHF, peripheral vasodilation in cirrhosis). Urine Na^+ concentration is typically very low, i.e., <10 m*M*, even after hydration with normal saline; this Na^+-avid state may be obscured by diuretic therapy. The degree of hyponatremia provides an indirect index of the associated neurohumoral activation and is an important prognostic indicator in hypervolemic hyponatremia.

Euvolemic Hyponatremia Euvolemic hyponatremia can occur in moderate to severe hypothyroidism, with correction after achieving a euthyroid state. Severe hyponatremia can also be a consequence of secondary adrenal insufficiency due to pituitary disease; whereas the deficit in circulating aldosterone in primary adrenal insufficiency causes *hypovolemic* hyponatremia, the predominant glucocorticoid deficiency in secondary adrenal failure is associated with *euvolemic* hyponatremia. Glucocorticoids exert a negative feedback on AVP release by the posterior pituitary such that hydrocortisone replacement in these patients will rapidly normalize the AVP response to osmolality, reducing circulating AVP.

The syndrome of inappropriate antidiuresis (SIAD) is the most frequent cause of euvolemic hyponatremia (Table 63-1). The generation of hyponatremia in SIAD requires an intake of free water, with persistent intake at serum osmolalities that are lower than the usual threshold for thirst; as one would expect, the osmotic threshold and osmotic response curves for the sensation of thirst are shifted downward in patients with SIAD. Four distinct patterns of AVP secretion have been recognized in patients with SIAD, independent for the most part of the underlying cause. Unregulated, erratic AVP secretion is seen in about a third of patients, with no obvious correlation between serum osmolality and circulating AVP levels. Other patients fail to suppress AVP secretion at lower serum osmolalities, with a normal response curve to hyperosmolar conditions; others have a "reset osmostat," with a lower threshold osmolality and a left-shifted osmotic response curve. Finally, the fourth subset of patients have essentially no detectable

TABLE 63-1 CAUSES OF THE SYNDROME OF INAPPROPRIATE ANTIDIURESIS (SIAD)

Malignant Diseases	Pulmonary Disorders	Disorders of the Central Nervous System	Drugs	Other Causes
Carcinoma	Infections	Infection	Drugs that stimulate release of AVP or enhance its action	Hereditary (gain-of-function mutations in the vasopressin V_2 receptor)
Lung	Bacterial pneumonia	Encephalitis	Chlorpropamide	Idiopathic
Small cell	Viral pneumonia	Meningitis	SSRIs	Transient
Mesothelioma	Pulmonary abscess	Brain abscess	Tricyclic antidepressants	Endurance exercise
Oropharynx	Tuberculosis	Rocky Mountain spotted fever	Clofibrate	General anesthesia
Gastrointestinal tract	Aspergillosis	AIDS	Carbamazepine	Nausea
Stomach	Asthma	Bleeding and masses	Vincristine	Pain
Duodenum	Cystic fibrosis	Subdural hematoma	Nicotine	Stress
Pancreas	Respiratory failure associated with positive-pressure breathing	Subarachnoid hemorrhage	Narcotics	
Genitourinary tract		Cerebrovascular accident	Antipsychotic drugs	
Ureter		Brain tumors	Ifosfamide	
Bladder		Head trauma	Cyclophosphamide	
Prostate		Hydrocephalus	Nonsteroidal anti-inflammatory drugs	
Endometrium		Cavernous sinus thrombosis	MDMA ("ecstasy")	
Endocrine thymoma		Other	AVP analogues	
Lymphomas		Multiple sclerosis	Desmopressin	
Sarcomas		Guillain-Barré syndrome	Oxytocin	
Ewing's sarcoma		Shy-Drager syndrome	Vasopressin	
		Delirium tremens		
		Acute intermittent porphyria		

Abbreviations: AVP, vasopressin; MDMA; 3,4-methylenedioxymethamphetamine; SSRI, selective serotonin reuptake inhibitor.

Source: From DH Ellison, T Berl: Syndrome of inappropriate antidiuresis. N Engl J Med 356:2064, 2007.

circulating AVP, suggesting either a gain in function in renal water reabsorption or a circulating antidiuretic substance that is distinct from AVP. Gain-in-function mutations of a single specific residue in the V_2 AVP receptor have been described in some of these patients, leading to constitutive activation of the receptor in the absence of AVP and "nephrogenic" SIAD.

Strictly speaking, patients with SIAD are not euvolemic but are subclinically volume-expanded, due to AVP-induced water and Na^+-Cl^- retention; "AVP escape" mechanisms invoked by sustained increases in AVP serve to limit distal renal tubular transport, preserving a modestly hypervolemic steady state. Serum uric acid is often low (<4 mg/dL) in patients with SIAD, consistent with suppressed proximal tubular transport in the setting of increased distal tubular Na^+-Cl^- and water transport; in contrast, patients with hypovolemic hyponatremia will often be hyperuricemic, due to a shared activation of proximal tubular Na^+-Cl^- and urate transport.

Common causes of SIAD include pulmonary disease (e.g., pneumonia, tuberculosis, pleural effusion) and central nervous system (CNS) diseases (e.g., tumor, subarachnoid hemorrhage, meningitis). SIAD also occurs with malignancies, most commonly with small-cell lung carcinoma (75% of malignancy-associated SIAD); ~10% of patients with this tumor will have a plasma Na^+ concentration of <130 m*M* at presentation. SIAD is also a frequent complication of certain drugs, most commonly the selective serotonin reuptake inhibitors (SSRIs). Other drugs can potentiate the renal effect of AVP, without exerting direct effects on circulating AVP levels (Table 63-1).

Low Solute Intake and Hyponatremia Hyponatremia can occasionally occur in patients with a very low intake of dietary solutes. Classically, this occurs in alcoholics whose sole nutrient is beer, hence the diagnostic label of *beer potomania*; beer is very low in protein and salt content, containing only 1–2 m*M* of Na^+. The syndrome has also been described in nonalcoholic patients with highly restricted solute intake due to nutrient-restricted diets, e.g., extreme vegetarian diets. Patients with hyponatremia due to low solute intake typically present with a very low urine osmolality (<100–200 mOsm/kg) with a urine Na^+ concentration that is <10–20 m*M*. The fundamental abnormality is the inadequate dietary intake of solutes; the reduced urinary solute excretion limits water excretion such that hyponatremia ensues after relatively modest polydipsia. AVP levels have not been reported in patients with beer potomania but are expected to be suppressed or rapidly suppressible with saline hydration; this fits with the overly rapid correction in plasma Na^+ concentration that can be seen with saline hydration. Resumption of a normal diet and/or saline hydration will also correct the causative deficit in urinary solute excretion, such that patients with beer potomania typically correct their plasma Na^+ concentration promptly after admission to the hospital.

Clinical Features of Hyponatremia Hyponatremia induces generalized cellular swelling, a consequence of water movement down the osmotic gradient from the hypotonic ECF to the ICF. The symptoms of hyponatremia are primarily neurologic, reflecting the development of cerebral edema within a rigid skull. The initial CNS response to acute hyponatremia is an increase in interstitial pressure, leading to shunting of ECF and solutes from the interstitial space into the cerebrospinal fluid and then on into the systemic circulation. This is accompanied by an efflux of the major intracellular ions, Na^+, K^+, and Cl^-, from brain cells. Acute hyponatremic encephalopathy ensues when these volume regulatory mechanisms are overwhelmed by a rapid decrease in tonicity, resulting in acute cerebral edema. Early symptoms can include nausea, headache, and vomiting. However, severe complications can rapidly evolve, including seizure activity, brainstem herniation, coma, and death. A key complication of acute hyponatremia is normocapneic or hypercapneic respiratory failure; the associated hypoxia may amplify the neurologic injury. Normocapneic respiratory failure in this setting is typically due to noncardiogenic, "neurogenic" pulmonary edema, with a normal pulmonary capillary wedge pressure.

Acute symptomatic hyponatremia is a medical emergency, occurring in a number of specific settings (Table 63-2). Women, particularly before menopause, are much more likely than men to develop encephalopathy and severe neurologic sequelae. Acute hyponatremia often has an iatrogenic component, e.g., when hypotonic intravenous fluids are given to postoperative patients with an increase in circulating AVP. Exercise-associated hyponatremia, an important clinical issue at

TABLE 63-2 CAUSES OF ACUTE HYPONATREMIA

Iatrogenic	
	Postoperative: premenopausal women
	Hypotonic fluids with cause of ↑ vasopressin
	Glycine irrigation: TURP, uterine surgery
	Colonoscopy preparation
Recent institution of thiazides	
Polydipsia	
MDMA ("ecstasy," "Molly") ingestion	
Exercise induced	
Multifactorial, e.g., thiazide and polydipsia	

Abbreviations: MDMA, 3,4-methylenedioxymethamphetamine; TURP, transurethral resection of the prostate.

marathons and other endurance events, has similarly been linked to both a "nonosmotic" increase in circulating AVP and excessive free water intake. The recreational drugs Molly and ecstasy, which share an active ingredient (MDMA, 3,4-methylenedioxymethamphetamine), cause a rapid and potent induction of both thirst and AVP, leading to severe acute hyponatremia.

Persistent, chronic hyponatremia results in an efflux of organic osmolytes (creatine, betaine, glutamate, myoinositol, and taurine) from brain cells; this response reduces intracellular osmolality and the osmotic gradient favoring water entry. This reduction in intracellular osmolytes is largely complete within 48 h, the time period that clinically defines chronic hyponatremia; this temporal definition has considerable relevance for the treatment of hyponatremia (see below). The cellular response to chronic hyponatremia does not fully protect patients from symptoms, which can include vomiting, nausea, confusion, and seizures, usually at plasma Na^+ concentration <125 m*M*. Even patients who are judged "asymptomatic" can manifest subtle gait and cognitive defects that reverse with correction of hyponatremia; notably, chronic "asymptomatic" hyponatremia increases the risk of falls. Chronic hyponatremia also increases the risk of bony fractures owing to the associated neurologic dysfunction and to a hyponatremia-associated reduction in bone density. Therefore, every attempt should be made to correct safely the plasma Na^+ concentration in patients with chronic hyponatremia, even in the absence of overt symptoms (see the section on treatment of hyponatremia below).

The management of chronic hyponatremia is complicated significantly by the asymmetry of the cellular response to correction of plasma Na^+ concentration. Specifically, the *reaccumulation* of organic osmolytes by brain cells is attenuated and delayed as osmolality increases after correction of hyponatremia, sometimes resulting in degenerative loss of oligodendrocytes and an osmotic demyelination syndrome (ODS). Overly rapid correction of hyponatremia (>8–10 m*M* in 24 h or 18 m*M* in 48 h) is also associated with a disruption in integrity of the blood-brain barrier, allowing the entry of immune mediators that may contribute to demyelination. The lesions of ODS classically affect the pons, a structure wherein the delay in the reaccumulation of osmotic osmolytes is particularly pronounced; clinically, patients with central pontine myelinolysis can present 1 or more days after overcorrection of hyponatremia with paraparesis or quadriparesis, dysphagia, dysarthria, diplopia, a "locked-in syndrome," and/or loss of consciousness. Other regions of the brain can also be involved in ODS, most commonly in association with lesions of the pons but occasionally in isolation; in order of frequency, the lesions of extrapontine myelinolysis can occur in the cerebellum, lateral geniculate body, thalamus, putamen, and cerebral cortex or subcortex. Clinical presentation of ODS can, therefore, vary as a function of the extent and localization of extrapontine myelinolysis, with the reported development of ataxia, mutism, parkinsonism, dystonia, and catatonia. Relowering of plasma Na^+ concentration after overly rapid correction can prevent or attenuate ODS (see the section on treatment of hyponatremia below). However, even appropriately slow correction can be associated with ODS, particularly in patients with additional risk factors; these include alcoholism, malnutrition, hypokalemia, and liver transplantation.

Diagnostic Evaluation of Hyponatremia Clinical assessment of hyponatremic patients should focus on the underlying cause; a detailed drug history is particularly crucial (Table 63-1). A careful clinical assessment of volume status is obligatory for the classical diagnostic approach to hyponatremia (Fig. 63-5). Hyponatremia is frequently multifactorial, particularly when severe; clinical evaluation should consider *all* the possible causes for excessive circulating AVP, including volume status, drugs, and the presence of nausea and/or pain. Radiologic imaging may also be appropriate to assess whether patients have a pulmonary or CNS cause for hyponatremia. A screening chest x-ray may fail to detect a small-cell carcinoma of the lung; computed tomography (CT) scanning of the thorax should be considered in patients at high risk for this tumor (e.g., patients with a smoking history).

Laboratory investigation should include a measurement of serum osmolality to exclude pseudohyponatremia, which is defined as the coexistence of hyponatremia with a normal or increased plasma tonicity. Most clinical laboratories measure plasma Na^+ concentration by testing diluted samples with automated ion-sensitive electrodes, correcting for this dilution by assuming that plasma is 93% water. This correction factor can be inaccurate in patients with pseudohyponatremia due to extreme hyperlipidemia and/or hyperproteinemia, in whom serum lipid or protein makes up a greater percentage of plasma volume. The measured osmolality should also be converted to the effective osmolality (tonicity) by subtracting the measured concentration of urea (divided by 2.8, if in mg/dL); patients with hyponatremia have an effective osmolality of <275 mOsm/kg.

Elevated BUN and creatinine in routine chemistries can also indicate renal dysfunction as a potential cause of hyponatremia, whereas hyperkalemia may suggest adrenal insufficiency or hypoaldosteronism. Serum glucose should also be measured; plasma Na^+ concentration falls by ~1.6–2.4 m*M* for every 100-mg/dL increase in glucose, due to glucose-induced water efflux from cells; this "true" hyponatremia resolves after correction of hyperglycemia. Measurement of serum uric acid should also be performed; whereas patients with SIAD-type physiology will typically be hypouricemic (serum uric acid <4 mg/dL), volume-depleted patients will often be hyperuricemic. In the appropriate clinical setting, thyroid, adrenal, and pituitary function should also be tested; hypothyroidism and secondary adrenal failure due to pituitary insufficiency are important causes of euvolemic hyponatremia, whereas primary adrenal failure causes hypovolemic hyponatremia. A cosyntropin stimulation test is necessary to assess for primary adrenal insufficiency.

Urine electrolytes and osmolality are crucial tests in the initial evaluation of hyponatremia. A urine Na^+ concentration <20–30 m*M* is consistent with hypovolemic hyponatremia, in the clinical absence of a hypervolemic, Na^+-avid syndrome such as CHF (Fig. 63-5). In contrast, patients with SIAD will typically excrete urine with an Na^+ concentration that is >30 m*M*. However, there can be substantial overlap in urine Na^+ concentration values in patients with SIAD and hypovolemic hyponatremia, particularly in the elderly; the ultimate "gold standard" for the diagnosis of hypovolemic hyponatremia is the demonstration that plasma Na^+ concentration corrects after hydration with normal saline. Patients with thiazide-associated hyponatremia may also present with higher than expected urine Na^+ concentration and other findings suggestive of SIAD; one should defer making a diagnosis of SIAD in these patients until 1–2 weeks after discontinuing the thiazide. A urine osmolality <100 mOsm/kg is suggestive of polydipsia; urine osmolality >400 mOsm/kg indicates that AVP excess is playing a more dominant role, whereas intermediate values are more consistent with multifactorial pathophysiology (e.g., AVP excess with a significant component of polydipsia). Patients with hyponatremia due to decreased solute intake (beer potomania) typically have urine Na^+ concentration <20 m*M* and urine osmolality in the range of <100 to the low 200s. Finally, the measurement of urine K^+ concentration is required to calculate the urine-to-plasma electrolyte ratio, which is useful to predict the response to fluid restriction (see the section on treatment of hyponatremia below).

TREATMENT HYPONATREMIA

Three major considerations guide the therapy of hyponatremia. First, the presence and/or severity of symptoms determine the urgency and goals of therapy. Patients with acute hyponatremia (Table 63-2) present with symptoms that can range from headache, nausea, and/or vomiting, to seizures, obtundation, and central herniation; patients with chronic hyponatremia, present for >48 h, are less likely to have severe symptoms. Second, patients with chronic hyponatremia are at risk for ODS if plasma Na^+ concentration is corrected by >8–10 m*M* within the first 24 h and/or by >18 m*M* within the first 48 h. Third, the response to interventions such as hypertonic saline, isotonic saline, or AVP antagonists can be highly unpredictable, such that frequent monitoring of plasma Na^+ concentration during corrective therapy is imperative.

Once the urgency in correcting the plasma Na^+ concentration has been established and appropriate therapy instituted, the focus should be on treatment or withdrawal of the underlying cause. Patients with euvolemic hyponatremia due to SIAD, hypothyroidism, or secondary adrenal failure will respond to successful treatment of the underlying cause, with an increase in plasma Na^+ concentration. However, not all causes of SIAD are immediately reversible, necessitating pharmacologic therapy to increase the plasma Na^+ concentration (see below). Hypovolemic hyponatremia will respond to intravenous hydration with isotonic normal saline, with a rapid reduction in circulating AVP and a brisk water diuresis; it may be necessary to reduce the rate of correction if the history suggests that hyponatremia has been chronic, i.e., present for more than 48 h (see below). Hypervolemic hyponatremia due to CHF will often respond to improved therapy of the underlying cardiomyopathy, e.g., following the institution or intensification of angiotensin-converting enzyme (ACE) inhibition. Finally, patients with hyponatremia due to beer potomania and low solute intake will respond very rapidly to intravenous saline and the resumption of a normal diet. Notably, patients with beer potomania have a very high risk of developing ODS, due to the associated hypokalemia, alcoholism, malnutrition, and high risk of overcorrecting the plasma Na^+ concentration.

Water deprivation has long been a cornerstone of the therapy of chronic hyponatremia. However, patients who are excreting minimal electrolyte-free water will require aggressive fluid restriction; this can be very difficult for patients with SIAD to tolerate, given that their thirst is also inappropriately stimulated. The urine-to-plasma electrolyte ratio (urinary $[Na^+] + [K^+]$/plasma $[Na^+]$) can be exploited as a quick indicator of electrolyte-free water excretion (Table 63-3); patients with a ratio of >1 should be more aggressively restricted (<500 mL/d), those with a ratio of ~1 should be restricted to 500–700 mL/d, and those with a ratio <1 should be restricted to <1 L/d. In hypokalemic patients, potassium replacement will serve to increase plasma Na^+ concentration, given that the plasma Na^+ concentration is a functional of both exchangeable Na^+ and exchangeable K^+ divided by total-body water; a corollary is that aggressive repletion of K^+ has the potential to overcorrect the plasma Na^+ concentration even in the absence of hypertonic saline. Plasma Na^+ concentration will also tend to respond to an increase in dietary solute intake, which increases the ability to excrete free water; however, the use of oral urea and/or salt tablets for this purpose is generally not practical or well tolerated.

Patients in whom therapy with fluid restriction, potassium replacement, and/or increased solute intake fails may merit pharmacologic therapy to increase their plasma Na^+ concentration. Many patients with SIAD respond to combined therapy with oral furosemide, 20 mg twice a day (higher doses may be necessary in renal insufficiency), and oral salt tablets; furosemide serves to inhibit the renal countercurrent mechanism and blunt urinary concentrating ability, whereas the salt tablets counteract diuretic-associated natriuresis. Demeclocycline is a potent inhibitor of principal cells and can be used in patients whose Na levels do not increase in response to furosemide and salt tablets. However, this agent can be associated with a reduction in GFR, due to excessive natriuresis and/or direct renal toxicity; it should be avoided in cirrhotic patients in particular, who are at higher risk of nephrotoxicity due to drug accumulation.

AVP antagonists (vaptans) are highly effective in SIAD and in hypervolemic hyponatremia due to heart failure or cirrhosis, reliably increasing plasma Na^+ concentration due to their "aquaretic" effects (augmentation of free water clearance). Most of these agents specifically antagonize the V_2 AVP receptor; tolvaptan is currently the only oral V_2 antagonist to be approved by the U.S. Food and Drug Administration. Conivaptan, the only available intravenous vaptan, is a mixed V_{1A}/V_2 antagonist, with a modest risk of hypotension due to V_{1A} receptor inhibition. Therapy with vaptans must be initiated in a hospital setting, with a liberalization of fluid restriction (>2 L/d) and close monitoring of plasma Na^+ concentration. Although approved for the management of all but hypovolemic hyponatremia and acute hyponatremia, the clinical indications for these agents are not completely clear. Oral tolvaptan is perhaps most appropriate for the management of significant and persistent SIAD (e.g., in small-cell lung carcinoma) that has not responded to water restriction and/or oral furosemide and salt tablets. Abnormalities in liver function tests have been reported with chronic tolvaptan therapy; hence, the use of this agent should be restricted to <1–2 months.

Treatment of acute symptomatic hyponatremia should include hypertonic 3% saline (513 m*M*) to acutely increase plasma Na^+ concentration by 1–2 m*M*/h to a total of 4–6 m*M*; this modest increase is typically sufficient to alleviate severe acute symptoms, after which corrective guidelines for chronic hyponatremia are appropriate (see below). A number of equations have been developed to estimate the required rate of hypertonic saline, which has an Na^+-Cl^- concentration of 513 m*M*. The traditional approach is to calculate an Na^+ deficit, where the Na^+ deficit = 0.6 × body weight × (target plasma Na^+ concentration – starting plasma Na^+ concentration), followed by a calculation of the required rate. Regardless of the method used to determine the rate of administration, the increase in plasma Na^+ concentration can be highly unpredictable during treatment with hypertonic saline, due to rapid changes in the underlying physiology; plasma Na^+ concentration should be monitored every 2–4 h during treatment, with appropriate changes in therapy based on the observed rate of change. The administration of supplemental oxygen and ventilatory support is also critical in acute hyponatremia, in the event that patients develop acute pulmonary edema or hypercapneic respiratory failure. Intravenous loop diuretics will help treat acute pulmonary edema and will also increase free water excretion, by interfering with the renal countercurrent multiplication system. AVP antagonists do *not* have an approved role in the management of acute hyponatremia.

TABLE 63-3 MANAGEMENT OF HYPERNATREMIA

Water Deficit
1. Estimate total-body water (TBW): 50% of body weight in women and 60% in men
2. Calculate free-water deficit: $[(Na^+ - 140)/140] \times TBW$
3. Administer deficit over 48–72 h, without decrease in plasma Na^+ concentration by >10 m*M*/24 h
Ongoing Water Losses
4. Calculate free-water clearance, C_eH_2O: $C_eH_2O = V \times \left(1 - \frac{U_{Na} + U_K}{P_{Na}}\right)$ where V is urinary volume, U_{Na} is urinary $[Na^+]$, U_K is urinary $[K^+]$, and P_{Na} is plasma $[Na^+]$
Insensible Losses
5. ~10 mL/kg per day: less if ventilated, more if febrile
Total
6. Add components to determine water deficit and ongoing water loss; correct the water deficit over 48–72 h and replace daily water loss. Avoid correction of plasma $[Na^+]$ by >10 m*M*/d.

The rate of correction should be comparatively slow in *chronic* hyponatremia (<8–10 m*M* in the first 24 h and <18 m*M* in the first 48 h), so as to avoid ODS; lower target rates are appropriate in patients at particular risk for ODS, such as alcoholics or hypokalemic patients. Overcorrection of the plasma Na^+ concentration can occur when AVP levels rapidly normalize, for example following the treatment of patients with chronic hypovolemic hyponatremia with intravenous saline or following glucocorticoid replacement of patients with hypopituitarism and secondary adrenal failure. Approximately 10% of patients treated with vaptans will overcorrect; the risk is increased if water intake is not liberalized. In the event that the plasma Na^+ concentration overcorrects following therapy, be it with hypertonic saline, isotonic saline, or a vaptan, hyponatremia can be safely reinduced or stabilized by the administration of the AVP *agonist* desmopressin acetate (DDAVP) and/or the administration of free water, typically intravenous D_5W; the goal is to prevent or reverse the development of ODS. Alternatively, the treatment of patients with marked hyponatremia can be initiated with the twice-daily administration of DDAVP to maintain constant AVP bioactivity, combined with the administration of hypertonic saline to slowly correct the serum sodium in a more controlled fashion, thus reducing upfront the risk of overcorrection.

HYPERNATREMIA

Etiology Hypernatremia is defined as an increase in the plasma Na^+ concentration to >145 m*M*. Considerably less common than hyponatremia, hypernatremia is nonetheless associated with mortality rates of as high as 40–60%, mostly due to the severity of the associated underlying disease processes. Hypernatremia is usually the result of a combined water and electrolyte deficit, with losses of H_2O in excess of Na^+. Less frequently, the ingestion or iatrogenic administration of excess Na^+ can be causative, for example after IV administration of excessive hypertonic Na^+-Cl^- or Na^+-HCO_3^- (Fig. 63-6).

Elderly individuals with reduced thirst and/or diminished access to fluids are at the highest risk of developing hypernatremia. Patients with hypernatremia may rarely have a central defect in hypothalamic osmoreceptor function, with a mixture of both decreased thirst and reduced AVP secretion. Causes of this adipsic diabetes insipidus include primary or metastatic tumor, occlusion or ligation of the anterior communicating artery, trauma, hydrocephalus, and inflammation.

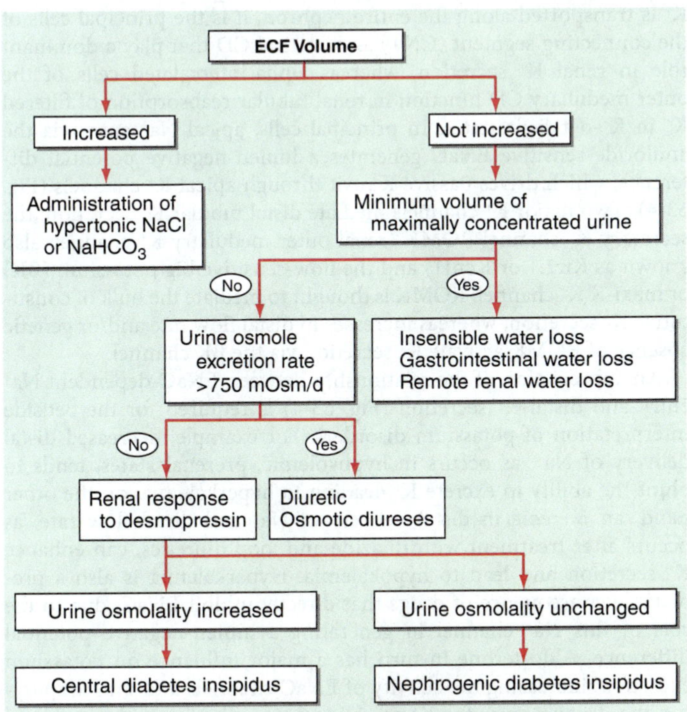

FIGURE 63-6 The diagnostic approach to hypernatremia. ECF, extracellular fluid.

Hypernatremia can develop following the loss of water via both renal and nonrenal routes. Insensible losses of water may increase in the setting of fever, exercise, heat exposure, severe burns, or mechanical ventilation. Diarrhea is, in turn, the most common gastrointestinal cause of hypernatremia. Notably, osmotic diarrhea and viral gastroenteritides typically generate stools with Na^+ and K^+ <100 m*M*, thus leading to water loss and hypernatremia; in contrast, secretory diarrhea typically results in isotonic stool and thus hypovolemia with or without hypovolemic hyponatremia.

Common causes of renal water loss include osmotic diuresis secondary to hyperglycemia, excess urea, postobstructive diuresis, or mannitol; these disorders share an increase in urinary solute excretion and urinary osmolality (see "Diagnostic Approach," below). Hypernatremia due to a water diuresis occurs in central or nephrogenic diabetes insipidus (DI).

Nephrogenic DI (NDI) is characterized by renal resistance to AVP, which can be partial or complete (see "Diagnostic Approach," below). Genetic causes include loss-of-function mutations in the X-linked V_2 receptor; mutations in the AVP-responsive aquaporin-2 water channel can cause autosomal recessive and autosomal dominant NDI, whereas recessive deficiency of the aquaporin-1 water channel causes a more modest concentrating defect (Fig. 63-2). Hypercalcemia can also cause polyuria and NDI; calcium signals directly through the calcium-sensing receptor to downregulate Na^+, K^+, and Cl^- transport by the TALH and water transport in principal cells, thus reducing renal concentrating ability in hypercalcemia. Another common acquired cause of NDI is hypokalemia, which inhibits the renal response to AVP and downregulates aquaporin-2 expression. Several drugs can cause acquired NDI, in particular lithium, ifosfamide, and several antiviral agents. Lithium causes NDI by multiple mechanisms, including direct inhibition of renal glycogen synthase kinase-3 (GSK3), a kinase thought to be the pharmacologic target of lithium in bipolar disease; GSK3 is required for the response of principal cells to AVP. The entry of lithium through the amiloride-sensitive Na^+ channel ENaC (Fig. 63-4) is required for the effect of the drug on principal cells, such that combined therapy within lithium and amiloride can mitigate lithium-associated NDI. However, lithium causes chronic tubulointerstitial scarring and chronic kidney disease after prolonged therapy, such that patients may have a persistent NDI long after stopping the drug, with a reduced therapeutic benefit from amiloride.

Finally, gestational DI is a rare complication of late-term pregnancy wherein increased activity of a circulating placental protease with "vasopressinase" activity leads to reduced circulating AVP and polyuria, often accompanied by hypernatremia. DDAVP is an effective therapy for this syndrome, given its resistance to the vasopressinase enzyme.

Clinical Features Hypernatremia increases osmolality of the ECF, generating an osmotic gradient between the ECF and ICF, an efflux of intracellular water, and cellular shrinkage. As in hyponatremia, the symptoms of hypernatremia are predominantly neurologic. Altered mental status is the most frequent manifestation, ranging from mild confusion and lethargy to deep coma. The sudden shrinkage of brain cells in acute hypernatremia may lead to parenchymal or subarachnoid hemorrhages and/or subdural hematomas; however, these vascular complications are primarily encountered in pediatric and neonatal patients. Osmotic damage to muscle membranes can also lead to hypernatremic rhabdomyolysis. Brain cells accommodate to a chronic increase in ECF osmolality (>48 h) by activating membrane transporters that mediate influx and intracellular accumulation of organic osmolytes (creatine, betaine, glutamate, myoinositol, and taurine); this results in an increase in ICF water and normalization of brain parenchymal volume. In consequence, patients with *chronic* hypernatremia are less likely to develop severe neurologic compromise. However, the cellular response to chronic hypernatremia predisposes these patients to the development of cerebral edema and seizures during overly rapid hydration (overcorrection of plasma Na^+ concentration by >10 m*M*/d).

Diagnostic Approach The history should focus on the presence or absence of thirst, polyuria, and/or an extrarenal source for water loss, such as diarrhea. The physical examination should include a detailed neurologic exam and an assessment of the ECFV; patients with a particularly large water deficit and/or a combined deficit in electrolytes and water may be hypovolemic, with reduced JVP and orthostasis. Accurate documentation of daily fluid intake and daily urine output is also critical for the diagnosis and management of hypernatremia.

Laboratory investigation should include a measurement of serum and urine osmolality, in addition to urine electrolytes. The appropriate response to hypernatremia and a serum osmolality >295 mOsm/kg is an increase in circulating AVP and the excretion of low volumes (<500 mL/d) of maximally concentrated urine, i.e., urine with osmolality >800 mOsm/kg; should this be the case, then an extrarenal source of water loss is primarily responsible for the generation of hypernatremia. Many patients with hypernatremia are polyuric; should an osmotic diuresis be responsible, with excessive excretion of Na^+-Cl^-, glucose, and/or urea, then daily solute excretion will be >750–1000 mOsm/d (>15 mOsm/kg body water per day) (Fig. 63-6). More commonly, patients with hypernatremia and polyuria will have a predominant water diuresis, with excessive excretion of hypotonic, dilute urine.

Adequate differentiation between nephrogenic and central causes of DI requires the measurement of the response in urinary osmolality to DDAVP, combined with measurement of circulating AVP in the setting of hypertonicity. By definition, patients with baseline hypernatremia are hypertonic, with an adequate stimulus for AVP by the posterior pituitary. Therefore, in contrast to polyuric patients with a normal or reduced baseline plasma Na^+ concentration and osmolality, a water deprivation test (Chap. 61) is unnecessary in hypernatremia; indeed, water deprivation is absolutely contraindicated in this setting, given the risk for worsening the hypernatremia. Patients with NDI will fail to respond to DDAVP, with a urine osmolality that increases by <50% or <150 mOsm/kg from baseline, in combination with a normal or high circulating AVP level; patients with central DI will respond to DDAVP, with a reduced circulating AVP. Patients may exhibit a partial response to DDAVP, with a >50% rise in urine osmolality that nonetheless fails to reach 800 mOsm/kg; the level of circulating AVP will help differentiate the underlying cause, i.e., NDI versus central DI. In pregnant patients, AVP assays should be drawn in tubes containing the protease inhibitor 1,10-phenanthroline, to prevent in vitro degradation of AVP by placental vasopressinase.

For patients with hypernatremia due to renal loss of water, it is critical to quantify *ongoing* daily losses using the calculated electrolyte-free water clearance, in addition to calculation of the baseline water deficit (the relevant formulas are discussed in Table 63-3). This requires daily measurement of urine electrolytes, combined with accurate measurement of daily urine volume.

TREATMENT HYPERNATREMIA

The underlying cause of hypernatremia should be withdrawn or corrected, be it drugs, hyperglycemia, hypercalcemia, hypokalemia, or diarrhea. The approach to the correction of hypernatremia is outlined in Table 63-3. It is imperative to correct hypernatremia slowly to avoid cerebral edema, typically replacing the calculated free water deficit over 48 h. Notably, the plasma Na^+ concentration should be corrected by no more than 10 m*M*/d, which may take longer than 48 h in patients with severe hypernatremia (>160 m*M*). A rare exception is patients with acute hypernatremia (<48 h) due to sodium loading, who can safely be corrected rapidly at a rate of 1 m*M*/h.

Water should ideally be administered by mouth or by nasogastric tube, as the most direct way to provide free water, i.e., water without electrolytes. Alternatively, patients can receive free water in dextrose-containing IV solutions, such as 5% dextrose (D_5W); blood glucose should be monitored in case hyperglycemia occurs. Depending on the history, blood pressure, or clinical volume status, it may be appropriate to initially treat with hypotonic saline solutions (1/4 or 1/2 normal saline); normal saline is usually inappropriate in the absence of very severe hypernatremia, where normal saline is proportionally more hypotonic relative to plasma, or frank hypotension. Calculation of urinary electrolyte-free water clearance (Table 63-3) is required to estimate daily, ongoing loss of free water in patients with NDI or central DI, which should be replenished daily.

Additional therapy may be feasible in specific cases. Patients with central DI should respond to the administration of intravenous, intranasal, or oral DDAVP. Patients with NDI due to lithium may reduce their polyuria with amiloride (2.5–10 mg/d), which decreases entry of lithium into principal cells by inhibiting ENaC (see above); in practice, however, most patients with lithium-associated DI are able to compensate for their polyuria by simply increasing their daily water intake. Thiazides may reduce polyuria due to NDI, ostensibly by inducing hypovolemia and increasing proximal tubular water reabsorption. Occasionally, nonsteroidal anti-inflammatory drugs (NSAIDs) have been used to treat polyuria associated with NDI, reducing the negative effect of intrarenal prostaglandins on urinary concentrating mechanisms; however, this assumes the risks of NSAID-associated gastric and/or renal toxicity. Furthermore, it must be emphasized that thiazides, amiloride, and NSAIDs are only appropriate for *chronic* management of polyuria from NDI and have *no* role in the acute management of associated hypernatremia, where the focus is on replacing free water deficits and ongoing free water loss.

POTASSIUM DISORDERS

Homeostatic mechanisms maintain plasma K^+ concentration between 3.5 and 5.0 m*M*, despite marked variation in dietary K^+ intake. In a healthy individual at steady state, the entire daily intake of potassium is excreted, approximately 90% in the urine and 10% in the stool; thus, the kidney plays a dominant role in potassium homeostasis. However, more than 98% of total-body potassium is intracellular, chiefly in muscle; buffering of extracellular K^+ by this large intracellular pool plays a crucial role in the regulation of plasma K^+ concentration. Changes in the exchange and distribution of intra- and extracellular K^+ can thus lead to marked hypo- or hyperkalemia. A corollary is that massive necrosis and the attendant release of tissue K^+ can cause severe hyperkalemia, particularly in the setting of acute kidney injury and reduced excretion of K^+.

Changes in whole-body K^+ content are primarily mediated by the kidney, which *reabsorbs* filtered K^+ in hypokalemic, K^+-deficient states and *secretes* K^+ in hyperkalemic, K^+-replete states. Although K^+ is transported along the entire nephron, it is the principal cells of the connecting segment (CNT) and cortical CD that play a dominant role in renal K^+ secretion, whereas alpha-intercalated cells of the outer medullary CD function in renal tubular reabsorption of filtered K^+ in K^+-deficient states. In principal cells, apical Na^+ entry via the amiloride-sensitive ENaC generates a lumen-negative potential difference, which drives passive K^+ exit through apical K^+ channels (Fig. 63-4). Two major K^+ channels mediate distal tubular K^+ secretion: the secretory K^+ channel ROMK (renal outer medullary K^+ channel; also known as Kir1.1 or KcnJ1) and the flow-sensitive big potassium (BK) or maxi-K K^+ channel. ROMK is thought to mediate the bulk of constitutive K^+ secretion, whereas increases in distal flow rate and/or genetic absence of ROMK activate K^+ secretion via the BK channel.

An appreciation of the relationship between ENaC-dependent Na^+ entry and distal K^+ secretion (Fig. 63-4) is required for the bedside interpretation of potassium disorders. For example, decreased distal delivery of Na^+, as occurs in hypovolemic, prerenal states, tends to blunt the ability to excrete K^+, leading to hyperkalemia; on the other hand, an *increase* in distal delivery of Na^+ and distal flow rate, as occurs after treatment with thiazide and loop diuretics, can enhance K^+ secretion and lead to hypokalemia. Hyperkalemia is also a predictable consequence of drugs that directly inhibit ENaC, due to the role of this Na^+ channel in generating a lumen-negative potential difference. Aldosterone in turn has a major influence on potassium excretion, increasing the activity of ENaC channels and thus amplifying the driving force for K^+ secretion across the luminal membrane of principal cells. Abnormalities in the renin-angiotensin-aldosterone system can thus cause both hypokalemia and hyperkalemia. Notably, however, potassium excess and potassium restriction have opposing, aldosterone-independent effects on the density and activity of apical K^+ channels in the distal nephron, i.e., factors other than aldosterone modulate the renal capacity to secrete K^+. In addition, potassium restriction and hypokalemia activates aldosterone-independent distal *reabsorption* of filtered K^+, activating apical H^+/K^+-ATPase activity in intercalated cells within the outer medullary CD. Reflective perhaps of this physiology, changes in plasma K^+ concentration are not universal in disorders associated with changes in aldosterone activity.

HYPOKALEMIA

Hypokalemia, defined as a plasma K^+ concentration of <3.5 m*M*, occurs in up to 20% of hospitalized patients. Hypokalemia is associated with a 10-fold increase in in-hospital mortality, due to adverse effects on cardiac rhythm, blood pressure, and cardiovascular morbidity. Mechanistically, hypokalemia can be caused by redistribution of K^+ between tissues and the ECF or by renal and nonrenal loss of K^+ (Table 63-4). Systemic hypomagnesemia can also cause treatment-resistant hypokalemia, due to a combination of reduced cellular uptake of K^+ and exaggerated renal secretion. Spurious hypokalemia or "pseudohypokalemia" can occasionally result from in vitro cellular uptake of K^+ after venipuncture, for example, due to profound leukocytosis in acute leukemia.

Redistribution and Hypokalemia Insulin, β_2-adrenergic activity, thyroid hormone, and alkalosis promote Na^+/K^+-ATPase-mediated cellular uptake of K^+, leading to hypokalemia. Inhibition of the passive *efflux* of K^+ can also cause hypokalemia, albeit rarely; this typically occurs in the setting of systemic inhibition of K^+ channels by toxic barium ions. Exogenous insulin can cause iatrogenic hypokalemia, particularly during the management of K^+-deficient states such as diabetic ketoacidosis. Alternatively, the stimulation of *endogenous* insulin can provoke hypokalemia, hypomagnesemia, and/or hypophosphatemia in malnourished patients given a carbohydrate load. Alterations in the activity of the endogenous sympathetic nervous system can cause hypokalemia in several settings, including alcohol withdrawal, hyperthyroidism, acute myocardial infarction, and severe head injury. β_2 agonists, including both bronchodilators and tocolytics (ritodrine), are powerful activators of cellular K^+ uptake; "hidden" sympathomimetics, such as pseudoephedrine and ephedrine in cough syrup or dieting agents, may also cause unexpected hypokalemia. Finally, xanthine-dependent activation of cAMP-dependent signaling, downstream of the β_2 receptor, can lead to hypokalemia, usually in the setting of overdose (theophylline) or marked overingestion (dietary caffeine).

Redistributive hypokalemia can also occur in the setting of hyperthyroidism, with periodic attacks of hypokalemic paralysis (thyrotoxic periodic paralysis [TPP]). Similar episodes of hypokalemic weakness in the absence of thyroid abnormalities occur in *familial* hypokalemic periodic paralysis, usually caused by missense mutations of voltage sensor domains within the α_1 subunit of L-type calcium channels or the skeletal Na^+ channel; these mutations generate an abnormal gating pore current activated by hyperpolarization. TPP develops more frequently in patients of Asian or Hispanic origin; this shared predisposition has been linked to genetic variation in Kir2.6, a muscle-specific, thyroid hormone–responsive K^+ channel. Patients with TPP typically present with weakness of the extremities and limb girdles, with paralytic episodes that occur most frequently between 1 and 6 AM. Signs and symptoms of hyperthyroidism are not invariably present. Hypokalemia is usually profound and almost invariably accompanied by hypophosphatemia and hypomagnesemia. The hypokalemia in TPP is attributed to both direct and indirect activation of the Na^+/K^+-ATPase, resulting in increased uptake of K^+ by muscle and other tissues. Increases in β-adrenergic activity play an important role in that high-dose propranolol (3 mg/kg) rapidly reverses the associated hypokalemia, hypophosphatemia, and paralysis.

Nonrenal Loss of Potassium The loss of K^+ in sweat is typically low, except under extremes of physical exertion. Direct gastric losses of K^+ due to vomiting or nasogastric suctioning are also minimal; however, the ensuing hypochloremic alkalosis results in persistent kaliuresis due to secondary hyperaldosteronism and bicarbonaturia, i.e., a *renal* loss of K^+. Diarrhea is a globally important cause of hypokalemia, given the worldwide prevalence of infectious diarrheal disease. Noninfectious gastrointestinal processes such as celiac disease, ileostomy, villous adenomas, inflammatory bowel disease, colonic pseudo-obstruction (Ogilvie's syndrome), VIPomas, and chronic laxative abuse can also cause significant hypokalemia; an exaggerated intestinal secretion of potassium by upregulated colonic BK channels has been directly implicated in the pathogenesis of hypokalemia in many of these disorders.

Renal Loss of Potassium Drugs can increase renal K^+ excretion by a variety of different mechanisms. Diuretics are a particularly common cause, due to associated increases in distal tubular Na^+ delivery and

TABLE 63-4 CAUSES OF HYPOKALEMIA

I. Decreased intake
  A. Starvation
  B. Clay ingestion
II. Redistribution into cells
  A. Acid-base
    1. Metabolic alkalosis
  B. Hormonal
    1. Insulin
    2. Increased β_2-adrenergic sympathetic activity: post–myocardial infarction, head injury
    3. β_2-Adrenergic agonists – bronchodilators, tocolytics
    4. α-Adrenergic antagonists
    5. Thyrotoxic periodic paralysis
    6. Downstream stimulation of Na^+/K^+-ATPase: theophylline, caffeine
  C. Anabolic state
    1. Vitamin B_{12} or folic acid administration (red blood cell production)
    2. Granulocyte-macrophage colony-stimulating factor (white blood cell production)
    3. Total parenteral nutrition
  D. Other
    1. Pseudohypokalemia
    2. Hypothermia
    3. Familial hypokalemic periodic paralysis
    4. Barium toxicity: systemic inhibition of "leak" K^+ channels
III. Increased loss
  A. Nonrenal
    1. Gastrointestinal loss (diarrhea)
    2. Integumentary loss (sweat)
  B. Renal
    1. Increased distal flow and distal Na^+ delivery: diuretics, osmotic diuresis, salt-wasting nephropathies
    2. Increased secretion of potassium
      a. Mineralocorticoid excess: primary hyperaldosteronism (aldosterone-producing adenomas, primary or unilateral adrenal hyperplasia, idiopathic hyperaldosteronism due to bilateral adrenal hyperplasia, and adrenal carcinoma), genetic hyperaldosteronism (familial hyperaldosteronism types I/II/III, congenital adrenal hyperplasias), secondary hyperaldosteronism (malignant hypertension, renin-secreting tumors, renal artery stenosis, hypovolemia), Cushing's syndrome, Bartter's syndrome, Gitelman's syndrome
      b. Apparent mineralocorticoid excess: genetic deficiency of 11β-dehydrogenase-2 (syndrome of apparent mineralocorticoid excess), inhibition of 11β-dehydrogenase-2 (glycyrrhetinic/glycyrrhizinic acid and/or carbenoxolone; licorice, food products, drugs), Liddle's syndrome (genetic activation of epithelial Na^+ channels)
      c. Distal delivery of nonreabsorbed anions: vomiting, nasogastric suction, proximal renal tubular acidosis, diabetic ketoacidosis, glue-sniffing (toluene abuse), penicillin derivatives (penicillin, nafcillin, dicloxacillin, ticarcillin, oxacillin, and carbenicillin)
    3. Magnesium deficiency

distal tubular flow rate, in addition to secondary hyperaldosteronism. Thiazides have a greater effect on plasma K^+ concentration than loop diuretics, despite their lesser natriuretic effect. The diuretic effect of thiazides is largely due to inhibition of the Na^+-Cl^- cotransporter NCC in DCT cells. This leads to a direct increase in the delivery of luminal Na^+ to the principal cells immediately downstream in the CNT and cortical CD, which augments Na^+ entry via ENaC, increases the lumen-negative potential difference, and amplifies K^+ secretion. The higher propensity of thiazides to cause hypokalemia may also be secondary to thiazide-associated hypocalciuria, versus the *hypercalciuria* seen with loop diuretics; the increases in downstream luminal calcium in response to loop diuretics inhibit ENaC in principal cells, thus reducing the lumen-negative potential difference and attenuating distal K^+ excretion. High doses of penicillin-related antibiotics (nafcillin, dicloxacillin, ticarcillin, oxacillin, and carbenicillin) can increase obligatory K^+ excretion by acting as nonreabsorbable anions in the distal nephron. Finally, several renal tubular toxins cause renal K^+ and magnesium wasting, leading to hypokalemia and hypomagnesemia; these drugs include aminoglycosides, amphotericin, foscarnet, cisplatin, and ifosfamide (see also "Magnesium Deficiency and Hypokalemia," below).

Aldosterone activates the ENaC channel in principal cells via multiple synergistic mechanisms, thus increasing the driving force for K^+ excretion. In consequence, increases in aldosterone bioactivity and/or gains in function of aldosterone-dependent signaling pathways are associated with hypokalemia. Increases in circulating aldosterone (hyperaldosteronism) may be primary or secondary. Increased levels of circulating renin in secondary forms of hyperaldosteronism lead to increased angiotensin II and thus aldosterone; renal artery stenosis is perhaps the most frequent cause (Table 63-4). Primary hyperaldosteronism may be genetic or acquired. Hypertension and hypokalemia, due to increases in circulating 11-deoxycorticosterone, occur in patients with congenital adrenal hyperplasia caused by defects in either steroid 11β-hydroxylase or steroid 17α-hydroxylase; deficient 11β-hydroxylase results in associated virilization and other signs of androgen excess, whereas reduced sex steroids in 17α-hydroxylase deficiency lead to hypogonadism.

The major forms of *isolated* primary genetic hyperaldosteronism are familial hyperaldosteronism type I (FH-I, also known as glucocorticoid-remediable hyperaldosteronism [GRA]) and familial hyperaldosteronism types II and III (FH-II and FH-III), in which aldosterone production is not repressible by exogenous glucocorticoids. FH-I is caused by a chimeric gene duplication between the homologous 11β-hydroxylase (*CYP11B1*) and aldosterone synthase (*CYP11B2*) genes, fusing the adrenocorticotropic hormone (ACTH)–responsive 11β-hydroxylase promoter to the coding region of aldosterone synthase; this chimeric gene is under the control of ACTH and thus repressible by glucocorticoids. FH-III is caused by mutations in the *KCNJ5* gene, which encodes the G-protein-activated inward rectifier K^+ channel 4 (GIRK4); these mutations lead to the acquisition of sodium permeability in the mutant GIRK4 channels, causing an exaggerated membrane depolarization in adrenal glomerulosa cells and the activation of voltage-gated calcium channels. The resulting calcium influx is sufficient to produce aldosterone secretion and cell proliferation, leading to adrenal adenomas and hyperaldosteronism.

Acquired causes of primary hyperaldosteronism include aldosterone-producing adenomas (APAs), primary or unilateral adrenal hyperplasia (PAH), idiopathic hyperaldosteronism (IHA) due to bilateral adrenal hyperplasia, and adrenal carcinoma; APA and IHA account for close to 60% and 40%, respectively, of diagnosed hyperaldosteronism. Acquired somatic mutations in *KCNJ5* or less frequently in the *ATP1A1* (an Na^+/K^+ ATPase α subunit) and *ATP2B3* (a Ca^{2+} ATPase) genes can be detected in APAs; as in FH-III (see above), the exaggerated depolarization of adrenal glomerulosa cells caused by these mutations is implicated in the excessive adrenal proliferation and the exaggerated release of aldosterone.

Random testing of plasma renin activity (PRA) and aldosterone is a helpful screening tool in hypokalemic and/or hypertensive patients, with an aldosterone:PRA ratio of >50 suggestive of primary hyperaldosteronism. Hypokalemia and multiple antihypertensive drugs may alter the aldosterone:PRA ratio by suppressing aldosterone or increasing PRA, leading to a ratio of <50 in patients who do in fact have primary hyperaldosteronism; therefore, the clinical context should always be considered when interpreting these results.

The glucocorticoid cortisol has equal affinity for the mineralocorticoid receptor (MLR) to that of aldosterone, with resultant "mineralocorticoid-like" activity. However, cells in the aldosterone-sensitive distal nephron are protected from this "illicit" activation by the enzyme 11β-hydroxysteroid dehydrogenase-2 (11βHSD-2), which converts cortisol to cortisone; cortisone has minimal affinity for the MLR. Recessive loss-of-function mutations in the *11βHSD-2* gene are thus associated with cortisol-dependent activation of the MLR and the syndrome of apparent mineralocorticoid excess (SAME), encompassing hypertension, hypokalemia, hypercalciuria, and metabolic alkalosis, with suppressed PRA and suppressed aldosterone. A similar syndrome is caused by biochemical inhibition of 11βHSD-2 by glycyrrhetinic/glycyrrhizinic acid and/or carbenoxolone. Glycyrrhizinic acid is a natural sweetener found in licorice root, typically encountered in licorice and its many guises or as a flavoring agent in tobacco and food products.

Finally, hypokalemia may also occur with systemic increases in glucocorticoids. In Cushing's syndrome caused by increases in pituitary ACTH (Chap. 406), the incidence of hypokalemia is only 10%, whereas it is 60–100% in patients with ectopic secretion of ACTH, despite a similar incidence of hypertension. Indirect evidence suggests that the activity of renal 11βHSD-2 is reduced in patients with ectopic ACTH compared with Cushing's syndrome, resulting in SAME.

Finally, defects in multiple renal tubular transport pathways are associated with hypokalemia. For example, loss-of-function mutations in subunits of the acidifying H^+-ATPase in alpha-intercalated cells cause hypokalemic distal renal tubular acidosis, as do many acquired disorders of the distal nephron. Liddle's syndrome is caused by autosomal dominant gain-in-function mutations of ENaC subunits. Disease-associated mutations either activate the channel directly or abrogate aldosterone-inhibited retrieval of ENaC subunits from the plasma membrane; the end result is increased expression of activated ENaC channels at the plasma membrane of principal cells. Patients with Liddle's syndrome classically manifest severe hypertension with hypokalemia, unresponsive to spironolactone yet sensitive to amiloride. Hypertension and hypokalemia are, however, variable aspects of the Liddle's phenotype; more consistent features include a blunted aldosterone response to ACTH and reduced urinary aldosterone excretion.

Loss of the transport functions of the TALH and DCT nephron segments causes hereditary hypokalemic alkalosis, Bartter's syndrome (BS) and Gitelman's syndrome (GS), respectively. Patients with classic BS typically suffer from polyuria and polydipsia, due to the reduction in renal concentrating ability. They may have an increase in urinary calcium excretion, and 20% are hypomagnesemic. Other features include marked activation of the renin-angiotensin-aldosterone axis. Patients with antenatal BS suffer from a severe systemic disorder characterized by marked electrolyte wasting, polyhydramnios, and hypercalciuria with nephrocalcinosis; renal prostaglandin synthesis and excretion are significantly increased, accounting for much of the systemic symptoms. There are five disease genes for BS, all of them functioning in some aspect of regulated Na^+, K^+, and Cl^- transport by the TALH. In contrast, GS is genetically homogeneous, caused almost exclusively by loss-of-function mutations in the thiazide-sensitive Na^+-Cl^- cotransporter of the DCT. Patients with GS are uniformly hypomagnesemic and exhibit marked hypocalciuria, rather than the hypercalciuria typically seen in BS; urinary calcium excretion is thus a critical diagnostic test in GS. GS is a milder phenotype than BS; however, patients with GS may suffer from chondrocalcinosis, an abnormal deposition of calcium pyrophosphate dihydrate (CPPD) in joint cartilage (Chap. 339).

Magnesium Deficiency and Hypokalemia Magnesium depletion has inhibitory effects on muscle Na^+/K^+-ATPase activity, reducing influx into muscle cells and causing a secondary kaliuresis. In addition, magnesium depletion causes exaggerated K^+ secretion by the distal nephron; this effect is attributed to a reduction in the magnesium-dependent, intracellular block of K^+ efflux through the secretory K^+ channel of principal cells (ROMK; Fig. 63-4). In consequence, hypomagnesemic patients are clinically refractory to K^+ replacement in the absence of Mg^{2+} repletion. Notably, magnesium deficiency is also a common concomitant of hypokalemia because many disorders of the distal nephron may cause both potassium and magnesium wasting (Chap. 339).

Clinical Features Hypokalemia has prominent effects on cardiac, skeletal, and intestinal muscle cells. In particular, hypokalemia is a major risk factor for both ventricular and atrial arrhythmias. Hypokalemia predisposes to digoxin toxicity by a number of mechanisms, including reduced competition between K^+ and digoxin for shared binding sites on cardiac Na^+/K^+-ATPase subunits. Electrocardiographic changes in hypokalemia include broad flat T waves, ST depression, and QT prolongation; these are most marked when serum K^+ is <2.7 mmol/L. Hypokalemia can thus be an important precipitant of arrhythmia in patients with additional genetic or acquired causes of QT prolongation. Hypokalemia also results in hyperpolarization of skeletal muscle, thus impairing the capacity to depolarize and contract; weakness and even paralysis may ensue. It also causes a skeletal myopathy and predisposes to rhabdomyolysis. Finally, the paralytic effects of hypokalemia on intestinal smooth muscle may cause intestinal ileus.

The functional effects of hypokalemia on the kidney can include Na^+-Cl^- and HCO_3^- retention, polyuria, phosphaturia, hypocitraturia, and an activation of renal ammoniagenesis. Bicarbonate retention and other acid-base effects of hypokalemia can contribute to the generation of metabolic alkalosis. Hypokalemic polyuria is due to a combination of central polydipsia and an AVP-resistant renal concentrating defect. Structural changes in the kidney due to hypokalemia include a relatively specific vacuolizing injury to proximal tubular cells, interstitial nephritis, and renal cysts. Hypokalemia also predisposes to acute kidney injury and can lead to end-stage renal disease in patients with longstanding hypokalemia due to eating disorders and/or laxative abuse.

Hypokalemia and/or reduced dietary K^+ are implicated in the pathophysiology and progression of hypertension, heart failure, and stroke. For example, short-term K^+ restriction in healthy humans and patients with essential hypertension induces Na^+-Cl^- retention and hypertension. Correction of hypokalemia is particularly important in hypertensive patients treated with diuretics, in whom blood pressure improves with the establishment of normokalemia.

Diagnostic Approach The cause of hypokalemia is usually evident from history, physical examination, and/or basic laboratory tests. The history should focus on medications (e.g., laxatives, diuretics, antibiotics), diet and dietary habits (e.g., licorice), and/or symptoms that suggest a particular cause (e.g., periodic weakness, diarrhea). The physical examination should pay particular attention to blood pressure, volume status, and signs suggestive of specific hypokalemic disorders, e.g., hyperthyroidism and Cushing's syndrome. Initial laboratory evaluation should include electrolytes, BUN, creatinine, serum osmolality, Mg^{2+}, Ca^{2+}, a complete blood count, and urinary pH, osmolality, creatinine, and electrolytes (Fig. 63-7). The presence of a non–anion gap acidosis suggests a distal, hypokalemic renal tubular acidosis or diarrhea; calculation of the urinary anion gap can help differentiate these two diagnoses. Renal K^+ excretion can be assessed with a 24-h urine collection; a 24-h K^+ excretion of <15 mmol is indicative of an extrarenal cause of hypokalemia (Fig. 63-7). If only a random, spot urine sample is available, serum and urine osmolality can be used to calculate the transtubular K^+ gradient (TTKG), which should be <3 in the presence of hypokalemia (see also "Hyperkalemia"). Alternatively, a urinary K^+-to-creatinine ratio of >13 mmol/g creatinine (>1.5 mmol/mmol creatinine) is compatible with excessive renal K^+ excretion. Urine Cl^- is usually decreased in patients with hypokalemia from a nonreabsorbable anion, such as antibiotics or HCO_3^-. The most common causes of chronic hypokalemic alkalosis are surreptitious vomiting, diuretic abuse, and GS; these can be distinguished by the pattern of urinary electrolytes. Hypokalemic patients with vomiting due to bulimia will thus have a urinary Cl^- <10 mmol/L; urine Na^+, K^+, and Cl^- are persistently elevated in GS, due to loss of function in the thiazide-sensitive Na^+-Cl^- cotransporter, but less elevated in diuretic abuse and with greater variability. Urine diuretic screens for loop diuretics and thiazides may be necessary to further exclude diuretic abuse.

Other tests, such as urinary Ca^{2+}, thyroid function tests, and/or PRA and aldosterone levels, may also be appropriate in specific cases. A plasma aldosterone:PRA ratio of >50, due to suppression of circulating renin and an elevation of circulating aldosterone, is suggestive of hyperaldosteronism. Patients with hyperaldosteronism or apparent mineralocorticoid excess may require further testing, for example adrenal vein sampling (Chap. 406) or the clinically available testing for specific genetic causes (e.g., FH-I, SAME, Liddle's syndrome). Patients with primary aldosteronism should thus be tested for the chimeric FH-I/GRA gene (see above) if they are younger than 20 years of age or have a family history of primary aldosteronism or stroke at a young age (<40 years). Preliminary differentiation of Liddle's syndrome due to mutant ENaC channels from SAME due to mutant 11βHSD-2 (see above), both of which cause hypokalemia and hypertension with aldosterone suppression, can be made on a clinical basis and then confirmed by genetic analysis; patients with Liddle's syndrome should respond to amiloride (ENaC inhibition) but not spironolactone, whereas patients with SAME will respond to spironolactone.

TREATMENT HYPOKALEMIA

The goals of therapy in hypokalemia are to prevent life-threatening and/or serious chronic consequences, to replace the associated K^+ deficit, and to correct the underlying cause and/or mitigate future hypokalemia. The urgency of therapy depends on the severity of hypokalemia, associated clinical factors (e.g., cardiac disease, digoxin therapy), and the rate of decline in serum K^+. Patients with a prolonged QT interval and/or other risk factors for arrhythmia should be monitored by continuous cardiac telemetry during repletion. Urgent but cautious K^+ replacement should be considered in patients with severe redistributive hypokalemia (plasma K^+ concentration <2.5 m*M*) and/or when serious complications ensue; however, this approach has a risk of rebound hyperkalemia following acute resolution of the underlying cause. When excessive activity of the sympathetic nervous system is thought to play a dominant role in redistributive hypokalemia, as in TPP, theophylline overdose, and acute head injury, high-dose propranolol (3 mg/kg) should be considered; this nonspecific b-adrenergic blocker will correct hypokalemia without the risk of rebound hyperkalemia.

Oral replacement with K^+-Cl^- is the mainstay of therapy in hypokalemia. Potassium phosphate, oral or IV, may be appropriate in patients with combined hypokalemia and hypophosphatemia. Potassium bicarbonate or potassium citrate should be considered in patients with concomitant metabolic acidosis. Notably, hypomagnesemic patients are refractory to K^+ replacement alone, such that concomitant Mg^{2+} deficiency should *always* be corrected with oral or intravenous repletion. The deficit of K^+ and the rate of correction should be estimated as accurately as possible; renal function, medications, and comorbid conditions such as diabetes should also be considered, so as to gauge the risk of overcorrection. In the absence of abnormal K^+ redistribution, the total deficit correlates with serum K^+, such that serum K^+ drops by approximately 0.27 m*M* for every 100-mmol reduction in total-body stores; loss of 400–800 mmol of total-body K^+ results in a reduction in serum K^+ by approximately 2.0 m*M*. Notably, given the delay in redistributing potassium into intracellular compartments, this deficit must be replaced gradually over 24-48 h, with frequent monitoring of plasma K^+ concentration to avoid transient overrepletion and transient hyperkalemia.

The use of intravenous administration should be limited to patients unable to use the enteral route or in the setting of severe complications (e.g., paralysis, arrhythmia). Intravenous K^+-Cl^- should always be administered in saline solutions, rather than dextrose, because the dextrose-induced increase in insulin can acutely

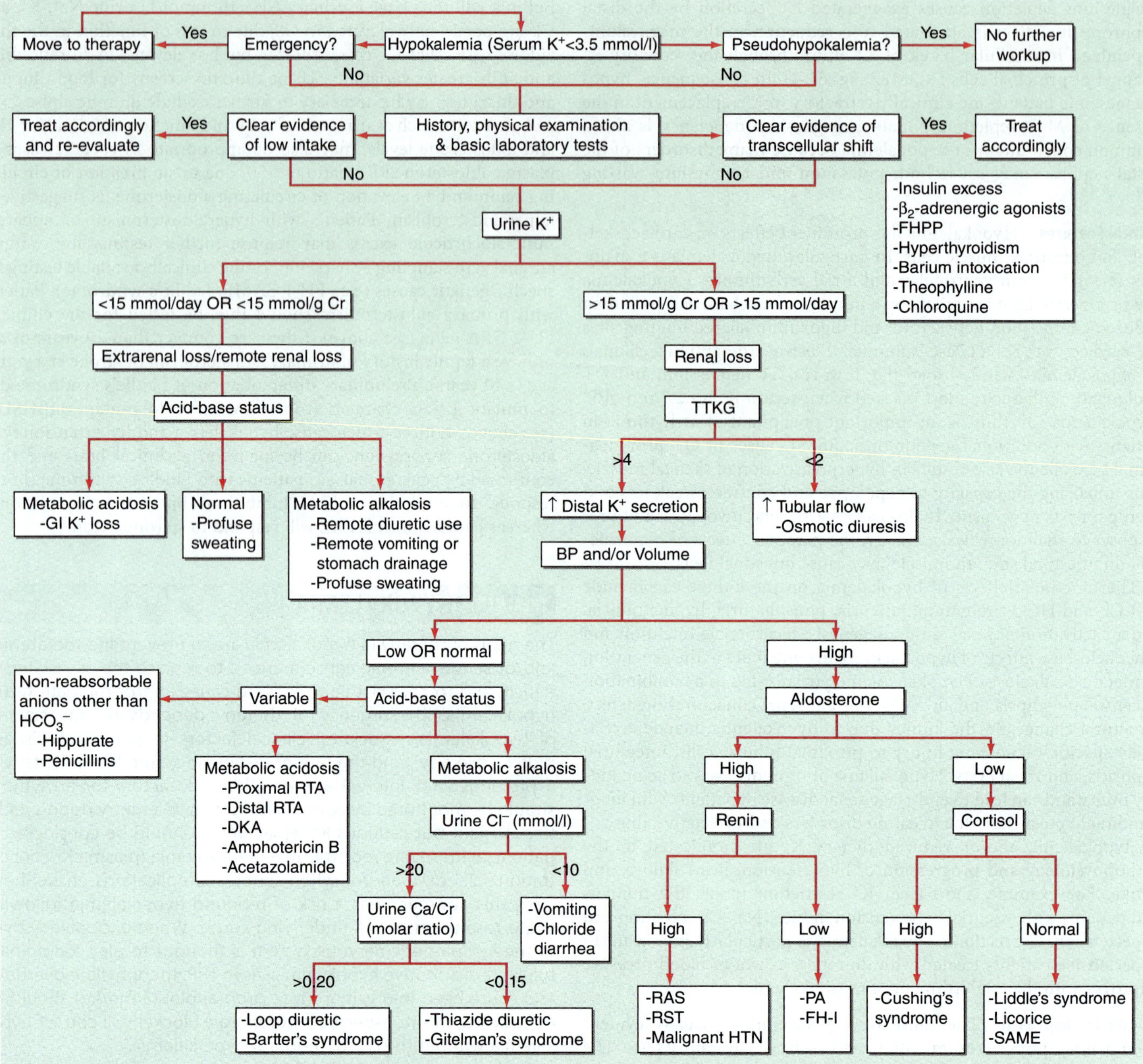

FIGURE 63-7 The diagnostic approach to hypokalemia. See text for details. AME, apparent mineralocorticoid excess; BP, blood pressure; CCD, cortical collecting duct; DKA, diabetic ketoacidosis; FH-I, familial hyperaldosteronism type I; FHPP, familial hypokalemic periodic paralysis; GI, gastrointestinal; GRA, glucocorticoid remediable aldosteronism; HTN, hypertension; PA, primary aldosteronism; RAS, renal artery stenosis; RST, renin-secreting tumor; RTA, renal tubular acidosis; SAME, syndrome of apparent mineralocorticoid excess; TTKG, transtubular potassium gradient. *(Used with permission from DB Mount, K Zandi-Nejad K: Disorders of potassium balance, in Brenner and Rector's The Kidney, 8th ed, BM Brenner [ed]. Philadelphia, W.B. Saunders & Company, 2008, pp 547-587.)*

exacerbate hypokalemia. The peripheral intravenous dose is usually 20–40 mmol of K^+-Cl^- per liter; higher concentrations can cause localized pain from chemical phlebitis, irritation, and sclerosis. If hypokalemia is severe (<2.5 mmol/L) and/or critically symptomatic, intravenous K^+-Cl^- can be administered through a central vein with cardiac monitoring in an intensive care setting, at rates of 10–20 mmol/h; higher rates should be reserved for acutely life-threatening complications. The absolute amount of administered K^+ should be restricted (e.g., 20 mmol in 100 mL of saline solution) to prevent inadvertent infusion of a large dose. Femoral veins are preferable, because infusion through internal jugular or subclavian central lines can acutely increase the local concentration of K^+ and affect cardiac conduction.

Strategies to minimize K^+ losses should also be considered. These measures may include minimizing the dose of non-K^+-sparing diuretics, restricting Na^+ intake, and using clinically appropriate combinations of non-K^+-sparing and K^+-sparing medications (e.g., loop diuretics with angiotensin-converting enzyme inhibitors).

HYPERKALEMIA

Hyperkalemia is defined as a plasma potassium level of 5.5 m*M*, occurring in up to 10% of hospitalized patients; severe hyperkalemia (>6.0 m*M*) occurs in approximately 1%, with a significantly increased risk of mortality. Although redistribution and reduced tissue uptake can acutely cause hyperkalemia, a decrease in renal K^+ excretion is the most frequent underlying cause (Table 63-5). Excessive intake of K^+ is a rare cause, given the adaptive capacity to increase renal secretion; however, dietary intake can have a major effect in susceptible patients, e.g., diabetics with hyporeninemic hypoaldosteronism and chronic kidney disease. Drugs that impact on the renin-angiotensin-aldosterone axis are also a major cause of hyperkalemia.

TABLE 63-5 CAUSES OF HYPERKALEMIA

I. Pseudohyperkalemia
  A. Cellular efflux; thrombocytosis, erythrocytosis, leukocytosis, in vitro hemolysis
  B. Hereditary defects in red cell membrane transport
II. Intra- to extracellular shift
  A. Acidosis
  B. Hyperosmolality; radiocontrast, hypertonic dextrose, mannitol
  C. β_2-Adrenergic antagonists (noncardioselective agents)
  D. Digoxin and related glycosides (yellow oleander, foxglove, bufadienolide)
  E. Hyperkalemic periodic paralysis
  F. Lysine, arginine, and ε-aminocaproic acid (structurally similar, positively charged)
  G. Succinylcholine; thermal trauma, neuromuscular injury, disuse atrophy, mucositis, or prolonged immobilization
  H. Rapid tumor lysis
III. Inadequate excretion
  A. Inhibition of the renin-angiotensin-aldosterone axis; ↑ risk of hyperkalemia when used in combination
    1. Angiotensin-converting enzyme (ACE) inhibitors
    2. Renin inhibitors; aliskiren (in combination with ACE inhibitors or angiotensin receptor blockers [ARBs])
    3. Angiotensin receptor blockers (ARBs)
    4. Blockade of the mineralocorticoid receptor: spironolactone, eplerenone, drospirenone
    5. Blockade of the epithelial sodium channel (ENaC): amiloride, triamterene, trimethoprim, pentamidine, nafamostat
  B. Decreased distal delivery
    1. Congestive heart failure
    2. Volume depletion
  C. Hyporeninemic hypoaldosteronism
    1. Tubulointerstitial diseases: systemic lupus erythematosus (SLE), sickle cell anemia, obstructive uropathy
    2. Diabetes, diabetic nephropathy
    3. Drugs: nonsteroidal anti-inflammatory drugs (NSAIDs), cyclooxygenase 2 (COX2) inhibitors, β-blockers, cyclosporine, tacrolimus
    4. Chronic kidney disease, advanced age
    5. Pseudohypoaldosteronism type II: defects in WNK1 or WNK4 kinases, Kelch-like 3 (KLHL3), or Cullin 3 (CUL3)
  D. Renal resistance to mineralocorticoid
    1. Tubulointerstitial diseases: SLE, amyloidosis, sickle cell anemia, obstructive uropathy, post–acute tubular necrosis
    2. Hereditary: pseudohypoaldosteronism type I; defects in the mineralocorticoid receptor *or* the epithelial sodium channel (ENaC)
  E. Advanced renal insufficiency
    1. Chronic kidney disease
    2. End-stage renal disease
    3. Acute oliguric kidney injury
  F. Primary adrenal insufficiency
    1. Autoimmune: Addison's disease, polyglandular endocrinopathy
    2. Infectious: HIV, cytomegalovirus, tuberculosis, disseminated fungal infection
    3. Infiltrative: amyloidosis, malignancy, metastatic cancer
    4. Drug-associated: heparin, low-molecular-weight heparin
    5. Hereditary: adrenal hypoplasia congenita, congenital lipoid adrenal hyperplasia, aldosterone synthase deficiency
    6. Adrenal hemorrhage or infarction, including in antiphospholipid syndrome

Pseudohyperkalemia Hyperkalemia should be distinguished from factitious hyperkalemia or "pseudohyperkalemia," an artifactual increase in serum K^+ due to the release of K^+ during or after venipuncture. Pseudohyperkalemia can occur in the setting of excessive muscle activity during venipuncture (e.g., fist clenching), a marked increase in cellular elements (thrombocytosis, leukocytosis, and/or erythrocytosis) with in vitro efflux of K^+, and acute anxiety during venipuncture with respiratory alkalosis and redistributive hyperkalemia. Cooling of blood following venipuncture is another cause, due to reduced cellular uptake; the converse is the increased uptake of K^+ by cells at high ambient temperatures, leading to normal values for hyperkalemic patients and/or to spurious hypokalemia in normokalemic patients. Finally, there are multiple genetic subtypes of hereditary pseudohyperkalemia, caused by increases in the passive K^+ permeability of erythrocytes. For example, causative mutations have been described in the red cell anion exchanger (AE1, encoded by the *SLC4A1* gene), leading to reduced red cell anion transport, hemolytic anemia, the acquisition of a novel AE1-mediated K^+ leak, and pseudohyperkalemia.

Redistribution and Hyperkalemia Several different mechanisms can induce an efflux of intracellular K^+ and hyperkalemia. Acidemia is associated with cellular uptake of H^+ and an associated efflux of K^+; it is thought that this effective K^+-H^+ exchange serves to help maintain extracellular pH. Notably, this effect of acidosis is limited to non–anion gap causes of metabolic acidosis and, to a lesser extent, respiratory causes of acidosis; hyperkalemia due to an acidosis-induced shift of potassium from the cells into the ECF does *not* occur in the anion gap acidoses lactic acidosis and ketoacidosis. Hyperkalemia due to hypertonic mannitol, hypertonic saline, and intravenous immune globulin is generally attributed to a "solvent drag" effect, as water moves out of cells along the osmotic gradient. Diabetics are also prone to osmotic hyperkalemia in response to intravenous hypertonic glucose, when given without adequate insulin. Cationic amino acids, specifically lysine, arginine, and the structurally related drug epsilon-aminocaproic acid, cause efflux of K^+ and hyperkalemia, through an effective cation-K^+ exchange of unknown identity and mechanism. Digoxin inhibits Na^+/K^+-ATPase and impairs the uptake of K^+ by skeletal muscle, such that digoxin overdose predictably results in hyperkalemia. Structurally related glycosides are found in specific plants (e.g., yellow oleander, foxglove) and in the cane toad, *Bufo marinus* (bufadienolide); ingestion of these substances and extracts thereof can also cause hyperkalemia. Finally, fluoride ions also inhibit Na^+/K^+-ATPase, such that fluoride poisoning is typically associated with hyperkalemia.

Succinylcholine depolarizes muscle cells, causing an efflux of K^+ through acetylcholine receptors (AChRs). The use of this agent is contraindicated in patients who have sustained thermal trauma, neuromuscular injury, disuse atrophy, mucositis, or prolonged immobilization. These disorders share a marked increase and redistribution of AChRs at the plasma membrane of muscle cells; depolarization of these upregulated AChRs by succinylcholine leads to an exaggerated efflux of K^+ through the receptor-associated cation channels, resulting in acute hyperkalemia.

Hyperkalemia Caused by Excess Intake or Tissue Necrosis Increased intake of even small amounts of K^+ may provoke severe hyperkalemia in patients with predisposing factors; hence, an assessment of dietary intake is crucial. Foods rich in potassium include tomatoes, bananas, and citrus fruits; occult sources of K^+, particularly K^+-containing salt substitutes, may also contribute significantly. Iatrogenic causes include simple overreplacement with K^+-Cl^- or the administration of a potassium-containing medication (e.g., K^+-penicillin) to a susceptible patient. Red cell transfusion is a well-described cause of hyperkalemia, typically in the setting of massive transfusions. Finally, severe tissue necrosis, as in acute tumor lysis syndrome and rhabdomyolysis, will predictably cause hyperkalemia from the release of intracellular K^+.

Hypoaldosteronism and Hyperkalemia Aldosterone release from the adrenal gland may be reduced by hyporeninemic hypoaldosteronism, medications, primary hypoaldosteronism, or isolated deficiency of ACTH (secondary hypoaldosteronism). Primary hypoaldosteronism may be genetic or acquired (Chap. 406) but is commonly caused by autoimmunity, either in Addison's disease or in the context of a polyglandular endocrinopathy. HIV has surpassed tuberculosis as the most important infectious cause of adrenal insufficiency. The adrenal involvement in HIV disease is usually subclinical; however, adrenal insufficiency may be precipitated by stress, drugs such as ketoconazole that inhibit steroidogenesis, or the acute withdrawal of steroid agents such as megestrol.

Hyporeninemic hypoaldosteronism is a very common predisposing factor in several overlapping subsets of hyperkalemic patients: diabetics, the elderly, and patients with renal insufficiency. Classically, patients should have suppressed PRA and aldosterone; approximately 50% have an associated acidosis, with a reduced renal excretion of NH_4^+, a positive urinary anion gap, and urine pH <5.5. Most patients are volume expanded, with secondary increases in circulating atrial natriuretic peptide (ANP) that inhibit both renal renin release and adrenal aldosterone release.

Renal Disease and Hyperkalemia Chronic kidney disease and end-stage kidney disease are very common causes of hyperkalemia, due to the associated deficit or absence of functioning nephrons. Hyperkalemia is more common in oliguric acute kidney injury; distal tubular flow rate and Na^+ delivery are less limiting factors in nonoliguric patients. Hyperkalemia out of proportion to GFR can also be seen in the context of tubulointerstitial disease that affects the distal nephron, such as amyloidosis, sickle cell anemia, interstitial nephritis, and obstructive uropathy.

Hereditary renal causes of hyperkalemia have overlapping clinical features with hypoaldosteronism, hence the diagnostic label *pseudohypoaldosteronism* (PHA). PHA type I (PHA-I) has both an autosomal recessive and an autosomal dominant form. The autosomal dominant form is due to loss-of-function mutations in the MLR; the recessive form is caused by various combinations of mutations in the three subunits of ENaC, resulting in impaired Na^+ channel activity in principal cells and other tissues. Patients with recessive PHA-I suffer from lifelong salt wasting, hypotension, and hyperkalemia, whereas the phenotype of autosomal dominant PHA-I due to MLR dysfunction improves in adulthood. PHA type II (PHA-II; also known as *hereditary hypertension with hyperkalemia*) is in every respect the mirror image of GS caused by loss of function in NCC, the thiazide-sensitive Na^+-Cl^- cotransporter (see above); the clinical phenotype includes hypertension, hyperkalemia, hyperchloremic metabolic acidosis, suppressed PRA and aldosterone, hypercalciuria, and reduced bone density. PHA-II thus behaves like a gain of function in NCC, and treatment with thiazides results in resolution of the entire clinical phenotype. However, the NCC gene is not directly involved in PHA-II, which is caused by mutations in the WNK1 and WNK4 serine-threonine kinases or the upstream Kelch-like 3 (KLHL3) and Cullin 3 (CUL3), two components of an E3 ubiquitin ligase complex that regulates these kinases; these proteins collectively regulate NCC activity, with PHA-II-associated activation of the transporter.

Medication-Associated Hyperkalemia Most medications associated with hyperkalemia cause inhibition of some component of the renin-angiotensin-aldosterone axis. ACE inhibitors, angiotensin receptor blockers, renin inhibitors, and MLRs are predictable and common causes of hyperkalemia, particularly when prescribed in combination. The oral contraceptive agent Yasmin-28 contains the progestin drospirenone, which inhibits the MLR and can cause hyperkalemia in susceptible patients. Cyclosporine, tacrolimus, NSAIDs, and cyclooxygenase 2 (COX2) inhibitors cause hyperkalemia by multiple mechanisms, but share the ability to cause hyporeninemic hypoaldosteronism. Notably, most drugs that affect the renin-angiotensin-aldosterone axis also block the local adrenal response to hyperkalemia, thus attenuating the *direct* stimulation of aldosterone release by increased plasma K^+ concentration.

Inhibition of apical ENaC activity in the distal nephron by amiloride and other K^+-sparing diuretics results in hyperkalemia, often with a voltage-dependent hyperchloremic acidosis and/or hypovolemic hyponatremia. Amiloride is structurally similar to the antibiotics trimethoprim (TMP) and pentamidine, which also block ENaC; risk factors for TMP-associated hyperkalemia include the administered dose, renal insufficiency, and hyporeninemic hypoaldosteronism. Indirect inhibition of ENaC at the plasma membrane is also a cause of drug-associated hyperkalemia; nafamostat, a protease inhibitor used in some countries for the management of pancreatitis, inhibits aldosterone-induced renal proteases that activate ENaC by proteolytic cleavage.

Clinical Features Hyperkalemia is a medical emergency due to its effects on the heart. Cardiac arrhythmias associated with hyperkalemia include sinus bradycardia, sinus arrest, slow idioventricular rhythms, ventricular tachycardia, ventricular fibrillation, and asystole. Mild increases in extracellular K^+ affect the repolarization phase of the cardiac action potential, resulting in changes in T-wave morphology; further increase in plasma K^+ concentration depresses intracardiac conduction, with progressive prolongation of the PR and QRS intervals. Severe hyperkalemia results in loss of the P wave and a progressive widening of the QRS complex; development of a sine-wave sinoventricular rhythm suggests impending ventricular fibrillation or asystole. Hyperkalemia can also cause a type I Brugada pattern in the electrocardiogram (ECG), with a pseudo–right bundle branch block and persistent coved ST segment elevation in at least two precordial leads. This hyperkalemic Brugada's sign occurs in critically ill patients with severe hyperkalemia and can be differentiated from genetic Brugada's syndrome by an absence of P waves, marked QRS widening, and an abnormal QRS axis. Classically, the electrocardiographic manifestations in hyperkalemia progress from tall peaked T waves (5.5–6.5 m*M*), to a loss of P waves (6.5–7.5 m*M*) to a widened QRS complex (7.0–8.0 m*M*), and, ultimately, a to a sine wave pattern (>8.0 m*M*). However, these changes are notoriously insensitive, particularly in patients with chronic kidney disease or end-stage renal disease.

Hyperkalemia from a variety of causes can also present with ascending paralysis, denoted *secondary hyperkalemic paralysis* to differentiate it from familial hyperkalemic periodic paralysis (HYPP). The presentation may include diaphragmatic paralysis and respiratory failure. Patients with familial HYPP develop myopathic weakness during hyperkalemia induced by increased K^+ intake or rest after heavy exercise. Depolarization of skeletal muscle by hyperkalemia unmasks an inactivation defect in skeletal Na^+ channel; autosomal dominant mutations in the *SCN4A* gene encoding this channel are the predominant cause.

Within the kidney, hyperkalemia has negative effects on the ability to excrete an acid load, such that hyperkalemia per se can contribute to metabolic acidosis. This defect appears to be due in part to competition between K^+ and NH_4^+ for reabsorption by the TALH and subsequent countercurrent multiplication, ultimately reducing the medullary gradient for NH_3/NH_4 excretion by the distal nephron. Regardless of the underlying mechanism, restoration of normokalemia can, in many instances, correct hyperkalemic metabolic acidosis.

Diagnostic Approach The first priority in the management of hyperkalemia is to assess the need for emergency treatment, followed by a comprehensive workup to determine the cause (Fig. 63-8). History and physical examination should focus on medications, diet and dietary supplements, risk factors for kidney failure, reduction in urine output, blood pressure, and volume status. Initial laboratory tests should include electrolytes, BUN, creatinine, serum osmolality, Mg^{2+} and Ca^{2+}, a complete blood count, and urinary pH, osmolality, creatinine, and electrolytes. A urine Na^+ concentration of <20 m*M* indicates that distal Na^+ delivery is a limiting factor in K^+ excretion; volume repletion with 0.9% saline or treatment with furosemide may be effective in reducing plasma K^+ concentration. Serum and urine osmolality are required for calculation of the transtubular K^+ gradient (TTKG) (Fig. 63-8). The expected values of the TTKG are largely based on historical data, and are <3 in the presence of hypokalemia and >7–8 in the presence of hyperkalemia.

$$TTKG = \frac{[K^+]_{urine} \times Osm_{serum}}{[K^+]_{serum} \times Osm_{urine}}$$

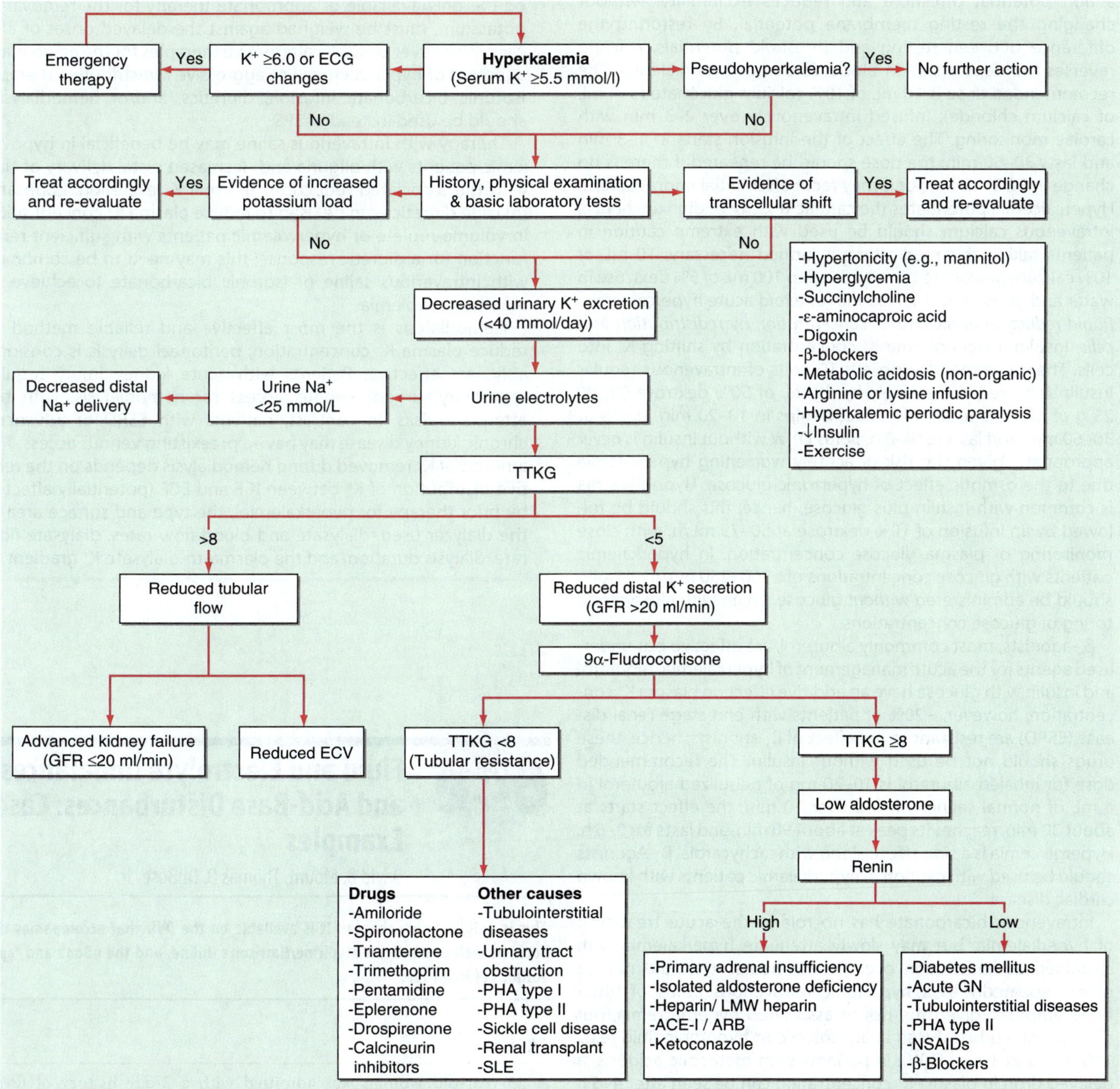

FIGURE 63-8 The diagnostic approach to hyperkalemia. See text for details. ACE-I, angiotensin-converting enzyme inhibitor; ARB, angiotensin II receptor blocker; CCD, cortical collecting duct; ECG, electrocardiogram; ECV, effective circulatory volume; GFR, glomerular filtration rate; GN, glomerulonephritis; HIV, human immunodeficiency virus; LMW heparin, low-molecular-weight heparin; NSAIDs, nonsteroidal anti-inflammatory drugs; PHA, pseudohypoaldosteronism; SLE, systemic lupus erythematosus; TTKG, transtubular potassium gradient. *(Used with permission from DB Mount, K Zandi-Nejad K: Disorders of potassium balance, in Brenner and Rector's The Kidney, 8th ed, BM Brenner [ed]. Philadelphia, W.B. Saunders & Company, 2008, pp 547-587.)*

TREATMENT HYPERKALEMIA

Electrocardiographic manifestations of hyperkalemia should be considered a medical emergency and treated urgently. However, patients with significant hyperkalemia (plasma K^+ concentration ≥6.5 m*M*) in the absence of ECG changes should also be aggressively managed, given the limitations of ECG changes as a predictor of cardiac toxicity. Urgent management of hyperkalemia includes admission to the hospital, continuous cardiac monitoring, and immediate treatment. The treatment of hyperkalemia is divided into three stages:

1. *Immediate antagonism of the cardiac effects of hyperkalemia.* Intravenous calcium serves to protect the heart, whereas other measures are taken to correct hyperkalemia. Calcium raises the action potential threshold and reduces excitability, without changing the resting membrane potential. By restoring the difference between resting and threshold potentials, calcium reverses the depolarization blockade due to hyperkalemia. The recommended dose is 10 mL of 10% calcium gluconate (3–4 mL of calcium chloride), infused intravenously over 2–3 min with cardiac monitoring. The effect of the infusion starts in 1–3 min and lasts 30–60 min; the dose should be repeated if there is no change in ECG findings or if they recur after initial improvement. Hypercalcemia potentiates the cardiac toxicity of digoxin; hence, intravenous calcium should be used with extreme caution in patients taking this medication; if judged necessary, 10 mL of 10% calcium gluconate can be added to 100 mL of 5% dextrose in water and infused over 20–30 min to avoid acute hypercalcemia.
2. *Rapid reduction in plasma K^+ concentration by redistribution into cells.* Insulin lowers plasma K^+ concentration by shifting K^+ into cells. The recommended dose is 10 units of intravenous regular insulin followed immediately by 50 mL of 50% dextrose ($D_{50}W$, 25 g of glucose total); the effect begins in 10–20 min, peaks at 30–60 min, and lasts for 4–6 h. Bolus $D_{50}W$ without insulin is *never* appropriate, given the risk of acutely worsening hyperkalemia due to the osmotic effect of hypertonic glucose. Hypoglycemia is common with insulin plus glucose; hence, this should be followed by an infusion of 10% dextrose at 50–75 mL/h, with close monitoring of plasma glucose concentration. In hyperkalemic patients with glucose concentrations of ≥200–250 mg/dL, insulin should be administered *without* glucose, again with close monitoring of glucose concentrations.

   β_2-agonists, most commonly albuterol, are effective but underused agents for the acute management of hyperkalemia. Albuterol and insulin with glucose have an additive effect on plasma K^+ concentration; however, ~20% of patients with end-stage renal disease (ESRD) are resistant to the effect of β_2-agonists; hence, these drugs should not be used without insulin. The recommended dose for inhaled albuterol is 10–20 mg of nebulized albuterol in 4 mL of normal saline, inhaled over 10 min; the effect starts at about 30 min, reaches its peak at about 90 min, and lasts for 2–6 h. Hyperglycemia is a side effect, along with tachycardia. β_2-Agonists should be used with caution in hyperkalemic patients with known cardiac disease.

   Intravenous bicarbonate has no role in the acute treatment of hyperkalemia, but may slowly attenuate hyperkalemia with sustained administration over several hours. It should not be given repeatedly as a hypertonic intravenous bolus of undiluted ampules, given the risk of associated hypernatremia, but should instead be infused in an isotonic or hypotonic fluid (e.g., 150 mEqu in 1 L of D_5W). In patients with metabolic acidosis, a delayed drop in plasma K^+ concentration can be seen after 4–6 h of isotonic bicarbonate infusion.
3. *Removal of potassium.* This is typically accomplished using cation exchange resins, diuretics, and/or dialysis. The cation exchange resin sodium polystyrene sulfonate (SPS) exchanges Na^+ for K^+ in the gastrointestinal tract and increases the fecal excretion of K^+; alternative calcium-based resins, when available, may be more appropriate in patients with an increased ECFV. The recommended dose of SPS is 15–30 g of powder, almost always given in a premade suspension with 33% sorbitol. The effect of SPS on plasma K^+ concentration is slow; the full effect may take up to 24 h and usually requires repeated doses every 4–6 h. Intestinal necrosis, typically of the colon or ileum, is a rare but usually fatal complication of SPS. Intestinal necrosis is more common in patients administered SPS via enema and/or in patients with reduced intestinal motility (e.g., in the postoperative state or after treatment with opioids). The coadministration of SPS with sorbitol appears to increase the risk of intestinal necrosis; however, this complication can also occur with SPS alone. If SPS without sorbitol is not available, clinicians must consider whether treatment with SPS in sorbitol is absolutely necessary. The low but real risk of intestinal necrosis with SPS, which can sometimes be the only available or appropriate therapy for the removal of potassium, must be weighed against the delayed onset of efficacy. Whenever possible, alternative therapies for the acute management of hyperkalemia (i.e., aggressive redistributive therapy, isotonic bicarbonate infusion, diuretics, and/or hemodialysis) should be used instead of SPS.

   Therapy with intravenous saline may be beneficial in hypovolemic patients with oliguria and decreased distal delivery of Na^+, with the associated reductions in renal K^+ excretion. Loop and thiazide diuretics can be used to reduce plasma K^+ concentration in volume-replete or hypervolemic patients with sufficient renal function for a diuretic response; this may need to be combined with intravenous saline or isotonic bicarbonate to achieve or maintain euvolemia.

   Hemodialysis is the most effective and reliable method to reduce plasma K^+ concentration; peritoneal dialysis is considerably less effective. Patients with acute kidney injury require temporary, urgent venous access for hemodialysis, with the attendant risks; in contrast, patients with ESRD or advanced chronic kidney disease may have a preexisting venous access. The amount of K^+ removed during hemodialysis depends on the relative distribution of K^+ between ICF and ECF (potentially affected by prior therapy for hyperkalemia), the type and surface area of the dialyzer used, dialysate and blood flow rates, dialysate flow rate, dialysis duration, and the plasma-to-dialysate K^+ gradient.

64e Fluid and Electrolyte Imbalances and Acid-Base Disturbances: Case Examples

David B. Mount, Thomas D. DuBose, Jr.

This is a digital-only chapter. It is available on the DVD that accompanies this book, as well as on Access Medicine/Harrison's Online, and the eBook and "app" editions of HPIM 19e.

CASE 1

A 23-year-old woman was admitted with a 3-day history of fever, cough productive of blood-tinged sputum, confusion, and orthostasis. Past medical history included type 1 diabetes mellitus. A physical examination in the emergency department indicated postural hypotension, tachycardia, and Kussmaul respiration. The breath was noted to smell of "acetone." Examination of the thorax suggested consolidation in the right lower lobe.

65 Hypercalcemia and Hypocalcemia

Sundeep Khosla

The calcium ion plays a critical role in normal cellular function and signaling, regulating diverse physiologic processes such as neuromuscular signaling, cardiac contractility, hormone secretion, and blood coagulation. Thus, extracellular calcium concentrations are maintained within an exquisitely narrow range through a series of feedback mechanisms that involve parathyroid hormone (PTH) and the active vitamin D metabolite 1,25-dihydroxyvitmin D [$1,25(OH)_2D$]. These feedback mechanisms are orchestrated by integrating signals between the parathyroid glands, kidney, intestine, and bone (Fig. 65-1; Chap. 423). Disorders of serum calcium concentration are relatively common and often serve as a harbinger of underlying disease. This chapter provides a brief summary of the approach to patients with altered serum calcium levels. See Chap. 424 for a detailed discussion of this topic.

HYPERCALCEMIA

ETIOLOGY

The causes of hypercalcemia can be understood and classified based on derangements in the normal feedback mechanisms that regulate serum calcium (Table 65-1). Excess PTH production, which is not appropriately suppressed by increased serum calcium concentrations, occurs in primary neoplastic disorders of the parathyroid glands (parathyroid adenomas; hyperplasia; or, rarely, carcinoma) that are associated with

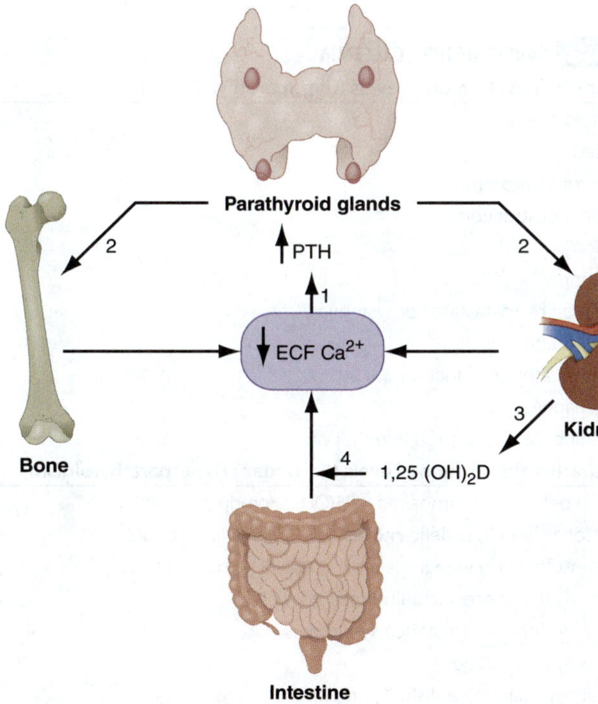

FIGURE 65-1 Feedback mechanisms maintaining extracellular calcium concentrations within a narrow, physiologic range (8.9–10.1 mg/dL [2.2–2.5 m*M*]). A decrease in extracellular (ECF) calcium (Ca^{2+}) triggers an increase in parathyroid hormone (PTH) secretion (1) via the calcium sensor receptor on parathyroid cells. PTH, in turn, results in increased tubular reabsorption of calcium by the kidney (2) and resorption of calcium from bone (2) and also stimulates renal $1,25(OH)_2D$ production (3). $1,25(OH)_2D$, in turn, acts principally on the intestine to increase calcium absorption (4). Collectively, these homeostatic mechanisms serve to restore serum calcium levels to normal.

TABLE 65-1 CAUSES OF HYPERCALCEMIA

Excessive PTH production
Primary hyperparathyroidism (adenoma, hyperplasia, rarely carcinoma)
Tertiary hyperparathyroidism (long-term stimulation of PTH secretion in renal insufficiency)
Ectopic PTH secretion (very rare)
Inactivating mutations in the CaSR or in G proteins (FHH)
Alterations in CaSR function (lithium therapy)
Hypercalcemia of malignancy
Overproduction of PTHrP (many solid tumors)
Lytic skeletal metastases (breast, myeloma)
Excessive $1,25(OH)_2D$ production
Granulomatous diseases (sarcoidosis, tuberculosis, silicosis)
Lymphomas
Vitamin D intoxication
Primary increase in bone resorption
Hyperthyroidism
Immobilization
Excessive calcium intake
Milk-alkali syndrome
Total parenteral nutrition
Other causes
Endocrine disorders (adrenal insufficiency, pheochromocytoma, VIPoma)
Medications (thiazides, vitamin A, antiestrogens)

Abbreviations: CaSR, calcium sensor receptor; FHH, familial hypocalciuric hypercalcemia; PTH, parathyroid hormone; PTHrP, PTH-related peptide.

increased parathyroid cell mass and impaired feedback inhibition by calcium. Inappropriate PTH secretion for the ambient level of serum calcium also occurs with heterozygous inactivating calcium sensor receptor (CaSR) or G protein mutations, which impair extracellular calcium sensing by the parathyroid glands and the kidneys, resulting in familial hypocalciuric hypercalcemia (FHH). Although PTH secretion by tumors is extremely rare, many solid tumors produce PTH-related peptide (PTHrP), which shares homology with PTH in the first 13 amino acids and binds the PTH receptor, thus mimicking effects of PTH on bone and the kidney. In PTHrP-mediated hypercalcemia of malignancy, PTH levels are suppressed by the high serum calcium levels. Hypercalcemia associated with granulomatous disease (e.g., sarcoidosis) or lymphomas is caused by enhanced conversion of 25(OH) D to the potent $1,25(OH)_2D$. In these disorders, $1,25(OH)_2D$ enhances intestinal calcium absorption, resulting in hypercalcemia and suppressed PTH. Disorders that directly increase calcium mobilization from bone, such as hyperthyroidism or osteolytic metastases, also lead to hypercalcemia with suppressed PTH secretion as does exogenous calcium overload, as in milk-alkali syndrome, or total parenteral nutrition with excessive calcium supplementation.

CLINICAL MANIFESTATIONS

Mild hypercalcemia (up to 11–11.5 mg/dL) is usually asymptomatic and recognized only on routine calcium measurements. Some patients may complain of vague neuropsychiatric symptoms, including trouble concentrating, personality changes, or depression. Other presenting symptoms may include peptic ulcer disease or nephrolithiasis, and fracture risk may be increased. More severe hypercalcemia (>12–13 mg/dL), particularly if it develops acutely, may result in lethargy, stupor, or coma, as well as gastrointestinal symptoms (nausea, anorexia, constipation, or pancreatitis). Hypercalcemia decreases renal concentrating ability, which may cause polyuria and polydipsia. With longstanding hyperparathyroidism, patients may present with bone pain or pathologic fractures. Finally, hypercalcemia can result in significant electrocardiographic changes, including bradycardia, AV block, and short QT interval; changes in serum calcium can be monitored by following the QT interval.

DIAGNOSTIC APPROACH

The first step in the diagnostic evaluation of hyper- or hypocalcemia is to ensure that the alteration in serum calcium levels is not due to abnormal albumin concentrations. About 50% of total calcium is ionized, and the rest is bound principally to albumin. Although direct measurements of ionized calcium are possible, they are easily influenced by collection methods and other artifacts; thus, it is generally preferable to measure total calcium and albumin to "correct" the serum calcium. When serum albumin concentrations are reduced, a corrected calcium concentration is calculated by adding 0.2 m*M* (0.8 mg/dL) to the total calcium level for every decrement in serum albumin of 1.0 g/dL below the reference value of 4.1 g/dL for albumin, and, conversely, for elevations in serum albumin.

A detailed history may provide important clues regarding the etiology of the hypercalcemia (Table 65-1). Chronic hypercalcemia is most commonly caused by primary hyperparathyroidism, as opposed to the second most common etiology of hypercalcemia, an underlying malignancy. The history should include medication use, previous neck surgery, and systemic symptoms suggestive of sarcoidosis or lymphoma.

Once true hypercalcemia is established, the second most important laboratory test in the diagnostic evaluation is a PTH level using a two-site assay for the intact hormone. Increases in PTH are often accompanied by hypophosphatemia. In addition, serum creatinine should be measured to assess renal function; hypercalcemia may impair renal function, and renal clearance of PTH may be altered depending on the fragments detected by the assay. If the PTH level is increased (or "inappropriately normal") in the setting of elevated calcium and low phosphorus, the diagnosis is almost always primary hyperparathyroidism. Because individuals with FHH may also present with mildly elevated PTH levels and hypercalcemia, this diagnosis should be considered and excluded because parathyroid surgery is ineffective in this condition. A calcium/creatinine clearance ratio (calculated as urine calcium/serum calcium divided by urine creatinine/serum creatinine) of <0.01 is suggestive of FHH, particularly when there is a family history of mild, asymptomatic hypercalcemia. In addition, sequence analysis of the CaSR gene is now commonly performed for the definitive diagnosis of FHH, although in some families, FHH may be caused by mutations in G proteins that mediate signaling by the CaSR. Ectopic PTH secretion is extremely rare.

A suppressed PTH level in the face of hypercalcemia is consistent with non-parathyroid-mediated hypercalcemia, most often due to underlying malignancy. Although a tumor that causes hypercalcemia is generally overt, a PTHrP level may be needed to establish the diagnosis of hypercalcemia of malignancy. Serum $1,25(OH)_2D$ levels are increased in granulomatous disorders, and clinical evaluation in combination with laboratory testing will generally provide a diagnosis for the various disorders listed in Table 65-1.

TREATMENT HYPERCALCEMIA

Mild, asymptomatic hypercalcemia does not require immediate therapy, and management should be dictated by the underlying diagnosis. By contrast, significant, symptomatic hypercalcemia usually requires therapeutic intervention independent of the etiology of hypercalcemia. Initial therapy of significant hypercalcemia begins with volume expansion because hypercalcemia invariably leads to dehydration; 4–6 L of intravenous saline may be required over the first 24 h, keeping in mind that underlying comorbidities (e.g., congestive heart failure) may require the use of loop diuretics to enhance sodium and calcium excretion. However, loop diuretics should not be initiated until the volume status has been restored to normal. If there is increased calcium mobilization from bone (as in malignancy or severe hyperparathyroidism), drugs that inhibit bone resorption should be considered. Zoledronic acid (e.g., 4 mg intravenously over ~30 min), pamidronate (e.g., 60–90 mg intravenously over 2–4 h), and ibandronate (2 mg intravenously over 2 h) are bisphosphonates that are commonly used for the treatment of hypercalcemia of malignancy in adults. Onset of action is within 1–3 days, with normalization of serum calcium levels occurring in 60–90% of patients. Bisphosphonate infusions may need to be repeated if hypercalcemia relapses. An alternative to the bisphosphonates is gallium nitrate (200 mg/m² intravenously daily for 5 days), which is also effective, but has potential nephrotoxicity. In rare instances, dialysis may be necessary. Finally, although intravenous phosphate chelates calcium and decreases serum calcium levels, this therapy can be toxic because calcium-phosphate complexes may deposit in tissues and cause extensive organ damage.

In patients with $1,25(OH)_2D$-mediated hypercalcemia, glucocorticoids are the preferred therapy, as they decrease $1,25(OH)_2D$ production. Intravenous hydrocortisone (100–300 mg daily) or oral prednisone (40–60 mg daily) for 3–7 days is used most often. Other drugs, such as ketoconazole, chloroquine, and hydroxychloroquine, may also decrease $1,25(OH)_2D$ production and are used occasionally.

HYPOCALCEMIA

ETIOLOGY

The causes of hypocalcemia can be differentiated according to whether serum PTH levels are low (hypoparathyroidism) or high (secondary hyperparathyroidism). Although there are many potential causes of hypocalcemia, impaired PTH production and impaired vitamin D production are the most common etiologies (Table 65-2) (Chap. 424). Because PTH is the main defense against hypocalcemia, disorders associated with deficient PTH production or secretion may be associated with profound, life-threatening hypocalcemia. In adults, hypoparathyroidism most commonly results from inadvertent damage to all four glands during thyroid or parathyroid gland surgery. Hypoparathyroidism is a cardinal feature of autoimmune endocrinopathies (Chap. 408); rarely, it

TABLE 65-2 CAUSES OF HYPOCALCEMIA

Low Parathyroid Hormone Levels (Hypoparathyroidism)
Parathyroid agenesis
Isolated
DiGeorge's syndrome
Parathyroid destruction
Surgical
Radiation
Infiltration by metastases or systemic diseases
Autoimmune
Reduced parathyroid function
Hypomagnesemia
Activating CaSR or G protein mutations
High Parathyroid Hormone Levels (Secondary Hyperparathyroidism)
Vitamin D deficiency or impaired $1,25(OH)_2D$ production/action
Nutritional vitamin D deficiency (poor intake or absorption)
Renal insufficiency with impaired $1,25(OH)_2D$ production
Vitamin D resistance, including receptor defects
Parathyroid hormone resistance syndromes
PTH receptor mutations
Pseudohypoparathyroidism (G protein mutations)
Drugs
Calcium chelators
Inhibitors of bone resorption (bisphosphonates, plicamycin)
Altered vitamin D metabolism (phenytoin, ketoconazole)
Miscellaneous causes
Acute pancreatitis
Acute rhabdomyolysis
Hungry bone syndrome after parathyroidectomy
Osteoblastic metastases with marked stimulation of bone formation (prostate cancer)

Abbreviations: CaSR, calcium sensor receptor; PTH, parathyroid hormone.

may be associated with infiltrative diseases such as sarcoidosis. Impaired PTH secretion may be secondary to magnesium deficiency or to activating mutations in the CaSR or in the G proteins that mediate CaSR signaling, which suppress PTH, leading to effects that are opposite to those that occur in FHH.

Vitamin D deficiency, impaired 1,25(OH)$_2$D production (primarily secondary to renal insufficiency), or vitamin D resistance also cause hypocalcemia. However, the degree of hypocalcemia in these disorders is generally not as severe as that seen with hypoparathyroidism because the parathyroids are capable of mounting a compensatory increase in PTH secretion. Hypocalcemia may also occur in conditions associated with severe tissue injury such as burns, rhabdomyolysis, tumor lysis, or pancreatitis. The cause of hypocalcemia in these settings may include a combination of low albumin, hyperphosphatemia, tissue deposition of calcium, and impaired PTH secretion.

CLINICAL MANIFESTATIONS

Patients with hypocalcemia may be asymptomatic if the decreases in serum calcium are relatively mild and chronic, or they may present with life-threatening complications. Moderate to severe hypocalcemia is associated with paresthesias, usually of the fingers, toes, and circumoral regions, and is caused by increased neuromuscular irritability. On physical examination, a Chvostek's sign (twitching of the circumoral muscles in response to gentle tapping of the facial nerve just anterior to the ear) may be elicited, although it is also present in ~10% of normal individuals. Carpal spasm may be induced by inflation of a blood pressure cuff to 20 mmHg above the patient's systolic blood pressure for 3 min (Trousseau's sign). Severe hypocalcemia can induce seizures, carpopedal spasm, bronchospasm, laryngospasm, and prolongation of the QT interval.

DIAGNOSTIC APPROACH

In addition to measuring serum calcium, it is useful to determine albumin, phosphorus, and magnesium levels. As for the evaluation of hypercalcemia, determining the PTH level is central to the evaluation of hypocalcemia. A suppressed (or "inappropriately low") PTH level in the setting of hypocalcemia establishes absent or reduced PTH secretion (hypoparathyroidism) as the cause of the hypocalcemia. Further history will often elicit the underlying cause (i.e., parathyroid agenesis vs. destruction). By contrast, an elevated PTH level (secondary hyperparathyroidism) should direct attention to the vitamin D axis as the cause of the hypocalcemia. Nutritional vitamin D deficiency is best assessed by obtaining serum 25-hydroxyvitamin D levels, which reflect vitamin D stores. In the setting of renal insufficiency or suspected vitamin D resistance, serum 1,25(OH)$_2$D levels are informative.

TREATMENT HYPOCALCEMIA

The approach to treatment depends on the severity of the hypocalcemia, the rapidity with which it develops, and the accompanying complications (e.g., seizures, laryngospasm). Acute, symptomatic hypocalcemia is initially managed with calcium gluconate, 10 mL 10% wt/vol (90 mg or 2.2 mmol) intravenously, diluted in 50 mL of 5% dextrose or 0.9% sodium chloride, given intravenously over 5 min. Continuing hypocalcemia often requires a constant intravenous infusion (typically 10 ampules of calcium gluconate or 900 mg of calcium in 1 L of 5% dextrose or 0.9% sodium chloride administered over 24 h). Accompanying hypomagnesemia, if present, should be treated with appropriate magnesium supplementation.

Chronic hypocalcemia due to hypoparathyroidism is treated with calcium supplements (1000–1500 mg/d elemental calcium in divided doses) and either vitamin D_2 or D_3 (25,000–100,000 U daily) or calcitriol [1,25(OH)$_2$D, 0.25–2 μg/d]. Other vitamin D metabolites (dihydrotachysterol, alfacalcidiol) are now used less frequently. Vitamin D deficiency, however, is best treated using vitamin D supplementation, with the dose depending on the severity of the deficit and the underlying cause. Thus, nutritional vitamin D deficiency generally responds to relatively low doses of vitamin D (50,000 U, 2–3 times per week for several months), whereas vitamin D deficiency due to malabsorption may require much higher doses (100,000 U/d or more). The treatment goal is to bring serum calcium into the low normal range and to avoid hypercalciuria, which may lead to nephrolithiasis.

GLOBAL CONSIDERATIONS

In countries with more limited access to health care or screening laboratory testing of serum calcium levels, primary hyperparathyroidism often presents in its severe form with skeletal complications (osteitis fibrosa cystica) in contrast to the asymptomatic form that is common in developed countries. In addition, vitamin D deficiency is paradoxically common in some countries despite extensive sunlight (e.g., India) due to avoidance of sun exposure and poor dietary vitamin D intake.

66 Acidosis and Alkalosis

Thomas D. DuBose, Jr.

NORMAL ACID-BASE HOMEOSTASIS

Systemic arterial pH is maintained between 7.35 and 7.45 by extracellular and intracellular chemical buffering together with respiratory and renal regulatory mechanisms. The control of arterial CO_2 tension (Pa$_{CO_2}$) by the central nervous system (CNS) and respiratory system and the control of plasma bicarbonate by the kidneys stabilize the arterial pH by excretion or retention of acid or alkali. The metabolic and respiratory components that regulate systemic pH are described by the Henderson-Hasselbalch equation:

$$P^H = 6.1 + \log \frac{HCO_3^-}{Pa_{co_2} \times 0.0301}$$

Under most circumstances, CO_2 production and excretion are matched, and the usual steady-state Pa$_{CO_2}$ is maintained at 40 mmHg. Underexcretion of CO_2 produces hypercapnia, and overexcretion causes hypocapnia. Nevertheless, production and excretion are again matched at a new steady-state Pa$_{CO_2}$. Therefore, the Pa$_{CO_2}$ is regulated primarily by neural respiratory factors and is not subject to regulation by the rate of CO_2 production. Hypercapnia is usually the result of hypoventilation rather than of increased CO_2 production. Increases or decreases in Pa$_{CO_2}$ represent derangements of neural respiratory control or are due to compensatory changes in response to a primary alteration in the plasma [HCO_3^-].

DIAGNOSIS OF GENERAL TYPES OF DISTURBANCES

The most common clinical disturbances are simple acid-base disorders; i.e., metabolic acidosis or alkalosis or respiratory acidosis or alkalosis.

SIMPLE ACID-BASE DISORDERS

Primary respiratory disturbances (primary changes in Pa$_{CO_2}$) invoke compensatory metabolic responses (secondary changes in [HCO_3^-]), and primary metabolic disturbances elicit predictable compensatory respiratory responses (secondary changes in Pa$_{CO_2}$). Physiologic compensation can be predicted from the relationships displayed in Table 66-1. In general, with one exception, compensatory responses return the pH toward, but not to, the normal value. Chronic respiratory alkalosis when prolonged is an exception to this rule and often returns the pH to a normal value. Metabolic acidosis due to an increase in endogenous acids (e.g., ketoacidosis) lowers extracellular fluid [HCO_3^-] and decreases extracellular pH. This stimulates the medullary chemoreceptors to increase ventilation and to return

TABLE 66-1 PREDICTION OF COMPENSATORY RESPONSES ON SIMPLE ACID-BASE DISTURBANCES AND PATTERN OF CHANGES

Disorder	Prediction of Compensation	Range of Values: pH	HCO_3^-	$Paco_2$
Metabolic acidosis	$Paco_2 = (1.5 \times HCO_3^-) + 8 \pm 2$	Low	Low	Low
	or			
	$Paco_2$ will ↓ 1.25 mmHg per mmol/L ↓ in $[HCO_3^-]$			
	or			
	$Paco_2 = [HCO_3^-] + 15$			
Metabolic alkalosis	$Paco_2$ will ↑ 0.75 mmHg per mmol/L ↑ in $[HCO_3^-]$	High	High	High
	or			
	$Paco_2$ will ↑ 6 mmHg per 10 mmol/L ↑ in $[HCO_3^-]$			
	or			
	$Paco_2 = [HCO_3^-] + 15$			
Respiratory alkalosis		High	Low	Low
Acute	$[HCO_3^-]$ will ↓ 0.2 mmol/L per mmHg ↓ in $Paco_2$			
Chronic	$[HCO_3^-]$ will ↓ 0.4 mmol/L per mmHg ↓ in $Paco_2$			
Respiratory acidosis		Low	High	High
Acute	$[HCO_3^-]$ will ↑ 0.1 mmol/L per mmHg ↑ in $Paco_2$			
Chronic	$[HCO_3^-]$ will ↑ 0.4 mmol/L per mmHg ↑ in $Paco_2$			

the ratio of $[HCO_3^-]$ to $Paco_2$, and thus pH, toward, but not to, normal. The degree of respiratory compensation expected in a simple form of metabolic acidosis can be predicted from the relationship: $Paco_2 = (1.5 \times [HCO_3^-]) + 8 \pm 2$. Thus, a patient with metabolic acidosis and $[HCO_3^-]$ of 12 mmol/L would be expected to have a $Paco_2$ between 24 and 28 mmHg. Values for $Paco_2$ <24 or >28 mmHg define a mixed disturbance (metabolic acidosis and respiratory alkalosis or metabolic alkalosis and respiratory acidosis, respectively). Compensatory responses for primary metabolic disorders move the $Paco_2$ in the same direction as the change in $[HCO_3^-]$, whereas, conversely, compensation for primary respiratory disorders moves the $[HCO_3^-]$ in the same direction as the primary change in $Paco_2$ (Table 66-1). Therefore, changes in $Paco_2$ and $[HCO_3^-]$ in **opposite directions** (i.e., $Paco_2$ or $[HCO_3^-]$ is increased, whereas the other value is decreased) indicate a **mixed disturbance**. Another way to judge the appropriateness of the response in $[HCO_3^-]$ or $Paco_2$ is to use an acid-base nomogram (Fig. 66-1). While the shaded areas of the nomogram show the 95% confidence limits for normal compensation in simple disturbances, finding acid-base values within the shaded area does not necessarily rule out a mixed disturbance. Imposition of one disorder over another may result in values lying within the area of a third. Thus, the nomogram, while convenient, is not a substitute for the equations in Table 66-1.

MIXED ACID-BASE DISORDERS

Mixed acid-base disorders—defined as independently coexisting disorders, not merely compensatory responses—are often seen in patients in critical care units and can lead to dangerous extremes of pH (Table 66-2). A patient with diabetic ketoacidosis (metabolic acidosis) may develop an independent respiratory problem (e.g.,

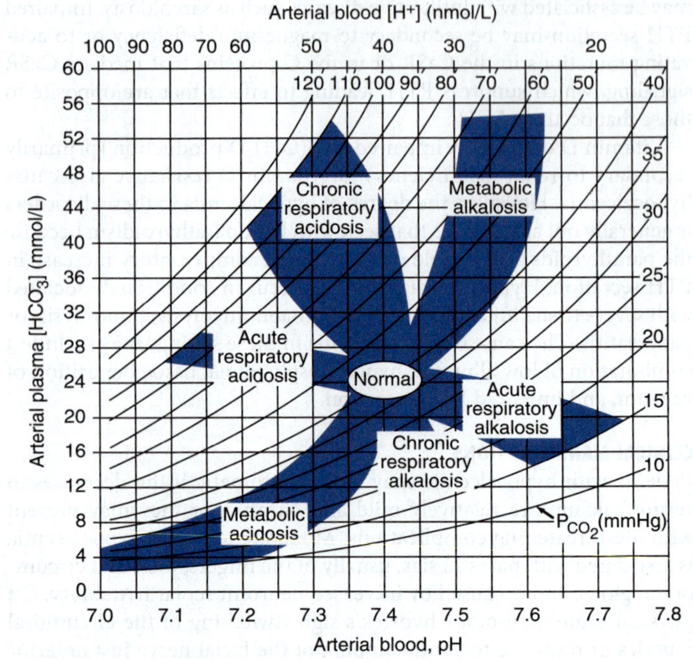

FIGURE 66-1 Acid-base nomogram. Shown are the 90% confidence limits (range of values) of the normal respiratory and metabolic compensations for primary acid-base disturbances. *(From TD DuBose Jr: Acid-base disorders, in Brenner and Rector's The Kidney, 8th ed, BM Brenner [ed]. Philadelphia, Saunders, 2008, pp 505–546, with permission.)*

TABLE 66-2 EXAMPLES OF MIXED ACID-BASE DISORDERS

Mixed Metabolic and Respiratory

Metabolic acidosis—respiratory alkalosis

- Key: High- or normal-AG metabolic acidosis; prevailing $Paco_2$ *below* predicted value (Table 66-1)
- Example: Na^+, 140; K^+, 4.0; Cl^-, 106; HCO_3^-, 14; AG, 20; $Paco_2$, 24; pH, 7.39 (lactic acidosis, sepsis in ICU)

Metabolic acidosis—respiratory acidosis

- Key: High- or normal-AG metabolic acidosis; prevailing $Paco_2$ *above* predicted value (Table 66-1)
- Example: Na^+, 140; K^+, 4.0; Cl^-, 102; HCO_3^-, 18; AG, 20; $Paco_2$, 38; pH, 7.30 (severe pneumonia, pulmonary edema)

Metabolic alkalosis—respiratory alkalosis

- Key: $Paco_2$ does not increase as predicted; pH higher than expected
- Example: Na^+, 140; K^+, 4.0; Cl^-, 91; HCO_3^-, 33; AG, 16; $Paco_2$, 38; pH, 7.55 (liver disease and diuretics)

Metabolic alkalosis—respiratory acidosis

- Key: $Paco_2$ higher than predicted; pH normal
- Example: Na^+, 140; K^+, 3.5; Cl^-, 88; HCO_3^-, 42; AG, 10; $Paco_2$, 67; pH, 7.42 (COPD on diuretics)

Mixed Metabolic Disorders

Metabolic acidosis—metabolic alkalosis

- Key: Only detectable with high-AG acidosis; $\Delta AG >> \Delta HCO_3^-$
- Example: Na^+, 140; K^+, 3.0; Cl^-, 95; HCO_3^-, 25; AG, 20; $Paco_2$, 40; pH, 7.42 (uremia with vomiting)

Metabolic acidosis—metabolic acidosis

- Key: Mixed high-AG—normal-AG acidosis; ΔHCO_3^- accounted for by combined change in ΔAG and ΔCl^-
- Example: Na^+, 135; K^+, 3.0; Cl^-, 110; HCO_3^-, 10; AG, 15; $Paco_2$, 25; pH, 7.20 (diarrhea and lactic acidosis, toluene toxicity, treatment of diabetic ketoacidosis)

Abbreviations: AG, anion gap; COPD, chronic obstructive pulmonary disease; ICU, intensive care unit.

pneumonia) leading to respiratory acidosis or alkalosis. Patients with underlying pulmonary disease (e.g., chronic obstructive pulmonary disease) may not respond to metabolic acidosis with an appropriate ventilatory response because of insufficient respiratory reserve. Such imposition of respiratory acidosis on metabolic acidosis can lead to severe acidemia. When metabolic acidosis and metabolic alkalosis coexist in the same patient, the pH may be normal or near normal. When the pH is normal, an elevated anion gap (AG; see below) reliably denotes the presence of an AG metabolic acidosis at a normal serum albumin of 4.5 g/dL. Assuming a normal AG of 10 mmol/L, a discrepancy in the ΔAG (prevailing minus normal AG) and the ΔHCO_3^- (normal value of 25 mmol/L minus abnormal HCO_3^- in the patient) indicates the presence of a mixed high-gap acidosis—metabolic alkalosis (see example below). A diabetic patient with ketoacidosis may have renal dysfunction resulting in simultaneous metabolic acidosis. Patients who have ingested an overdose of drug combinations such as sedatives and salicylates may have mixed disturbances as a result of the acid-base response to the individual drugs (metabolic acidosis mixed with respiratory acidosis or respiratory alkalosis, respectively). Triple acid-base disturbances are more complex. For example, patients with metabolic acidosis due to alcoholic ketoacidosis may develop metabolic alkalosis due to vomiting and superimposed respiratory alkalosis due to the hyperventilation of hepatic dysfunction or alcohol withdrawal.

APPROACH TO THE PATIENT: Acid-Base Disorders

A stepwise approach to the diagnosis of acid-base disorders follows (Table 66-3). Care should be taken when measuring blood gases to obtain the arterial blood sample without using excessive heparin. Blood for electrolytes and arterial blood gases should be drawn simultaneously prior to therapy, because an increase in $[HCO_3^-]$ occurs with metabolic alkalosis and respiratory acidosis. Conversely, a decrease in $[HCO_3^-]$ occurs in metabolic acidosis and respiratory alkalosis. In the determination of arterial blood gases by the clinical laboratory, both pH and $Paco_2$ are measured, and the $[HCO_3^-]$ is calculated from the Henderson-Hasselbalch equation. This calculated value should be compared with the measured $[HCO_3^-]$ (total CO_2) on the electrolyte panel. These two values should agree within 2 mmol/L. If they do not, the values may not have been drawn simultaneously, a laboratory error may be present, or an error could have been made in calculating the $[HCO_3^-]$. After verifying the blood acid-base values, the precise acid-base disorder can then be identified.

CALCULATE THE ANION GAP

All evaluations of acid-base disorders should include a simple calculation of the AG; it represents those unmeasured anions in plasma (normally 8–10 mmol/L) and is calculated as follows: $AG = Na^+ - (Cl^- + HCO_3^-)$. The unmeasured anions include anionic proteins (e.g., albumin), phosphate, sulfate, and organic anions. When acid anions, such as acetoacetate and lactate, accumulate in extracellular fluid, the AG increases, causing a high-AG acidosis. An increase in the AG is most often due to an increase in unmeasured anions and, less commonly, is due to a decrease in unmeasured cations (calcium, magnesium, potassium). In addition, the AG may increase with an increase in anionic albumin, because of either increased albumin concentration or alkalosis, which alters albumin charge. A decrease in the AG can be due to (1) an increase in unmeasured cations; (2) the addition to the blood of abnormal cations, such as lithium (lithium intoxication) or cationic immunoglobulins (plasma cell dyscrasias); (3) a reduction in the major plasma anion albumin concentration (nephrotic syndrome); (4) a decrease in the effective anionic charge on albumin by acidosis; or (5) hyperviscosity and severe hyperlipidemia, which can lead to an underestimation of sodium and chloride concentrations. A fall in serum albumin by 1 g/dL from the normal value (4.5 g/dL) decreases the AG by 2.5 meq/L. Know the common causes of a high-AG acidosis (Table 66-3).

In the face of a normal serum albumin, a high AG is usually due to non–chloride-containing acids that contain inorganic (phosphate, sulfate), organic (ketoacids, lactate, uremic organic anions), exogenous (salicylate or ingested toxins with organic acid production), or unidentified anions. The high AG is significant even if an additional acid-base disorder is superimposed to modify the $[HCO_3^-]$ independently. Simultaneous metabolic acidosis of the high-AG variety plus either chronic respiratory acidosis or metabolic alkalosis represents such a situation in which $[HCO_3^-]$ may be normal or even high (Table 66-3). Compare the change in $[HCO_3^-]$ (ΔHCO_3^-) and the change in the AG (ΔAG).

Similarly, normal values for $[HCO_3^-]$, $Paco_2$, and pH do not ensure the absence of an acid-base disturbance. For instance, an alcoholic who has been vomiting may develop a metabolic alkalosis with a pH of 7.55, $Paco_2$ of 47 mmHg, $[HCO_3^-]$ of 40 mmol/L, $[Na^+]$ of 135, $[Cl^-]$ of 80, and $[K^+]$ of 2.8. If such a patient were then to develop a superimposed alcoholic ketoacidosis with a β-hydroxybutyrate concentration of 15 m*M*, arterial pH would fall to 7.40, $[HCO_3^-]$ to 25 mmol/L, and the $Paco_2$ to 40 mmHg. Although these blood gases are normal, the AG is elevated at 30 mmol/L, indicating a mixed metabolic alkalosis and metabolic acidosis. A mixture of high-gap acidosis and metabolic alkalosis is recognized easily by comparing the differences (Δ values) in the normal to prevailing patient values. In this example, the ΔHCO_3^- is 0 (25 – 25 mmol/L), but the ΔAG is 20 (30 – 10 mmol/L). Therefore, 20 mmol/L is unaccounted for in the Δ/Δ value (ΔAG to ΔHCO_3^-).

TABLE 66-3 STEPS IN ACID-BASE DIAGNOSIS

1. Obtain arterial blood gas (ABG) and electrolytes simultaneously.
2. Compare $[HCO_3^-]$ on ABG and electrolytes to verify accuracy.
3. Calculate anion gap (AG).
4. Know four causes of high-AG acidosis (ketoacidosis, lactic acid acidosis, renal failure, and toxins).
5. Know two causes of hyperchloremic or nongap acidosis (bicarbonate loss from gastrointestinal tract, renal tubular acidosis).
6. Estimate compensatory response (Table 66-1).
7. Compare ΔAG and ΔHCO_3^-.
8. Compare change in $[Cl^-]$ with change in $[Na^+]$.

METABOLIC ACIDOSIS

Metabolic acidosis can occur because of an increase in endogenous acid production (such as lactate and ketoacids), loss of bicarbonate (as in diarrhea), or accumulation of endogenous acids (as in renal failure). Metabolic acidosis has profound effects on the respiratory, cardiac, and nervous systems. The fall in blood pH is accompanied by a characteristic increase in ventilation, especially the tidal volume (Kussmaul respiration). Intrinsic cardiac contractility may be depressed, but inotropic function can be normal because of catecholamine release. Both peripheral arterial vasodilation and central venoconstriction can be present; the decrease in central and pulmonary vascular compliance predisposes to pulmonary edema with even minimal volume overload. CNS function is depressed, with headache, lethargy, stupor, and, in some cases, even coma. Glucose intolerance may also occur.

There are two major categories of clinical metabolic acidosis: high-AG and non-AG, or hyperchloremic, acidosis (Table 66-3 and Table 66-4).

TREATMENT METABOLIC ACIDOSIS

Treatment of metabolic acidosis with alkali should be reserved for severe acidemia except when the patient has no "potential HCO_3^-" in plasma. Potential $[HCO_3^-]$ can be estimated from the increment (Δ) in the AG (ΔAG = patient's AG – 10). It must be determined if

TABLE 66-4 CAUSES OF HIGH-ANION GAP METABOLIC ACIDOSIS

Lactic acidosis	Toxins
Ketoacidosis	Ethylene glycol
Diabetic	Methanol
Alcoholic	Salicylates
Starvation	Propylene glycol
	Pyroglutamic acid (5-oxoproline)
	Renal failure (acute and chronic)

the acid anion in plasma is metabolizable (i.e., β-hydroxybutyrate, acetoacetate, and lactate) or nonmetabolizable (anions that accumulate in chronic renal failure and after toxin ingestion). The latter requires return of renal function to replenish the [HCO_3^-] deficit, a slow and often unpredictable process. Consequently, patients with a normal AG acidosis (hyperchloremic acidosis), a slightly elevated AG (mixed hyperchloremic and AG acidosis), or an AG attributable to a nonmetabolizable anion in the face of renal failure should receive alkali therapy, either PO ($NaHCO_3$ or Shohl's solution) or IV ($NaHCO_3$), in an amount necessary to slowly increase the plasma [HCO_3^-] into the 20–22 mmol/L range. Overcorrection must be avoided.

Controversy exists, however, in regard to the use of alkali in patients with a pure AG acidosis owing to accumulation of a metabolizable organic acid anion (ketoacidosis or lactic acidosis). In general, severe acidosis (pH <7.10) warrants the IV administration of 50–100 meq of $NaHCO_3$, over 30–45 min, during the initial 1–2 h of therapy. Provision of such modest quantities of alkali in this situation seems to provide an added measure of safety, but it is essential to monitor plasma electrolytes during the course of therapy, because the [K^+] may decline as pH rises. The goal is to increase the [HCO_3^-] to 10 meq/L and the pH to approximately 7.20, not to increase these values to normal.

HIGH-ANION GAP ACIDOSES

APPROACH TO THE PATIENT: High-Anion Gap Acidoses

There are four principal causes of a high-AG acidosis: (1) lactic acidosis, (2) ketoacidosis, (3) ingested toxins, and (4) acute and chronic renal failure (Table 66-4). Initial screening to differentiate the high-AG acidoses should include (1) a probe of the history for evidence of drug and toxin ingestion and measurement of arterial blood gas to detect coexistent respiratory alkalosis (salicylates); (2) determination of whether diabetes mellitus is present (diabetic ketoacidosis); (3) a search for evidence of alcoholism or increased levels of β-hydroxybutyrate (alcoholic ketoacidosis); (4) observation for clinical signs of uremia and determination of the blood urea nitrogen (BUN) and creatinine (uremic acidosis); (5) inspection of the urine for oxalate crystals (ethylene glycol); and (6) recognition of the numerous clinical settings in which lactate levels may be increased (hypotension, shock, cardiac failure, leukemia, cancer, and drug or toxin ingestion).

Lactic Acidosis An increase in plasma l-lactate may be secondary to poor tissue perfusion (type A)—circulatory insufficiency (shock, cardiac failure), severe anemia, mitochondrial enzyme defects, and inhibitors (carbon monoxide, cyanide)—or to aerobic disorders (type B)—malignancies, nucleoside analogue reverse transcriptase inhibitors in HIV, diabetes mellitus, renal or hepatic failure, thiamine deficiency, severe infections (cholera, malaria), seizures, or drugs/toxins (biguanides, ethanol, methanol, propylene glycol, isoniazid, and fructose). Unrecognized bowel ischemia or infarction in a patient with severe atherosclerosis or cardiac decompensation receiving vasopressors is a common cause of lactic acidosis. Pyroglutamic acidemia has been reported in critically ill patients receiving acetaminophen, which is associated with depletion of glutathione. D-Lactic acid acidosis, which may be associated with jejunoileal bypass, short bowel syndrome, or intestinal obstruction, is due to formation of D-lactate by gut bacteria.

APPROACH TO THE PATIENT: L-Lactic Acid Acidosis

The underlying condition that disrupts lactate metabolism must first be corrected; tissue perfusion must be restored when inadequate. Vasoconstrictors should be avoided, if possible, because they may worsen tissue perfusion. Alkali therapy is generally advocated for acute, severe acidemia (pH <7.15) to improve cardiac function and lactate use. However, $NaHCO_3$ therapy may paradoxically depress cardiac performance and exacerbate acidosis by enhancing lactate production (HCO_3^- stimulates phosphofructokinase). While the use of alkali in moderate lactic acidosis is controversial, it is generally agreed that attempts to return the pH or [HCO_3^-] to normal by administration of exogenous $NaHCO_3$ are deleterious. A reasonable approach is to infuse sufficient $NaHCO_3$ to raise the arterial pH to no more than 7.2 over 30–40 min.

$NaHCO_3$ therapy can cause fluid overload and hypertension because the amount required can be massive when accumulation of lactic acid is relentless. Fluid administration is poorly tolerated because of central venoconstriction, especially in the oliguric patient. When the underlying cause of the lactic acidosis can be remedied, blood lactate will be converted to HCO_3^- and may result in an overshoot alkalosis.

Ketoacidosis • ***DIABETIC KETOACIDOSIS (DKA)*** This condition is caused by increased fatty acid metabolism and the accumulation of ketoacids (acetoacetate and β-hydroxybutyrate). DKA usually occurs in insulin-dependent diabetes mellitus in association with cessation of insulin or an intercurrent illness such as an infection, gastroenteritis, pancreatitis, or myocardial infarction, which increases insulin requirements temporarily and acutely. The accumulation of ketoacids accounts for the increment in the AG and is accompanied most often by hyperglycemia (glucose >17 mmol/L [300 mg/dL]). The relationship between the ΔAG and ΔHCO_3^- is typically ~1:1 in DKA. It should be noted that, because insulin prevents production of ketones, bicarbonate therapy is rarely needed except with extreme acidemia (pH < 7.1), and then in only limited amounts. Patients with DKA are typically volume depleted and require fluid resuscitation with isotonic saline. Volume overexpansion with IV fluid administration is not uncommon, however, and contributes to the development of a hyperchloremic acidosis during treatment of DKA. The mainstay for treatment of this condition is IV regular insulin and is described in Chap. 417 in more detail.

ALCOHOLIC KETOACIDOSIS (AKA) Chronic alcoholics can develop ketoacidosis when alcohol consumption is abruptly curtailed and nutrition is poor. AKA is usually associated with binge drinking, vomiting, abdominal pain, starvation, and volume depletion. The glucose concentration is variable, and acidosis may be severe because of elevated ketones, predominantly β-hydroxybutyrate. Hypoperfusion may enhance lactic acid production, chronic respiratory alkalosis may accompany liver disease, and metabolic alkalosis can result from vomiting (refer to the relationship between ΔAG and ΔHCO_3^-). Thus, mixed acid-base disorders are common in AKA. As the circulation is restored by administration of isotonic saline, the preferential accumulation of β-hydroxybutyrate is then shifted to acetoacetate. This explains the common clinical observation of an increasingly positive nitroprusside reaction as the patient improves. The nitroprusside ketone reaction (Acetest) can detect acetoacetic acid but not β-hydroxybutyrate, so that the degree of ketosis and ketonuria can not only change with therapy, but can be underestimated initially. Patients with AKA usually present with relatively normal renal function, as opposed to DKA, where renal function is often compromised because of volume depletion (osmotic diuresis) or diabetic nephropathy. The AKA patient with normal renal function may excrete relatively large quantities of ketoacids in the urine and, therefore, may have a relatively normal AG and a discrepancy in the $\Delta AG/\Delta HCO_3^-$ relationship.

TREATMENT ALCOHOLIC KETOACIDOSIS

Extracellular fluid deficits almost always accompany AKA and should be repleted by IV administration of saline and glucose (5% dextrose in 0.9% NaCl). Hypophosphatemia, hypokalemia, and hypomagnesemia may coexist and should be corrected. Hypophosphatemia usually emerges 12–24 h after admission, may be exacerbated by glucose infusion, and, if severe, may induce rhabdomyolysis or even respiratory arrest. Upper gastrointestinal hemorrhage, pancreatitis, and pneumonia may accompany this disorder.

Drug- and Toxin-Induced Acidosis • ***SALICYLATES*** (See also Chap. 472e) Salicylate intoxication in adults usually causes respiratory alkalosis or a mixture of high-AG metabolic acidosis and respiratory alkalosis. Only a portion of the AG is due to salicylates. Lactic acid production is also often increased.

TREATMENT SALICYLATE-INDUCED ACIDOSIS

Vigorous gastric lavage with isotonic saline (not $NaHCO_3$) should be initiated immediately, followed by administration of activated charcoal per nasogastric tube. In the acidotic patient, to facilitate removal of salicylate, IV $NaHCO_3$ is administered in amounts adequate to alkalinize the urine and to maintain urine output (urine pH >7.5). While this form of therapy is straightforward in acidotic patients, a coexisting respiratory alkalosis may make this approach hazardous. Alkalemic patients should not receive $NaHCO_3$. Acetazolamide may be administered in the face of alkalemia, when an alkaline diuresis cannot be achieved, or to ameliorate volume overload associated with $NaHCO_3$ administration, but this drug can cause systemic metabolic acidosis if HCO_3^- is not replaced. Hypokalemia should be anticipated with an alkaline diuresis and should be treated promptly and aggressively. Glucose-containing fluids should be administered because of the danger of hypoglycemia. Excessive insensible fluid losses may cause severe volume depletion and hypernatremia. If renal failure prevents rapid clearance of salicylate, hemodialysis can be performed against a bicarbonate dialysate.

ALCOHOLS Under most physiologic conditions, sodium, urea, and glucose generate the osmotic pressure of blood. Plasma osmolality is calculated according to the following expression: $P_{osm} = 2Na^+ + Glu + BUN$ (all in mmol/L), or, using conventional laboratory values in which glucose and BUN are expressed in milligrams per deciliter: $P_{osm} = 2Na^+ + Glu/18 + BUN/2.8$. The calculated and determined osmolality should agree within 10–15 mmol/kg H_2O. When the measured osmolality exceeds the calculated osmolality by >10–15 mmol/kg H_2O, one of two circumstances prevails. Either the serum sodium is spuriously low, as with hyperlipidemia or hyperproteinemia (pseudohyponatremia), or osmolytes other than sodium salts, glucose, or urea have accumulated in plasma. Examples of such osmolytes include mannitol, radiocontrast media, ethanol, isopropyl alcohol, ethylene glycol, propylene glycol, methanol, and acetone. In this situation, the difference between the calculated osmolality and the measured osmolality (*osmolar gap*) is proportional to the concentration of the unmeasured solute. With an appropriate clinical history and index of suspicion, identification of an osmolar gap is helpful in identifying the presence of poison-associated AG acidosis. Three alcohols may cause fatal intoxications: ethylene glycol, methanol, and isopropyl alcohol. All cause an elevated osmolal gap, but only the first two cause a high-AG acidosis.

ETHYLENE GLYCOL (See also Chap. 472e) Ingestion of ethylene glycol (commonly used in antifreeze) leads to a metabolic acidosis and severe damage to the CNS, heart, lungs, and kidneys. The increased AG and osmolar gap are attributable to ethylene glycol and its metabolites, oxalic acid, glycolic acid, and other organic acids. Lactic acid production increases secondary to inhibition of the tricarboxylic acid cycle and altered intracellular redox state. Diagnosis is facilitated by recognizing oxalate crystals in the urine, the presence of an osmolar gap in serum, and a high-AG acidosis. Although use of a Wood's lamp to visualize the fluorescent additive to commercial antifreeze in the urine of patients with ethylene glycol ingestion, this is rarely reproducible. The combination of a high AG and high osmolar gap in a patient suspected of ethylene glycol ingestion should be taken as evidence of ethylene glycol toxicity. Treatment should not be delayed while awaiting measurement of ethylene glycol levels in this setting.

TREATMENT ETHYLENE GLYCOL-INDUCED ACIDOSIS

This includes the prompt institution of a saline or osmotic diuresis, thiamine and pyridoxine supplements, fomepizole, and usually, hemodialysis. The IV administration of the alcohol dehydrogenase inhibitor fomepizole (4-methylpyrazole; 15 mg/kg as a loading dose) is the agent of choice and offers the advantages of a predictable decline in ethylene glycol levels without excessive obtundation as seen during ethyl alcohol infusion. If used, ethanol IV should be infused to achieve a blood level of 22 mmol/L (100 mg/dL). Both fomepizole and ethanol reduce toxicity because they compete with ethylene glycol for metabolism by alcohol dehydrogenase. Hemodialysis is indicated when the arterial pH is <7.3 or the osmolar gap exceeds 20 mOsm/kg.

METHANOL (See also Chap. 472e) The ingestion of methanol (wood alcohol) causes metabolic acidosis, and its metabolites formaldehyde and formic acid cause severe optic nerve and CNS damage. Lactic acid, ketoacids, and other unidentified organic acids may contribute to the acidosis. Due to its low molecular mass (32 Da), an osmolar gap is usually present.

TREATMENT METHANOL-INDUCED ACIDOSIS

This is similar to that for ethylene glycol intoxication, including general supportive measures, fomepizole, and hemodialysis (as above).

PROPYLENE GLYCOL Propylene glycol is the vehicle used in IV administration of diazepam, lorazepam, phenobarbital, nitroglycerine, etomidate, enoximone, and phenytoin. Propylene glycol is generally safe for limited use in these IV preparations, but toxicity has been reported, most often in the setting of the intensive care unit in patients receiving frequent or continuous therapy. This form of high-gap acidosis should be considered in patients with unexplained high-gap acidosis, hyperosmolality, and clinical deterioration. Propylene glycol, like ethylene glycol and methanol, is metabolized by alcohol dehydrogenase. With intoxication by propylene glycol, the first response is to stop the offending infusion. Additionally, fomepizole should also be administered in acidotic patients.

ISOPROPYL ALCOHOL Ingested isopropanol is absorbed rapidly and may be fatal when as little as 150 mL of rubbing alcohol, solvent, or deicer is consumed. A plasma level >400 mg/dL is life-threatening. Isopropyl alcohol is metabolized by alcohol dehydrogenase to acetone. The characteristic features differ from ethylene glycol and methanol in that the parent compound, not the metabolites, causes toxicity, and an AG acidosis is *not* present because acetone is rapidly excreted. Both isopropyl alcohol and acetone increase the osmolal gap, and hypoglycemia is common. Alternative diagnoses should be considered if the patient does not improve significantly within a few hours. Patients with hemodynamic instability with plasma levels above 400 mg/dL should be considered for hemodialysis.

TREATMENT ISOPROPYL ALCOHOL TOXICITY

Isopropanol alcohol toxicity is treated by watchful waiting and supportive therapy, IV fluids, pressors, ventilatory support if needed, and occasionally hemodialysis for prolonged coma, hemodynamic instability, or levels >400 mg/dL.

PYROGLUTAMIC ACID Acetaminophen-induced high-AG metabolic acidosis is uncommon but is being recognized more often in either patients with acetaminophen overdose or malnourished or critically ill patients receiving acetaminophen in typical dosage. 5-Oxoproline accumulation after acetaminophen should be suspected in the setting of an unexplained high-AG acidosis without elevation of the osmolar gap in patients receiving acetaminophen. The first step in treatment is to immediately discontinue the drug. Additionally, sodium bicarbonate IV should be given. Although *N*-acetylcysteine has been suggested, it is not known if it hastens the metabolism of 5-oxoproline by increasing intracellular glutathione concentrations in this setting.

Renal Failure (See also Chap. 335) The hyperchloremic acidosis of moderate renal insufficiency is eventually converted to the high-AG acidosis of advanced renal failure. Poor filtration and reabsorption of organic anions contribute to the pathogenesis. As renal disease progresses, the number of functioning nephrons eventually becomes insufficient to keep pace with net acid production. Uremic acidosis is characterized, therefore, by a reduced rate of NH_4^+ production and excretion. The acid retained in chronic renal disease is buffered by alkaline salts from bone. Despite significant retention of acid (up to 20 mmol/d), the serum [HCO_3^-] does not decrease further, indicating participation of buffers outside the extracellular compartment. Chronic metabolic acidosis results in significant loss of bone mass due to reduction in bone calcium carbonate. Chronic acidosis also increases urinary calcium excretion, proportional to cumulative acid retention.

TREATMENT RENAL FAILURE

Because of the association of renal failure acidosis with muscle catabolism and bone disease, both uremic acidosis and the hyperchloremic acidosis of renal failure require oral alkali replacement to maintain the [HCO_3^-] >22 mmol/L. This can be accomplished with relatively modest amounts of alkali (1.0–1.5 mmol/kg body weight per day). Sodium citrate (Shohl's solution) or $NaHCO_3$ tablets (650-mg tablets contain 7.8 meq) are equally effective alkalinizing salts. Citrate enhances the absorption of aluminum from the gastrointestinal tract and should never be given together with aluminum-containing antacids because of the risk of aluminum intoxication.

NON–ANION GAP METABOLIC ACIDOSES

Alkali can be lost from the gastrointestinal tract from diarrhea or from the kidneys (renal tubular acidosis, RTA). In these disorders (Table 66-5), reciprocal changes in [Cl^-] and [HCO_3^-] result in a normal AG. In pure non–AG acidosis, therefore, the increase in [Cl^-] above the normal value approximates the decrease in [HCO_3^-]. The absence of such a relationship suggests a mixed disturbance.

TREATMENT NON–ANION GAP METABOLIC ACIDOSES

In diarrhea, stools contain a higher [HCO_3^-] and decomposed HCO_3^- than plasma so that metabolic acidosis develops along with volume depletion. Instead of an acid urine pH (as anticipated with systemic acidosis), urine pH is usually >6 because metabolic acidosis and hypokalemia increase renal synthesis and excretion of NH_4^+, thus providing a urinary buffer that increases urine pH. Metabolic acidosis due to gastrointestinal losses with a high urine pH can be differentiated from RTA because urinary NH_4^+ excretion is typically low in RTA and high with diarrhea. Urinary NH_4^+ levels can be estimated by calculating the urine anion gap (UAG): UAG = $[Na^+ + K^+]_u - [Cl^-]_u$. When $[Cl^-]_u > [Na^+ + K^+]_u$, the UAG is negative by definition. This indicates that the urine ammonium level is appropriately increased, suggesting an extrarenal cause of the acidosis. Conversely, when the UAG is positive, the urine ammonium level is low, suggesting a renal cause of the acidosis.

TABLE 66-5 CAUSES OF NON–ANION GAP ACIDOSIS

I. Gastrointestinal bicarbonate loss
   - A. Diarrhea
   - B. External pancreatic or small-bowel drainage
   - C. Ureterosigmoidostomy, jejunal loop, ileal loop
   - D. Drugs
     1. Calcium chloride (acidifying agent)
     2. Magnesium sulfate (diarrhea)
     3. Cholestyramine (bile acid diarrhea)

II. Renal acidosis
   - A. Hypokalemia
     1. Proximal RTA (type 2)
        Drug-induced: acetazolamide, topiramate
     2. Distal (classic) RTA (type 1)
        Drug induced: amphotericin B, ifosfamide
   - B. Hyperkalemia
     1. Generalized distal nephron dysfunction (type 4 RTA)
        - a. Mineralocorticoid deficiency
        - b. Mineralocorticoid resistance (PHA I, autosomal dominant)
        - c. Voltage defect (PHA I, autosomal recessive, and PHA II)
        - d. Tubulointerstitial disease
   - C. Normokalemia
     1. Chronic progressive kidney disease

III. Drug-induced hyperkalemia (with renal insufficiency)
   - A. Potassium-sparing diuretics (amiloride, triamterene, spironolactone, eplerenone)
   - B. Trimethoprim
   - C. Pentamidine
   - D. ACE-Is and ARBs
   - E. Nonsteroidal anti-inflammatory drugs
   - F. Calcineurin inhibitors

IV. Other
   - A. Acid loads (ammonium chloride, hyperalimentation)
   - B. Loss of potential bicarbonate: ketosis with ketone excretion
   - C. Expansion acidosis (rapid saline administration)
   - D. Hippurate
   - E. Cation exchange resins

Abbreviations: ACE-I, angiotensin-converting enzyme inhibitor; ARB, angiotensin receptor blocker; PHA, pseudohypoaldosteronism; RTA, renal tubular acidosis.

Proximal RTA (type 2 RTA) (Chap. 339) is most often due to generalized proximal tubular dysfunction manifested by glycosuria, generalized aminoaciduria, and phosphaturia (Fanconi syndrome). With a low plasma [HCO_3^-], the urine pH is acid (pH <5.5). The fractional excretion of [HCO_3^-] may exceed 10–15% when the serum HCO_3^- >20 mmol/L. Because HCO_3^- is not reabsorbed normally in the proximal tubule, therapy with $NaHCO_3$ will enhance renal potassium wasting and hypokalemia.

The typical findings in acquired or inherited forms of **classic distal RTA** (type 1 RTA) include hypokalemia, non-AG metabolic acidosis, low urinary NH_4^+ excretion (positive UAG, low urine [NH_4^+]), and inappropriately high urine pH (pH > 5.5). Most patients have hypocitraturia and hypercalciuria, so nephrolithiasis, nephrocalcinosis, and bone disease are common. In **generalized distal RTA** (type 4 RTA), hyperkalemia is disproportionate to the reduction in glomerular filtration rate (GFR) because of coexisting dysfunction of potassium and acid secretion. Urinary ammonium excretion is invariably depressed, and renal function may be compromised, for example, due to diabetic nephropathy, obstructive uropathy, or chronic tubulointerstitial disease.

Hyporeninemic hypoaldosteronism typically causes non-AG metabolic acidosis, most commonly in older adults with diabetes mellitus or tubulointerstitial disease and renal insufficiency. Patients usually have mild to moderate CKD (GFR, 20–50 mL/min) and acidosis, with elevation in serum [K+] (5.2–6.0 mmol/L), concurrent hypertension, and congestive heart failure. Both the metabolic acidosis and the hyperkalemia are out of proportion to impairment in GFR. Nonsteroidal anti-inflammatory drugs, trimethoprim, pentamidine, and angiotensin-converting enzyme (ACE) inhibitors can also cause non-AG metabolic acidosis in patients with renal insufficiency (Table 66-5).

METABOLIC ALKALOSIS

Metabolic alkalosis is manifested by an elevated arterial pH, an increase in the serum [HCO_3^-], and an increase in $Paco_2$ as a result of compensatory alveolar hypoventilation (Table 66-1). It is often accompanied by hypochloremia and hypokalemia. The arterial pH establishes the diagnosis, because it is increased in metabolic alkalosis and decreased or normal in respiratory acidosis. Metabolic alkalosis frequently occurs in association with other disorders such as respiratory acidosis or alkalosis or metabolic acidosis.

PATHOGENESIS

Metabolic alkalosis occurs as a result of net gain of [HCO_3^-] or loss of nonvolatile acid (usually HCl by vomiting) from the extracellular fluid. For HCO_3^- to be added to the extracellular fluid, it must be administered exogenously or synthesized endogenously, in part or entirely by the kidneys. Because it is unusual for alkali to be added to the body, the disorder involves a generative stage, in which the loss of acid usually causes alkalosis, and a maintenance stage, in which the kidneys fail to compensate by excreting HCO_3^-.

Maintenance of metabolic alkalosis represents a failure of the kidneys to eliminate HCO_3^- in the usual manner. The kidneys will retain, rather than excrete, the excess alkali and maintain the alkalosis if (1) volume deficiency, chloride deficiency, and K^+ deficiency exist in combination with a reduced GFR; or (2) hypokalemia exists because of autonomous hyperaldosteronism. In the first example, alkalosis is corrected by administration of NaCl and KCl, whereas, in the latter, it may be necessary to repair the alkalosis by pharmacologic or surgical intervention, not with saline administration.

DIFFERENTIAL DIAGNOSIS

To establish the cause of metabolic alkalosis (Table 66-6), it is necessary to assess the status of the extracellular fluid volume (ECFV), the recumbent and upright blood pressure, the serum [K^+], and the renin-aldosterone system. For example, the presence of chronic hypertension and chronic hypokalemia in an alkalotic patient suggests either mineralocorticoid excess or that the hypertensive patient is receiving diuretics. Low plasma renin activity and normal urine [Na^+] and [Cl^-] in a patient who is not taking diuretics indicate a primary mineralocorticoid excess syndrome. The combination of hypokalemia and alkalosis in a normotensive, nonedematous patient can be due to Bartter's or Gitelman's syndrome, magnesium deficiency, vomiting, exogenous alkali, or diuretic ingestion. Determination of urine electrolytes (especially the urine [Cl^-]) and screening of the urine for diuretics may be helpful. If the urine is alkaline, with an elevated [Na^+] and [K^+] but low [Cl^-], the diagnosis is usually either vomiting (overt or surreptitious) or alkali ingestion. If the urine is relatively acid and has low concentrations of Na^+, K^+, and Cl^-, the most likely possibilities are prior vomiting, the posthypercapnic state, or prior diuretic ingestion. If, on the other hand, neither the urine sodium, potassium, nor chloride concentrations are depressed, magnesium deficiency, Bartter's or Gitelman's syndrome, or current diuretic ingestion should be considered. Bartter's syndrome is distinguished from Gitelman's syndrome because of hypocalciuria and hypomagnesemia in the latter disorder.

Alkali Administration Chronic administration of alkali to individuals with normal renal function rarely causes alkalosis. However, in patients with coexistent hemodynamic disturbances, alkalosis can develop because the normal capacity to excrete HCO_3^- may be exceeded or there may be enhanced reabsorption of HCO_3^-. Such patients include those who receive HCO_3^- (PO or IV), acetate loads (parenteral hyperalimentation solutions), citrate loads (transfusions), or antacids plus cation-exchange resins (aluminum hydroxide and sodium polystyrene sulfonate). Nursing home patients receiving tube feedings have a higher incidence of metabolic alkalosis than nursing home patients receiving oral feedings.

TABLE 66-6 CAUSES OF METABOLIC ALKALOSIS

I. Exogenous HCO_3^- loads
  - A. Acute alkali administration
  - B. Milk-alkali syndrome

II. Effective ECFV contraction, normotension, K^+ deficiency, and secondary hyperreninemic hyperaldosteronism
  - A. Gastrointestinal origin
    1. Vomiting
    2. Gastric aspiration
    3. Congenital chloridorrhea
    4. Villous adenoma
  - B. Renal origin
    1. Diuretics
    2. Posthypercapnic state
    3. Hypercalcemia/hypoparathyroidism
    4. Recovery from lactic acidosis or ketoacidosis
    5. Nonreabsorbable anions including penicillin, carbenicillin
    6. Mg^{2+} deficiency
    7. K^+ depletion
    8. Bartter's syndrome (loss of function mutations of transporters and ion channels in TALH)
    9. Gitelman's syndrome (loss of function mutation in Na^+-Cl^- cotransporter in DCT)

III. ECFV expansion, hypertension, K^+ deficiency, and mineralocorticoid excess
  - A. High renin
    1. Renal artery stenosis
    2. Accelerated hypertension
    3. Renin-secreting tumor
    4. Estrogen therapy
  - B. Low renin
    1. Primary aldosteronism
       a. Adenoma
       b. Hyperplasia
       c. Carcinoma
    2. Adrenal enzyme defects
       a. 11β-Hydroxylase deficiency
       b. 17α-Hydroxylase deficiency
    3. Cushing's syndrome or disease
    4. Other
       a. Licorice
       b. Carbenoxolone
       c. Chewer's tobacco

IV. Gain-of-function mutation of renal sodium channel with ECFV expansion, hypertension, K^+ deficiency, and hyporeninemic-hypoaldosteronism
  - A. Liddle's syndrome

Abbreviations: DCT, distal convoluted tubule; ECFV, extracellular fluid volume; TALH, thick ascending limb of Henle's loop.

METABOLIC ALKALOSIS ASSOCIATED WITH ECFV CONTRACTION, K^+ DEPLETION, AND SECONDARY HYPERRENINEMIC HYPERALDOSTERONISM

Gastrointestinal Origin Gastrointestinal loss of H^+ from vomiting or gastric aspiration results in retention of HCO_3^-. During active vomiting, the filtered load of bicarbonate is acutely increased to exceed the reabsorptive capacity of the proximal tubule for HCO_3^- so that the urine becomes alkaline and high in potassium. When vomiting ceases, the persistence of volume, potassium, and chloride depletion causes maintenance of the alkalosis because of an enhanced capacity of the nephron to reabsorb HCO_3^-. Correction of the contracted ECFV with NaCl and repair of K^+ deficits corrects the acid-base disorder by restoring the ability of the kidney to excrete the excess bicarbonate.

Renal Origin • ***DIURETICS*** (See also Chap. 279) Drugs that induce chloruresis, such as thiazides and loop diuretics (furosemide, bumetanide, torsemide, and ethacrynic acid), acutely diminish the ECFV without altering the total body bicarbonate content. The serum $[HCO_3^-]$ increases because the reduced ECFV "contracts" the $[HCO_3^-]$ in the plasma (contraction alkalosis). The chronic administration of diuretics tends to generate an alkalosis by increasing distal salt delivery, so that K^+ and H^+ secretion are stimulated. The alkalosis is maintained by persistence of the contraction of the ECFV, secondary hyperaldosteronism, K^+ deficiency, and the direct effect of the diuretic (as long as diuretic administration continues). Repair of the alkalosis is achieved by providing isotonic saline to correct the ECFV deficit.

SOLUTE LOSING DISORDERS: BARTTER'S SYNDROME AND GITELMAN'S SYNDROME See Chap. 339.

NONREABSORBABLE ANIONS AND MAGNESIUM DEFICIENCY Administration of large quantities of nonreabsorbable anions, such as penicillin or carbenicillin, can enhance distal acidification and K^+ secretion by increasing the transepithelial potential difference. Mg^{2+} deficiency results in hypokalemic alkalosis by enhancing distal acidification through stimulation of renin and hence aldosterone secretion.

POTASSIUM DEPLETION Chronic K^+ depletion may cause metabolic alkalosis by increasing urinary acid excretion. Both NH_4^+ production and absorption are enhanced and HCO_3^- reabsorption is stimulated. Chronic K^+ deficiency upregulates the renal H^+, K^+-ATPase to increase K^+ absorption at the expense of enhanced H^+ secretion. Alkalosis associated with severe K^+ depletion is resistant to salt administration, but repair of the K^+ deficiency corrects the alkalosis.

AFTER TREATMENT OF LACTIC ACIDOSIS OR KETOACIDOSIS When an underlying stimulus for the generation of lactic acid or ketoacid is removed rapidly, as with repair of circulatory insufficiency or with insulin therapy, the lactate or ketones are metabolized to yield an equivalent amount of HCO_3^-. Other sources of new HCO_3^- are additive with the original amount generated by organic anion metabolism to create a surfeit of HCO_3^-. Such sources include (1) new HCO_3^- added to the blood by the kidneys as a result of enhanced acid excretion during the preexisting period of acidosis, and (2) alkali therapy during the treatment phase of the acidosis. Acidosis-induced contraction of the ECFV and K^+ deficiency act to sustain the alkalosis.

POSTHYPERCAPNIA Prolonged CO_2 retention with chronic respiratory acidosis enhances renal HCO_3^- absorption and the generation of new HCO_3^- (increased net acid excretion). Metabolic alkalosis results from the effect of the persistently elevated $[HCO_3^-]$ when the elevated Pa_{CO_2} is abruptly returned toward normal.

METABOLIC ALKALOSIS ASSOCIATED WITH ECFV EXPANSION, HYPERTENSION, AND HYPERALDOSTERONISM

Increased aldosterone levels may be the result of autonomous primary adrenal overproduction or of secondary aldosterone release due to renal overproduction of renin. Mineralocorticoid excess increases net acid excretion and may result in metabolic alkalosis, which may be worsened by associated K^+ deficiency. ECFV expansion from salt retention causes hypertension. The kaliuresis persists because of mineralocorticoid excess and distal Na^+ absorption causing enhanced K^+ excretion, continued K^+ depletion with polydipsia, inability to concentrate the urine, and polyuria.

Liddle's syndrome (Chap. 339) results from increased activity of the collecting duct Na^+ channel (ENaC) and is a rare monogenic form of hypertension due to volume expansion manifested as hypokalemic alkalosis and normal aldosterone levels.

Symptoms With metabolic alkalosis, changes in CNS and peripheral nervous system function are similar to those of hypocalcemia (Chap. 423); symptoms include mental confusion; obtundation; and a predisposition to seizures, paresthesia, muscular cramping, tetany, aggravation of arrhythmias, and hypoxemia in chronic obstructive pulmonary disease. Related electrolyte abnormalities include hypokalemia and hypophosphatemia.

TREATMENT METABOLIC ALKALOSIS

This is primarily directed at correcting the underlying stimulus for HCO_3^- generation. If primary aldosteronism, renal artery stenosis, or Cushing's syndrome is present, correction of the underlying cause will reverse the alkalosis. $[H^+]$ loss by the stomach or kidneys can be mitigated by the use of proton pump inhibitors or the discontinuation of diuretics. The second aspect of treatment is to remove the factors that sustain the inappropriate increase in HCO_3^- reabsorption, such as ECFV contraction or K^+ deficiency. K^+ deficits should always be repaired. Isotonic saline is usually sufficient to reverse the alkalosis if ECFV contraction is present.

If associated conditions preclude infusion of saline, renal HCO_3^- loss can be accelerated by administration of acetazolamide, a carbonic anhydrase inhibitor, which is usually effective in patients with adequate renal function but can worsen K^+ losses. Dilute hydrochloric acid (0.1 *N* HCl) is also effective but can cause hemolysis, and must be delivered slowly in a central vein.

RESPIRATORY ACIDOSIS

Respiratory acidosis can be due to severe pulmonary disease, respiratory muscle fatigue, or abnormalities in ventilatory control and is recognized by an increase in Pa_{CO_2} and decrease in pH (Table 66-7). In acute respiratory acidosis, there is an immediate compensatory elevation (due to cellular buffering mechanisms) in HCO_3^-, which increases 1 mmol/L for every 10-mmHg increase in Pa_{CO_2}. In chronic respiratory acidosis (>24 h), renal adaptation increases the $[HCO_3^-]$ by 4 mmol/L for every 10-mmHg increase in Pa_{CO_2}. The serum HCO_3^- usually does not increase above 38 mmol/L.

The clinical features vary according to the severity and duration of the respiratory acidosis, the underlying disease, and whether there is accompanying hypoxemia. A rapid increase in Pa_{CO_2} may cause anxiety, dyspnea, confusion, psychosis, and hallucinations and may progress to coma. Lesser degrees of dysfunction in chronic hypercapnia include sleep disturbances; loss of memory; daytime somnolence; personality changes; impairment of coordination; and motor disturbances such as tremor, myoclonic jerks, and asterixis. Headaches and other signs that mimic raised intracranial pressure, such as papilledema, abnormal reflexes, and focal muscle weakness, are due to vasoconstriction secondary to loss of the vasodilator effects of CO_2.

Depression of the respiratory center by a variety of drugs, injury, or disease can produce respiratory acidosis. This may occur acutely with general anesthetics, sedatives, and head trauma or chronically with sedatives, alcohol, intracranial tumors, and the syndromes of sleep-disordered breathing including the primary alveolar and obesity-hypoventilation syndromes (Chaps. 318 and 319). Abnormalities or disease in the motor neurons, neuromuscular junction, and skeletal muscle can cause hypoventilation via respiratory muscle fatigue. Mechanical ventilation, when not properly adjusted and supervised, may result in respiratory acidosis, particularly if CO_2 production suddenly rises (because of fever, agitation, sepsis, or overfeeding) or alveolar ventilation falls because of worsening pulmonary function. High levels of positive end-expiratory pressure in the presence of reduced cardiac output may cause hypercapnia as a result of large increases in alveolar dead space (Chap. 306e). Permissive hypercapnia is being used with increasing frequency because of studies suggesting lower mortality rates than with conventional mechanical ventilation, especially with severe CNS or heart disease. The respiratory acidosis associated with permissive hypercapnia may require administration of $NaHCO_3$ to increase the arterial pH to 7.25, but overcorrection of the acidemia may be deleterious.

Acute hypercapnia follows sudden occlusion of the upper airway or generalized bronchospasm as in severe asthma, anaphylaxis,

TABLE 66-7 RESPIRATORY ACID-BASE DISORDERS

I. Alkalosis
- A. Central nervous system stimulation
  1. Pain
  2. Anxiety, psychosis
  3. Fever
  4. Cerebrovascular accident
  5. Meningitis, encephalitis
  6. Tumor
  7. Trauma
- B. Hypoxemia or tissue hypoxia
  1. High altitude
  2. Pneumonia, pulmonary edema
  3. Aspiration
  4. Severe anemia
- C. Drugs or hormones
  1. Pregnancy, progesterone
  2. Salicylates
  3. Cardiac failure
- D. Stimulation of chest receptors
  1. Hemothorax
  2. Flail chest
  3. Cardiac failure
  4. Pulmonary embolism
- E. Miscellaneous
  1. Septicemia
  2. Hepatic failure
  3. Mechanical hyperventilation
  4. Heat exposure
  5. Recovery from metabolic acidosis

II. Acidosis
- A. Central
  1. Drugs (anesthetics, morphine, sedatives)
  2. Stroke
  3. Infection
- B. Airway
  1. Obstruction
  2. Asthma
- C. Parenchyma
  1. Emphysema
  2. Pneumoconiosis
  3. Bronchitis
  4. Adult respiratory distress syndrome
  5. Barotrauma
- D. Neuromuscular
  1. Poliomyelitis
  2. Kyphoscoliosis
  3. Myasthenia
  4. Muscular dystrophies
- E. Miscellaneous
  1. Obesity
  2. Hypoventilation
  3. Permissive hypercapnia

inhalational burn, or toxin injury. Chronic hypercapnia and respiratory acidosis occur in end-stage obstructive lung disease. Restrictive disorders involving both the chest wall and the lungs can cause respiratory acidosis because the high metabolic cost of respiration causes ventilatory muscle fatigue. Advanced stages of intrapulmonary and extrapulmonary restrictive defects present as chronic respiratory acidosis.

The diagnosis of respiratory acidosis requires the measurement of Pa_{CO_2} and arterial pH. A detailed history and physical examination often indicate the cause. Pulmonary function studies (Chap. 306e), including spirometry, diffusion capacity for carbon monoxide, lung volumes, and arterial Pa_{CO_2} and O_2 saturation, usually make it possible to determine if respiratory acidosis is secondary to lung disease. The workup for nonpulmonary causes should include a detailed drug history, measurement of hematocrit, and assessment of upper airway, chest wall, pleura, and neuromuscular function.

TREATMENT RESPIRATORY ACIDOSIS

The management of respiratory acidosis depends on its severity and rate of onset. Acute respiratory acidosis can be life-threatening, and measures to reverse the underlying cause should be undertaken simultaneously with restoration of adequate alveolar ventilation. This may necessitate tracheal intubation and assisted mechanical ventilation. Oxygen administration should be titrated carefully in patients with severe obstructive pulmonary disease and chronic CO_2 retention who are breathing spontaneously (Chap. 314). When oxygen is used injudiciously, these patients may experience progression of the respiratory acidosis. Aggressive and rapid correction of hypercapnia should be avoided, because the falling Pa_{CO_2} may provoke the same complications noted with acute respiratory alkalosis (i.e., cardiac arrhythmias, reduced cerebral perfusion, and seizures). The Pa_{CO_2} should be lowered gradually in chronic respiratory acidosis, aiming to restore the Pa_{CO_2} to baseline levels and to provide sufficient Cl^- and K^+ to enhance the renal excretion of HCO_3^-.

Chronic respiratory acidosis is frequently difficult to correct, but measures aimed at improving lung function (Chap. 314) can help some patients and forestall further deterioration in most.

RESPIRATORY ALKALOSIS

Alveolar hyperventilation decreases Pa_{CO_2} and increases the HCO_3^-/Pa_{CO_2} ratio, thus increasing pH (Table 66-7). Nonbicarbonate cellular buffers respond by consuming HCO_3^-. Hypocapnia develops when a sufficiently strong ventilatory stimulus causes CO_2 output in the lungs to exceed its metabolic production by tissues. Plasma pH and $[HCO_3^-]$ appear to vary proportionately with Pa_{CO_2} over a range from 40–15 mmHg. The relationship between arterial $[H^+]$ concentration and Pa_{CO_2} is ~0.7 mmol/L per mmHg (or 0.01 pH unit/mmHg), and that for plasma $[HCO_3^-]$ is 0.2 mmol/L per mmHg. Hypocapnia sustained for >2–6 h is further compensated by a decrease in renal ammonium and titratable acid excretion and a reduction in filtered HCO_3^- reabsorption. Full renal adaptation to respiratory alkalosis may take several days and requires normal volume status and renal function. The kidneys appear to respond directly to the lowered Pa_{CO_2} rather than to alkalosis per se. In chronic respiratory alkalosis a 1-mmHg decrease in Pa_{CO_2} causes a 0.4-to 0.5-mmol/L drop in $[HCO_3^-]$ and a 0.3-mmol/L decrease (or 0.003 increase in pH) in $[H^+]$.

The effects of respiratory alkalosis vary according to duration and severity but are primarily those of the underlying disease. Reduced cerebral blood flow as a consequence of a rapid decline in Pa_{CO_2} may cause dizziness, mental confusion, and seizures, even in the absence of hypoxemia. The cardiovascular effects of acute hypocapnia in the conscious human are generally minimal, but in the anesthetized or mechanically ventilated patient, cardiac output and blood pressure may fall because of the depressant effects of anesthesia and positive-pressure ventilation on heart rate, systemic resistance, and venous return. Cardiac arrhythmias may occur in patients with heart disease as a result of changes in oxygen unloading by blood from a left shift in the hemoglobin-oxygen dissociation curve (Bohr effect). Acute respiratory alkalosis causes intracellular shifts of Na^+, K^+, and PO_4^{2-} and reduces free $[Ca^{2+}]$ by increasing the protein-bound fraction. Hypocapnia-induced hypokalemia is usually minor.

Chronic respiratory alkalosis is the most common acid-base disturbance in critically ill patients and, when severe, portends a poor prognosis. Many cardiopulmonary disorders manifest respiratory alkalosis in their early to intermediate stages, and the finding of normocapnia and hypoxemia in a patient with hyperventilation may herald the onset of rapid respiratory failure and should prompt an assessment to determine if the patient is becoming fatigued. Respiratory alkalosis is common during mechanical ventilation.

The hyperventilation syndrome may be disabling. Paresthesia; circumoral numbness; chest wall tightness or pain; dizziness; inability to take an adequate breath; and, rarely, tetany may be sufficiently stressful to perpetuate the disorder. Arterial blood-gas analysis demonstrates an acute or chronic respiratory alkalosis, often with hypocapnia in the range of 15–30 mmHg and no hypoxemia. CNS diseases or injury can produce several patterns of hyperventilation and sustained $Pa{CO_2}$ levels of 20–30 mmHg. Hyperthyroidism, high caloric loads, and exercise raise the basal metabolic rate, but ventilation usually rises in proportion so that arterial blood gases are unchanged and respiratory alkalosis does not develop. Salicylates are the most common cause of drug-induced respiratory alkalosis as a result of direct stimulation of the medullary chemoreceptor (Chap. 472e). The methylxanthines, theophylline, and aminophylline stimulate ventilation and increase the ventilatory response to CO_2. Progesterone increases ventilation and lowers arterial $Pa{CO_2}$ by as much as 5–10 mmHg. Therefore, chronic respiratory alkalosis is a common feature of pregnancy. Respiratory alkalosis is also prominent in liver failure, and the severity correlates with the degree of hepatic insufficiency. Respiratory alkalosis is often an early finding in gram-negative septicemia, before fever, hypoxemia, or hypotension develops.

The diagnosis of respiratory alkalosis depends on measurement of arterial pH and $Pa{CO_2}$. The plasma $[K^+]$ is often reduced and the $[Cl^-]$ increased. In the acute phase, respiratory alkalosis is not associated with increased renal HCO_3^- excretion, but within hours net acid excretion is reduced. In general, the HCO_3^- concentration falls by 2.0 mmol/L for each 10-mmHg decrease in $Pa{CO_2}$. Chronic hypocapnia reduces the serum $[HCO_3^-]$ by 4.0 mmol/L for each 10-mmHg decrease in $Pa{CO_2}$. It is unusual to observe a plasma HCO_3^- <12 mmol/L as a result of a pure respiratory alkalosis.

When a diagnosis of respiratory alkalosis is made, its cause should be investigated. The diagnosis of hyperventilation syndrome is made by exclusion. In difficult cases, it may be important to rule out other conditions such as pulmonary embolism, coronary artery disease, and hyperthyroidism.

TREATMENT RESPIRATORY ALKALOSIS

The management of respiratory alkalosis is directed toward alleviation of the underlying disorder. If respiratory alkalosis complicates ventilator management, changes in dead space, tidal volume, and frequency can minimize the hypocapnia. Patients with the hyperventilation syndrome may benefit from reassurance, rebreathing from a paper bag during symptomatic attacks, and attention to underlying psychological stress. Antidepressants and sedatives are not recommended. β-Adrenergic blockers may ameliorate peripheral manifestations of the hyperadrenergic state.

SECTION 8 ALTERATIONS IN SEXUAL FUNCTION AND REPRODUCTION

67 Sexual Dysfunction

Kevin T. McVary

Male sexual dysfunction affects 10–25% of middle-aged and elderly men, and female sexual dysfunction occurs with similar frequency. Demographic changes, the popularity of newer treatments, and greater awareness of sexual dysfunction by patients and society have led to increased diagnosis and associated health care expenditures for the management of this common disorder. Because many patients are reluctant to initiate discussion of their sex lives, physicians should address this topic directly to elicit a history of sexual dysfunction.

MALE SEXUAL DYSFUNCTION

PHYSIOLOGY OF MALE SEXUAL RESPONSE

Normal male sexual function requires (1) an intact libido, (2) the ability to achieve and maintain penile erection, (3) ejaculation, and (4) detumescence. *Libido* refers to sexual desire and is influenced by a variety of visual, olfactory, tactile, auditory, imaginative, and hormonal stimuli. Sex steroids, particularly testosterone, act to increase libido. Libido can be diminished by hormonal or psychiatric disorders and by medications.

Penile tumescence leading to erection depends on an increased flow of blood into the lacunar network accompanied by complete relaxation of the arteries and corporal smooth muscle. The microarchitecture of the corpora is composed of a mass of smooth muscle (trabecula) that contains a network of endothelial-lined vessels (lacunar spaces). Subsequent compression of the trabecular smooth muscle against the fibroelastic tunica albuginea causes a passive closure of the emissary veins and accumulation of blood in the corpora. In the presence of a full erection and a competent valve mechanism, the corpora become noncompressible cylinders from which blood does not escape.

The central nervous system (CNS) exerts an important influence by either stimulating or antagonizing spinal pathways that mediate erectile function and ejaculation. The erectile response is mediated by a combination of central (psychogenic) innervation and peripheral (reflexogenic) innervation. Sensory nerves that originate from receptors in the penile skin and glans converge to form the dorsal nerve of the penis, which travels to the S2-S4 dorsal root ganglia via the pudendal nerve. Parasympathetic nerve fibers to the penis arise from neurons in the intermediolateral columns of the S2-S4 sacral spinal segments. Sympathetic innervation originates from the T11 to the L2 spinal segments and descends through the hypogastric plexus.

Neural input to smooth-muscle tone is crucial to the initiation and maintenance of an erection. There is also an intricate interaction between the corporal smooth-muscle cell and its overlying endothelial cell lining (Fig. 67-1). Nitric oxide, which induces vascular relaxation, promotes erection and is opposed by endothelin 1 (ET-1) and Rho kinase, which mediate vascular contraction. Nitric oxide is synthesized from l-arginine by nitric oxide synthase and is released from the nonadrenergic, noncholinergic (NANC) autonomic nerve supply to act postjunctionally on smooth-muscle cells. Nitric oxide increases the production of cyclic 3′,5′-guanosine monophosphate (cyclic GMP), which induces relaxation of smooth muscle (Fig. 67-2). Cyclic GMP is gradually broken down by phosphodiesterase type 5 (PDE-5). Inhibitors of PDE-5, such as the oral medications sildenafil, vardenafil, and tadalafil, maintain erections by reducing the breakdown of cyclic GMP. However, if nitric oxide is not produced at some level, PDE-5 inhibitors are ineffective, as these drugs facilitate, but do not initiate, the initial enzyme cascade. In addition to nitric oxide, vasoactive prostaglandins (PGE_1, $PGF_{2\alpha}$) are synthesized within the cavernosal tissue and increase cyclic AMP levels, also leading to relaxation of cavernosal smooth-muscle cells.

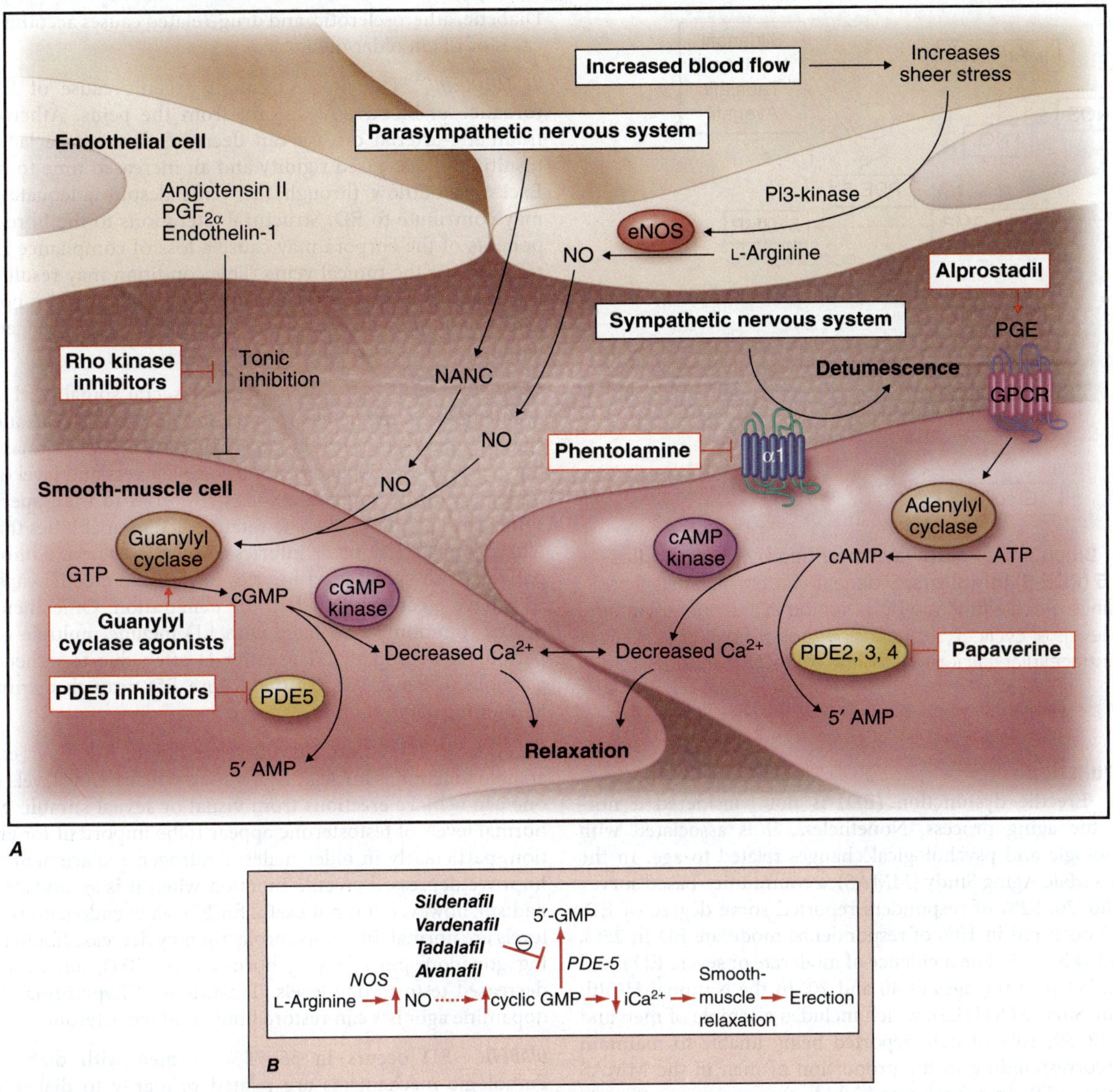

FIGURE 67-1 Pathways that regulate penile smooth-muscle relaxation and erection. *A.* Outflow from the parasympathetic nervous system leads to relaxation of the cavernous sinusoids in two ways, both of which increase the concentration of nitric oxide (NO) in smooth-muscle cells. First, NO is the neurotransmitter in nonadrenergic, noncholinergic (NANC) fibers; second, stimulation of endothelial nitric oxide synthase (eNOS) through cholinergic output causes increased production of NO. The NO produced in the endothelium then diffuses into the smooth-muscle cells and decreases its intracellular calcium concentration through a pathway mediated by cyclic guanosine monophosphate (cGMP), leading to relaxation. A separate mechanism that decreases the intracellular calcium level is mediated by cyclic adenosine monophosphate (cAMP). With increased cavernosal blood flow, as well as increased levels of vascular endothelial growth factor (VEGF), the endothelial release of NO is further sustained through the phosphatidylinositol 3 (PI3) kinase pathway. Active treatments (red boxes) include drugs that affect the cGMP pathway (phosphodiesterase [PDE] type 5 inhibitors and guanylyl cyclase agonists), the cAMP pathway (alprostadil), or both pathways (papaverine), along with neural-tone mediators (phentolamine and Rho kinase inhibitors). Agents that are being developed include guanylyl cyclase agonists (to bypass the need for endogenous NO) and Rho kinase inhibitors (to inhibit tonic contraction of smooth-muscle cells mediated through endothelin). α1, α-adrenergic receptor; GPCR, G-protein–coupled receptor, GTP, guanosine triphosphate; PGE, prostaglandin E; PGF, prostaglandin F. ***B.*** Biochemical pathways of NO synthesis and action. Sildenafil, vardenafil, and tadalafil enhance erectile function by inhibiting phosphodiesterase type 5 (PDE-5), thereby maintaining high levels of cyclic 3′,5′-guanosine monophosphate (cyclic GMP). iCa^{2+}, intracellular calcium; NOS, nitric oxide synthase. *(Part A from K McVary: N Engl J Med 357:2472, 2007; with permission.)*

Ejaculation is stimulated by the sympathetic nervous system; this results in contraction of the epididymis, vas deferens, seminal vesicles, and prostate, causing seminal fluid to enter the urethra. Seminal fluid emission is followed by rhythmic contractions of the bulbocavernosus and ischiocavernosus muscles, leading to ejaculation. *Premature ejaculation* usually is related to anxiety or a learned behavior and is amenable to behavioral therapy or treatment with medications such as selective serotonin reuptake inhibitors (SSRIs). *Retrograde ejaculation* results when the internal urethral sphincter does not close; it may occur in men with diabetes or after surgery involving the bladder neck.

Detumescence is mediated by norepinephrine from the sympathetic nerves, endothelin from the vascular surface, and smooth-muscle contraction induced by postsynaptic α-adrenergic receptors and activation of Rho kinase. These events increase venous outflow and restore the flaccid state. Venous leak can cause premature detumescence and is caused by insufficient relaxation of the corporal smooth muscle rather than a specific anatomic defect. *Priapism* refers to a persistent and painful erection and may be associated with sickle cell anemia, hypercoagulable states, spinal cord injury, or injection of vasodilator agents into the penis.

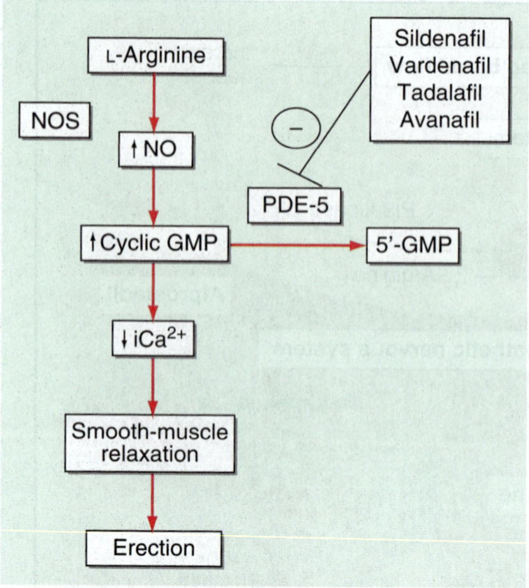

FIGURE 67-2 Biochemical pathways modified by phosphodiesterase type 5 (PDE-5) inhibitors. Sildenafil, vardenafil, tadalafil and avanafil enhance erectile function by inhibiting PDE-5, thereby maintaining high levels of cyclic 3′,5′-guanosine monophosphate (cyclic GMP). iCa^{2+}, intracellular calcium; NO, nitric oxide; NOS, nitric oxide synthase.

ERECTILE DYSFUNCTION

Epidemiology Erectile dysfunction (ED) is not considered a normal part of the aging process. Nonetheless, it is associated with certain physiologic and psychological changes related to age. In the Massachusetts Male Aging Study (MMAS), a community-based survey of men age 40–70, 52% of responders reported some degree of ED. Complete ED occurred in 10% of respondents, moderate ED in 25%, and minimal ED in 17%. The incidence of moderate or severe ED more than doubled between the ages of 40 and 70. In the National Health and Social Life Survey (NHSLS), which included a sample of men and women age 18–59, 10% of men reported being unable to maintain an erection (corresponding to the proportion of men in the MMAS reporting severe ED). Incidence was highest among men in the age group 50–59 (21%) and men who were poor (14%), divorced (14%), and less educated (13%).

The incidence of ED is also higher among men with certain medical disorders, such as diabetes mellitus, obesity, lower urinary tract symptoms secondary to benign prostatic hyperplasia (BPH), heart disease, hypertension, decreased high-density lipoprotein (HDL) levels, and diseases associated with general systemic inflammation (e.g., rheumatoid arthritis). Cardiovascular disease and ED share etiologies as well as pathophysiology (e.g., endothelial dysfunction), and the degree of ED appears to correlate with the severity of cardiovascular disease. Consequently, ED represents a "sentinel symptom" in patients with occult cardiovascular and peripheral vascular disease.

Smoking is also a significant risk factor in the development of ED. Medications used in treating diabetes or cardiovascular disease are additional risk factors (see below). There is a higher incidence of ED among men who have undergone radiation or surgery for prostate cancer and in those with a lower spinal cord injury. Psychological causes of ED include depression, anger, stress from unemployment, and other stress-related causes.

Pathophysiology ED may result from three basic mechanisms: (1) failure to initiate (psychogenic, endocrinologic, or neurogenic), (2) failure to fill (arteriogenic), and (3) failure to store adequate blood volume within the lacunar network (venoocclusive dysfunction). These categories are not mutually exclusive, and multiple factors contribute to ED in many patients. For example, diminished filling pressure can lead secondarily to venous leak. Psychogenic factors frequently coexist with other etiologic factors and should be considered in all cases. Diabetic, atherosclerotic, and drug-related causes account for >80% of cases of ED in older men.

VASCULOGENIC The most common organic cause of ED is a disturbance of blood flow to and from the penis. Atherosclerotic or traumatic arterial disease can decrease flow to the lacunar spaces, resulting in decreased rigidity and an increased time to full erection. Excessive outflow through the veins despite adequate inflow also may contribute to ED. Structural alterations to the fibroelastic components of the corpora may cause a loss of compliance and inability to compress the tunical veins. This condition may result from aging, increased cross-linking of collagen fibers induced by nonenzymatic glycosylation, hypoxemia, or altered synthesis of collagen associated with hypercholesterolemia.

NEUROGENIC Disorders that affect the sacral spinal cord or the autonomic fibers to the penis preclude nervous system relaxation of penile smooth muscle, thus leading to ED. In patients with spinal cord injury, the degree of ED depends on the completeness and level of the lesion. Patients with incomplete lesions or injuries to the upper part of the spinal cord are more likely to retain erectile capabilities than are those with complete lesions or injuries to the lower part. Although 75% of patients with spinal cord injuries have some erectile capability, only 25% have erections sufficient for penetration. Other neurologic disorders commonly associated with ED include multiple sclerosis and peripheral neuropathy. The latter is often due to either diabetes or alcoholism. Pelvic surgery may cause ED through disruption of the autonomic nerve supply.

ENDOCRINOLOGIC Androgens increase libido, but their exact role in erectile function is unclear. Individuals with castrate levels of testosterone can achieve erections from visual or sexual stimuli. Nonetheless, normal levels of testosterone appear to be important for erectile function, particularly in older males. Androgen replacement therapy can improve depressed erectile function when it is secondary to hypogonadism; however, it is not useful for ED when endogenous testosterone levels are normal. Increased prolactin may decrease libido by suppressing gonadotropin-releasing hormone (GnRH), and it also leads to decreased testosterone levels. Treatment of hyperprolactinemia with dopamine agonists can restore libido and testosterone.

DIABETIC ED occurs in 35–75% of men with diabetes mellitus. Pathologic mechanisms are related primarily to diabetes-associated vascular and neurologic complications. Diabetic macrovascular complications are related mainly to age, whereas microvascular complications correlate with the duration of diabetes and the degree of glycemic control (Chap. 417). Individuals with diabetes also have reduced amounts of nitric oxide synthase in both endothelial and neural tissues.

PSYCHOGENIC Two mechanisms contribute to the inhibition of erections in psychogenic ED. First, psychogenic stimuli to the sacral cord may inhibit reflexogenic responses, thereby blocking activation of vasodilator outflow to the penis. Second, excess sympathetic stimulation in an anxious man may increase penile smooth-muscle tone. The most common causes of psychogenic ED are performance anxiety, depression, relationship conflict, loss of attraction, sexual inhibition, conflicts over sexual preference, sexual abuse in childhood, and fear of pregnancy or sexually transmitted disease. Almost all patients with ED, even when it has a clear-cut organic basis, develop a psychogenic component as a reaction to ED.

MEDICATION-RELATED Medication-induced ED (Table 67-1) is estimated to occur in 25% of men seen in general medical outpatient clinics. The adverse effects related to drug therapy are additive, especially in older men. In addition to the drug itself, the disease being treated is likely to contribute to sexual dysfunction. Among the antihypertensive agents, the thiazide diuretics and beta blockers have been implicated most frequently. Calcium channel blockers and angiotensin converting-enzyme inhibitors are cited less frequently. These drugs may act directly at the corporal level (e.g., calcium channel blockers) or indirectly by reducing pelvic blood pressure, which is important in the development of penile rigidity. α-Adrenergic blockers are less likely to

TABLE 67-1 DRUGS ASSOCIATED WITH ERECTILE DYSFUNCTION

Classification	Drugs
Diuretics	Thiazides
	Spironolactone
Antihypertensives	Calcium channel blockers
	Methyldopa
	Clonidine
	Reserpine
	Beta blockers
	Guanethidine
Cardiac/antihyperlipidemics	Digoxin
	Gemfibrozil
	Clofibrate
Antidepressants	Selective serotonin reuptake inhibitors
	Tricyclic antidepressants
	Lithium
	Monoamine oxidase inhibitors
Tranquilizers	Butyrophenones
	Phenothiazines
H_2 antagonists	Ranitidine
	Cimetidine
Hormones	Progesterone
	Estrogens
	Corticosteroids
	GnRH agonists
	5α-Reductase inhibitors
	Cyproterone acetate
Cytotoxic agents	Cyclophosphamide
	Methotrexate
	Roferon-A
Anticholinergics	Disopyramide
	Anticonvulsants
Recreational	Ethanol
	Cocaine
	Marijuana

Abbreviation: GnRH, gonadotropin-releasing hormone.

cause ED. Estrogens, GnRH agonists, H_2 antagonists, and spironolactone cause ED by suppressing gonadotropin production or by blocking androgen action. Antidepressant and antipsychotic agents—particularly neuroleptics, tricyclics, and SSRIs—are associated with erectile, ejaculatory, orgasmic, and sexual desire difficulties.

If there is a strong association between the institution of a drug and the onset of ED, alternative medications should be considered. Otherwise, it is often practical to treat the ED without attempting multiple changes in medications, as it may be difficult to establish a causal role for a drug.

APPROACH TO THE PATIENT: Erectile Dysfunction

A good physician-patient relationship helps unravel the possible causes of ED, many of which require discussion of personal and sometimes embarrassing topics. For this reason, a primary care provider is often ideally suited to initiate the evaluation. However, a significant percentage of men experience ED and remain undiagnosed unless specifically questioned about this issue. By far the two most common reasons for underreporting of ED are patient embarrassment and perceptions of physicians' inattention to the disease. Once the topic is initiated by the physician, patients are more willing to discuss their potency issues. A complete medical and sexual history should be taken in an effort to assess whether the cause of ED is organic, psychogenic, or multifactorial (Fig. 67-3).

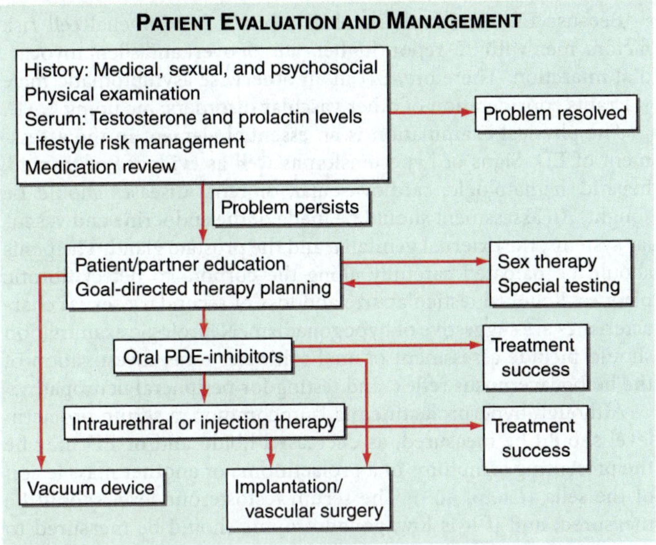

FIGURE 67-3 Algorithm for the evaluation and management of patients with erectile dysfunction. PDE, phosphodiesterase.

Both the patient and his sexual partner should be interviewed regarding sexual history. ED should be distinguished from other sexual problems, such as premature ejaculation. Lifestyle factors such as sexual orientation, the patient's distress from ED, performance anxiety, and details of sexual techniques should be addressed. Standardized questionnaires are available to assess ED, including the International Index of Erectile Function (IIEF) and the more easily administered Sexual Health Inventory for Men (SHIM), a validated abridged version of the IIEF.

The initial evaluation of ED begins with a review of the patient's medical, surgical, sexual, and psychosocial histories. The history should note whether the patient has experienced pelvic trauma, surgery, or radiation. In light of the increasing recognition of the relationship between lower urinary tract symptoms and ED, it is advisable to evaluate for the presence of symptoms of bladder outlet obstruction. Questions should focus on the onset of symptoms, the presence and duration of partial erections, and the progression of ED. A history of nocturnal or early morning erections is useful for distinguishing physiologic ED from psychogenic ED. Nocturnal erections occur during rapid eye movement (REM) sleep and require intact neurologic and circulatory systems. Organic causes of ED generally are characterized by a gradual and persistent change in rigidity or the inability to sustain nocturnal, coital, or self-stimulated erections. The patient should be questioned about the presence of penile curvature or pain with coitus. It is also important to address libido, as decreased sexual drive and ED are sometimes the earliest signs of endocrine abnormalities (e.g., increased prolactin, decreased testosterone levels). It is useful to ask whether the problem is confined to coitus with one partner or also involves other partners; ED not uncommonly arises in association with new or extramarital sexual relationships. Situational ED, as opposed to consistent ED, suggests psychogenic causes. Ejaculation is much less commonly affected than erection, but questions should be asked about whether ejaculation is normal, premature, delayed, or absent. Relevant risk factors should be identified, such as diabetes mellitus, coronary artery disease (CAD), and neurologic disorders. The patient's surgical history should be explored with an emphasis on bowel, bladder, prostate, and vascular procedures. A complete drug history is also important. Social changes that may precipitate ED are also crucial to the evaluation, including health worries, spousal death, divorce, relationship difficulties, and financial concerns.

Because ED commonly involves a host of endothelial cell risk factors, men with ED report higher rates of overt and silent myocardial infarction. Therefore, ED in an otherwise asymptomatic male warrants consideration of other vascular disorders, including CAD.

The physical examination is an essential element in the assessment of ED. Signs of hypertension as well as evidence of thyroid, hepatic, hematologic, cardiovascular, or renal diseases should be sought. An assessment should be made of the endocrine and vascular systems, the external genitalia, and the prostate gland. The penis should be palpated carefully along the corpora to detect fibrotic plaques. Reduced testicular size and loss of secondary sexual characteristics are suggestive of hypogonadism. Neurologic examination should include assessment of anal sphincter tone, investigation of the bulbocavernosus reflex, and testing for peripheral neuropathy.

Although hyperprolactinemia is uncommon, a serum prolactin level should be measured, as decreased libido and/or ED may be the presenting symptoms of a prolactinoma or another mass lesion of the sella (Chap. 403). The serum testosterone level should be measured, and if it is low, gonadotropins should be measured to determine whether hypogonadism is primary (testicular) or secondary (hypothalamic-pituitary) in origin (Chap. 411). If not performed recently, serum chemistries, complete blood count (CBC), and lipid profiles may be of value, as they can yield evidence of anemia, diabetes, hyperlipidemia, or other systemic diseases associated with ED. Determination of serum prostate-specific antigen (PSA) should be conducted according to recommended clinical guidelines (Chap. 115).

Additional diagnostic testing is rarely necessary in the evaluation of ED. However, in selected patients, specialized testing may provide insight into pathologic mechanisms of ED and aid in the selection of treatment options. Optional specialized testing includes (1) studies of nocturnal penile tumescence and rigidity, (2) vascular testing (in-office injection of vasoactive substances, penile Doppler ultrasound, penile angiography, dynamic infusion cavernosography/cavernosometry), (3) neurologic testing (biothesiometry-graded vibratory perception, somatosensory evoked potentials), and (4) psychological diagnostic tests. The information potentially gained from these procedures must be balanced against their invasiveness and cost.

TREATMENT MALE SEXUAL DYSFUNCTION

PATIENT EDUCATION

Patient and partner education is essential in the treatment of ED. In goal-directed therapy, education facilitates understanding of the disease, the results of the tests, and the selection of treatment. Discussion of treatment options helps clarify how treatment is best offered and stratify first- and second-line therapies. Patients with high-risk lifestyle issues such as obesity, smoking, alcohol abuse, and recreational drug use should be counseled on the role those factors play in the development of ED.

Therapies currently employed for the treatment of ED include oral PDE-5 inhibitor therapy (most commonly used), injection therapies, testosterone therapy, penile devices, and psychological therapy. In addition, limited data suggest that treatments for underlying risk factors and comorbidities—for example, weight loss, exercise, stress reduction, and smoking cessation—may improve erectile function. Decisions regarding therapy should take into account the preferences and expectations of patients and their partners.

ORAL AGENTS

Sildenafil, tadalafil, vardenafil, and avanafil are the only approved and effective oral agents for the treatment of ED. These four medications have markedly improved the management of ED because they are effective for the treatment of a broad range of causes, including psychogenic, diabetic, vasculogenic, post-radical prostatectomy (nerve-sparing procedures), and spinal cord injury. They belong to a class of medications that are selective and potent inhibitors of PDE-5, the predominant phosphodiesterase isoform found in the penis. They are administered in graduated doses and enhance erections after sexual stimulation. The onset of action is approximately 30–120 min, depending on the medication used and other factors, such as recent food intake. Reduced initial doses should be considered for patients who are elderly, are taking concomitant alpha blockers, have renal insufficiency, or are taking medications that inhibit the CYP3A4 metabolic pathway in the liver (e.g., erythromycin, cimetidine, ketoconazole, and possibly itraconazole and mibefradil), as they may increase the serum concentration of the PDE-5 inhibitors (PDE-5i) or promote hypotension.

Initially, there were concerns about the cardiovascular safety of PDE-5i drugs. These agents can act as a mild vasodilator, and warnings exist about orthostatic hypotension with concomitant use of alpha blockers. The use of PDE-5i is not contraindicated in men who are also receiving alpha blockers, but they must be stabilized on this blood pressure medication prior to initiating therapy. Concerns also existed that use of PDE-5i would increase cardiovascular events. However, the safety of these drugs has been confirmed in several controlled trials with no increase in myocardial ischemic events or overall mortality compared to the general population.

Several randomized trials have demonstrated the efficacy of this class of medications. There are no compelling data to support the superiority of one PDE-5i over another. Subtle differences between agents have variable clinical relevance (Table 67-2).

Patients may fail to respond to a PDE-5i for several reasons (Table 67-3). Some patients may not tolerate PDE-5i secondary to adverse events from vasodilation in nonpenile tissues expressing PDE-5 or from the inhibition of homologous nonpenile isozymes (i.e., PDE-6 found in the retina). Abnormal vision attributed to the effects of PDE-5i on retinal PDE-6 is of short duration, reported only with sildenafil and not thought to be clinically significant. A more serious concern is the possibility that PDE-5i may cause nonarteritic anterior ischemic optic neuropathy; although data to support that association are limited, it is prudent to avoid the use of these agents in men with a prior history of nonarteritic anterior ischemic optic neuropathy.

Testosterone supplementation combined with a PDE-5i may be beneficial in improving erectile function in hypogonadal men with ED who are unresponsive to PDE-5i alone. These drugs do not affect ejaculation, orgasm, or sexual drive. Side effects associated with PDE-5i include headaches (19%), facial flushing (9%), dyspepsia (6%), and nasal congestion (4%). Approximately 7% of men using sildenafil may experience transient altered color vision (blue halo effect), and 6% of men taking tadalafil may experience loin pain. PDE-5i is contraindicated in men receiving nitrate therapy for cardiovascular disease, including agents delivered by the oral, sublingual, transnasal, and topical routes. These agents can potentiate its hypotensive effect and may result in profound shock. Likewise, amyl/butyl nitrate "poppers" may have a fatal synergistic effect on blood pressure. PDE-5i also should be avoided in patients with congestive heart failure and cardiomyopathy because of the risk of vascular collapse. Because sexual activity leads to an increase in physiologic expenditure (5–6 metabolic equivalents [METS]), physicians have been advised to exercise caution in prescribing any drug for sexual activity to those with active coronary disease, heart failure, borderline hypotension, or hypovolemia and to those on complex antihypertensive regimens.

Although the various forms of PDE-5i have a common mechanism of action, there are a few differences among the four agents (Table 67-2). Tadalafil is unique in its longer half-life, whereas avanafil appears to have the most rapid onset of action. All four drugs are effective for patients with ED of all ages, severities, and etiologies. Although there are pharmacokinetic and pharmacodynamic differences among these agents, clinically relevant differences are not clear.

ANDROGEN THERAPY

Testosterone replacement is used to treat both primary and secondary causes of hypogonadism (Chap. 411). Androgen supplementation

TABLE 67-2 CHARACTERISTICS OF PDE-5i MEDICATIONS

Drug	Onset of Action	Half-Life	Dose	Adverse Effects	Contraindications
Sildenafil	T_{max}, 30-120 min Duration, 4 h High-fat meal decreases absorption ETOH may affect efficacy	2–5 h	25–100 mg Starting dose, 50 mg	Headache, flushing, dyspepsia, nasal congestion, altered vision	Nitrates Hypotension Cardiovascular risk factors Retinitis pigmentosa Change dose with some antiretrovirals Should be on stable dose of alpha blockers
Vardenafil	T_{max}, 30–120 min Duration, 4–5 h High-fat meal decreases absorption ETOH may affect efficacy	4.5 h	5–10 mg	Headache, flushing, rhinitis, dyspepsia	Same as sildenafil May have minor prolongation of QT interval Concomitant use of Class I antiarrhythmic
Tadalafil	T_{max}, 30–60 min Duration, 12–36 h Plasma concentration Not affected by food or ETOH	17.5 h	10 mg, 20 mg; 2.5 or 5 mg for daily dose	Headache, dyspepsia, back pain, nasal congestion, myalgia	Same as sildenafil
Avanafil	T_{max}, 30 min Duration, 2 h Plasma concentration not affected by food	3–5 h	50, 100, and 200 mg	Headache, flushing, nasal congestion, nasopharyngitis, back pain	Same as sildenafil

Abbreviations: ETOH, alcohol; T_{max}, time to maximum plasma concentration.

in the setting of normal testosterone is rarely efficacious in the treatment of ED and is discouraged. Methods of androgen replacement include transdermal patches and gels, parenteral administration of long-acting testosterone esters (enanthate and cypionate), and oral preparations (17 α-alkylated derivatives) (Chap. 411). Oral androgen preparations have the potential for hepatotoxicity and should be avoided.

Men who receive testosterone should be reevaluated after 1–3 months and at least annually thereafter for testosterone levels, erectile function, and adverse effects, which may include gynecomastia, sleep apnea, development or exacerbation of lower urinary tract symptoms or BPH, prostate cancer, lowering of HDL, erythrocytosis, elevations of liver function tests, and reduced fertility. Periodic reevaluation should include measurement of CBC and PSA and digital rectal exam. Therapy should be discontinued in patients who do not respond within 3 months.

VACUUM CONSTRICTION DEVICES

Vacuum constriction devices (VCDs) are a well-established noninvasive therapy. They are a reasonable treatment alternative for select patients who cannot take sildenafil or do not desire other interventions. VCDs draw venous blood into the penis and use a constriction ring to restrict venous return and maintain tumescence. Adverse events with VCD include pain, numbness, bruising, and altered ejaculation. Additionally, many patients complain that the devices are cumbersome and that the induced erections have a nonphysiologic appearance and feel.

INTRAURETHRAL ALPROSTADIL

If a patient fails to respond to oral agents, a reasonable next choice is intraurethral or self-injection of vasoactive substances.

TABLE 67-3 ISSUES TO CONSIDER IF PATIENTS REPORT FAILURE OF PDE-5i TO IMPROVE ERECTILE DYSFUNCTION

- A trial of medication on at least 6 different days at the maximal dose should be made before declaring patient nonresponsive to PDE-5i use
- Confirm that patient did not take medication after a high-fat meal
- Failure to include physical and psychic stimulation at the time of foreplay to induce endogenous NO
- Unrecognized hypogonadism

Abbreviations: NO, nitric oxide; PDE-5i, phosphodiesterase type 5 inhibitor.

Intraurethral prostaglandin E_1 (alprostadil), in the form of a semisolid pellet (doses of 125–1000 μg), is delivered with an applicator. Approximately 65% of men receiving intraurethral alprostadil respond with an erection when tested in the office, but only 50% achieve successful coitus at home. Intraurethral insertion is associated with a markedly reduced incidence of priapism in comparison to intracavernosal injection.

INTRACAVERNOSAL SELF-INJECTION

Injection of synthetic formulations of alprostadil is effective in 70–80% of patients with ED, but discontinuation rates are high because of the invasive nature of administration. Doses range between 1 and 40 μg. Injection therapy is contraindicated in men with a history of hypersensitivity to the drug and men at risk for priapism (hypercoagulable states, sickle cell disease). Side effects include local adverse events, prolonged erections, pain, and fibrosis with chronic use. Various combinations of alprostadil, phentolamine, and/or papaverine sometimes are used.

SURGERY

A less frequently used form of therapy for ED involves the surgical implantation of a semirigid or inflatable penile prosthesis. The choice of prosthesis is dependent on patient preference and should take into account body habitus and manual dexterity, which may affect the ability of the patient to manipulate the device. Because of the permanence of prosthetic devices, patients should be advised to first consider less invasive options for treatment. These surgical treatments are invasive, are associated with potential complications, and generally are reserved for treatment of refractory ED. Despite their high cost and invasiveness, penile prostheses are associated with high rates of patient and partner satisfaction.

SEX THERAPY

A course of sex therapy may be useful for addressing specific interpersonal factors that may affect sexual functioning. Sex therapy generally consists of in-session discussion and at-home exercises specific to the person and the relationship. Psychosexual therapy involves techniques such as sensate focus (nongenital massage), sensory awareness exercises, correction of misconceptions about sexuality, and interpersonal difficulties therapy (e.g., open communication about sexual issues, physical intimacy scheduling, and behavioral interventions). These approaches may be useful in patients who have psychogenic or social components to their ED, although data from randomized trials are scanty and inconsistent. It is preferable if therapy includes both partners if the patient is involved in an ongoing relationship.

FEMALE SEXUAL DYSFUNCTION

Female sexual dysfunction (FSD) has traditionally included disorders of desire, arousal, pain, and muted orgasm. The associated risk factors for FSD are similar to those in males: cardiovascular disease, endocrine disorders, hypertension, neurologic disorders, and smoking (Table 67-4).

EPIDEMIOLOGY

Epidemiologic data are limited, but the available estimates suggest that as many as 43% of women complain of at least one sexual problem. Despite the recent interest in organic causes of FSD, desire and arousal phase disorders (including lubrication complaints) remain the most common presenting problems when surveyed in a community-based population.

PHYSIOLOGY OF THE FEMALE SEXUAL RESPONSE

The female sexual response requires the presence of estrogens. A role for androgens is also likely but less well established. In the CNS, estrogens and androgens work synergistically to enhance sexual arousal and response. A number of studies report enhanced libido in women during preovulatory phases of the menstrual cycle, suggesting that hormones involved in the ovulatory surge (e.g., estrogens) increase desire.

Sexual motivation is heavily influenced by context, including the environment and partner factors. Once sufficient sexual desire is reached, sexual arousal is mediated by the central and autonomic nervous systems. Cerebral sympathetic outflow is thought to increase desire, and peripheral parasympathetic activity results in clitoral vasocongestion and vaginal secretion (lubrication).

The neurotransmitters for clitoral corporal engorgement are similar to those in the male, with a prominent role for neural, smooth-muscle, and endothelial released nitric oxide (NO). A fine network of vaginal nerves and arterioles promotes a vaginal transudate. The major transmitters of this complex vaginal response are not certain, but roles for NO and vasointestinal polypeptide (VIP) are suspected. Investigators studying the normal female sexual response have challenged the long-held construct of a linear and unmitigated relationship between initial desire, arousal, vasocongestion, lubrication, and eventual orgasm. Caregivers should consider a paradigm of a positive emotional and physical outcome with one, many, or no orgasmic peak and release.

Although there are anatomic differences as well as variation in the density of vascular and neural beds in males and females, the primary effectors of sexual response are strikingly similar. Intact sensation is important for arousal. Thus, reduced levels of sexual functioning are more common in women with peripheral neuropathies (e.g., diabetes). Vaginal lubrication is a transudate of serum that results from the increased pelvic blood flow associated with arousal. Vascular insufficiency from a variety of causes may compromise adequate lubrication and result in dyspareunia. Cavernosal and arteriole smooth-muscle relaxation occurs via increased nitric oxide synthase (NOS) activity and produces engorgement in the clitoris and the surrounding vestibule. Orgasm requires an intact sympathetic outflow tract; hence, orgasmic disorders are common in female patients with spinal cord injuries.

TABLE 67-4 RISK FACTORS FOR FEMALE SEXUAL DYSFUNCTION

Neurologic disease: stroke, spinal cord injury, parkinsonism
Trauma, genital surgery, radiation
Endocrinopathies: diabetes, hyperprolactinemia
Liver and/or renal failure
Cardiovascular disease
Psychological factors and interpersonal relationship disorders: sexual abuse, life stressors
Medications
Antiandrogens: cimetidine, spironolactone
Antidepressants, alcohol, hypnotics, sedatives
Antiestrogens or GnRH antagonists
Antihistamines, sympathomimetic amines
Antihypertensives: diuretics, calcium channel blockers
Alkylating agents
Anticholinergics

Abbreviation: GnRH, gonadotropin-releasing hormone.

APPROACH TO THE PATIENT: Female Sexual Dysfunction

Many women do not volunteer information about their sexual response. Open-ended questions in a supportive atmosphere are helpful in initiating a discussion of sexual fitness in women who are reluctant to discuss such issues. Once a complaint has been voiced, a comprehensive evaluation should be performed, including a medical history, a psychosocial history, a physical examination, and limited laboratory testing.

The history should include the usual medical, surgical, obstetric, psychological, gynecologic, sexual, and social information. Past experiences, intimacy, knowledge, and partner availability should also be ascertained. Medical disorders that may affect sexual health should be delineated. They include diabetes, cardiovascular disease, gynecologic conditions, obstetric history, depression, anxiety disorders, and neurologic disease. Medications should be reviewed as they may affect arousal, libido, and orgasm. The need for counseling and recognizing life stresses should be identified. The physical examination should assess the genitalia, including the clitoris. Pelvic floor examination may identify prolapse or other disorders. Laboratory studies are needed, especially if menopausal status is uncertain. Estradiol, follicle-stimulating hormone (FSH), and luteinizing hormone (LH) are usually obtained, and dehydroepiandrosterone (DHEA) should be considered as it reflects adrenal androgen secretion. A CBC, liver function assessment, and lipid studies may be useful, if not otherwise obtained. Complicated diagnostic evaluations such as clitoral Doppler ultrasonography and biothesiometry require expensive equipment and are of uncertain utility. It is important for the patient to identify which symptoms are most distressing.

The evaluation of FSD previously occurred mainly in a psychosocial context. However, inconsistencies between diagnostic categories based only on psychosocial considerations and the emerging recognition of organic etiologies have led to a new classification of FSD. This diagnostic scheme is based on four components that are not mutually exclusive: (1) *hypoactive sexual desire*—the persistent or recurrent lack of sexual thoughts and/or receptivity to sexual activity, which causes personal distress; hypoactive sexual desire may result from endocrine failure or may be associated with psychological or emotional disorders; (2) *sexual arousal disorder*—the persistent or recurrent inability to attain or maintain sexual excitement, which causes personal distress; (3) *orgasmic disorder*—the persistent or recurrent loss of orgasmic potential after sufficient sexual stimulation and arousal, which causes personal distress; and (4) *sexual pain disorder*—persistent or recurrent genital pain associated with noncoital sexual stimulation, which causes personal distress. This newer classification emphasizes "personal distress" as a requirement for dysfunction and provides clinicians with an organized framework for evaluation before or in conjunction with more traditional counseling methods.

TREATMENT FEMALE SEXUAL DYSFUNCTION

GENERAL

An open discussion with the patient is important as couples may need to be educated about normal anatomy and physiologic responses, including the role of orgasm, in sexual encounters. Physiologic changes associated with aging and/or disease should be explained. Couples may need to be reminded that clitoral stimulation rather than coital intromission may be more beneficial.

Behavioral modification and nonpharmacologic therapies should be a first step. Patient and partner counseling may improve communication and relationship strains. Lifestyle changes involving known risk factors can be an important part of the treatment process. Emphasis on maximizing physical health and avoiding lifestyles (e.g., smoking, alcohol abuse) and medications likely to produce FSD is important (Table 67-4). The use of topical lubricants may address complaints of dyspareunia and dryness. Contributing medications such as antidepressants may need to be altered, including the use of medications with less impact on sexual function, dose reduction, medication switching, or drug holidays.

HORMONAL THERAPY

In postmenopausal women, estrogen replacement therapy may be helpful in treating vaginal atrophy, decreasing coital pain, and improving clitoral sensitivity (Chap. 413). Estrogen replacement in the form of local cream is the preferred method, as it avoids systemic side effects. Androgen levels in women decline substantially before menopause. However, low levels of testosterone or DHEA are not effective predictors of a positive therapeutic outcome with androgen therapy. The widespread use of exogenous androgens is not supported by the literature except in select circumstances (premature ovarian failure or menopausal states) and in secondary arousal disorders.

ORAL AGENTS

The efficacy of PDE-5i in FDS has been a marked disappointment in light of the proposed role of nitric oxide–dependent physiology in the normal female sexual response. The use of PDE-5i for FSD should be discouraged pending proof that it is effective.

CLITORAL VACUUM DEVICE

In patients with arousal and orgasmic difficulties, the option of using a clitoral vacuum device may be explored. This handheld battery-operated device has a small soft plastic cup that applies a vacuum over the stimulated clitoris. This causes increased cavernosal blood flow, engorgement, and vaginal lubrication.

68 Hirsutism

David A. Ehrmann

Hirsutism, which is defined as androgen-dependent excessive male-pattern hair growth, affects approximately 10% of women. Hirsutism is most often idiopathic or the consequence of androgen excess associated with the polycystic ovarian syndrome (PCOS). Less frequently, it may result from adrenal androgen overproduction as occurs in nonclassic congenital adrenal hyperplasia (CAH) (Table 68-1). Rarely, it is a sign of a serious underlying condition. Cutaneous manifestations commonly associated with hirsutism include acne and male-pattern balding (androgenic alopecia). *Virilization* refers to a condition in which androgen levels are sufficiently high to cause additional signs and symptoms, such as deepening of the voice, breast atrophy, increased muscle bulk, clitoromegaly, and increased libido; virilization is an ominous sign that suggests the possibility of an ovarian or adrenal neoplasm.

TABLE 68-1 CAUSES OF HIRSUTISM

Gonadal hyperandrogenism
Ovarian hyperandrogenism
Polycystic ovary syndrome/functional ovarian hyperandrogenism
Ovarian steroidogenic blocks
Syndromes of extreme insulin resistance (e.g., lipodystrophy)
Ovarian neoplasms
Adrenal hyperandrogenism
Premature adrenarche
Functional adrenal hyperandrogenism
Congenital adrenal hyperplasia (nonclassic and classic)
Abnormal cortisol action/metabolism
Adrenal neoplasms
Other endocrine disorders
Cushing's syndrome
Hyperprolactinemia
Acromegaly
Peripheral androgen overproduction
Obesity
Idiopathic
Pregnancy-related hyperandrogenism
Hyperreactio luteinalis
Thecoma of pregnancy
Drugs
Androgens
Oral contraceptives containing androgenic progestins
Minoxidil
Phenytoin
Diazoxide
Cyclosporine
True hermaphroditism

HAIR FOLLICLE GROWTH AND DIFFERENTIATION

Hair can be categorized as either *vellus* (fine, soft, and not pigmented) or *terminal* (long, coarse, and pigmented). The number of hair follicles does not change over an individual's lifetime, but the follicle size and type of hair can change in response to numerous factors, particularly androgens. Androgens are necessary for terminal hair and sebaceous gland development and mediate differentiation of pilosebaceous units (PSUs) into either a terminal hair follicle or a sebaceous gland. In the former case, androgens transform the vellus hair into a terminal hair; in the latter case, the sebaceous component proliferates and the hair remains vellus.

There are three phases in the cycle of hair growth: (1) *anagen* (growth phase), (2) *catagen* (involution phase), and (3) *telogen* (rest phase). Depending on the body site, hormonal regulation may play an important role in the hair growth cycle. For example, the eyebrows, eyelashes, and vellus hairs are androgen-insensitive, whereas the axillary and pubic areas are sensitive to low levels of androgens. Hair growth on the face, chest, upper abdomen, and back requires higher levels of androgens and is therefore more characteristic of the pattern typically seen in men. Androgen excess in women leads to increased hair growth in most androgen-sensitive sites except in the scalp region, where hair loss occurs because androgens cause scalp hairs to spend less time in the anagen phase.

Although androgen excess underlies most cases of hirsutism, there is only a modest correlation between androgen levels and the quantity of hair growth. This is due to the fact that hair growth from the follicle also depends on local growth factors, and there is variability in end organ (PSU) sensitivity. Genetic factors and ethnic background also influence hair growth. In general, dark-haired individuals tend to be more hirsute than blond or fair individuals. Asians and Native Americans have relatively sparse hair in regions sensitive to high androgen levels, whereas people of Mediterranean descent are more hirsute.

CLINICAL ASSESSMENT

Historic elements relevant to the assessment of hirsutism include the age at onset and rate of progression of hair growth and associated symptoms or signs (e.g., acne). Depending on the cause, excess hair growth typically is first noted during the second and third decades of life. The growth is usually slow but progressive. Sudden development and rapid progression of hirsutism suggest the possibility of an androgen-secreting neoplasm, in which case virilization also may be present.

The age at onset of menstrual cycles (menarche) and the pattern of the menstrual cycle should be ascertained; irregular cycles from the time of menarche onward are more likely to result from ovarian rather than adrenal androgen excess. Associated symptoms such as galactorrhea should prompt evaluation for hyperprolactinemia (Chap. 403) and possibly hypothyroidism (Chap. 405). Hypertension, striae, easy bruising, centripetal weight gain, and weakness suggest hypercortisolism (Cushing's syndrome; Chap. 406). Rarely, patients with growth hormone excess (i.e., acromegaly) present with hirsutism. Use of medications such as phenytoin, minoxidil, and cyclosporine may be associated with androgen-independent excess hair growth (i.e., hypertrichosis). A family history of infertility and/or hirsutism may indicate disorders such as nonclassic CAH (Chap. 406). Lipodystrophy is often associated with increased ovarian androgen production that occurs as a consequence of insulin resistance. Patients with lipodystrophy have a preponderance of central fat distribution together with scant subcutaneous adipose tissue in the upper and lower extremities.

Physical examination should include measurement of height and weight and calculation of body mass index (BMI). A BMI >25 kg/m^2 is indicative of excess weight for height, and values >30 kg/m^2 are often seen in association with hirsutism, probably the result of increased conversion of androgen precursors to testosterone. Notation should be made of blood pressure, as adrenal causes may be associated with hypertension. Cutaneous signs sometimes associated with androgen excess and insulin resistance include acanthosis nigricans and skin tags. Body fat distribution should also be noted.

An objective clinical assessment of hair distribution and quantity is central to the evaluation in any woman presenting with hirsutism. This assessment permits the distinction between hirsutism and hypertrichosis and provides a baseline reference point to gauge the response to treatment. A simple and commonly used method to grade hair growth is the modified scale of Ferriman and Gallwey (Fig. 68-1), in which each of nine androgen-sensitive sites is graded from 0 to 4. Approximately 95% of white women have a score below 8 on this scale; thus, it is normal for most women to have some hair growth in androgen-sensitive sites. Scores above 8 suggest excess androgen-mediated hair growth, a finding that should be assessed further by means of hormonal evaluation (see below). In racial/ethnic groups that are less likely to manifest hirsutism (e.g., Asian women), additional cutaneous evidence of androgen excess should be sought, including pustular acne and thinning scalp hair.

HORMONAL EVALUATION

Androgens are secreted by the ovaries and adrenal glands in response to their respective tropic hormones: luteinizing hormone (LH) and adrenocorticotropic hormone (ACTH). The principal circulating steroids involved in the etiology of hirsutism are testosterone, androstenedione, and dehydroepiandrosterone (DHEA) and its sulfated form (DHEAS). The ovaries and adrenal glands normally contribute about equally to testosterone production. Approximately half of the total testosterone originates from direct glandular secretion, and the remainder is derived from the peripheral conversion of androstenedione and DHEA (Chap. 411).

Although it is the most important circulating androgen, testosterone is in effect the penultimate androgen in mediating hirsutism; it is converted to the more potent dihydrotestosterone (DHT) by the enzyme 5α-reductase, which is located in the PSU. DHT has a higher affinity for, and slower dissociation from, the androgen receptor. The local production of DHT allows it to serve as the primary mediator of androgen action at the level of the pilosebaceous unit. There are two isoenzymes of 5α-reductase: Type 2 is found in the prostate gland and in hair follicles, and type 1 is found primarily in sebaceous glands.

One approach to the evaluation of hirsutism is depicted in Fig. 68-2. In addition to measuring blood levels of testosterone and DHEAS, it is important to measure the level of free (or unbound) testosterone. The fraction of testosterone that is not bound to its carrier protein, sex hormone–binding globulin (SHBG), is biologically available for conversion to DHT and binding to androgen receptors. Hyperinsulinemia and/or androgen excess decrease hepatic production of SHBG, resulting in levels of total testosterone within the high-normal range, whereas the unbound hormone is elevated more substantially. Although there is a decline in ovarian testosterone production after menopause, ovarian estrogen production decreases to an even greater extent, and the concentration of SHBG is reduced. Consequently, there is an increase in the relative proportion of unbound testosterone, and it may exacerbate hirsutism after menopause.

A baseline plasma total testosterone level >12 nmol/L (>3.5 ng/mL) usually indicates a virilizing tumor, whereas a level >7 nmol/L (>2 ng/mL) is suggestive. A basal DHEAS level >18.5 μmol/L (>7000 μg/L) suggests an adrenal tumor. Although DHEAS has been proposed as a "marker" of predominant adrenal androgen excess, it is not unusual to find modest elevations in DHEAS among women with PCOS. Computed tomography (CT) or magnetic resonance imaging (MRI) should be used to localize an adrenal mass, and transvaginal ultrasound usually suffices to identify an ovarian mass if clinical evaluation and hormonal levels suggest these possibilities.

PCOS is the most common cause of ovarian androgen excess (Chap. 412). An increased ratio of LH to follicle-stimulating hormone (FSH) is characteristic in carefully studied patients with PCOS. However, because of the pulsatile nature of gonadotropin secretion, this finding may be absent in up to half of women with PCOS. Therefore, measurement of plasma LH and FSH is not needed to make a diagnosis of PCOS. Transvaginal ultrasound classically shows enlarged ovaries and increased stroma in women with PCOS. However, cystic ovaries also may be found in women without clinical or laboratory features of PCOS.

It has been suggested that the measurement of circulating levels of antimüllerian hormone (AMH) may help in making the diagnosis of PCOS; however, this remains controversial. AMH levels reflect ovarian reserve and correlate with follicular number. Measurement of AMH can be useful when considering premature ovarian insufficiency in a patient who presents with oligomenorrhea, in which case a subnormal level of AMH will be present.

Because adrenal androgens are readily suppressed by low doses of glucocorticoids, the dexamethasone androgen-suppression test may broadly distinguish ovarian from adrenal androgen overproduction. A blood sample is obtained before and after the administration of dexamethasone (0.5 mg orally every 6 h for 4 days). An adrenal source is suggested by suppression of unbound testosterone into the normal range; incomplete suppression suggests ovarian androgen excess. An overnight 1-mg dexamethasone suppression test, with measurement of 8:00 a.m. serum cortisol, is useful when there is clinical suspicion of Cushing's syndrome (Chap. 406).

Nonclassic CAH is most commonly due to 21-hydroxylase deficiency but also can be caused by autosomal recessive defects in other steroidogenic enzymes necessary for adrenal corticosteroid synthesis (Chap. 406). Because of the enzyme defect, the adrenal gland cannot secrete glucocorticoids (especially cortisol) efficiently. This results in diminished negative feedback inhibition of ACTH, leading to compensatory adrenal hyperplasia and the accumulation of steroid precursors that subsequently are converted to androgen. Deficiency

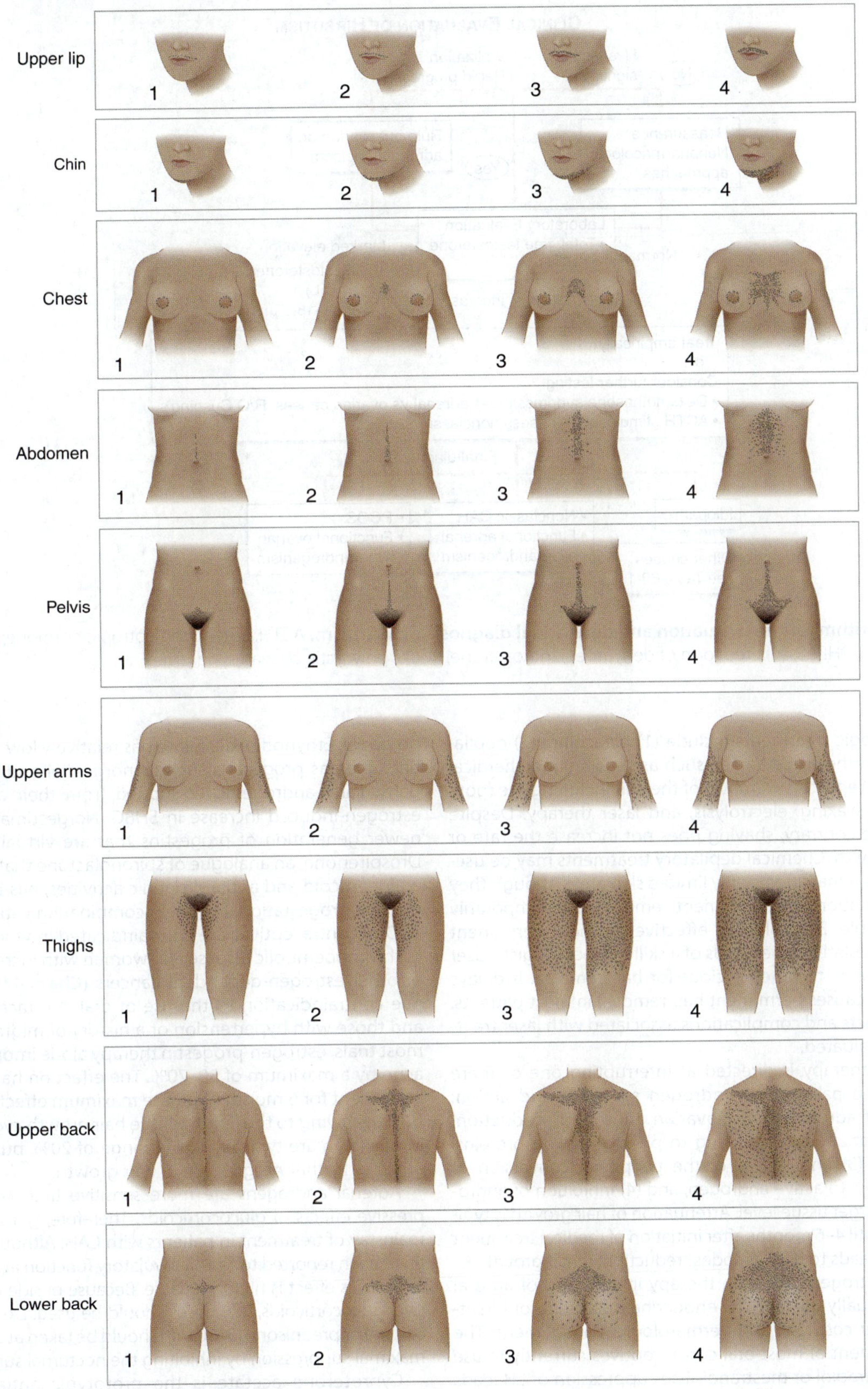

FIGURE 68-1 Hirsutism scoring scale of Ferriman and Gallwey. The nine body areas that have androgen-sensitive areas are graded from 0 (no terminal hair) to 4 (frankly virile) to obtain a total score. A normal hirsutism score is <8. *(Modified from DA Ehrmann et al: Hyperandrogenism, hirsutism, and polycystic ovary syndrome, in LJ DeGroot and JL Jameson [eds], Endocrinology, 5th ed. Philadelphia, Saunders, 2006; with permission.)*

of 21-hydroxylase can be reliably excluded by determining a morning 17-hydroxyprogesterone level <6 nmol/L (<2 μg/L) (drawn in the follicular phase). Alternatively, 21-hydroxylase deficiency can be diagnosed by measurement of 17-hydroxyprogesterone 1 h after the administration of 250 μg of synthetic ACTH (cosyntropin) intravenously.

TREATMENT HIRSUTISM

Treatment of hirsutism may be accomplished pharmacologically or by mechanical means of hair removal. Nonpharmacologic treatments should be considered in all patients either as the only treatment or as an adjunct to drug therapy.

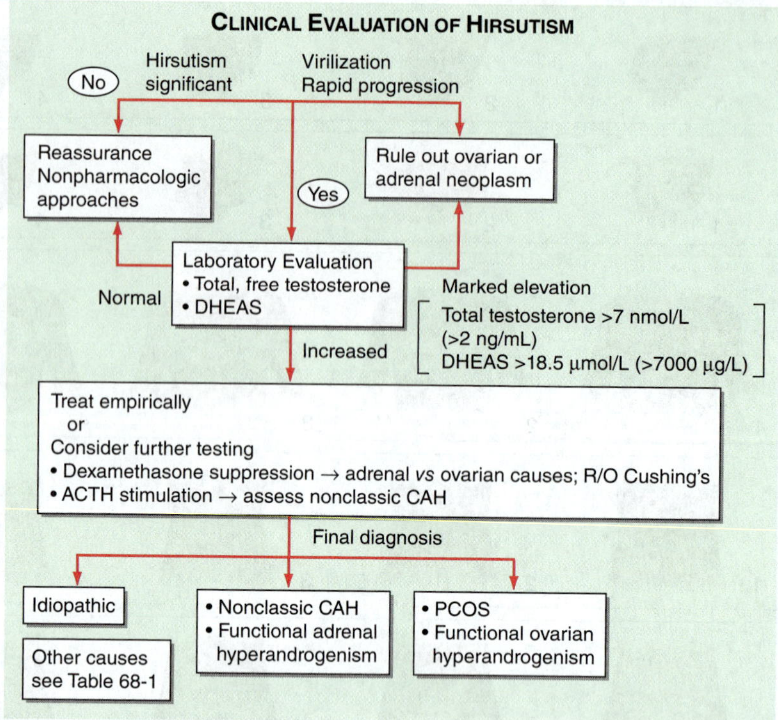

FIGURE 68-2 Algorithm for the evaluation and differential diagnosis of hirsutism. ACTH, adrenocorticotropic hormone; CAH, congenital adrenal hyperplasia; DHEAS, sulfated form of dehydroepiandrosterone; PCOS, polycystic ovarian syndrome.

Nonpharmacologic treatments include (1) bleaching; (2) depilatory (removal from the skin surface), such as shaving and chemical treatments; and (3) epilatory (removal of the hair including the root), such as plucking, waxing, electrolysis, and laser therapy. Despite perceptions to the contrary, shaving does not increase the rate or density of hair growth. Chemical depilatory treatments may be useful for mild hirsutism that affects only limited skin areas, though they can cause skin irritation. Wax treatment removes hair temporarily but is uncomfortable. Electrolysis is effective for more permanent hair removal, particularly in the hands of a skilled electrologist. Laser phototherapy appears to be efficacious for hair removal. It delays hair regrowth and causes permanent hair removal in most patients. The long-term effects and complications associated with laser treatment are being evaluated.

Pharmacologic therapy is directed at interrupting one or more of the steps in the pathway of androgen synthesis and action: (1) suppression of adrenal and/or ovarian androgen production; (2) enhancement of androgen-binding to plasma-binding proteins, particularly SHBG; (3) impairment of the peripheral conversion of androgen precursors to active androgen; and (4) inhibition of androgen action at the target tissue level. Attenuation of hair growth is typically not evident until 4–6 months after initiation of medical treatment and in most cases leads to only a modest reduction in hair growth.

Combination estrogen-progestin therapy in the form of an oral contraceptive is usually the first-line endocrine treatment for hirsutism and acne, after cosmetic and dermatologic management. The estrogenic component of most oral contraceptives currently in use is either ethinyl estradiol or mestranol. The suppression of LH leads to reduced production of ovarian androgens. The reduced androgen levels also result in a dose-related increase in SHBG, thus lowering the fraction of unbound plasma testosterone. Combination therapy also has been demonstrated to decrease DHEAS, perhaps by reducing ACTH levels. Estrogens also have a direct, dose-dependent suppressive effect on sebaceous cell function.

The choice of a specific oral contraceptive should be predicated on the progestational component, as progestins vary in their suppressive effect on SHBG levels and in their androgenic potential. Ethynodiol diacetate has relatively low androgenic potential, whereas progestins such as norgestrel and levonorgestrel are particularly androgenic, as judged from their attenuation of the estrogen-induced increase in SHBG. Norgestimate exemplifies the newer generation of progestins that are virtually nonandrogenic. Drospirenone, an analogue of spironolactone that has both antimineralocorticoid and antiandrogenic activities, has been approved for use as a progestational agent in combination with ethinyl estradiol.

Oral contraceptives are contraindicated in women with a history of thromboembolic disease and women with increased risk of breast or other estrogen-dependent cancers (Chap. 413). There is a relative contraindication to the use of oral contraceptives in smokers and those with hypertension or a history of migraine headaches. In most trials, estrogen-progestin therapy alone improves the extent of acne by a maximum of 50–70%. The effect on hair growth may not be evident for 6 months, and the maximum effect may require 9–12 months owing to the length of the hair growth cycle. Improvements in hirsutism are typically in the range of 20%, but there may be an arrest of further progression of hair growth.

Adrenal androgens are more sensitive than cortisol to the suppressive effects of glucocorticoids. Therefore, glucocorticoids are the mainstay of treatment in patients with CAH. Although glucocorticoids have been reported to restore ovulatory function in some women with PCOS, this effect is highly variable. Because of side effects from excessive glucocorticoids, low doses should be used. Dexamethasone (0.2–0.5 mg) or prednisone (5–10 mg) should be taken at bedtime to achieve maximal suppression by inhibiting the nocturnal surge of ACTH.

Cyproterone acetate is the prototypic antiandrogen. It acts mainly by competitive inhibition of the binding of testosterone and DHT to the androgen receptor. In addition, it may enhance the metabolic clearance of testosterone by inducing hepatic enzymes. Although not available for use in the United States, cyproterone acetate is widely used in Canada, Mexico, and Europe. Cyproterone (50–100 mg) is given on days 1–15 and ethinyl estradiol (50 μg) is given on days 5–26 of the menstrual cycle. Side effects include irregular uterine bleeding, nausea, headache, fatigue, weight gain, and decreased libido.

Spironolactone, which usually is used as a mineralocorticoid antagonist, is also a weak antiandrogen. It is almost as effective as cyproterone acetate when used at high enough doses (100–200 mg daily). Patients should be monitored intermittently for hyperkalemia or hypotension, although these side effects are uncommon. Pregnancy should be avoided because of the risk of feminization of a male fetus. Spironolactone can also cause menstrual irregularity. It often is used in combination with an oral contraceptive, which suppresses ovarian androgen production and helps prevent pregnancy.

Flutamide is a potent nonsteroidal antiandrogen that is effective in treating hirsutism, but concerns about the induction of hepatocellular dysfunction have limited its use. Finasteride is a competitive inhibitor of 5α-reductase type 2. Beneficial effects on hirsutism have been reported, but the predominance of 5α-reductase type 1 in the PSU appears to account for its limited efficacy. Finasteride would also be expected to impair sexual differentiation in a male fetus, and it should not be used in women who may become pregnant.

Eflornithine cream (Vaniqa) has been approved as a novel treatment for unwanted facial hair in women, but long-term efficacy remains to be established. It can cause skin irritation under exaggerated conditions of use. Ultimately, the choice of any specific agent(s) must be tailored to the unique needs of the patient being treated. As noted previously, pharmacologic treatments for hirsutism should be used in conjunction with nonpharmacologic approaches. It is also helpful to review the pattern of female hair distribution in the normal population to dispel unrealistic expectations.

69 Menstrual Disorders and Pelvic Pain

Janet E. Hall

Menstrual dysfunction can signal an underlying abnormality that may have long-term health consequences. Although frequent or prolonged bleeding usually prompts a woman to seek medical attention, infrequent or absent bleeding may seem less troubling and the patient may not bring it to the attention of the physician. Thus, a focused menstrual history is a critical part of every encounter with a female patient. Pelvic pain is a common complaint that may relate to an abnormality of the reproductive organs but also may be of gastrointestinal, urinary tract, or musculoskeletal origin. Depending on its cause, pelvic pain may require urgent surgical attention.

MENSTRUAL DISORDERS

DEFINITION AND PREVALENCE

Amenorrhea refers to the absence of menstrual periods. Amenorrhea is classified as *primary* if menstrual bleeding has never occurred in the absence of hormonal treatment or *secondary* if menstrual periods cease for 3–6 months. Primary amenorrhea is a rare disorder that occurs in <1% of the female population. However, between 3 and 5% of women experience at least 3 months of secondary amenorrhea in any specific year. There is no evidence that race or ethnicity influences the prevalence of amenorrhea. However, because of the importance of adequate nutrition for normal reproductive function, both the age at menarche and the prevalence of secondary amenorrhea vary significantly in different parts of the world.

Oligomenorrhea is defined as a cycle length >35 days or <10 menses per year. Both the frequency and the amount of vaginal bleeding are irregular in oligomenorrhea, and moliminal symptoms (premenstrual breast tenderness, food cravings, mood lability), suggestive of ovulation, are variably present. Anovulation can also present with intermenstrual intervals <24 days or vaginal bleeding for >7 days. Frequent or heavy irregular bleeding is termed *dysfunctional uterine bleeding* if anatomic uterine and outflow tract lesions or a bleeding diathesis has been excluded.

Primary Amenorrhea The absence of menses by age 16 has been used traditionally to define primary amenorrhea. However, other factors, such as growth, secondary sexual characteristics, the presence of cyclic pelvic pain, and the secular trend toward an earlier age of menarche, particularly in African-American girls, also influence the age at which primary amenorrhea should be investigated. Thus, an evaluation for amenorrhea should be initiated by age 15 or 16 in the presence of normal growth and secondary sexual characteristics; age 13 in the absence of secondary sexual characteristics or if height is less than the third percentile; age 12 or 13 in the presence of breast development and cyclic pelvic pain; or within 2 years of breast development if menarche, defined by the first menstrual period, has not occurred.

Secondary Amenorrhea or Oligomenorrhea Anovulation and irregular cycles are relatively common for up to 2 years after menarche and for 1–2 years before the final menstrual period. In the intervening years, menstrual cycle length is ~28 days, with an intermenstrual interval normally ranging between 25 and 35 days. Cycle-to-cycle variability in an individual woman who is ovulating consistently is generally +/– 2 days. Pregnancy is the most common cause of amenorrhea and should be excluded early in any evaluation of menstrual irregularity. However, many women occasionally miss a single period. Three or more months of secondary amenorrhea should prompt an evaluation, as should a history of intermenstrual intervals >35 or <21 days or bleeding that persists for >7 days.

DIAGNOSIS

Evaluation of menstrual dysfunction depends on understanding the interrelationships between the four critical components of the reproductive tract: (1) the hypothalamus, (2) the pituitary, (3) the ovaries, and (4) the uterus and outflow tract (Fig. 69-1; Chap. 412). This system is maintained by complex negative and positive feedback loops involving the ovarian steroids (estradiol and progesterone) and peptides (inhibin B and inhibin A) and the hypothalamic (gonadotropin-releasing hormone [GnRH]) and pituitary (follicle-stimulating hormone [FSH] and luteinizing hormone [LH]) components of this system (Fig. 69-1).

Disorders of menstrual function can be thought of in two main categories: disorders of the uterus and outflow tract and disorders of ovulation. Many of the conditions that cause primary amenorrhea are congenital but go unrecognized until the time of normal puberty (e.g., genetic, chromosomal, and anatomic abnormalities). All causes of secondary amenorrhea also can cause primary amenorrhea.

Disorders of the Uterus or Outflow Tract Abnormalities of the uterus and outflow tract typically present as primary amenorrhea. In patients with normal pubertal development and a blind vagina, the differential diagnosis includes *obstruction* by a transverse vaginal septum or imperforate hymen; *müllerian agenesis* (Mayer-Rokitansky-Kuster-Hauser syndrome), which has been associated with mutations in the *WNT4* gene; and *androgen insensitivity syndrome* (AIS), which is an X-linked recessive disorder that accounts for ~10% of all cases of primary amenorrhea (Chap. 411). Patients with AIS have a 46,XY karyotype, but because of the lack of androgen receptor responsiveness, those with complete AIS have severe underandrogenization and female external genitalia. The absence of pubic and axillary hair distinguishes them clinically from patients with müllerian agenesis, as does an elevated testosterone level. *Asherman's syndrome* presents as secondary amenorrhea or hypomenorrhea and results from partial or complete obliteration of the uterine cavity by adhesions that prevent normal growth and shedding of the endometrium. Curettage performed for pregnancy complications accounts for >90% of cases; genital tuberculosis is an important cause in regions where it is endemic.

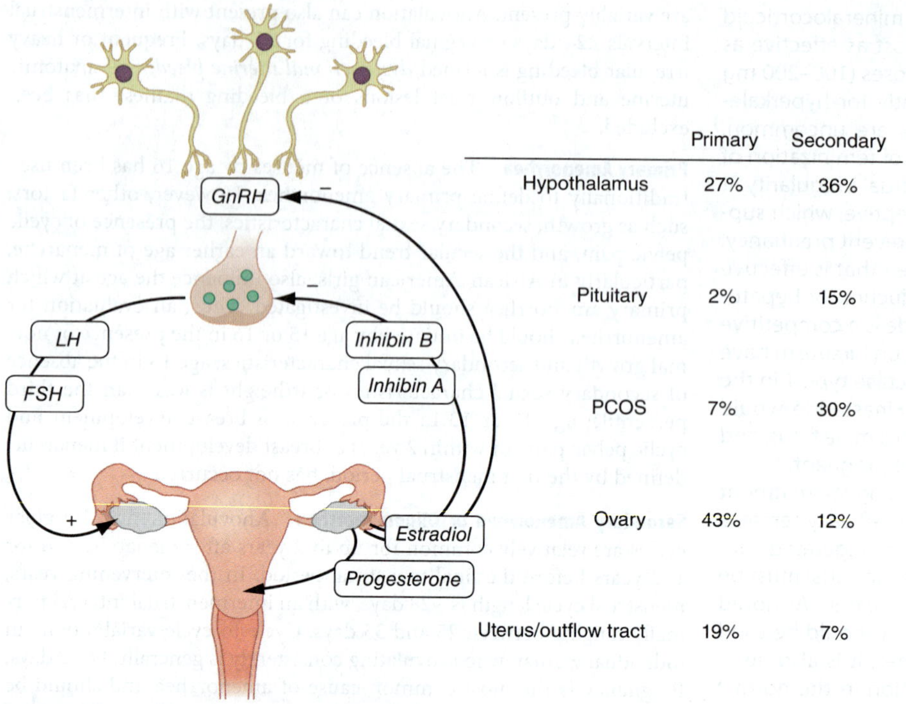

FIGURE 69-1 Role of the hypothalamic-pituitary-gonadal axis in the etiology of amenorrhea. Gonadotropin-releasing hormone (GnRH) secretion from the hypothalamus stimulates follicle-stimulating hormone (FSH) and luteinizing hormone (LH) secretion from the pituitary to induce ovarian folliculogenesis and steroidogenesis. Ovarian secretion of estradiol and progesterone controls the shedding of the endometrium, resulting in menses, and, in combination with the inhibins, provides feedback regulation of the hypothalamus and pituitary to control secretion of FSH and LH. The prevalence of amenorrhea resulting from abnormalities at each level of the reproductive system (hypothalamus, pituitary, ovary, uterus, and outflow tract) varies depending on whether amenorrhea is primary or secondary. PCOS, polycystic ovarian syndrome.

TREATMENT DISORDERS OF THE UTERUS OR OUTFLOW TRACT

Obstruction of the outflow tract requires surgical correction. The risk of endometriosis is increased with this condition, perhaps because of retrograde menstrual flow. *Müllerian agenesis* also may require surgical intervention to allow sexual intercourse, although vaginal dilatation is adequate in some patients. Because ovarian function is normal, assisted reproductive techniques can be used with a surrogate carrier. *Androgen resistance syndrome* requires gonadectomy because there is risk of gonadoblastoma in the dysgenetic gonads. Whether this should be performed in early childhood or after completion of breast development is controversial. Estrogen replacement is indicated after gonadectomy, and vaginal dilatation may be required to allow sexual intercourse.

Disorders of Ovulation Once uterus and outflow tract abnormalities have been excluded, other causes of amenorrhea involve disorders of ovulation. The differential diagnosis is based on the results of initial tests, including a pregnancy test, an FSH level (to determine whether the cause is likely to be ovarian or central), and assessment of hyperandrogenism (Fig. 69-2).

HYPOGONADOTROPIC HYPOGONADISM Low estrogen levels in combination with normal or low levels of LH and FSH are seen with anatomic, genetic, or functional abnormalities that interfere with hypothalamic GnRH secretion or normal pituitary responsiveness to GnRH. Although relatively uncommon, tumors and infiltrative diseases should be considered in the differential diagnosis of hypogonadotropic hypogonadism (Chap. 403). These disorders may present with primary or secondary amenorrhea. They may occur in association with other features suggestive of hypothalamic or pituitary dysfunction, such as short stature, diabetes insipidus, galactorrhea, and headache. Hypogonadotropic hypogonadism also may be seen after cranial irradiation. In the postpartum period, it may be caused by pituitary necrosis (Sheehan's syndrome) or lymphocytic hypophysitis. Because reproductive dysfunction is commonly associated with hyperprolactinemia from neuroanatomic lesions or medications, prolactin should be measured in all patients with hypogonadotropic hypogonadism (Chap. 403).

Isolated hypogonadotropic hypogonadism (IHH) occurs in women, although it is three times more common in men. IHH generally presents with primary amenorrhea, although 50% have some degree of breast development, and one to two menses have been described in ~10%. IHH is associated with anosmia in about 50% of women (termed Kallmann's syndrome). Genetic causes of IHH have been identified in ~60% of patients (Chaps. 411 and 412).

Functional hypothalamic amenorrhea (HA) is caused by a mismatch between energy expenditure and energy intake. Recent studies suggest that variants in genes associated with IHH may increase susceptibility to these environmental inputs, accounting in part for the clinical variability in this disorder. Leptin secretion may play a key role in transducing the signals from the periphery to the hypothalamus in HA. The hypothalamic-pituitary-adrenal axis also may play a role. The diagnosis of HA generally can be made on the basis of a careful history, a physical examination, and the demonstration of low levels of gonadotropins and normal prolactin levels. Eating disorders and chronic disease must be specifically excluded. An atypical history, headache, signs of other hypothalamic dysfunction, or hyperprolactinemia, even if mild, necessitates cranial imaging with computed tomography (CT) or magnetic resonance imaging (MRI) to exclude a neuroanatomic cause.

HYPERGONADOTROPIC HYPOGONADISM Ovarian failure is considered premature when it occurs in women <40 years old and accounts for ~10% of secondary amenorrhea. *Primary ovarian insufficiency* (POI) has generally replaced the terms *premature menopause* and *premature ovarian failure* in recognition that this disorder represents a continuum of impaired ovarian function. Ovarian insufficiency is associated with the loss of negative-feedback restraint on the hypothalamus and pituitary, resulting in increased FSH and LH levels. FSH is a better marker of ovarian failure as its levels are less variable than those of LH. Antimüllerian hormone (AMH) levels will also be low in patients with POI, but are more frequently used in management of infertility. As with natural menopause, POI may wax and wane, and serial measurements may be necessary to establish the diagnosis.

Once the diagnosis of POI has been established, further evaluation is indicated because of other health problems that may be associated with POI. For example, POI occurs in association with a variety of chromosomal abnormalities, including Turner's syndrome, autoimmune polyglandular failure syndromes, radio- and chemotherapy, and galactosemia. The recognition that early ovarian failure occurs in premutation carriers of the fragile X syndrome is important because of the increased risk of severe mental retardation in male children with *FMR1* mutations. In the majority of cases, a cause for POI is not determined. Although there are increasing reports of genetic mutations in individuals and families with POI, testing for other than chromosomal abnormalities and *FMR1* mutations is not recommended.

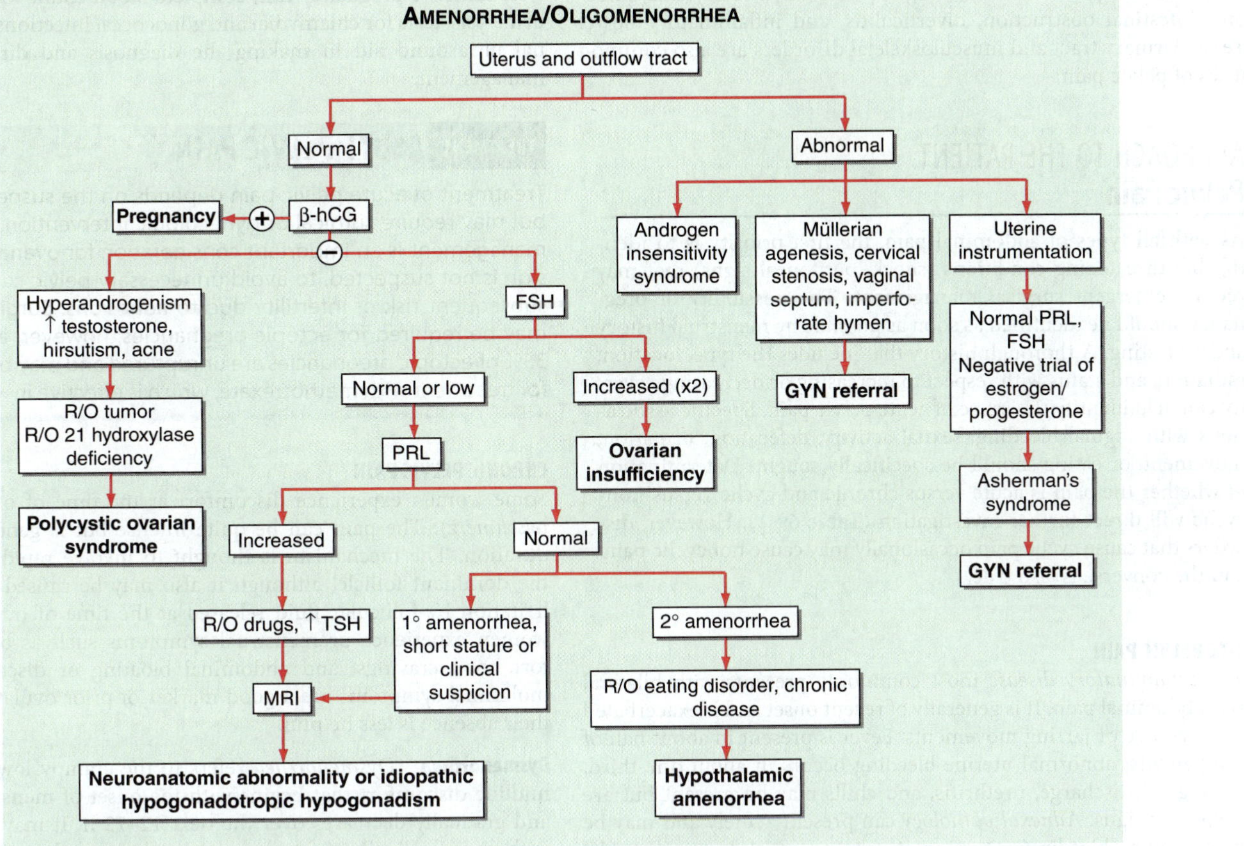

FIGURE 69-2 Algorithm for evaluation of amenorrhea. β-hCG, human chorionic gonadotropin; FSH, follicle-stimulating hormone; GYN, gynecologist; MRI, magnetic resonance imaging; PRL, prolactin; R/O, rule out; TSH, thyroid-stimulating hormone.

Hypergonadotropic hypogonadism occurs rarely in other disorders, such as mutations in the FSH or LH receptors. Aromatase deficiency and 17α-hydroxylase deficiency are associated with decreased estrogen and elevated gonadotropins and with hyperandrogenism and hypertension, respectively. Gonadotropin-secreting tumors in women of reproductive age generally present with high, rather than low, estrogen levels and cause ovarian hyperstimulation or dysfunctional bleeding.

TREATMENT HYPO- AND HYPERGONADOTROPIC CAUSES OF AMENORRHEA

Amenorrhea almost always is associated with chronically low levels of estrogen, whether it is caused by hypogonadotropic hypogonadism or ovarian insufficiency. Development of secondary sexual characteristics requires gradual titration of estradiol replacement with eventual addition of progestin. Hormone replacement with either low-dose estrogen/progesterone regimens or oral contraceptive pills is recommended until the usual age of menopause for bone and cardiovascular protection. Patients with hypogonadotropic hypogonadism who are interested in fertility require treatment with exogenous FSH combined with LH or pulsatile GnRH. Patients with ovarian failure can consider oocyte donation, which has a high rate of success in this population, although its use in women with Turner's syndrome is limited by significant maternal cardiovascular risk.

POLYCYSTIC OVARIAN SYNDROME (PCOS) PCOS is diagnosed based on a combination of clinical or biochemical evidence of hyperandrogenism, amenorrhea or oligomenorrhea, and the ultrasound appearance of polycystic ovaries. Approximately half of patients with PCOS are obese, and abnormalities in insulin dynamics are common, as is metabolic syndrome. Symptoms generally begin shortly after menarche and are slowly progressive. Lean oligo-ovulatory patients with PCOS generally have high LH levels in the presence of normal to low levels of FSH and estradiol. The LH/FSH ratio is less pronounced in obese patients in whom insulin resistance is a more prominent feature.

TREATMENT POLYCYSTIC OVARIAN SYNDROME

A major abnormality in patients with PCOS is the failure of regular, predictable ovulation. Thus, these patients are at risk for the development of dysfunctional bleeding and endometrial hyperplasia associated with unopposed estrogen exposure. Endometrial protection can be achieved with the use of oral contraceptives or progestins (medroxyprogesterone acetate, 5–10 mg, or prometrium, 200 mg daily for 10–14 days of each month). Oral contraceptives are also useful for management of hyperandrogenic symptoms, as are spironolactone and cyproterone acetate (not available in the United States), which function as weak androgen receptor blockers. Management of the associated metabolic syndrome may be appropriate for some patients (Chap. 422). For patients interested in fertility, weight control is a critical first step. Clomiphene citrate is highly effective as a first-line treatment, and there is increasing evidence that the aromatase inhibitor letrozole may also be effective. Exogenous gonadotropins can be used by experienced practitioners; a diagnosis of polycystic ovaries in the presence or absence of cycle abnormalities increases the risk of hyperstimulation.

PELVIC PAIN

The mechanisms that cause pelvic pain are similar to those that cause abdominal pain (Chap. 20) and include inflammation of the parietal peritoneum, obstruction of hollow viscera, vascular disturbances, and pain originating in the abdominal wall. Pelvic pain may reflect pelvic disease per se but also may reflect extrapelvic disorders that refer pain to the pelvis. In up to 60% of cases, pelvic pain can be attributed to gastrointestinal problems, including appendicitis, cholecystitis, infections, intestinal obstruction, diverticulitis, and inflammatory bowel disease. Urinary tract and musculoskeletal disorders are also common causes of pelvic pain.

APPROACH TO THE PATIENT: Pelvic Pain

As with all types of abdominal pain, the first priority is to identify life-threatening conditions (shock, peritoneal signs) that may require emergent surgical management. The possibility of pregnancy should be identified as soon as possible by menstrual history and/or testing. A thorough history that includes the type, location, radiation, and status with respect to increasing or decreasing severity can help identify the cause of acute pelvic pain. Specific associations with vaginal bleeding, sexual activity, defecation, urination, movement, or eating should be specifically sought. Determination of whether the pain is acute versus chronic and cyclic versus noncyclic will direct further investigation (Table 69-1). However, disorders that cause cyclic pain occasionally may cause noncyclic pain, and the converse is also true.

ACUTE PELVIC PAIN

Pelvic inflammatory disease most commonly presents with bilateral lower abdominal pain. It is generally of recent onset and is exacerbated by intercourse or jarring movements. Fever is present in about half of these patients; abnormal uterine bleeding occurs in about one-third. New vaginal discharge, urethritis, and chills may be present but are less specific signs. *Adnexal pathology* can present acutely and may be due to rupture, bleeding or torsion of cysts, or, much less commonly, neoplasms of the ovary, fallopian tubes, or paraovarian areas. Fever may be present with ovarian torsion. *Ectopic pregnancy* is associated with right- or left-sided lower abdominal pain, with clinical signs generally appearing 6–8 weeks after the last normal menstrual period. Amenorrhea is present in ~75% of cases and vaginal bleeding in ~50% of cases. Orthostatic signs and fever may be present. Risk factors include the presence of known tubal disease, previous ectopic pregnancies, a history of infertility, diethylstilbestrol (DES) exposure of the mother in utero, or a history of pelvic infections. *Threatened abortion* may also present with amenorrhea, abdominal pain, and vaginal bleeding. Although more common than ectopic pregnancy, it is rarely associated with systemic signs. *Uterine pathology* includes endometritis and, less frequently, degenerating leiomyomas (fibroids). Endometritis often is associated with vaginal bleeding and systemic signs of infection. It occurs in the setting of sexually transmitted infections, uterine instrumentation, or postpartum infection.

TABLE 69-1 CAUSES OF PELVIC PAIN

	Acute	Chronic
Cyclic pelvic pain		Premenstrual symptoms
		Mittelschmerz
		Dysmenorrhea
		Endometriosis
Noncyclic pelvic pain	Pelvic inflammatory disease	Pelvic congestion syndrome
	Ruptured or hemorrhagic ovarian cyst, endometrioma, or ovarian torsion	Adhesions and retroversion of the uterus
	Ectopic pregnancy	Pelvic malignancy
	Endometritis	Vulvodynia
	Acute growth or degeneration of uterine myoma	Chronic pelvic inflammatory disease
	Threatened abortion	Tuberculous salpingitis
		History of sexual abuse

A sensitive pregnancy test, complete blood count with differential, urinalysis, tests for chlamydial and gonococcal infections, and abdominal ultrasound aid in making the diagnosis and directing further management.

TREATMENT ACUTE PELVIC PAIN

Treatment of acute pelvic pain depends on the suspected etiology but may require surgical or gynecologic intervention. Conservative management is an important consideration for ovarian cysts, if torsion is not suspected, to avoid unnecessary pelvic surgery and the subsequent risk of infertility due to adhesions. Surgical treatment may be required for ectopic pregnancies; however, approximately 35% of ectopic pregnancies are unruptured and may be appropriate for treatment with methotrexate, which is effective in ~90% of cases.

CHRONIC PELVIC PAIN

Some women experience discomfort at the time of ovulation (*mittelschmerz*). The pain can be quite intense but is generally of short duration. The mechanism is thought to involve rapid expansion of the dominant follicle, although it also may be caused by peritoneal irritation by follicular fluid released at the time of ovulation. Many women experience premenstrual symptoms such as breast discomfort, food cravings, and abdominal bloating or discomfort. These moliminal symptoms are a good marker of prior ovulation, although their absence is less helpful.

Dysmenorrhea *Dysmenorrhea* refers to the crampy lower abdominal midline discomfort that begins with the onset of menstrual bleeding and gradually decreases over the next 12–72 h. It may be associated with nausea, diarrhea, fatigue, and headache and occurs in 60–93% of adolescents, beginning with the establishment of regular ovulatory cycles. Its prevalence decreases after pregnancy and with the use of oral contraceptives.

Primary dysmenorrhea results from increased stores of prostaglandin precursors, which are generated by sequential stimulation of the uterus by estrogen and progesterone. During menstruation, these precursors are converted to prostaglandins, which cause intense uterine contractions, decreased blood flow, and increased peripheral nerve hypersensitivity, resulting in pain.

Secondary dysmenorrhea is caused by underlying pelvic pathology. *Endometriosis* results from the presence of endometrial glands and stroma outside the uterus. These deposits of ectopic endometrium respond to hormonal stimulation and cause dysmenorrhea, which begins several days before menses. Endometriosis also may be associated with painful intercourse, painful bowel movements, and tender nodules in the uterosacral ligament. Fibrosis and adhesions can produce lateral displacement of the cervix. Transvaginal pelvic ultrasound is part of the initial workup and may detect an endometrioma within the ovary, rectovaginal or bladder nodules, or ureteral involvement. The CA125 level may be increased, but it has low negative predictive value. Definitive diagnosis requires laparoscopy. Symptomatology does not always predict the extent of endometriosis. The prevalence is lower in black and Hispanic women than in Caucasians and Asians. *Other secondary causes* of dysmenorrhea include adenomyosis, a condition caused by the presence of ectopic endometrial glands and stroma within the myometrium. Cervical stenosis may result from trauma, infection, or surgery.

TREATMENT DYSMENORRHEA

Local application of heat; dietary dairy intake; use of vitamins B_1, B_6, and E and fish oil; acupuncture; yoga; and exercise are of some benefit for the treatment of dysmenorrhea. Studies of vitamin D_3 are not yet adequate to provide a recommendation. However, nonsteroidal anti-inflammatory drugs (NSAIDs) are the most effective treatment and provide >80% sustained response rates. Ibuprofen, naproxen, ketoprofen, mefanamic acid, and nimesulide are all superior to placebo. Treatment should be started a day before expected menses and generally is continued for 2–3 days. Oral contraceptives also reduce symptoms of dysmenorrhea. The use of tocolytics, antiphosphodiesterase inhibitors, and magnesium has been suggested, but there are insufficient data to recommend them. Failure of response to NSAIDs and/or oral contraceptives is suggestive of a pelvic disorder such as endometriosis, and diagnostic laparoscopy should be considered to guide further treatment.

SECTION 9 ALTERATIONS IN THE SKIN

70 Approach to the Patient with a Skin Disorder

Thomas J. Lawley, Kim B. Yancey

The challenge of examining the skin lies in distinguishing normal from abnormal findings, distinguishing significant findings from trivial ones, and integrating pertinent signs and symptoms into an appropriate differential diagnosis. The fact that the largest organ in the body is visible is both an advantage and a disadvantage to those who examine it. It is advantageous because no special instrumentation is necessary and because the skin can be biopsied with little morbidity. However, the casual observer can be misled by a variety of stimuli and overlook important, subtle signs of skin or systemic disease. For instance, the sometimes minor differences in color and shape that distinguish a melanoma **(Fig. 70-1)** from a benign nevomelanocytic nevus **(Fig. 70-2)** can be difficult to recognize. A variety of descriptive terms have been developed that characterize cutaneous lesions **(Tables 70-1, 70-2, and Tables 70-3; Fig. 70-3)**, thereby aiding in their interpretation and in the formulation of a differential diagnosis **(Table 70-4)**. For example, the finding of scaling papules, which are present in psoriasis or atopic dermatitis, places the patient in a different diagnostic category than would hemorrhagic papules, which may indicate vasculitis or sepsis **(Figs. 70-4 and 70-5, respectively)**. It is also important to differentiate primary from secondary skin lesions. If the examiner focuses on linear erosions overlying an area of erythema and scaling, he or she may incorrectly assume that the erosion is the primary lesion and that the redness and scale are secondary, whereas the correct interpretation would be that the patient has a pruritic eczematous dermatitis with erosions caused by scratching.

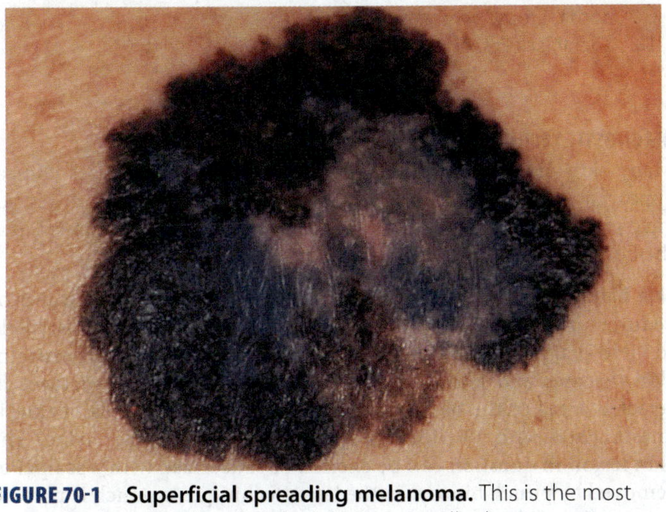

FIGURE 70-1 Superficial spreading melanoma. This is the most common type of melanoma. Such lesions usually demonstrate asymmetry, border irregularity, color variegation (black, blue, brown, pink, and white), a diameter >6 mm, and a history of change (e.g., an increase in size or development of associated symptoms such as pruritus or pain).

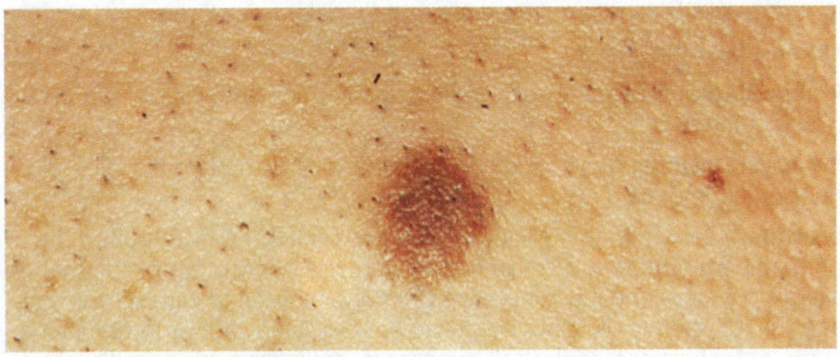

FIGURE 70-2 Nevomelanocytic nevus. Nevi are benign proliferations of nevomelanocytes characterized by regularly shaped hyperpigmented macules or papules of a uniform color.

TABLE 70-1 DESCRIPTION OF PRIMARY SKIN LESIONS

Macule: A flat, colored lesion, <2 cm in diameter, not raised above the surface of the surrounding skin. A "freckle," or ephelid, is a prototypical pigmented macule.
Patch: A large (>2-cm) flat lesion with a color different from the surrounding skin. This differs from a macule only in size.
Papule: A small, solid lesion, <0.5 cm in diameter, raised above the surface of the surrounding skin and thus palpable (e.g., a closed comedone, or whitehead, in acne).
Nodule: A larger (0.5- to 5.0-cm), firm lesion raised above the surface of the surrounding skin. This differs from a papule only in size (e.g., a large dermal nevomelanocytic nevus).
Tumor: A solid, raised growth >5 cm in diameter.
Plaque: A large (>1-cm), flat-topped, raised lesion; edges may either be distinct (e.g., in psoriasis) or gradually blend with surrounding skin (e.g., in eczematous dermatitis).
Vesicle: A small, fluid-filled lesion, <0.5 cm in diameter, raised above the plane of surrounding skin. Fluid is often visible, and the lesions are translucent (e.g., vesicles in allergic contact dermatitis caused by *Toxicodendron* [poison ivy]).
Pustule: A vesicle filled with leukocytes. Note: The presence of pustules does not necessarily signify the existence of an infection.
Bulla: A fluid-filled, raised, often translucent lesion >0.5 cm in diameter.
Wheal: A raised, erythematous, edematous papule or plaque, usually representing short-lived vasodilation and vasopermeability.
Telangiectasia: A dilated, superficial blood vessel.

TABLE 70-2 DESCRIPTION OF SECONDARY SKIN LESIONS

Lichenification: A distinctive thickening of the skin that is characterized by accentuated skin-fold markings.
Scale: Excessive accumulation of stratum corneum.
Crust: Dried exudate of body fluids that may be either yellow (i.e., serous crust) or red (i.e., hemorrhagic crust).
Erosion: Loss of epidermis without an associated loss of dermis.
Ulcer: Loss of epidermis and at least a portion of the underlying dermis.
Excoriation: Linear, angular erosions that may be covered by crust and are caused by scratching.
Atrophy: An acquired loss of substance. In the skin, this may appear as a depression with intact epidermis (i.e., loss of dermal or subcutaneous tissue) or as sites of shiny, delicate, wrinkled lesions (i.e., epidermal atrophy).
Scar: A change in the skin secondary to trauma or inflammation. Sites may be erythematous, hypopigmented, or hyperpigmented depending on their age or character. Sites on hair-bearing areas may be characterized by destruction of hair follicles.

TABLE 70-3 COMMON DERMATOLOGIC TERMS

Alopecia: Hair loss, partial or complete.

Annular: Ring-shaped.

Cyst: A soft, raised, encapsulated lesion filled with semisolid or liquid contents.

Herpetiform: In a grouped configuration.

Lichenoid eruption: Violaceous to purple, polygonal lesions that resemble those seen in lichen planus.

Milia: Small, firm, white papules filled with keratin.

Morbilliform rash: Generalized, small erythematous macules and/or papules that resemble lesions seen in measles.

Nummular: Coin-shaped.

Poikiloderma: Skin that displays variegated pigmentation, atrophy, and telangiectases.

Polycyclic lesions: A configuration of skin lesions formed from coalescing rings or incomplete rings.

Pruritus: A sensation that elicits the desire to scratch. Pruritus is often the predominant symptom of inflammatory skin diseases (e.g., atopic dermatitis, allergic contact dermatitis); it is also commonly associated with xerosis and aged skin. Systemic conditions that can be associated with pruritus include chronic renal disease, cholestasis, pregnancy, malignancy, thyroid disease, polycythemia vera, and delusions of parasitosis.

APPROACH TO THE PATIENT: Skin Disorder

In examining the skin it is usually advisable to assess the patient before taking an extensive history. This approach ensures that the entire cutaneous surface will be evaluated, and objective findings can be integrated with relevant historical data. Four basic features of a skin lesion must be noted and considered during a physical examination: the *distribution* of the eruption, the *types* of primary and secondary lesions, the *shape* of individual lesions, and the *arrangement* of the lesions. An ideal skin examination includes evaluation of the skin, hair, and nails as well as the mucous membranes of the mouth, eyes, nose, nasopharynx, and anogenital region. In the initial examination, it is important that the patient be disrobed as completely as possible to minimize chances of missing important individual skin lesions and permit accurate assessment of the distribution of the eruption. The patient should first be viewed from a distance of about 1.5–2 m (4–6 ft) so that the general character of the skin and the distribution of lesions can be evaluated. Indeed, the distribution of lesions often correlates highly with diagnosis (Fig. 70-6). For example, a hospitalized patient with a generalized erythematous exanthem is more likely to have a drug eruption than is a patient with a similar rash limited to the sun-exposed portions of the face. Once the distribution of the lesions has been established, the nature of the primary lesion must be determined. Thus, when lesions are distributed on elbows, knees, and scalp, the most likely possibility based solely on distribution is psoriasis or dermatitis herpetiformis (Figs. 70-7 and 70-8, respectively). The primary lesion in psoriasis is a scaly papule that soon forms erythematous plaques covered with a white scale, whereas that of dermatitis herpetiformis is an urticarial papule that quickly becomes a small vesicle. In this manner, identification of the primary lesion directs the examiner toward the proper diagnosis. Secondary changes in skin can also be quite helpful. For example, scale represents excessive epidermis, while crust is the result of a discontinuous epithelial cell layer. Palpation of skin lesions can yield insight into the character of an eruption. Thus, red papules on the lower extremities that blanch with pressure can be a manifestation of many different diseases, but hemorrhagic red papules that do not blanch with pressure indicate palpable purpura characteristic of necrotizing vasculitis (Fig. 70-4).

The shape of lesions is also an important feature. Flat, round, erythematous papules and plaques are common in many cutaneous diseases. However, target-shaped lesions that consist in part of erythematous plaques are specific for erythema multiforme (Fig. 70-9). Likewise, the arrangement of individual lesions is important. Erythematous papules and vesicles can occur in many conditions, but their arrangement in a specific linear array suggests an external etiology such as allergic contact dermatitis (Fig. 70-10) or primary irritant dermatitis. In contrast, lesions with a generalized arrangement are common and suggest a systemic etiology.

As in other branches of medicine, a complete history should be obtained to emphasize the following features:

1. Evolution of lesions
   a. Site of onset
   b. Manner in which the eruption progressed or spread
   c. Duration
   d. Periods of resolution or improvement in chronic eruptions
2. Symptoms associated with the eruption
   a. Itching, burning, pain, numbness
   b. What, if anything, has relieved symptoms
   c. Time of day when symptoms are most severe
3. Current or recent medications (prescribed as well as over-the-counter)
4. Associated systemic symptoms (e.g., malaise, fever, arthralgias)
5. Ongoing or previous illnesses
6. History of allergies
7. Presence of photosensitivity
8. Review of systems
9. Family history (particularly relevant for patients with melanoma, atopy, psoriasis, or acne)
10. Social, sexual, or travel history

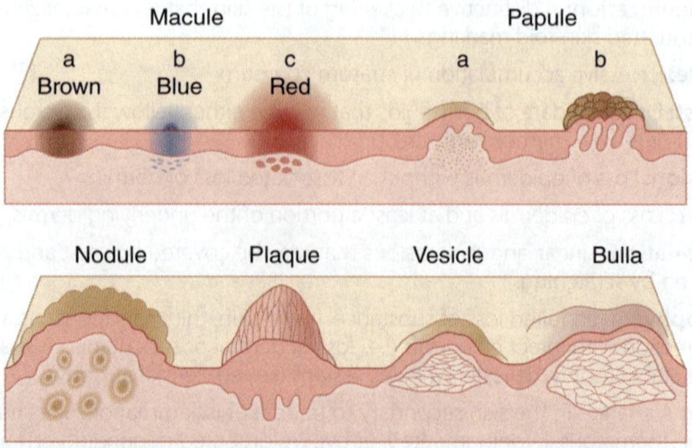

FIGURE 70-3 A schematic representation of several common primary skin lesions (see Table 70-1).

DIAGNOSTIC TECHNIQUES

Many skin diseases can be diagnosed on the basis of gross clinical appearance, but sometimes relatively simple diagnostic procedures can yield valuable information. In most instances, they can be performed at the bedside with a minimum of equipment.

Skin Biopsy A skin biopsy is a straightforward minor surgical procedure; however, it is important to biopsy a lesion that is most likely to yield diagnostic findings. This decision may require expertise in skin diseases and knowledge of superficial anatomic structures in selected areas of the body. In this procedure, a small area of skin is anesthetized with 1% lidocaine with or without epinephrine. The skin lesion in question can be excised or saucerized with a scalpel or removed by punch biopsy. In the latter technique, a punch is pressed against the surface of the skin and rotated with downward pressure until it penetrates to the subcutaneous tissue. The circular biopsy is then lifted with forceps, and the bottom is cut with iris scissors. Biopsy sites may or may not need suture closure, depending on size and location.

TABLE 70-4 SELECTED COMMON DERMATOLOGIC CONDITIONS

Diagnosis	Common Distribution	Usual Morphology	Diagnosis	Common Distribution	Usual Morphology
Acne vulgaris	Face, upper back, chest	Open and closed comedones, erythematous papules, pustules, cysts	Seborrheic keratosis	Trunk, face	Brown plaques with adherent, greasy scale; "stuck on" appearance
Rosacea	Blush area of cheeks, nose, forehead, chin	Erythema, telangiectases, papules, pustules	Folliculitis	Any hair-bearing area	Follicular pustules
			Impetigo	Anywhere	Papules, vesicles, pustules, often with honey-colored crusts
Seborrheic dermatitis	Scalp, eyebrows, perinasal areas	Erythema with greasy yellow-brown scale	Herpes simplex	Lips, genitalia	Grouped vesicles progressing to crusted erosions
Atopic dermatitis	Antecubital and popliteal fossae; may be widespread	Patches and plaques of erythema, scaling, and lichenification; pruritus	Herpes zoster	Dermatomal, usually trunk but may be anywhere	Vesicles limited to a dermatome (often painful)
Stasis dermatitis	Ankles, lower legs over medial malleoli	Patches of erythema and scaling on background of hyperpigmentation associated with signs of venous insufficiency	Varicella	Face, trunk, relative sparing of extremities	Lesions arise in crops and quickly progress from erythematous macules, to papules, to vesicles, to pustules, to crusted sites.
Dyshidrotic eczema	Palms, soles, sides of fingers and toes	Deep vesicles	Pityriasis rosea	Trunk (Christmas tree pattern); herald patch followed by multiple smaller lesions	Symmetric erythematous patches with a collarette of scale
Allergic contact dermatitis	Anywhere	Localized erythema, vesicles, scale, and pruritus (e.g., fingers, earlobes—nickel; dorsal aspect of foot—shoe; exposed surfaces—poison ivy)	Tinea versicolor	Chest, back, abdomen, proximal extremities	Scaly hyper- or hypopigmented macules
Psoriasis	Elbows, knees, scalp, lower back, fingernails (may be generalized)	Papules and plaques covered with silvery scale; nails have pits	Candidiasis	Groin, beneath breasts, vagina, oral cavity	Erythematous macerated areas with satellite pustules; white, friable patches on mucous membranes
Lichen planus	Wrists, ankles, mouth (may be widespread)	Violaceous flat-topped papules and plaques	Dermatophytosis	Feet, groin, beard, or scalp	Varies with site, (e.g., tinea corporis—scaly annular plaque)
Keratosis pilaris	Extensor surfaces of arms and thighs, buttocks	Keratotic follicular papules with surrounding erythema	Scabies	Groin, axillae, between fingers and toes, beneath breasts	Excoriated papules, burrows, pruritus
Melasma	Forehead, cheeks, temples, upper lip	Tan to brown patches	Insect bites	Anywhere	Erythematous papules with central puncta
Vitiligo	Periorificial, trunk, extensor surfaces of extremities, flexor wrists, axillae	Chalk-white macules	Cherry angioma	Trunk	Red, blood-filled papules
			Keloid	Anywhere (site of previous injury)	Firm tumor, pink, purple, or brown
			Dermatofibroma	Anywhere	Firm red to brown nodule that shows dimpling of overlying skin with lateral compression
Actinic keratosis	Sun-exposed areas	Skin-colored or red-brown macule or papule with dry, rough, adherent scale	Acrochordons (skin tags)	Groin, axilla, neck	Fleshy papules
Basal cell carcinoma	Face	Papule with pearly, telangiectatic border on sun-damaged skin	Urticaria	Anywhere	Wheals, sometimes with surrounding flare; pruritus
Squamous cell carcinoma	Face, especially lower lip, ears	Indurated and possibly hyperkeratotic lesions often showing ulceration and/or crusting	Transient acantholytic dermatosis	Trunk, especially anterior chest	Erythematous papules
			Xerosis	Extensor extremities, especially legs	Dry, erythematous, scaling patches; pruritus

KOH Preparation A potassium hydroxide (KOH) preparation is performed on scaling skin lesions where a fungal infection is suspected. The edge of such a lesion is scraped gently with a no. 15 scalpel blade. The removed scale is collected on a glass microscope slide and then treated with 1 or 2 drops of a solution of 10–20% KOH. KOH dissolves keratin and allows easier visualization of fungal elements. Brief heating of the slide accelerates dissolution of keratin. When the preparation is viewed under the microscope, the refractile hyphae are seen more easily when the light intensity is reduced and the condenser is lowered. This technique can be used to identify hyphae in dermatophyte infections, pseudohyphae and budding yeasts in *Candida* infections, and "spaghetti and meatballs" yeast forms in tinea versicolor. The same sampling technique can be used to obtain scale for culture of selected pathogenic organisms.

Tzanck Smear A Tzanck smear is a cytologic technique most often used in the diagnosis of herpesvirus infections (herpes simplex virus [HSV] or varicella zoster virus [VZV]) (see Figs. 217-1 and 217-3). An early vesicle, not a pustule or crusted lesion, is unroofed, and the base of the lesion is scraped gently with a scalpel

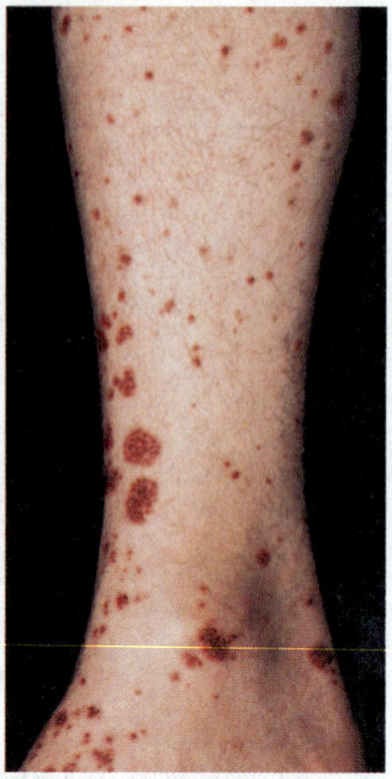

FIGURE 70-4 **Necrotizing vasculitis.** Palpable purpuric papules on the lower legs are seen in this patient with cutaneous small-vessel vasculitis. *(Courtesy of Robert Swerlick, MD; with permission.)*

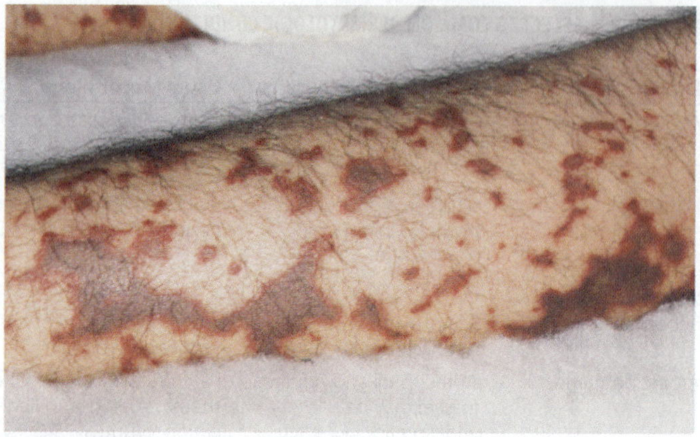

FIGURE 70-5 **Meningococcemia.** An example of fulminant meningococcemia with extensive angular purpuric patches. *(Courtesy of Stephen E. Gellis, MD; with permission.)*

blade. The material is placed on a glass slide, air-dried, and stained with Giemsa or Wright's stain. Multinucleated epithelial giant cells suggest the presence of HSV or VZV; culture, immunofluorescence microscopy, or genetic testing must be performed to identify the specific virus.

Diascopy Diascopy is designed to assess whether a skin lesion will blanch with pressure as, for example, in determining whether a red lesion is hemorrhagic or simply blood-filled. Urticaria (Fig. 70-11) will blanch with pressure, whereas a purpuric lesion caused by necrotizing vasculitis (Fig. 70-4) will not. Diascopy is performed by pressing a microscope slide or magnifying lens against a lesion and noting the amount of blanching that occurs. Granulomas often have an opaque to transparent, brown-pink "apple jelly" appearance on diascopy.

Wood's Light A Wood's lamp generates 360-nm ultraviolet ("black") light that can be used to aid the evaluation of certain skin disorders.

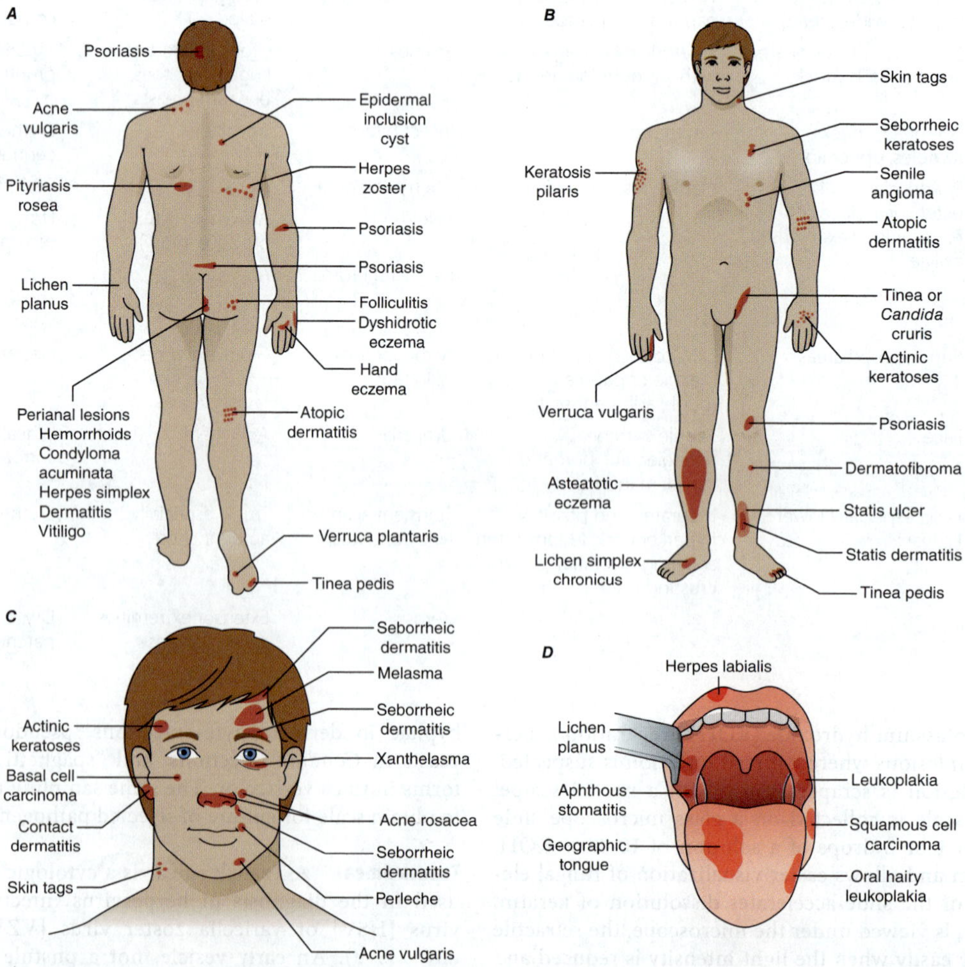

FIGURE 70-6 **Distribution of some common dermatologic diseases and lesions.**

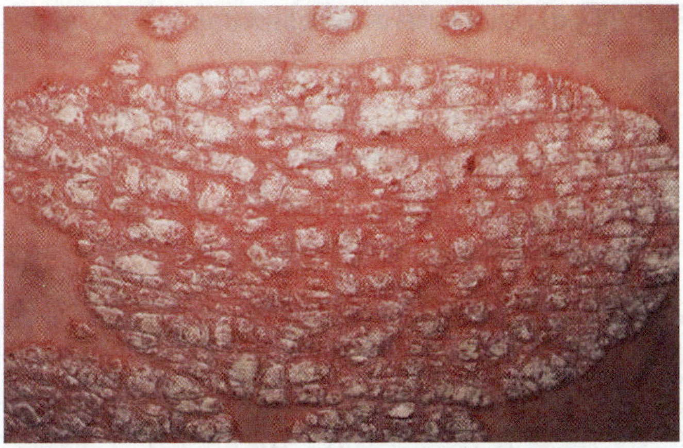

FIGURE 70-7 Psoriasis. This papulosquamous skin disease is characterized by small and large erythematous papules and plaques with overlying adherent silvery scale.

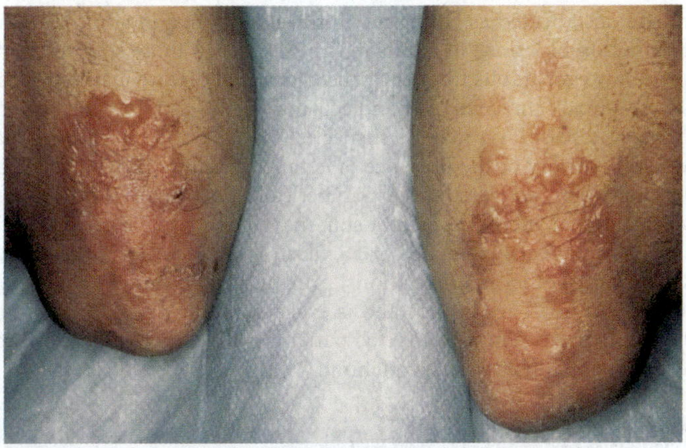

FIGURE 70-8 Dermatitis herpetiformis. This disorder typically displays pruritic, grouped papulovesicles on elbows, knees, buttocks, and posterior scalp. Vesicles are often excoriated due to associated pruritus.

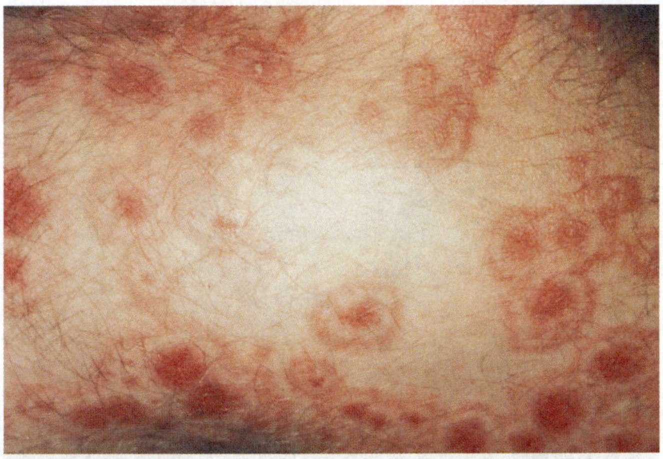

FIGURE 70-9 Erythema multiforme. This eruption is characterized by multiple erythematous plaques with a target or iris morphology. It usually represents a hypersensitivity reaction to drugs (e.g., sulfonamides) or infections (e.g., HSV). *(Courtesy of the Yale Resident's Slide Collection; with permission.)*

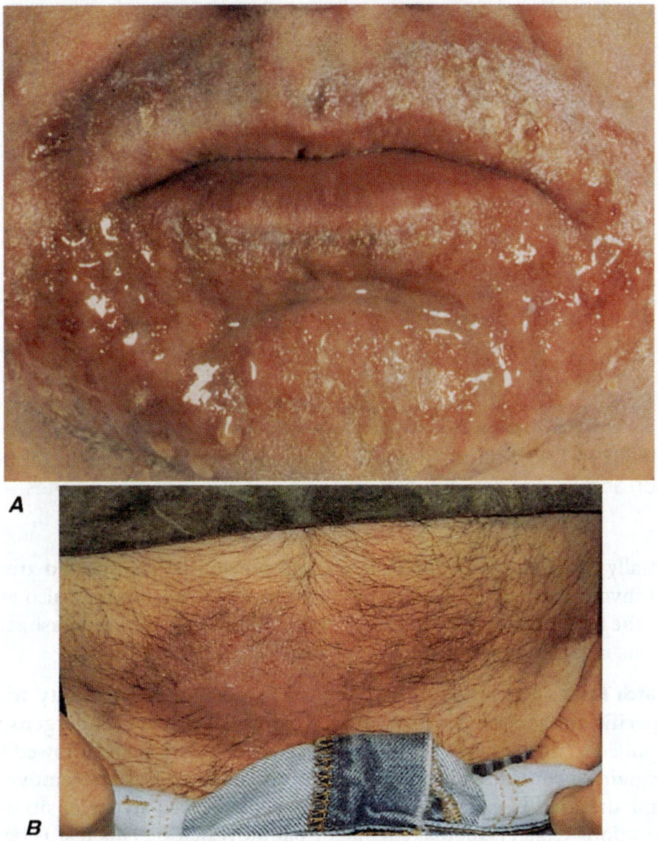

A

B

FIGURE 70-10 Allergic contact dermatitis (ACD). ***A.*** An example of ACD in its acute phase, with sharply demarcated, weeping, eczematous plaques in a perioral distribution. ***B.*** ACD in its chronic phase, with an erythematous, lichenified, weeping plaque on skin chronically exposed to nickel in a metal snap. *(B, Courtesy of Robert Swerlick, MD; with permission.)*

For example, a Wood's lamp will cause erythrasma (a superficial, intertriginous infection caused by *Corynebacterium minutissimum*) to show a characteristic coral pink color, and wounds colonized by *Pseudomonas* will appear pale blue. Tinea capitis caused by certain dermatophytes (e.g., *Microsporum canis* or *M. audouinii*) exhibits a yellow fluorescence. Pigmented lesions of the epidermis such as freckles are accentuated, while dermal pigment such as postinflammatory hyperpigmentation fades under a Wood's light. Vitiligo (Fig. 70-12) appears

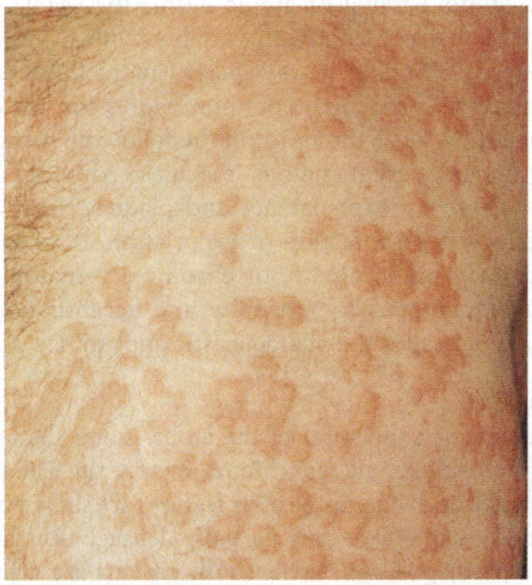

FIGURE 70-11 Urticaria. Discrete and confluent, edematous, erythematous papules and plaques are characteristic of this whealing eruption.

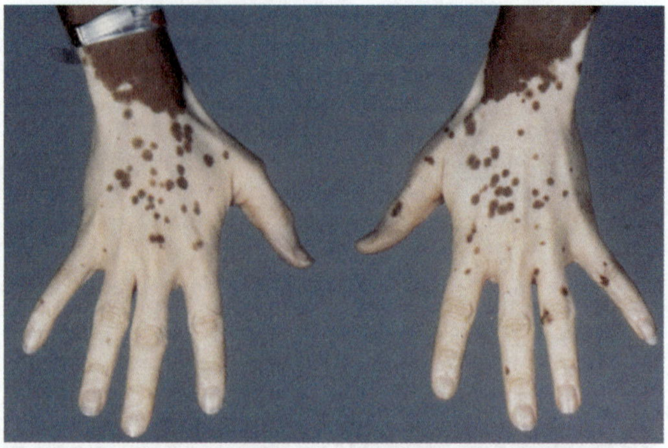

FIGURE 70-12 Vitiligo. Characteristic lesions display an acral distribution and striking depigmentation as a result of loss of melanocytes.

totally white under a Wood's lamp, and previously unsuspected areas of involvement often become apparent. A Wood's lamp may also aid in the demonstration of tinea versicolor and in recognition of ash leaf spots in patients with tuberous sclerosis.

Patch Tests Patch testing is designed to document sensitivity to a specific antigen. In this procedure, a battery of suspected allergens is applied to the patient's back under occlusive dressings and allowed to remain in contact with the skin for 48 h. The dressings are removed, and the area is examined for evidence of delayed hypersensitivity reactions (e.g., erythema, edema, or papulovesicles). This test is best performed by physicians with special expertise in patch testing and is often helpful in the evaluation of patients with chronic dermatitis.

71 Eczema, Psoriasis, Cutaneous Infections, Acne, and Other Common Skin Disorders

Leslie P. Lawley, Calvin O. McCall, Thomas J. Lawley

ECZEMA AND DERMATITIS

Eczema is a type of dermatitis, and these terms are often used synonymously (e.g., atopic eczema or atopic dermatitis [AD]). Eczema is a reaction pattern that presents with variable clinical findings and the common histologic finding of *spongiosis* (intercellular edema of the epidermis). Eczema is the final common expression for a number of disorders, including those discussed in the following sections. Primary lesions may include erythematous macules, papules, and vesicles, which can coalesce to form patches and plaques. In severe eczema, secondary lesions from infection or excoriation, marked by weeping and crusting, may predominate. In chronic eczematous conditions, *lichenification* (cutaneous hypertrophy and accentuation of normal skin markings) may alter the characteristic appearance of eczema.

ATOPIC DERMATITIS

AD is the cutaneous expression of the atopic state, characterized by a family history of asthma, allergic rhinitis, or eczema. The prevalence of AD is increasing worldwide. Some of its features are shown in Table 71-1. The etiology of AD is only partially defined, but there is a clear genetic predisposition. When both parents are affected by AD, >80% of their children manifest the disease. When only one parent is affected, the prevalence drops to slightly over 50%. A characteristic defect in AD that contributes to the pathophysiology is an impaired epidermal barrier. In many patients, a mutation in the gene encoding filaggrin, a structural protein in the stratum corneum, is responsible. Patients with AD may display a variety of immunoregulatory abnormalities, including increased IgE synthesis; increased serum IgE levels; and impaired, delayed-type hypersensitivity reactions.

TABLE 71-1 CLINICAL FEATURES OF ATOPIC DERMATITIS

1. Pruritus and scratching
2. Course marked by exacerbations and remissions
3. Lesions typical of eczematous dermatitis
4. Personal or family history of atopy (asthma, allergic rhinitis, food allergies, or eczema)
5. Clinical course lasting >6 weeks
6. Lichenification of skin

The clinical presentation often varies with age. Half of patients with AD present within the first year of life, and 80% present by 5 years of age. About 80% ultimately coexpress allergic rhinitis or asthma. The infantile pattern is characterized by weeping inflammatory patches and crusted plaques on the face, neck, and extensor surfaces. The childhood and adolescent pattern is typified by dermatitis of flexural skin, particularly in the antecubital and popliteal fossae (Fig. 71-1). AD may resolve spontaneously, but approximately 40% of all individuals affected as children will have dermatitis in adult life. The distribution of lesions in adults may be similar to those seen in childhood; however, adults frequently have localized disease manifesting as lichen simplex chronicus or hand eczema (see below). In patients with localized disease, AD may be suspected because of a typical personal or family history or the presence of cutaneous stigmata of AD such as perioral pallor, an extra fold of skin beneath the lower eyelid (Dennie-Morgan folds), increased palmar skin markings, and an increased incidence of cutaneous infections, particularly with *Staphylococcus aureus*. Regardless of other manifestations, pruritus is a prominent characteristic of AD in all age groups and is exacerbated by dry skin. Many of the cutaneous findings in affected patients, such as lichenification, are secondary to rubbing and scratching.

TREATMENT ATOPIC DERMATITIS

Therapy for AD should include avoidance of cutaneous irritants, adequate moisturizing through the application of emollients, judicious use of topical anti-inflammatory agents, and prompt treatment of secondary infection. Patients should be instructed to bathe no more often than daily, using warm or cool water, and to use only mild bath soap. Immediately after bathing, while the skin is still moist, a topical anti-inflammatory agent in a cream or ointment base should be applied to areas of dermatitis, and all other skin

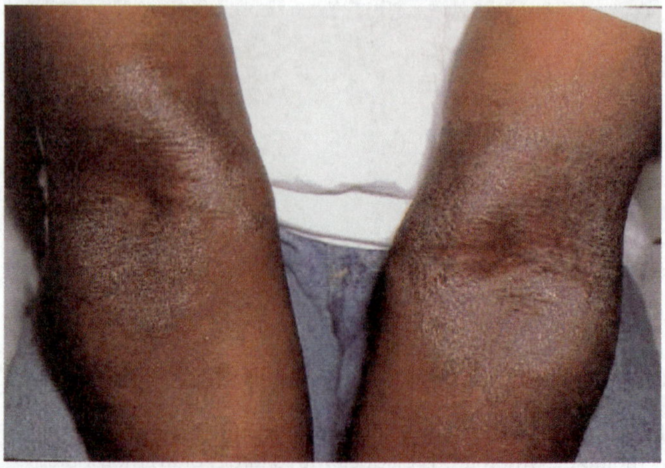

FIGURE 71-1 Atopic dermatitis. Hyperpigmentation, lichenification, and scaling in the antecubital fossae are seen in this patient with atopic dermatitis. *(Courtesy of Robert Swerlick, MD; with permission.)*

areas should be lubricated with a moisturizer. Approximately 30 g of a topical agent is required to cover the entire body surface of an average adult.

Low- to mid-potency topical glucocorticoids are employed in most treatment regimens for AD. Skin atrophy and the potential for systemic absorption are constant concerns, especially with more potent agents. Low-potency topical glucocorticoids or nonglucocorticoid anti-inflammatory agents should be selected for use on the face and in intertriginous areas to minimize the risk of skin atrophy. Two nonglucocorticoid anti-inflammatory agents are available: tacrolimus ointment and pimecrolimus cream. These agents are macrolide immunosuppressants that are approved by the U.S. Food and Drug Administration (FDA) for topical use in AD. Reports of broader effectiveness appear in the literature. These agents do not cause skin atrophy, nor do they suppress the hypothalamic-pituitary-adrenal axis. However, concerns have emerged regarding the potential for lymphomas in patients treated with these agents. Thus, caution should be exercised when these agents are considered. Currently, they are also more costly than topical glucocorticoids. Barrier-repair products that attempt to restore the impaired epidermal barrier are also nonglucocorticoid agents and are gaining popularity in the treatment of AD.

Secondary infection of eczematous skin may lead to exacerbation of AD. Crusted and weeping skin lesions may be infected with *S. aureus*. When secondary infection is suspected, eczematous lesions should be cultured and patients treated with systemic antibiotics active against *S. aureus*. The initial use of penicillinase-resistant penicillins or cephalosporins is preferable. Dicloxacillin or cephalexin (250 mg qid for 7–10 days) is generally adequate for adults; however, antibiotic selection must be directed by culture results and clinical response. More than 50% of *S. aureus* isolates are now methicillin resistant in some communities. Current recommendations for the treatment of infection with these community-acquired methicillin-resistant *S. aureus* (CA-MRSA) strains in adults include trimethoprim-sulfamethoxazole (1 double-strength tablet bid), minocycline (100 mg bid), doxycycline (100 mg bid), or clindamycin (300–450 mg qid). Duration of therapy should be 7–10 days. Inducible resistance may limit clindamycin's usefulness. Such resistance can be detected by the double-disk diffusion test, which should be ordered if the isolate is erythromycin resistant and clindamycin sensitive. As an adjunct, antibacterial washes or dilute sodium hypochlorite baths (0.005% bleach) and intermittent nasal mupirocin may be useful.

Control of pruritus is essential for treatment, because AD often represents "an itch that rashes." Antihistamines are most often used to control pruritus. Diphenhydramine (25 mg every 4–6 h), hydroxyzine (10–25mg every 6 h), or doxepin (10–25 mg at bedtime) are useful primarily due to their sedating action. Higher doses of these agents may be required, but sedation can become bothersome. Patients need to be counseled about driving or operating heavy equipment after taking these medications. When used at bedtime, sedating antihistamines may improve the patient's sleep. Although they are effective in urticaria, non-sedating antihistamines and selective H_2 blockers are of little use in controlling the pruritus of AD.

Treatment with systemic glucocorticoids should be limited to severe exacerbations unresponsive to topical therapy. In the patient with chronic AD, therapy with systemic glucocorticoids will generally clear the skin only briefly, and cessation of the systemic therapy will invariably be accompanied by a return, if not a worsening, of the dermatitis. Patients who do not respond to conventional therapies should be considered for patch testing to rule out allergic contact dermatitis (ACD). The role of dietary allergens in AD is controversial, and there is little evidence that they play any role outside of infancy, during which a small percentage of patients with AD may be affected by food allergens.

LICHEN SIMPLEX CHRONICUS

Lichen simplex chronicus may represent the end stage of a variety of pruritic and eczematous disorders, including AD. It consists of a circumscribed plaque or plaques of lichenified skin due to chronic scratching or rubbing. Common areas involved include the posterior nuchal region, dorsum of the feet, and ankles. Treatment of lichen simplex chronicus centers on breaking the cycle of chronic itching and scratching. High-potency topical glucocorticoids are helpful in most cases, but, in recalcitrant cases, application of topical glucocorticoids under occlusion, or intralesional injection of glucocorticoids may be required.

CONTACT DERMATITIS

Contact dermatitis is an inflammatory skin process caused by an exogenous agent or agents that directly or indirectly injure the skin. In *irritant* contact dermatitis (ICD), this injury is caused by an inherent characteristic of a compound—for example, a concentrated acid or base. Agents that cause ACD induce an antigen-specific immune response (e.g., poison ivy dermatitis). The clinical lesions of contact dermatitis may be acute (wet and edematous) or chronic (dry, thickened, and scaly), depending on the persistence of the insult (see Fig. 70-10).

Irritant Contact Dermatitis ICD is generally well demarcated and often localized to areas of thin skin (eyelids, intertriginous areas) or to areas where the irritant was occluded. Lesions may range from minimal skin erythema to areas of marked edema, vesicles, and ulcers. Prior exposure to the offending agent is not necessary, and the reaction develops in minutes to a few hours. Chronic low-grade irritant dermatitis is the most common type of ICD, and the most common area of involvement is the hands (see below). The most common irritants encountered are chronic wet work, soaps, and detergents. Treatment should be directed toward the avoidance of irritants and the use of protective gloves or clothing.

Allergic Contact Dermatitis ACD is a manifestation of delayed-type hypersensitivity mediated by memory T lymphocytes in the skin. Prior exposure to the offending agent is necessary to develop the hypersensitivity reaction, which may take as little as 12 h or as much as 72 h to develop. The most common cause of ACD is exposure to plants, especially to members of the family Anacardiaceae, including the genus *Toxicodendron*. Poison ivy, poison oak, and poison sumac are members of this genus and cause an allergic reaction marked by erythema, vesiculation, and severe pruritus. The eruption is often linear or angular, corresponding to areas where plants have touched the skin. The sensitizing antigen common to these plants is urushiol, an oleoresin containing the active ingredient pentadecylcatechol. The oleoresin may adhere to skin, clothing, tools, and pets, and contaminated articles may cause dermatitis even after prolonged storage. Blister fluid does not contain urushiol and is not capable of inducing skin eruption in exposed subjects.

TREATMENT CONTACT DERMATITIS

If contact dermatitis is suspected and an offending agent is identified and removed, the eruption will resolve. Usually, treatment with high-potency topical glucocorticoids is enough to relieve symptoms while the dermatitis runs its course. For those patients who require systemic therapy, daily oral prednisone—beginning at 1 mg/kg, but usually ≤60 mg/d—is sufficient. The dose should be tapered over 2–3 weeks, and each daily dose should be taken in the morning with food.

Identification of a contact allergen can be a difficult and time-consuming task. Allergic contact dermatitis should be suspected in patients with dermatitis unresponsive to conventional therapy or with an unusual and patterned distribution. Patients should be questioned carefully regarding occupational exposures and topical medications. Common sensitizers include preservatives in topical preparations, nickel sulfate, potassium dichromate, thimerosal, neomycin sulfate, fragrances, formaldehyde, and rubber-curing agents. Patch testing is helpful in identifying these agents but should not be attempted when patients have widespread active dermatitis or are taking systemic glucocorticoids.

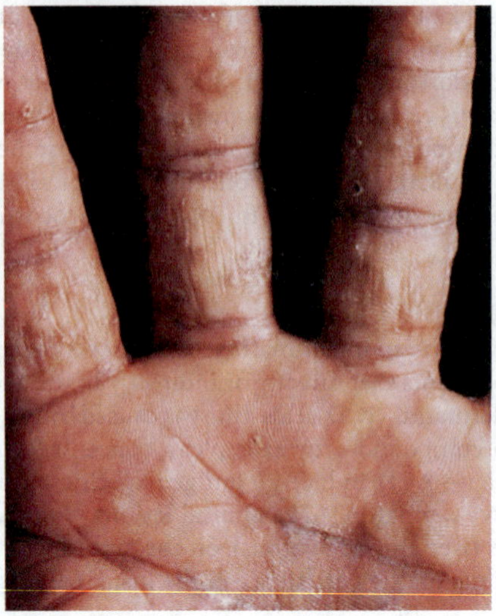

FIGURE 71-2 Dyshidrotic eczema. This example is characterized by deep-seated vesicles and scaling on palms and lateral fingers, and the disease is often associated with an atopic diathesis.

HAND ECZEMA

Hand eczema is a very common, chronic skin disorder in which both exogenous and endogenous factors play important roles. It may be associated with other cutaneous disorders such as AD, and contact with various agents may be involved. Hand eczema represents a large proportion of cases of occupation-associated skin disease. Chronic, excessive exposure to water and detergents, harsh chemicals, or allergens may initiate or aggravate this disorder. It may present with dryness and cracking of the skin of the hands as well as with variable amounts of erythema and edema. Often, the dermatitis will begin under rings, where water and irritants are trapped. *Dyshidrotic* eczema, a variant of hand eczema, presents with multiple, intensely pruritic, small papules and vesicles on the thenar and hypothenar eminences and the sides of the fingers (Fig. 71-2). Lesions tend to occur in crops that slowly form crusts and then heal.

The evaluation of a patient with hand eczema should include an assessment of potential occupation-associated exposures. The history should be directed to identifying possible irritant or allergen exposures.

TREATMENT HAND ECZEMA

Therapy for hand eczema is directed toward avoidance of irritants, identification of possible contact allergens, treatment of coexistent infection, and application of topical glucocorticoids. Whenever possible, the hands should be protected by gloves, preferably vinyl. The use of rubber gloves (latex) to protect dermatitic skin is sometimes associated with the development of hypersensitivity reactions to components of the gloves. Patients can be treated with cool moist compresses followed by application of a mid- to high-potency topical glucocorticoid in a cream or ointment base. As in AD, treatment of secondary infection is essential for good control. In addition, patients with hand eczema should be examined for dermatophyte infection by KOH preparation and culture (see below).

NUMMULAR ECZEMA

Nummular eczema is characterized by circular or oval "coinlike" lesions, beginning as small edematous papules that become crusted and scaly. The etiology of nummular eczema is unknown, but dry skin is a contributing factor. Common locations are the trunk or the extensor surfaces of the extremities, particularly on the pretibial areas or dorsum of the hands. Nummular eczema occurs more frequently in men and is most common in middle age. The treatment of nummular eczema is similar to that for AD.

ASTEATOTIC ECZEMA

Asteatotic eczema, also known as *xerotic eczema* or *"winter itch,"* is a mildly inflammatory dermatitis that develops in areas of extremely dry skin, especially during the dry winter months. Clinically, there may be considerable overlap with nummular eczema. This form of eczema accounts for a large number of physician visits because of the associated pruritus. Fine cracks and scale, with or without erythema, characteristically develop in areas of dry skin, especially on the anterior surfaces of the lower extremities in elderly patients. Asteatotic eczema responds well to topical moisturizers and the avoidance of cutaneous irritants. Overbathing and the use of harsh soaps exacerbate asteatotic eczema.

STASIS DERMATITIS AND STASIS ULCERATION

Stasis dermatitis develops on the lower extremities secondary to venous incompetence and chronic edema. Patients may give a history of deep venous thrombosis and may have evidence of vein removal or varicose veins. Early findings in stasis dermatitis consist of mild erythema and scaling associated with pruritus. The typical initial site of involvement is the medial aspect of the ankle, often over a distended vein (Fig. 71-3).

Stasis dermatitis may become acutely inflamed, with crusting and exudate. In this state, it is easily confused with cellulitis. Chronic stasis dermatitis is often associated with dermal fibrosis that is recognized clinically as brawny edema of the skin. As the disorder progresses, the dermatitis becomes progressively pigmented due to chronic erythrocyte extravasation leading to cutaneous hemosiderin deposition. Stasis dermatitis may be complicated by secondary infection and contact dermatitis. Severe stasis dermatitis may precede the development of stasis ulcers.

TREATMENT STASIS DERMATITIS AND STASIS ULCERATION

Patients with stasis dermatitis and stasis ulceration benefit greatly from leg elevation and the routine use of compression stockings with a gradient of at least 30–40 mmHg. Stockings providing less compression, such as antiembolism hose, are poor substitutes. Use of emollients and/or mid-potency topical glucocorticoids and avoidance of irritants are also helpful in treating stasis dermatitis. Protection of the legs from injury, including scratching, and control of chronic edema are essential to prevent ulcers. Diuretics may be required to adequately control chronic edema.

Stasis ulcers are difficult to treat, and resolution is slow. It is extremely important to elevate the affected limb as much as possible. The ulcer should be kept clear of necrotic material by gentle debridement and covered with a semipermeable dressing and a compression dressing or compression stocking. Glucocorticoids

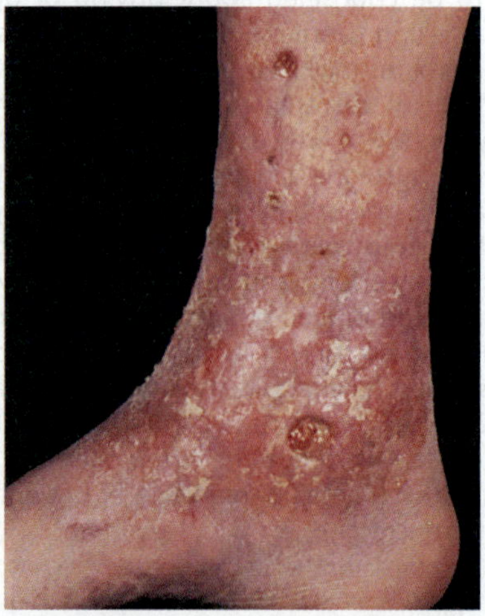

FIGURE 71-3 Stasis dermatitis. An example of stasis dermatitis showing erythematous, scaly, and oozing patches over the lower leg. Several stasis ulcers are also seen in this patient.

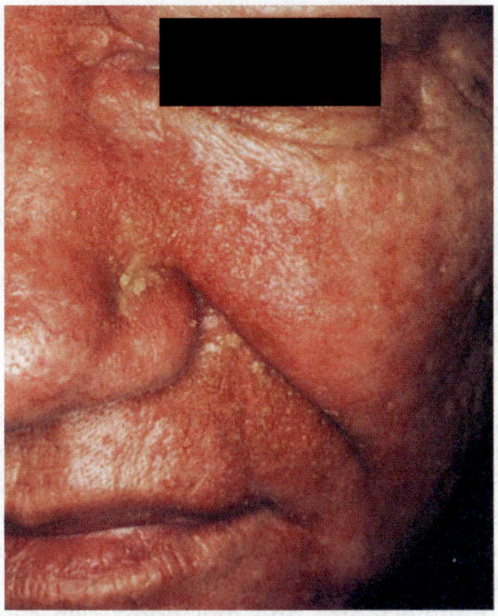

FIGURE 71-4 Seborrheic dermatitis. Central facial erythema with overlying greasy, yellowish scale is seen in this patient. *(Courtesy of Jean Bolognia, MD; with permission.)*

should not be applied to ulcers, because they may retard healing; however, they may be applied to the surrounding skin to control itching, scratching, and additional trauma. Secondarily infected lesions should be treated with appropriate oral antibiotics, but it should be noted that all ulcers will become colonized with bacteria, and the purpose of antibiotic therapy should not be to clear all bacterial growth. Care must be taken to exclude treatable causes of leg ulcers (hypercoagulation, vasculitis) before beginning the chronic management outlined above.

SEBORRHEIC DERMATITIS

Seborrheic dermatitis is a common, chronic disorder characterized by greasy scales overlying erythematous patches or plaques. Induration and scale are generally less prominent than in psoriasis, but clinical overlap exists between these diseases ("sebopsoriasis"). The most common location is in the scalp, where it may be recognized as severe dandruff. On the face, seborrheic dermatitis affects the eyebrows, eyelids, glabella, and nasolabial folds (Fig. 71-4). Scaling of the external auditory canal is common in seborrheic dermatitis. In addition, the postauricular areas often become macerated and tender. Seborrheic dermatitis may also develop in the central chest, axilla, groin, submammary folds, and gluteal cleft. Rarely, it may cause widespread generalized dermatitis. Pruritus is variable.

Seborrheic dermatitis may be evident within the first few weeks of life, and within this context it typically occurs in the scalp ("cradle cap"), face, or groin. It is rarely seen in children beyond infancy but becomes evident again during adult life. Although it is frequently seen in patients with Parkinson's disease, in those who have had cerebrovascular accidents, and in those with HIV infection, the overwhelming majority of individuals with seborrheic dermatitis have no underlying disorder.

TREATMENT SEBORRHEIC DERMATITIS

Treatment with low-potency topical glucocorticoids in conjunction with a topical antifungal agent, such as ketoconazole cream or ciclopirox cream, is often effective. The scalp and beard areas may benefit from antidandruff shampoos, which should be left in place 3–5 min before rinsing. High-potency topical glucocorticoid solutions (betamethasone or clobetasol) are effective for control of severe scalp involvement. High-potency glucocorticoids should not be used on the face because this treatment is often associated with steroid-induced rosacea or atrophy.

PAPULOSQUAMOUS DISORDERS (TABLE 71-2)

PSORIASIS

Psoriasis is one of the most common dermatologic diseases, affecting up to 2% of the world's population. It is an immune-mediated disease clinically characterized by erythematous, sharply demarcated papules and rounded plaques covered by silvery micaceous scale. The skin lesions of psoriasis are variably pruritic. Traumatized areas often develop lesions of psoriasis (the *Koebner* or isomorphic phenomenon). In addition, other external factors may exacerbate psoriasis, including infections, stress, and medications (lithium, beta blockers, and antimalarial drugs).

The most common variety of psoriasis is called *plaque-type*. Patients with plaque-type psoriasis have stable, slowly enlarging plaques, which remain basically unchanged for long periods of time. The most commonly involved areas are the elbows, knees, gluteal cleft, and scalp. Involvement tends to be symmetric. Plaque psoriasis generally develops slowly and runs an indolent course. It rarely remits spontaneously. *Inverse psoriasis* affects the intertriginous regions, including the axilla, groin, submammary region, and navel; it also tends to affect the scalp, palms, and soles. The individual lesions are sharply demarcated plaques (see Fig. 70-7), but they may be moist and without scale due to their locations.

Guttate psoriasis (eruptive psoriasis) is most common in children and young adults. It develops acutely in individuals without psoriasis or in those with chronic plaque psoriasis. Patients present with many small erythematous, scaling papules, frequently after upper respiratory tract infection with β-hemolytic streptococci. The differential diagnosis should include pityriasis rosea and secondary syphilis.

In *pustular psoriasis*, patients may have disease localized to the palms and soles, or the disease may be generalized. Regardless of the extent of disease, the skin is erythematous, with pustules and variable scale. Localized to the palms and soles, it is easily confused with eczema. When it is generalized, episodes are characterized by fever (39°–40°C [102.2°–104.0°F]) lasting several days, an accompanying generalized eruption of sterile pustules, and a background of intense erythema; patients may become erythrodermic. Episodes of fever and pustules are recurrent. Local irritants, pregnancy, medications, infections, and systemic glucocorticoid withdrawal can precipitate this form of psoriasis. Oral retinoids are the treatment of choice in nonpregnant patients.

TABLE 71-2 PAPULOSQUAMOUS DISORDERS

	Clinical Features	Other Notable Features	Histologic Features
Psoriasis	Sharply demarcated, erythematous plaques with mica-like scale; predominantly on elbows, knees, and scalp; atypical forms may localize to intertriginous areas; eruptive forms may be associated with infection	May be aggravated by certain drugs, infection; severe forms seen in association with HIV	Acanthosis, vascular proliferation
Lichen planus	Purple polygonal papules marked by severe pruritus; lacy white markings, especially associated with mucous membrane lesions	Certain drugs may induce: thiazides, antimalarial drugs	Interface dermatitis
Pityriasis rosea	Rash often preceded by herald patch; oval to round plaques with trailing scale; most often affects trunk; eruption lines up in skinfolds giving a "fir tree–like" appearance; generally spares palms and soles	Variable pruritus; self-limited, resolving in 2–8 weeks; may be imitated by secondary syphilis	Pathologic features often nonspecific
Dermatophytosis	Polymorphous appearance depending on dermatophyte, body site, and host response; sharply defined to ill-demarcated scaly plaques with or without inflammation; may be associated with hair loss	KOH preparation may show branching hyphae; culture helpful	Hyphae and neutrophils in stratum corneum

TABLE 71-3 FDA-APPROVED SYSTEMIC THERAPY FOR PSORIASIS

Agent	Medication Class	Administration: Route	Administration: Frequency	Adverse Events (Selected)
Methotrexate	Antimetabolite	Oral	Weekly	Hepatotoxicity, pulmonary toxicity, pancytopenia, potential for increased malignancies, ulcerative stomatitis, nausea, diarrhea, teratogenicity
Acitretin	Retinoid	Oral	Daily	Teratogenicity, hepatotoxicity, hyperostosis, hyperlipidemia/pancreatitis, depression, ophthalmologic effects, pseudotumor cerebri
Cyclosporine	Calcineurin inhibitor	Oral	Twice daily	Renal dysfunction, hypertension, hyperkalemia, hyperuricemia, hypomagnesemia, hyperlipidemia, increased risk of malignancies

Fingernail involvement, appearing as punctate pitting, onycholysis, nail thickening, or subungual hyperkeratosis, may be a clue to the diagnosis of psoriasis when the clinical presentation is not classic.

According to the National Psoriasis Foundation, up to 30% of patients with psoriasis have psoriatic arthritis (PsA). There are five subtypes of PsA: symmetric, asymmetric, distal interphalangeal predominant (DIP), spondylitis, and arthritis mutilans. Symmetric arthritis resembles rheumatoid arthritis, but is usually milder. Asymmetric arthritis can involve any joint and may present as "sausage digits." DIP is the classic form, but occurs in only about 5% of patients with PsA. It may involve fingers and toes. Spondylitis also occurs in about 5% of patients with PsA. Arthritis mutilans is severe and deforming. It affects primarily the small joints of the hands and feet. It accounts for fewer than 5% of PsA cases.

An increased risk of metabolic syndrome, including increased morbidity and mortality from cardiovascular events, has been demonstrated in psoriasis patients. Appropriate screening tests should be performed. The etiology of psoriasis is still poorly understood, but there is clearly a genetic component to the disease. In various studies, 30–50% of patients with psoriasis report a positive family history. Psoriatic lesions contain infiltrates of activated T cells that are thought to elaborate cytokines responsible for keratinocyte hyperproliferation, which results in the characteristic clinical findings. Agents inhibiting T cell activation, clonal expansion, or release of proinflammatory cytokines are often effective for the treatment of severe psoriasis (see below).

TREATMENT PSORIASIS

Treatment of psoriasis depends on the type, location, and extent of disease. All patients should be instructed to avoid excess drying or irritation of their skin and to maintain adequate cutaneous hydration. Most cases of localized, plaque-type psoriasis can be managed with mid-potency topical glucocorticoids, although their long-term use is often accompanied by loss of effectiveness (tachyphylaxis) and atrophy of the skin. A topical vitamin D analogue (calcipotriene) and a retinoid (tazarotene) are also efficacious in the treatment of limited psoriasis and have largely replaced other topical agents such as coal tar, salicylic acid, and anthralin.

Ultraviolet (UV) light, natural or artificial, is an effective therapy for many patients with widespread psoriasis. Ultraviolet B (UVB), narrowband UVB, and ultraviolet A (UVA) light with either oral or topical psoralens (PUVA) is used clinically. UV light's immunosuppressive properties are thought to be responsible for its therapeutic activity in psoriasis. It is also mutagenic, potentially leading to an increased incidence of nonmelanoma and melanoma skin cancer. UV-light therapy is contraindicated in patients receiving cyclosporine and should be used with great care in all immunocompromised patients due to the increased risk of skin cancer.

Various systemic agents can be used for severe, widespread psoriatic disease (Table 71-3). Oral glucocorticoids should not be used for the treatment of psoriasis due to the potential for development of life-threatening pustular psoriasis when therapy is discontinued. Methotrexate is an effective agent, especially in patients with psoriatic arthritis. The synthetic retinoid acitretin is useful, especially when immunosuppression must be avoided; however, teratogenicity limits its use.

The evidence implicating psoriasis as a T cell–mediated disorder has directed therapeutic efforts to immunoregulation. Cyclosporine and other immunosuppressive agents can be very effective in the treatment of psoriasis, and much attention is currently directed toward the development of biologic agents with more selective immunosuppressive properties and better safety profiles (Table 71-4). Experience with these biologic agents is limited, and information regarding combination therapy and adverse events continues to emerge. Use of tumor necrosis factor (TNF-α) inhibitors may worsen congestive heart failure (CHF), and they should be used with caution in patients at risk for or known to have CHF. Further, none of the immunosuppressive agents used in the treatment of psoriasis should be initiated if the patient has a severe infection; patients on such therapy should be routinely screened for tuberculosis. There have been reports of progressive multifocal leukoencephalopathy in association with treatment with the TNF-α inhibitors. Malignancies, including a risk or history of certain malignancies, may limit the use of these systemic agents.

TABLE 71-4 BIOLOGICS APPROVED FOR PSORIASIS OR PSORIATIC ARTHRITIS

Agent	Mechanism of Action	Administration: Indication	Administration: Route	Frequency	Warnings
Etanercept	Anti-TNF-α	Ps, PsA	SC	Once or twice weekly	Serious infections, hepatotoxicity, CHF, hematologic events, hypersensitivity reactions, neurologic events, potential for increased malignancies
Adalimumab	Anti-TNF-α	Ps, PsA	SC	Every other week	Serious infections, hepatotoxicity, CHF, hematologic events, hypersensitivity reactions, neurologic events, potential for increased malignancies
Infliximab	Anti-TNF-α	Ps, PsA	IV	Initial infusion followed by infusions at weeks 2 and 6, then every 8 weeks	Serious infections, hepatotoxicity, CHF, hematologic events, hypersensitivity reactions, neurologic events, potential for increased malignancies
Golimumab	Anti-TNF-α	PsA	SC	Monthly	Serious infections, hepatotoxicity, CHF, hypersensitivity reactions, neurologic events, potential for increased malignancies
Ustekinumab	Anti-IL-12 and anti-IL-23	Ps	SC	2 doses 4 weeks apart, then every 12 weeks	Serious infections, neurologic events, potential for increased malignancies

Abbreviations: CHF, congestive heart failure; IL, interleukin; IM, intramuscular; Ps, psoriasis; PsA, psoriatic arthritis; SC, subcutaneous; TNF, tumor necrosis factor.

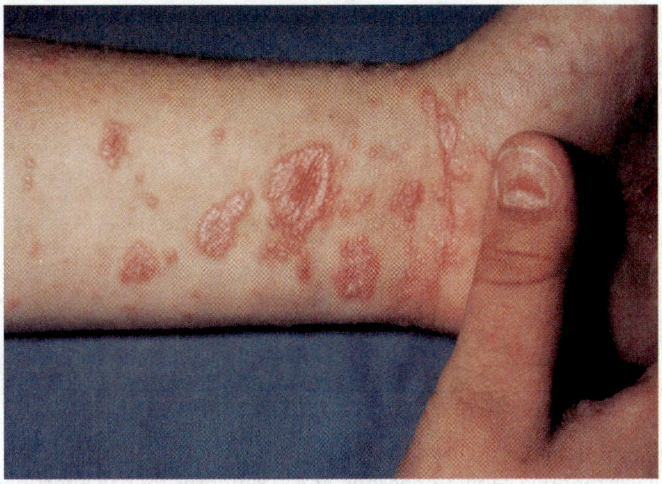

FIGURE 71-5 Lichen planus. An example of lichen planus showing multiple flat-topped, violaceous papules and plaques. Nail dystrophy, as seen in this patient's thumbnail, may also be a feature. *(Courtesy of Robert Swerlick, MD; with permission.)*

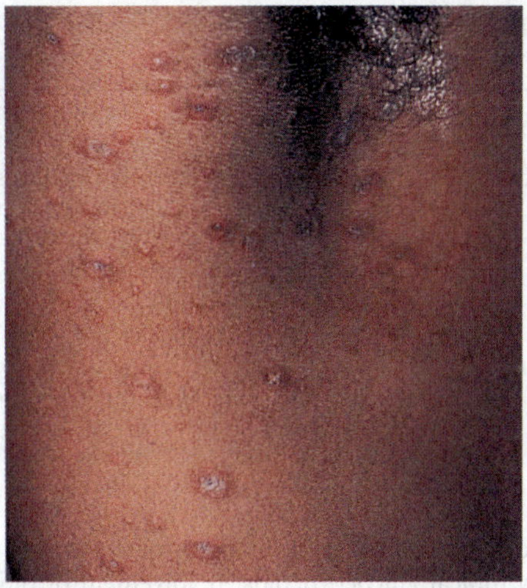

FIGURE 71-6 Pityriasis rosea. In this patient with pityriasis rosea, multiple round to oval erythematous patches with fine central scale are distributed along the skin tension lines on the trunk.

LICHEN PLANUS

Lichen planus (LP) is a papulosquamous disorder that may affect the skin, scalp, nails, and mucous membranes. The primary cutaneous lesions are pruritic, polygonal, flat-topped, violaceous papules. Close examination of the surface of these papules often reveals a network of gray lines (*Wickham's striae*). The skin lesions may occur anywhere but have a predilection for the wrists, shins, lower back, and genitalia (Fig. 71-5). Involvement of the scalp (*lichen planopilaris*) may lead to scarring alopecia, and nail involvement may lead to permanent deformity or loss of fingernails and toenails. LP commonly involves mucous membranes, particularly the buccal mucosa, where it can present on a spectrum ranging from a mild, white, reticulate eruption of the mucosa to a severe, erosive stomatitis. Erosive stomatitis may persist for years and may be linked to an increased risk of oral squamous cell carcinoma. Cutaneous eruptions clinically resembling LP have been observed after administration of numerous drugs, including thiazide diuretics, gold, antimalarial agents, penicillamine, and phenothiazines, and in patients with skin lesions of chronic graft-versus-host disease. In addition, LP may be associated with hepatitis C infection. The course of LP is variable, but most patients have spontaneous remissions 6 months to 2 years after the onset of disease. Topical glucocorticoids are the mainstay of therapy.

PITYRIASIS ROSEA

Pityriasis rosea (PR) is a papulosquamous eruption of unknown etiology occurring more commonly in the spring and fall. Its first manifestation is the development of a 2- to 6-cm annular lesion (the herald patch). This is followed in a few days to a few weeks by the appearance of many smaller annular or papular lesions with a predilection to occur on the trunk (Fig. 71-6). The lesions are generally oval, with their long axis parallel to the skinfold lines. Individual lesions may range in color from red to brown and have a trailing scale. PR shares many clinical features with the eruption of secondary syphilis, but palm and sole lesions are extremely rare in PR and common in secondary syphilis. The eruption tends to be moderately pruritic and lasts 3–8 weeks. Treatment is directed at alleviating pruritus and consists of oral antihistamines; mid-potency topical glucocorticoids; and, in some cases, UVB phototherapy.

CUTANEOUS INFECTIONS (TABLE 71-5)

IMPETIGO, ECTHYMA, AND FURUNCULOSIS

Impetigo is a common superficial bacterial infection of skin caused most often by *S. aureus* (Chap. 172) and in some cases by group A β-hemolytic streptococci (Chap. 173). The primary lesion is a superficial pustule that ruptures and forms a characteristic yellow-brown honey-colored crust (see Fig. 173-3). Lesions may occur on normal skin (primary infection) or in areas already affected by another skin disease (secondary infection). Lesions caused by staphylococci may be tense, clear bullae, and this less common form of the disease is called *bullous impetigo*. Blisters are caused by the production of exfoliative toxin by *S. aureus* phage type II. This is the same toxin responsible for staphylococcal scalded-skin syndrome, often resulting in dramatic loss of the superficial epidermis due to blistering. The latter syndrome is much more common in children than in adults; however, it should be considered along with toxic epidermal necrolysis and severe drug eruptions in patients with widespread blistering of the skin. *Ecthyma* is a deep non-bullous variant of impetigo that causes punched-out ulcerative lesions. It is more often caused by a primary or secondary infection with *Streptococcus pyogenes*. Ecthyma is a deeper infection than typical impetigo and resolves with scars. Treatment of both ecthyma and impetigo involves gentle debridement of adherent crusts, which is facilitated by the use of soaks and topical antibiotics in conjunction with appropriate oral antibiotics.

Furunculosis is also caused by *S. aureus*, and this disorder has gained prominence in the last decade because of CA-MRSA. A furuncle, or boil, is a painful, erythematous nodule that can occur on any cutaneous surface. The lesions may be solitary but are most often multiple. Patients frequently believe they have been bitten by spiders or insects. Family members or close contacts may also be affected. Furuncles can rupture and drain spontaneously or may need incision and drainage, which may be adequate therapy for small solitary furuncles without cellulitis or systemic symptoms. Whenever possible, lesional material should be sent for culture. Current recommendations for methicillin-sensitive infections are β-lactam antibiotics. Therapy for CA-MRSA was discussed previously (see "Atopic Dermatitis"). Warm compresses and nasal mupirocin are helpful therapeutic additions. Severe infections may require IV antibiotics.

ERYSIPELAS AND CELLULITIS

See Chap. 156.

DERMATOPHYTOSIS

Dermatophytes are fungi that infect skin, hair, and nails and include members of the genera *Trichophyton*, *Microsporum*, and *Epidermophyton* (Chap. 243). *Tinea corporis*, or infection of the relatively hairless skin of the body (glabrous skin), may have a variable appearance depending on the extent of the associated inflammatory reaction. Typical infections consist of erythematous, scaly plaques, with an annular appearance that accounts for the common name "ringworm." Deep inflammatory nodules or granulomas occur in

TABLE 71-5 COMMON SKIN INFECTIONS

	Clinical Features	Etiologic Agent	Treatment
Impetigo	Honey-colored crusted papules, plaques, or bullae	Group A *Streptococcus* and *Staphylococcus aureus*	Systemic or topical antistaphylococcal and antistreptoccal antibiotics
Dermatophytosis	Inflammatory or noninflammatory annular scaly plaques; may involve hair loss; groin involvement spares scrotum; hyphae on KOH preparation	*Trichophyton, Epidermophyton*, or *Microsporum* spp.	Topical azoles, systemic griseofulvin, terbinafine, or azoles
Candidiasis	Inflammatory papules and plaques with satellite pustules, frequently in intertriginous areas; may involve scrotum; pseudohyphae on KOH preparation	*Candida albicans* and other *Candida* spp.	Topical nystatin or azoles; systemic azoles for resistant disease
Tinea versicolor	Hyper- or hypopigmented scaly patches on trunk; characteristic mixture of hyphae and spores ("spaghetti and meatballs") on KOH preparation	*Malassezia furfur*	Topical selenium sulfide lotion or azoles

some infections, most often those inappropriately treated with mid- to high-potency topical glucocorticoids. Involvement of the groin (*tinea cruris*) is more common in males than in females. It presents as a scaling, erythematous eruption sparing the scrotum. Infection of the foot (*tinea pedis*) is the most common dermatophyte infection and is often chronic; it is characterized by variable erythema, edema, scaling, pruritus, and occasionally vesiculation. The infection may be widespread or localized but generally involves the web space between the fourth and fifth toes. Infection of the nails (*tinea unguium* or *onychomycosis*) occurs in many patients with tinea pedis and is characterized by opacified, thickened nails and subungual debris. The distal-lateral variant is most common. Proximal subungual onychomycosis may be a marker for HIV infection or other immunocompromised states. Dermatophyte infection of the scalp (*tinea capitis*) continues to be common, particularly affecting inner-city children but also affecting adults. The predominant organism is *Trichophyton tonsurans*, which can produce a relatively noninflammatory infection with mild scale and hair loss that is diffuse or localized. *T. tonsurans* can also cause a markedly inflammatory dermatosis with edema and nodules. This latter presentation is a *kerion*.

The diagnosis of tinea can be made from skin scrapings, nail scrapings, or hair by culture or direct microscopic examination with potassium hydroxide (KOH). Nail clippings may be sent for histologic examination with periodic acid–Schiff (PAS) stain.

TREATMENT DERMATOPHYTOSIS

Both topical and systemic therapies may be used in dermatophyte infections. Treatment depends on the site involved and the type of infection. Topical therapy is generally effective for uncomplicated tinea corporis, tinea cruris, and limited tinea pedis. Topical agents are not effective as monotherapy for tinea capitis or onychomycosis (see below). Topical imidazoles, triazoles, and allylamines may be effective therapies for dermatophyte infections, but nystatin is not active against dermatophytes. Topicals are generally applied twice daily, and treatment should continue for 1 week beyond clinical resolution of the infection. Tinea pedis often requires longer treatment courses and frequently relapses. Oral antifungal agents may be required for recalcitrant tinea pedis or tinea corporis.

Oral antifungal agents are required for dermatophyte infections involving the hair and nails and for other infections unresponsive to topical therapy. A fungal etiology should be confirmed by direct microscopic examination or by culture before oral antifungal agents are prescribed. All of the oral agents may cause hepatotoxicity. They should not be used in women who are pregnant or breast-feeding.

Griseofulvin is approved in the United States for dermatophyte infections involving the skin, hair, or nails. When griseofulvin is used, a daily dose of 500 mg microsized or 375 mg ultramicrosized, administered with a fatty meal, is adequate for most dermatophyte infections. Higher doses are required for some cases of tinea pedis and tinea capitis. Markedly inflammatory tinea capitis may result in scarring and hair loss, and systemic or topical glucocorticoids may be helpful in preventing these sequelae. The duration of griseofulvin therapy may be 2 weeks for uncomplicated tinea corporis, 8–12 weeks for tinea capitis, or as long as 6–18 months for nail infections. Due to high relapse rates, griseofulvin is seldom used for nail infections. Common side effects of griseofulvin include gastrointestinal distress, headache, and urticaria.

Oral itraconazole is approved for onychomycosis. Itraconazole is given with food as either continuous daily therapy (200 mg/d) or pulses (200 mg bid for 1 week per month). Fingernails require 2 months of continuous therapy or two pulses. Toenails require 3 months of continuous therapy or three pulses. Itraconazole has the potential for serious interactions with other drugs requiring the P450 enzyme system for metabolism. Itraconazole should not be administered to patients with evidence of ventricular dysfunction or patients with known CHF. Terbinafine (250 mg/d) is also effective for onychomycosis, and the granule version is approved for treatment of tinea capitis. Therapy with terbinafine is continued for 6 weeks for fingernail and scalp infections and 12 weeks for toenail infections. Terbinafine has fewer interactions with other drugs than itraconazole, but caution should be used with patients who are on multiple medications. The risk/benefit ratio should be considered when an asymptomatic toenail infection is treated with systemic agents.

TINEA VERSICOLOR

Tinea versicolor is caused by a nondermatophytic, dimorphic fungus, *Malassezia furfur*, a normal inhabitant of the skin. The expression of infection is promoted by heat and humidity. The typical lesions consist of oval scaly macules, papules, and patches concentrated on the chest, shoulders, and back but only rarely on the face or distal extremities. On dark skin the lesions often appear as hypopigmented areas, while on light skin they are slightly erythematous or hyperpigmented. A KOH preparation from scaling lesions will demonstrate a confluence of short hyphae and round spores ("spaghetti and meatballs"). Lotions or shampoos containing sulfur, salicylic acid, or selenium sulfide will clear the infection if used daily for 1–2 weeks and then weekly thereafter. These preparations are irritating if left on the skin for >10 min; thus, they should be washed off completely. Treatment with some oral antifungal agents is also effective, but they do not provide lasting results and are not FDA approved for this indication. A very short course of ketoconazole has been used, as have itraconazole and fluconazole. The patient must sweat after taking the medication if it is to be effective. Griseofulvin is not effective and terbinafine is not reliably effective for tinea versicolor.

CANDIDIASIS

Candidiasis is a fungal infection caused by a related group of yeasts whose manifestations may be localized to the skin and mucous membranes or, rarely, may be systemic and life-threatening (Chap. 240). The causative organism is usually *Candida albicans*. These organisms are normal saprophytic inhabitants of the gastrointestinal tract but may overgrow due to broad-spectrum antibiotic therapy, diabetes mellitus, or immunosuppression and cause disease. Candidiasis is a very common infection in HIV-infected individuals (Chap. 226). The oral cavity is commonly involved. Lesions may occur on the tongue or buccal mucosa (*thrush*) and appear as white plaques. Fissured, macerated lesions at the corners of the mouth (*perléche*) are often seen in individuals with poorly fitting dentures and may also be associated with candidal infection. In addition, candidal infections have an affinity for sites that are chronically wet and macerated, including the skin around nails (onycholysis and paronychia), and in intertriginous areas. Intertriginous lesions are characteristically edematous, erythematous, and scaly, with scattered "satellite pustules." In males, there is often involvement of the penis and scrotum as well as the inner aspect of the thighs. In contrast to dermatophyte infections, candidal infections are frequently painful and accompanied by a marked inflammatory response. Diagnosis of candidal infection is based upon the clinical pattern and demonstration of yeast on KOH preparation or culture.

TREATMENT CANDIDIASIS

Treatment involves removal of any predisposing factors such as antibiotic therapy or chronic wetness and the use of appropriate topical or systemic antifungal agents. Effective topicals include nystatin or azoles (miconazole, clotrimazole, econazole, or ketoconazole). The associated inflammatory response accompanying candidal infection on glabrous skin can be treated with a mild glucocorticoid lotion or cream (2.5% hydrocortisone). Systemic therapy is usually reserved for immunosuppressed patients or individuals with chronic or recurrent disease who fail to respond to appropriate topical therapy. Oral agents approved for the treatment of candidiasis include itraconazole and fluconazole. Oral nystatin is effective only for candidiasis of the gastrointestinal tract. Griseofulvin and terbinafine are not effective.

WARTS

Warts are cutaneous neoplasms caused by papillomaviruses. More than 100 different human papillomaviruses (HPVs) have been described. A typical wart, *verruca vulgaris*, is sessile, dome-shaped, and usually about a centimeter in diameter. Its surface is hyperkeratotic, consisting of many small filamentous projections. The HPV types that cause typical verruca vulgaris also cause typical plantar warts, flat warts (*verruca plana*), and filiform warts. Plantar warts are endophytic and are covered by thick keratin. Paring of the wart will generally reveal a central core of keratinized debris and punctate bleeding points. Filiform warts are most commonly seen on the face, neck, and skinfolds and present as papillomatous lesions on a narrow base. Flat warts are only slightly elevated and have a velvety, nonverrucous surface. They have a propensity for the face, arms, and legs and are often spread by shaving.

Genital warts begin as small papillomas that may grow to form large, fungating lesions. In women, they may involve the labia, perineum, or perianal skin. In addition, the mucosa of the vagina, urethra, and anus can be involved as well as the cervical epithelium. In men, the lesions often occur initially in the coronal sulcus but may be seen on the shaft of the penis, the scrotum, or the perianal skin or in the urethra.

Appreciable evidence has accumulated indicating that HPV plays a role in the development of neoplasia of the uterine cervix and anogenital skin (Chap. 117). HPV types 16 and 18 have been most intensely studied and are the major risk factors for intraepithelial neoplasia and squamous cell carcinoma of the cervix, anus, vulva, and penis. The risk is higher among patients immunosuppressed after solid organ transplantation and among those infected with HIV. Recent evidence also implicates other HPV types. Histologic examination of biopsied samples from affected sites may reveal changes associated with typical warts and/or features typical of intraepidermal carcinoma (Bowen's disease). Squamous cell carcinomas associated with HPV infections have also been observed in extragenital skin (Chap. 105), most commonly in patients immunosuppressed after organ transplantation. Patients on long-term immunosuppression should be monitored for the development of squamous cell carcinoma and other cutaneous malignancies.

TREATMENT WARTS

Treatment of warts, other than anogenital warts, should be tempered by the observation that a majority of warts in normal individuals resolve spontaneously within 1–2 years. There are many modalities available to treat warts, but no single therapy is universally effective. Factors that influence the choice of therapy include the location of the wart, the extent of disease, the age and immunologic status of the patient, and the patient's desire for therapy. Perhaps the most useful and convenient method for treating warts in almost any location is cryotherapy with liquid nitrogen. Equally effective for nongenital warts, but requiring much more patient compliance, is the use of keratolytic agents such as salicylic acid plasters or solutions. For genital warts, in-office application of a podophyllin solution is moderately effective but may be associated with marked local reactions. Prescription preparations of dilute, purified podophyllin are available for home use. Topical imiquimod, a potent inducer of local cytokine release, has been approved for treatment of genital warts. A new topical compound composed of green tea extracts (sinecatechins) is also available. Conventional and laser surgical procedures may be required for recalcitrant warts. Recurrence of warts appears to be common to all these modalities. A highly effective vaccine for selected types of HPV has been approved by the FDA, and its use appears to reduce the incidence of anogenital and cervical carcinoma.

HERPES SIMPLEX

See Chap. 216.

HERPES ZOSTER

See Chap. 217.

ACNE

ACNE VULGARIS

Acne vulgaris is a self-limited disorder primarily of teenagers and young adults, although perhaps 10–20% of adults may continue to experience some form of the disorder. The permissive factor for the expression of the disease in adolescence is the increase in sebum production by sebaceous glands after puberty. Small cysts, called *comedones*, form in hair follicles due to blockage of the follicular orifice by retention of keratinous material and sebum. The activity of bacteria (*Propionibacterium acnes*) within the comedones releases free fatty acids from sebum, causes inflammation within the cyst, and results in rupture of the cyst wall. An inflammatory foreign-body reaction develops as result of extrusion of oily and keratinous debris from the cyst.

The clinical hallmark of acne vulgaris is the comedone, which may be closed (*whitehead*) or open (*blackhead*). Closed comedones appear as 1- to 2-mm pebbly white papules, which are accentuated when the skin is stretched. They are the precursors of inflammatory lesions of acne vulgaris. The contents of closed comedones are not easily expressed. Open comedones, which rarely result in inflammatory acne lesions, have a large dilated follicular orifice and are filled with easily expressible oxidized, darkened, oily debris. Comedones are usually accompanied by inflammatory lesions: papules, pustules, or nodules.

The earliest lesions seen in adolescence are generally mildly inflamed or noninflammatory comedones on the forehead. Subsequently, more typical inflammatory lesions develop on the cheeks, nose, and chin (Fig. 71-7). The most common location for acne is the face, but involvement of the chest and back is common. Most disease remains mild and does not lead to scarring. A small number of patients develop large inflammatory cysts and nodules, which may drain and result in significant scarring. Regardless of the severity, acne may affect a patient's quality of life. With adequate treatment, this effect may be transient. In the case of severe, scarring acne, the effects can be permanent and profound. Early therapeutic intervention in severe acne is essential.

Exogenous and endogenous factors can alter the expression of acne vulgaris. Friction and trauma (from headbands or chin straps of athletic helmets), application of comedogenic topical agents (cosmetics

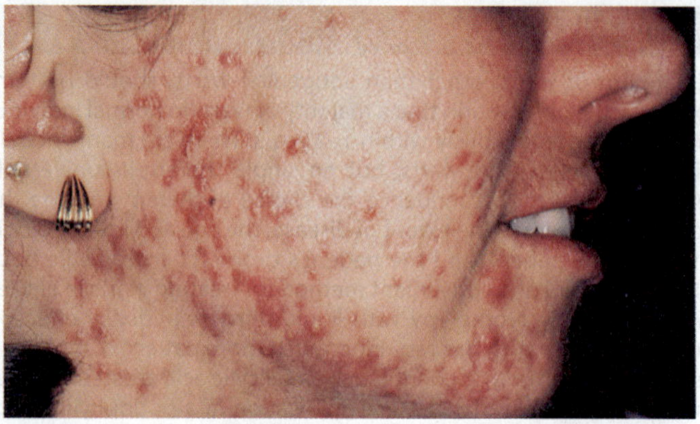

FIGURE 71-7 Acne vulgaris. An example of acne vulgaris with inflammatory papules, pustules, and comedones. *(Courtesy of Kalman Watsky, MD; with permission.)*

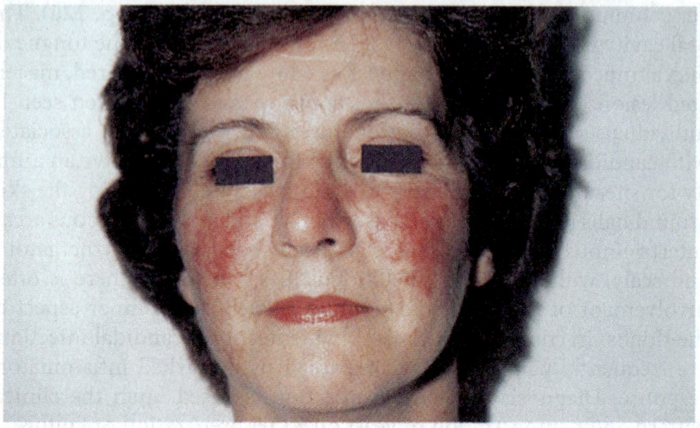

FIGURE 71-8 Acne rosacea. Prominent facial erythema, telangiectasia, scattered papules, and small pustules are seen in this patient with acne rosacea. *(Courtesy of Robert Swerlick, MD; with permission.)*

or hair preparations), or chronic topical exposure to certain industrial compounds may elicit or aggravate acne. Glucocorticoids, topical or systemic, may also elicit acne. Other systemic medications such as oral contraceptive pills, lithium, isoniazid, androgenic steroids, halogens, phenytoin, and phenobarbital may produce acneiform eruptions or aggravate preexisting acne. Genetic factors and polycystic ovary disease may also play a role.

TREATMENT ACNE VULGARIS

Treatment of acne vulgaris is directed toward elimination of comedones by normalizing follicular keratinization, decreasing sebaceous gland activity, decreasing the population of *P. acnes*, and decreasing inflammation. Minimal to moderate pauci-inflammatory disease may respond adequately to local therapy alone. Although areas affected with acne should be kept clean, overly vigorous scrubbing may aggravate acne due to mechanical rupture of comedones. Topical agents such as retinoic acid, benzoyl peroxide, or salicylic acid may alter the pattern of epidermal desquamation, preventing the formation of comedones and aiding in the resolution of preexisting cysts. Topical antibacterial agents (such as azelaic acid, erythromycin, clindamycin, or dapsone) are also useful adjuncts to therapy.

Patients with moderate to severe acne with a prominent inflammatory component will benefit from the addition of systemic therapy, such as tetracycline in doses of 250–500 mg bid or doxycycline in doses of 100 mg bid. Minocycline is also useful. Such antibiotics appear to have anti-inflammatory effects independent of their antibacterial effects. Female patients who do not respond to oral antibiotics may benefit from hormonal therapy. Several oral contraceptives are now approved by the FDA for use in the treatment of acne vulgaris.

Patients with severe nodulocystic acne unresponsive to the therapies discussed above may benefit from treatment with the synthetic retinoid isotretinoin. Its dose is based on the patient's weight, and it is given once daily for 5 months. Results are excellent in appropriately selected patients. Its use is highly regulated due to its potential for severe adverse events, primarily teratogenicity and depression. In addition, patients receiving this medication develop extremely dry skin and cheilitis and must be followed for development of hypertriglyceridemia.

At present, prescribers must enroll in a program designed to prevent pregnancy and adverse events while patients are taking isotretinoin. These measures are imposed to ensure that all prescribers are familiar with the risks of isotretinoin; that all female patients have two negative pregnancy tests prior to initiation of therapy and a negative pregnancy test prior to each refill; and that all patients have been warned about the risks associated with isotretinoin.

ACNE ROSACEA

Acne rosacea, commonly referred to simply as rosacea, is an inflammatory disorder predominantly affecting the central face. Persons most often affected are Caucasians of northern European background, but rosacea also occurs in patients with dark skin. Rosacea is seen almost exclusively in adults, only rarely affecting patients <30 years old. Rosacea is more common in women, but those most severely affected are men. It is characterized by the presence of erythema, telangiectases, and superficial pustules (Fig. 71-8) but is not associated with the presence of comedones. Rosacea rarely involves the chest or back.

There is a relationship between the tendency for facial flushing and the subsequent development of acne rosacea. Often, individuals with rosacea initially demonstrate a pronounced flushing reaction. This may be in response to heat, emotional stimuli, alcohol, hot drinks, or spicy foods. As the disease progresses, the flush persists longer and longer and may eventually become permanent. Papules, pustules, and telangiectases can become superimposed on the persistent flush. Rosacea of very long standing may lead to connective tissue overgrowth, particularly of the nose (*rhinophyma*). Rosacea may also be complicated by various inflammatory disorders of the eye, including keratitis, blepharitis, iritis, and recurrent chalazion. These ocular problems are potentially sight-threatening and warrant ophthalmologic evaluation.

TREATMENT ACNE ROSACEA

Acne rosacea can be treated topically or systemically. Mild disease often responds to topical metronidazole, sodium sulfacetamide, or azaleic acid. More severe disease requires oral tetracyclines: tetracycline, 250–500 mg bid; doxycycline, 100 mg bid; or minocycline, 50–100 mg bid. Residual telangiectasia may respond to laser therapy. Topical glucocorticoids, especially potent agents, should be avoided because chronic use of these preparations may elicit rosacea. Application of topical agents to the skin is not effective treatment for ocular disease.

SKIN DISEASES AND SMALLPOX VACCINATION

Although smallpox vaccinations were discontinued several decades ago for the general population, they are still required for certain military personnel and first responders. In the absence of a bioterrorism attack and a real or potential exposure to smallpox, such vaccination is contraindicated in persons with a history of skin diseases such as AD, eczema, and psoriasis, who have a higher incidence of adverse events associated with smallpox vaccination. In the case of such exposure, the risk of smallpox infection outweighs the risk of adverse events from the vaccine (Chap. 261e).

72 Skin Manifestations of Internal Disease

Jean L. Bolognia, Irwin M. Braverman

It is a generally accepted concept in medicine that the skin can develop signs of internal disease. Therefore, in textbooks of medicine, one finds a chapter describing in detail the major systemic disorders that can be identified by cutaneous signs. The underlying assumption of such a chapter is that the clinician has been able to identify the specific disorder in the patient and needs only to read about it in the textbook. In reality, concise differential diagnoses and the identification of these disorders are actually difficult for the nondermatologist because he or she is not well-versed in the recognition of cutaneous lesions or their spectrum of presentations. Therefore, this chapter covers this particular topic of cutaneous medicine not by simply focusing on individual diseases, but by describing the various presenting clinical signs and symptoms that point to specific disorders. Concise differential diagnoses will be generated in which the significant diseases will be distinguished from the more common cutaneous disorders that have minimal or no significance with regard to associated internal disease. The latter disorders are reviewed in table form and always need to be excluded when considering the former. For a detailed description of individual diseases, the reader should consult a dermatologic text.

PAPULOSQUAMOUS SKIN LESIONS

(Table 72-1) When an eruption is characterized by elevated lesions, either papules (<1 cm) or plaques (>1 cm), in association with scale, it is referred to as *papulosquamous*. The most common papulosquamous diseases—*tinea*, *psoriasis*, *pityriasis rosea*, and *lichen planus*—are primary cutaneous disorders (Chap. 71). When psoriatic lesions are accompanied by arthritis, the possibility of psoriatic arthritis or reactive arthritis (formerly known as Reiter's syndrome) should be considered. A history of oral ulcers, conjunctivitis, uveitis, and/or urethritis points to the latter diagnosis. Lithium, beta blockers, HIV or streptococcal infections, and a rapid taper of systemic glucocorticoids are known to exacerbate psoriasis. Comorbidities in patients with psoriasis include cardiovascular disease and metabolic syndrome.

Whenever the diagnosis of pityriasis rosea or lichen planus is made, it is important to review the patient's medications because the eruption may resolve by simply discontinuing the offending agent. Pityriasis rosea–like drug eruptions are seen most commonly with beta blockers, angiotensin-converting enzyme (ACE) inhibitors, and metronidazole, whereas the drugs that can produce a lichenoid eruption include thiazides, antimalarials, quinidine, beta blockers, and ACE inhibitors. In some populations, there is a higher prevalence of hepatitis C viral infection in patients with lichen planus. Lichen planus–like lesions are also observed in chronic graft-versus-host disease.

In its early stages, the mycosis fungoides (MF) form of *cutaneous T cell lymphoma* (CTCL) may be confused with eczema or psoriasis, but it often fails to respond to the appropriate therapy for those inflammatory diseases. MF can develop within lesions of large-plaque parapsoriasis and is suggested by an increase in the thickness of the lesions. The diagnosis of MF is established by skin biopsy in which collections of atypical T lymphocytes are found in the epidermis and dermis. As the disease progresses, cutaneous tumors and lymph node involvement may appear.

In *secondary syphilis*, there are scattered red-brown papules with thin scale. The eruption often involves the palms and soles and can resemble pityriasis rosea. Associated findings are helpful in making the diagnosis and include annular plaques on the face, nonscarring alopecia, condyloma lata (broad-based and moist), and mucous patches as well as lymphadenopathy, malaise, fever, headache, and myalgias. The interval between the primary chancre and the secondary stage is usually 4–8 weeks, and spontaneous resolution without appropriate therapy occurs.

TABLE 72-1 SELECTED CAUSES OF PAPULOSQUAMOUS SKIN LESIONS

1. Primary cutaneous disorders
   a. Tinea[a]
   b. Psoriasis[a]
   c. Pityriasis rosea[a]
   d. Lichen planus[a]
   e. Parapsoriasis, small plaque and large plaque
   f. Bowen's disease (squamous cell carcinoma in situ)[b]
2. Drugs
3. Systemic diseases
   a. Lupus erythematosus, primarily subacute or chronic (discoid) lesions[c]
   b. Cutaneous T cell lymphoma, in particular, mycosis fungoides[d]
   c. Secondary syphilis
   d. Reactive arthritis (formerly known as Reiter's syndrome)
   e. Sarcoidosis[e]

[a]Discussed in detail in Chap. 71; cardiovascular disease and the metabolic syndrome are comorbidities in psoriasis; primarily in Europe, hepatitis C virus is associated with oral lichen planus. [b]Associated with chronic sun exposure more often than exposure to arsenic; usually one or a few lesions. [c]See also Red Lesions in "Papulonodular Skin Lesions." [d]Also cutaneous lesions of HTLV-1-associated adult T cell leukemia/lymphoma. [e]See also Red-Brown Lesions in "Papulonodular Skin Lesions."

ERYTHRODERMA

(Table 72-2) *Erythroderma* is the term used when the majority of the skin surface is erythematous (red in color). There may be associated scale, erosions, or pustules as well as shedding of the hair and nails. Potential systemic manifestations include fever, chills, hypothermia, reactive lymphadenopathy, peripheral edema, hypoalbuminemia, and high-output cardiac failure. The major etiologies of erythroderma are (1) cutaneous diseases such as psoriasis and dermatitis (Table 72-3); (2) drugs; (3) systemic diseases, most commonly CTCL; and (4) idiopathic. In the first three groups, the location and description of the initial lesions, prior to the development of the erythroderma, aid in the diagnosis. For example, a history of red scaly plaques on the elbows and knees would point to psoriasis. It is also important to examine the skin carefully for a migration of the erythema and associated secondary changes such as pustules or erosions. Migratory waves of erythema studded with superficial pustules are seen in *pustular psoriasis*.

Drug-induced erythroderma (exfoliative dermatitis) may begin as an exanthematous (morbilliform) eruption (Chap. 74) or may arise as diffuse erythema. A number of drugs can produce an erythroderma, including penicillins, sulfonamides, carbamazepine, phenytoin, and allopurinol. Fever and peripheral eosinophilia often accompany the eruption, and there may also be facial swelling, hepatitis, myocarditis, thyroiditis, and allergic interstitial nephritis; this constellation is frequently referred to as *drug reaction with eosinophilia and systemic symptoms* (DRESS) or *drug-induced hypersensitivity reaction* (DIHS). In addition, these reactions, especially to aromatic anticonvulsants, can lead to a pseudolymphoma syndrome (with adenopathy and

TABLE 72-2 CAUSES OF ERYTHRODERMA

1. Primary cutaneous disorders
   a. Psoriasis[a]
   b. Dermatitis (atopic > contact >> stasis [with autosensitization] or seborrheic)[a]
   c. Pityriasis rubra pilaris
2. Drugs
3. Systemic diseases
   a. Cutaneous T cell lymphoma (Sézary syndrome, erythrodermic mycosis fungoides)
   b. Other lymphomas
4. Idiopathic (usually older men)

[a]Discussed in detail in Chap. 71.

TABLE 72-3 ERYTHRODERMA (PRIMARY CUTANEOUS DISORDERS)

	Initial Lesions	Location of Initial Lesions	Other Findings	Diagnostic Aids	Treatment
Psoriasis[a]	Pink-red, silvery scale, sharply demarcated	Elbows, knees, scalp, presacral area, intergluteal fold	Nail dystrophy, arthritis, pustules; SAPHO syndrome, especially with palmoplantar pustulosis	Skin biopsy	Topical glucocorticoids, vitamin D; UV-B (narrowband) > PUVA; oral retinoid; MTX, cyclosporine, anti-TNF agents, anti-IL-12/23 Ab
Dermatitis[a]					
Atopic	Acute: Erythema, fine scale, crust, indistinct borders, excoriations Chronic: Lichenification (increased skin markings), excoriations	Antecubital and popliteal fossae, neck, hands, eyelids	Pruritus Personal and/or family history of atopy, including asthma, allergic rhinitis or conjunctivitis, and atopic dermatitis Exclude secondary infection with *Staphylococcus aureus* or HSV Exclude superimposed irritant or allergic contact dermatitis	Skin biopsy	Topical glucocorticoids, tacrolimus, pimecrolimus, tar, and antipruritics; oral antihistamines; open wet dressings; UV-B ± UV-A > PUVA; oral/IM glucocorticoids (short-term); MTX; mycophenolate mofetil; azathioprine; cyclosporine Topical or oral antibiotics
Contact	Local: Erythema, crusting, vesicles, and bullae	Depends on offending agent	Irritant—onset often within hours Allergic—delayed-type hypersensitivity; lag time of 48 h	Patch testing; open use test	Remove irritant or allergen; topical glucocorticoids; oral antihistamines; oral/IM glucocorticoids (short-term)
	Systemic: Erythema, fine scale, crust	Generalized vs major intertriginous zones (especially groin)	Patient has history of allergic contact dermatitis to topical agent and then receives systemic medication that is structurally related, e.g., thiuram (skin), disulfiram (oral)	Patch testing	Same as local
Seborrheic (rare in adults)	Pink-red to pink-orange, greasy scale	Scalp, nasolabial folds, eyebrows, intertriginous zones	Flares with stress, HIV infection Associated with Parkinson's disease	Skin biopsy	Topical glucocorticoids and imidazoles
Stasis (with autosensitization)	Erythema, crusting, excoriations	Lower extremities	Pruritus, lower extremity edema, varicosities, hemosiderin deposits History of venous ulcers, thrombophlebitis, and/or cellulitis Exclude cellulitis Exclude superimposed contact dermatitis, e.g., topical neomycin	Skin biopsy	Topical glucocorticoids; open wet dressings; leg elevation; pressure stockings; pressure wraps if associated ulcers
Pityriasis rubra pilaris	Orange-red (salmon-colored), perifollicular papules	Generalized, but characteristic "skip" areas of normal skin	Wax-like palmoplantar keratoderma Exclude cutaneous T cell lymphoma	Skin biopsy	Isotretinoin or acitretin; MTX; perhaps anti-IL-12/23 Ab, IV anti-TNF agent

[a]Discussed in detail in Chap. 71.

Abbreviations: Ab, antibody; HSV, herpes simplex virus; IL, interleukin; IM, intramuscular; IV, intravenous; MTX, methotrexate; PUVA, psoralens + ultraviolet A irradiation; SAPHO, synovitis, *a*cne, *p*ustulosis, *h*yperostosis, and *o*steitis (also referred to as chronic recurrent multifocal osteomyelitis); TNF, tumor necrosis factor; UV-A, ultraviolet A irradiation; UV-B, ultraviolet B irradiation.

circulating atypical lymphocytes), while reactions to allopurinol may be accompanied by gastrointestinal bleeding.

The most common malignancy that is associated with erythroderma is CTCL; in some series, up to 25% of the cases of erythroderma were due to CTCL. The patient may progress from isolated plaques and tumors, but more commonly, the erythroderma is present throughout the course of the disease (Sézary syndrome). In the Sézary syndrome, there are circulating clonal atypical T lymphocytes, pruritus, and lymphadenopathy. In cases of erythroderma where there is no apparent cause (idiopathic), longitudinal evaluation is mandatory to monitor for the possible development of CTCL. There have been isolated case reports of erythroderma secondary to some solid tumors—lung, liver, prostate, thyroid, and colon—but it is primarily during a late stage of the disease.

ALOPECIA

(Table 72-4) The two major forms of alopecia are scarring and nonscarring. *Scarring alopecia* is associated with fibrosis, inflammation, and loss of hair follicles. A smooth scalp with a decreased number of follicular openings is usually observed clinically, but in some patients, the changes are seen only in biopsy specimens from affected areas. In *nonscarring alopecia*, the hair shafts are absent or miniaturized, but the hair follicles are preserved, explaining the reversible nature of nonscarring alopecia.

The most common causes of nonscarring alopecia include *androgenetic alopecia*, *telogen effluvium*, *alopecia areata*, *tinea capitis*, and the early phase of *traumatic alopecia* (Table 72-5). In women with androgenetic alopecia, an elevation in circulating levels of androgens may be seen as a result of ovarian or adrenal gland dysfunction or neoplasm. When there are signs of virilization, such as a deepened voice and enlarged clitoris, the possibility of an ovarian or adrenal gland tumor should be considered.

Exposure to various drugs can also cause diffuse hair loss, usually by inducing a telogen effluvium. An exception is the anagen effluvium observed with antimitotic agents such as daunorubicin. Alopecia is a side effect of the following drugs: warfarin, heparin, propylthiouracil, carbimazole, isotretinoin, acitretin, lithium, beta blockers, interferons, colchicine, and amphetamines. Fortunately, spontaneous regrowth usually follows discontinuation of the offending agent.

Less commonly, nonscarring alopecia is associated with *lupus erythematosus* and *secondary syphilis*. In systemic lupus there are two forms of alopecia—one is scarring secondary to discoid lesions (see below), and the other is nonscarring. The latter form coincides with flares of systemic disease and may involve the entire scalp or just the frontal scalp, with the appearance of multiple short hairs ("lupus hairs") as a sign of initial regrowth. Scattered, poorly circumscribed patches of alopecia with a "moth-eaten" appearance are a manifestation

TABLE 72-4 CAUSES OF ALOPECIA

I. Nonscarring alopecia
  A. Primary cutaneous disorders
    1. Androgenetic alopecia
    2. Telogen effluvium
    3. Alopecia areata
    4. Tinea capitis
    5. Traumatic alopecia[a]
  B. Drugs
  C. Systemic diseases
    1. Systemic lupus erythematosus
    2. Secondary syphilis
    3. Hypothyroidism
    4. Hyperthyroidism
    5. Hypopituitarism
    6. Deficiencies of protein, biotin, zinc, and perhaps iron
II. Scarring alopecia
  A. Primary cutaneous disorders
    1. Cutaneous lupus (chronic discoid lesions)[b]
    2. Lichen planus
    3. Central centrifugal cicatricial alopecia
    4. Folliculitis decalvans
    5. Linear scleroderma (morphea)[c]
  B. Systemic diseases
    1. Discoid lesions in the setting of systemic lupus erythematosus[b]
    2. Sarcoidosis
    3. Cutaneous metastases

[a]Most patients with trichotillomania, pressure-induced alopecia, or early stages of traction alopecia. [b]While the majority of patients with discoid lesions have only cutaneous disease, these lesions do represent one of the 11 American College of Rheumatology criteria (1982) for systemic lupus erythematosus. [c]Can involve underlying muscles and osseous structures.

of the secondary stage of syphilis. Diffuse thinning of the hair is also associated with hypothyroidism and hyperthyroidism (Table 72-4).

Scarring alopecia is more frequently the result of a primary cutaneous disorder such as *lichen planus, folliculitis decalvans, chronic cutaneous (discoid) lupus*, or *linear scleroderma (morphea)* than it is a sign of systemic disease. Although the scarring lesions of *discoid lupus* can be seen in patients with systemic lupus, in the majority of patients, the disease process is limited to the skin. Less common causes of scarring alopecia include *sarcoidosis* (see "Papulonodular Skin Lesions," below) and *cutaneous metastases*.

In the early phases of discoid lupus, lichen planus, and folliculitis decalvans, there are circumscribed areas of alopecia. Fibrosis and subsequent loss of hair follicles are observed primarily in the center of these alopecic patches, whereas the inflammatory process is most prominent at the periphery. The areas of active inflammation in discoid lupus are erythematous with scale, whereas the areas of previous inflammation are often hypopigmented with a rim of hyperpigmentation. In lichen planus, perifollicular macules at the periphery are usually violet-colored. A complete examination of the skin and oral mucosa combined with a biopsy and direct immunofluorescence microscopy of inflamed skin will aid in distinguishing these two entities. The peripheral active lesions in folliculitis decalvans are follicular pustules; these patients can develop a reactive arthritis.

FIGURATE SKIN LESIONS

(Table 72-6) In *figurate eruptions*, the lesions form rings and arcs that are usually erythematous but can be skin-colored to brown. Most commonly, they are due to primary cutaneous diseases such as *tinea, urticaria, granuloma annulare*, and *erythema annulare centrifugum* (Chaps. 71 and 73). An underlying systemic illness is found in a second, less common group of migratory annular erythemas. It includes *erythema migrans, erythema gyratum repens, erythema marginatum*, and *necrolytic migratory erythema*.

In erythema gyratum repens, one sees numerous mobile concentric arcs and wavefronts that resemble the grain in wood. A search for an

TABLE 72-5 NONSCARRING ALOPECIA (PRIMARY CUTANEOUS DISORDERS)

	Clinical Characteristics	Pathogenesis	Treatment
Telogen effluvium	Diffuse shedding of normal hairs Follows major stress (high fever, severe infection) or change in hormone levels (postpartum) Reversible without treatment	Stress causes more of the asynchronous growth cycles of individual hairs to become synchronous; therefore, larger numbers of growing (anagen) hairs simultaneously enter the dying (telogen) phase	Observation; discontinue any drugs that have alopecia as a side effect; must exclude underlying metabolic causes, e.g., hypothyroidism, hyperthyroidism
Androgenetic alopecia (male pattern; female pattern)	Miniaturization of hairs along the midline of the scalp Recession of the anterior scalp line in men and some women	Increased sensitivity of affected hairs to the effects of androgens Increased levels of circulating androgens (ovarian or adrenal source in women)	If no evidence of hyperandrogenemia, then topical minoxidil; finasteride[a]; spironolactone (women); hair transplant
Alopecia areata	Well-circumscribed, circular areas of hair loss, 2–5 cm in diameter In extensive cases, coalescence of lesions and/or involvement of other hair-bearing surfaces of the body Pitting or sandpapered appearance of the nails	The germinative zones of the hair follicles are surrounded by T lymphocytes Occasional associated diseases: hyperthyroidism, hypothyroidism, vitiligo, Down syndrome	Topical anthralin or tazarotene; intralesional glucocorticoids; topical contact sensitizers
Tinea capitis	Varies from scaling with minimal hair loss to discrete patches with "black dots" (broken infected hairs) to boggy plaque with pustules (kerion)[b]	Invasion of hairs by dermatophytes, most commonly *Trichophyton tonsurans*	Oral griseofulvin or terbinafine plus 2.5% selenium sulfide or ketoconazole shampoo; examine family members
Traumatic alopecia[c]	Broken hairs, often of varying lengths Irregular outline	Traction with curlers, rubber bands, braiding Exposure to heat or chemicals (e.g., hair straighteners) Mechanical pulling (trichotillomania)	Discontinuation of offending hair style or chemical treatments; diagnosis of trichotillomania may require observation of shaved hairs (for growth) or biopsy, possibly followed by psychotherapy

[a]To date, Food and Drug Administration–approved for men. [b]Scarring alopecia can occur at sites of kerions. [c]May also be scarring, especially late-stage traction alopecia.

TABLE 72-6 CAUSES OF FIGURATE SKIN LESIONS

I. Primary cutaneous disorders
  A. Tinea
  B. Urticaria (primary in ≥90% of patients)
  C. Granuloma annulare
  D. Erythema annulare centrifugum
  E. Psoriasis
II. Systemic diseases
  A. Migratory
    1. Erythema migrans (CDC case definition is ≥5 cm in diameter)
    2. Urticaria (≤10% of patients)
    3. Erythema gyratum repens
    4. Erythema marginatum
    5. Pustular psoriasis (generalized)
    6. Necrolytic migratory erythema (glucagonoma syndrome)[a]
  B. Nonmigratory
    1. Sarcoidosis
    2. Subacute cutaneous lupus erythematosus
    3. Secondary syphilis
    4. Cutaneous T cell lymphoma (especially mycosis fungoides)

[a]Migratory erythema with erosions; favors lower extremities and girdle area.

Abbreviation: CDC, Centers for Disease Control and Prevention.

underlying malignancy is mandatory in a patient with this eruption. Erythema migrans is the cutaneous manifestation of Lyme disease, which is caused by the spirochete *Borrelia burgdorferi*. In the initial stage (3–30 days after tick bite), a single annular lesion is usually seen, which can expand to ≥10 cm in diameter. Within several days, up to half of the patients develop multiple smaller erythematous lesions at sites distant from the bite. Associated symptoms include fever, headache, photophobia, myalgias, arthralgias, and malar rash. Erythema marginatum is seen in patients with rheumatic fever, primarily on the trunk. Lesions are pink-red in color, flat to minimally elevated, and transient.

There are additional cutaneous diseases that present as annular eruptions but lack an obvious migratory component. Examples include *CTCL*, *subacute cutaneous lupus*, *secondary syphilis*, and *sarcoidosis* (see "Papulonodular Skin Lesions," below).

ACNE

(Table 72-7) In addition to *acne vulgaris* and *acne rosacea*, the two major forms of acne (Chap. 71), there are drugs and systemic diseases that can lead to acneiform eruptions.

Patients with the *carcinoid syndrome* have episodes of flushing of the head, neck, and sometimes the trunk. Resultant skin changes of the face, in particular telangiectasias, may mimic the clinical appearance of acne rosacea.

TABLE 72-7 CAUSES OF ACNEIFORM ERUPTIONS

I. Primary cutaneous disorders
  A. Acne vulgaris
  B. Acne rosacea
II. Drugs, e.g., anabolic steroids, glucocorticoids, lithium, EGFR[a] inhibitors, iodides
III. Systemic diseases
  A. Increased androgen production
    1. Adrenal origin, e.g., Cushing's disease, 21-hydroxylase deficiency
    2. Ovarian origin, e.g., polycystic ovary syndrome, ovarian hyperthecosis
  B. Cryptococcosis, disseminated
  C. Dimorphic fungal infections
  D. Behçet's disease

[a]EGFR, epidermal growth factor receptor.

PUSTULAR LESIONS

Acneiform eruptions (see "Acne," above) and *folliculitis* represent the most common pustular dermatoses. An important consideration in the evaluation of follicular pustules is a determination of the associated pathogen, e.g., normal flora, *Staphylococcus aureus*, *Pseudomonas aeruginosa* ("hot tub" folliculitis), *Malassezia*, dermatophytes (Majocchi's granuloma), and *Demodex* spp. Noninfectious forms of folliculitis include HIV- or immunosuppression-associated eosinophilic folliculitis and folliculitis secondary to drugs such as glucocorticoids, lithium, and epidermal growth factor receptor (EGFR) inhibitors. Administration of high-dose systemic glucocorticoids can result in a widespread eruption of follicular pustules on the trunk, characterized by lesions in the same stage of development. With regard to underlying systemic diseases, nonfollicular-based pustules are a characteristic component of pustular psoriasis (sterile) and can be seen in septic emboli of bacterial or fungal origin (see "Purpura," below). In patients with acute generalized exanthematous pustulosis (AGEP) due primarily to medications (e.g., cephalosporins), there are large areas of erythema studded with multiple sterile pustules in addition to neutrophilia.

TELANGIECTASIAS

(Table 72-8) To distinguish the various types of telangiectasias, it is important to examine the shape and configuration of the dilated blood vessels. *Linear telangiectasias* are seen on the face of patients

TABLE 72-8 CAUSES OF TELANGIECTASIAS

I. Primary cutaneous disorders
  A. Linear/branching
    1. Acne rosacea
    2. Actinically damaged skin
    3. Venous hypertension
    4. Generalized essential telangiectasia
    5. Cutaneous collagenous vasculopathy
    6. Within basal cell carcinomas or cutaneous lymphoma
  B. Poikiloderma
    1. Ionizing radiation[a]
    2. Parapsoriasis, large plaque
  C. Spider angioma
    1. Idiopathic
    2. Pregnancy
II. Systemic diseases
  A. Linear/branching
    1. Carcinoid
    2. Ataxia-telangiectasia
    3. Mastocytosis
  B. Poikiloderma
    1. Dermatomyositis
    2. Mycosis fungoides
    3. Xeroderma pigmentosum
  C. Mat
    1. Systemic sclerosis (scleroderma)
  D. Periungual/cuticular
    1. Lupus erythematosus
    2. Systemic sclerosis (scleroderma)
    3. Dermatomyositis
    4. Hereditary hemorrhagic telangiectasia
  E. Papular
    1. Hereditary hemorrhagic telangiectasia
  F. Spider angioma
    1. Cirrhosis

[a]Becoming less common.

with *actinically damaged skin* and *acne rosacea*, and they are found on the legs of patients with *venous hypertension* and *generalized essential telangiectasia*. Patients with an unusual form of *mastocytosis* (telangiectasia macularis eruptiva perstans) and the *carcinoid syndrome* (see "Acne," above) also have linear telangiectasias. Lastly, linear telangiectasias are found in areas of cutaneous inflammation. For example, lesions of discoid lupus frequently have telangiectasias within them.

Poikiloderma is a term used to describe a patch of skin with: (1) reticulated hypo- and hyperpigmentation, (2) wrinkling secondary to epidermal atrophy, and (3) telangiectasias. Poikiloderma does not imply a single disease entity—although it is becoming less common, it is seen in skin damaged by *ionizing radiation* as well as in patients with autoimmune connective tissue diseases, primarily *dermatomyositis* (DM), and rare genodermatoses (e.g., Kindler syndrome).

In *systemic sclerosis (scleroderma)* the dilated blood vessels have a unique configuration and are known as *mat telangiectasias*. The lesions are broad macules that usually measure 2–7 mm in diameter but occasionally are larger. Mats have a polygonal or oval shape, and their erythematous color may appear uniform, but, upon closer inspection, the erythema is the result of delicate telangiectasias. The most common locations for mat telangiectasias are the face, oral mucosa, and hands—peripheral sites that are prone to intermittent ischemia. The limited form of systemic sclerosis, often referred to as the CREST (*c*alcinosis cutis, *R*aynaud's phenomenon, *e*sophageal dysmotility, *s*clerodactyly, and *t*elangiectasia) variant (Chap. 382), is associated with a chronic course and anticentromere antibodies. Mat telangiectasias are an important clue to the diagnosis of this variant as well as the diffuse form of systemic sclerosis because they may be the only cutaneous finding.

Periungual telangiectasias are pathognomonic signs of the three major autoimmune connective tissue diseases: *lupus erythematosus*, *systemic sclerosis*, and *DM*. They are easily visualized by the naked eye and occur in at least two-thirds of these patients. In both DM and lupus, there is associated nailfold erythema, and in DM, the erythema is often accompanied by "ragged" cuticles and fingertip tenderness. Under 10× magnification, the blood vessels in the nailfolds of lupus patients are tortuous and resemble "glomeruli," whereas in systemic sclerosis and DM, there is a loss of capillary loops and those that remain are markedly dilated.

In *hereditary hemorrhagic telangiectasia* (Osler-Rendu-Weber disease), the lesions usually appear during adolescence (mucosal) and adulthood (cutaneous) and are most commonly seen on the mucous membranes (nasal, orolabial), face, and distal extremities, including under the nails. They represent arteriovenous (AV) malformations of the dermal microvasculature, are dark red in color, and are usually slightly elevated. When the skin is stretched over an individual lesion, an eccentric punctum with radiating legs is seen. Although the degree of systemic involvement varies in this autosomal dominant disease (due primarily to mutations in either the endoglin or activin receptor-like kinase gene), the major symptoms are recurrent epistaxis and gastrointestinal bleeding. The fact that these mucosal telangiectasias are actually AV communications helps to explain their tendency to bleed.

HYPOPIGMENTATION

(Table 72-9) Disorders of hypopigmentation are often classified as either diffuse or localized. The classic example of *diffuse hypopigmentation* is *oculocutaneous albinism* (OCA). The most common forms are due to mutations in the tyrosinase gene (type I) or the *P* gene (type II); patients with type IA OCA have a total lack of enzyme activity. At birth, different forms of OCA can appear similar—white hair, gray-blue eyes, and pink-white skin. However, the patients with no tyrosinase activity maintain this phenotype, whereas those with decreased activity will acquire some pigmentation of the eyes, hair, and skin as they age. The degree of pigment formation is also a function of racial background, and the pigmentary dilution is more readily apparent when patients are compared to their first-degree relatives. The ocular findings in OCA correlate with the degree of hypopigmentation and include decreased visual acuity, nystagmus, photophobia, strabismus, and a lack of normal binocular vision.

TABLE 72-9 CAUSES OF HYPOPIGMENTATION

- I. Primary cutaneous disorders
  - A. Diffuse
    1. Generalized vitiligo[a]
  - B. Localized
    1. Idiopathic guttate hypomelanosis
    2. Postinflammatory
    3. Tinea (pityriasis) versicolor
    4. Vitiligo[a]
    5. Chemical- or drug-induced leukoderma
    6. Nevus depigmentosus
    7. Piebaldism[a]
- II. Systemic diseases
  - A. Diffuse
    1. Oculocutaneous albinism[b]
    2. Hermansky-Pudlak syndrome[b,c]
    3. Chédiak-Higashi syndrome[b,d]
    4. Phenylketonuria
  - B. Localized
    1. Systemic sclerosis (scleroderma)
    2. Melanoma-associated leukoderma, spontaneous or immunotherapy-induced
    3. Vogt-Koyanagi-Harada syndrome
    4. Onchocerciasis
    5. Sarcoidosis
    6. Cutaneous T cell lymphoma (especially mycosis fungoides)
    7. Tuberculoid and indeterminate leprosy
    8. Linear nevoid hypopigmentation (hypomelanosis of Ito)[e]
    9. Incontinentia pigmenti (stage IV)
    10. Tuberous sclerosis
    11. Waardenburg syndrome and Shah-Waardenburg syndrome

[a]Absence of melanocytes in areas of leukoderma. [b]Normal number of melanocytes. [c]Platelet storage defect and restrictive lung disease secondary to deposits of ceroid-like material or immunodeficiency; due to mutations in β subunit of adaptor protein 3 as well as subunits of *b*iogenesis of *l*ysosome-related *o*rganelles *c*omplex (BLOC)-1, -2, and -3. [d]Giant lysosomal granules and recurrent infections. [e]Minority of patients in a nonreferral setting have systemic abnormalities (musculoskeletal, central nervous system, ocular).

The differential diagnosis of *localized hypomelanosis* includes the following primary cutaneous disorders: *idiopathic guttate hypomelanosis, postinflammatory hypopigmentation, tinea (pityriasis) versicolor, vitiligo, chemical- or drug-induced leukoderma, nevus depigmentosus* (see below), and *piebaldism* (Table 72-10). In this group of diseases, the areas of involvement are macules or patches with a decrease or absence of pigmentation. Patients with vitiligo also have an increased incidence of several autoimmune disorders, including Hashimoto's thyroiditis, Graves' disease, pernicious anemia, Addison's disease, uveitis, alopecia areata, chronic mucocutaneous candidiasis, and the autoimmune polyendocrine syndromes (types I and II). Diseases of the thyroid gland are the most frequently associated disorders, occurring in up to 30% of patients with vitiligo. Circulating autoantibodies are often found, and the most common ones are antithyroglobulin, antimicrosomal, and antithyroid-stimulating hormone receptor antibodies.

There are four systemic diseases that should be considered in a patient with skin findings suggestive of vitiligo—*Vogt-Koyanagi-Harada syndrome, systemic sclerosis, onchocerciasis*, and *melanoma-associated leukoderma*. A history of aseptic meningitis, nontraumatic uveitis, tinnitus, hearing loss, and/or dysacousia points to the diagnosis of the Vogt-Koyanagi-Harada syndrome. In these patients, the face and scalp are the most common locations of pigment loss. The

TABLE 72-10 HYPOPIGMENTATION (PRIMARY CUTANEOUS DISORDERS, LOCALIZED)

	Clinical Characteristics	Wood's Lamp Examination (UV-A; Peak = 365 nm)	Skin Biopsy Specimen	Pathogenesis	Treatment
Idiopathic guttate hypomelanosis	Common; acquired; 1–4 mm in diameter Shins and extensor forearms	Less enhancement than vitiligo	Abrupt decrease in epidermal melanin content	Possible somatic mutations as a reflection of aging or UV exposure	None
Postinflammatory hypopigmentation	Can develop within active lesions, as in subacute cutaneous lupus, or after the lesion fades, as in atopic dermatitis	Depends on particular disease Usually less enhancement than in vitiligo	Type of inflammatory infiltrate depends on specific disease	Block in transfer of melanin from melanocytes to keratinocytes could be secondary to edema or decrease in contact time Destruction of melanocytes if inflammatory cells attack basal layer of epidermis	Treat underlying inflammatory disease
Pityriasis (tinea) versicolor	Common disorder Upper trunk and neck (shawl-like distribution), groin Young adults Macules have fine white scale when scratched	Golden fluorescence	Hyphal forms and budding yeast in stratum corneum	Invasion of stratum corneum by the yeast *Malassezia* Yeast is lipophilic and produces C_9 and C_{11} dicarboxylic acids, which in vitro inhibit tyrosinase	Selenium sulfide 2.5%; topical imidazoles; oral triazoles
Vitiligo	Acquired; progressive Symmetric areas of complete pigment loss Periorificial—around mouth, nose, eyes, nipples, umbilicus, anus Other areas—flexor wrists, extensor distal extremities Segmental form is less common—unilateral, dermatomal-like	More apparent Chalk-white	Absence of melanocytes Mild inflammation	Autoimmune phenomenon that results in destruction of melanocytes—primarily cellular (circulating skin-homing autoreactive T cells)	Topical glucocorticoids; topical calcineurin inhibitors; NBUV-B; PUVA; transplants, if stable; depigmentation (topical MBEH), if widespread
Chemical- or drug-induced leukoderma	Similar appearance to vitiligo Often begins on hands when associated with chemical exposure Satellite lesions in areas not exposed to chemicals	More apparent Chalk-white	Decreased number or absence of melanocytes	Exposure to chemicals that selectively destroy melanocytes, in particular phenols and catechols (germicides; adhesives) or ingestion of drugs such as imatinib Release of cellular antigens and activation of circulating lymphocytes may explain satellite phenomenon Possible inhibition of KIT receptor	Avoid exposure to offending agent, then treat as vitiligo Drug-induced variant may undergo repigmentation when medication is discontinued
Piebaldism	Autosomal dominant Congenital, stable White forelock Areas of amelanosis contain normally pigmented and hyperpigmented macules of various sizes Symmetric involvement of central forehead, ventral trunk, and mid regions of upper and lower extremities	Enhancement of leukoderma and hyperpigmented macules	Amelanotic areas—few to no melanocytes	Defect in migration of melanoblasts from neural crest to involved skin or failure of melanoblasts to survive or differentiate in these areas Mutations within the *c-kit* protooncogene that encodes the tyrosine kinase receptor for stem cell growth factor (kit ligand)	None; occasionally transplants

Abbreviations: MBEH, monobenzylether of hydroquinone; NBUV-B, narrow band ultraviolet B; PUVA, psoralens + ultraviolet A irradiation.

vitiligo-like leukoderma seen in patients with systemic sclerosis has a clinical resemblance to idiopathic vitiligo that has begun to repigment as a result of treatment; that is, perifollicular macules of normal pigmentation are seen within areas of depigmentation. The basis of this leukoderma is unknown; there is no evidence of inflammation in areas of involvement, but it can resolve if the underlying connective tissue disease becomes inactive. In contrast to idiopathic vitiligo, melanoma-associated leukoderma often begins on the trunk, and its appearance, if spontaneous, should prompt a search for metastatic disease. It is also seen in patients undergoing immunotherapy for melanoma, including ipilimumab, with cytotoxic T lymphocytes presumably recognizing cell surface antigens common to melanoma cells and melanocytes, and is associated with a greater likelihood of a clinical response.

There are two systemic disorders (neurocristopathies) that may have the cutaneous findings of piebaldism (Table 72-9). They are *Shah-Waardenburg syndrome* and *Waardenburg syndrome*. A possible explanation for both disorders is an abnormal embryonic migration or survival of two neural crest–derived elements, one of them being melanocytes and the other myenteric ganglion cells (leading to Hirschsprung disease in Shah-Waardenburg syndrome) or auditory nerve cells (Waardenburg syndrome). The latter syndrome is characterized by congenital sensorineural hearing loss, dystopia canthorum (lateral displacement of the inner canthi but normal interpupillary distance), heterochromic irises, and a broad nasal root, in addition to the piebaldism. The facial dysmorphism can be explained by the neural crest origin of the connective tissues of the head and neck. Patients with Waardenburg syndrome have been shown to have mutations in four genes, including *PAX-3* and *MITF*, all of which encode DNA-binding proteins, whereas patients with Hirschsprung disease plus white spotting have mutations in one of three genes—endothelin 3, endothelin B receptor, and *SOX-10*.

In *tuberous sclerosis*, the earliest cutaneous sign is macular hypomelanosis, referred to as an ash leaf spot. These lesions are often present at birth and are usually multiple; however, detection may require Wood's lamp examination, especially in fair-skinned individuals. The pigment within them is reduced, but not absent. The average size is 1–3 cm, and the common shapes are polygonal and lance-ovate. Examination of the patient for additional cutaneous signs such as multiple angiofibromas of the face (adenoma sebaceum), ungual and gingival fibromas, fibrous plaques of the forehead, and connective tissue nevi (shagreen patches) is recommended. It is important to remember that an ash leaf spot on the scalp will result in a circumscribed patch of lightly pigmented hair. Internal manifestations include seizures, mental retardation, central nervous system (CNS) and retinal hamartomas, pulmonary lymphangioleiomyomatosis (women), renal angiomyolipomas, and cardiac rhabdomyomas. The latter can be detected in up to 60% of children (<18 years) with tuberous sclerosis by echocardiography.

Nevus depigmentosus is a stable, well-circumscribed hypomelanosis that is present at birth. There is usually a single oval or rectangular lesion, but when there are multiple lesions, the possibility of tuberous sclerosis needs to be considered. In *linear nevoid hypopigmentation*, a term that is replacing hypomelanosis of Ito and segmental or systematized nevus depigmentosus, streaks and swirls of hypopigmentation are observed. Up to a third of patients in a tertiary care setting had associated abnormalities involving the musculoskeletal system (asymmetry), the CNS (seizures and mental retardation), and the eyes (strabismus and hypertelorism). Chromosomal mosaicism has been detected in these patients, lending support to the hypothesis that the cutaneous pattern is the result of the migration of two clones of primordial melanocytes, each with a different pigment potential.

Localized areas of decreased pigmentation are commonly seen as a result of cutaneous inflammation (Table 72-10) and have been observed in the skin overlying active lesions of sarcoidosis (see "Papulonodular Skin Lesions," below) as well as in CTCL. Cutaneous infections also present as disorders of hypopigmentation, and in *tuberculoid leprosy*, there are a few asymmetric patches of hypomelanosis that have associated anesthesia, anhidrosis, and alopecia. Biopsy specimens of the palpable border show dermal granulomas that contain rare, if any, *Mycobacterium leprae* organisms.

HYPERPIGMENTATION

(Table 72-11) Disorders of hyperpigmentation are also divided into two groups—localized and diffuse. The localized forms are due to an epidermal alteration, a proliferation of melanocytes, or an increase in pigment production. Both seborrheic keratoses and acanthosis nigricans belong to the first group. *Seborrheic keratoses* are common lesions, but in one rare clinical setting, they are a sign of systemic disease, and that setting is the sudden appearance of multiple lesions, often with an inflammatory base and in association with acrochordons (skin tags) and acanthosis nigricans. This is termed the *sign of Leser-Trélat* and alerts the clinician to search for an internal malignancy. *Acanthosis nigricans* can also be a reflection of an internal malignancy, most commonly of the gastrointestinal tract, and it appears as velvety hyperpigmentation, primarily in flexural areas. However, in the majority of patients, acanthosis nigricans is associated with obesity and insulin resistance, although it may be a reflection of an endocrinopathy such as acromegaly, Cushing's syndrome, polycystic ovary syndrome, or insulin-resistant diabetes mellitus (type A, type B, and lipodystrophic forms).

A proliferation of melanocytes results in the following pigmented lesions: *lentigo*, *melanocytic nevus*, and *melanoma* (Chap. 105). In an adult, the majority of lentigines are related to sun exposure, which explains their distribution. However, in the Peutz-Jeghers and LEOPARD (*l*entigines; *E*CG abnormalities, primarily conduction defects; *o*cular hypertelorism; *p*ulmonary stenosis and subaortic valvular stenosis; *a*bnormal genitalia [cryptorchidism, hypospadias]; *r*etardation of growth; and *d*eafness [sensorineural]) syndromes, lentigines do serve as a clue to systemic disease. In *LEOPARD syndrome*, hundreds of lentigines develop during childhood and are scattered over the entire surface of the body. The lentigines in patients with *Peutz-Jeghers syndrome* are located primarily around the nose and mouth, on the hands and feet, and within the oral cavity. While the pigmented macules on the face may fade with age, the oral lesions persist. However, similar intraoral lesions are also seen in Addison's disease, in Laugier-Hunziker syndrome (no internal manifestations), and as a normal finding in darkly pigmented individuals. Patients with this autosomal dominant syndrome (due to mutations in a novel serine threonine kinase gene) have multiple benign polyps of the gastrointestinal tract, testicular or ovarian tumors, and an increased risk of developing gastrointestinal (primarily colon) and pancreatic cancers.

In the *Carney complex*, numerous lentigines are also seen, but they are in association with cardiac myxomas. This autosomal dominant disorder is also known as the *LAMB* (*l*entigines, *a*trial myxomas, *m*ucocutaneous myxomas, and *b*lue nevi) *syndrome* or *NAME* (*n*evi, *a*trial myxoma, *m*yxoid neurofibroma, and *e*phelides [freckles]) *syndrome*. These patients can also have evidence of endocrine overactivity in the form of Cushing's syndrome (pigmented nodular adrenocortical disease) and acromegaly.

The third type of localized hyperpigmentation is due to a local increase in pigment production, and it includes *ephelides* and *café au lait macules* (CALMs). While a single CALM can be seen in up to 10% of the normal population, the presence of multiple or large-sized CALMs raises the possibility of an associated genodermatosis, e.g., neurofibromatosis (NF) or McCune-Albright syndrome. *CALMs* are flat, uniformly brown in color (usually two shades darker than uninvolved skin), and can vary in size from 0.5–12 cm. Approximately 80–90% of adult patients with *type I NF* will have six or more CALMs measuring ≥1.5 cm in diameter. Additional findings are discussed in the section on neurofibromas (see "Papulonodular Skin Lesions," below). In comparison with NF, the CALMs in patients with *McCune-Albright syndrome* (polyostotic fibrous dysplasia with precocious puberty in females due to mosaicism for an activating mutation in a G protein [$G_s\alpha$] gene) are usually larger, are more irregular in outline, and tend to respect the midline.

In incontinentia pigmenti, dyskeratosis congenita, and bleomycin pigmentation, the areas of localized hyperpigmentation form a pattern—swirled in the first, reticulated in the second, and flagellate in the third. In *dyskeratosis congenita*, atrophic reticulated

TABLE 72-11 CAUSES OF HYPERPIGMENTATION

I. Primary cutaneous disorders
  A. Localized
    1. Epidermal alteration
      a. Seborrheic keratosis
      b. Pigmented actinic keratosis
    2. Proliferation of melanocytes
      a. Lentigo
      b. Melanocytic nevus (mole)
      c. Melanoma
    3. Increased pigment production
      a. Ephelide (freckle)
      b. Café au lait macule
      c. Postinflammatory hyperpigmentation
  B. Localized and diffuse
    1. Drugs (e.g., minocycline, hydroxychloroquine, bleomycin)
II. Systemic diseases
  A. Localized
    1. Epidermal alteration
      a. Seborrheic keratoses (sign of Leser-Trélat)
      b. Acanthosis nigricans (insulin resistance, other endocrine disorders, paraneoplastic)
    2. Proliferation of melanocytes
      a. Lentigines (Peutz-Jeghers and LEOPARD syndromes; xeroderma pigmentosum)
      b. Melanocytic nevi (Carney complex [LAMB and NAME syndromes])[a]
    3. Increased pigment production
      a. Café au lait macules (neurofibromatosis, McCune-Albright syndrome[b])
      b. Urticaria pigmentosa[c]
    4. Dermal pigmentation
      a. Incontinentia pigmenti (stage III)
      b. Dyskeratosis congenita
  B. Diffuse
    1. Endocrinopathies
      a. Addison's disease
      b. Nelson syndrome
      c. Ectopic ACTH syndrome
      d. Hyperthyroidism
    2. Metabolic
      a. Porphyria cutanea tarda
      b. Hemochromatosis
      c. Vitamin B_{12}, folate deficiency
      d. Pellagra
      e. Malabsorption, including Whipple's disease
    3. Melanosis secondary to metastatic melanoma
    4. Autoimmune
      a. Biliary cirrhosis
      b. Systemic sclerosis (scleroderma)
      c. POEMS syndrome
      d Eosinophilia-myalgia syndrome[d]
    5. Drugs and metals (e.g., arsenic)

[a]Also lentigines. [b]Polyostotic fibrous dysplasia. [c]See also "Papulonodular Skin Lesions." [d]Late 1980s.

Abbreviations: LAMB, *l*entigines, *a*trial *m*yxomas, *m*ucocutaneous myxomas, and *b*lue nevi; LEOPARD, *l*entigines, *E*CG abnormalities, *o*cular hypertelorism, *p*ulmonary stenosis and subaortic valvular stenosis, *a*bnormal genitalia, *r*etardation of growth, and *d*eafness (sensorineural); NAME, *n*evi, *a*trial myxoma, *m*yxoid neurofibroma, and *e*phelides (freckles); POEMS, *p*olyneuropathy, *o*rganomegaly, *e*ndocrinopathies, *M*-protein, and *s*kin changes.

hyperpigmentation is seen on the neck, trunk, and thighs and is accompanied by nail dystrophy, pancytopenia, and leukoplakia of the oral and anal mucosae. The latter often develops into squamous cell carcinoma. In addition to the flagellate pigmentation (linear streaks) on the trunk, patients receiving bleomycin often have hyperpigmentation overlying the elbows, knees, and small joints of the hand.

Localized hyperpigmentation is seen as a side effect of several other *systemic medications*, including those that produce fixed drug reactions (nonsteroidal anti-inflammatory drugs [NSAIDs], sulfonamides, barbiturates, and tetracyclines) and those that can complex with melanin (antimalarials) or iron (minocycline). Fixed drug eruptions recur in the exact same location as circular areas of erythema that can become bullous and then resolve as brown macules. The eruption usually appears within hours of administration of the offending agent, and common locations include the genitalia, distal extremities, and perioral region. Chloroquine and hydroxychloroquine produce gray-brown to blue-black discoloration of the shins, hard palate, and face, while blue macules (often misdiagnosed as bruises) can be seen on the lower extremities and in sites of inflammation with prolonged minocycline administration. Estrogen in oral contraceptives can induce melasma—symmetric brown patches on the face, especially the cheeks, upper lip, and forehead. Similar changes are seen in pregnancy and in patients receiving phenytoin.

In the diffuse forms of hyperpigmentation, the darkening of the skin may be of equal intensity over the entire body or may be accentuated in sun-exposed areas. The causes of diffuse hyperpigmentation can be divided into four major groups—endocrine, metabolic, autoimmune, and drugs. The endocrinopathies that frequently have associated hyperpigmentation include *Addison's disease*, *Nelson syndrome*, and *ectopic ACTH syndrome*. In these diseases, the increased pigmentation is diffuse but is accentuated in sun-exposed areas, the palmar creases, sites of friction, and scars. An overproduction of the pituitary hormones α-MSH (melanocyte-stimulating hormone) and ACTH can lead to an increase in melanocyte activity. These peptides are products of the proopiomelanocortin gene and exhibit homology; e.g., α-MSH and ACTH share 13 amino acids. A minority of patients with Cushing's disease or hyperthyroidism have generalized hyperpigmentation.

The metabolic causes of hyperpigmentation include *porphyria cutanea tarda* (PCT), *hemochromatosis*, *vitamin* B_{12} *deficiency*, *folic acid deficiency*, *pellagra*, and *malabsorption*, including *Whipple's disease*. In patients with PCT (see "Vesicles/Bullae," below), the skin darkening is seen in sun-exposed areas and is a reflection of the photoreactive properties of porphyrins. The increased level of iron in the skin of patients with type 1 hemochromatosis stimulates melanin pigment production and leads to the classic bronze color. Patients with pellagra have a brown discoloration of the skin, especially in sun-exposed areas, as a result of nicotinic acid (niacin) deficiency. In the areas of increased pigmentation, there is a thin, varnish-like scale. These changes are also seen in patients who are vitamin B_6 deficient, have functioning carcinoid tumors (increased consumption of niacin), or take isoniazid. Approximately 50% of the patients with Whipple's disease have an associated generalized hyperpigmentation in association with diarrhea, weight loss, arthritis, and lymphadenopathy. A diffuse, slate-blue to gray-brown color is seen in patients with *melanosis secondary to metastatic melanoma*. The color reflects widespread deposition of melanin within the dermis as a result of the high concentration of circulating melanin precursors.

Of the autoimmune diseases associated with diffuse hyperpigmentation, *biliary cirrhosis* and *systemic sclerosis* are the most common, and occasionally, both disorders are seen in the same patient. The skin is dark brown in color, especially in sun-exposed areas. In biliary cirrhosis, the hyperpigmentation is accompanied by pruritus, jaundice, and xanthomas, whereas in systemic sclerosis, it is accompanied by sclerosis of the extremities, face, and, less commonly, the trunk. Additional clues to the diagnosis of systemic sclerosis are mat and periungual telangiectasias, calcinosis cutis, Raynaud's phenomenon, and distal ulcerations (see "Telangiectasias," above). The differential diagnosis of cutaneous sclerosis with hyperpigmentation includes the POEMS (*p*olyneuropathy; *o*rganomegaly [liver, spleen, lymph nodes]; *e*ndocrinopathies [impotence, gynecomastia]; *M*-protein; and *s*kin changes) syndrome. The skin changes include hyperpigmentation, induration, hypertrichosis, angiomas, clubbing, and facial lipoatrophy.

Diffuse hyperpigmentation that is due to drugs or metals can result from one of several mechanisms—induction of melanin pigment formation, complexing of the drug or its metabolites to melanin, and deposits of the drug in the dermis. Busulfan, cyclophosphamide, 5-fluorouracil, and inorganic arsenic induce pigment production. Complexes containing melanin or iron plus the drug or its metabolites are seen in patients receiving minocycline, and a diffuse, blue-gray, muddy appearance within sun-exposed areas may develop, in addition to pigmentation of the mucous membranes, teeth, nails, bones, and thyroid. Administration of amiodarone can result in both a phototoxic eruption (exaggerated sunburn) and/or a slate-gray to violaceous discoloration of sun-exposed skin. Biopsy specimens of the latter show yellow-brown granules in dermal macrophages, which represent intralysosomal accumulations of lipids, amiodarone, and its metabolites. Actual deposits of a particular drug or metal in the skin are seen with silver (argyria), where the skin appears blue-gray in color; gold (chrysiasis), where the skin has a brown to blue-gray color; and clofazimine, where the skin appears reddish brown. The associated pigmentation is accentuated in sun-exposed areas, and discoloration of the eye is seen with gold (sclerae) and clofazimine (conjunctivae).

VESICLES/BULLAE

(Table 72-12) Depending on their size, cutaneous blisters are referred to as *vesicles* (<1 cm) or *bullae* (>1 cm). The primary autoimmune blistering disorders include *pemphigus vulgaris*, *pemphigus foliaceus*, *paraneoplastic pemphigus*, *bullous pemphigoid*, *gestational pemphigoid*, *cicatricial pemphigoid*, *epidermolysis bullosa acquisita*, *linear IgA bullous dermatosis* (LABD), and *dermatitis herpetiformis* (Chap. 73).

Vesicles and bullae are also seen in *contact dermatitis*, both allergic and irritant forms (Chap. 71). When there is a linear arrangement of vesicular lesions, an exogenous cause or herpes zoster should be suspected. Bullous disease secondary to the ingestion of drugs can take one of several forms, including phototoxic eruptions, isolated bullae, Stevens-Johnson syndrome (SJS), and toxic epidermal necrolysis (TEN) (Chap. 74). Clinically, phototoxic eruptions resemble an exaggerated sunburn with diffuse erythema and bullae in sun-exposed areas. The most commonly associated drugs are doxycycline, quinolones, thiazides, NSAIDs, voriconazole, and psoralens. The development of a phototoxic eruption is dependent on the doses of both the drug and ultraviolet (UV)-A irradiation.

Toxic epidermal necrolysis is characterized by bullae that arise on widespread areas of tender erythema and then slough. This results in large areas of denuded skin. The associated morbidity, such as sepsis, and mortality rates are relatively high and are a function of the extent of epidermal necrosis. In addition, these patients may also have involvement of the mucous membranes and respiratory and intestinal tracts. Drugs are the primary cause of TEN, and the most common offenders are aromatic anticonvulsants (phenytoin, barbiturates, carbamazepine), sulfonamides, aminopenicillins, allopurinol, and NSAIDs. Severe acute graft-versus-host disease (grade 4), vancomycin-induced LABD, and the acute syndrome of apoptotic panepidermolysis (ASAP) in patients with lupus can also resemble TEN.

In *erythema multiforme* (EM), the primary lesions are pink-red macules and edematous papules, the centers of which may become vesicular. In contrast to a morbilliform exanthem, the clue to the diagnosis of EM, and especially SJS, is the development of a "dusky" violet color in the center of the lesions. Target lesions are also characteristic of EM and arise as a result of active centers and borders in combination with centrifugal spread. However, target lesions need not be present to make the diagnosis of EM.

EM has been subdivided into two major groups: (1) EM minor due to herpes simplex virus (HSV) and (2) EM major due to HSV; *Mycoplasma pneumoniae*; or, occasionally, drugs. Involvement of the mucous membranes (ocular, nasal, oral, and genital) is seen more commonly in the latter form. Hemorrhagic crusts of the lips are characteristic of EM major and SJS as well as herpes simplex, pemphigus vulgaris, and paraneoplastic pemphigus. Fever, malaise, myalgias, sore throat, and cough may precede or accompany the eruption. The lesions of EM usually resolve over 2–4 weeks but may be recurrent, especially when due to HSV. In addition to HSV (in which lesions usually appear 7–12 days after the viral eruption), EM can also follow vaccinations, radiation therapy, and exposure to environmental toxins, including the oleoresin in poison ivy.

Induction of SJS is most often due to drugs, especially sulfonamides, phenytoin, barbiturates, lamotrigine, aminopenicillins, nonnucleoside reverse transcriptase inhibitors (e.g., nevirapine), and carbamazepine. Widespread dusky macules and significant mucosal involvement are characteristic of SJS, and the cutaneous lesions may or may not develop epidermal detachment. If the latter occurs, by definition, it is limited to <10% of the body surface area (BSA). Greater involvement leads to the diagnosis of SJS/TEN overlap (10–30% BSA) or TEN (>30% BSA).

In addition to primary blistering disorders and hypersensitivity reactions, bacterial and viral infections can lead to vesicles and bullae. The most common infectious agents are HSV (Chap. 216), varicella-zoster virus (Chap. 217), and *S. aureus* (Chap. 172).

TABLE 72-12 CAUSES OF VESICLES/BULLAE

I. Primary mucocutaneous diseases
A. Primary blistering diseases (autoimmune)
1. Pemphigus, foliaceus and vulgaris[a]
2. Bullous pemphigoid[b]
3. Gestational pemphigoid[b]
4. Cicatricial pemphigoid[b]
5. Dermatitis herpetiformis[b,c]
6. Linear IgA bullous dermatosis[b]
7. Epidermolysis bullosa acquisita[b,d]
B. Secondary blistering diseases
1. Contact dermatitis[a,b]
2. Erythema multiforme[e]
3. Stevens-Johnson syndrome[e]
4. Toxic epidermal necrolysis[e]
C. Infections
1. Varicella-zoster virus[a,f]
2. Herpes simplex virus[a,f]
3. Enteroviruses, e.g., hand-foot-and-mouth disease[f]
4. Staphylococcal scalded-skin syndrome[a,g]
5. Bullous impetigo[a]
II. Systemic diseases
A. Autoimmune
1. Paraneoplastic pemphigus[a]
B. Infections
1. Cutaneous emboli[b]
C. Metabolic
1. Diabetic bullae[a,b]
2. Porphyria cutanea tarda[b]
3. Porphyria variegata[b]
4. Pseudoporphyria[b]
5. Bullous dermatosis of hemodialysis[b]
D. Ischemia
1. Coma bullae

[a]Intraepidermal. [b]Subepidermal. [c]Associated with gluten enteropathy. [d]Associated with inflammatory bowel disease. [e]Degeneration of cells within the basal layer of the epidermis can give impression split is subepidermal. [f]Also systemic. [g]In adults, associated with renal failure and immunocompromised state.

Staphylococcal scalded-skin syndrome (SSSS) and *bullous impetigo* are two blistering disorders associated with staphylococcal (phage group II) infection. In SSSS, the initial findings are redness and tenderness of the central face, neck, trunk, and intertriginous zones. This is followed by short-lived flaccid bullae and a slough or exfoliation of the superficial epidermis. Crusted areas then develop, characteristically around the mouth in a radial pattern. SSSS is distinguished from TEN by the following features: younger age group (primarily infants), more superficial site of blister formation, no oral lesions, shorter course, lower morbidity and mortality rates, and an association with staphylococcal exfoliative toxin ("exfoliatin"), not drugs. A rapid diagnosis of SSSS versus TEN can be made by a frozen section of the blister roof or exfoliative cytology of the blister contents. In SSSS, the site of staphylococcal infection is usually extracutaneous (conjunctivitis, rhinorrhea, otitis media, pharyngitis, tonsillitis), and the cutaneous lesions are sterile, whereas in bullous impetigo, the skin lesions are the site of infection. Impetigo is more localized than SSSS and usually presents with honey-colored crusts. Occasionally, superficial purulent blisters also form. *Cutaneous emboli* from gram-negative infections may present as isolated bullae, but the base of the lesion is purpuric or necrotic, and it may develop into an ulcer (see "Purpura," below).

Several metabolic disorders are associated with blister formation, including diabetes mellitus, renal failure, and porphyria. Local hypoxemia secondary to decreased cutaneous blood flow can also produce blisters, which explains the presence of bullae over pressure points in comatose patients (coma bullae). In *diabetes mellitus*, tense bullae with clear sterile viscous fluid arise on normal skin. The lesions can be as large as 6 cm in diameter and are located on the distal extremities. There are several types of porphyria, but the most common form with cutaneous findings is *porphyria cutanea tarda* (PCT). In sun-exposed areas (primarily the face and hands), the skin is very fragile, with trauma leading to erosions mixed with tense vesicles. These lesions then heal with scarring and formation of milia; the latter are firm, 1- to 2-mm white or yellow papules that represent epidermoid inclusion cysts. Associated findings can include hypertrichosis of the lateral malar region (men) or face (women) and, in sun-exposed areas, hyperpigmentation and firm sclerotic plaques. An elevated level of urinary uroporphyrins confirms the diagnosis and is due to a decrease in uroporphyrinogen decarboxylase activity. PCT can be exacerbated by alcohol, hemochromatosis and other forms of iron overload, chlorinated hydrocarbons, hepatitis C and HIV infections, and hepatomas.

The differential diagnosis of PCT includes (1) *porphyria variegata*—the skin signs of PCT plus the systemic findings of acute intermittent porphyria; it has a diagnostic plasma porphyrin fluorescence emission at 626 nm; (2) *drug-induced* pseudoporphyria—the clinical and histologic findings are similar to PCT, but porphyrins are normal; etiologic agents include naproxen and other NSAIDs, furosemide, tetracycline, and voriconazole; (3) *bullous dermatosis of hemodialysis*—the same appearance as PCT, but porphyrins are usually normal or occasionally borderline elevated; patients have chronic renal failure and are on hemodialysis; (4) PCT associated with hepatomas and hemodialysis; and (5) *epidermolysis bullosa acquisita* (Chap. 73).

EXANTHEMS

(Table 72-13) Exanthems are characterized by an acute generalized eruption. The most common presentation is erythematous macules and papules (morbilliform) and less often confluent blanching erythema (scarlatiniform). *Morbilliform* eruptions are usually due to either drugs or viral infections. For example, up to 5% of patients receiving penicillins, sulfonamides, phenytoin, or nevirapine will develop a maculopapular eruption. Accompanying signs may include pruritus, fever, eosinophilia, and transient lymphadenopathy. Similar maculopapular eruptions are seen in the classic childhood viral exanthems, including (1) *rubeola* (measles)—a prodrome of coryza, cough, and conjunctivitis followed by Koplik's spots on the buccal mucosa; the eruption begins behind the ears, at the hairline, and on the forehead and then spreads down the body, often becoming confluent; (2) *rubella*—the eruption begins on the forehead and face and then spreads down the body; it resolves in the same order and is associated with retroauricular and suboccipital lymphadenopathy; and (3) *erythema infectiosum* (fifth disease)—erythema of the cheeks is followed by a reticulated pattern on the extremities; it is secondary to a parvovirus B19 infection, and an associated arthritis is seen in adults.

TABLE 72-13 CAUSES OF EXANTHEMS

I. Morbilliform
   - A. Drugs
   - B. Viral
     1. Rubeola (measles)
     2. Rubella
     3. Erythema infectiosum (erythema of cheeks; reticulated on extremities)
     4. Epstein-Barr virus, echovirus, coxsackievirus, CMV, adenovirus, HHV-6/HHV-7[a], dengue virus, and West Nile virus infections
     5. HIV seroconversion exanthem (plus mucosal ulcerations)
   - C. Bacterial
     1. Typhoid fever
     2. Early secondary syphilis
     3. Early *Rickettsia* infections
     4. Early meningococcemia
     5. Ehrlichiosis
   - D. Acute graft-versus-host disease
   - E. Kawasaki disease

II. Scarlatiniform
   - A. Scarlet fever
   - B. Toxic shock syndrome
   - C. Kawasaki disease
   - D. Early staphylococcal scalded-skin syndrome

[a]Primary infection in infants and reactivation in the setting of immunosuppression.

Abbreviations: CMV, cytomegalovirus; HHV, human herpesvirus; HIV, human immunodeficiency virus.

Both measles and rubella can occur in unvaccinated adults, and an atypical form of measles is seen in adults immunized with either killed measles vaccine or killed vaccine followed in time by live vaccine. In contrast to classic measles, the eruption of atypical measles begins on the palms, soles, wrists, and ankles, and the lesions may become purpuric. The patient with atypical measles can have pulmonary involvement and be quite ill. Rubelliform and roseoliform eruptions are also associated with *Epstein-Barr virus* (5–15% of patients), *echovirus, coxsackievirus, cytomegalovirus, adenovirus, dengue virus*, and *West Nile virus* infections. Detection of specific IgM antibodies or fourfold elevations in IgG antibodies allow the proper diagnosis, but polymerase chain reaction (PCR) is gradually replacing serologic assays. Occasionally, a maculopapular drug eruption is a reflection of an underlying viral infection. For example, ~95% of the patients with infectious mononucleosis who are given ampicillin will develop a rash.

Of note, early in the course of infections with *Rickettsia* and meningococcus, prior to the development of petechiae and purpura, the lesions may be erythematous macules and papules. This is also the case in chickenpox prior to the development of vesicles. Maculopapular eruptions are associated with early *HIV infection*, early secondary *syphilis, typhoid fever*, and *acute graft-versus-host disease*. In the last, lesions frequently begin on the dorsal hands and forearms; the macular rose spots of typhoid fever involve primarily the anterior trunk.

The prototypic *scarlatiniform* eruption is seen in *scarlet fever* and is due to an erythrogenic toxin produced by bacteriophage-containing group A β-hemolytic streptococci, most commonly in the setting of pharyngitis. This eruption is characterized by diffuse erythema, which begins on the neck and upper trunk, and red follicular puncta. Additional findings include a white strawberry tongue (white coating with red papillae) followed by a red strawberry tongue (red tongue with red papillae); petechiae of the palate; a facial flush with circumoral pallor; linear petechiae in the antecubital fossae; and desquamation of the involved skin, palms, and soles 5–20 days after onset of the eruption. A similar desquamation of the palms and soles is seen in toxic shock syndrome (TSS), in Kawasaki disease, and after severe febrile illnesses. Certain strains of staphylococci also produce an erythrotoxin that leads to the same clinical findings as in streptococcal scarlet fever, except that the anti-streptolysin O or -DNase B titers are not elevated.

In *toxic shock syndrome*, staphylococcal (phage group I) infections produce an exotoxin (TSST-1) that causes the fever and rash as well as enterotoxins. Initially, the majority of cases were reported in menstruating women who were using tampons. However, other sites of infection, including wounds and nasal packing, can lead to TSS. The diagnosis of TSS is based on clinical criteria (Chap. 172), and three of these involve mucocutaneous sites (diffuse erythema of the skin, desquamation of the palms and soles 1–2 weeks after onset of illness, and involvement of the mucous membranes). The latter is characterized as hyperemia of the vagina, oropharynx, or conjunctivae. Similar systemic findings have been described in *streptococcal toxic shock syndrome* (Chap. 173), and although an exanthem is seen less often than in TSS due to a staphylococcal infection, the underlying infection is often in the soft tissue (e.g., cellulitis).

The cutaneous eruption in *Kawasaki disease* (Chap. 385) is polymorphous, but the two most common forms are morbilliform and scarlatiniform. Additional mucocutaneous findings include bilateral conjunctival injection; erythema and edema of the hands and feet followed by desquamation; and diffuse erythema of the oropharynx, red strawberry tongue, and dry fissured lips. This clinical picture can resemble TSS and scarlet fever, but clues to the diagnosis of Kawasaki disease are cervical lymphadenopathy, cheilitis, and thrombocytosis. The most serious associated systemic finding in this disease is coronary aneurysms secondary to arteritis. Scarlatiniform eruptions are also seen in the early phase of SSSS (see "Vesicles/Bullae," above), in young adults with *Arcanobacterium haemolyticum* infection, and as reactions to drugs.

URTICARIA

(Table 72-14) *Urticaria* (hives) are transient lesions that are composed of a central wheal surrounded by an erythematous halo or flare. Individual lesions are round, oval, or figurate and are often pruritic. Acute and chronic urticaria have a wide variety of allergic etiologies and reflect edema in the dermis. Urticarial lesions can also be seen in patients with mastocytosis (urticaria pigmentosa), hypo- or hyperthyroidism, and systemic-onset juvenile idiopathic arthritis (Still's disease). In both juvenile- and adult-onset Still's disease, the lesions coincide with the fever spike, are transient, and are due to dermal infiltrates of neutrophils.

The common *physical urticarias* include dermatographism, solar urticaria, cold urticaria, and cholinergic urticaria. Patients with *dermatographism* exhibit linear wheals following minor pressure or scratching of the skin. It is a common disorder, affecting ~5% of the population. *Solar urticaria* characteristically occurs within minutes of sun exposure and is a skin sign of one systemic disease—erythropoietic protoporphyria. In addition to the urticaria, these patients have subtle pitted scarring of the nose and hands. *Cold urticaria* is precipitated by exposure to the cold, and therefore exposed areas are usually affected. In occasional patients, the disease is associated with abnormal circulating proteins—more commonly cryoglobulins and less commonly cryofibrinogens. Additional systemic symptoms include wheezing and syncope, thus explaining the need for these patients to avoid swimming in cold water. Autosomal dominantly inherited cold urticaria is associated with dysfunction of cryopyrin. *Cholinergic urticaria* is precipitated by heat, exercise, or emotion and is characterized by small wheals with relatively large flares. It is occasionally associated with wheezing.

Whereas urticarias are the result of dermal edema, subcutaneous edema leads to the clinical picture of *angioedema*. Sites of involvement include the eyelids, lips, tongue, larynx, and gastrointestinal tract as well as the subcutaneous tissue. Angioedema occurs alone or in combination with urticaria, including urticarial vasculitis and the physical urticarias. Both acquired and hereditary (autosomal dominant) forms of angioedema occur (Chap. 376), and in the latter, urticaria is rarely, if ever, seen.

Urticarial vasculitis is an immune complex disease that may be confused with simple urticaria. In contrast to simple urticaria, individual lesions tend to last longer than 24 h and usually develop central petechiae that can be observed even after the urticarial phase has resolved. The patient may also complain of burning rather than pruritus. On biopsy, there is a leukocytoclastic vasculitis of the small dermal blood vessels. Although many cases of urticarial vasculitis are idiopathic in origin, it can be a reflection of an underlying systemic illness such as lupus erythematosus, Sjögren's syndrome, or hereditary complement deficiency. There is a spectrum of urticarial vasculitis that ranges from purely cutaneous to multisystem involvement. The most common systemic signs and symptoms are arthralgias and/or arthritis, nephritis, and crampy abdominal pain, with asthma and chronic obstructive lung disease seen less often. Hypocomplementemia occurs in one- to two-thirds of patients, even in the idiopathic cases. Urticarial vasculitis can also be seen in patients with *hepatitis B* and *hepatitis C* infections, *serum sickness*, and *serum sickness–like illnesses* (e.g., due to cefaclor, minocycline).

TABLE 72-14 CAUSES OF URTICARIA AND ANGIOEDEMA

- I. Primary cutaneous disorders
  - A. Acute and chronic urticaria[a]
  - B. Physical urticaria
    1. Dermatographism
    2. Solar urticaria[b]
    3. Cold urticaria[b]
    4. Cholinergic urticaria[b]
  - C. Angioedema (hereditary and acquired)[b,c]
- II. Systemic diseases
  - A. Urticarial vasculitis
  - B. Hepatitis B or C infection
  - C. Serum sickness
  - D. Angioedema (hereditary and acquired)

[a]A small minority develop anaphylaxis. [b]Also systemic. [c]Acquired angioedema can be idiopathic, associated with a lymphoproliferative disorder, or due to a drug, e.g., angiotensin-converting enzyme (ACE) inhibitors.

PAPULONODULAR SKIN LESIONS

(Table 72-15) In the *papulonodular diseases*, the lesions are elevated above the surface of the skin and may coalesce to form larger plaques. The location, consistency, and color of the lesions are the keys to their diagnosis; this section is organized on the basis of color.

WHITE LESIONS

In *calcinosis cutis*, there are firm white to white-yellow papules with an irregular surface. When the contents are expressed, a chalky white material is seen. *Dystrophic calcification* is seen at sites of previous inflammation or damage to the skin. It develops in acne scars as well as on the distal extremities of patients with systemic sclerosis and in the subcutaneous tissue and intermuscular fascial planes in DM. The latter is more extensive and is more commonly seen in children. An elevated calcium phosphate product, most commonly due to secondary hyperparathyroidism in the setting of renal failure, can lead to nodules of *metastatic calcinosis cutis*, which tend to be subcutaneous and periarticular. These patients can also develop calcification of muscular arteries and subsequent ischemic necrosis (calciphylaxis). *Osteoma cutis*, in the form of small papules, most commonly occurs on the face

TABLE 72-15 PAPULONODULAR SKIN LESIONS ACCORDING TO COLOR GROUPS

I. White
- A. Calcinosis cutis
- B. Osteoma cutis (also skin-colored or blue)

II. Skin-colored
- A. Rheumatoid nodules
- B. Neurofibromas (von Recklinghausen's disease)
- C. Angiofibromas (tuberous sclerosis, MEN syndrome, type 1)
- D. Neuromas (MEN syndrome, type 2b)
- E. Adnexal tumors
  1. Basal cell carcinomas (nevoid basal cell carcinoma syndrome)
  2. Tricholemmomas (Cowden disease)
- F. Osteomas (arise in skull and jaw in Gardner syndrome)
- G. Primary cutaneous disorders
  1. Epidermal inclusion cysts[a]
  2. Lipomas

III. Pink/translucent[b]
- A. Amyloidosis, primary systemic
- B. Papular mucinosis/scleromyxedema
- C. Multicentric reticulohistiocytosis

IV. Yellow
- A. Xanthomas
- B. Tophi
- C. Necrobiosis lipoidica
- D. Pseudoxanthoma elasticum
- E. Sebaceous adenomas (Muir-Torre syndrome)

V. Red[b]
- A. Papules
  1. Angiokeratomas (Fabry disease)
  2. Bacillary angiomatosis (primarily in AIDS)
- B. Papules/plaques
  1. Cutaneous lupus
  2. Lymphoma cutis
  3. Leukemia cutis
  4. Sweet syndrome
- C. Nodules
  1. Panniculitis
  2. Medium-sized vessel vasculitis (e.g., cutaneous polyarteritis nodosa)
- D. Primary cutaneous disorders
  1. Arthropod bites
  2. Cherry hemangiomas
  3. Infections, e.g., streptococcal cellulitis, sporotrichosis
  4. Polymorphous light eruption
  5. Lymphocytoma cutis (pseudolymphoma)

VI. Red-brown[b]
- A. Sarcoidosis
- B. Urticaria pigmentosa
- C. Erythema elevatum diutinum (chronic leukocytoclastic vasculitis)
- D. Lupus vulgaris

VII. Blue[b]
- A. Venous malformations (e.g., blue rubber bleb syndrome)
- B. Primary cutaneous disorders
  1. Venous lake
  2. Blue nevus

VIII. Violaceous
- A. Lupus pernio (sarcoidosis)
- B. Lymphoma cutis
- C. Cutaneous lupus

IX. Purple
- A. Kaposi's sarcoma
- B. Angiosarcoma
- C. Palpable purpura (see Table 72-16)

X. Brown-black[c]

XI. Any color
- A. Metastases

[a]If multiple with childhood onset, consider Gardner syndrome. [b]May have darker hue in more darkly pigmented individuals. [c]See also "Hyperpigmentation."

Abbreviation: MEN, multiple endocrine neoplasia.

of individuals with a history of acne vulgaris, whereas plate-like lesions occur in rare genetic syndromes (Chap. 82).

SKIN-COLORED LESIONS

There are several types of skin-colored lesions, including epidermoid inclusion cysts, lipomas, rheumatoid nodules, neurofibromas, angiofibromas, neuromas, and adnexal tumors such as tricholemmomas. Both *epidermoid inclusion cysts* and *lipomas* are very common mobile subcutaneous nodules—the former are rubbery and drain cheese-like material (sebum and keratin) if incised. Lipomas are firm and somewhat lobulated on palpation. When extensive facial epidermoid inclusion cysts develop during childhood or there is a family history of such lesions, the patient should be examined for other signs of Gardner syndrome, including osteomas and desmoid tumors. *Rheumatoid nodules* are firm 0.5- to 4-cm nodules that favor the extensor aspect of joints, especially the elbows. They are seen in ~20% of patients with rheumatoid arthritis and 6% of patients with Still's disease. Biopsies of the nodules show palisading granulomas. Similar lesions that are smaller and shorter-lived are seen in rheumatic fever.

Neurofibromas (benign Schwann cell tumors) are soft papules or nodules that exhibit the "button-hole" sign; that is, they invaginate into the skin with pressure in a manner similar to a hernia. Single lesions are seen in normal individuals, but multiple neurofibromas, usually in combination with six or more CALMs measuring >1.5 cm (see "Hyperpigmentation," above), axillary freckling, and multiple Lisch nodules, are seen in von Recklinghausen's disease (NF type I) (Chap. 118). In some patients, the neurofibromas are localized and unilateral due to somatic mosaicism.

Angiofibromas are firm pink to skin-colored papules that measure from 3 mm to a few centimeters in diameter. When multiple lesions are located on the central cheeks (adenoma sebaceum), the patient has tuberous sclerosis or multiple endocrine neoplasia (MEN) syndrome, type 1. The former is an autosomal disorder due to mutations in two different genes, and the associated findings are discussed in the section on ash leaf spots as well as in Chap. 118.

Neuromas (benign proliferations of nerve fibers) are also firm, skin-colored papules. They are more commonly found at sites of amputation and as rudimentary supernumerary digits. However, when there are multiple neuromas on the eyelids, lips, distal tongue, and/or oral mucosa, the patient should be investigated for other signs of the MEN syndrome, type 2b. Associated findings include marfanoid habitus, protuberant lips, intestinal ganglioneuromas, and medullary thyroid carcinoma (>75% of patients; Chap. 408).

Adnexal tumors are derived from pluripotent cells of the epidermis that can differentiate toward hair, sebaceous, apocrine, or eccrine glands or remain undifferentiated. *Basal cell carcinomas* (BCCs) are examples of adnexal tumors that have little or no evidence of differentiation. Clinically, they are translucent papules with rolled borders, telangiectasias, and central erosion. BCCs commonly arise in sun-damaged skin of the head and neck as well as the upper trunk. When a patient has multiple BCCs, especially prior to age 30, the possibility of the nevoid basal cell carcinoma syndrome should be raised. It is inherited as an autosomal dominant trait and is associated with jaw cysts, palmar and plantar pits, frontal bossing, medulloblastomas, and calcification of the falx cerebri and diaphragma sellae. *Tricholemmomas* are also skin-colored adnexal tumors but differentiate toward hair follicles and can have a wartlike appearance. The presence of multiple tricholemmomas on the face and cobblestoning of the oral mucosa points to the diagnosis of Cowden disease (multiple hamartoma syndrome) due to mutations in the phosphatase and tensin homolog (*PTEN*) gene. Internal organ involvement (in decreasing order of frequency) includes fibrocystic disease and carcinoma of the breast, adenomas and carcinomas of the thyroid, and gastrointestinal polyposis. Keratoses of the palms, soles, and dorsal aspect of the hands are also seen.

PINK LESIONS

The cutaneous lesions associated with primary systemic *amyloidosis* are often pink in color and translucent. Common locations are the face, especially the periorbital and perioral regions, and flexural areas. On biopsy, homogeneous deposits of amyloid are seen in the dermis and in the walls of blood vessels; the latter lead to an increase in vessel wall fragility. As a result, petechiae and purpura develop in clinically normal skin as well as in lesional skin following minor trauma, hence the term *pinch purpura*. Amyloid deposits are also seen in the striated muscle of the tongue and result in macroglossia.

Even though specific mucocutaneous lesions are present in only ~30% of the patients with primary systemic (AL) amyloidosis, the diagnosis can be made via histologic examination of abdominal subcutaneous fat, in conjunction with a serum free light chain assay. By special staining, amyloid deposits are seen around blood vessels or individual fat cells in 40–50% of patients. There are also three forms of amyloidosis that are limited to the skin and that should not be construed as cutaneous lesions of systemic amyloidosis. They are macular amyloidosis (upper back), lichen amyloidosis (usually lower extremities), and nodular amyloidosis. In macular and lichen amyloidosis, the deposits are composed of altered epidermal keratin. Early-onset macular and lichen amyloidosis have been associated with MEN syndrome, type 2a.

Patients with *multicentric reticulohistiocytosis* also have pink-colored papules and nodules on the face and mucous membranes as well as on the extensor surface of the hands and forearms. They have a polyarthritis that can mimic rheumatoid arthritis clinically. On histologic examination, the papules have characteristic giant cells that are not seen in biopsies of rheumatoid nodules. Pink to skin-colored papules that are firm, 2–5 mm in diameter, and often in a linear arrangement are seen in patients with *papular mucinosis*. This disease is also referred to as *generalized lichen myxedematosus* or *scleromyxedema*. The latter name comes from the induration of the face and extremities that may accompany the papular eruption. Biopsy specimens of the papules show localized mucin deposition, and serum protein electrophoresis plus immunofixation electrophoresis demonstrates a monoclonal spike of IgG, usually with a λ light chain.

YELLOW LESIONS

Several systemic disorders are characterized by yellow-colored cutaneous papules or plaques—hyperlipidemia (xanthomas), gout (tophi), diabetes (necrobiosis lipoidica), pseudoxanthoma elasticum, and Muir-Torre syndrome (sebaceous tumors). Eruptive xanthomas are the most common form of *xanthomas* and are associated with hypertriglyceridemia (primarily hyperlipoproteinemia types I, IV, and V). Crops of yellow papules with erythematous halos occur primarily on the extensor surfaces of the extremities and the buttocks, and they spontaneously involute with a fall in serum triglycerides. Types II and III result in one or more of the following types of xanthoma: xanthelasma, tendon xanthomas, and plane xanthomas. Xanthelasma are found on the eyelids, whereas tendon xanthomas are frequently associated with the Achilles and extensor finger tendons; plane xanthomas are flat and favor the palmar creases, neck, upper trunk, and flexural folds. Tuberous xanthomas are frequently associated with hypertriglyceridemia, but they are also seen in patients with hypercholesterolemia and are found most frequently over the large joints or hand. Biopsy specimens of xanthomas show collections of lipid-containing macrophages (foam cells).

Patients with several disorders, including biliary cirrhosis, can have a secondary form of hyperlipidemia with associated tuberous and plane xanthomas. However, patients with plasma cell dyscrasias have *normolipemic plane xanthomas*. This latter form of xanthoma may be ≥12 cm in diameter and is most frequently seen on the upper trunk or side of the neck. It is important to note that the most common setting for eruptive xanthomas is uncontrolled diabetes mellitus. The least specific sign for hyperlipidemia is xanthelasma, because at least 50% of the patients with this finding have normal lipid profiles.

In *tophaceous gout*, there are deposits of monosodium urate in the skin around the joints, particularly those of the hands and feet. Additional sites of *tophi* formation include the helix of the ear and the olecranon and prepatellar bursae. The lesions are firm, yellow in color, and occasionally discharge a chalky material. Their size varies from 1 mm to 7 cm, and the diagnosis can be established by polarized light microscopy of the aspirated contents of a lesion. Lesions of *necrobiosis lipoidica* are found primarily on the shins (90%), and patients can have diabetes mellitus or develop it subsequently. Characteristic findings include a central yellow color, atrophy (transparency), telangiectasias, and a red to red-brown border. Ulcerations can also develop within the plaques. Biopsy specimens show necrobiosis of collagen and granulomatous inflammation.

In *pseudoxanthoma elasticum* (PXE), due to mutations in the gene *ABCC6*, there is an abnormal deposition of calcium on the elastic fibers of the skin, eye, and blood vessels. In the skin, the flexural areas such as the neck, axillae, antecubital fossae, and inguinal area are the primary sites of involvement. Yellow papules coalesce to form reticulated plaques that have an appearance similar to that of plucked chicken skin. In severely affected skin, hanging, redundant folds develop. Biopsy specimens of involved skin show swollen and irregularly clumped elastic fibers with deposits of calcium. In the eye, the calcium deposits in Bruch's membrane lead to angioid streaks and choroiditis; in the arteries of the heart, kidney, gastrointestinal tract, and extremities, the deposits lead to angina, hypertension, gastrointestinal bleeding, and claudication, respectively.

Adnexal tumors that have differentiated toward sebaceous glands include sebaceous adenoma, sebaceous carcinoma, and sebaceous hyperplasia. Except for sebaceous hyperplasia, which is commonly seen on the face, these tumors are fairly rare. Patients with Muir-Torre syndrome have one or more *sebaceous adenoma(s)*, and they can also have sebaceous carcinomas and sebaceous hyperplasia as well as keratoacanthomas. The internal manifestations of Muir-Torre syndrome include *multiple* carcinomas of the gastrointestinal tract (primarily colon) as well as cancers of the larynx, genitourinary tract, and breast.

RED LESIONS

Cutaneous lesions that are red in color have a wide variety of etiologies; in an attempt to simplify their identification, they will be subdivided into papules, papules/plaques, and subcutaneous nodules. Common red papules include *arthropod bites* and *cherry hemangiomas*; the latter are small, bright-red, dome-shaped papules that represent a benign proliferation of capillaries. In patients with AIDS (Chap. 226), the development of multiple red hemangioma-like lesions points to bacillary angiomatosis, and biopsy specimens show clusters of bacilli that stain positive with the Warthin-Starry stain; the pathogens have been identified as *Bartonella henselae* and *Bartonella quintana*. Disseminated visceral disease is seen primarily in immunocompromised hosts but can occur in immunocompetent individuals.

Multiple *angiokeratomas* are seen in Fabry disease, an X-linked recessive lysosomal storage disease that is due to a deficiency of α-galactosidase A. The lesions are red to red-blue in color and can be quite small in size (1–3 mm), with the most common location being the lower trunk. Associated findings include chronic renal disease, peripheral neuropathy, and corneal opacities (cornea verticillata). Electron photomicrographs of angiokeratomas and clinically normal skin demonstrate lamellar lipid deposits in fibroblasts, pericytes, and endothelial cells that are diagnostic of this disease. Widespread acute eruptions of erythematous papules are discussed in the section on exanthems.

There are several infectious diseases that present as erythematous papules or nodules in a lymphocutaneous or sporotrichoid pattern, i.e., in a linear arrangement along the lymphatic channels. The two most common etiologies are *Sporothrix schenckii* (sporotrichosis) and the atypical mycobacterium *Mycobacterium marinum*. The organisms are introduced as a result of trauma, and a primary inoculation site is often seen in addition to the lymphatic nodules. Additional causes include *Nocardia*, *Leishmania*, and other atypical mycobacteria and dimorphic fungi; culture of lesional tissue will aid in the diagnosis.

The diseases that are characterized by erythematous plaques with scale are reviewed in the papulosquamous section, and the various forms of dermatitis are discussed in the section on erythroderma. Additional disorders in the differential diagnosis of red papules/plaques include *cellulitis*, *polymorphous light eruption* (PMLE), *cutaneous lymphoid hyperplasia* (lymphocytoma cutis), *cutaneous lupus*, *lymphoma cutis*, and *leukemia cutis*. The first three diseases represent primary cutaneous disorders, although cellulitis may be accompanied by a bacteremia. PMLE is characterized by erythematous papules and plaques in a primarily sun-exposed distribution—dorsum of the hand, extensor forearm, and upper trunk. Lesions follow exposure to UV-B and/or UV-A, and in higher latitudes, PMLE is most severe in the late spring and early summer. A process referred to as "hardening" occurs with continued UV exposure, and the eruption fades, but in temperate climates, it will recur in the spring. PMLE must be differentiated from cutaneous lupus, and this is accomplished by observation of the natural history, histologic examination, and direct immunofluorescence of the lesions. Cutaneous lymphoid hyperplasia (pseudolymphoma) is a *benign* polyclonal proliferation of lymphocytes in the skin that presents as infiltrated pink-red to red-purple papules and plaques; it must be distinguished from lymphoma cutis.

Several types of red plaques are seen in patients with systemic *lupus*, including (1) erythematous urticarial plaques across the cheeks and nose in the classic butterfly rash; (2) erythematous discoid lesions with fine or "carpet-tack" scale, telangiectasias, central hypopigmentation, peripheral hyperpigmentation, follicular plugging, and atrophy located on the face, scalp, external ears, arms, and upper trunk; and (3) psoriasiform or annular lesions of subacute cutaneous lupus with hypopigmented centers located primarily on the extensor arms and upper trunk. Additional mucocutaneous findings include (1) a violaceous flush on the face and V of the neck; (2) photosensitivity; (3) urticarial vasculitis (see "Urticaria," above); (4) lupus panniculitis (see below); (5) diffuse alopecia; (6) alopecia secondary to discoid lesions; (7) periungual telangiectasias and erythema; (8) EM-like lesions that may become bullous; (9) oral ulcers; and (10) distal ulcerations secondary to Raynaud's phenomenon, vasculitis, or livedoid vasculopathy. Patients with only discoid lesions usually have the form of lupus that is limited to the skin. However, up to 10% of these patients eventually develop systemic lupus. Direct immunofluorescence of involved skin, in particular discoid lesions, shows deposits of IgG or IgM and C3 in a granular distribution along the dermal-epidermal junction.

In *lymphoma cutis*, there is a proliferation of malignant lymphocytes in the skin, and the clinical appearance resembles that of cutaneous lymphoid hyperplasia—infiltrated pink-red to red-purple papules and plaques. Lymphoma cutis can occur anywhere on the surface of the skin, whereas the sites of predilection for lymphocytomas include the malar ridge, tip of the nose, and earlobes. Patients with non-Hodgkin's lymphomas have specific cutaneous lesions more often than those with Hodgkin's disease, and, occasionally, the skin nodules precede the development of extracutaneous non-Hodgkin's lymphoma or represent the only site of involvement (e.g., primary cutaneous B cell lymphoma). Arcuate lesions are sometimes seen in lymphoma and lymphocytoma cutis as well as in CTCL. *Adult T cell leukemia/lymphoma* that develops in association with HTLV-1 infection is characterized by cutaneous plaques, hypercalcemia, and circulating CD25+ lymphocytes. *Leukemia cutis* has the same appearance as lymphoma cutis, and specific lesions are seen more commonly in monocytic leukemias than in lymphocytic or granulocytic leukemias. Cutaneous chloromas (granulocytic sarcomas) may precede the appearance of circulating blasts in acute myelogenous leukemia and, as such, represent a form of aleukemic leukemia cutis.

Sweet syndrome is characterized by pink-red to red-brown edematous plaques that are frequently painful and occur primarily on the head, neck, and upper (and, less often, lower) extremities. The patients also have fever, neutrophilia, and a dense dermal infiltrate of neutrophils in the lesions. In ~10% of the patients, there is an associated malignancy, most commonly acute myelogenous leukemia. Sweet syndrome has also been reported with inflammatory bowel disease, systemic lupus erythematosus, and solid tumors (primarily of the genitourinary tract) as well as drugs (e.g., all-*trans*-retinoic acid, granulocyte colony-stimulating factor [G-CSF]). The differential diagnosis includes neutrophilic eccrine hidradenitis; bullous forms of pyoderma gangrenosum; and, occasionally, cellulitis. Extracutaneous sites of involvement include joints, muscles, eye, kidney (proteinuria, occasionally glomerulonephritis), and lung (neutrophilic infiltrates). The idiopathic form of Sweet syndrome is seen more often in women, following a respiratory tract infection.

Common causes of erythematous subcutaneous nodules include inflamed epidermoid inclusion cysts, acne cysts, and furuncles. *Panniculitis*, an inflammation of the fat, also presents as subcutaneous nodules and is frequently a sign of systemic disease. There are several forms of panniculitis, including erythema nodosum, erythema induratum/nodular vasculitis, lupus panniculitis, lipodermatosclerosis, α_1-antitrypsin deficiency, factitial, and fat necrosis secondary to pancreatic disease. Except for erythema nodosum, these lesions may break down and ulcerate or heal with a scar. The shin is the most common location for the nodules of erythema nodosum, whereas the calf is the most common location for lesions of erythema induratum. In erythema nodosum, the nodules are initially red but then develop a blue color as they resolve. Patients with erythema nodosum but no underlying systemic illness can still have fever, malaise, leukocytosis, arthralgias, and/or arthritis. However, the possibility of an underlying illness should be excluded, and the most common associations are streptococcal infections, upper respiratory viral infections, sarcoidosis, and inflammatory bowel disease, in addition to drugs (oral contraceptives, sulfonamides, penicillins, bromides, iodides). Less common associations include bacterial gastroenteritis (*Yersinia*, *Salmonella*) and coccidioidomycosis followed by tuberculosis, histoplasmosis, brucellosis, and infections with *Chlamydophila pneumoniae* or *Chlamydia trachomatis*, *Mycoplasma pneumoniae*, or hepatitis B virus.

Erythema induratum and nodular vasculitis have overlapping features clinically and histologically, and whether they represent two separate entities or the ends of a single disease spectrum is a point of debate; in general, the latter is usually idiopathic and the former is associated with the presence of *Mycobacterium tuberculosis* DNA by PCR within skin lesions. The lesions of lupus panniculitis are found primarily on the cheeks, upper arms, and buttocks (sites of abundant fat) and are seen in both the cutaneous and systemic forms of lupus. The overlying skin may be normal, erythematous, or have the changes of discoid lupus. The subcutaneous fat necrosis that is associated with pancreatic disease is presumably secondary to circulating lipases and is seen in patients with pancreatic carcinoma as well as in patients with acute and chronic pancreatitis. In this disorder, there may be an associated arthritis, fever, and inflammation of visceral fat. Histologic examination of deep incisional biopsy specimens will aid in the diagnosis of the particular type of panniculitis.

Subcutaneous erythematous nodules are also seen in cutaneous polyarteritis nodosa and as a manifestation of *systemic vasculitis* when there is involvement of medium-sized vessels, e.g., systemic polyarteritis nodosa, allergic granulomatosis, or granulomatosis with polyangiitis (Wegener's) (Chap. 385). Cutaneous polyarteritis nodosa presents with painful subcutaneous nodules and ulcers within a red-purple, netlike pattern of livedo reticularis. The latter is due to slowed blood flow through the superficial horizontal venous plexus. The majority of lesions are found on the lower extremities, and while arthralgias and myalgias may accompany cutaneous polyarteritis nodosa, there is no evidence of systemic involvement. In both the cutaneous and systemic forms of vasculitis, skin biopsy specimens of the associated nodules will show the changes characteristic of a necrotizing vasculitis and/or granulomatous inflammation.

RED-BROWN LESIONS

The cutaneous lesions in *sarcoidosis* (Chap. 390) are classically red to red-brown in color, and with diascopy (pressure with a glass slide), a yellow-brown residual color is observed that is secondary to the granulomatous infiltrate. The waxy papules and plaques may be found anywhere on the skin, but the face is the most common location. Usually there are no surface changes, but occasionally the lesions will have scale. Biopsy specimens of the papules show "naked" granulomas in the dermis, i.e., granulomas surrounded by a minimal number of lymphocytes. Other cutaneous findings in sarcoidosis include annular lesions with an atrophic or scaly center, papules within scars, hypopigmented papules and patches, alopecia, acquired ichthyosis, erythema nodosum, and lupus pernio (see below).

The differential diagnosis of sarcoidosis includes foreign-body granulomas produced by chemicals such as beryllium and zirconium, late secondary syphilis, and *lupus vulgaris.* Lupus vulgaris is a form of cutaneous tuberculosis that is seen in previously infected and sensitized individuals. There is often underlying active tuberculosis elsewhere, usually in the lungs or lymph nodes. Lesions occur primarily in the head and neck region and are red-brown plaques with a yellow-brown color on diascopy. Secondary scarring and squamous cell carcinomas can develop within the plaques. Cultures or PCR analysis of the lesions should be performed, along with an interferon γ release assay of peripheral blood, because it is rare for the acid-fast stain to show bacilli within the dermal granulomas.

A generalized distribution of red-brown macules and papules is seen in the form of mastocytosis known as *urticaria pigmentosa* (Chap. 376). Each lesion represents a collection of mast cells in the dermis, with hyperpigmentation of the overlying epidermis. Stimuli such as rubbing cause these mast cells to degranulate, and this leads to the formation of localized urticaria (Darier's sign). Additional symptoms can result from mast cell degranulation and include headache, flushing, diarrhea, and pruritus. Mast cells also infiltrate various organs such as the liver, spleen, and gastrointestinal tract, and accumulations of mast cells in the bones may produce either osteosclerotic or osteolytic lesions on radiographs. In the majority of these patients, however, the internal involvement remains indolent. A subtype of chronic cutaneous small-vessel vasculitis, *erythema elevatum diutinum* (EED), also presents with papules that are red-brown in color. The papules coalesce into plaques on the extensor surfaces of knees, elbows, and the small joints of the hand. Flares of EED have been associated with streptococcal infections.

BLUE LESIONS

Lesions that are blue in color are the result of vascular ectasias, hyperplasias and tumors or melanin pigment within the dermis. *Venous lakes* (ectasias) are compressible dark-blue lesions that are found commonly in the head and neck region. *Venous malformations* are also compressible blue papulonodules and plaques that can occur anywhere on the body, including the oral mucosa. When there are multiple rather than single congenital lesions, the patient may have the blue rubber bleb syndrome or Maffucci's syndrome. Patients with the blue rubber bleb syndrome also have vascular anomalies of the gastrointestinal tract that may bleed, whereas patients with Maffucci's syndrome have associated osteochondromas. *Blue nevi* (moles) are seen when there are collections of pigment-producing nevus cells in the dermis. These benign papular lesions are dome-shaped and occur most commonly on the dorsum of the hand or foot or in the head and neck region.

VIOLACEOUS LESIONS

Violaceous papules and plaques are seen in *lupus pernio, lymphoma cutis,* and *cutaneous lupus.* Lupus pernio is a particular type of sarcoidosis that involves the tip and alar rim of the nose as well as the earlobes, with lesions that are violaceous in color rather than red-brown. This form of sarcoidosis is associated with involvement of the upper respiratory tract. The plaques of lymphoma cutis and cutaneous lupus may be red or violaceous in color and were discussed above.

PURPLE LESIONS

Purple-colored papules and plaques are seen in vascular tumors, such as *Kaposi's sarcoma* (Chap. 226) and *angiosarcoma,* and when there is extravasation of red blood cells into the skin in association with inflammation, as in *palpable purpura* (see "Purpura," below). Patients with congenital or acquired AV fistulas and venous hypertension can develop purple papules on the lower extremities that can resemble Kaposi's sarcoma clinically and histologically; this condition is referred to as pseudo-Kaposi's sarcoma (acral angiodermatitis). Angiosarcoma is found most commonly on the scalp and face of elderly patients or within areas of chronic lymphedema and presents as purple papules and plaques. In the head and neck region, the tumor often extends beyond the clinically defined borders and may be accompanied by facial edema.

BROWN AND BLACK LESIONS

Brown- and black-colored papules are reviewed in "Hyperpigmentation," above.

CUTANEOUS METASTASES

These are discussed last because they can have a wide range of colors. Most commonly, they present as either firm, skin-colored subcutaneous nodules or firm, red to red-brown papulonodules. The lesions of lymphoma cutis range from pink-red to plum in color, whereas metastatic melanoma can be pink, blue, or black in color. Cutaneous metastases develop from hematogenous or lymphatic spread and are most often due to the following primary carcinomas: in men, melanoma, oropharynx, lung, and colon; and in women, breast, melanoma, and ovary. These metastatic lesions may be the initial presentation of the carcinoma, especially when the primary site is the lung.

PURPURA

(Table 72-16) *Purpura* are seen when there is an extravasation of red blood cells into the dermis and, as a result, the lesions do not blanch with pressure. This is in contrast to those erythematous or violet-colored lesions that are due to localized vasodilatation—they do blanch with pressure. Purpura ($\geq$3 mm) and petechiae ($\leq$2 mm) are divided into two major groups: palpable and nonpalpable. The most frequent causes of *nonpalpable* petechiae and purpura are primary cutaneous disorders such as *trauma, solar (actinic) purpura,* and *capillaritis.* Less common causes are *steroid purpura* and *livedoid vasculopathy* (see "Ulcers," below). Solar purpura are seen primarily on the extensor forearms, whereas steroid purpura secondary to potent topical glucocorticoids or endogenous or exogenous Cushing's syndrome can be more widespread. In both cases, there is alteration of the supporting connective tissue that surrounds the dermal blood vessels. In contrast, the petechiae that result from capillaritis are found primarily on the lower extremities. In capillaritis, there is an extravasation of erythrocytes as a result of perivascular lymphocytic inflammation. The petechiae are bright red, 1–2 mm in size, and scattered within yellow-brown patches. The yellow-brown color is caused by hemosiderin deposits within the dermis.

Systemic causes of nonpalpable purpura fall into several categories, and those secondary to clotting disturbances and vascular fragility will be discussed first. The former group includes *thrombocytopenia* (Chap. 140), *abnormal platelet function* as is seen in uremia, and *clotting factor defects.* The initial site of presentation for thrombocytopenia-induced petechiae is the distal lower extremity. Capillary fragility leads to nonpalpable purpura in patients with systemic *amyloidosis* (see "Papulonodular Skin Lesions," above), disorders of collagen production such as *Ehlers-Danlos syndrome,* and *scurvy.* In scurvy, there are flattened corkscrew hairs with surrounding hemorrhage on the lower extremities, in addition to gingivitis. Vitamin C is a cofactor for lysyl hydroxylase, an enzyme involved in the posttranslational modification of procollagen that is necessary for cross-link formation.

TABLE 72-16 CAUSES OF PURPURA

- I. Primary cutaneous disorders
  - A. Nonpalpable
    1. Trauma
    2. Solar (actinic, senile) purpura
    3. Steroid purpura
    4. Capillaritis
    5. Livedoid vasculopathy in the setting of venous hypertension[a]
- II. Systemic diseases
  - A. Nonpalpable
    1. Clotting disturbances
       - a. Thrombocytopenia (including ITP)
       - b. Abnormal platelet function
       - c. Clotting factor defects
    2. Vascular fragility
       - a. Amyloidosis (within normal-appearing skin)
       - b. Ehlers-Danlos syndrome
       - c. Scurvy
    3. Thrombi
       - a. Disseminated intravascular coagulation
       - b. Warfarin (Coumadin)-induced necrosis
       - c. Heparin-induced thrombocytopenia and thrombosis
       - d. Antiphospholipid antibody syndrome
       - e. Monoclonal cryoglobulinemia
       - f. Vasculopathy induced by levamisole-adulterated cocaine
       - g. Thrombotic thrombocytopenic purpura
       - h. Thrombocytosis
       - i Homozygous protein C or protein S deficiency
    4. Emboli
       - a. Cholesterol
       - b. Fat
    5. Possible immune complex
       - a. Gardner-Diamond syndrome (autoerythrocyte sensitivity)
       - b. Waldenström's hypergammaglobulinemic purpura
  - B. Palpable
    1. Vasculitis
       - a. Cutaneous small-vessel vasculitis, including in the setting of systemic vasculitides
       - b. Polyarteritis nodosa
    2. Emboli[b]
       - a. Acute meningococcemia
       - b. Disseminated gonococcal infection
       - c. Rocky Mountain spotted fever
       - d. Ecthyma gangrenosum

[a]Also associated with underlying disorders that lead to hypercoagulability, e.g., factor V Leiden, protein C dysfunction/deficiency. [b]Bacterial (including rickettsial), fungal, or parasitic.

Abbreviation: ITP, idiopathic thrombocytopenic purpura.

In contrast to the previous group of disorders, the purpura (noninflammatory with a retiform outline) seen in the following group of diseases are associated with thrombi formation within vessels. It is important to note that these thrombi are demonstrable in skin biopsy specimens. This group of disorders includes disseminated intravascular coagulation (DIC), monoclonal cryoglobulinemia, thrombocytosis, thrombotic thrombocytopenic purpura, antiphospholipid antibody syndrome, and reactions to warfarin and heparin (heparin-induced thrombocytopenia and thrombosis). DIC is triggered by several types of infection (gram-negative, gram-positive, viral, and rickettsial) as well as by tissue injury and neoplasms. Widespread purpura and hemorrhagic infarcts of the distal extremities are seen. Similar lesions are found in purpura fulminans, which is a form of DIC associated with fever and hypotension that occurs more commonly in children following an infectious illness such as varicella, scarlet fever, or an upper respiratory tract infection. In both disorders, hemorrhagic bullae can develop in involved skin.

Monoclonal cryoglobulinemia is associated with plasma cell dyscrasias, chronic lymphocytic leukemia, and lymphoma. Purpura, primarily of the lower extremities, and hemorrhagic infarcts of the fingers, toes, and ears are seen in these patients. Exacerbations of disease activity can follow cold exposure or an increase in serum viscosity. Biopsy specimens show precipitates of the cryoglobulin within dermal vessels. Similar deposits have been found in the lung, brain, and renal glomeruli. Patients with *thrombotic thrombocytopenic purpura* can also have hemorrhagic infarcts as a result of intravascular thromboses. Additional signs include microangiopathic hemolytic anemia and fluctuating neurologic abnormalities, especially headaches and confusion.

Administration of *warfarin* can result in painful areas of erythema that become purpuric and then necrotic with an adherent black eschar; the condition is referred to as warfarin-induced necrosis. This reaction is seen more often in women and in areas with abundant subcutaneous fat—breasts, abdomen, buttocks, thighs, and calves. The erythema and purpura develop between the third and tenth day of therapy, most likely as a result of a transient imbalance in the levels of anticoagulant and procoagulant vitamin K–dependent factors. Continued therapy does not exacerbate preexisting lesions, and patients with an inherited or acquired deficiency of protein C are at increased risk for this particular reaction as well as for purpura fulminans and calciphylaxis.

Purpura secondary to *cholesterol emboli* are usually seen on the lower extremities of patients with atherosclerotic vascular disease. They often follow anticoagulant therapy or an invasive vascular procedure such as an arteriogram but also occur spontaneously from disintegration of atheromatous plaques. Associated findings include livedo reticularis, gangrene, cyanosis, and ischemic ulcerations. Multiple step sections of the biopsy specimen may be necessary to demonstrate the cholesterol clefts within the vessels. Petechiae are also an important sign of *fat embolism* and occur primarily on the upper body 2–3 days after a major injury. By using special fixatives, the emboli can be demonstrated in biopsy specimens of the petechiae. Emboli of tumor or thrombus are seen in patients with atrial myxomas and marantic endocarditis.

In the *Gardner-Diamond syndrome* (autoerythrocyte sensitivity), female patients develop large ecchymoses within areas of painful, warm erythema. Intradermal injections of autologous erythrocytes or phosphatidyl serine derived from the red cell membrane can reproduce the lesions in some patients; however, there are instances where a reaction is seen at an injection site of the forearm but not in the midback region. The latter has led some observers to view Gardner-Diamond syndrome as a cutaneous manifestation of severe emotional stress. More recently, the possibility of platelet dysfunction (as assessed via aggregation studies) has been raised. *Waldenström's hypergammaglobulinemic purpura* is a chronic disorder characterized by petechiae on the lower extremities. There are circulating complexes of IgG–anti-IgG molecules, and exacerbations are associated with prolonged standing or walking.

Palpable purpura are further subdivided into vasculitic and embolic. In the group of vasculitic disorders, cutaneous small-vessel vasculitis, also known as *leukocytoclastic vasculitis* (LCV), is the one most commonly associated with palpable purpura (Chap. 385). Underlying etiologies include drugs (e.g., antibiotics), infections (e.g., hepatitis C virus), and autoimmune connective tissue diseases (e.g., rheumatoid arthritis, Sjögren's syndrome, lupus). *Henoch-Schönlein purpura* (HSP) is a subtype of acute LCV that is seen more commonly in children and adolescents following an upper respiratory infection. The majority of lesions are found on the lower extremities and buttocks. Systemic manifestations include fever, arthralgias (primarily of the knees and ankles), abdominal pain, gastrointestinal bleeding, and nephritis. Direct immunofluorescence examination shows deposits of IgA within dermal blood vessel walls. Renal disease is of particular concern in adults with HSP. In *polyarteritis nodosa*, specific cutaneous lesions result from a vasculitis of arterial vessels (arteritis), or there may be an associated LCV. Arteritis leads to an infarct of the skin, and this explains the irregular outline of the purpura (see below).

Several types of infectious emboli can give rise to palpable purpura. These embolic lesions are usually *irregular* in outline as opposed to the lesions of LCV, which are *circular* in outline. The irregular outline is indicative of a cutaneous infarct, and the size corresponds to the area of skin that received its blood supply from that particular arteriole or artery. The palpable purpura in LCV are circular because the erythrocytes simply diffuse out evenly from the postcapillary venules as a result of inflammation. Infectious emboli are most commonly due to gram-negative cocci (meningococcus, gonococcus), gram-negative rods (Enterobacteriaceae), and gram-positive cocci (*Staphylococcus*). Additional causes include *Rickettsia* and, in immunocompromised patients, *Aspergillus* and other opportunistic fungi.

The embolic lesions in *acute meningococcemia* are found primarily on the trunk, lower extremities, and sites of pressure, and a gunmetal-gray color often develops within them. Their size varies from a few millimeters to several centimeters, and the organisms can be cultured from the lesions. Associated findings include a preceding upper respiratory tract infection; fever; meningitis; DIC; and, in some patients, a deficiency of the terminal components of complement. In *disseminated gonococcal infection* (arthritis-dermatitis syndrome), a small number of inflammatory papules and vesicopustules, often with central purpura or hemorrhagic necrosis, are found on the distal extremities. Additional symptoms include arthralgias, tenosynovitis, and fever. To establish the diagnosis, a Gram stain of these lesions should be performed. *Rocky Mountain spotted fever* is a tick-borne disease that is caused by *Rickettsia rickettsii*. A several-day history of fever, chills, severe headache, and photophobia precedes the onset of the cutaneous eruption. The initial lesions are erythematous macules and papules on the wrists, ankles, palms, and soles. With time, the lesions spread centripetally and become purpuric.

Lesions of *ecthyma gangrenosum* begin as edematous, erythematous papules or plaques and then develop central purpura and necrosis. Bullae formation also occurs in these lesions, and they are frequently found in the girdle region. The organism that is classically associated with ecthyma gangrenosum is *Pseudomonas aeruginosa*, but other gram-negative rods such as *Klebsiella*, *Escherichia coli*, and *Serratia* can produce similar lesions. In immunocompromised hosts, the list of potential pathogens is expanded to include *Candida* and other opportunistic fungi (e.g., *Aspergillus*, *Fusarium*).

ULCERS

The approach to the patient with a cutaneous ulcer is outlined in Table 72-17. Peripheral vascular diseases of the extremities are reviewed in Chap. 302, as is Raynaud's phenomenon.

Livedoid vasculopathy (livedoid vasculitis; atrophie blanche) represents a combination of a vasculopathy plus intravascular thrombosis. Purpuric lesions and livedo reticularis are found in association with *painful* ulcerations of the lower extremities. These ulcers are often slow to heal, but when they do, irregularly shaped white scars form. The majority of cases are secondary to venous hypertension, but possible underlying illnesses include cryofibrinogenemia and disorders of hypercoagulability, e.g., the antiphospholipid syndrome (Chaps. 142 and 379).

In *pyoderma gangrenosum*, the border of untreated active ulcers has a characteristic appearance consisting of an undermined necrotic violaceous edge and a peripheral erythematous halo. The ulcers often begin as pustules that then expand rather rapidly to a size as large as 20 cm. Although these lesions are most commonly found on the lower extremities, they can arise anywhere on the surface of the body, including sites of trauma (pathergy). An estimated 30–50% of cases are idiopathic, and the most common associated disorders are ulcerative colitis and Crohn's disease. Less commonly, pyoderma gangrenosum is associated with seropositive rheumatoid arthritis, acute and chronic myelogenous leukemia, hairy cell leukemia, myelofibrosis, or a monoclonal gammopathy, usually IgA. Because the histology of pyoderma gangrenosum may be nonspecific (dermal infiltrate of neutrophils when in untreated state), the diagnosis requires clinicopathologic correlation, in particular, the exclusion of similar-appearing ulcers such as necrotizing vasculitis, Meleney's ulcer (synergistic infection at a site of trauma or surgery), dimorphic fungi, cutaneous amebiasis, spider bites, and factitial. In the myeloproliferative disorders, the ulcers may be more superficial with a pustulobullous border, and these lesions provide a connection between classic pyoderma gangrenosum and acute febrile neutrophilic dermatosis (Sweet syndrome).

TABLE 72-17 CAUSES OF MUCOCUTANEOUS ULCERS

I. Primary cutaneous disorders
  A. Peripheral vascular disease (Chap. 302)
    1. Venous
    2. Arterial[a]
  B. Livedoid vasculopathy in the setting of venous hypertension[b]
  C. Squamous cell carcinoma, e.g., within scars, basal cell carcinomas
  D. Infections, e.g., ecthyma caused by *Streptococcus* (Chap. 173)
  E. Physical, e.g., trauma, pressure
  F. Drugs, e.g., hydroxyurea
II. Systemic diseases
  A. Lower legs
    1. Small-vessel and medium-vessel vasculitis[c]
    2. Hemoglobinopathies (Chap. 127)
    3. Cryoglobulinemia,[c] cryofibrinogenemia
    4. Cholesterol emboli[c]
    5. Necrobiosis lipoidica[d]
    6. Antiphospholipid syndrome (Chap. 141)
    7. Neuropathic[e] (Chap. 417)
    8. Panniculitis
    9. Kaposi's sarcoma, acral angiodermatitis
    10. Diffuse dermal angiomatosis
  B. Hands and feet
    1. Raynaud's phenomenon (Chap. 302)
    2. Buerger disease
  C. Generalized
    1. Pyoderma gangrenosum, but most commonly legs
    2. Calciphylaxis (Chap. 424)
    3. Infections, e.g., dimorphic fungi, leishmaniasis
    4. Lymphoma
  D. Face, especially perioral, and anogenital
    1. Chronic herpes simplex[f]
III. Mucosal
  A. Behçet's syndrome (Chap. 387)
  B. Erythema multiforme major, Stevens-Johnson syndrome, TEN
  C. Primary blistering disorders (Chap. 73)
  D. Lupus erythematosus, lichen planus
  E. Inflammatory bowel disease
  F. Acute HIV infection
  G. Reactive arthritis (formerly known as Reiter's syndrome)

[a]Underlying atherosclerosis. [b]Also associated with underlying disorders that lead to hypercoagulability, e.g., factor V Leiden, protein C dysfunction/deficiency, antiphospholipid antibodies. [c]Reviewed in section on Purpura. [d]Reviewed in section on Papulonodular Skin Lesions. [e]Favors plantar surface of the foot. [f]Sign of immunosuppression.

Abbreviation: TEN, toxic epidermal necrolysis.

FEVER AND RASH

The major considerations in a patient with a fever and a rash are inflammatory diseases versus infectious diseases. In the hospital setting, the most common scenario is a patient who has a drug rash plus a fever secondary to an underlying infection. However, it should be emphasized that a drug reaction can lead to both a cutaneous eruption and a fever ("drug fever"), especially in the setting of DRESS, AGEP, or serum sickness–like reaction. Additional inflammatory diseases that are often associated with a fever include pustular psoriasis, erythroderma, and Sweet syndrome. Lyme disease, secondary syphilis, and viral and bacterial exanthems (see "Exanthems," above) are examples of infectious diseases that produce a rash and a fever. Lastly, it is important to determine whether or not the cutaneous lesions represent septic emboli (see "Purpura," above). Such lesions usually have evidence of ischemia in the form of purpura, necrosis, or impending necrosis (gunmetal-gray color). In the patient with thrombocytopenia, however, purpura can be seen in inflammatory reactions such as morbilliform drug eruptions and infectious lesions.

73 Immunologically Mediated Skin Diseases

Kim B. Yancey, Thomas J. Lawley

A number of immunologically mediated skin diseases and immunologically mediated systemic disorders with cutaneous manifestations are now recognized as distinct entities with consistent clinical, histologic, and immunopathologic findings. Clinically, these disorders are characterized by morbidity (pain, pruritus, disfigurement) and, in some instances, result in death (largely due to loss of epidermal barrier function and/or secondary infection). The major features of the more common immunologically mediated skin diseases are summarized in this chapter (Table 73-1), as are the autoimmune systemic disorders with cutaneous manifestations.

AUTOIMMUNE CUTANEOUS DISEASES

PEMPHIGUS VULGARIS

Pemphigus refers to a group of autoantibody-mediated intraepidermal blistering diseases characterized by loss of cohesion between epidermal cells (a process termed *acantholysis*). Manual pressure to the skin of these patients may elicit the separation of the epidermis (*Nikolsky's sign*). This finding, while characteristic of pemphigus, is not specific to this group of disorders and is also seen in toxic epidermal necrolysis, Stevens-Johnson syndrome, and a few other skin diseases.

Pemphigus vulgaris (PV) is a mucocutaneous blistering disease that predominantly occurs in patients >40 years of age. PV typically begins on mucosal surfaces and often progresses to involve the skin. This disease is characterized by fragile, flaccid blisters that rupture to produce extensive denudation of mucous membranes and skin (Fig. 73-1). The mouth, scalp, face, neck, axilla, groin, and trunk are typically involved. PV may be associated with severe skin pain; some patients experience pruritus as well. Lesions usually heal without scarring except at sites complicated by secondary infection or mechanically induced dermal wounds. Postinflammatory hyperpigmentation is usually present for some time at sites of healed lesions.

Biopsies of early lesions demonstrate intraepidermal vesicle formation secondary to loss of cohesion between epidermal cells (i.e., acantholytic blisters). Blister cavities contain acantholytic epidermal cells, which appear as round homogeneous cells containing hyperchromatic nuclei. Basal keratinocytes remain attached to the epidermal basement membrane; hence, blister formation takes place within the suprabasal portion of the epidermis. Lesional skin may contain focal collections of intraepidermal eosinophils within blister cavities; dermal alterations are slight, often limited to an eosinophil-predominant leukocytic infiltrate. Direct immunofluorescence microscopy of lesional or intact patient skin shows deposits of IgG on the surface of keratinocytes; deposits of complement components are typically found in lesional but not in uninvolved skin. Deposits of IgG on keratinocytes are derived from circulating autoantibodies to cell-surface autoantigens. Such circulating autoantibodies

TABLE 73-1 IMMUNOLOGICALLY MEDIATED BLISTERING DISEASES

Disease	Clinical Manifestations	Histology	Immunopathology	Autoantigens[a]
Pemphigus vulgaris	Flaccid blisters, denuded skin, oromucosal lesions	Acantholytic blister formed in suprabasal layer of epidermis	Cell surface deposits of IgG on keratinocytes	Dsg3 (plus Dsg1 in patients with skin involvement)
Pemphigus foliaceus	Crusts and shallow erosions on scalp, central face, upper chest, and back	Acantholytic blister formed in superficial layer of epidermis	Cell surface deposits of IgG on keratinocytes	Dsg1
Paraneoplastic pemphigus	Painful stomatitis with papulosquamous or lichenoid eruptions that may progress to blisters	Acantholysis, keratinocyte necrosis, and vacuolar interface dermatitis	Cell surface deposits of IgG and C3 on keratinocytes and (variably) similar immunoreactants in epidermal BMZ	Plakin protein family members and desmosomal cadherins (see text for details)
Bullous pemphigoid	Large tense blisters on flexor surfaces and trunk	Subepidermal blister with eosinophil-rich infiltrate	Linear band of IgG and/or C3 in epidermal BMZ	BPAG1, BPAG2
Pemphigoid gestationis	Pruritic, urticarial plaques rimmed by vesicles and bullae on the trunk and extremities	Teardrop-shaped, subepidermal blisters in dermal papillae; eosinophil-rich infiltrate	Linear band of C3 in epidermal BMZ	BPAG2 (plus BPAG1 in some patients)
Dermatitis herpetiformis	Extremely pruritic small papules and vesicles on elbows, knees, buttocks, and posterior neck	Subepidermal blister with neutrophils in dermal papillae	Granular deposits of IgA in dermal papillae	Epidermal transglutaminase
Linear IgA disease	Pruritic small papules on extensor surfaces; occasionally larger, arciform blisters	Subepidermal blister with neutrophil-rich infiltrate	Linear band of IgA in epidermal BMZ	BPAG2 (see text for specific details)
Epidermolysis bullosa acquisita	Blisters, erosions, scars, and milia on sites exposed to trauma; widespread, inflammatory, tense blisters may be seen initially	Subepidermal blister that may or may not include a leukocytic infiltrate	Linear band of IgG and/or C3 in epidermal BMZ	Type VII collagen
Mucous membrane pemphigoid	Erosive and/or blistering lesions of mucous membranes and possibly the skin; scarring of some sites	Subepidermal blister that may or may not include a leukocytic infiltrate	Linear band of IgG, IgA, and/or C3 in epidermal BMZ	BPAG2, laminin-332, or others

[a]Autoantigens bound by these patients' autoantibodies are defined as follows: Dsg1, desmoglein 1; Dsg3, desmoglein 3; BPAG1, bullous pemphigoid antigen 1; BPAG2, bullous pemphigoid antigen 2.

Abbreviation: BMZ, basement membrane zone.

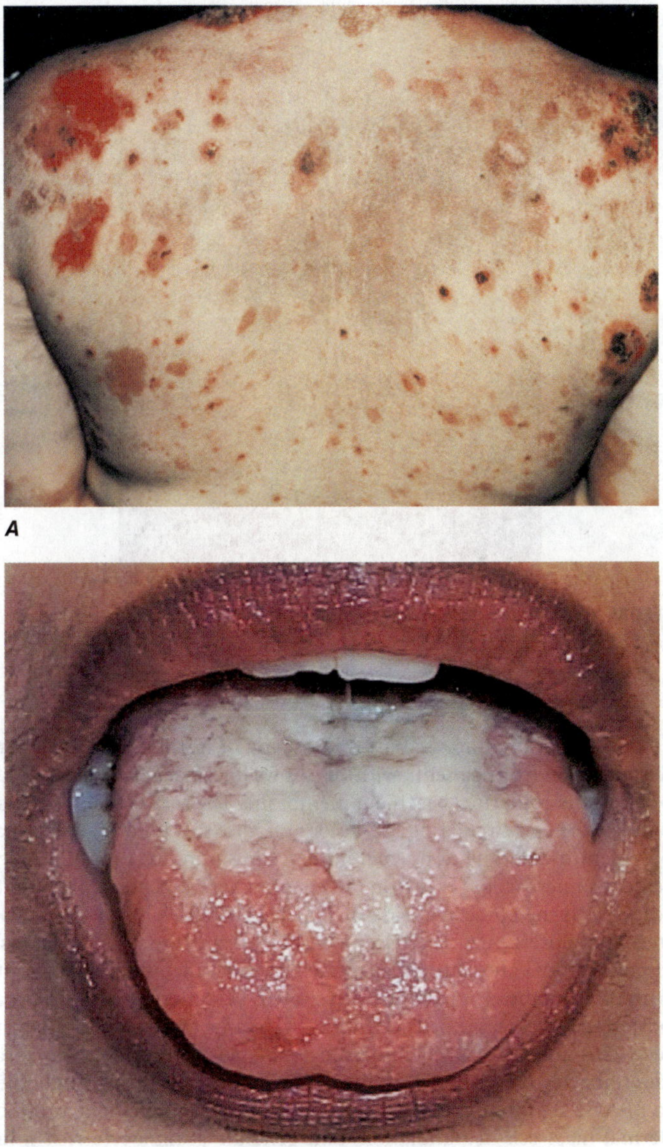

FIGURE 73-1 **Pemphigus vulgaris. *A.*** Flaccid bullae are easily ruptured, resulting in multiple erosions and crusted plaques. ***B.*** Involvement of the oral mucosa, which is almost invariable, may present with erosions on the gingiva, buccal mucosa, palate, posterior pharynx, or tongue. *(B, Courtesy of Robert Swerlick, MD; with permission.)*

can be demonstrated in 80–90% of PV patients by indirect immunofluorescence microscopy; monkey esophagus is the optimal substrate for these studies. Patients with PV have IgG autoantibodies to *desmogleins* (Dsgs), transmembrane desmosomal glycoproteins that belong to the cadherin family of calcium-dependent adhesion molecules. Such autoantibodies can be precisely quantitated by enzyme-linked immunosorbent assay (ELISA). Patients with early PV (i.e., mucosal disease) have IgG autoantibodies to Dsg3; patients with advanced PV (i.e., mucocutaneous disease) have IgG autoantibodies to both Dsg3 and Dsg1. Experimental studies have shown that autoantibodies from patients with PV are pathogenic (i.e., responsible for blister formation) and that their titer correlates with disease activity. Recent studies have shown that the anti-Dsg autoantibody profile in these patients' sera as well as the tissue distribution of Dsg3 and Dsg1 determine the site of blister formation in patients with PV. Coexpression of Dsg3 and Dsg1 by epidermal cells protects against pathogenic IgG antibodies to either of these cadherins but not against pathogenic autoantibodies to both.

PV can be life-threatening. Prior to the availability of glucocorticoids, mortality rates ranged from 60% to 90%; the current figure is ~5%. Common causes of morbidity and death are infection and complications of treatment with glucocorticoids. Bad prognostic factors include advanced age, widespread involvement, and the requirement for high doses of glucocorticoids (with or without other immunosuppressive agents) for control of disease. The course of PV in individual patients is variable and difficult to predict. Some patients experience remission, while others may require long-term treatment or succumb to complications of their disease or its treatment. The mainstay of treatment is systemic glucocorticoids. Patients with moderate to severe PV are usually started on prednisone at 1 mg/kg per day. If new lesions continue to appear after 1–2 weeks of treatment, the dose may need to be increased and/or prednisone may need to be combined with other immunosuppressive agents such as azathioprine (2–2.5 mg/kg per day), mycophenolate mofetil (20–35 mg/kg per day), or cyclophosphamide (1–2 mg/kg per day). Patients with severe, treatment-resistant disease may derive benefit from plasmapheresis (six high-volume exchanges [i.e., 2–3 L per exchange] over ~2 weeks), IV immunoglobulin (IVIg) (2 g/kg over 3–5 days every 6–8 weeks), or rituximab (375 mg/m^2 per week × 4, or 1000 mg on days 1 and 15). It is important to bring severe or progressive disease under control quickly in order to lessen the severity and/or duration of this disorder. Accordingly, some have suggested that rituximab and daily glucocorticoids should be used early in PV patients to avert the development of treatment-resistant disease.

PEMPHIGUS FOLIACEUS

Pemphigus foliaceus (PF) is distinguished from PV by several features. In PF, acantholytic blisters are located high within the epidermis, usually just beneath the stratum corneum. Hence, PF is a more superficial blistering disease than PV. The distribution of lesions in the two disorders is much the same, except that in PF mucous membranes are almost always spared. Patients with PF rarely have intact blisters but rather exhibit shallow erosions associated with erythema, scale, and crust formation. Mild cases of PF resemble severe seborrheic dermatitis; severe PF may cause extensive exfoliation. Sun exposure (ultraviolet irradiation) may be an aggravating factor.

PF has immunopathologic features in common with PV. Specifically, direct immunofluorescence microscopy of perilesional skin demonstrates IgG on the surface of keratinocytes. Similarly, patients with PF have circulating IgG autoantibodies directed against the surface of keratinocytes. In PF, autoantibodies are directed against Dsg1, a 160-kDa desmosomal cadherin. These autoantibodies can be quantitated by ELISA. As noted for PV, the autoantibody profile in patients with PF (i.e., anti-Dsg1 IgG) and the tissue distribution of this autoantigen (i.e., expression in oral mucosa that is compensated by coexpression of Dsg3) are thought to account for the distribution of lesions in this disease.

Endemic forms of PF are found in south-central rural Brazil, where the disease is known as *fogo salvagem* (FS), as well as in selected sites in Latin America and Tunisia. Endemic PF, like other forms of this disease, is mediated by IgG autoantibodies to Dsg1. Clusters of FS overlap with those of leishmaniasis, a disease transmitted by bites of the sand fly *Lutzomyia longipalis*. Recent studies have shown that sand-fly salivary antigens (specifically, the LJM11 salivary protein) are recognized by IgG autoantibodies from FS patients (as well as by monoclonal antibodies to Dsg1 derived from these patients). Moreover, mice immunized with LJM11 produce antibodies to Dsg1. Thus, these findings suggest that insect bites may deliver salivary antigens that initiate a cross-reactive humoral immune response, which may lead to FS in genetically susceptible individuals.

Although pemphigus has been associated with several autoimmune diseases, its association with thymoma and/or myasthenia gravis is particularly notable. To date, >30 cases of thymoma and/or myasthenia gravis have been reported in association with pemphigus, usually with PF. Patients may also develop pemphigus as a consequence of drug exposure; drug-induced pemphigus usually resembles PF rather than PV. Drugs containing a thiol group in their chemical structure (e.g., penicillamine, captopril, enalapril) are most commonly associated with drug-induced pemphigus. Nonthiol drugs linked to pemphigus include penicillins, cephalosporins, and piroxicam. It has been suggested that thiol-containing and non-thiol-containing drugs induce pemphigus via biochemical and immunologic mechanisms, respectively—hence, the better prognosis upon drug withdrawal in cases of pemphigus induced by thiol-containing medications. Some cases of drug-induced pemphigus are durable and require treatment with systemic glucocorticoids and/or immunosuppressive agents.

PF is generally a less severe disease than PV and carries a better prognosis. Localized disease can sometimes be treated with topical or intralesional glucocorticoids; more active cases can usually be controlled with systemic glucocorticoids. Patients with severe, treatment-resistant disease may require more aggressive interventions, as described above for patients with PV.

PARANEOPLASTIC PEMPHIGUS

Paraneoplastic pemphigus (PNP) is an autoimmune acantholytic mucocutaneous disease associated with an occult or confirmed neoplasm. Patients with PNP typically have painful mucosal erosive lesions in association with papulosquamous and/or lichenoid eruptions that often progress to blisters. Palm and sole involvement are common in these patients and raise the possibility that prior reports of neoplasia-associated erythema multiforme actually may have represented unrecognized cases of PNP. Biopsies of lesional skin from these patients show varying combinations of acantholysis, keratinocyte necrosis, and vacuolar-interface dermatitis. Direct immunofluorescence microscopy of a patient's skin shows deposits of IgG and complement on the surface of keratinocytes and (variably) similar immunoreactants in the epidermal basement membrane zone. Patients with PNP have IgG autoantibodies to cytoplasmic proteins that are members of the plakin family (e.g., desmoplakins I and II, bullous pemphigoid antigen [BPAG]1, envoplakin, periplakin, and plectin) and to cell-surface proteins that are members of the cadherin family (e.g., Dsg1 and Dsg3). Passive transfer studies have shown that autoantibodies from patients with PNP are pathogenic in animal models.

The predominant neoplasms associated with PNP are non-Hodgkin's lymphoma, chronic lymphocytic leukemia, thymoma, spindle cell tumors, Waldenström's macroglobulinemia, and Castleman's disease; the last-mentioned neoplasm is particularly common among children with PNP. Rare cases of seronegative PNP have been reported in patients with B cell malignancies previously treated with rituximab. In addition to severe skin lesions, many patients with PNP develop life-threatening bronchiolitis obliterans. PNP is generally resistant to conventional therapies (i.e., those used to treat PV); rarely, a patient's disease may ameliorate or even remit following ablation or removal of underlying neoplasms.

BULLOUS PEMPHIGOID

Bullous pemphigoid (BP) is a polymorphic autoimmune subepidermal blistering disease usually seen in the elderly. Initial lesions may consist of urticarial plaques; most patients eventually display tense blisters on either normal-appearing or erythematous skin (Fig. 73-2). The lesions are usually distributed over the lower abdomen, groin, and flexor surface of the extremities; oral mucosal lesions are found in some patients. Pruritus may be nonexistent or severe. As lesions evolve, tense blisters tend to rupture and be replaced by erosions with or without surmounting crust. Nontraumatized blisters heal without scarring. The major histocompatibility complex class II allele HLA-DQβ1*0301 is prevalent in patients with BP. Despite isolated reports, several studies have shown that patients with BP do not have a higher incidence of malignancy than appropriately age- and gender-matched controls.

Biopsies of early lesional skin demonstrate subepidermal blisters and histologic features that roughly correlate with the clinical character of the particular lesion under study. Lesions on normal-appearing skin generally contain a sparse perivascular leukocytic infiltrate with some eosinophils; conversely, biopsies of inflammatory lesions typically show an eosinophil-rich infiltrate at sites of vesicle formation and in perivascular areas. In addition to eosinophils, cell-rich lesions also contain mononuclear cells and neutrophils. It is not possible to distinguish BP from other subepidermal blistering diseases by routine histologic studies alone.

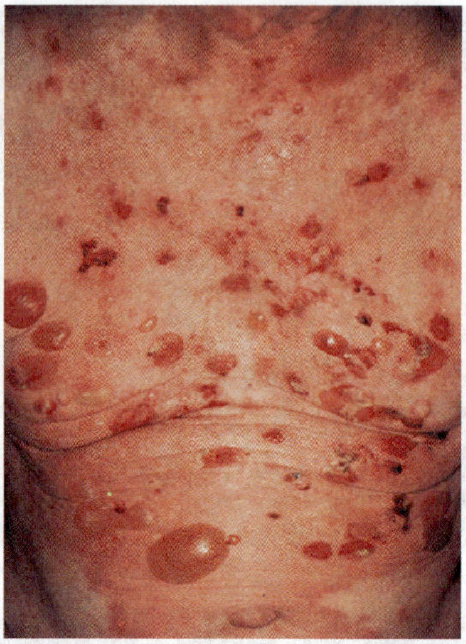

FIGURE 73-2 Bullous pemphigoid with tense vesicles and bullae on erythematous, urticarial bases. *(Courtesy of the Yale Resident's Slide Collection; with permission.)*

Direct immunofluorescence microscopy of normal-appearing perilesional skin from patients with BP shows linear deposits of IgG and/or C3 in the epidermal basement membrane. The sera of ~70% of these patients contain circulating IgG autoantibodies that bind the epidermal basement membrane of normal human skin in indirect immunofluorescence microscopy. IgG from an even higher percentage of patients reacts with the epidermal side of 1 *M* NaCl split skin (an alternative immunofluorescence microscopy test substrate used to distinguish circulating IgG autoantibodies to the basement membrane in patients with BP from those in patients with similar, yet different, subepidermal blistering diseases; see below). In BP, circulating autoantibodies recognize 230- and 180-kDa hemidesmosome-associated proteins in basal keratinocytes (i.e., BPAG1 and BPAG2, respectively). Autoantibodies to BPAG2 are thought to deposit in situ, activate complement, produce dermal mast-cell degranulation, and generate granulocyte-rich infiltrates that cause tissue damage and blister formation.

BP may persist for months to years, with exacerbations or remissions. Extensive involvement may result in widespread erosions and compromise cutaneous integrity; elderly and/or debilitated patients may die. The mainstay of treatment is systemic glucocorticoids. Local or minimal disease can sometimes be controlled with topical glucocorticoids alone; more extensive lesions generally respond to systemic glucocorticoids either alone or in combination with immunosuppressive agents. Patients usually respond to prednisone (0.75–1 mg/kg per day). In some instances, azathioprine (2–2.5 mg/kg per day), mycophenolate mofetil (20–35 mg/kg per day), or cyclophosphamide (1–2 mg/kg per day) are necessary adjuncts.

PEMPHIGOID GESTATIONIS

Pemphigoid gestationis (PG), also known as *herpes gestationis*, is a rare, nonviral, subepidermal blistering disease of pregnancy and the puerperium. PG may begin during any trimester of pregnancy or present shortly after delivery. Lesions are usually distributed over the abdomen, trunk, and extremities; mucous membrane lesions are rare. Skin lesions in these patients may be quite polymorphic and consist of erythematous urticarial papules and plaques, vesiculopapules, and/or frank bullae. Lesions are almost always extremely pruritic. Severe exacerbations of PG frequently follow delivery, typically within 24–48 h. PG tends to recur in subsequent pregnancies, often beginning earlier during such gestations. Brief flare-ups of disease may occur with resumption of menses and may develop in patients later exposed to oral contraceptives. Occasionally, infants of affected mothers have transient skin lesions.

Biopsies of early lesional skin show teardrop-shaped subepidermal vesicles forming in dermal papillae in association with an eosinophil-rich leukocytic infiltrate. Differentiation of PG from other subepidermal bullous diseases by light microscopy is difficult. However, direct immunofluorescence microscopy of perilesional skin from PG patients reveals the immunopathologic hallmark of this disorder: linear deposits of C3 in the epidermal basement membrane. These deposits develop as a consequence of complement activation produced by low-titer IgG anti–basement membrane autoantibodies directed against BPAG2, the same hemidesmosome-associated protein that is targeted by autoantibodies in patients with BP—a subepidermal bullous disease that resembles PG clinically, histologically, and immunopathologically.

The goals of therapy in patients with PG are to prevent the development of new lesions, relieve intense pruritus, and care for erosions at sites of blister formation. Many patients require treatment with moderate doses of daily glucocorticoids (i.e., 20–40 mg of prednisone) at some point in their course. Mild cases (or brief flare-ups) may be controlled by vigorous use of potent topical glucocorticoids. Infants born of mothers with PG appear to be at increased risk of being born slightly premature or "small for dates." Current evidence suggests that there is no difference in the incidence of uncomplicated live births between PG patients treated with systemic glucocorticoids and those managed more conservatively. If systemic glucocorticoids are administered, newborns are at risk for development of reversible adrenal insufficiency.

DERMATITIS HERPETIFORMIS

Dermatitis herpetiformis (DH) is an intensely pruritic, papulovesicular skin disease characterized by lesions symmetrically distributed over extensor surfaces (i.e., elbows, knees, buttocks, back, scalp, and posterior neck) (see Fig. 70-8). Primary lesions in this disorder consist of papules, papulovesicles, or urticarial plaques. Because pruritus is prominent, patients may present with excoriations and crusted papules but no observable primary lesions. Patients sometimes report that their pruritus has a distinctive burning or stinging component; the onset of such local symptoms reliably heralds the development of distinct clinical lesions 12–24 h later. Almost all DH patients have associated, usually subclinical, gluten-sensitive enteropathy (Chap. 349), and >90% express the HLA-B8/DRw3 and HLA-DQw2 haplotypes. DH may present at any age, including in childhood; onset in the second to fourth decades is most common. The disease is typically chronic.

Biopsy of early lesional skin reveals neutrophil-rich infiltrates within dermal papillae. Neutrophils, fibrin, edema, and microvesicle formation at these sites are characteristic of early disease. Older lesions may demonstrate nonspecific features of a subepidermal bulla or an excoriated papule. Because the clinical and histologic features of this disease can be variable and resemble those of other subepidermal blistering disorders, the diagnosis is confirmed by direct immunofluorescence microscopy of normal-appearing perilesional skin. Such studies demonstrate granular deposits of IgA (with or without complement components) in the papillary dermis and along the epidermal basement membrane zone. IgA deposits in the skin are unaffected by control of disease with medication; however, these immunoreactants diminish in intensity or disappear in patients maintained for long periods on a strict gluten-free diet (see below). Patients with DH have granular deposits of IgA in their epidermal basement membrane zone and should be distinguished from individuals with linear IgA deposits at this site (see below).

Although most DH patients do not report overt gastrointestinal symptoms or have laboratory evidence of malabsorption, biopsies of the small bowel usually reveal blunting of intestinal villi and a lymphocytic infiltrate in the lamina propria. As is true for patients with celiac disease, this gastrointestinal abnormality can be reversed by a gluten-free diet. Moreover, if maintained, this diet alone may control the skin disease and eventuate in clearance of IgA deposits from these patients' epidermal basement membrane zones. Subsequent gluten exposure in such patients alters the morphology of their small bowel, elicits a flare-up of their skin disease, and is associated with the reappearance of IgA in their epidermal basement membrane zones. As in patients with celiac disease, dietary gluten sensitivity in patients with DH is associated with IgA endomysial autoantibodies that target tissue transglutaminase. Studies indicate that patients with DH also have high-avidity IgA autoantibodies to epidermal transglutaminase 3 and that the latter is co-localized with granular deposits of IgA in the papillary dermis of DH patients. Patients with DH also have an increased incidence of thyroid abnormalities, achlorhydria, atrophic gastritis, and autoantibodies to gastric parietal cells. These associations likely relate to the high frequency of the HLA-B8/DRw3 haplotype in these patients, because this marker is commonly linked to autoimmune disorders. The mainstay of treatment of DH is dapsone, a sulfone. Patients respond rapidly (24–48 h) to dapsone (50–200 mg/d), but require careful pretreatment evaluation and close follow-up to ensure that complications are avoided or controlled. All patients taking dapsone at >100 mg/d will have some hemolysis and methemoglobinemia, which are expected pharmacologic side effects of this agent. Gluten restriction can control DH and lessen dapsone requirements; this diet must rigidly exclude gluten to be of maximal benefit. Many months of dietary restriction may be necessary before a beneficial result is achieved. Good dietary counseling by a trained dietitian is essential.

LINEAR IgA DISEASE

Linear IgA disease, once considered a variant form of DH, is actually a separate and distinct entity. Clinically, patients with linear IgA disease may resemble individuals with DH, BP, or other subepidermal blistering diseases. Lesions typically consist of papulovesicles, bullae, and/or urticarial plaques that develop predominantly on central or flexural sites. Oral mucosal involvement occurs in some patients. Severe pruritus resembles that seen in patients with DH. Patients with linear IgA disease do not have an increased frequency of the HLA-B8/DRw3 haplotype or an associated enteropathy and therefore are not candidates for treatment with a gluten-free diet.

Histologic alterations in early lesions may be virtually indistinguishable from those in DH. However, direct immunofluorescence microscopy of normal-appearing perilesional skin reveals a linear band of IgA (and often C3) in the epidermal basement membrane zone. Most patients with linear IgA disease have circulating IgA basement membrane autoantibodies directed against neoepitopes in the proteolytically processed extracellular domain of BPAG2. These patients generally respond to treatment with dapsone (50–200 mg/d).

EPIDERMOLYSIS BULLOSA ACQUISITA

Epidermolysis bullosa acquisita (EBA) is a rare, noninherited, polymorphic, chronic, subepidermal blistering disease. (The inherited form is discussed in Chap. 427.) Patients with classic or noninflammatory EBA have blisters on noninflamed skin, atrophic scars, milia, nail dystrophy, and oral lesions. Because lesions generally occur at sites exposed to minor trauma, classic EBA is considered a mechanobullous disease. Other patients with EBA have widespread inflammatory scarring and bullous lesions that resemble severe BP. Inflammatory EBA may evolve into the classic, noninflammatory form of this disease. Rarely, patients present with lesions that predominate on mucous membranes. The HLA-DR2 haplotype is found with increased frequency in EBA patients. Studies suggest that EBA is sometimes associated with inflammatory bowel disease (especially Crohn's disease).

The histology of lesional skin varies with the character of the lesion being studied. Noninflammatory bullae are subepidermal, feature a sparse leukocytic infiltrate, and resemble the lesions in patients with porphyria cutanea tarda. Inflammatory lesions consist of neutrophil-rich subepidermal blisters. EBA patients have continuous deposits of IgG (and frequently C3) in a linear pattern within the epidermal basement membrane zone. Ultrastructurally, these immunoreactants are found in the sublamina densa region in association with anchoring fibrils. Approximately 50% of EBA patients have demonstrable circulating IgG basement membrane autoantibodies directed against type VII collagen—the collagen species that makes up anchoring fibrils. Such IgG autoantibodies bind the dermal side of 1 *M* NaCl split skin (in contrast to IgG autoantibodies in patients with BP). Studies have shown that passive transfer of experimental or clinical IgG against type

VII collagen can produce lesions in mice that clinically, histologically, and immunopathologically resemble those in patients with inflammatory EBA.

Treatment of EBA is generally unsatisfactory. Some patients with inflammatory EBA may respond to systemic glucocorticoids, either alone or in combination with immunosuppressive agents. Other patients (especially those with neutrophil-rich inflammatory lesions) may respond to dapsone. The chronic, noninflammatory form of EBA is largely resistant to treatment, although some patients may respond to cyclosporine, azathioprine, or IVIg.

MUCOUS MEMBRANE PEMPHIGOID

Mucous membrane pemphigoid (MMP) is a rare, acquired, subepithelial immunobullous disease characterized by erosive lesions of mucous membranes and skin that result in scarring of at least some sites of involvement. Common sites include the oral mucosa (especially the gingiva) and conjunctiva; other sites that may be affected include the nasopharyngeal, laryngeal, esophageal, and anogenital mucosa. Skin lesions (present in about one-third of patients) tend to predominate on the scalp, face, and upper trunk and generally consist of a few scattered erosions or tense blisters on an erythematous or urticarial base. MMP is typically a chronic and progressive disorder. Serious complications may arise as a consequence of ocular, laryngeal, esophageal, or anogenital lesions. Erosive conjunctivitis may result in shortened fornices, symblepharon, ankyloblepharon, entropion, corneal opacities, and (in severe cases) blindness. Similarly, erosive lesions of the larynx may cause hoarseness, pain, and tissue loss that, if unrecognized and untreated, may eventuate in complete destruction of the airway. Esophageal lesions may result in stenosis and/or strictures that could place patients at risk for aspiration. Strictures may also complicate anogenital involvement.

Biopsies of lesional tissue generally show subepithelial vesiculobullae and a mononuclear leukocytic infiltrate. Neutrophils and eosinophils may be seen in biopsies of early lesions; older lesions may demonstrate a scant leukocytic infiltrate and fibrosis. Direct immunofluorescence microscopy of perilesional tissue typically reveals deposits of IgG, IgA, and/or C3 in the epidermal basement membrane. Because many patients with MMP exhibit no evidence of circulating basement membrane autoantibodies, testing of perilesional skin is important diagnostically. Although MMP was once thought to be a single nosologic entity, it is now largely regarded as a disease phenotype that may develop as a consequence of an autoimmune reaction to a variety of molecules in the epidermal basement membrane (e.g., BPAG2, laminin-332, type VII collagen, and other antigens yet to be completely defined). Studies suggest that MMP patients with autoantibodies to laminin-332 have an increased relative risk for cancer. Treatment of MMP is largely dependent upon the sites of involvement. Due to potentially severe complications, patients with ocular, laryngeal, esophageal, and/or anogenital involvement require aggressive systemic treatment with dapsone, prednisone, or the latter in combination with another immunosuppressive agent (e.g., azathioprine, mycophenolate mofetil, cyclophosphamide, or rituximab) or IVIg. Less threatening forms of the disease may be managed with topical or intralesional glucocorticoids.

AUTOIMMUNE SYSTEMIC DISEASES WITH PROMINENT CUTANEOUS FEATURES

DERMATOMYOSITIS

The cutaneous manifestations of dermatomyositis (Chap. 388) are often distinctive but at times may resemble those of systemic lupus erythematosus (SLE) (Chap. 378), scleroderma (Chap. 382), or other overlapping connective tissue diseases (Chap. 382). The extent and severity of cutaneous disease may or may not correlate with the extent and severity of the myositis. The cutaneous manifestations of dermatomyositis are similar, whether the disease appears in children or in the elderly, except that calcification of subcutaneous tissue is a common late sequela in childhood dermatomyositis.

The cutaneous signs of dermatomyositis may precede or follow the development of myositis by weeks to years. Cases lacking muscle involvement (i.e., *dermatomyositis sine myositis*) have also been reported. The most common manifestation is a purple-red discoloration of the upper eyelids, sometimes associated with scaling ("heliotrope" erythema; Fig. 73-3) and periorbital edema. Erythema on the cheeks and nose in a "butterfly" distribution may resemble the malar eruption of SLE. Erythematous or violaceous scaling patches are common on the upper anterior chest, posterior neck, scalp, and the extensor surfaces of the arms, legs, and hands. Erythema and scaling may be particularly prominent over the elbows, knees, and dorsal interphalangeal joints. Approximately one-third of patients have violaceous, flat-topped papules over the dorsal interphalangeal joints that are pathognomonic of dermatomyositis (Gottron's papules). Thin violaceous papules and plaques on the elbows and knees of patients with dermatomyositis are referred to as *Gottron's sign* (Fig. 73-4). These lesions can be contrasted with the erythema and scaling on the dorsum of the fingers that spares the skin over the interphalangeal joints of some SLE patients. Periungual telangiectasia may be prominent in patients with dermatomyositis. Lacy or reticulated erythema may be associated with fine scaling on the extensor and lateral surfaces of the thighs and upper arms. Other patients, particularly those with long-standing disease, develop areas of hypopigmentation, hyperpigmentation, mild atrophy, and telangiectasia known as *poikiloderma*. Poikiloderma is rare in both SLE and scleroderma and thus can serve as a clinical sign that distinguishes dermatomyositis from these two diseases. Cutaneous changes may

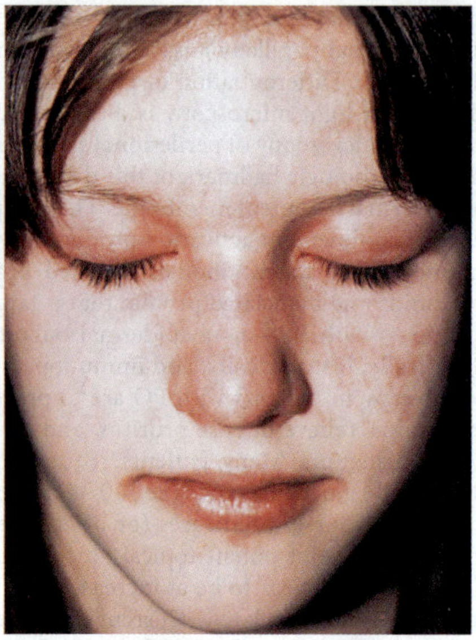

FIGURE 73-3 Dermatomyositis. Periorbital violaceous erythema characterizes the classic heliotrope rash. *(Courtesy of James Krell, MD; with permission.)*

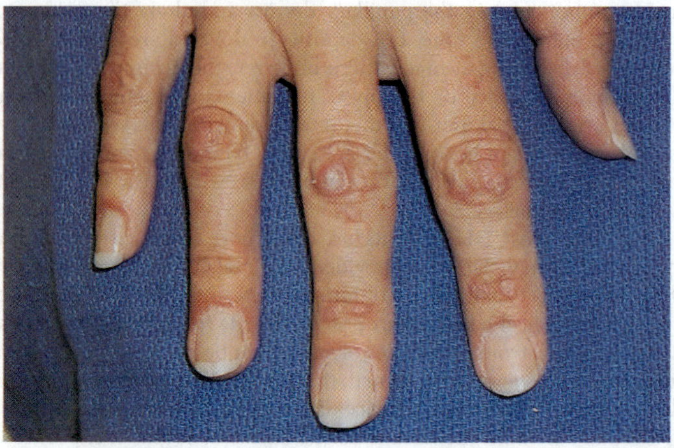

FIGURE 73-4 Gottron's papules. Dermatomyositis often involves the hands as erythematous flat-topped papules over the knuckles. Periungual telangiectases are also evident.

be similar in dermatomyositis and various overlap syndromes where thickening and binding down of the skin of the hands (*sclerodactyly*) as well as Raynaud's phenomenon can be seen. However, the presence of severe muscle disease, Gottron's papules, heliotrope erythema, and poikiloderma serves to distinguish patients with dermatomyositis. Skin biopsy of the erythematous, scaling lesions of dermatomyositis may reveal only mild nonspecific inflammation but sometimes may show changes indistinguishable from those found in SLE, including epidermal atrophy, hydropic degeneration of basal keratinocytes, edema of the upper dermis, and a mild mononuclear cell infiltrate. Direct immunofluorescence microscopy of lesional skin is usually negative, although granular deposits of immunoglobulin(s) and complement in the epidermal basement membrane zone have been described in some patients. Treatment should be directed at the systemic disease. Topical glucocorticoids are sometimes useful; patients should avoid exposure to ultraviolet irradiation and aggressively use photoprotective measures, including broad-spectrum sunscreens.

LUPUS ERYTHEMATOSUS

The cutaneous manifestations of lupus erythematosus (LE) (Chap. 378) can be divided into acute, subacute, and chronic or discoid types. *Acute cutaneous LE* is characterized by erythema of the nose and malar eminences in a "butterfly" distribution (Fig. 73-5*A*). The erythema is often sudden in onset, accompanied by edema and fine scale, and correlated with systemic involvement. Patients may have widespread involvement of the face as well as erythema and scaling of the extensor surfaces of the extremities and upper chest (Fig. 73-5*B*). These acute lesions, while sometimes evanescent, usually last for days and are often associated with exacerbations of systemic disease. Skin biopsy of acute lesions may show only a sparse dermal infiltrate of mononuclear cells and dermal edema. In some instances, cellular infiltrates around blood vessels and hair follicles are notable, as is hydropic degeneration of basal cells of the epidermis. Direct immunofluorescence microscopy of lesional skin frequently reveals deposits of immunoglobulin(s) and complement in the epidermal basement membrane zone. Treatment is aimed at control of systemic disease. Photoprotection is very important in this as well as in other forms of LE.

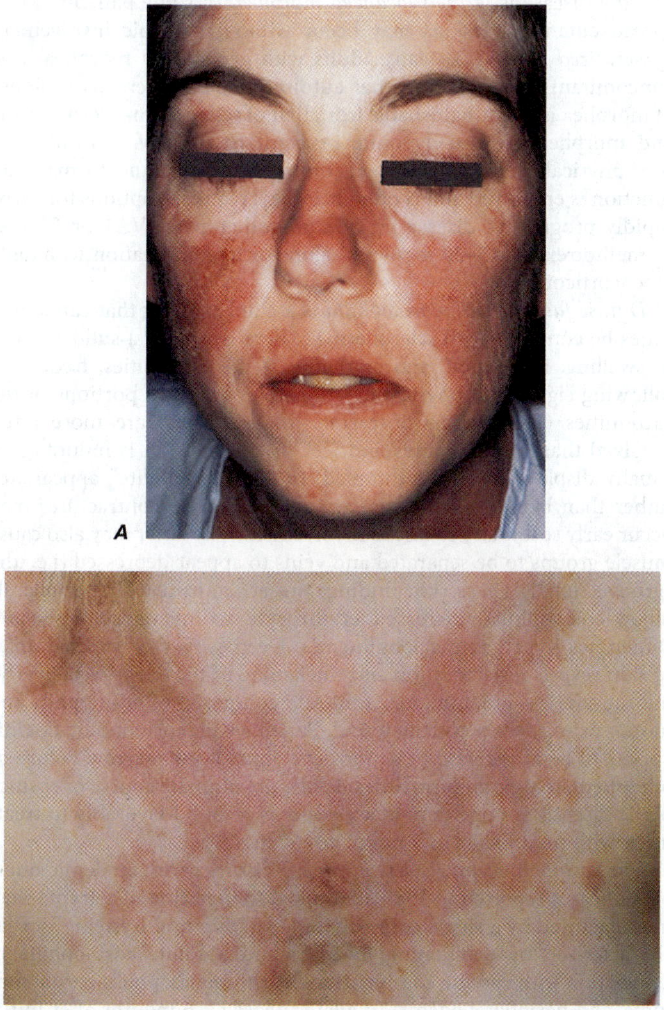

FIGURE 73-5 Acute cutaneous lupus erythematosus (LE). *A.* Acute cutaneous LE on the face, showing prominent, scaly, malar erythema. Involvement of other sun-exposed sites is also common. ***B.*** Acute cutaneous LE on the upper chest, demonstrating brightly erythematous and slightly edematous papules and plaques. *(B, Courtesy of Robert Swerlick, MD; with permission.)*

Subacute cutaneous lupus erythematosus (SCLE) is characterized by a widespread photosensitive, nonscarring eruption. In most patients, renal and central nervous system involvement is mild or absent. SCLE may present as a papulosquamous eruption that resembles psoriasis or as annular polycyclic lesions that resemble those seen in erythema multiforme. In the papulosquamous form, discrete erythematous papules arise on the back, chest, shoulders, extensor surfaces of the arms, and dorsum of the hands; lesions are uncommon on the central face and the flexor surfaces of the arms as well as below the waist. These slightly scaling papules tend to merge into large plaques, some with a reticulate appearance. The annular form involves the same areas and presents with erythematous papules that evolve into oval, circular, or polycyclic lesions. The lesions of SCLE are more widespread but have less tendency for scarring than lesions of discoid LE. Skin biopsy reveals a dense mononuclear cell infiltrate around hair follicles and blood vessels in the superficial dermis, combined with hydropic degeneration of basal cells in the epidermis. Direct immunofluorescence microscopy of lesional skin reveals deposits of immunoglobulin(s) in the epidermal basement membrane zone in about one-half of these cases. A particulate pattern of IgG deposition throughout the epidermis has been associated with SCLE. Most SCLE patients have anti-Ro autoantibodies. Local therapy alone is usually unsuccessful. Most patients require treatment with aminoquinoline antimalarial drugs. Low-dose therapy with oral glucocorticoids is sometimes necessary. Photoprotective measures against both ultraviolet B and ultraviolet A wavelengths are very important.

Discoid lupus erythematosus (DLE, also called *chronic cutaneous LE*) is characterized by discrete lesions, most often found on the face, scalp, and/or external ears. The lesions are erythematous papules or plaques with a thick, adherent scale that occludes hair follicles (follicular plugging). When the scale is removed, its underside shows small excrescences that correlate with the openings of hair follicles (so-called "carpet tacking"), a finding relatively specific for DLE. Long-standing lesions develop central atrophy, scarring, and hypopigmentation but frequently have erythematous, sometimes raised borders (Fig. 73-6). These lesions persist for years and tend to expand slowly. Up to 15% of patients with DLE eventually meet the American College of Rheumatology criteria for SLE. However, typical discoid lesions are frequently seen in patients with SLE. Biopsy of DLE lesions shows hyperkeratosis, follicular plugging, atrophy of the epidermis, hydropic degeneration of basal keratinocytes, and a mononuclear cell infiltrate adjacent to epidermal, adnexal, and microvascular basement membranes. Direct immunofluorescence microscopy demonstrates immunoglobulin(s) and complement deposits at the basement membrane zone in ~90% of cases. Treatment is focused on control of local cutaneous disease and consists mainly of photoprotection and topical or intralesional glucocorticoids. If local therapy is ineffective, use of aminoquinoline antimalarial agents may be indicated.

SCLERODERMA AND MORPHEA

The skin changes of scleroderma (Chap. 382) usually begin on the hands, feet, and face, with episodes of recurrent nonpitting edema. Sclerosis of the skin commences distally on the fingers (sclerodactyly) and spreads proximally, usually accompanied by resorption of bone of the fingertips, which may have punched out ulcers, stellate scars, or areas of hemorrhage (Fig. 73-7). The fingers may actually shrink and

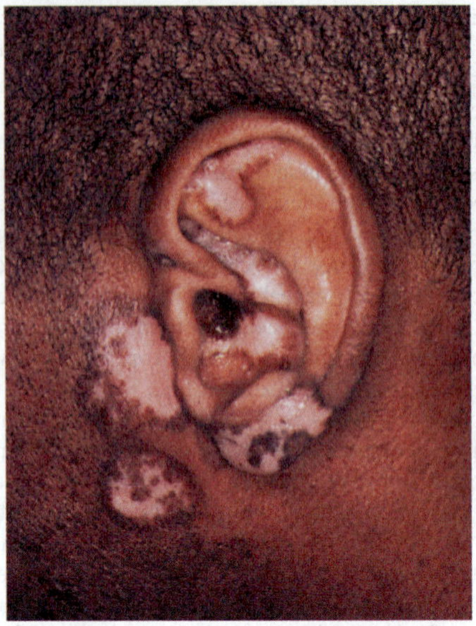

FIGURE 73-6 Discoid (chronic cutaneous) lupus erythematosus. Violaceous, hyperpigmented, atrophic plaques, often with evidence of follicular plugging that may result in scarring, are typical.

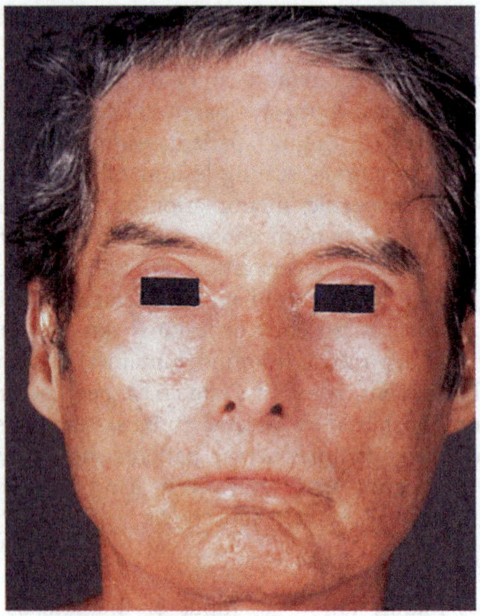

FIGURE 73-8 Scleroderma often eventuates in development of an expressionless, masklike facies.

become sausage-shaped, and, because the fingernails are usually unaffected, they may curve over the end of the fingertips. Periungual telangiectases are usually present, but periungual erythema is rare. In advanced cases, the extremities show contractures and calcinosis cutis. Facial involvement includes a smooth, unwrinkled brow, taut skin over the nose, shrinkage of tissue around the mouth, and perioral radial furrowing (Fig. 73-8). Matlike telangiectases are often present, particularly on the face and hands. Involved skin feels indurated, smooth, and bound to underlying structures; hyper- and hypopigmentation are common as well. *Raynaud's phenomenon* (i.e., cold-induced blanching, cyanosis, and reactive hyperemia) is documented in almost all patients and can precede development of scleroderma by many years. *Linear scleroderma* is a limited form of disease that presents in a linear, bandlike distribution and tends to involve deep as well as superficial layers of skin. The combination of calcinosis cutis, Raynaud's phenomenon, esophageal dysmotility, sclerodactyly, and telangiectasia has been termed the *CREST syndrome.* Centromere antibodies have been reported in a very high percentage of patients with the CREST syndrome but in only a small minority of patients with scleroderma. Skin biopsy reveals thickening of the dermis and homogenization of collagen bundles. Direct immunofluorescence microscopy of lesional skin is usually negative.

Morphea is characterized by localized thickening and sclerosis of skin; it dominates on the trunk. This disorder may affect children or adults. Morphea begins as erythematous or flesh-colored plaques that become sclerotic, develop central hypopigmentation, and have an

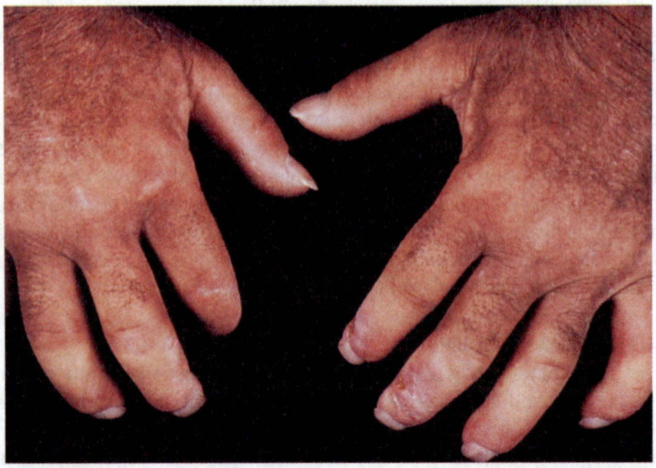

FIGURE 73-7 Scleroderma showing acral sclerosis and focal digital ulcers.

erythematous border. In most cases, patients have one or a few lesions, and the disease is termed *localized morphea.* In some patients, widespread cutaneous lesions may occur without systemic involvement (*generalized morphea*). Many adults with generalized morphea have concomitant rheumatic or other autoimmune disorders. Skin biopsy of morphea is indistinguishable from that of scleroderma. Scleroderma and morphea are usually quite resistant to therapy. For this reason, physical therapy to prevent joint contractures and to maintain function is employed and is often helpful. Treatment options for early, rapidly progressive disease include phototherapy (UVA1 or PUVA) or methotrexate (15–20 mg/week) alone or in combination with daily glucocorticoids.

Diffuse fasciitis with eosinophilia is a clinical entity that can sometimes be confused with scleroderma. There is usually a sudden onset of swelling, induration, and erythema of the extremities, frequently following significant physical exertion. The proximal portions of the extremities (upper arms, forearms, thighs, calves) are more often involved than are the hands and feet. While the skin is indurated, it usually displays a woody, dimpled, or "pseudocellulite" appearance rather than being bound down as in scleroderma; contractures may occur early secondary to fascial involvement. The latter may also cause muscle groups to be separated and veins to appear depressed (i.e., the "groove sign"). These skin findings are accompanied by peripheral-blood eosinophilia, increased erythrocyte sedimentation rate, and sometimes hypergammaglobulinemia. Deep biopsy of affected areas of skin reveals inflammation and thickening of the deep fascia overlying muscle. An inflammatory infiltrate composed of eosinophils and mononuclear cells is usually found. Patients with eosinophilic fasciitis appear to be at increased risk for developing bone marrow failure or other hematologic abnormalities. While the ultimate course of eosinophilic fasciitis is uncertain, many patients respond favorably to treatment with prednisone in doses of 40–60 mg/d.

The *eosinophilia-myalgia syndrome*, a disorder with epidemic numbers of cases reported in 1989 and linked to ingestion of L-tryptophan manufactured by a single company in Japan, is a multisystem disorder characterized by debilitating myalgias and absolute eosinophilia in association with varying combinations of arthralgias, pulmonary symptoms, and peripheral edema. In a later phase (3–6 months after initial symptoms), these patients often develop localized sclerodermatous skin changes, weight loss, and/or neuropathy (Chap. 382). The precise cause of this syndrome, which may resemble other sclerotic skin conditions, is unknown. However, the implicated lots of L-tryptophan contained the contaminant 1,1-ethylidene bis[tryptophan]. This contaminant may be pathogenic or may be a marker for another substance that provokes the disorder.

74 Cutaneous Drug Reactions

Kanade Shinkai, Robert S. Stern, Bruce U. Wintroub

Cutaneous reactions are among the most frequent adverse reactions to drugs. Most are benign, but a few can be life threatening. Prompt recognition of severe reactions, drug withdrawal, and appropriate therapeutic interventions can minimize toxicity. This chapter focuses on adverse cutaneous reactions to systemic medications; it covers their incidence, patterns, and pathogenesis and provides some practical guidelines on treatment, assessment of causality, and future use of drugs.

USE OF PRESCRIPTION DRUGS IN THE UNITED STATES

In the United States, more than 3 billion prescriptions for over 60,000 drug products, which include more than 2000 different active agents, are dispensed annually. Hospital inpatients alone annually receive about 120 million courses of drug therapy, and half of adult Americans receive prescription drugs on a regular outpatient basis. Many patients use over-the-counter medicines that may cause adverse cutaneous reactions.

INCIDENCE OF CUTANEOUS REACTIONS

Several large cohort studies established that acute cutaneous reaction to drugs affected about 3% of hospital inpatients. Reactions usually occur a few days to 4 weeks after initiation of therapy.

Many drugs of common use are associated with a 1–2% rate of rashes during premarketing clinical trials. The risk is often higher when medications are used in general, unselected populations. The rate may reach 3–7% for amoxicillin, sulfamethoxazole, many anticonvulsants, and anti-HIV agents.

In addition to acute eruptions, a variety of skin diseases can be induced or exacerbated by prolonged use of drugs (e.g., pruritus, pigmentation, nail or hair disorders, psoriasis, bullous pemphigoid, photosensitivity, and even cutaneous neoplasms). These drug reactions are not frequent, but neither their incidence nor their impact on public health has been evaluated.

In a series of 48,005 inpatients over a 20-year period, morbilliform rash (91%) and urticaria (6%) were the most frequent skin reactions. Severe reactions are actually too rare to be detected in such cohorts. Although rare, severe cutaneous reactions to drugs have an important impact on health because of significant sequelae, including mortality. Adverse drug rashes are responsible for hospitalization, increase the duration of hospital stay, and are life threatening. Some populations are at increased risk of drug reactions, including patients with collagen vascular diseases, bone marrow graft recipients, and those with acute Epstein-Barr virus infection. The pathophysiology underlying this association is unknown, but may be related to immunocompromise or immune dysregulation. Risk of drug allergy, including severe hypersensitivity reactions, is increased with HIV infection; individuals with advanced HIV disease (e.g., CD4 T lymphocyte count <200 cells/μL) have a forty- to fiftyfold increased risk of adverse reactions to sulfamethoxazole (Chap. 226).

PATHOGENESIS OF DRUG REACTIONS

Adverse cutaneous responses to drugs can arise as a result of immunologic or nonimmunologic mechanisms.

NONIMMUNOLOGIC DRUG REACTIONS

Examples of responses that arise from nonimmunologic mechanisms are pigmentary changes related to dermal accumulation of medications or their metabolites; alteration of hair follicles by antimetabolites and signaling inhibitors; and lipodystrophy associated with metabolic effects of anti-HIV medications. These side effects are mostly toxic, predictable, and sometimes can be avoided in part by simple preventive measures.

IMMUNOLOGIC DRUG REACTIONS

Evidence suggests an immunologic basis for most acute drug eruptions. Drug reactions may result from immediate release of preformed mediators (e.g., urticaria, anaphylaxis), antibody-mediated reactions, immune complex deposition, and antigen-specific responses. Drug-specific T cell clones can be derived from the blood or from skin lesions of patients with a variety of drug allergies, strongly suggesting that these T cells play a role in drug allergy in an antigen-specific manner. Specific clones were obtained with penicillin G, amoxicillin, cephalosporins, sulfamethoxazole, phenobarbital, carbamazepine, and lamotrigine (medications that are frequently a cause of drug eruptions). Both CD4 and CD8 clones have been obtained; however, their specific roles in the manifestations of allergy have not been elucidated. Drug presentation to T cells was major histocompatibility complex (MHC)-restricted and may involve drug-peptide complex recognition by specific T cell receptors (TCRs).

Once a drug has induced an immune response, the final phenotype of the reaction probably depends on the nature of effectors: cytotoxic (CD8+) T cells in blistering and certain hypersensitivity reactions, chemokines for reactions mediated by neutrophils or eosinophils, and collaboration with B cells for production of specific antibodies for urticarial reaction. Immunologic reactions have recently been classified into further subtypes that provide a useful framework for designating adverse drug reactions based on involvement of specific immune pathways (Table 74-1).

Immediate Reactions Immediate reactions depend on the release of mediators of inflammation by tissue mast cells or circulating basophils. These mediators include histamine, leukotrienes, prostaglandins, bradykinins, platelet-activating factor, enzymes, and proteoglycans. Drugs can trigger mediator release either directly ("anaphylactoid" reaction) or through IgE-specific antibodies. These reactions usually manifest in the skin and gastrointestinal, respiratory, and cardiovascular systems (Chap. 376). Primary symptoms and signs include pruritus, urticaria, nausea, vomiting, abdominal cramps, bronchospasm, laryngeal edema, and, occasionally, anaphylactic shock with hypotension and death. They occur within minutes of drug exposure. Nonsteroidal anti-inflammatory drugs (NSAIDs), including aspirin, and radiocontrast media are frequent causes of direct mast cell degranulation or anaphylactoid reactions, which can occur on first exposure. Penicillins and muscle relaxants used in general anesthesia are the most frequent causes of IgE-dependent reactions to drugs, which require prior sensitization. Release of mediators is triggered when polyvalent drug protein conjugates cross-link IgE molecules fixed to sensitized cells. Certain routes of administration favor different clinical patterns (e.g., gastrointestinal effects from oral route, circulatory effects from intravenous route).

Immune Complex–Dependent Reactions Serum sickness is produced by tissue deposition of circulating immune complexes with consumption of complement. It is characterized by fever, arthritis, nephritis, neuritis, edema, and a urticarial, papular, or purpuric rash (Chap. 385). First described following administration of nonhuman sera, it currently occurs in the setting of monoclonal antibodies and other similar medications. In classic serum sickness, symptoms develop 6 days or more after exposure to a drug, the latent period representing the time needed to synthesize antibody. Cutaneous or systemic vasculitis, a relatively rare complication of drugs, may also be a result of immune complex deposition (Chap. 385). Cephalosporin and other medications, including monoclonal antibodies such as infliximab, rituximab, and omalizumab, may be associated with clinically similar "serum sickness–like" reactions. The mechanism of this reaction is unknown but is unrelated to complement activation and immune complex formation.

Delayed Hypersensitivity While not completely understood, delayed hypersensitivity directed by drug-specific T cells is an important mechanism underlying the most common drug eruptions, i.e., morbilliform eruptions, and also rare and severe forms such as drug-induced hypersensitivity syndrome (DIHS) (also known

TABLE 74-1 CLASSIFICATION OF ADVERSE DRUG REACTIONS BASED ON IMMUNE PATHWAY

Type	Key Pathway	Key Immune Mediators	Adverse Drug Reaction Type
Type I	IgE	IgE	Urticaria, angioedema, anaphylaxis
Type II	IgG-mediated cytotoxicity	IgG	Drug-induced hemolysis, thrombocytopenia (e.g., penicillin)
Type III	Immune complex	IgG + antigen	Vasculitis, serum sickness, drug-induced lupus
Type IVa	T lymphocyte–mediated macrophage inflammation	IFN-γ, TNF-α T_H1 cells	Tuberculin skin test, contact dermatitis
Type IVb	T lymphocyte–mediated eosinophil inflammation	IL-4, IL-5, IL-13 T_H2 cells Eosinophils	Drug-induced hypersensitivity syndrome (DIHS) Morbilliform eruption
Type IVc	T lymphocyte–mediated cytotoxic T lymphocyte inflammation	Cytotoxic T lymphocytes Granzyme Perforin Granulysin (Stevens-Johnson syndrome [SJS]/toxic epidermal necrolysis [TEN]) only)	SJS/TEN Morbilliform eruption
Type IVd	T lymphocyte–mediated neutrophil inflammation	CXCL8, IL-17, GM-CSF Neutrophils	Acute generalized exanthematous pustulosis (AGEP)

Abbreviations: GM-CSF, granulocyte-macrophage colony-stimulating factor; IFN, interferon; IL, interleukin; TNF, tumor necrosis factor.

as drug rash with eosinophilia and systemic symptoms [DRESS]), acute generalized exanthematous pustulosis (AGEP), Stevens-Johnson syndrome (SJS), and toxic epidermal necrolysis (TEN) (Table 74-1). Drug-specific T cells have been detected in these types of drug eruptions. For example, drug-specific cytotoxic T cells have been detected in the skin lesions of fixed drug eruptions and of TEN. In TEN, skin lesions contain T lymphocytes reactive to autologous lymphocytes and keratinocytes in a drug-specific, HLA-restricted, and perforin/granzyme-mediated pathway.

The mechanism(s) by which medications result in T cell activation is unknown. Two hypotheses prevail: first, that the antigens driving these reactions may be the native drug itself or components of the drug covalently complexed with endogenous proteins, presented in association with HLA molecules to T cells through the classical antigen presentation pathway, or alternatively, through direct interaction of the drug/metabolite with the T cell receptor or peptide-loaded HLA (e.g., the pharmacologic interaction of drugs with immune receptors, or p-i hypothesis). Recent x-ray crystallography data characterizing binding between specific HLA molecules to particular drugs known to cause hypersensitivity reactions demonstrates unique alterations to the MHC peptide-binding groove, suggesting a molecular basis for T cell activation and the development of hypersensitivity reactions.

GENETIC FACTORS AND CUTANEOUS DRUG REACTIONS

Genetic determinants may predispose individuals to severe drug reactions by affecting either drug metabolism or immune responses to drugs. Polymorphisms in cytochrome P450 enzymes, drug acetylation, methylation (such as thiopurine methyltransferase activity and azathioprine), and other forms of metabolism (such as glucose-6-phosphate dehydrogenase) may increase susceptibility to drug toxicity or underdosing, highlighting a role for differential pharmacokinetic or pharmacodynamic effects.

Associations between drug hypersensitivities and HLA haplotypes also suggest a key role for immune mechanisms. Hypersensitivity to the anti-HIV medication abacavir is strongly associated with HLA-B*57:01 (Chap. 226). In Taiwan, within a homogeneous Han Chinese population, a 100% association was observed between SJS/TEN (but not DIHS) related to carbamazepine and HLA-B*15:02. In the same population, another 100% association was found between SJS, TEN, or DIHS related to allopurinol and HLA-B*58:01. These associations are drug and phenotype specific; that is, HLA-specific T cell stimulation by medications leads to distinct reactions and may explain why the reaction patterns are so clinically diverse. However, the strong associations found in Taiwan have not been observed in other countries with more heterogeneous populations.

GLOBAL CONSIDERATIONS

Recognition of the HLA associations with drug hypersensitivity has been acknowledged by recommendations to screen high-risk populations. Genetic screening for HLA-B*57:01 to prevent abacavir hypersensitivity, which carries a 100% negative predictive value when patch test confirmed and 55% positive predictive value generalizable across races, is becoming the clinical standard of care worldwide (number needed to treat = 13). The U.S. Food and Drug Administration recently mandated new labeling of carbamazepine recommending HLA-B*15:02 screening of Asian individuals prior to receiving a new prescription of the medication. The American College of Rheumatology has recommended HLA-B*58:01 screening of Han Chinese patients prescribed allopurinol. To date, screening for a single HLA (but not multiple HLA haplotypes) in specific populations has been determined to be cost-effective.

Several investigators have proposed that specific HLA haplotypes associated with drug hypersensitivity indeed play a pathogenic role; stimulation of carbamazepine-specific cytotoxic T lymphocytes (CTL) in the context of HLA-B*15:02 results in production of a putative mediator of keratinocyte necrosis in TEN. Other studies have identified CTLs reactive to carbamazepine that use highly restricted V-alpha and V-beta TCR repertoires in patients with carbamazepine hypersensitivity that are not found in carbamazepine-tolerant individuals. Although not yet clinically available, some investigators have suggested combined genetic testing for specific HLA haplotypes and functional screening for TCR repertoire to best identify patients at risk.

CLINICAL PRESENTATION OF CUTANEOUS DRUG REACTIONS

NONIMMUNE CUTANEOUS REACTIONS

Exacerbation or Induction of Dermatologic Diseases A variety of drugs can exacerbate preexisting diseases or sometimes induce a disease that may or may not disappear after withdrawal of the inducing medication. For example, NSAIDs, lithium, beta blockers, tumor necrosis factor (TNF) α cytokine antagonists, interferon (IFN) α, and angiotensin-converting enzyme (ACE) inhibitors can exacerbate plaque psoriasis, whereas antimalarials and withdrawal of systemic glucocorticoids can worsen pustular psoriasis. The situation of TNF-α inhibitors is unusual, as this class of medications is used to treat psoriasis; however, in other cases, they may induce psoriasis (especially palmar-plantar) in patients being treated for other conditions. Acne may be induced by glucocorticoids, androgens, lithium, and antidepressants. Follicular papular or pustular eruptions of the face and trunk, sometimes mimicking acne, frequently occur with epidermal growth factor (EGF) receptor antagonists. In the case of EGF-receptor antagonists, the severity of the eruption correlates with a better anticancer effect. It may be secondarily impetiginized and often spares areas of prior or active radiation. Tetracycline antibiotics, topical corticosteroids, and topical anti-acne treatments (such as benzoyl peroxide and clindamycin lotion) are helpful.

Several medications induce or exacerbate autoimmune disease. Interleukin (IL) 2, IFN-α, and anti-TNF-α are associated with new-onset systemic lupus erythematosus (SLE). Drug-induced lupus is classically marked by antinuclear and antihistone antibodies and, in some cases, anti-double-stranded DNA (D-penicillamine, anti-TNF-α) or p-ANCA (minocycline) antibodies. Minocycline and thiazide diuretics may exacerbate subacute SLE; pemphigus can be induced by D-penicillamine and ACE inhibitors. Furosemide is associated with drug-induced bullous pemphigoid. Vancomycin is associated with linear IgA bullous dermatitis, a transient blistering disorder.

Other medications may cause highly selective cutaneous reactions. Gadolinium contrast has been associated with nephrogenic systemic fibrosis, a condition of sclerosing skin with rare internal organ involvement; advanced renal compromise may be an important risk factor. Granulocyte colony-stimulating factor may induce various neutrophilic dermatoses, including Sweet syndrome and pyoderma gangrenosum. Both systemic and topical glucocorticoids cause a variety of atrophic skin changes, including atrophy and striae, and, in sufficiently high doses, can impede wound healing.

The hypothesis that a drug may be responsible should always be considered, especially in cases with atypical clinical presentation. Resolution of the cutaneous reaction may be delayed upon discontinuation of the medication (e.g., lichenoid drug eruptions may take years to resolve).

Photosensitivity Eruptions Photosensitivity eruptions are usually most marked in sun-exposed areas but may extend to sun-protected areas. The mechanism is almost always phototoxicity. Phototoxic reactions resemble sunburn and can occur with first exposure to a drug. Blistering may occur in drug-related pseudoporphyria, most commonly with NSAIDs (Fig. 74-1). The severity of the reactions depends on the tissue level of the drug, its efficiency as a photosensitizer, and the extent of exposure to the activating wavelengths of ultraviolet (UV) light (Chap. 75).

Common orally administered photosensitizing drugs include fluoroquinolones and tetracycline antibiotics. Other drugs less frequently encountered are chlorpromazine, thiazides, and NSAIDs. Voriconazole may result in severe photosensitivity, accelerated photo-induced aging, and cutaneous carcinogenesis in organ transplant recipients.

Because UV-A and visible light, which trigger these reactions, are not easily absorbed by nonopaque sunscreens and are transmitted through window glass, photosensitivity reactions may be difficult to block. Photosensitivity reactions abate with removal of either the drug or UV radiation, use of sunscreens that block UV-A light, and treating the reaction as one would a sunburn. Rarely, individuals develop persistent reactivity to light, necessitating long-term avoidance of sun exposure.

Pigmentation Changes Drugs, either systemic or topical, may cause a variety of pigmentary changes in the skin. Oral contraceptives may induce melasma. Long-term minocycline, pefloxacin, and amiodarone may cause blue-gray pigmentation. Phenothiazine, gold, and bismuth result in gray-brown pigmentation of sun-exposed areas. Numerous cancer chemotherapeutic agents may be associated with characteristic patterns of pigmentation (e.g., bleomycin, busulfan, daunorubicin, cyclophosphamide, hydroxyurea, and methotrexate). Clofazimine causes a drug-induced lipofuscinosis with characteristic red-brown coloration. Hyperpigmentation of the face, mucous membranes, and pretibial and subungual areas occurs with antimalarials. Quinacrine causes generalized, cutaneous yellow discoloration. Pigmentation changes may also occur in mucous membranes (busulfan, bismuth), conjunctiva (chlorpromazine, thioridazine, imipramine, clomipramine), nails (zidovudine, doxorubicin, cyclophosphamide, bleomycin, fluorouracil, hydroxyurea), hair, and teeth (tetracyclines).

Warfarin Necrosis of Skin This rare reaction (0.01–0.1%) usually occurs between the third and tenth days of therapy with warfarin, usually in women. Common sites are breasts, thighs, and buttocks (Fig. 74-2). Lesions are sharply demarcated, indurated, and erythematous or purpuric and may progress to form large, hemorrhagic bullae with eventual necrosis and slow-healing eschar formation. These lesions can be life threatening.

Development of the syndrome is unrelated to drug dose, and the course is not altered by discontinuation of the drug after onset of the eruption. Warfarin anticoagulation in heterozygous protein C deficiency causes a precipitous fall in circulating levels of protein C, permitting hypercoagulability and thrombosis in the cutaneous microvasculature, with consequent areas of necrosis. Heparin-induced necrosis may have clinically similar features but is probably due to heparin-induced platelet aggregation with subsequent occlusion of blood vessels; it can affect areas adjacent to the injection site or more distant sites if infused.

Warfarin-induced cutaneous necrosis is treated with vitamin K, heparin, surgical debridement, and intensive wound care. Treatment with protein C concentrates may also be helpful. Newer agents such as dabigatran etexilate may avoid warfarin necrosis in high-risk patients.

Drug-Induced Hair Disorders • ***DRUG-INDUCED HAIR LOSS*** Medications may affect hair follicles at two different phases of their growth cycle: anagen (growth) or telogen (resting). *Anagen effluvium* occurs within days of drug administration, especially with antimetabolite or other chemotherapeutic drugs. In contrast, in *telogen effluvium*, the delay is 2 to 4 months following initiation of a new medication. Both present as diffuse nonscarring alopecia most often reversible after discontinuation

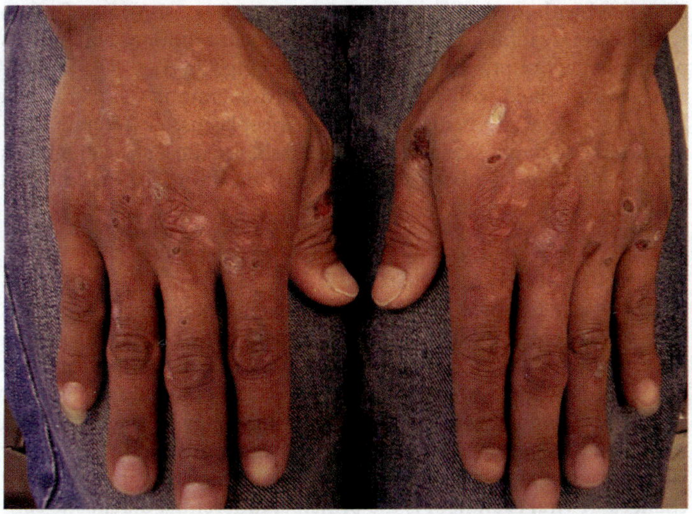

FIGURE 74-1 Pseudoporphyria due to nonsteroidal anti-inflammatory drugs.

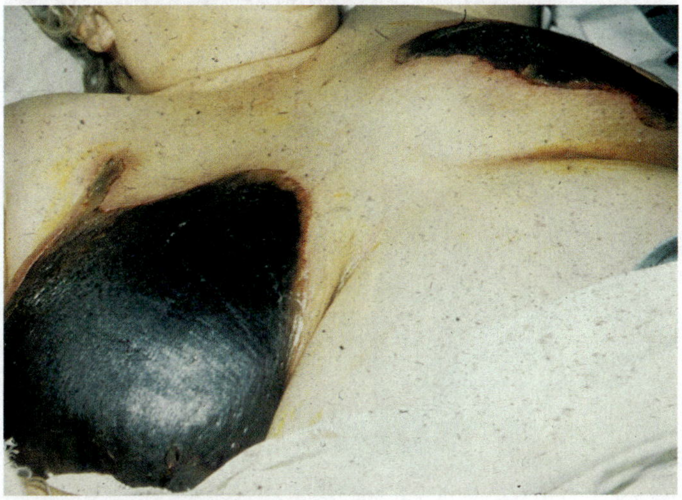

FIGURE 74-2 Warfarin necrosis.

of the responsible agent. The prevalence and severity of alopecia depend on the drug as well as on an individual's predisposition.

A considerable number of drugs have been reported to induce hair loss. These include antineoplastic agents (alkylating agents, bleomycin, vinca alkaloids, platinum compounds), anticonvulsants (carbamazepine, valproate), antihypertensive drugs (beta blockers), antidepressants, antithyroid drugs, IFNs (especially IFN-α), oral contraceptives, and cholesterol-lowering agents.

DRUG-INDUCED HAIR GROWTH Medications may also cause hair growth. Hirsutism is an excessive growth of terminal hair with masculine hair growth pattern in a female, most often on the face and trunk, due to androgenic stimulation of hormone-sensitive hair follicles (anabolic steroids, oral contraceptives, testosterone, corticotropin). Hypertrichosis is a distinct pattern of hair growth, not in a masculine pattern, typically located on the forehead and temporal regions of the face. Drugs responsible for hypertrichosis include anti-inflammatory drugs, glucocorticoids, vasodilators (diazoxide, minoxidil), diuretics (acetazolamide), anticonvulsants (phenytoin), immunosuppressive agents (cyclosporine A), psoralens, and zidovudine.

Changes in hair color or structure are uncommon adverse effects from medications. Hair discoloration may occur with chloroquine, IFN-α, chemotherapeutic agents, and tyrosine kinase inhibitors. Changes in hair structure have been observed in patients given epidermal growth factor receptor (EGFR) inhibitors, tyrosine kinase inhibitors (Fig. 74-3), and acitretin.

Drug-Induced Nail Disorders Drug-related nail disorders usually involve all 20 nails and need months to resolve after withdrawal of the offending agent. The pathogenesis is most often toxic. Drug-induced nail changes include Beau's line (transverse depression of the nail plate), onycholysis (detachment of the distal part of the nail plate), onychomadesis (detachment of the proximal part of the nail plate), pigmentation, and paronychia (inflammation of periungual skin).

ONYCHOLYSIS Onycholysis occurs with tetracyclines, fluoroquinolones, phenothiazines, and psoralens, as well as in persons taking NSAIDs, captopril, retinoids, sodium valproate, and many chemotherapeutic agents such as anthracyclines or taxanes including paclitaxel and docetaxel. The risk of onycholysis in patients receiving cytotoxic drugs, tetracyclines, quinolones, phenothiazines, and psoralens can be increased by exposure to sunlight.

ONYCHOMADESIS Onychomadesis is caused by temporary arrest of nail matrix mitotic activity. Common drugs reported to induce onychomadesis include carbamazepine, lithium, retinoids, and chemotherapeutic agents such as cyclophosphamide and vincristine.

PARONYCHIA Paronychia and multiple pyogenic granuloma (Fig. 74-4) with progressive and painful periungual abscess of fingers and toes

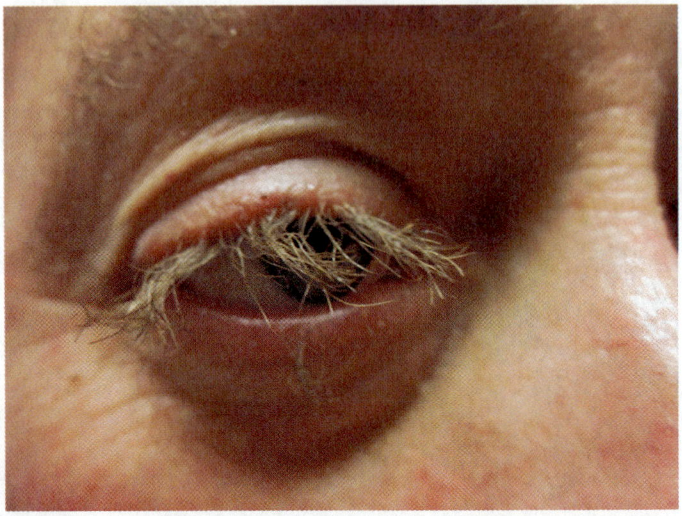

FIGURE 74-3 Dysmorphic eyelashes in association with erlotinib.

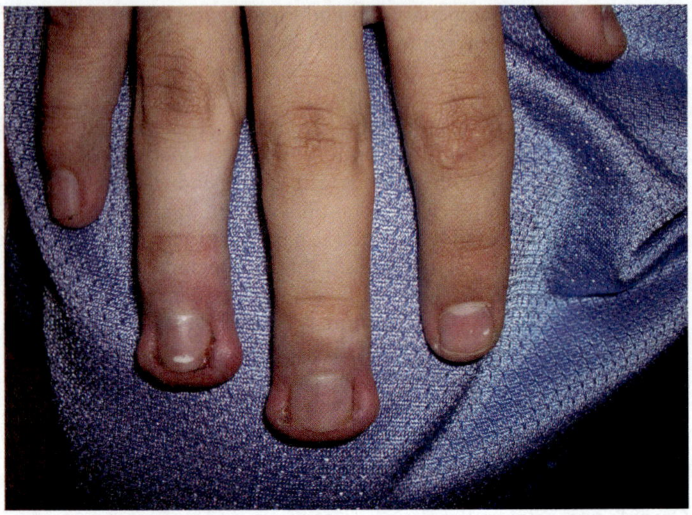

FIGURE 74-4 Pyogenic granuloma in association with isotretinoin.

are side effects of systemic retinoids, lamivudine, indinavir, and anti-EGFR monoclonal antibodies (cetuximab, gefitinib).

NAIL DISCOLORATION Some drugs—including anthracyclines, taxanes, fluorouracil, psoralens, and zidovudine—may induce nail bed hyperpigmentation through melanocyte stimulation. It appears to be reversible and dose-dependent.

Toxic Erythema of Chemotherapy and Other Chemotherapy Reactions Because many agents used in cancer chemotherapy inhibit cell division, rapidly proliferating elements of the skin, including hair, mucous membranes, and appendages, are sensitive to their effects. A broad spectrum of chemotherapy-related skin toxicities have been reported, including neutrophilic eccrine hidradenitis, sterile cellulitis, exfoliative dermatitis, and flexural erythema; although previously designated as distinct skin eruptions, recent nomenclature classifies these under the unifying diagnosis of toxic erythema of chemotherapy (TEC). Acral erythema, marked by dysesthesia and an erythematous, edematous eruption of the palms and soles, is caused by cytarabine, doxorubicin, methotrexate, hydroxyurea, and fluorouracil and may be alleviated by pyridoxine supplementation.

The recent introduction of many new monoclonal antibody and small molecular signaling inhibitors for the treatment of cancer has been accompanied by numerous reports of skin and hair toxicity; only the most common of these are mentioned here. Cetuximab and other EGFR antagonists induce follicular eruptions and nail toxicity after a mean interval of 10 days in a majority of patients. Xerosis, eczematous eruptions, acneiform eruptions, and pruritus are common. Erlotinib is associated with marked hair textural changes (Fig. 74-3). Sorafenib, a tyrosine kinase inhibitor, may result in follicular eruptions and bullous palmoplantar eruptions with dysesthesia (Fig. 74-5). BRAF inhibitors are associated with photosensitivity, dyskeratotic (Grover's-like) rash, hyperkeratotic benign cutaneous neoplasms, and keratoacanthoma-like squamous cell carcinomas. Rash, pruritus, and vitiliginous depigmentation have been reported in association with ipilimumab (anti-CTLA4) treatment.

IMMUNE CUTANEOUS REACTIONS: COMMON

Maculopapular Eruptions Morbilliform or maculopapular eruptions (Fig. 74-6) are the most common of all drug-induced reactions, often start on the trunk or intertriginous areas, and consist of erythematous macules and papules that are symmetric and confluent. Involvement of mucous membranes is unusual; the eruption may be associated with moderate to severe pruritus and fever. Diagnosis is rarely assisted by laboratory testing. Skin biopsy often shows nonspecific inflammatory changes. A viral exanthem is the principal differential diagnostic consideration, especially in children, and graft-versus-host disease is also a consideration in the proper clinical setting. Absence of enanthems;

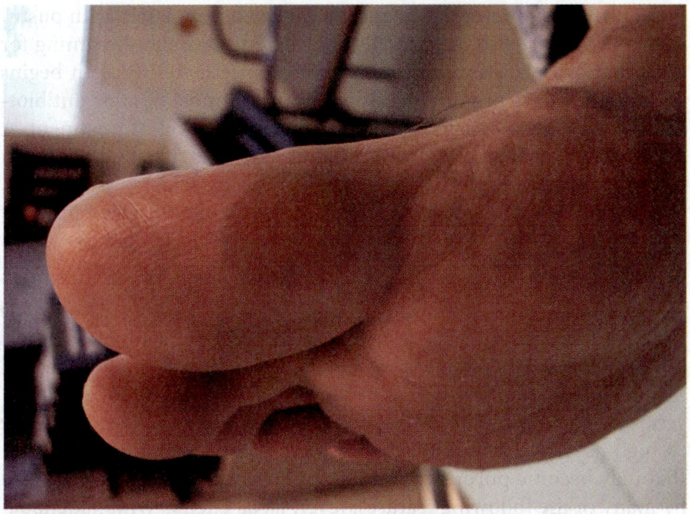

FIGURE 74-5 Sorafenib-associated hand-foot syndrome.

absence of ear, nose, throat, and upper respiratory tract symptoms; and polymorphism of the skin lesions support a drug rather than a viral eruption. Certain medications carry very high rates of morbilliform eruption, including nevirapine and lamotrigine, even in the absence of hypersensitivity reactions. Lamotrigine morbilliform rash is associated with higher starting doses, rapid dose escalation, concomitant use of valproate (which increases lamotrigine levels and half-life) and use in children, especially with seizure disorder.

Maculopapular reactions usually develop within 1 week of initiation of therapy and last less than 2 weeks. Occasionally, these eruptions resolve despite continued use of the responsible drug. Because the eruption may also worsen, the suspect drug should be discontinued unless it is essential; it is important to note that the rash may continue to progress for a few days to up to one week following medication discontinuation. Oral antihistamines and emollients may help relieve pruritus. Short courses of potent topical glucocorticoids can reduce inflammation and symptoms. Systemic glucocorticoid treatment is rarely indicated.

Pruritus Pruritus is associated with almost all drug eruptions and, in some cases, may represent the only symptom of the adverse cutaneous reaction. It is usually alleviated by antihistamines such as hydroxyzine or diphenhydramine. Pruritus stemming from specific medications may require distinct treatment; opiate-related pruritus may require selective opiate antagonists to gain relief. Pruritus is a common complication of antimalarial therapy, occurring in up to 50% of black patients receiving chloroquine, and may be severe enough to lead to discontinuation of treatment. It is much rarer in Caucasians taking chloroquine. Intense pruritus, sometimes accompanied by an eczematous rash, may occur in 20% of patients receiving IFN and ribavirin for

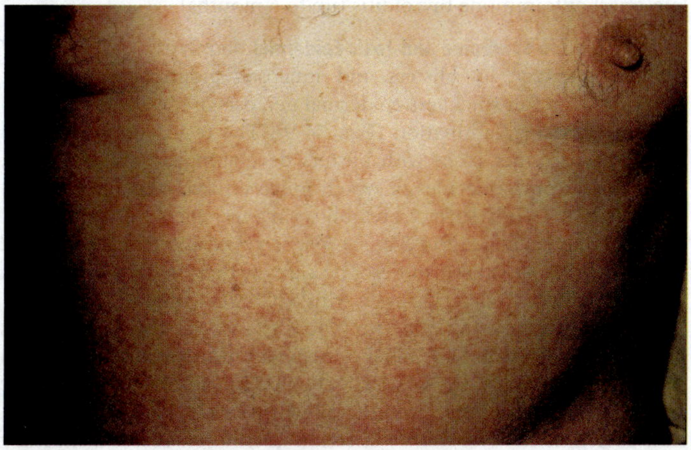

FIGURE 74-6 Morbilliform drug eruption.

hepatitis C; addition of the protease inhibitor telaprevir may increase this occurrence to 50% of treated patients.

Urticaria/Angioedema/Anaphylaxis Urticaria, the second most frequent type of cutaneous reaction to drugs, is characterized by pruritic, red wheals of varying size rarely lasting more than 24 h. It has been observed in association with nearly all drugs, most frequently ACE inhibitors, aspirin, NSAIDs, penicillin, and blood products. However, medications account for no more than 10–20% of acute urticaria cases. Deep edema within dermal and subcutaneous tissues is known as angioedema and may involve respiratory and gastrointestinal mucous membranes as well. Urticaria and angioedema may be part of a life-threatening anaphylactic reaction.

Drug-induced urticaria may be caused by three mechanisms: an IgE-dependent mechanism, circulating immune complexes (serum sickness), and nonimmunologic activation of effector pathways. IgE-dependent urticarial reactions usually occur within 36 h of drug exposure but can occur within minutes. Immune complex–induced urticaria associated with serum sickness–like reactions usually occurs 6–12 days after first exposure. In this syndrome, the urticarial eruption (typically polycyclic plaques) may be accompanied by fever, hematuria, arthralgias, hepatic dysfunction, and neurologic symptoms. Certain drugs, such as NSAIDs, ACE inhibitors, angiotensin II antagonists, radiographic dye, and opiates, may induce urticarial reactions, angioedema, and anaphylaxis in the absence of drug-specific antibody through direct mast-cell degranulation.

Radiocontrast agents are a common cause of urticaria and, in rare cases, can cause anaphylaxis. High-osmolality radiocontrast media were about five times more likely to induce urticaria (1%) or anaphylaxis than were newer low-osmolality media. About one-third of those with mild reactions to previous exposure react on reexposure. Pretreatment with prednisone and diphenhydramine reduces reaction rates. Persons with a reaction to a high-osmolality contrast media may be given low-osmolality media if later contrast studies are required.

The treatment of urticaria or angioedema depends on the severity of the reaction. In severe cases with respiratory or cardiovascular compromise, epinephrine is the mainstay of therapy, but its effect is reduced in patients using beta blockers. Treatment with intravenous systemic glucocorticoids is helpful. For patients with urticaria without symptoms of angioedema or anaphylaxis, drug withdrawal and oral antihistamines are usually sufficient. Future drug avoidance is recommended; rechallenge, especially in individuals with severe reactions, should only occur in an intensive care setting.

Anaphylactoid Reactions Vancomycin is associated with red man syndrome, a histamine-related anaphylactoid reaction characterized by flushing, diffuse maculopapular eruption, and hypotension. In rare cases, cardiac arrest may be associated with rapid IV infusion of the medication.

Irritant/Allergic Contact Dermatitis Patients using topical medications may develop an irritant or allergic contact dermatitis to the medication itself or to a preservative or other component of the formulation. Reactions to chlorhexidine, neomycin sulfate, and polymyxin B are common. Allergic contact dermatitis to topical glucocorticoids may also occur and is paradoxically partially masked by the anti-inflammatory nature of the medication itself; typically this allergy is selective for one of the four classes of glucocorticoid types, as subdivided by allergenic properties. Patch testing can be useful to determine whether a patient is steroid allergic. Desoximetasone is rarely allergenic.

Fixed Drug Eruptions These less common reactions are characterized by one or more sharply demarcated, dull red to brown lesions, sometimes with central bulla (Fig. 74-7). Hyperpigmentation often results after resolution of the acute inflammation. With rechallenge, the lesion recurs in the same (e.g., fixed) location. Lesions often involve the lips, hands, legs, face, genitalia, and oral mucosa and cause a burning sensation. Most patients have multiple lesions. Fixed drug eruptions have been associated with pseudoephedrine (frequently a nonpigmented reaction), phenolphthalein (in laxatives), sulfonamides, tetracyclines, NSAIDs, and barbiturates.

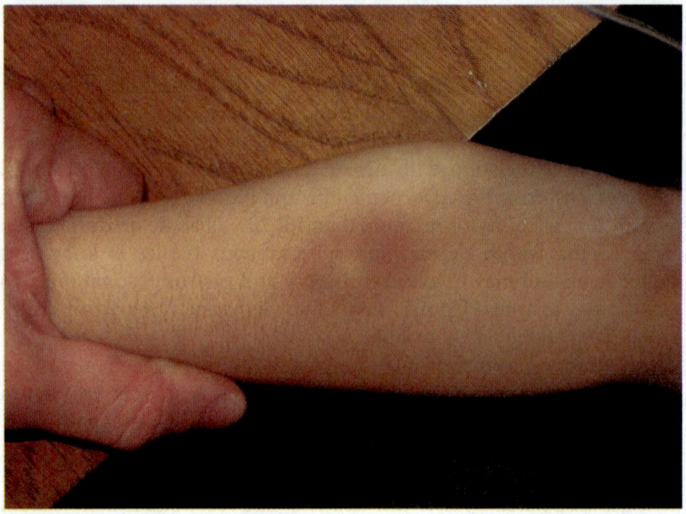

FIGURE 74-7 Fixed drug eruption.

IMMUNE CUTANEOUS REACTIONS: RARE AND SEVERE

Vasculitis Cutaneous small-vessel vasculitis often presents as palpable purpuric lesions that may be generalized or limited to the lower extremities or other dependent areas (Chap. 385). Pustular lesions and hemorrhagic blisters also occur. Vasculitis may involve other organs, including the liver, kidney, brain, and joints. Drugs are implicated as a cause of 10–15% of all cases of small-vessel vasculitides. Infection, malignancy, and collagen vascular disease are responsible for the majority of non-drug-related cases.

Propylthiouracil induces a cutaneous vasculitis that is accompanied by leukopenia and splenomegaly. Direct immunofluorescent changes in these lesions suggest immune-complex deposition. Common drugs implicated in vasculitis include allopurinol, thiazides, sulfonamides, antimicrobials, and NSAIDs. The presence of eosinophils in the perivascular infiltrate of skin biopsy suggests a drug etiology.

Pustular Eruptions AGEP is a rare reaction pattern (3–5 cases per million per year) that is often associated with exposure to drugs (Fig. 74-8). Usually beginning on the face or intertriginous areas, small nonfollicular pustules overlying erythematous and edematous skin may coalesce and lead to superficial erosion. Differentiating this eruption from TEN in its initial stages may be difficult. A skin biopsy is important and shows neutrophil collections and sparse necrotic keratinocytes in the upper part of the epidermis instead of the full-thickness epidermal necrosis that characterizes TEN. Fever and leukocytosis are common, and eosinophilia occurs in one-third of cases. Acute pustular psoriasis is the principal differential diagnostic consideration. DIHS with pustular features must also be clinically considered, although the timing for the onset of DIHS is distinct (much later onset). AGEP often begins within a few days of initiating drug treatment, most notably antibiotics, but may occur as late as 7–14 days after initiation of treatment. A broad range of drug classes (anticonvulsants, mercury, radiocontrast dye) and infections (viral, *Mycoplasma*) are also associated with AGEP. Patch testing with the responsible drug results in a localized pustular eruption.

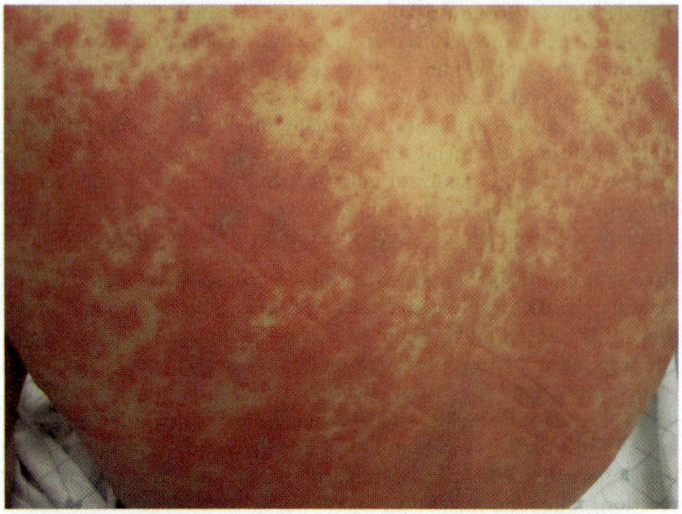

FIGURE 74-8 Acute generalized exanthematous pustulosis.

Drug-induced Hypersensitivity Syndrome Drug-induced hypersensitivity syndrome (DIHS) is a multiorgan drug reaction previously known as DRESS (drug reaction with eosinophilia and systemic symptoms); since eosinophilia is not always present, the term *DIHS* is now preferred. Allopurinol is the most common cause. Although less frequently prescribed, abacavir has been reported to cause DIHS with an incidence as high as 4–8%. It presents as a widespread erythematous eruption that may become purpuric, pustular, or lichenoid and is accompanied by many of the following features: fever, facial edema, lymphadenopathy, leukocytosis (often with atypical lymphocytes and eosinophilia), hepatitis, myositis (including myocarditis), and sometimes nephritis (with proteinuria) or pneumonitis. Distinct patterns of timing of onset and organ involvement may exist; e.g., allopurinol classically induces DIHS with renal involvement. Cardiac and lung involvement is more common with minocycline; gastrointestinal involvement is almost exclusively seen with abacavir, and some medications typically lack eosinophilia (abacavir, dapsone, lamotrigine). The cutaneous reaction usually begins 2–8 weeks after the drug is started and lasts longer than mild eruptions after drug cessation. Signs and symptoms may persist for several weeks, especially those associated with hepatitis. The eruption recurs with rechallenge, and cross-reactions among aromatic anticonvulsants, including phenytoin, carbamazepine, and barbiturates, are frequent. Other drugs causing this syndrome include sulfonamides and other antibiotics. Hypersensitivity to reactive drug metabolites, hydroxylamine for sulfamethoxazole, and arene oxide for aromatic anticonvulsants may be involved in the pathogenesis of DIHS. Reactivation of herpes viruses, especially herpesvirus 6 and Epstein-Barr virus (EBV), has been frequently reported in this syndrome, although the causal role of viral infection has been debated. Recent research suggests that inciting drugs may reactivate quiescent herpes viruses, resulting in expansion of viral-specific CD8+ T lymphocytes with subsequent end-organ damage. Viral reactivation may be associated with a worse clinical prognosis. Mortality rates as high as 10% have been reported; mortality is highest in association with hepatitis. Systemic glucocorticoids (prednisone, 1–2 mg/kg daily) should be started with slow taper over 8–12 weeks. A steroid-sparing agent, such as mycophenolate mofetil, may be indicated in cases of rapid recurrence upon steroid taper. In all cases, rapid withdrawal of the suspected drug is required. Given the severe long-term complications of myocarditis, patients should undergo cardiac evaluation if heart involvement is suspected by hypotension or arrhythmia. Patients should be closely monitored for resolution of organ dysfunction and for development of late-onset autoimmune thyroiditis (up to 6 months).

Stevens-Johnson Syndrome and Toxic Epidermal Necrolysis *SJS* and *TEN* are characterized by blisters and mucosal/epidermal detachment resulting from full-thickness epidermal necrosis in the absence of substantial dermal inflammation (Fig. 74-9). The term *Stevens-Johnson syndrome* describes cases with blisters developing on target lesions, dusky or purpuric macules in which mucosal involvement is significant, and total body surface area blistering and eventual detachment in <10% of cases. The term *Stevens-Johnson syndrome/toxic epidermal necrolysis overlap* is used to describe cases with 10–30% detachment, and *TEN* is used to describe cases with >30% detachment.

Other blistering eruptions with mucositis associated with infections may be confused with SJS/TEN. Erythema multiforme (EM) associated with herpes simplex virus is characterized by mucosal involvement and target lesions often more acrally distributed and with limited skin detachment. *Mycoplasma* infection in children causes a clinically distinct presentation with prominent mucositis and limited blistering

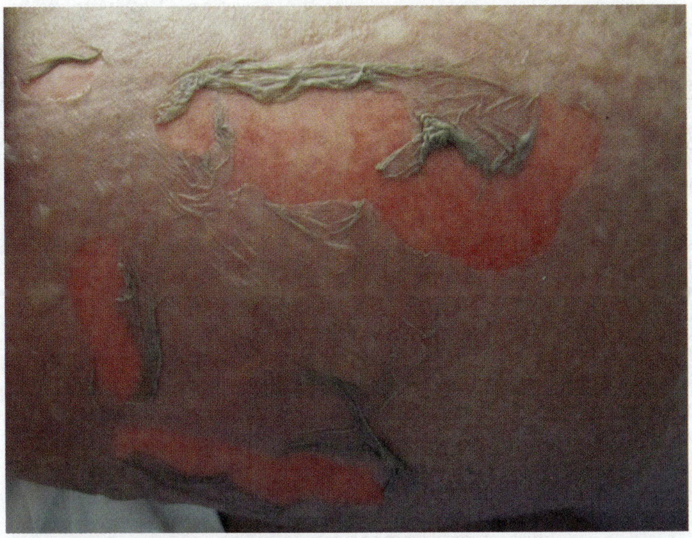

FIGURE 74-9 Toxic epidermal necrolysis. *(Photo credit: Lindy Peta Fox, MD, and Jubin Ryu, MD, PhD.)*

lesions; some believe that this clinical entity is the syndrome originally described by Stevens and Johnson.

Patients with SJS, SJS/TEN, or TEN initially present with acute onset of painful skin lesions, fever >39°C (102.2°F), sore throat, and conjunctivitis resulting from mucosal lesions. Intestinal and pulmonary involvement is associated with a poor prognosis, as are a greater extent of epidermal detachment and older age. About 10% and 30% of SJS- and TEN-affected persons die from their disease, respectively. Drugs that most commonly cause SJS or TEN are sulfonamides, nevirapine (1 in 1000 risk of SJS or TEN), allopurinol, lamotrigine, aromatic anticonvulsants, and NSAIDs, specifically oxicam. Frozen-section skin biopsy may aid in rapid diagnosis. At this time, SJS and TEN have no proven effective treatment. The best results come from early diagnosis, immediate discontinuation of any suspected drug, supportive therapy, and paying close attention to ocular complications and infection. Systemic glucocorticoid therapy (prednisone 1–2 mg/kg) may be useful early in the evolution of the disease, but long-term systemic glucocorticoid use has been associated with higher mortality. Cyclosporine may be a possible therapy for SJS/TEN. After initial enthusiasm for the use of intravenous immunoglobulin (IVIG) in the treatment of SJS/TEN, some recent data questions whether IVIG benefits these patients. Randomized studies to more definitively assess the potential benefit of systemic glucocorticoids and IVIG are lacking and difficult to perform but are necessary.

Overlap Hypersensitivity Syndromes An important emerging concept in the clinical approach to severe drug eruptions is the presence of overlap syndromes, most notably DIHS with TEN-like features, DIHS with pustular eruption (AGEP-like), and AGEP with TEN-like features. In several case series of AGEP, 50% of cases had TEN-like or DRESS-like features, and 20% of cases had mucosal involvement resembling SJS/TEN. In one study, up to 20% of all severe drug eruptions had overlap features, suggesting that AGEP, DIHS, and SJS/TEN represent a clinical spectrum with common pathophysiologic mechanisms. Designation of a single diagnosis based on cutaneous and extracutaneous involvement may not always be possible in cases of hypersensitivity.

MANAGEMENT OF A PATIENT WITH A DRUG ERUPTION

There are four main questions to answer regarding an eruption:

1. Is it a drug reaction?
2. Is it a severe eruption or the onset of a form that may become severe?
3. Which drug(s) is (are) suspected, and which drug(s) should be withdrawn?
4. What is recommended for future use of drugs?

TABLE 74-2 CLINICAL AND LABORATORY FINDINGS ASSOCIATED WITH MORE SERIOUS DRUG-INDUCED CUTANEOUS CLINICAL FINDINGS

Cutaneous
Generalized erythema
Facial edema
Skin pain
Palpable purpura
Target lesions
Skin necrosis
Blisters or epidermal detachment
Positive Nikolsky's sign
Mucous membrane erosions
Urticaria
Swelling of tongue
General
High fever (temperature >40°C [>104°F])
Enlarged lymph nodes
Arthralgias or arthritis
Shortness of breath, wheezing, hypotension
Laboratory Results
Eosinophil count >1000/μL
Lymphocytosis with atypical lymphocytes
Abnormal liver or kidney function tests

Source: Adapted from JC Roujeau, RS Stern: N Engl J Med 331:1272, 1994.

EARLY DIAGNOSIS OF SEVERE ERUPTIONS

Rapid recognition of adverse drug reactions that may become serious or life threatening is paramount. Table 74-2 lists clinical and laboratory features that, if present, suggest that the reaction may be serious. Table 74-3 provides key features of the most serious adverse cutaneous reactions. Intensity of symptoms and rapid progression of signs should raise the suspicion of a severe eruption. Any doubt should lead to prompt consultation with a dermatologist and/or referral of the patient to a specialized center.

CONFIRMATION OF DRUG REACTION

The probability of drug etiology varies with the pattern of the reaction. Only fixed drug eruptions are always drug-induced. Morbilliform eruptions are usually viral in children and drug-induced in adults. Among severe reactions, drugs account for 10–20% of anaphylaxis and vasculitis and between 70–90% of AGEP, DIHS, SJS, or TEN. Skin biopsy helps in characterizing the reaction but does not indicate drug causality. Blood counts and liver and renal function tests are important for evaluating organ involvement. The association of mild elevation of liver enzymes and high eosinophil count is frequent but not specific for a drug reaction. Blood tests that could identify an alternative cause, antihistone antibody tests (to rule out drug-induced lupus), and serology or polymerase chain reaction for infections may be of great importance to determine a cause.

WHAT DRUG(S) TO SUSPECT AND WITHDRAW

Most cases of drug eruptions occur during the first course of treatment with a new medication. A notable exception is IgE-mediated urticaria and anaphylaxis that need presensitization and develop a few minutes to a few hours after rechallenge. Characteristic times of onset to drug reaction are as follows: 4–14 days for morbilliform eruptions, 2–4 days for AGEP, 5–28 days for SJS/TEN, and 14–48 days for DIHS. A drug chart, compiling information of all current and past medications/supplements and the timing of administration relative to the rash, is a key diagnostic tool to identifying the inciting drug. Medications introduced for the first time in the relevant time frame are prime suspects. Two other important elements to suspect causality at this stage are (1) previous experience with the drug in the population and (2) alternative etiologic candidates.

TABLE 74-3 CLINICAL FEATURES OF SEVERE CUTANEOUS DRUG REACTIONS

Diagnosis	Mucosal Lesions	Typical Skin Lesions	Frequent Signs and Symptoms	Alternative Causes Not Related to Drugs
Stevens-Johnson syndrome	Erosions usually at two or more sites	Small blisters on dusky purpuric macules or atypical targets; rare areas of confluence; detachment ≤10% of body surface area	Most cases involve fever	10–20% cause not determined
Toxic epidermal necrolysis[a]	Erosions usually at two or more sites	Individual lesions like those seen in Stevens-Johnson syndrome; confluent erythema; outer layer of epidermis separates readily from basal layer with lateral pressure; large sheet of necrotic epidermis; total detachment of >30% of body surface area	Nearly all cases involve fever, "acute skin failure," leukopenia	10–20% cause not determined
Hypersensitivity syndrome	Infrequent	Severe exanthematous rash (may become purpuric), exfoliative dermatitis, facial edema	30–50% of cases involve fever, lymphadenopathy, hepatitis, nephritis, myocarditis, eosinophilia, atypical lymphocytes	Cutaneous lymphoma
Acute generalized exanthematous pustulosis	About 20% erosions (mouth, tongue)	Initially nonfollicular, small pustules overlying edematous erythema, sometimes leading to superficial erosions	Fever, burning, pruritus, facial swelling, leukocytosis, hypocalcemia	Infection
Serum sickness or reactions resembling serum sickness	Absent	Morbilliform lesions, sometimes with urticarial plaques (typically polycyclic)	Fever, arthralgias	Infection
Anticoagulant-induced necrosis	Infrequent	Erythema then purpura and necrosis, especially of fatty areas	Pain in affected areas	Disseminated intravascular coagulopathy, septicemia
Angioedema	Often involved	Urticaria or swelling of central part of face	Respiratory distress, cardiovascular collapse	Insect stings, foods

[a]Overlap of Stevens-Johnson syndrome and toxic epidermal necrolysis have features of both and attachment of 10–30% of body surface area may occur.

Source: Adapted from JC Roujeau, RS Stern: N Engl J Med 331:1272, 1994.

The decision to continue or discontinue any medication will depend on the severity of the reaction, the severity of the primary disease, the degree of suspicion of causality, and the feasibility of an alternative safer treatment. In any potentially fatal drug reaction, elimination of all possible suspect drugs or unnecessary medications should be attempted. Some rashes may resolve when "treating through" a benign drug-related eruption. The decision to treat through an eruption should, however, remain the exception and withdrawal of every suspect drug the general rule. On the other hand, drugs that are not suspected and are important for the patient (e.g., antihypertensive agents) generally should not be quickly withdrawn. This approach prevents reluctance to future use of these agents.

RECOMMENDATION FOR FUTURE USE OF DRUGS

The aims are (1) to prevent the recurrence of the drug eruption and (2) not to compromise future treatments by contraindicating otherwise useful medications.

Begin with thorough assessment of drug causality. Drug causality is evaluated based on timing of the reaction, evaluation of other possible causes, effect of drug withdrawal or continuation, and knowledge of medications that have been associated with the observed reaction. Combination of these criteria leads to considering the causality as definite, probable, possible, or unlikely. The RegiSCAR group has proposed a useful algorithm called Algorithm of Drug Causality for Epidermal Necrolysis (ALDEN) to determine drug causality in SJS/TEN. A drug with a "definite" or "probable" causality should be contraindicated, a warning card or medical alert tag (e.g., wristband) should be given to the patient, and the drugs should be listed in the patient's medical chart as an allergy.

A drug with a "possible" causality may be submitted to further investigations depending on the expected need for future treatment.

A drug with "unlikely" causality or that has been continued when the reaction improved or was reintroduced without a reaction can be administered safely.

The usefulness of laboratory tests to determine causality is still debated. Many in vitro immunologic assays have been developed, but the predictive value of these tests has not been validated in any large series of affected patients; these tests exist primarily for research and not clinical purposes.

In some cases, diagnostic rechallenge may be appropriate, even for drugs with high rates of adverse reactions. Desensitization is often successful in HIV-infected patients with morbilliform eruptions to sulfonamides but is not recommended in HIV-infected patients who manifested erythroderma or a bullous reaction in response to their earlier sulfonamide exposure.

In patients with history suggesting immediate IgE-mediated reactions to penicillin, skin-prick testing with penicillins or cephalosporins has proved useful for identifying patients at risk of anaphylactic reactions to these agents. However, skin tests themselves carry a small risk of anaphylaxis. Negative skin tests do not totally rule out IgE-mediated reactivity, but the risk of anaphylaxis in response to penicillin administration in patients with negative skin tests is about 1%. In contrast, two-thirds of patients with a positive skin test experience an allergic response upon rechallenge.

For patients with delayed-type hypersensitivity, the clinical utility of skin tests is more questionable. At least one of a combination of several tests (prick, patch, and intradermal) is positive in 50–70% of patients with a reaction "definitely" attributed to a single medication. This low sensitivity corresponds to the observation that readministration of drugs with negative skin testing resulted in eruptions in 17% of cases.

CROSS-SENSITIVITY

Because of the possibility of cross-sensitivity among chemically related drugs, many physicians recommend avoidance of not only the medication that induced the reaction but also all drugs of the same pharmacologic class.

There are two types of cross-sensitivity. Reactions that depend on a pharmacologic interaction may occur with all drugs that target the same pathway, whether they are structurally similar or not. This is the case with angioedema caused by NSAIDs and ACE inhibitors. In this situation, the risk of recurrence varies from drug to drug in a particular class; however, avoidance of all drugs in the class is usually recommended. Immune recognition of structurally related drugs is the second mechanism by which cross-sensitivity occurs. A classic example is hypersensitivity to aromatic antiepileptics (barbiturates, phenytoin, carbamazepine) with up to 50% reaction to a second drug in patients who reacted to one. For other drugs, in vitro as well as in vivo data have suggested that cross-reactivity existed only between compounds with very similar chemical structures. Sulfamethoxazole-specific lymphocytes may be activated by other antibacterial sulfonamides but not diuretics, antidiabetic drugs, or anti-COX2 NSAIDs with a sulfonamide group. Approximately 10% of patients with penicillin allergies will also develop allergic reactions to cephalosporin class antibiotics.

Recent data suggest that although the risk of a drug eruption to another drug was increased in persons with a prior reaction, "cross-sensitivity" was probably not the explanation. As an example, persons with a history of an allergic-like reaction to penicillin were at higher risk to develop a reaction to antibacterial sulfonamides than to cephalosporins.

These data suggest that the list of drugs to avoid after a drug reaction should be limited to the causative one(s) and to a few very similar medications.

Because of growing evidence that some severe cutaneous reactions to drugs are associated with HLA genes, it is recommended that first-degree family members of patients with severe cutaneous reactions also should avoid these causative medications. This may be most relevant to sulfonamides and antiseizure medications.

Desensitization can be considered in those with a history of reaction to a medication that must be used again. Efficacy of such procedures has been demonstrated in cases of immediate reaction to penicillin and positive skin tests, anaphylactic reactions to platinum chemotherapy, and delayed reactions to sulfonamides in patients with AIDS. Various protocols are available, including oral and parenteral approaches. Oral desensitization appears to have a lower risk of serious anaphylactic reactions. However, desensitization carries the risk of anaphylaxis regardless of how it is performed and should be performed in monitored clinical settings such as an intensive care unit. After desensitization, many patients experience non-life-threatening reactions during therapy with the culprit drug.

REPORTING

Any severe reaction to drugs should be reported to a regulatory agency or to pharmaceutical companies (e.g., MedWatch, *http://www.fda.gov/Safety/MedWatch/default.htm*). Because severe reactions are too rare to be detected in premarketing clinical trials, spontaneous reports are of critical importance for early detection of unexpected life-threatening events. To be useful, the report should contain enough details to permit ascertainment of severity and drug causality. This enables recognition of similar cases that may be reported from several different sources.

Acknowledgment

We acknowledge the contribution of Dr. Jean-Claude Roujeau to this chapter in the 17th edition.

75 Photosensitivity and Other Reactions to Light

Alexander G. Marneros, David R. Bickers

SOLAR RADIATION

Sunlight is the most visible and obvious source of comfort in the environment. The sun provides the beneficial effects of warmth and vitamin D synthesis. However, acute and chronic sun exposure also has pathologic consequences. Few effects of sun exposure beyond those affecting the skin have been identified, but cutaneous exposure to sunlight is the major cause of human skin cancer and can have immunosuppressive effects as well.

The sun's energy reaching the earth's surface is limited to components of the ultraviolet (UV) spectrum, the visible spectrum, and portions of the infrared spectrum. The cutoff at the short end of the UV spectrum at ~290 nm is due primarily to stratospheric ozone—formed by highly energetic ionizing radiation—that prevents penetration to the earth's surface of the shorter, more energetic, potentially more harmful wavelengths of solar radiation. Indeed, concern about destruction of the ozone layer by chlorofluorocarbons released into the atmosphere has led to international agreements to reduce production of those chemicals.

Measurements of solar flux showed a twentyfold regional variation in the amount of energy at 300 nm that reaches the earth's surface. This variability relates to seasonal effects, the path that sunlight traverses through ozone and air, the altitude (a 4% increase for each 300 m of elevation), the latitude (increasing intensity with decreasing latitude), and the amount of cloud cover, fog, and pollution.

The major components of the photobiologic action spectrum that are capable of affecting human skin include the UV and visible wavelengths between 290 and 700 nm. In addition, the wavelengths beyond 700 nm in the infrared spectrum primarily emit heat and in certain circumstances may exacerbate the pathologic effects of energy in the UV and visible spectra.

The UV spectrum reaching the earth represents <10% of total incident solar energy and is arbitrarily divided into two major segments, UV-B and UV-A, which constitute the wavelengths from 290 to 400 nm. UV-B consists of wavelengths between 290 and 320 nm. This portion of the photobiologic action spectrum is the most efficient in producing redness or erythema in human skin and thus is sometimes known as the "sunburn spectrum." UV-A includes wavelengths between 320 and 400 nm and is ~1000-fold less efficient in producing skin redness than is UV-B.

The wavelengths between 400 and 700 nm are visible to the human eye. The photon energy in the visible spectrum is not capable of damaging human skin in the absence of a photosensitizing chemical. Without the absorption of energy by a molecule, there can be no photosensitivity. Thus, the *absorption spectrum* of a molecule is defined as the range of wavelengths it absorbs, whereas the *action spectrum* for an effect of incident radiation is defined as the range of wavelengths that evoke the response.

Photosensitivity occurs when a photon-absorbing chemical (*chromophore*) present in the skin absorbs incident energy, becomes excited, and transfers the absorbed energy to various structures or to molecular oxygen.

UV RADIATION (UVR) AND SKIN STRUCTURE AND FUNCTION

Human skin consists of two major compartments: the outer epidermis, which is a stratified squamous epithelium, and the underlying dermis, which is rich in matrix proteins such as collagens and elastin. Both compartments are susceptible to damage from sun exposure. The epidermis and the dermis contain several chromophores capable of absorbing incident solar energy, including nucleic acids, proteins, and lipids. The outermost epidermal layer, the stratum corneum, is a major absorber of UV-B, and <10% of incident UV-B wavelengths penetrate through the epidermis to the dermis. Approximately 3% of radiation below 300 nm, 20% of radiation below 360 nm, and 33% of short visible radiation reach the basal cell layer in untanned human skin. In contrast, UV-A readily penetrates to the dermis and is capable of altering structural and matrix proteins that contribute to photoaging of chronically sun-exposed skin, particularly in individuals of light complexion. Thus, longer wavelengths can penetrate more deeply into the skin.

Molecular Targets for UVR-Induced Skin Effects Epidermal DNA—predominantly in keratinocytes and in Langerhans cells, which are dendritic antigen-presenting cells—absorbs UV-B and undergoes structural changes between adjacent pyrimidine bases (thymine or cytosine), including the formation of cyclobutane dimers and 6,4-photoproducts. These structural changes are potentially mutagenic and are found in most basal cell and squamous cell carcinomas (BCCs and SCCs, respectively). They can be repaired by cellular mechanisms that result in their recognition and excision and the restoration of normal base sequences. The efficient repair of these structural aberrations is crucial, since individuals with defective DNA repair are at high risk for the development of cutaneous cancer. For example, patients with xeroderma pigmentosum, an autosomal recessive disorder, have a variably deficient repair of UV-induced photoproducts. The skin of these patients often shows the dry, leathery appearance of prematurely photoaged skin, and these patients have an increased frequency of skin cancer already in the first two decades of life. Studies in transgenic mice have verified the importance of functional genes that regulate these repair pathways in preventing the development of UV-induced skin cancer. DNA damage in Langerhans cells may also contribute to the known immunosuppressive effects of UV-B (see "Photoimmunology," below).

In addition to DNA, molecular oxygen is a target for incident solar UVR, leading to the generation of reactive oxygen species (ROS). These ROS can damage skin components, such as epidermal lipids—either free lipids in the stratum corneum or cell membrane lipids. UVR also can target proteins, leading to increased cross-linking and degradation of matrix proteins in the dermis and accumulation of abnormal dermal elastin leading to photoaging changes known as *solar elastosis.*

Cutaneous Optics and Chromophores *Chromophores* are endogenous or exogenous chemical components that can absorb physical energy. Endogenous chromophores are of two types: (1) normal components of skin, including nucleic acids, proteins, lipids, and 7-dehydrocholesterol (the precursor of vitamin D); and (2) components that are synthesized elsewhere in the body and that circulate in the bloodstream and diffuse into the skin, such as porphyrins. Normally, only trace amounts of porphyrins are present in the skin, but, in selected diseases known as the *porphyrias* (Chap. 430), porphyrins are released into the circulation in increased amounts from the bone marrow and the liver and are transported to the skin, where they absorb incident energy both in the Soret band (around 400 nm; short visible) and, to a lesser extent, in the red portion of the visible spectrum (580–660 nm). This energy absorption results in the generation of ROS that can mediate structural damage to the skin, manifested as erythema, edema, urticaria, or blister formation. It is of interest that photoexcited porphyrins are currently used in the treatment of nonmelanoma skin cancers and their precursor lesions, actinic keratoses. Known as *photodynamic therapy*, this modality generates ROS in the skin, leading to cell death. Topical photosensitizers used in photodynamic therapy are the porphyrin precursors 5-aminolevulinic acid and methyl aminolevulinate, which are converted to porphyrins in the skin. It is believed that photodynamic therapy targets tumor cells for destruction more selectively than it targets adjacent nonneoplastic cells. The efficacy of such therapy requires appropriate timing of the application of methyl aminolevulinate or 5-aminolevulinic acid to the affected skin followed by exposure to artificial sources of visible light. High-intensity blue light has been used successfully for the treatment of thin actinic keratoses. Red light has a longer wavelength, penetrates more deeply into the skin, and is more beneficial in the treatment of superficial BCCs.

Acute Effects of Sun Exposure The acute effects of skin exposure to sunlight include sunburn and vitamin D synthesis.

SUNBURN This painful skin condition is an acute inflammatory response of the skin, predominantly to UV-B. Generally, an individual's ability to tolerate sunlight is inversely proportional to that individual's degree of melanin pigmentation. Melanin, a complex polymer of tyrosine derivatives, is synthesized in specialized epidermal dendritic cells known as *melanocytes* and is packaged into *melanosomes* that are transferred via dendritic processes into *keratinocytes*, thereby providing photoprotection and simultaneously darkening the skin. Sun-induced melanogenesis is a consequence of increased tyrosinase activity in melanocytes. Central to the suntan response is the melanocortin-1 receptor (*MC1R*), and mutations in this gene contribute to the wide variation in human skin and hair color; individuals with red hair and fair skin typically have low MC1R activity. Genetic studies have revealed additional genes that influence skin color variation in humans, such as the gene for tyrosinase (*TYR*) and the genes *APBA2[OCA2]*, *SLC45A2*, and *SLC24A5*. The human *MC1R* gene encodes a G protein–coupled receptor that binds α-melanocyte-stimulating hormone, which is secreted in the skin mainly by keratinocytes in response to UVR. The UV-induced expression of this hormone is controlled by the tumor suppressor p53, and absence of functional p53 attenuates the tanning response. Activation of the melanocortin receptor leads to increased intracellular cyclic adenosine 5′-monophosphate (cAMP) and protein kinase A activation, resulting in an increased transcription of the microphthalmia-associated transcription factor (MITF), which stimulates melanogenesis. Since the precursor of α-melanocyte-stimulating hormone, proopiomelanocortin, is also the precursor of β-endorphins, UVR may result in not only increased pigmentation but also in increased β-endorphin production, an effect that has been hypothesized to promote sun-seeking behaviors.

The Fitzpatrick classification of human skin phototypes is based on the efficiency of the epidermal-melanin unit, which usually can be ascertained by asking an individual two questions: (1) Do you burn after sun exposure? (2) Do you tan after sun exposure? The answers to these questions permit division of the population into six skin types, varying from type I (always burn, never tan) to type VI (never burn, always tan) (Table 75-1).

Sunburn erythema is due to vasodilation of dermal blood vessels. There is a lag time (usually 4–12 h) between skin exposure to sunlight and the development of visible redness. The action spectrum for sunburn erythema includes UV-B and UV-A, although UV-B is much more efficient than UV-A in evoking the response. However, UV-A may contribute to sunburn erythema at midday, when much more UV-A than UV-B is present in the solar spectrum. The erythema that accompanies the inflammatory response induced by UVR results from the orchestrated release of cytokines along with growth factors and the generation of ROS. Furthermore, UV-induced activation of nuclear factor κB–dependent gene transcription can augment release of several proinflammatory cytokines and vasoactive mediators. These cytokines and mediators accumulate locally in sunburned skin, providing chemotactic factors that attract neutrophils, macrophages, and T lymphocytes, which promote the inflammatory response. UVR also stimulates infiltration of inflammatory cells through induced expression of adhesion molecules such as E-selectin and intercellular adhesion molecule 1 on endothelial cells and keratinocytes. UVR also has been shown to activate phospholipase A_2, resulting in increases in eicosanoids such as prostaglandin E_2, which is known to be a potent inducer of sunburn erythema. The role

TABLE 75-1 SKIN TYPE AND SUNBURN SENSITIVITY (FITZPATRICK CLASSIFICATION)

Type	Description
I	Always burn, never tan
II	Always burn, sometimes tan
III	Sometimes burn, sometimes tan
IV	Sometimes burn, always tan
V	Never burn, sometimes tan
VI	Never burn, always tan

of eicosanoids in this reaction has been verified by studies showing that nonsteroidal anti-inflammatory drugs (NSAIDs) can reduce it.

Epidermal changes in sunburn include the induction of "sunburn cells," which are keratinocytes undergoing p53-dependent apoptosis as a defense, with elimination of cells that harbor UV-B-induced structural DNA damage.

VITAMIN D SYNTHESIS AND PHOTOCHEMISTRY Cutaneous exposure to UV-B causes photolysis of epidermal 7-dehydrocholesterol, converting it to pre–vitamin D_3, which then undergoes temperature-dependent isomerization to form the stable hormone vitamin D_3. This compound diffuses to the dermal vasculature and circulates to the liver and kidney, where it is converted to the dihydroxylated functional hormone 1,25-dihydroxyvitamin D_3. Vitamin D metabolites from the circulation and those produced in the skin itself can augment epidermal differentiation signaling and inhibit keratinocyte proliferation. These effects are exploited therapeutically in psoriasis with the topical application of synthetic vitamin D analogues. In addition, vitamin D is increasingly thought to have beneficial effects in several other inflammatory conditions, and some evidence suggests that—besides its classic physiologic effects on calcium metabolism and bone homeostasis—it is associated with a reduced risk of various internal malignancies. There is controversy regarding the risk-to-benefit ratio of sun exposure in vitamin D homeostasis. At present, it is important to emphasize that no clear-cut evidence suggests that the use of sunscreens substantially diminishes vitamin D levels. Since aging also substantially decreases the ability of human skin to photocatalytically produce vitamin D_3, the widespread use of sunscreens that filter out UV-B has led to concerns that the elderly might be unduly susceptible to vitamin D deficiency. However, the amount of sunlight needed to produce sufficient vitamin D is small and does not justify the risks of skin cancer and other types of photodamage linked to increased sun exposure or tanning behavior. Nutritional supplementation of vitamin D is a preferable strategy for patients with vitamin D deficiency.

Chronic Effects of Sun Exposure: Nonmalignant The clinical features of photoaging (*dermatoheliosis*) consist of wrinkling, blotchiness, and telangiectasia as well as a roughened, irregular, "weather-beaten" leathery appearance.

UVR is important in the pathogenesis of photoaging in human skin, and ROS are likely involved. The dermis and its connective tissue matrix are major targets for sun-associated chronic damage that manifests as solar elastosis, a massive increase in thickened irregular masses of abnormal-appearing elastic fibers. Collagen fibers are also abnormally clumped in the deeper dermis of sun-damaged skin. The chromophore(s), the action spectra, and the specific biochemical events orchestrating these changes are only partially understood, although more deeply penetrating UV-A seems to be primarily involved. Chronologically aged sun-protected skin and photoaged skin share important molecular features, including connective tissue damage and elevated levels of matrix metalloproteinases (MMPs). MMPs are enzymes involved in the degradation of the extracellular matrix. UV-A induces expression of some MMPs, including MMP-1 and MMP-3, leading to increased collagen breakdown. In addition, UV-A reduces type I procollagen mRNA expression. Thus, chronic UVR alters the structure and function of dermal collagen. On the basis of these observations, it is not surprising that high-dose UV-A phototherapy may have beneficial effects in some patients with localized fibrotic diseases of the skin, such as localized scleroderma.

Chronic Effects of Sun Exposure: Malignant One of the major known consequences of chronic excessive skin exposure to sunlight is nonmelanoma skin cancer. The two most common types of nonmelanoma skin cancer are BCC and SCC (Chap. 105). A model for skin cancer induction involves three major steps: initiation, promotion, and progression. Exposure of human skin to sunlight results in *initiation*, a step by which structural (mutagenic) changes in DNA evoke an irreversible alteration in the target cell (keratinocyte) that begins the tumorigenic process. Exposure to a tumor initiator such as UV-B is believed to be a necessary but not a sufficient step in the malignant process, since initiated skin cells not exposed to tumor promoters generally do not develop tumors. The second stage in tumor development is *promotion*, a multistep process by which chronic exposure to sunlight evokes further changes that culminate in the clonal expansion of initiated cells and cause the development, over many years, of premalignant growths known as *actinic keratoses*, a minority of which may progress to form SCCs. As a result of extensive studies, it seems clear that UV-B is a *complete carcinogen*, meaning that it can act as both a tumor initiator and a tumor promoter. The third and final step in the malignant process is *malignant conversion* of benign precursors into malignant lesions, a process thought to require additional genetic alterations.

On a molecular level, skin carcinogenesis results from the accumulation of gene mutations that cause inactivation of tumor suppressors, activation of oncogenes, or reactivation of cellular signaling pathways that normally are expressed only during epidermal embryologic development. Accumulation of mutations in the tumor-suppressor gene *p53* secondary to UV-induced DNA damage occurs in both SCCs and BCCs and is important in promoting skin carcinogenesis. Indeed, the majority of both human and murine UV-induced skin cancers have characteristic *p53* mutations (C $\rightarrow$ T and CC $\rightarrow$ TT transitions). Studies in mice have shown that sunscreens can substantially reduce the frequency of these signature mutations in *p53* and inhibit the induction of tumors.

BCCs also harbor inactivating mutations in the tumor-suppressor gene *patched*, which result in activation of the sonic hedgehog signaling pathway and increased cell proliferation. Thus, these tumors can manifest mutations in tumor suppressors (*p53* and *patched)* or oncogenes (*smoothened)*. New evidence links alterations in the Wnt/β-catenin signaling pathway, which is known to be critical for hair follicle development, to skin cancer as well. Thus interactions between this pathway and the hedgehog signaling pathway appear to be involved in both skin carcinogenesis and embryologic development of the skin and hair follicles.

Clonal analysis in mouse models of BCC revealed that tumor cells arise from long-term resident progenitor cells of the interfollicular epidermis and the upper infundibulum of the hair follicle. These BCC-initiating cells are reprogrammed to resemble embryonic hair follicle progenitors, whose tumor-initiating ability depends on activation of the Wnt/β-catenin signaling pathway.

SCC initiation occurs both in the interfollicular epidermis and in the hair follicle bulge stem cell populations. In mouse models, the combination of mutant K-Ras and p53 is sufficient to induce invasive SCCs from these cell populations.

The transcription factor Myc is important for stem cell maintenance in the skin, and oncogenic activation of Myc has been implicated in the development of BCCs and SCCs. Thus, nonmelanoma skin cancer involves mutations and alterations in multiple genes and pathways that occur as a result of their chronic accumulation driven by exposure to environmental factors such as UVR.

Epidemiologic studies have linked excessive sun exposure to an increased risk of nonmelanoma cancers and melanoma of the skin; the evidence is far more direct for nonmelanoma skin cancers (BCCs and SCCs) than for melanoma. Approximately 80% of nonmelanoma skin cancers develop on sun-exposed body areas, including the face, neck, and hands. Major risk factors include male sex, childhood sun exposures, older age, fair skin, and residence at latitudes relatively close to the equator. Individuals with darker-pigmented skin have a lower risk of skin cancer than do fair-skinned individuals. More than 2 million individuals in the United States develop nonmelanoma skin cancer annually, and the lifetime risk that a fair-skinned individual will develop such a neoplasm is estimated at ~15%. The incidence of nonmelanoma skin cancer in the population is increasing at a rate of 2–3% per year. One potential explanation is the widespread use of indoor tanning. It is estimated that 30 million people tan indoors in the United States annually, including >2 million adolescents.

The relationship of sun exposure to melanoma development is less direct, but strong evidence supports an association. Clear-cut risk factors include a positive family or personal history of melanoma and multiple dysplastic nevi. Melanomas can occur during adolescence; the implication is that the latent period for tumor growth is shorter than that for nonmelanoma skin cancer. For reasons that are only partially understood, melanomas are among the most rapidly increasing human malignancies (Chap. 105). Epidemiologic studies indicate that indoor tanning is a risk factor for melanoma, which may contribute to the increasing incidence of melanoma formation. Furthermore, epidemiologic studies suggest that life in a sunny climate from birth or early childhood may increase the risk of melanoma development. In general, risk does not correlate with cumulative sun exposure but may be related to the duration and extent of exposure in childhood.

However, in contrast to nonmelanoma skin cancers, melanoma frequently develops in sun-protected skin, and oncogenic mutations in melanoma may also not be UVR-signature mutations; these observations suggest that UVR-independent factors contribute to melanomagenesis. Low MC1R activity leads to production of the red/yellow pheomelanin pigment in individuals with red hair and fair skin, while high MC1R activity results in increased production of the black/brown eumelanin. Experiments in mice suggest that high pheomelanin content in skin (as in individuals with red hair and fair skin) leads to a UVR-independent increase in the risk of melanoma through a mechanism that involves oxidative damage. Thus, both UVR-dependent and UVR-independent factors are likely to contribute to melanoma formation.

Photoimmunology Exposure to solar radiation causes both local immunosuppression (through inhibition of immune responses to antigens applied at the irradiated site) and systemic immunosuppression (through inhibition of immune responses to antigens applied at remote, unirradiated sites). For example, human skin exposure to modest doses of UV-B can deplete the epidermal antigen-presenting cells known as Langerhans cells, thereby reducing the degree of allergic sensitization to application of the potent contact allergen dinitrochlorobenzene at the irradiated skin site.

An example of the systemic immunosuppressive effects of higher doses of UVR is the diminished immunologic response to antigens introduced either epicutaneously or intracutaneously at sites distant from the irradiated site. Various immunomodulatory factors and immune cells have been implicated in UVR-induced systemic immunosuppression, including tumor necrosis factor α, interleukin 4, interleukin 10, *cis*-urocanic acid, and eicosanoids. Experimental evidence suggests that prostaglandin E_2 signaling through prostaglandin E receptor subtype 4 mediates UVR-induced systemic immunosuppression by elevating the number of regulatory T cells, and this effect can be inhibited with NSAIDs.

The major chromophores in the upper epidermis that are known to initiate UV-mediated immunosuppression include DNA, *trans*-urocanic acid, and membrane components. The action spectrum for UV-induced immunosuppression closely mimics the absorption spectrum of DNA. Pyrimidine dimers in Langerhans cells may inhibit antigen presentation. The absorption spectrum of epidermal urocanic acid closely mimics the action spectrum for UV-B-induced immunosuppression. Urocanic acid is a metabolic product of the essential amino acid histidine and accumulates in the upper epidermis through breakdown of the histidine-rich protein filaggrin due to the absence of its catabolizing enzyme in keratinocytes. Urocanic acid is synthesized as a *trans*-isomer, and UV-induced *trans-cis* isomerization of urocanic acid in the stratum corneum drives immunosuppression. *Cis*-urocanic acid may exert its immunosuppressive effects through a variety of mechanisms, including inhibition of antigen presentation by Langerhans cells.

One important consequence of chronic sun exposure and associated immunosuppression is an enhanced risk of skin cancer. In part, UV-B activates regulatory T cells that suppress antitumor immune responses via interleukin 10 expression, whereas, in the absence of high UV-B exposure, epidermal Langerhans cells present tumor-associated antigens and induce protective immunity, thereby inhibiting skin tumorigenesis. UV-induced DNA damage is a major molecular trigger of this immunosuppressive effect.

Perhaps the most graphic demonstration of the role of immunosuppression in enhancing the risk of nonmelanoma skin cancer comes from studies of organ transplant recipients who require lifelong immunosuppressive/antirejection drug regimens. More than 50% of organ transplant recipients develop BCCs and SCCs, and these cancers are the most common types of malignancies arising in these patients. Rates of BCC and SCC increase with the duration and degree of immunosuppression. These patients ideally should be screened prior to organ transplantation, be monitored closely thereafter, and adhere to rigorous photoprotection measures, including the use of sunscreens and protective clothing as well as sun avoidance. Notably, immunosuppressive drugs that target the mTOR pathway, such as sirolimus and everolimus, may reduce the risk of nonmelanoma skin cancer in organ transplant recipients from that associated with the use of calcineurin inhibitors (cyclosporine and tacrolimus), which may contribute to nonmelanoma skin cancer formation not only through their immunosuppressive effects but also through suppression of p53-dependent cancer cell senescence pathways independent of host immunity.

PHOTOSENSITIVITY DISEASES

The diagnosis of photosensitivity requires elicitation of a careful history in order to define the duration of signs and symptoms, the length of time between exposure to sunlight and the development of subjective symptoms, and visible changes in the skin. The age of onset can also be a helpful diagnostic clue; for example, the acute photosensitivity of erythropoietic protoporphyria almost always begins in childhood, whereas the chronic photosensitivity of porphyria cutanea tarda (PCT) typically begins in the fourth and fifth decades of life. A patient's history of exposure to topical and systemic drugs and chemicals may provide important diagnostic clues. Many classes of drugs can cause photosensitivity on the basis of either phototoxicity or photoallergy. Fragrances such as musk ambrette that were previously present in numerous cosmetic products are also potent photosensitizers.

Examination of the skin may offer important clues. Anatomic areas that are naturally protected from direct sunlight, such as the hairy scalp, the upper eyelids, the retroauricular areas, and the infranasal and submental regions, may be spared, whereas exposed areas show characteristic features of the pathologic process. These anatomic localization patterns are often helpful, but not infallible, in making the diagnosis. For example, airborne contact sensitizers that are blown onto the skin may produce dermatitis that can be difficult to distinguish from photosensitivity despite the fact that such material may trigger skin reactivity in areas shielded from direct sunlight.

Many dermatologic conditions may be caused or aggravated by sunlight (Table 75-2). The role of light in evoking these responses may be dependent on genetic abnormalities ranging from well-described defects in DNA repair that occur in xeroderma pigmentosum to the inherited abnormalities in heme synthesis that characterize the porphyrias. The chromophore has been identified in certain photosensitivity diseases, but the energy-absorbing agent remains unknown in the majority.

Polymorphous Light Eruption A common type of photosensitivity disease is *polymorphous light eruption* (PMLE). Many affected individuals never seek medical attention because the condition is often transient, becoming manifest in the spring with initial sun exposure but then subsiding spontaneously with continuing exposure, a phenomenon known as "hardening." The major manifestations of PMLE include (often intensely) pruritic erythematous papules that may coalesce into plaques in a patchy distribution on exposed areas of the trunk and forearms. The face is usually less seriously involved. Whereas the morphologic skin findings remain similar for each patient with subsequent recurrences, significant interindividual variations in skin findings are characteristic (hence the term "polymorphous").

A skin biopsy and phototest procedures in which skin is exposed to multiple erythemal doses of UV-A and UV-B may aid in the diagnosis. The action spectrum for PMLE is usually within these portions of the solar spectrum.

Whereas the treatment of an acute flare of PMLE may require topical or systemic glucocorticoids, approaches to preventing PMLE are

TABLE 75-2 CLASSIFICATION OF PHOTOSENSITIVITY DISEASES

Type	Disease
Genetic	Erythropoietic porphyria
	Erythropoietic protoporphyria
	Porphyria cutanea tarda—familial
	Variegate porphyria
	Hepatoerythropoietic porphyria
	Albinism
	Xeroderma pigmentosum
	Rothmund-Thomson syndrome
	Bloom syndrome
	Cockayne syndrome
	Kindler syndrome
	Phenylketonuria
Metabolic	Porphyria cutanea tarda—sporadic
	Hartnup disease
	Kwashiorkor
	Pellagra
	Carcinoid syndrome
Phototoxic	
Internal	Drugs
External	Drugs, plants, food
Photoallergic	
Immediate	Solar urticaria
Delayed	Drug photoallergy
	Persistent light reaction/chronic actinic dermatitis
Neoplastic and degenerative	Photoaging
	Actinic keratosis
	Melanoma and nonmelanoma skin cancer
Idiopathic	Polymorphous light eruption
	Hydroa aestivale
	Actinic prurigo
Photoaggravated	Lupus erythematosus
	Systemic
	Subacute cutaneous
	Discoid
	Dermatomyositis
	Herpes simplex
	Lichen planus actinicus
	Acne vulgaris (aestivale)

important and include the use of high-SPF and high UVA-protection broad-spectrum sunscreens as well as the induction of "hardening" by the cautious administration of artificial UV-B (broad-band or narrow-band) and/or UV-A radiation or the use of psoralen plus UV-A (PUVA) photochemotherapy for 2–4 weeks before initial sun exposure. Such prophylactic phototherapy or photochemotherapy at the beginning of spring may prevent the occurrence of PMLE throughout the summer.

Phototoxicity and Photoallergy These photosensitivity disorders are related to the topical or systemic administration of drugs and other chemicals. Both reactions require the absorption of energy by a drug or chemical with consequent production of an excited-state photosensitizer that can transfer its absorbed energy to a bystander molecule or to molecular oxygen, thereby generating tissue-destructive chemical species, including ROS.

Phototoxicity is a nonimmunologic reaction that can be caused by drugs and chemicals, a few of which are listed in Table 75-3. The usual clinical manifestations include erythema resembling a sunburn reaction that quickly desquamates, or "peels," within several days. In addition, edema, vesicles, and bullae may occur.

TABLE 75-3 DRUGS THAT MAY CAUSE A PHOTOTOXIC REACTION

Drug	Topical	Systemic
Amiodarone		+
Dacarbazine		+
Fluoroquinolones		+
5-Fluorouracil	+	+
Furosemide		+
Nalidixic acid		+
Phenothiazines		+
Psoralens	+	+
Retinoids	+/–	+
Sulfonamides		+
Sulfonylureas		+
Tetracyclines		+
Thiazides		+
Vinblastine		+

Photoallergy is much less common and is distinct in that it is an immunopathologic process. The excited-state photosensitizer may create highly unstable haptenic free radicals that bind covalently to macromolecules to form a functional antigen capable of evoking a delayed-type hypersensitivity response. Some drugs and chemicals that can produce photoallergy are listed in Table 75-4. The clinical manifestations typically differ from those of phototoxicity in that an intensely pruritic eczematous dermatitis tends to predominate and evolves into lichenified, thickened, "leathery" changes in sun-exposed areas. A small subset (perhaps 5–10%) of patients with photoallergy may develop a persistent exquisite hypersensitivity to light even when the offending drug or chemical is identified and eliminated, a condition known as *persistent light reaction.*

A very uncommon type of persistent photosensitivity is known as *chronic actinic dermatitis*. The affected patients are typically elderly men with a long history of preexisting allergic contact dermatitis or photosensitivity. These individuals are usually exquisitely sensitive to UV-B, UV-A, and visible wavelengths.

Phototoxicity and photoallergy often can be diagnostically confirmed by phototest procedures. In patients with suspected phototoxicity, determining the minimal erythemal dose (MED) while the patient is exposed to a suspected agent and then repeating the MED after discontinuation of the agent may provide a clue to the causative drug or chemical. Photopatch testing can be performed to confirm the diagnosis of photoallergy. In this simple variant of ordinary patch testing, a series of known photoallergens is applied to the skin in duplicate, and one set is irradiated with a suberythemal dose of UV-A. The development of eczematous changes at sites exposed to sensitizer and light is a positive result. The characteristic abnormality in patients with persistent light reaction is a diminished threshold to erythema evoked

TABLE 75-4 DRUGS THAT MAY CAUSE A PHOTOALLERGIC REACTION

Drug	Topical	Systemic
6-Methylcoumarin	+	
Aminobenzoic acid and esters	+	
Bithionol	+	
Chlorpromazine		+
Diclofenac		+
Fluoroquinolones		+
Halogenated salicylanilides	+	
Hypericin (St. John's wort)	+	+
Musk ambrette	+	
Piroxicam		+
Promethazine		+
Sulfonamides		+
Sulfonylureas		+

by UV-B. Patients with chronic actinic dermatitis usually manifest a broad spectrum of UV hyperresponsiveness and require meticulous photoprotection, including avoidance of sun exposure, use of high-SPF (>30) sunscreens, and, in severe cases, systemic immunosuppression, such as with azathioprine.

The management of drug photosensitivity involves first and foremost the elimination of exposure to the chemical agents responsible for the reaction and the minimization of sun exposure. The acute symptoms of phototoxicity may be ameliorated by cool moist compresses, topical glucocorticoids, and systemically administered NSAIDs. In severely affected individuals, a rapidly tapered course of systemic glucocorticoids may be useful. Judicious use of analgesics may be necessary.

Photoallergic reactions require a similar management approach. Furthermore, patients with persistent light reaction and chronic actinic dermatitis must be meticulously protected against light exposure. In selected patients to whom chronic systemic high-dose glucocorticoids pose unacceptable risks, it may be necessary to employ an immunosuppressive drug such as azathioprine, cyclophosphamide, cyclosporine, or mycophenolate mofetil.

Porphyria The porphyrias (Chap. 430) are a group of diseases that have in common inherited or acquired derangements in the synthesis of heme. Heme is an iron-chelated tetrapyrrole or porphyrin, and the nonmetal chelated porphyrins are potent photosensitizers that absorb light intensely in both the short (400–410 nm) and the long (580–650 nm) portions of the visible spectrum.

Heme cannot be reutilized and must be synthesized continuously. The two body compartments with the largest capacity for its production are the bone marrow and the liver. Accordingly, the porphyrias originate in one or the other of these organs, with an end result of excessive endogenous production of potent photosensitizing porphyrins. The porphyrins circulate in the bloodstream and diffuse into the skin, where they absorb solar energy, become photoexcited, generate ROS, and evoke cutaneous photosensitivity. The mechanism of porphyrin photosensitization is known to be photodynamic, or oxygen-dependent, and is mediated by ROS such as singlet oxygen and superoxide anions.

Porphyria cutanea tarda is the most common type of porphyria and is associated with decreased activity of the enzyme uroporphyrinogen decarboxylase. There are two basic types of PCT: (1) the sporadic or acquired type, generally seen in individuals ingesting ethanol or receiving estrogens; and (2) the inherited type, in which there is autosomal dominant transmission of deficient enzyme activity. Both forms are associated with increased hepatic iron stores.

In both types of PCT, the predominant feature is chronic photosensitivity characterized by increased fragility of sun-exposed skin, particularly areas subject to repeated trauma such as the dorsa of the hands, the forearms, the face, and the ears. The predominant skin lesions are vesicles and bullae that rupture, producing moist erosions (often with a hemorrhagic base) that heal slowly, with crusting and purplish discoloration of the affected skin. Hypertrichosis, mottled pigmentary change, and scleroderma-like induration are associated features. The diagnosis can be confirmed biochemically by measurement of urinary porphyrin excretion, plasma porphyrin assay, and assay of erythrocyte and/or hepatic uroporphyrinogen decarboxylase. Multiple mutations of the uroporphyrinogen decarboxylase gene have been identified in human populations. Some patients with PCT have associated mutations in the *HFE* gene, which is linked to hemochromatosis; these mutations could contribute to the iron overload seen in PCT, although iron status as measured by serum ferritin, iron levels, and transferrin saturation is no different from that in PCT patients without *HFE* mutations. Prior hepatitis C virus infection appears to be an independent risk factor for PCT.

Treatment of PCT consists of repeated phlebotomies to diminish the excessive hepatic iron stores and/or intermittent low doses of chloroquine and hydroxychloroquine. Long-term remission of the disease can be achieved if the patient eliminates exposure to porphyrinogenic agents and prolonged exposure to sunlight.

Erythropoietic protoporphyria originates in the bone marrow and is due to a decrease in the mitochondrial enzyme ferrochelatase secondary to numerous gene mutations. The major clinical features include acute photosensitivity characterized by subjective burning and stinging of exposed skin that often develops during or just after sun exposure. There may be associated skin swelling and, after repeated episodes, a waxlike scarring.

The diagnosis is confirmed by demonstration of elevated levels of free erythrocyte protoporphyrin. Detection of increased plasma protoporphyrin helps distinguish erythropoietic protoporphyria from lead poisoning and iron-deficiency anemia, in both of which erythrocyte protoporphyrin levels are elevated in the absence of cutaneous photosensitivity and elevated plasma protoporphyrin levels.

Treatment includes reduction of sun exposure and oral administration of the carotenoid β-carotene, which is an effective scavenger of free radicals. This drug increases tolerance to sun exposure in some affected individuals, although it has no effect on deficient ferrochelatase.

An algorithm for managing patients with photosensitivity is presented in Fig. 75-1.

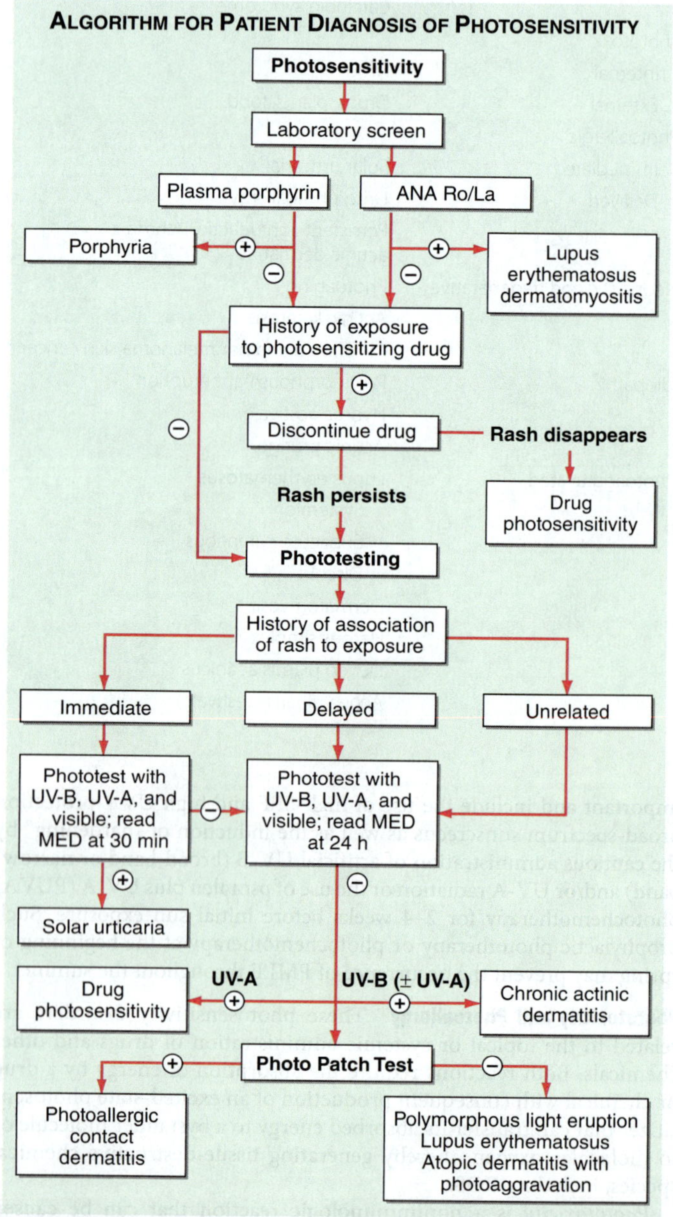

FIGURE 75-1 Algorithm for the diagnosis of a patient with photosensitivity. ANA, antinuclear antibody; MED, minimal erythemal dose; UV-A and UV-B, ultraviolet spectrum segments including wavelengths of 320–400 nm and 290–320 nm, respectively.

PHOTOPROTECTION

Since photosensitivity of the skin results from exposure to sunlight, it follows that absolute avoidance of sunlight will eliminate these disorders. However, contemporary lifestyles make this approach impractical for most individuals. Thus better approaches to photoprotection have been sought.

Natural photoprotection is provided by structural proteins in the epidermis, particularly keratins and melanin. The amount of melanin and its distribution in cells are genetically regulated, and individuals of darker complexion (skin types IV–VI) are at decreased risk for the development of acute sunburn and cutaneous malignancy.

Other forms of photoprotection include clothing and sunscreens. Clothing constructed of tightly woven sun-protective fabrics, irrespective of color, affords substantial protection. Wide-brimmed hats, long sleeves, and trousers all reduce direct exposure. Sunscreens are now considered over-the-counter drugs, and a monograph from the U.S. Food and Drug Administration (FDA) has recognized category I ingredients as safe and effective. Those ingredients are listed in Table 75-5. Sunscreens are rated for their photoprotective effect by their sun protection factor (SPF). The SPF is simply a ratio of the time required to produce sunburn erythema with and without sunscreen application. The SPF of most sunscreens reflects protection from UV-B but not from UV-A. The FDA monograph stipulates that sunscreens must be rated on a scale ranging from minimal (SPF ≥2 and <12) to moderate (SPF ≥12 and <30) to high (SPF ≥30, labeled as 30+).

Broad-spectrum sunscreens contain both UV-B-absorbing and UV-A-absorbing chemicals, the latter including avobenzone and ecamsule (terephthalylidene dicamphor sulfonic acid). These chemicals absorb UVR and transfer the absorbed energy to surrounding cells. In contrast, physical UV blockers (zinc oxide and titanium dioxide) scatter or reflect UVR.

In addition to light absorption, a critical determinant of the sustained photoprotective effect of sunscreens is their water resistance. The FDA monograph has defined strict testing criteria for sunscreens that claim to possess a high degree of water resistance.

Some degree of photoprotection can be achieved by limiting the time of sun exposure during the day. Since a large part of an individual's total lifetime sun exposure may occur by age 18, it is important to educate parents and young children about the hazards of sunlight. Simply eliminating exposure at midday will substantially reduce lifetime UVR exposure.

TABLE 75-5 FDA CATEGORY I MONOGRAPHED SUNSCREEN INGREDIENTS[a]

Ingredients	Maximum Concentration, %
p-Aminobenzoic acid (PABA)	15
Avobenzone	3
Cinoxate	3
Dioxybenzone (benzophenone-8)	3
Ecamsule	15
Homosalate	15
Methyl anthranilate	5
Octocrylene	10
Octyl methoxycinnamate	7.5
Octyl salicylate	5
Oxybenzone (benzophenone-3)	6
Padimate O (octyl dimethyl PABA)	8
Phenylbenzimidazole sulfonic acid	4
Sulisobenzone (benzophenone-4)	10
Titanium dioxide	25
Trolamine salicylate	12
Zinc oxide	25

[a]FDA, U.S. Food and Drug Administration.

PHOTOTHERAPY AND PHOTOCHEMOTHERAPY

UVR can be used therapeutically. The administration of UV-B alone or in combination with topically applied agents can induce remissions of many dermatologic diseases, including psoriasis and atopic dermatitis. In particular, narrow-band UV-B treatments (with fluorescent bulbs emitting radiation at ~311 nm) have enhanced efficacy over that obtained with broad-band UV-B in the treatment of psoriasis.

Photochemotherapy in which topically applied or systemically administered psoralens are combined with UV-A (PUVA) is effective in treating psoriasis and the early stages of cutaneous T cell lymphoma and vitiligo. Psoralens are tricyclic furocoumarins that, when intercalated into DNA and exposed to UV-A, form adducts with pyrimidine bases and eventually form DNA cross-links. These structural changes are thought to decrease DNA synthesis and to be related to the amelioration of psoriasis. Why PUVA photochemotherapy is effective in cutaneous T cell lymphoma is only partially understood, but it has been shown to induce apoptosis of atypical T lymphocyte populations in the skin. Consequently, direct treatment of circulating atypical lymphocytes by extracorporeal photochemotherapy (photopheresis) has been used in Sézary syndrome as well as in other severe systemic diseases with circulating atypical lymphocytes, such as graft-versus-host disease.

In addition to its effects on DNA, PUVA photochemotherapy stimulates epidermal thickening and melanin synthesis; the latter property, together with its anti-inflammatory effects, provides the rationale for use of PUVA in the depigmenting disease vitiligo. Oral 8-methoxypsoralen and UV-A appear to be most effective in this regard, but as many as 100 treatments extending over 12–18 months may be required for satisfactory repigmentation.

Not surprisingly, the major side effects of long-term UV-B phototherapy and PUVA photochemotherapy mimic those seen in individuals with chronic sun exposure and include skin dryness, actinic keratoses, and an increased risk of skin cancer. Despite these risks, the therapeutic index of these modalities continues to be excellent. It is important to choose the most appropriate phototherapeutic approach for a specific dermatologic disease. For example, narrow-band UV-B has been reported in several studies to be as effective as PUVA photochemotherapy in the treatment of psoriasis but to pose a lower risk of skin cancer development than PUVA.

76e Atlas of Skin Manifestations of Internal Disease

Thomas J. Lawley, Calvin O. McCall, Robert A. Swerlick

This is a digital-only chapter. It is available on the DVD that accompanies this book, as well as on Access Medicine/Harrison's Online, and the eBook and "app" editions of HPIM 19e.

In the practice of medicine, virtually every clinician encounters patients with skin disease. Physicians of all specialties face the daily task of determining the nature and clinical implication of dermatologic disease. In patients with skin disease, the physician must confront the question of whether the cutaneous process is confined to the skin, representing a purely dermatologic event, or whether it is a manifestation of internal disease related to the patient's overall medical condition. Evaluation and accurate diagnosis of skin lesions are particularly critical given the marked rise in both melanoma and nonmelanoma skin cancer. Dermatologic conditions can be classified and categorized in many ways. In this atlas, a selected group of inflammatory skin eruptions and neoplastic conditions are grouped in the following manner: (1) common skin diseases and lesions, (2) nonmelanoma skin cancer, (3) melanoma and benign pigmented lesions, (4) infectious disease and the skin, (5) immunologically mediated skin disease, and (6) skin manifestations of internal disease.

77 Anemia and Polycythemia

John W. Adamson, Dan L. Longo

HEMATOPOIESIS AND THE PHYSIOLOGIC BASIS OF RED CELL PRODUCTION

Hematopoiesis is the process by which the formed elements of blood are produced. The process is regulated through a series of steps beginning with the hematopoietic stem cell. Stem cells are capable of producing red cells, all classes of granulocytes, monocytes, platelets, and the cells of the immune system. The precise molecular mechanism—either intrinsic to the stem cell itself or through the action of extrinsic factors—by which the stem cell becomes committed to a given lineage is not fully defined. However, experiments in mice suggest that erythroid cells come from a common erythroid/megakaryocyte progenitor that does not develop in the absence of expression of the GATA-1 and FOG-1 (friend of GATA-1) transcription factors (Chap. 89e). Following lineage commitment, hematopoietic progenitor and precursor cells come increasingly under the regulatory influence of growth factors and hormones. For red cell production, erythropoietin (EPO) is the primary regulatory hormone. EPO is required for the maintenance of committed erythroid progenitor cells that, in the absence of the hormone, undergo programmed cell death (*apoptosis*). The regulated process of red cell production is *erythropoiesis*, and its key elements are illustrated in Fig. 77-1.

In the bone marrow, the first morphologically recognizable erythroid precursor is the pronormoblast. This cell can undergo four to five cell divisions, which result in the production of 16–32 mature red cells. With increased EPO production, or the administration of EPO as a drug, early progenitor cell numbers are amplified and, in turn, give rise to increased numbers of erythrocytes. The regulation of EPO production itself is linked to tissue oxygenation.

In mammals, O_2 is transported to tissues bound to the hemoglobin contained within circulating red cells. The mature red cell is 8 μm in diameter, anucleate, discoid in shape, and extremely pliable in order to traverse the microcirculation successfully; its membrane integrity is maintained by the intracellular generation of ATP. Normal red cell production results in the daily replacement of 0.8–1% of all circulating red cells in the body, since the average red cell lives 100–120 days. The organ responsible for red cell production is called the *erythron*. The erythron is a dynamic organ made up of a rapidly proliferating pool of marrow erythroid precursor cells and a large mass of mature circulating red blood cells. The size of the red cell mass reflects the balance of red cell production and destruction. The physiologic basis of red cell production and destruction provides an understanding of the mechanisms that can lead to anemia.

The physiologic regulator of red cell production, the glycoprotein hormone EPO, is produced and released by peritubular capillary lining cells within the kidney. These cells are highly specialized epithelial-like cells. A small amount of EPO is produced by hepatocytes. The fundamental stimulus for EPO production is the availability of O_2 for tissue metabolic needs. Key to EPO gene regulation is hypoxia-inducible factor (HIF)-1α. In the presence of O_2, HIF-1α is hydroxylated at a key proline, allowing HIF-1α to be ubiquitinated and degraded via the proteasome pathway. If O_2 becomes limiting, this critical hydroxylation step does not occur, allowing HIF-1α to partner with other proteins, translocate to the nucleus, and upregulate the expression of the EPO gene, among others.

Impaired O_2 delivery to the kidney can result from a decreased red cell mass (*anemia*), impaired O_2 loading of the hemoglobin molecule or a high O_2 affinity mutant hemoglobin (*hypoxemia*), or, rarely, impaired blood flow to the kidney (renal artery stenosis). EPO governs the day-to-day production of red cells, and ambient levels of the hormone can be measured in the plasma by sensitive immunoassays—the normal level being 10–25 U/L. When the hemoglobin concentration falls below 100–120 g/L (10–12 g/dL), plasma EPO levels increase in proportion to the severity of the anemia (Fig. 77-2). In circulation, EPO has a half-clearance time of 6–9 h. EPO acts by binding to specific receptors on the surface of marrow erythroid precursors, inducing them to proliferate and to mature. With EPO stimulation, red cell production can increase four- to fivefold within a 1- to 2-week period, but only in the presence of adequate nutrients, especially iron. The functional capacity of the erythron, therefore, requires normal renal production of EPO, a functioning erythroid marrow, and an adequate supply of substrates for hemoglobin synthesis. A defect in any of these key components can lead to anemia. Generally, anemia is recognized in the laboratory when a patient's hemoglobin level or hematocrit is reduced below an expected value (the normal range). The likelihood and severity of anemia are defined based on the deviation of the patient's hemoglobin/hematocrit from values expected for age- and sex-matched normal subjects. The hemoglobin concentration in adults has a Gaussian distribution. The

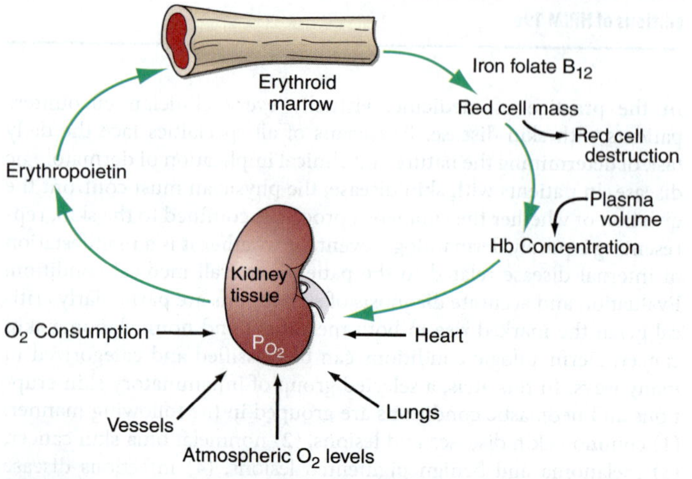

FIGURE 77-1 The physiologic regulation of red cell production by tissue oxygen tension. Hb, hemoglobin.

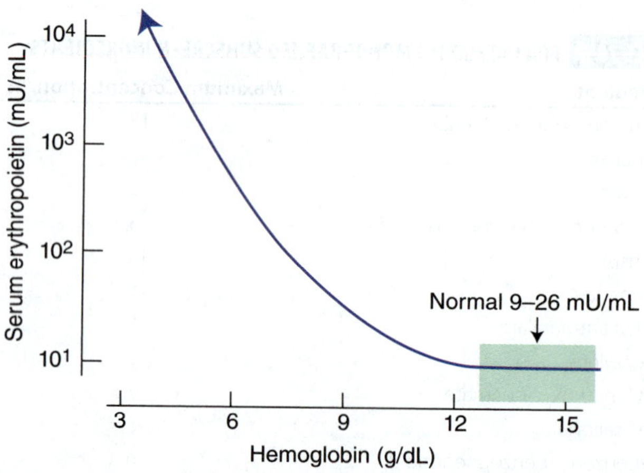

FIGURE 77-2 Erythropoietin (EPO) levels in response to anemia. When the hemoglobin level falls to 120 g/L (12 g/dL), plasma EPO levels increase logarithmically. In the presence of chronic kidney disease or chronic inflammation, EPO levels are typically lower than expected for the degree of anemia. As individuals age, the level of EPO needed to sustain normal hemoglobin levels appears to increase. *(From RS Hillman et al: Hematology in Clinical Practice, 5th ed. New York, McGraw-Hill, 2010.)*

mean hematocrit value for adult males is 47% (standard deviation, ±7%) and that for adult females is 42% (±5%). Any single hematocrit or hemoglobin value carries with it a likelihood of associated anemia. Thus, a hematocrit of <39% in an adult male or <35% in an adult female has only about a 25% chance of being normal. Hematocrit levels are less useful than hemoglobin levels in assessing anemia because they are calculated rather than measured directly. Suspected low hemoglobin or hematocrit values are more easily interpreted if previous values for the same patient are known for comparison. The World Health Organization (WHO) defines anemia as a hemoglobin level <130 g/L (13 g/dL) in men and <120 g/L (12 g/dL) in women.

The critical elements of erythropoiesis—EPO production, iron availability, the proliferative capacity of the bone marrow, and effective maturation of red cell precursors—are used for the initial classification of anemia (see below).

ANEMIA

CLINICAL PRESENTATION OF ANEMIA

Signs and Symptoms Anemia is most often recognized by abnormal screening laboratory tests. Patients less commonly present with advanced anemia and its attendant signs and symptoms. Acute anemia is due to blood loss or hemolysis. If blood loss is mild, enhanced O_2 delivery is achieved through changes in the O_2–hemoglobin dissociation curve mediated by a decreased pH or increased CO_2 (*Bohr effect*). With acute blood loss, hypovolemia dominates the clinical picture, and the hematocrit and hemoglobin levels do not reflect the volume of blood lost. Signs of vascular instability appear with acute losses of 10–15% of the total blood volume. In such patients, the issue is not anemia but hypotension and decreased organ perfusion. When >30% of the blood volume is lost suddenly, patients are unable to compensate with the usual mechanisms of vascular contraction and changes in regional blood flow. The patient prefers to remain supine and will show postural hypotension and tachycardia. If the volume of blood lost is >40% (i.e., >2 L in the average-sized adult), signs of hypovolemic shock including confusion, dyspnea, diaphoresis, hypotension, and tachycardia appear (Chap. 129). Such patients have significant deficits in vital organ perfusion and require immediate volume replacement.

With acute hemolysis, the signs and symptoms depend on the mechanism that leads to red cell destruction. Intravascular hemolysis with release of free hemoglobin may be associated with acute back pain, free hemoglobin in the plasma and urine, and renal failure. Symptoms associated with more chronic or progressive anemia depend on the age of the patient and the adequacy of blood supply to critical organs. Symptoms associated with moderate anemia include fatigue, loss of stamina, breathlessness, and tachycardia (particularly with physical exertion). However, because of the intrinsic compensatory mechanisms that govern the O_2–hemoglobin dissociation curve, the gradual onset of anemia—particularly in young patients—may not be associated with signs or symptoms until the anemia is severe (hemoglobin <70–80 g/L [7–8 g/dL]). When anemia develops over a period of days or weeks, the total blood volume is normal to slightly increased, and changes in cardiac output and regional blood flow help compensate for the overall loss in O_2-carrying capacity. Changes in the position of the O_2–hemoglobin dissociation curve account for some of the compensatory response to anemia. With chronic anemia, intracellular levels of 2,3-bisphosphoglycerate rise, shifting the dissociation curve to the right and facilitating O_2 unloading. This compensatory mechanism can only maintain normal tissue O_2 delivery in the face of a 20–30 g/L (2–3 g/dL) deficit in hemoglobin concentration. Finally, further protection of O_2 delivery to vital organs is achieved by the shunting of blood away from organs that are relatively rich in blood supply, particularly the kidney, gut, and skin.

Certain disorders are commonly associated with anemia. Chronic inflammatory states (e.g., infection, rheumatoid arthritis, cancer) are associated with mild to moderate anemia, whereas lymphoproliferative disorders, such as chronic lymphocytic leukemia and certain other B cell neoplasms, may be associated with autoimmune hemolysis.

APPROACH TO THE PATIENT: Anemia

The evaluation of the patient with anemia requires a careful history and physical examination. Nutritional history related to drugs or alcohol intake and family history of anemia should always be assessed. Certain geographic backgrounds and ethnic origins are associated with an increased likelihood of an inherited disorder of the hemoglobin molecule or intermediary metabolism. Glucose-6-phosphate dehydrogenase (G6PD) deficiency and certain hemoglobinopathies are seen more commonly in those of Middle Eastern or African origin, including African Americans who have a high frequency of G6PD deficiency. Other information that may be useful includes exposure to certain toxic agents or drugs and symptoms related to other disorders commonly associated with anemia. These include symptoms and signs such as bleeding, fatigue, malaise, fever, weight loss, night sweats, and other systemic symptoms. Clues to the mechanisms of anemia may be provided on physical examination by findings of infection, blood in the stool, lymphadenopathy, splenomegaly, or petechiae. Splenomegaly and lymphadenopathy suggest an underlying lymphoproliferative disease, whereas petechiae suggest platelet dysfunction. Past laboratory measurements are helpful to determine a time of onset.

In the anemic patient, physical examination may demonstrate a forceful heartbeat, strong peripheral pulses, and a systolic "flow" murmur. The skin and mucous membranes may be pale if the hemoglobin is <80–100 g/L (8–10 g/dL). This part of the physical examination should focus on areas where vessels are close to the surface such as the mucous membranes, nail beds, and palmar creases. If the palmar creases are lighter in color than the surrounding skin when the hand is hyperextended, the hemoglobin level is usually <80 g/L (8 g/dL).

LABORATORY EVALUATION

Table 77-1 lists the tests used in the initial workup of anemia. A routine complete blood count (CBC) is required as part of the evaluation and includes the hemoglobin, hematocrit, and red cell indices: the mean cell volume (MCV) in femtoliters, mean cell hemoglobin (MCH) in picograms per cell, and mean concentration of hemoglobin per volume of red cells (MCHC) in grams per liter (non-SI: grams per deciliter). The red cell indices are calculated as shown in Table 77-2, and the normal variations in the hemoglobin and hematocrit with age are shown in Table 77-3. A number of physiologic factors affect the CBC, including age, sex, pregnancy, smoking, and altitude. High-normal hemoglobin values may be seen in men and women who live at altitude or smoke heavily. Hemoglobin elevations due to smoking reflect normal compensation due to the displacement of O_2 by CO in hemoglobin binding. Other important information is provided by the reticulocyte count and measurements of iron supply including *serum iron, total iron-binding capacity* (TIBC; an indirect measure of serum transferrin), and *serum ferritin*. Marked alterations in the red cell indices usually reflect disorders of maturation or iron deficiency. A careful evaluation of the peripheral blood smear is important, and clinical laboratories often provide a description of both the red and white cells, a white cell differential count, and the platelet count. In patients with severe anemia and abnormalities in red blood cell morphology and/or low reticulocyte counts, a bone marrow aspirate or biopsy can assist in the diagnosis. Other tests of value in the diagnosis of specific anemias are discussed in chapters on specific disease states.

The components of the CBC also help in the classification of anemia. *Microcytosis* is reflected by a lower than normal MCV (<80), whereas high values (>100) reflect *macrocytosis*. The MCH and MCHC reflect defects in hemoglobin synthesis (*hypochromia*). Automated cell counters describe the red cell volume distribution width (RDW). The MCV (representing the peak of the distribution curve) is insensitive to the appearance of small populations of macrocytes or microcytes. An experienced laboratory technician

TABLE 77-1 LABORATORY TESTS IN ANEMIA DIAGNOSIS

I. Complete blood count (CBC)
  A. Red blood cell count
    1. Hemoglobin
    2. Hematocrit
    3. Reticulocyte count
  B. Red blood cell indices
    1. Mean cell volume (MCV)
    2. Mean cell hemoglobin (MCH)
    3. Mean cell hemoglobin concentration (MCHC)
    4. Red cell distribution width (RDW)
  C. White blood cell count
    1. Cell differential
    2. Nuclear segmentation of neutrophils
  D. Platelet count
  E. Cell morphology
    1. Cell size
    2. Hemoglobin content
    3. Anisocytosis
    4. Poikilocytosis
    5. Polychromasia
II. Iron supply studies
  A. Serum iron
  B. Total iron-binding capacity
  C. Serum ferritin
III. Marrow examination
  A. Aspirate
    1. M/E ratio[a]
    2. Cell morphology
    3. Iron stain
  B. Biopsy
    1. Cellularity
    2. Morphology

[a]M/E ratio, ratio of myeloid to erythroid precursors.

TABLE 77-2 RED BLOOD CELL INDICES

Index	Normal Value
Mean cell volume (MCV) = (hematocrit × 10)/(red cell count × 10[6])	90 ± 8 fL
Mean cell hemoglobin (MCH) = (hemoglobin × 10)/(red cell count × 10[6])	30 ± 3 pg
Mean cell hemoglobin concentration = (hemoglobin × 10)/hematocrit, or MCH/MCV	33 ± 2%

TABLE 77-3 CHANGES IN NORMAL HEMOGLOBIN/HEMATOCRIT VALUES WITH AGE, SEX, AND PREGNANCY

Age/Sex	Hemoglobin, g/dL	Hematocrit, %
At birth	17	52
Childhood	12	36
Adolescence	13	40
Adult man	16 (±2)	47 (±6)
Adult woman (menstruating)	13 (±2)	40 (±6)
Adult woman (postmenopausal)	14 (±2)	42 (±6)
During pregnancy	12 (±2)	37 (±6)

Source: From RS Hillman et al: *Hematology in Clinical Practice*, 5th ed. New York, McGraw-Hill, 2010.

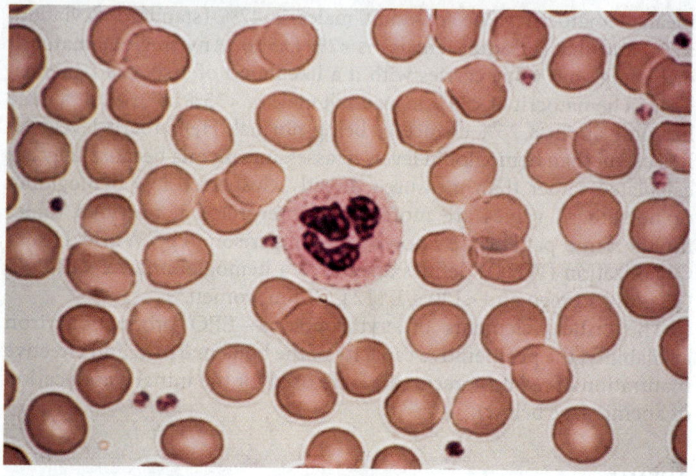

FIGURE 77-3 Normal blood smear (Wright stain). High-power field showing normal red cells, a neutrophil, and a few platelets. *(From RS Hillman et al: Hematology in Clinical Practice, 5th ed. New York, McGraw-Hill, 2010.)*

will be able to identify minor populations of large or small cells or hypochromic cells before the red cell indices change.

Peripheral Blood Smear The peripheral blood smear provides important information about defects in red cell production (Chap. 81e). As a complement to the red cell indices, the blood smear also reveals variations in cell size (*anisocytosis*) and shape (*poikilocytosis*). The degree of anisocytosis usually correlates with increases in the RDW or the range of cell sizes. Poikilocytosis suggests a defect in the maturation of red cell precursors in the bone marrow or fragmentation of circulating red cells. The blood smear may also reveal *polychromasia*—red cells that are slightly larger than normal and grayish blue in color on the Wright-Giemsa stain. These cells are reticulocytes that have been prematurely released from the bone marrow, and their color represents residual amounts of ribosomal RNA. These cells appear in circulation in response to EPO stimulation or to architectural damage of the bone marrow (fibrosis, infiltration of the marrow by malignant cells, etc.) that results in their disordered release from the marrow. The appearance of nucleated red cells, Howell-Jolly bodies, target cells, sickle cells, and others may provide clues to specific disorders (Figs. 77-3 to 77-11).

Reticulocyte Count An accurate reticulocyte count is key to the initial classification of anemia. Reticulocytes are red cells that

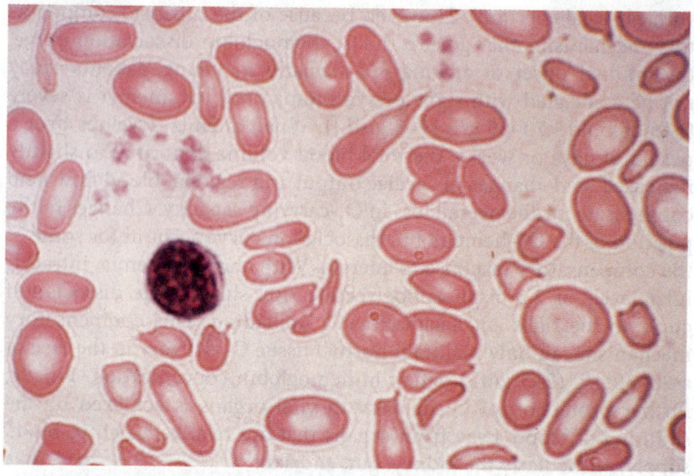

FIGURE 77-4 Severe iron-deficiency anemia. Microcytic and hypochromic red cells smaller than the nucleus of a lymphocyte associated with marked variation in size (anisocytosis) and shape (poikilocytosis). *(From RS Hillman et al: Hematology in Clinical Practice, 5th ed. New York, McGraw-Hill, 2010.)*

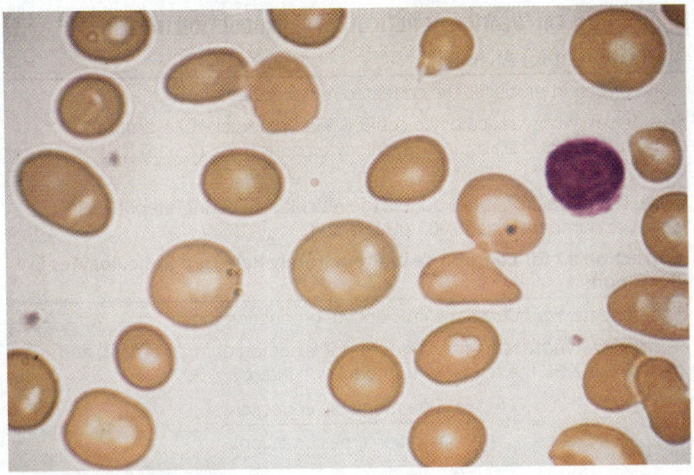

FIGURE 77-5 Macrocytosis. Red cells are larger than a small lymphocyte and well hemoglobinized. Often macrocytes are oval shaped (macro-ovalocytes).

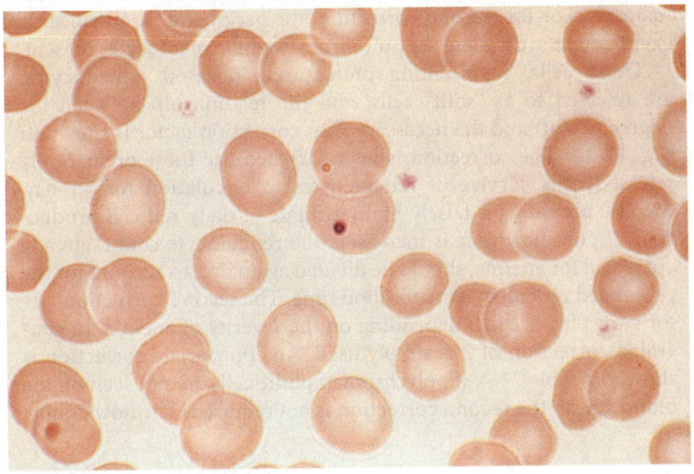

FIGURE 77-6 Howell-Jolly bodies. In the absence of a functional spleen, nuclear remnants are not culled from the red cells and remain as small homogeneously staining blue inclusions on Wright stain. *(From RS Hillman et al: Hematology in Clinical Practice, 5th ed. New York, McGraw-Hill, 2010.)*

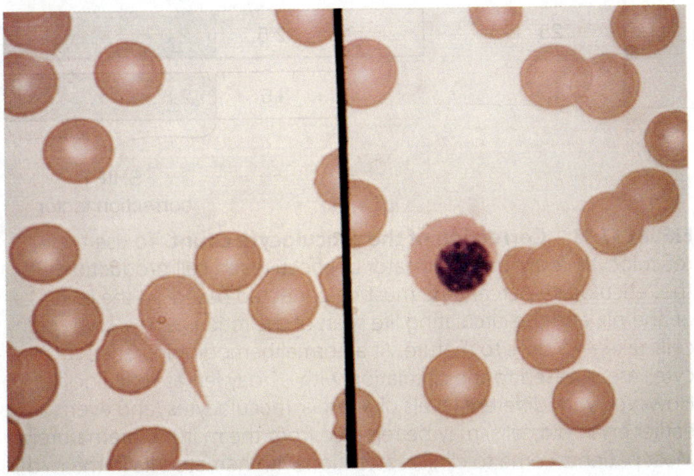

FIGURE 77-7 Red cell changes in myelofibrosis. The left panel shows a teardrop-shaped cell. The right panel shows a nucleated red cell. These forms can be seen in myelofibrosis.

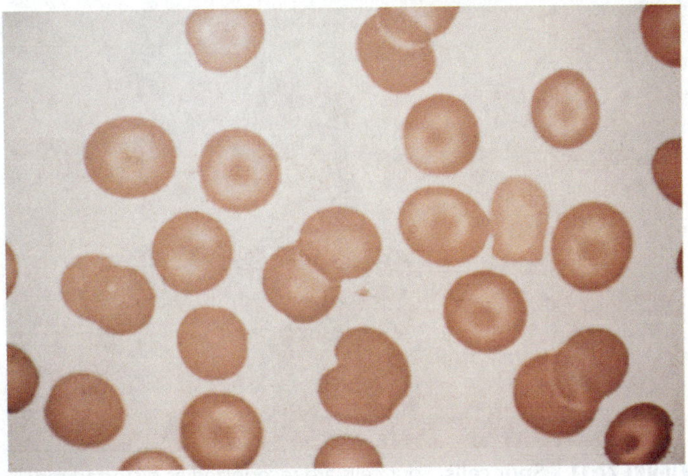

FIGURE 77-8 Target cells. Target cells have a bull's-eye appearance and are seen in thalassemia and in liver disease. *(From RS Hillman et al: Hematology in Clinical Practice, 5th ed. New York, McGraw-Hill, 2010.)*

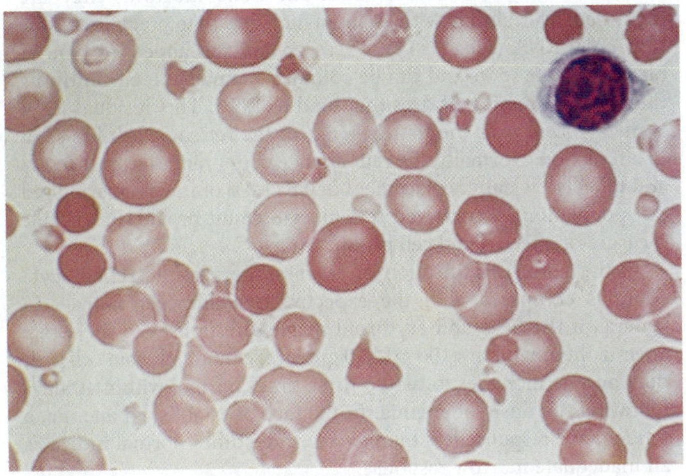

FIGURE 77-9 Red cell fragmentation. Red cells may become fragmented in the presence of foreign bodies in the circulation, such as mechanical heart valves, or in the setting of thermal injury. *(From RS Hillman et al: Hematology in Clinical Practice, 5th ed. New York, McGraw-Hill, 2010.)*

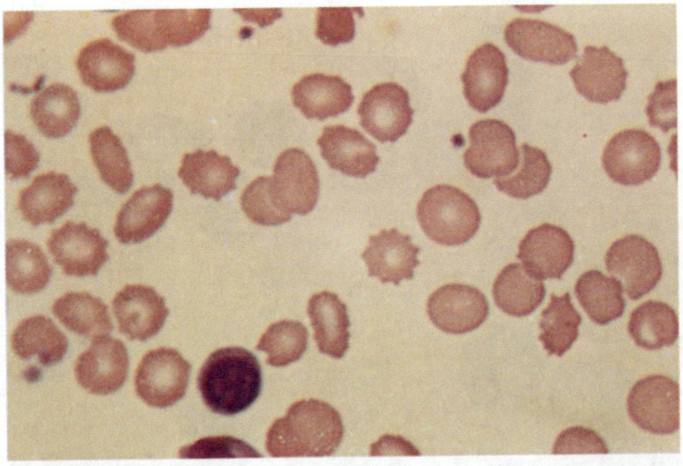

FIGURE 77-10 Uremia. The red cells in uremia may acquire numerous regularly spaced, small, spiny projections. Such cells, called burr cells or echinocytes, are readily distinguishable from irregularly spiculated acanthocytes shown in Fig. 77-11.

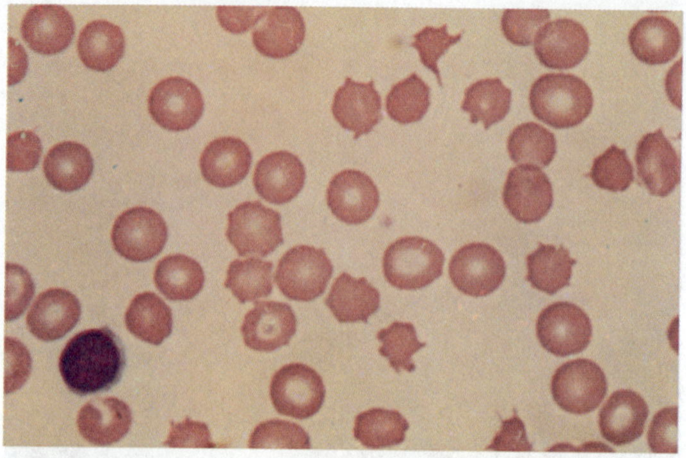

FIGURE 77-11 Spur cells. Spur cells are recognized as distorted red cells containing several irregularly distributed thornlike projections. Cells with this morphologic abnormality are also called acanthocytes. *(From RS Hillman et al: Hematology in Clinical Practice, 5th ed. New York, McGraw-Hill, 2010.)*

have been recently released from the bone marrow. They are identified by staining with a supravital dye that precipitates the ribosomal RNA (Fig. 77-12). These precipitates appear as blue or black punctate spots and can be counted manually or, currently, by fluorescent emission of dyes that bind to RNA. This residual RNA is metabolized over the first 24–36 h of the reticulocyte's life span in circulation. Normally, the reticulocyte count ranges from 1 to 2% and reflects the daily replacement of 0.8–1.0% of the circulating red cell population. A corrected reticulocyte count provides a reliable measure of effective red cell production.

In the initial classification of anemia, the patient's reticulocyte count is compared with the expected reticulocyte response. In general, if the EPO and erythroid marrow responses to moderate anemia [hemoglobin <100 g/L (10 g/dL)] are intact, the red cell production rate increases to two to three times normal within 10 days following the onset of anemia. In the face of established anemia, a reticulocyte response less than two to three times normal indicates an inadequate marrow response.

To use the reticulocyte count to estimate marrow response, two corrections are necessary. The first correction adjusts the reticulocyte count based on the reduced number of circulating red cells. With anemia, the percentage of reticulocytes may be increased while the absolute number is unchanged. To correct for this effect, the reticulocyte percentage is multiplied by the ratio of the patient's hemoglobin or hematocrit to the expected hemoglobin/hematocrit for the age and sex of the patient (Table 77-4). This provides an estimate of the reticulocyte count corrected for anemia. To convert the corrected reticulocyte count to an index of marrow production, a further correction is required, depending on whether some of the reticulocytes in circulation have been released from the marrow prematurely. For this second correction, the peripheral blood smear is examined to see if there are polychromatophilic macrocytes present.

These cells, representing prematurely released reticulocytes, are referred to as "shift" cells, and the relationship between the degree of shift and the necessary shift correction factor is shown in Fig. 77-13. The correction is necessary because these prematurely released cells survive as reticulocytes in circulation for >1 day, thereby providing a falsely high estimate of daily red cell production. If polychromasia is increased, the reticulocyte count, already corrected for anemia, should be divided again by 2 to account for the prolonged reticulocyte maturation time. The second correction factor varies from 1 to 3 depending on the severity of anemia. In general, a correction of 2 is simply used. An appropriate correction is shown in Table 77-4. If polychromatophilic cells are not seen on the blood smear, the second correction is not required. The now doubly

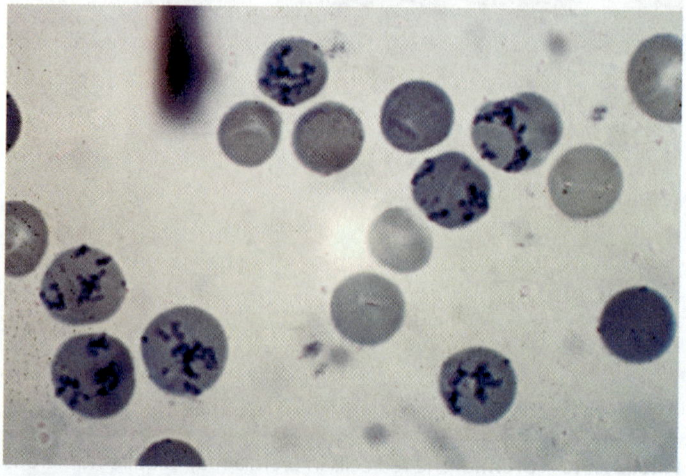

FIGURE 77-12 Reticulocytes. Methylene blue stain demonstrates residual RNA in newly made red cells. *(From RS Hillman et al: Hematology in Clinical Practice, 5th ed. New York, McGraw-Hill, 2010.)*

TABLE 77-4 CALCULATION OF RETICULOCYTE PRODUCTION INDEX

Correction #1 for Anemia:
This correction produces the corrected reticulocyte count.
In a person whose reticulocyte count is 9%, hemoglobin 7.5 g/dL, and hematocrit 23%, the absolute reticulocyte count = 9 × (7.5/15) [or × (23/45)] = 4.5%
Note. This correction is not done if the reticulocyte count is reported in absolute numbers (e.g., 50,000/μL of blood)
Correction #2 for Longer Life of Prematurely Released Reticulocytes in the Blood:
This correction produces the reticulocyte production index.
In a person whose reticulocyte count is 9%, hemoglobin 7.5 gm/dL, and hematocrit 23%, the reticulocyte production index
$= 9 \times \frac{(7.5/15)(\text{hemoglobin correction})}{2(\text{maturation time correction})} = 2.25$

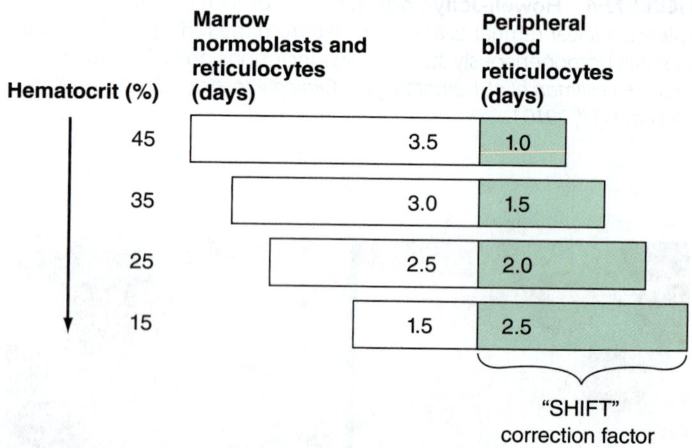

FIGURE 77-13 Correction of the reticulocyte count. To use the reticulocyte count as an indicator of effective red cell production, the reticulocyte percentage must be corrected based on the level of anemia and the circulating life span of the reticulocytes. Erythroid cells take ~4.5 days to mature. At a normal hemoglobin, reticulocytes are released to the circulation with ~1 day left as reticulocytes. However, with different levels of anemia, reticulocytes (and even earlier erythroid cells) may be released from the marrow prematurely. Most patients come to clinical attention with hematocrits in the mid-20s, and thus a correction factor of 2 is commonly used because the observed reticulocytes will live for 2 days in the circulation before losing their RNA.

TABLE 77-5 NORMAL MARROW RESPONSE TO ANEMIA

Hemoglobin	Production Index	Reticulocyte Count
15 g/dL	1	50,000/μL
11 g/dL	2.0–2.5	100–150,000/μL
8 g/dL	3.0–4.0	300–400,000/μL

corrected reticulocyte count is the *reticulocyte production index*, and it provides an estimate of marrow production relative to normal. In many hospital laboratories, the reticulocyte count is reported not only as a percentage but also in absolute numbers. If so, no correction for dilution is required. A summary of the appropriate marrow response to varying degrees of anemia is shown in Table 77-5.

Premature release of reticulocytes is normally due to increased EPO stimulation. However, if the integrity of the bone marrow release process is lost through tumor infiltration, fibrosis, or other disorders, the appearance of nucleated red cells or polychromatophilic macrocytes should still invoke the second reticulocyte correction. The shift correction should always be applied to a patient with anemia and a very high reticulocyte count to provide a true index of effective red cell production. Patients with severe chronic hemolytic anemia may increase red cell production as much as six- to sevenfold. This measure alone confirms the fact that the patient has an appropriate EPO response, a normally functioning bone marrow, and sufficient iron available to meet the demands for new red cell formation. If the reticulocyte production index is <2 in the face of established anemia, a defect in erythroid marrow proliferation or maturation must be present.

Tests of Iron Supply and Storage The laboratory measurements that reflect the availability of iron for hemoglobin synthesis include the serum iron, the TIBC, and the percent transferrin saturation. The percent transferrin saturation is derived by dividing the serum iron level (× 100) by the TIBC. The normal serum iron ranges from 9 to 27 μmol/L (50–150 μg/dL), whereas the normal TIBC is 54–64 μmol/L (300–360 μg/dL); the normal transferrin saturation ranges from 25 to 50%. A diurnal variation in the serum iron leads to a variation in the percent transferrin saturation. The serum ferritin is used to evaluate total body iron stores. Adult males have serum ferritin levels that average ~100 μg/L, corresponding to iron stores of ~1 g. Adult females have lower serum ferritin levels averaging 30 μg/L, reflecting lower iron stores (~300 mg). A serum ferritin level of 10–15 μg/L indicates depletion of body iron stores. However, ferritin is also an acute-phase reactant and, in the presence of acute or chronic inflammation, may rise several-fold above baseline levels. As a rule, a serum ferritin >200 μg/L means there is at least some iron in tissue stores.

Bone Marrow Examination A bone marrow aspirate and smear or a needle biopsy can be useful in the evaluation of some patients with anemia. In patients with hypoproliferative anemia and normal iron status, a bone marrow is indicated. Marrow examination can diagnose primary marrow disorders such as myelofibrosis, a red cell maturation defect, or an infiltrative disease (Figs. 77-14 to 77-16). The increase or decrease of one cell lineage (myeloid vs erythroid) compared to another is obtained by a differential count of nucleated cells in a bone marrow smear (the myeloid/erythroid [M/E] ratio). A patient with a hypoproliferative anemia (see below) and a reticulocyte production index <2 will demonstrate an M/E ratio of 2 or 3:1. In contrast, patients with hemolytic disease and a production index >3 will have an M/E ratio of at least 1:1. Maturation disorders are identified from the discrepancy between the M/E ratio and the reticulocyte production index (see below). Either the marrow smear or biopsy can be stained for the presence of iron stores or iron in developing red cells. The storage iron is in the form of ferritin or *hemosiderin*. On carefully prepared bone marrow smears, small ferritin granules can normally be seen under oil immersion in 20–40% of developing erythroblasts. Such cells are called *sideroblasts*.

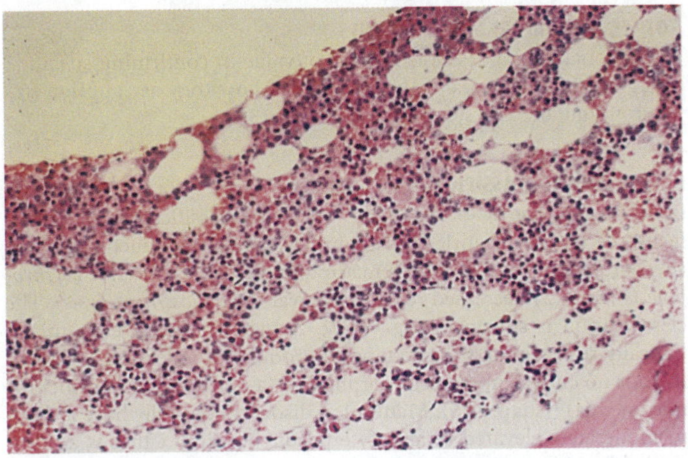

FIGURE 77-14 Normal bone marrow. This is a low-power view of a section of a normal bone marrow biopsy stained with hematoxylin and eosin (H&E). Note that the nucleated cellular elements account for ~40–50% and the fat (clear areas) accounts for ~50–60% of the area. *(From RS Hillman et al: Hematology in Clinical Practice, 5th ed. New York, McGraw-Hill, 2010.)*

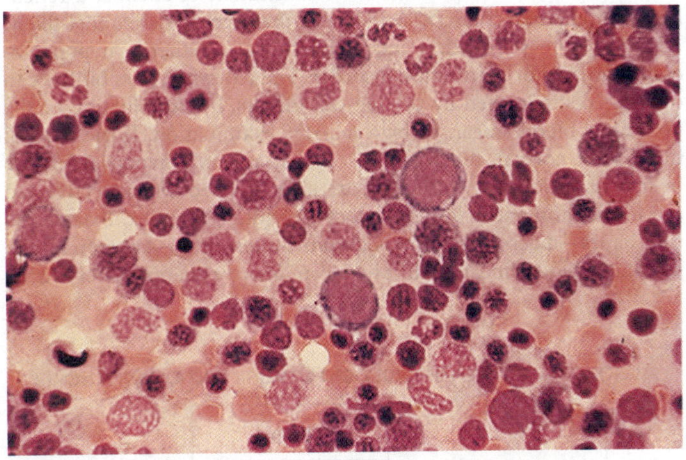

FIGURE 77-15 Erythroid hyperplasia. This marrow shows an increase in the fraction of cells in the erythroid lineage as might be seen when a normal marrow compensates for acute blood loss or hemolysis. The myeloid/erythroid (M/E) ratio is about 1:1. *(From RS Hillman et al: Hematology in Clinical Practice, 5th ed. New York, McGraw-Hill, 2010.)*

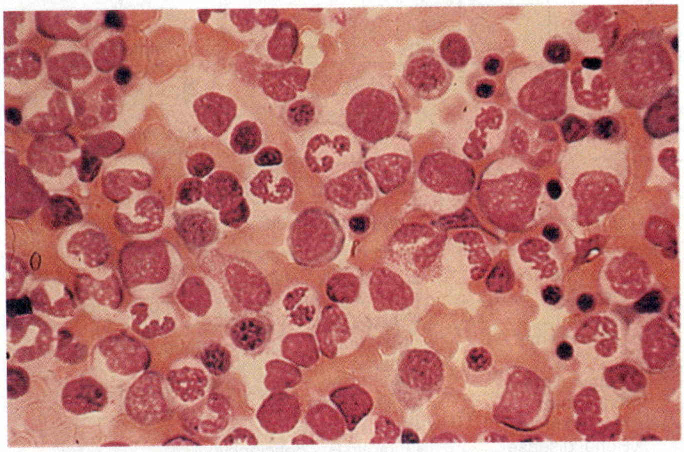

FIGURE 77-16 Myeloid hyperplasia. This marrow shows an increase in the fraction of cells in the myeloid or granulocytic lineage as might be seen in a normal marrow responding to infection. The myeloid/erythroid (M/E) ratio is >3:1. *(From RS Hillman et al: Hematology in Clinical Practice, 5th ed. New York, McGraw-Hill, 2010.)*

OTHER LABORATORY MEASUREMENTS

Additional laboratory tests may be of value in confirming specific diagnoses. For details of these tests and how they are applied in individual disorders, see Chaps. 126 to 130.

DEFINITION AND CLASSIFICATION OF ANEMIA

Initial Classification of Anemia The functional classification of anemia has three major categories. These are (1) marrow production defects (*hypoproliferation*), (2) red cell maturation defects (*ineffective erythropoiesis*), and (3) decreased red cell survival (*blood loss/hemolysis*). The classification is shown in Fig. 77-17. A hypoproliferative anemia is typically seen with a low reticulocyte production index together with little or no change in red cell morphology (a normocytic, normochromic anemia) (Chap. 126). Maturation disorders typically have a slight to moderately elevated reticulocyte production index that is accompanied by either macrocytic (Chap. 128) or microcytic (Chaps. 126, 127) red cell indices. Increased red blood cell destruction secondary to hemolysis results in an increase in the reticulocyte production index to at least three times normal (Chap. 129), provided sufficient iron is available. Hemorrhagic anemia does not typically result in production indices of more than 2.0–2.5 times normal because of the limitations placed on expansion of the erythroid marrow by iron availability.

In the first branch point of the classification of anemia, a reticulocyte production index >2.5 indicates that hemolysis is most likely. A reticulocyte production index <2 indicates either a hypoproliferative anemia or maturation disorder. The latter two possibilities can often be distinguished by the red cell indices, by examination of the peripheral blood smear, or by a marrow examination. If the red cell indices are normal, the anemia is almost certainly hypoproliferative in nature. Maturation disorders are characterized by ineffective red cell production and a low reticulocyte production index. Bizarre red cell shapes—macrocytes or hypochromic microcytes—are seen on the peripheral blood smear. With a hypoproliferative anemia, no erythroid

ALGORITHM OF THE PHYSIOLOGIC CLASSIFICATION OF ANEMIA

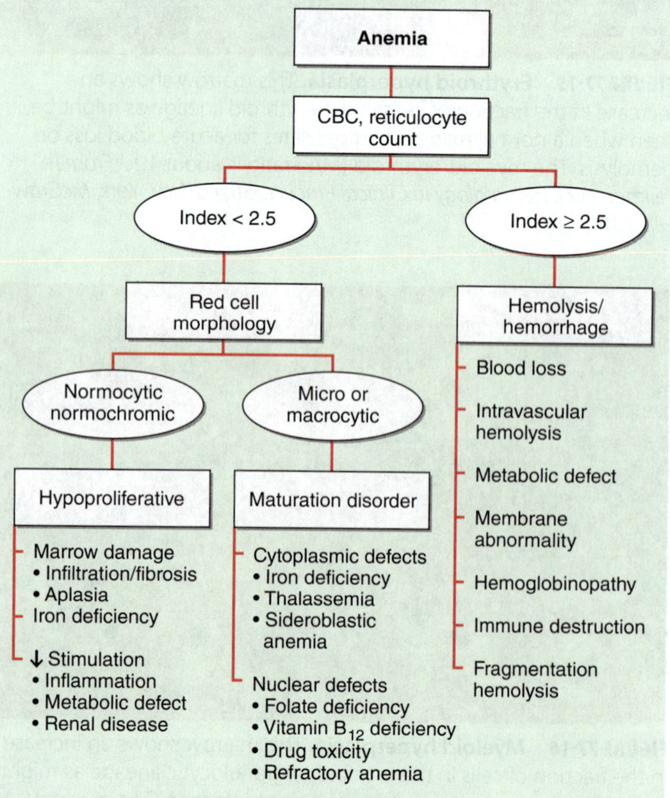

FIGURE 77-17 The physiologic classification of anemia. CBC, complete blood count.

hyperplasia is noted in the marrow, whereas patients with ineffective red cell production have erythroid hyperplasia and an M/E ratio <1:1.

Hypoproliferative Anemias At least 75% of all cases of anemia are hypoproliferative in nature. A hypoproliferative anemia reflects absolute or relative marrow failure in which the erythroid marrow has not proliferated appropriately for the degree of anemia. The majority of hypoproliferative anemias are due to mild to moderate iron deficiency or inflammation. A hypoproliferative anemia can result from marrow damage, iron deficiency, or inadequate EPO stimulation. The last may reflect impaired renal function, suppression of EPO production by inflammatory cytokines such as interleukin 1, or reduced tissue needs for O_2 from metabolic disease such as hypothyroidism. Only occasionally is the marrow unable to produce red cells at a normal rate, and this is most prevalent in patients with renal failure. With diabetes mellitus or myeloma, the EPO deficiency may be more marked than would be predicted by the degree of renal insufficiency. In general, hypoproliferative anemias are characterized by normocytic, normochromic red cells, although microcytic, hypochromic cells may be observed with mild iron deficiency or long-standing chronic inflammatory disease. The key laboratory tests in distinguishing between the various forms of hypoproliferative anemia include the serum iron and iron-binding capacity, evaluation of renal and thyroid function, a marrow biopsy or aspirate to detect marrow damage or infiltrative disease, and serum ferritin to assess iron stores. An iron stain of the marrow will determine the pattern of iron distribution. Patients with the anemia of acute or chronic inflammation show a distinctive pattern of serum iron (low), TIBC (normal or low), percent transferrin saturation (low), and serum ferritin (normal or high). These changes in iron values are brought about by hepcidin, the iron regulatory hormone that is produced by the liver and is increased in inflammation (Chap. 126). A distinct pattern of results is noted in mild to moderate iron deficiency (low serum iron, high TIBC, low percent transferrin saturation, low serum ferritin) (Chap. 126). Marrow damage by drugs, infiltrative disease such as leukemia or lymphoma, or marrow aplasia is diagnosed from the peripheral blood and bone marrow morphology. With infiltrative disease or fibrosis, a marrow biopsy is required.

Maturation Disorders The presence of anemia with an inappropriately low reticulocyte production index, macro- or microcytosis on smear, and abnormal red cell indices suggests a maturation disorder. Maturation disorders are divided into two categories: nuclear maturation defects, associated with macrocytosis, and cytoplasmic maturation defects, associated with microcytosis and hypochromia usually from defects in hemoglobin synthesis. The inappropriately low reticulocyte production index is a reflection of the ineffective erythropoiesis that results from the destruction within the marrow of developing erythroblasts. Bone marrow examination shows erythroid hyperplasia.

Nuclear maturation defects result from vitamin B_{12} or folic acid deficiency, drug damage, or myelodysplasia. Drugs that interfere with cellular DNA synthesis, such as methotrexate or alkylating agents, can produce a nuclear maturation defect. Alcohol, alone, is also capable of producing macrocytosis and a variable degree of anemia, but this is usually associated with folic acid deficiency. Measurements of folic acid and vitamin B_{12} are critical not only in identifying the specific vitamin deficiency but also because they reflect different pathogenetic mechanisms (Chap. 128).

Cytoplasmic maturation defects result from severe iron deficiency or abnormalities in globin or heme synthesis. Iron deficiency occupies an unusual position in the classification of anemia. If the iron-deficiency anemia is mild to moderate, erythroid marrow proliferation is blunted and the anemia is classified as hypoproliferative. However, if the anemia is severe and prolonged, the erythroid marrow will become hyperplastic despite the inadequate iron supply, and the anemia will be classified as ineffective erythropoiesis with a cytoplasmic maturation defect. In either case, an inappropriately low reticulocyte production index, microcytosis, and a classic pattern of iron values make the diagnosis clear and easily distinguish iron deficiency from other cytoplasmic maturation defects such as the thalassemias. Defects in heme synthesis, in contrast to globin synthesis, are less common and may be acquired or inherited (Chap. 430). Acquired abnormalities are usually associated with myelodysplasia, may lead to either a macro- or microcytic anemia, and are frequently associated with mitochondrial iron loading. In these cases, iron is taken up by the mitochondria of the developing erythroid cell but not incorporated into heme. The iron-encrusted mitochondria surround the nucleus of the erythroid cell, forming a ring. Based on the distinctive finding of so-called ringed sideroblasts on the marrow iron stain, patients are diagnosed as having a sideroblastic anemia—almost always reflecting myelodysplasia. Again, studies of iron parameters are helpful in the differential diagnosis of these patients.

Blood Loss/Hemolytic Anemia In contrast to anemias associated with an inappropriately low reticulocyte production index, hemolysis is associated with red cell production indices ≥2.5 times normal. The stimulated erythropoiesis is reflected in the blood smear by the appearance of increased numbers of polychromatophilic macrocytes. A marrow examination is rarely indicated if the reticulocyte production index is increased appropriately. The red cell indices are typically normocytic or slightly macrocytic, reflecting the increased number of reticulocytes. Acute blood loss is not associated with an increased reticulocyte production index because of the time required to increase EPO production and, subsequently, marrow proliferation. Subacute blood loss may be associated with modest reticulocytosis. Anemia from chronic blood loss presents more often as iron deficiency than with the picture of increased red cell production.

The evaluation of blood loss anemia is usually not difficult. Most problems arise when a patient presents with an increased red cell production index from an episode of acute blood loss that went unrecognized. The cause of the anemia and increased red cell production may not be obvious. The confirmation of a recovering state may require observations over a period of 2–3 weeks, during which the hemoglobin concentration will rise and the reticulocyte production index fall (Chap. 129).

Hemolytic disease, while dramatic, is among the least common forms of anemia. The ability to sustain a high reticulocyte production index reflects the ability of the erythroid marrow to compensate for hemolysis and, in the case of extravascular hemolysis, the efficient recycling of iron from the destroyed red cells to support red cell production. With intravascular hemolysis, such as paroxysmal nocturnal hemoglobinuria, the loss of iron may limit the marrow response. The level of response depends on the severity of the anemia and the nature of the underlying disease process.

Hemoglobinopathies, such as sickle cell disease and the thalassemias, present a mixed picture. The reticulocyte index may be high but is inappropriately low for the degree of marrow erythroid hyperplasia (Chap. 127).

Hemolytic anemias present in different ways. Some appear suddenly as an acute, self-limited episode of intravascular or extravascular hemolysis, a presentation pattern often seen in patients with autoimmune hemolysis or with inherited defects of the Embden-Meyerhof pathway or the glutathione reductase pathway. Patients with inherited disorders of the hemoglobin molecule or red cell membrane generally have a lifelong clinical history typical of the disease process. Those with chronic hemolytic disease, such as hereditary spherocytosis, may actually present not with anemia but with a complication stemming from the prolonged increase in red cell destruction such as symptomatic bilirubin gallstones or splenomegaly. Patients with chronic hemolysis are also susceptible to aplastic crises if an infectious process interrupts red cell production.

The differential diagnosis of an acute or chronic hemolytic event requires the careful integration of family history, the pattern of clinical presentation, and—whether the disease is congenital or acquired—careful examination of the peripheral blood smear. Precise diagnosis may require more specialized laboratory tests, such as hemoglobin electrophoresis or a screen for red cell enzymes. Acquired defects in red cell survival are often immunologically mediated and require a direct or indirect antiglobulin test or a cold agglutinin titer to detect the presence of hemolytic antibodies or complement-mediated red cell destruction (Chap. 129).

TREATMENT ANEMIA

An overriding principle is to initiate treatment of mild to moderate anemia only when a specific diagnosis is made. Rarely, in the acute setting, anemia may be so severe that red cell transfusions are required before a specific diagnosis is available. Whether the anemia is of acute or gradual onset, the selection of the appropriate treatment is determined by the documented cause(s) of the anemia. Often, the cause of the anemia is multifactorial. For example, a patient with severe rheumatoid arthritis who has been taking anti-inflammatory drugs may have a hypoproliferative anemia associated with chronic inflammation as well as chronic blood loss associated with intermittent gastrointestinal bleeding. In every circumstance, it is important to evaluate the patient's iron status fully before and during the treatment of any anemia. **Transfusion is discussed in Chap. 138e; iron therapy is discussed in Chap. 126; treatment of megaloblastic anemia is discussed in Chap. 128; treatment of other entities is discussed in their respective chapters (sickle cell anemia, Chap. 127; hemolytic anemias, Chap. 129; aplastic anemia and myelodysplasia, Chap. 130).**

Therapeutic options for the treatment of anemias have expanded dramatically during the past 30 years. Blood component therapy is available and safe. Recombinant EPO as an adjunct to anemia management has transformed the lives of patients with chronic renal failure on dialysis and reduced transfusion needs of anemic cancer patients receiving chemotherapy. Eventually, patients with inherited disorders of globin synthesis or mutations in the globin gene, such as sickle cell disease, may benefit from the successful introduction of targeted genetic therapy (Chap. 91e).

POLYCYTHEMIA

Polycythemia is defined as an increase in the hemoglobin above normal. This increase may be real or only apparent because of a decrease in plasma volume (spurious or relative polycythemia). The term *erythrocytosis* may be used interchangeably with polycythemia, but some draw a distinction between them: erythrocytosis implies documentation of increased red cell mass, whereas polycythemia refers to any increase in red cells. Often patients with polycythemia are detected through an incidental finding of elevated hemoglobin or hematocrit levels. Concern that the hemoglobin level may be abnormally high is usually triggered at 170 g/L (17 g/dL) for men and 150 g/L (15 g/dL) for women. Hematocrit levels >50% in men or >45% in women may be abnormal. Hematocrits >60% in men and >55% in women are almost invariably associated with an increased red cell mass. Given that the machine that quantitates red cell parameters actually measures hemoglobin concentrations and calculates hematocrits, hemoglobin levels may be a better index.

Features of the clinical history that are useful in the differential diagnosis include smoking history; current living at high altitude; or a history of congenital heart disease, sleep apnea, or chronic lung disease.

Patients with polycythemia may be asymptomatic or experience symptoms related to the increased red cell mass or the underlying disease process that leads to the increased red cell mass. The dominant symptoms from an increased red cell mass are related to hyperviscosity and thrombosis (both venous and arterial), because the blood viscosity increases logarithmically at hematocrits >55%. Manifestations range from digital ischemia to Budd-Chiari syndrome with hepatic vein thrombosis. Abdominal vessel thromboses are particularly common. Neurologic symptoms such as vertigo, tinnitus, headache, and visual disturbances may occur. Hypertension is often present. Patients with *polycythemia vera* may have aquagenic pruritus and symptoms related to hepatosplenomegaly. Patients may have easy bruising, epistaxis, or bleeding from the gastrointestinal tract. Peptic ulcer disease is common. Patients with hypoxemia may develop cyanosis on minimal exertion or have headache, impaired mental acuity, and fatigue.

The physical examination usually reveals a ruddy complexion. Splenomegaly favors polycythemia vera as the diagnosis (Chap. 131).

The presence of cyanosis or evidence of a right-to-left shunt suggests congenital heart disease presenting in the adult, particularly tetralogy of Fallot or Eisenmenger's syndrome (Chap. 236). Increased blood viscosity raises pulmonary artery pressure; hypoxemia can lead to increased pulmonary vascular resistance. Together, these factors can produce cor pulmonale.

Polycythemia can be spurious (related to a decrease in plasma volume; Gaisbock's syndrome), primary, or secondary in origin. The secondary causes are all associated with increases in EPO levels: either a physiologically adapted appropriate elevation based on tissue hypoxia (lung disease, high altitude, CO poisoning, high-affinity hemoglobinopathy) or an abnormal overproduction (renal cysts, renal artery stenosis, tumors with ectopic EPO production). A rare familial form of polycythemia is associated with normal EPO levels but hyperresponsive EPO receptors due to mutations.

APPROACH TO THE PATIENT: Polycythemia

As shown in Fig. 77-18, the first step is to document the presence of an increased red cell mass using the principle of isotope dilution by administering ^{51}Cr-labeled autologous red blood cells to the patient and sampling blood radioactivity over a 2-h period. If the red cell mass is normal (<36 mL/kg in men, <32 mL/kg in women), the patient has spurious or relative polycythemia. If the red cell mass is increased (>36 mL/kg in men, >32 mL/kg in women), serum EPO levels should be measured. If EPO levels are low or unmeasurable, the patient most likely has polycythemia vera. A mutation in *JAK2* (Val617Phe), a key member of the cytokine intracellular signaling pathway, can be found in 90–95% of patients with polycythemia vera. Many of those without this particular *JAK2* mutation have mutations in exon 12. As a practical matter, few centers assess red cell mass in the setting of an increased hematocrit. The short workup is to measure EPO levels, check for *JAK2* mutation, and perform an abdominal ultrasound to assess spleen size. Tests that support the diagnosis of polycythemia vera include elevated white blood cell count, increased absolute basophil count, and thrombocytosis.

If serum EPO levels are elevated, one needs to distinguish whether the elevation is a physiologic response to hypoxia or related to autonomous EPO production. Patients with low arterial O_2 saturation (<92%) should be further evaluated for the presence of heart or lung disease, if they are not living at high altitude. Patients with normal O_2 saturation who are smokers may have elevated EPO levels because of CO displacement of O_2. If carboxyhemoglobin (COHb) levels are high, the diagnosis is "smoker's polycythemia." Such patients should be urged to stop smoking. Those who cannot stop smoking require phlebotomy to control their polycythemia. Patients with normal O_2 saturation who do not smoke either have an abnormal hemoglobin that does not deliver O_2 to the tissues (evaluated by finding elevated O_2–hemoglobin affinity) or have a source of EPO production that is not responding to the normal feedback inhibition. Further workup is dictated by the differential diagnosis of EPO-producing neoplasms. Hepatoma, uterine leiomyoma, and renal cancer or cysts are all detectable with abdominopelvic computed tomography scans. Cerebellar hemangiomas may produce EPO, but they present with localizing neurologic signs and symptoms rather than polycythemia-related symptoms.

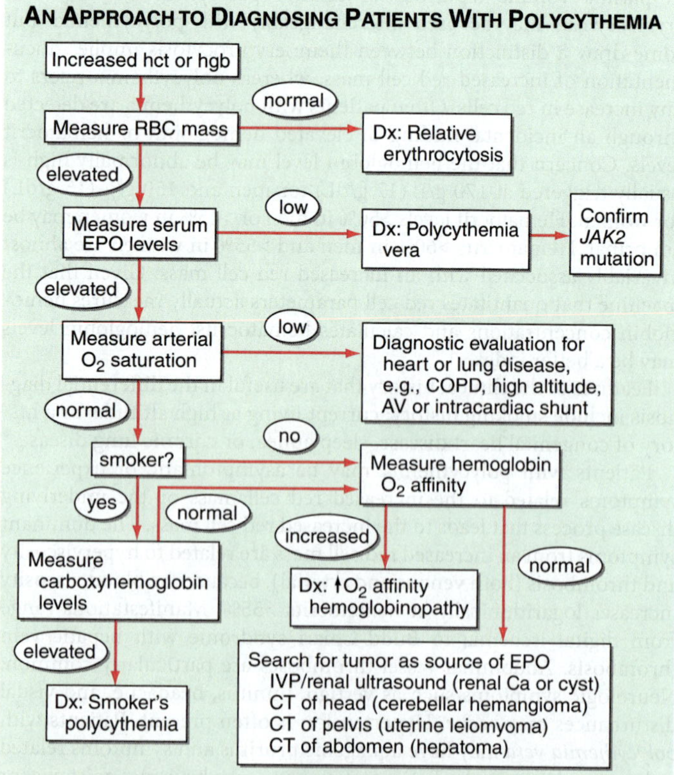

FIGURE 77-18 An approach to the differential diagnosis of patients with an elevated hemoglobin (possible polycythemia). AV, atrioventricular; COPD, chronic obstructive pulmonary disease; CT, computed tomography; EPO, erythropoietin; hct, hematocrit; hgb, hemoglobin; IVP, intravenous pyelogram; RBC, red blood cell.

78 Bleeding and Thrombosis

Barbara A. Konkle

The human hemostatic system provides a natural balance between procoagulant and anticoagulant forces. The procoagulant forces include platelet adhesion and aggregation and fibrin clot formation; anticoagulant forces include the natural inhibitors of coagulation and fibrinolysis. Under normal circumstances, hemostasis is regulated to promote blood flow; however, it is also prepared to clot blood rapidly to arrest blood flow and prevent exsanguination. After bleeding is successfully halted, the system remodels the damaged vessel to restore normal blood flow. The major components of the hemostatic system, which function in concert, are (1) platelets and other formed elements of blood, such as monocytes and red cells; (2) plasma proteins (the coagulation and fibrinolytic factors and inhibitors); and (3) the vessel wall.

STEPS OF NORMAL HEMOSTASIS

PLATELET PLUG FORMATION

On vascular injury, platelets adhere to the site of injury, usually the denuded vascular intimal surface. Platelet adhesion is mediated primarily by Von Willebrand factor (VWF), a large multimeric protein present in both plasma and the extracellular matrix of the subendothelial vessel wall, which serves as the primary "molecular glue," providing sufficient strength to withstand the high levels of shear stress that would tend to detach them with the flow of blood. Platelet adhesion is also facilitated by direct binding to subendothelial collagen through specific platelet membrane collagen receptors.

Platelet adhesion results in subsequent platelet activation and aggregation. This process is enhanced and amplified by humoral mediators in plasma (e.g., epinephrine, thrombin); mediators released from activated platelets (e.g., adenosine diphosphate, serotonin); and vessel wall extracellular matrix constituents that come in contact with adherent platelets (e.g., collagen, VWF). Activated platelets undergo the release reaction, during which they secrete contents that further promote aggregation and inhibit the naturally anticoagulant endothelial cell factors. During platelet aggregation (platelet-platelet interaction), additional platelets are recruited from the circulation to the site of vascular injury, leading to the formation of an occlusive platelet thrombus. The platelet plug is anchored and stabilized by the developing fibrin mesh.

The platelet glycoprotein (Gp) IIb/IIIa ($\alpha_{IIb}\beta_3$) complex is the most abundant receptor on the platelet surface. Platelet activation converts the normally inactive Gp IIb/IIIa receptor into an active receptor, enabling binding to fibrinogen and VWF. Because the surface of each platelet has about 50,000 Gp IIb/IIIa–binding sites, numerous activated platelets recruited to the site of vascular injury can rapidly form an occlusive aggregate by means of a dense network of intercellular fibrinogen bridges. Because this receptor is the key mediator of platelet aggregation, it has become an effective target for antiplatelet therapy.

FIBRIN CLOT FORMATION

Plasma coagulation proteins (*clotting factors*) normally circulate in plasma in their inactive forms. The sequence of coagulation protein reactions that culminate in the formation of fibrin was originally described as a *waterfall* or a *cascade*. Two pathways of blood coagulation have been described in the past: the so-called extrinsic, or tissue factor, pathway and the so-called intrinsic, or contact activation, pathway. We now know that coagulation is normally initiated through tissue factor (TF) exposure and activation through the classic *extrinsic pathway* but with critically important amplification through elements of the classic *intrinsic pathway*, as illustrated in Fig. 78-1. These reactions take place on phospholipid surfaces, usually the activated platelet surface. Coagulation testing in the laboratory can reflect other influences due to the artificial nature of the in vitro systems used (see below).

The immediate trigger for coagulation is vascular damage that exposes blood to TF that is constitutively expressed on the surfaces of subendothelial cellular components of the vessel wall, such as smooth muscle cells and fibroblasts. TF is also present in circulating microparticles, presumably shed from cells including monocytes and platelets. TF binds the serine protease factor VIIa; the complex activates factor X to factor Xa. Alternatively, the complex can indirectly activate factor X by initially converting factor IX to factor IXa, which then activates factor X. The participation of factor XI in hemostasis is not dependent on its activation by factor XIIa but rather on its positive feedback activation by thrombin. Thus, factor XIa functions in the propagation and amplification, rather than in the initiation, of the coagulation cascade.

Factor Xa can be formed through the actions of either the TF/factor VIIa complex or factor IXa (with factor VIIIa as a cofactor) and converts prothrombin to thrombin, the pivotal protease of the coagulation system. The essential cofactor for this reaction is factor Va. Like the homologous factor VIIIa, factor Va is produced by thrombin-induced limited proteolysis of factor V. Thrombin is a multifunctional enzyme that converts soluble plasma fibrinogen to an insoluble fibrin matrix. Fibrin polymerization involves an orderly process of intermolecular associations (Fig. 78-2). Thrombin also activates factor XIII (fibrin-stabilizing factor) to factor XIIIa, which covalently cross-links and thereby stabilizes the fibrin clot.

The assembly of the clotting factors on activated cell membrane surfaces greatly accelerates their reaction rates and also serves to localize blood clotting to sites of vascular injury. The critical cell membrane components, acidic phospholipids, are not normally exposed on resting cell membrane surfaces. However, when platelets, monocytes, and endothelial cells are activated by vascular injury or inflammatory stimuli, the procoagulant head groups of the membrane anionic phospholipids become translocated to the surfaces of these cells or released as part of microparticles, making them available to support and promote the plasma coagulation reactions.

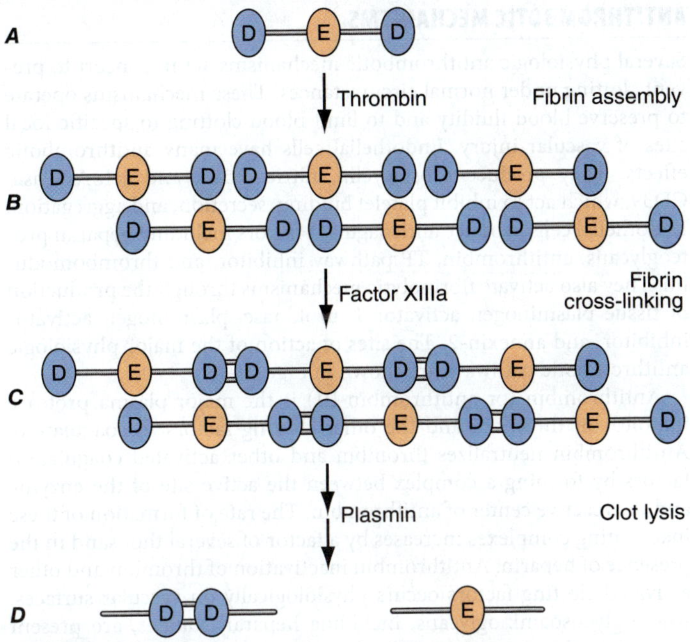

FIGURE 78-2 Fibrin formation and dissolution. (***A***) Fibrinogen is a trinodular structure consisting of two D domains and one E domain. Thrombin activation results in an ordered lateral assembly of protofibrils (***B***) with noncovalent associations. Factor XIIIa cross-links the D domains on adjacent molecules (***C***). Fibrin and fibrinogen (not shown) lysis by plasmin occurs at discrete sites and results in intermediary fibrin(ogen) degradation products (not shown). D-Dimers are the product of complete lysis of fibrin (***D***), maintaining the cross-linked D domains.

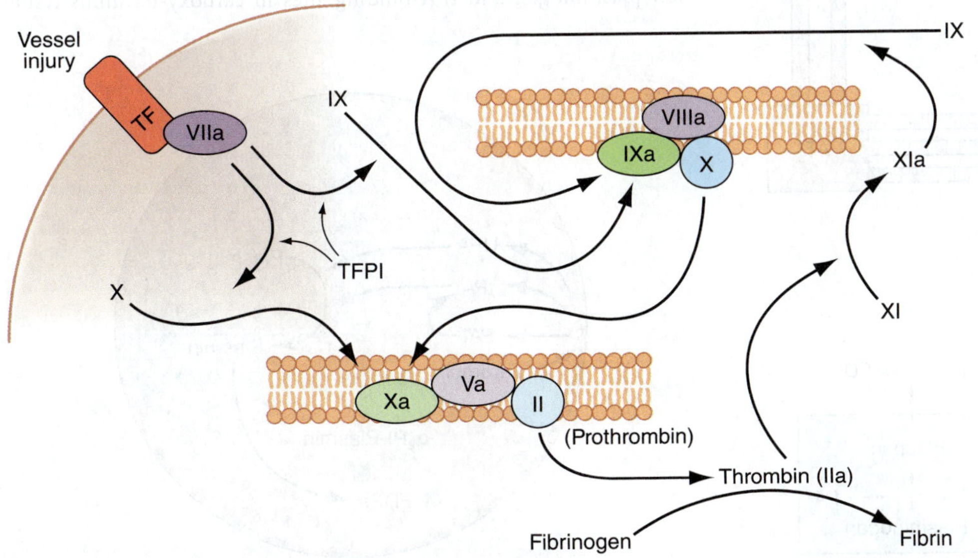

FIGURE 78-1 Coagulation is initiated by tissue factor (TF) exposure, which, with factor (F) VIIa, activates FIX and FX, which in turn, with FVIII and FV as cofactors, respectively, results in thrombin formation and subsequent conversion of fibrinogen to fibrin. Thrombin activates FXI, FVIII, and FV, amplifying the coagulation signal. Once the TF/FVIIa/FXa complex is formed, tissue factor pathway inhibitor (TFPI) inhibits the TF/FVIIa pathway, making coagulation dependent on the amplification loop through FIX/FVIII. Coagulation requires calcium (not shown) and takes place on phospholipid surfaces, usually the activated platelet membrane.

ANTITHROMBOTIC MECHANISMS

Several physiologic antithrombotic mechanisms act in concert to prevent clotting under normal circumstances. These mechanisms operate to preserve blood fluidity and to limit blood clotting to specific focal sites of vascular injury. Endothelial cells have many antithrombotic effects. They produce prostacyclin, nitric oxide, and ectoADPase/CD39, which act to inhibit platelet binding, secretion, and aggregation. Endothelial cells produce anticoagulant factors including heparan proteoglycans, antithrombin, TF pathway inhibitor, and thrombomodulin. They also activate fibrinolytic mechanisms through the production of tissue plasminogen activator 1, urokinase, plasminogen activator inhibitor, and annexin-2. The sites of action of the major physiologic antithrombotic pathways are shown in Fig. 78-3.

Antithrombin (or antithrombin III) is the major plasma protease inhibitor of thrombin and the other clotting factors in coagulation. Antithrombin neutralizes thrombin and other activated coagulation factors by forming a complex between the active site of the enzyme and the reactive center of antithrombin. The rate of formation of these inactivating complexes increases by a factor of several thousand in the presence of heparin. Antithrombin inactivation of thrombin and other activated clotting factors occurs physiologically on vascular surfaces, where glycosoaminoglycans, including heparan sulfates, are present to catalyze these reactions. Inherited quantitative or qualitative deficiencies of antithrombin lead to a lifelong predisposition to venous thromboembolism.

Protein C is a plasma glycoprotein that becomes an anticoagulant when it is activated by thrombin. The thrombin-induced activation of protein C occurs physiologically on thrombomodulin, a transmembrane proteoglycan-binding site for thrombin on endothelial cell surfaces. The binding of protein C to its receptor on endothelial cells places it in proximity to the thrombin-thrombomodulin complex, thereby enhancing its activation efficiency. Activated protein C acts as an anticoagulant by cleaving and inactivating activated factors V and VIII. This reaction is accelerated by a cofactor, protein S, which, like protein C, is a glycoprotein that undergoes vitamin K–dependent posttranslational modification. Quantitative or qualitative deficiencies of protein C or protein S, or resistance to the action of activated protein C by a specific mutation at its target cleavage site in factor Va (factor V Leiden), lead to hypercoagulable states.

Tissue factor pathway inhibitor (TFPI) is a plasma protease inhibitor that regulates the TF-induced extrinsic pathway of coagulation. TFPI inhibits the TF/factor VIIa/factor Xa complex, essentially turning off the TF/factor VIIa initiation of coagulation, which then becomes dependent on the "amplification loop" via factor XI and factor VIII activation by thrombin. TFPI is bound to lipoprotein and can also be released by heparin from endothelial cells, where it is bound to glycosaminoglycans, and from platelets. The heparin-mediated release of TFPI may play a role in the anticoagulant effects of unfractionated and low-molecular-weight heparins.

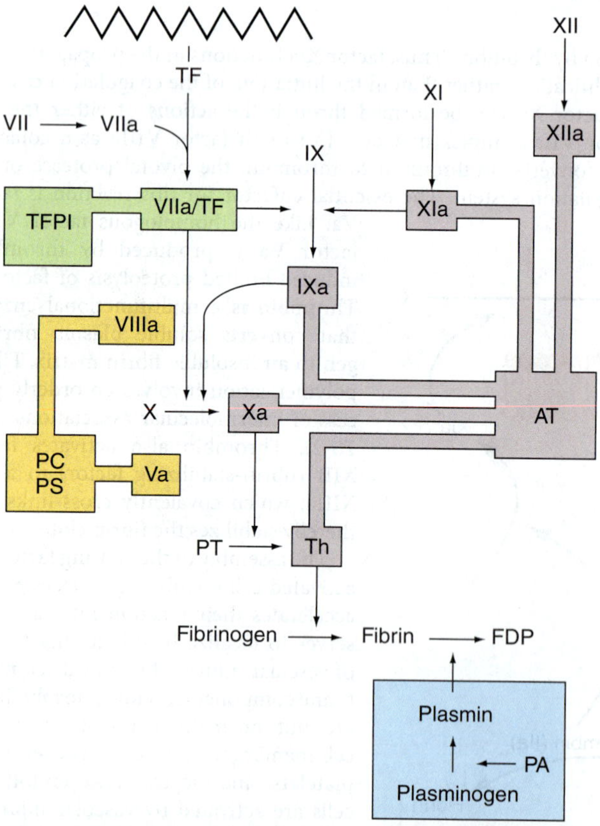

FIGURE 78-3 Sites of action of the four major physiologic antithrombotic pathways: antithrombin (AT); protein C/S (PC/PS); tissue factor pathway inhibitor (TFPI); and the fibrinolytic system, consisting of plasminogen, plasminogen activator (PA), and plasmin. PT, prothrombin; Th, thrombin; FDP, fibrin(ogen) degradation products. *(Modified from BA Konkle, AI Schafer, in DP Zipes et al [eds]: Braunwald's Heart Disease, 7th ed. Philadelphia, Saunders, 2005.)*

THE FIBRINOLYTIC SYSTEM

Any thrombin that escapes the inhibitory effects of the physiologic anticoagulant systems is available to convert fibrinogen to fibrin. In response, the endogenous fibrinolytic system is then activated to dispose of intravascular fibrin and thereby maintain or reestablish the patency of the circulation. Just as thrombin is the key protease enzyme of the coagulation system, plasmin is the major protease enzyme of the fibrinolytic system, acting to digest fibrin to fibrin degradation products. The general scheme of fibrinolysis and its control is shown in Fig. 78-4.

The plasminogen activators, tissue type plasminogen activator (tPA) and the urokinase-type plasminogen activator (uPA), cleave the Arg560-Val561 bond of plasminogen to generate the active enzyme plasmin. The lysine-binding sites of plasmin (and plasminogen) permit it to bind to fibrin, so that physiologic fibrinolysis is "fibrin specific." Both plasminogen (through its lysine-binding sites) and tPA possess specific affinity for fibrin and thereby bind selectively to clots. The assembly of a ternary complex, consisting of fibrin, plasminogen, and tPA, promotes the localized interaction between plasminogen and tPA and greatly accelerates the rate of plasminogen activation to plasmin. Moreover, partial degradation of fibrin by plasmin exposes new plasminogen and tPA-binding sites in carboxy-terminus lysine

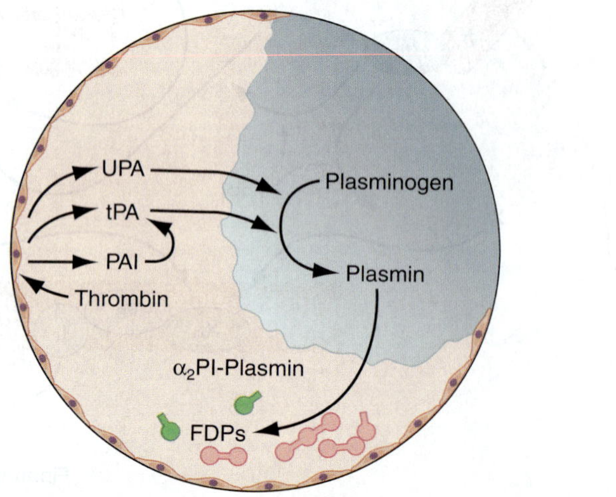

FIGURE 78-4 A schematic diagram of the fibrinolytic system. Tissue plasminogen activator (tPA) is released from endothelial cells, binds the fibrin clot, and activates plasminogen to plasmin. Excess fibrin is degraded by plasmin to distinct degradation products (FDPs). Any free plasmin is complexed with α_2-antiplasmin (α_2PI). PAI, plasminogen activator inhibitor; UPA, urokinase-type plasminogen activator.

residues of fibrin fragments to enhance these reactions further. This creates a highly efficient mechanism to generate plasmin focally on the fibrin clot, which then becomes plasmin's substrate for digestion to fibrin degradation products.

Plasmin cleaves fibrin at distinct sites of the fibrin molecule, leading to the generation of characteristic fibrin fragments during the process of fibrinolysis (Fig. 78-2). The sites of plasmin cleavage of fibrin are the same as those in fibrinogen. However, when plasmin acts on covalently cross-linked fibrin, D-dimers are released; hence, D-dimers can be measured in plasma as a relatively specific test of fibrin (rather than fibrinogen) degradation. D-Dimer assays can be used as sensitive markers of blood clot formation and have been validated for clinical use to exclude the diagnosis of deep venous thrombosis (DVT) and pulmonary embolism in selected populations. In addition, D-dimer measurement can be used to stratify patients, particularly women, for risk of recurrent venous thromboembolism (VTE) when measured 1 month after discontinuation of anticoagulation given for treatment of an initial idiopathic event. D-Dimer levels may be elevated in the absence of VTE in elderly people.

Physiologic regulation of fibrinolysis occurs primarily at three levels: (1) plasminogen activator inhibitors (PAIs), specifically PAI-1 and PAI-2, inhibit the physiologic plasminogen activators; (2) the thrombin-activatable fibrinolysis inhibitor (TAFI) limits fibrinolysis; and (3) α_2-antiplasmin inhibits plasmin. PAI-1 is the primary inhibitor of tPA and uPA in plasma. TAFI cleaves the N-terminal lysine residues of fibrin, which aid in localization of plasmin activity. α_2-Antiplasmin is the main inhibitor of plasmin in human plasma, inactivating any nonfibrin clot-associated plasmin.

TABLE 78-1 PRIMARY HEMOSTATIC (PLATELET PLUG) DISORDERS

Defects of Platelet Adhesion	
Von Willebrand disease	
Bernard-Soulier syndrome (absence or dysfunction of platelet Gp Ib-IX-V)	
Defects of Platelet Aggregation	
Glanzmann's thrombasthenia (absence or dysfunction of platelet glycoprotein [Gp] IIb/IIIa)	
Afibrinogenemia	
Defects of Platelet Secretion	
Decreased cyclooxygenase activity	
	Drug-induced (aspirin, nonsteroidal anti-inflammatory agents, thienopyridines)
	Inherited
Granule storage pool defects	
	Inherited
	Acquired
Nonspecific inherited secretory defects	
Nonspecific drug effects	
Uremia	
Platelet coating (e.g., paraprotein, penicillin)	
Defect of Platelet Coagulant Activity	
Scott's syndrome	

APPROACH TO THE PATIENT: Bleeding and Thrombosis

CLINICAL PRESENTATION

Disorders of hemostasis may be either inherited or acquired. A detailed personal and family history is key in determining the chronicity of symptoms and the likelihood of the disorder being inherited, as well as providing clues to underlying conditions that have contributed to the bleeding or thrombotic state. In addition, the history can give clues as to the etiology by determining (1) the bleeding (mucosal and/or joint) or thrombosis (arterial and/or venous) site and (2) whether an underlying bleeding or clotting tendency was enhanced by another medical condition or the introduction of medications or dietary supplements.

History of Bleeding A history of bleeding is the most important predictor of bleeding risk. In evaluating a patient for a bleeding disorder, a history of at-risk situations, including the response to past surgeries, should be assessed. Does the patient have a history of spontaneous or trauma/surgery-induced bleeding? Spontaneous hemarthroses are a hallmark of moderate and severe factor VIII and IX deficiency and, in rare circumstances, of other clotting factor deficiencies. Mucosal bleeding symptoms are more suggestive of underlying platelet disorders or Von Willebrand disease (VWD), termed *disorders of primary hemostasis or platelet plug formation.* Disorders affecting primary hemostasis are shown in Table 78-1.

A bleeding score has been validated as a tool to predict patients more likely to have type 1 VWD (International Society on Thrombosis and Haemostasis Bleeding Assessment Tool [*www.isth.org/resource/resmgr/ssc/isth-ssc_bleeding_assessment.pdf*]). This is most useful tool in excluding the diagnosis of a bleeding disorder, and thus avoiding unnecessary testing. One study found that a low bleeding score (≤3) and a normal activated partial thromboplastin time (aPTT) had 99.6% negative predictive value for the diagnosis of VWD. Bleeding symptoms that appear to be more common in patients with bleeding disorders include prolonged bleeding with surgery, dental procedures and extractions, and/or trauma, menorrhagia or postpartum hemorrhage, and large bruises (often described with lumps).

Easy bruising and menorrhagia are common complaints in patients with and without bleeding disorders. Easy bruising can also be a sign of medical conditions in which there is no identifiable coagulopathy; instead, the conditions are caused by an abnormality of blood vessels or their supporting tissues. In Ehlers-Danlos syndrome, there may be posttraumatic bleeding and a history of joint hyperextensibility. Cushing's syndrome, chronic steroid use, and aging result in changes in skin and subcutaneous tissue, and subcutaneous bleeding occurs in response to minor trauma. The latter has been termed *senile purpura.*

Epistaxis is a common symptom, particularly in children and in dry climates, and may not reflect an underlying bleeding disorder. However, it is the most common symptom in hereditary hemorrhagic telangiectasia and in boys with VWD. Clues that epistaxis is a symptom of an underlying bleeding disorder include lack of seasonal variation and bleeding that requires medical evaluation or treatment, including cauterization. Bleeding with eruption of primary teeth is seen in children with more severe bleeding disorders, such as moderate and severe hemophilia. It is uncommon in children with mild bleeding disorders. Patients with disorders of primary hemostasis (platelet adhesion) may have increased bleeding after dental cleanings and other procedures that involve gum manipulation.

Menorrhagia is defined quantitatively as a loss of >80 mL of blood per cycle, based on the quantity of blood loss required to produce iron-deficiency anemia. A complaint of heavy menses is subjective and has a poor correlation with excessive blood loss. Predictors of menorrhagia include bleeding resulting in iron-deficiency anemia or a need for blood transfusion, passage of clots >1 inch in diameter, and changing a pad or tampon more than hourly. Menorrhagia is a common symptom in women with underlying bleeding disorders and is reported in the majority of women with VWD, women with factor XI deficiency, and symptomatic carriers of hemophilia. Women with underlying bleeding disorders are more likely to have other bleeding symptoms, including bleeding after dental extractions, postoperative bleeding, and postpartum bleeding, and are much more likely to have menorrhagia beginning at menarche than women with menorrhagia due to other causes.

Postpartum hemorrhage (PPH) is a common symptom in women with underlying bleeding disorders. In women with type 1 VWD and symptomatic carriers of hemophilia A in whom levels of VWF and factor VIII usually normalize during pregnancy, PPH may be delayed. Women with a history of PPH have a high risk of recurrence with subsequent pregnancies. Rupture of ovarian cysts with intraabdominal hemorrhage has also been reported in women with underlying bleeding disorders.

Tonsillectomy is a major hemostatic challenge, because intact hemostatic mechanisms are essential to prevent excessive bleeding from the tonsillar bed. Bleeding may occur early after surgery or after approximately 7 days postoperatively, with loss of the eschar at the operative site. Similar delayed bleeding is seen after colonic polyp resection. Gastrointestinal (GI) bleeding and hematuria are usually due to underlying pathology, and procedures to identify and treat the bleeding site should be undertaken, even in patients with known bleeding disorders. VWD, particularly types 2 and 3, has been associated with angiodysplasia of the bowel and GI bleeding.

Hemarthroses and spontaneous muscle hematomas are characteristic of moderate or severe congenital factor VIII or IX deficiency. They can also be seen in moderate and severe deficiencies of fibrinogen, prothrombin, and factors V, VII, and X. Spontaneous hemarthroses occur rarely in other bleeding disorders except for severe VWD, with associated factor VIII levels <5%. Muscle and soft tissue bleeds are also common in acquired factor VIII deficiency. Bleeding into a joint results in severe pain and swelling, as well as loss of function, but is rarely associated with discoloration from bruising around the joint. Life-threatening sites of bleeding include bleeding into the oropharynx, where bleeding can obstruct the airway, into the central nervous system, and into the retroperitoneum. Central nervous system bleeding is the major cause of bleeding-related deaths in patients with severe congenital factor deficiencies.

Prohemorrhagic Effects of Medications and Dietary Supplements Aspirin and other nonsteroidal anti-inflammatory drugs (NSAIDs) that inhibit cyclooxygenase 1 impair primary hemostasis and may exacerbate bleeding from another cause or even unmask a previously occult mild bleeding disorder such as VWD. All NSAIDs, however, can precipitate GI bleeding, which may be more severe in patients with underlying bleeding disorders. The aspirin effect on platelet function as assessed by aggregometry can persist for up to 7 days, although it has frequently returned to normal by 3 days after the last dose. The effect of other NSAIDs is shorter, as the inhibitor effect is reversed when the drug is removed. Thienopyridines (clopidogrel and prasugrel) inhibit ADP-mediated platelet aggregation and, like NSAIDs, can precipitate or exacerbate bleeding symptoms.

Many herbal supplements can impair hemostatic function (Table 78-2). Some are more convincingly associated with a bleeding risk than others. Fish oil or concentrated omega-3 fatty acid supplements impair platelet function. They alter platelet biochemistry to produce more PGI_3, a more potent platelet inhibitor than prostacyclin (PGI_2), and more thromboxane A_3, a less potent platelet activator than thromboxane A_2. In fact, diets naturally rich in omega-3 fatty acids can result in a prolonged bleeding time and abnormal platelet aggregation studies, but the actual associated bleeding risk is unclear. Vitamin E appears to inhibit protein kinase C–mediated platelet aggregation and nitric oxide production. In patients with unexplained bruising or bleeding, it is prudent to review any new medications or supplements and discontinue those that may be associated with bleeding.

TABLE 78-2 HERBAL SUPPLEMENTS ASSOCIATED WITH INCREASED BLEEDING

Herbs with Potential Antiplatelet Activity
Ginkgo (*Ginkgo biloba L.*)
Garlic (*Allium sativum*)
Bilberry (*Vaccinium myrtillus*)
Ginger (*Gingiber officinale*)
Dong quai (*Angelica sinensis*)
Feverfew (*Tanacetum parthenium*)
Asian ginseng (*Panax ginseng*)
American ginseng (*Panax quinquefolius*)
Siberian ginseng/eleuthero (*Eleutherococcus senticosus*)
Turmeric (*Circuma longa*)
Meadowsweet (*Filipendula ulmaria*)
Willow (*Salix* spp.)
Coumarin-Containing Herbs
Motherwort (*Leonurus cardiaca*)
Chamomile (*Matricaria recutita, Chamaemelum mobile*)
Horse chestnut (*Aesculus hippocastanum*)
Red clover (*Trifolium pratense*)
Fenugreek (*Trigonella foenum-graecum*)

Underlying Systemic Diseases That Cause or Exacerbate a Bleeding Tendency Acquired bleeding disorders are commonly secondary to, or associated with, systemic disease. The clinical evaluation of a patient with a bleeding tendency must therefore include a thorough assessment for evidence of underlying disease. Bruising or mucosal bleeding may be the presenting complaint in liver disease, severe renal impairment, hypothyroidism, paraproteinemias or amyloidosis, and conditions causing bone marrow failure. All coagulation factors are synthesized in the liver, and hepatic failure results in combined factor deficiencies. This is often compounded by thrombocytopenia from splenomegaly due to portal hypertension. Coagulation factors II, VII, IX, and X and proteins C, S, and Z are dependent on vitamin K for posttranslational modification. Although vitamin K is required in both procoagulant and anticoagulant processes, the phenotype of vitamin K deficiency or the warfarin effect on coagulation is bleeding.

The normal blood platelet count is 150,000–450,000/μL. Thrombocytopenia results from decreased production, increased destruction, and/or sequestration. Although the bleeding risk varies somewhat by the reason for the thrombocytopenia, bleeding rarely occurs in isolated thrombocytopenia at counts <50,000/μL and usually not until <10,000–20,000/μL. Coexisting coagulopathies, as is seen in liver failure or disseminated coagulation; infection; platelet-inhibitory drugs; and underlying medical conditions can all increase the risk of bleeding in the thrombocytopenic patient. Most procedures can be performed in patients with a platelet count of 50,000/μL. The level needed for major surgery will depend on the type of surgery and the patient's underlying medical state, although a count of approximately 80,000/μL is likely sufficient.

HISTORY OF THROMBOSIS

The risk of thrombosis, like that of bleeding, is influenced by both genetic and environmental influences. The major risk factor for arterial thrombosis is atherosclerosis, whereas for venous thrombosis, the risk factors are immobility, surgery, underlying medical conditions such as malignancy, medications such as hormonal therapy, obesity, and genetic predispositions. Factors that increase risks for venous and for both venous and arterial thromboses are shown in Table 78-3.

The most important point in a history related to venous thrombosis is determining whether the thrombotic event was idiopathic (meaning there was no clear precipitating factor) or was a precipitated event. In patients without underlying malignancy, having an idiopathic event is the strongest predictor of recurrence of VTE. In patients who have a vague history of thrombosis, a history of being treated with warfarin suggests a past DVT. Age is an important risk factor for venous thrombosis—the risk of DVT increases per decade, with an approximate incidence of 1/100,000 per year in early childhood to 1/200 per year among octogenarians. Family history is helpful in determining if there is a genetic predisposition and how strong that predisposition appears to be. A genetic thrombophilia that confers a relatively small increased risk, such as being a heterozygote for the prothrombin G20210A or factor V Leiden mutation, may be a minor determinant of risk in an elderly individual

TABLE 78-3 RISK FACTORS FOR THROMBOSIS

Venous	Venous and Arterial
Inherited	**Inherited**
Factor V Leiden	Homocystinuria
Prothrombin G20210A	Dysfibrinogenemia
Antithrombin deficiency	**Mixed (inherited and acquired)**
Protein C deficiency	Hyperhomocysteinemia
Protein S deficiency	**Acquired**
Elevated factor VIII	Malignancy
Acquired	Antiphospholipid antibody syndrome
Age	Hormonal therapy
Previous thrombosis	Polycythemia vera
Immobilization	Essential thrombocythemia
Major surgery	Paroxysmal nocturnal hemoglobinuria
Pregnancy and puerperium	Thrombotic thrombocytopenic purpura
Hospitalization	Heparin-induced thrombocytopenia
Obesity	Disseminated intravascular coagulation
Infection	
APC resistance, nongenetic	
Smoking	
Unknown[a]	
Elevated factor II, IX, XI	
Elevated TAFI levels	
Low levels of TFPI	

[a]Unknown whether risk is inherited or acquired.

Abbreviations: APC, activated protein C; TAFI, thrombin-activatable fibrinolysis inhibitor; TFPI, tissue factor pathway inhibitor.

undergoing a high-risk surgical procedure. As illustrated in Fig. 78-5, a thrombotic event usually has more than one contributing factor. Predisposing factors must be carefully assessed to determine the risk of recurrent thrombosis and, with consideration of the patient's bleeding risk, determine the length of anticoagulation.

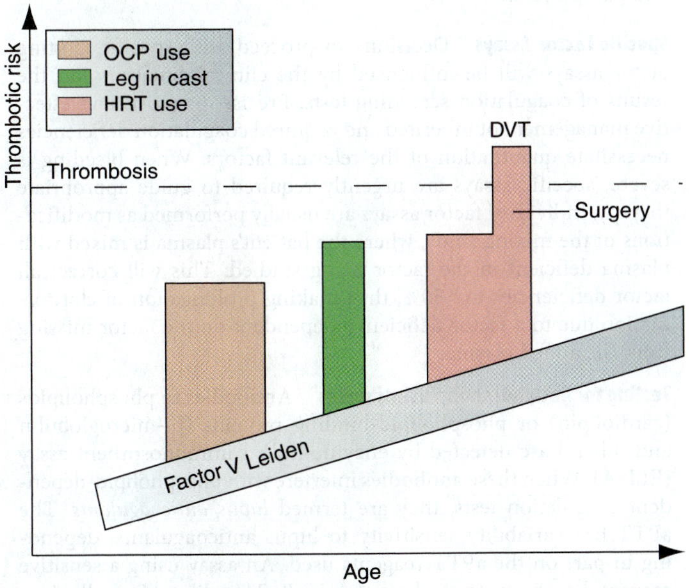

FIGURE 78-5 Thrombotic risk over time. Shown schematically is an individual's thrombotic risk over time. An underlying factor V Leiden mutation provides a "theoretically" constant increased risk. The thrombotic risk increases with age and, intermittently, with oral contraceptive (OCP) or hormone replacement therapy (HRT) use; other events may increase the risk further. At some point, the cumulative risk may increase to the threshold for thrombosis and result in deep venous thrombosis (DVT). Note: The magnitude and duration of risk portrayed in the figure are meant for example only and may not precisely reflect the relative risk determined by clinical study. *(From BA Konkle, A Schafer, in DP Zipes et al [eds]: Braunwald's Heart Disease, 7th ed. Philadelphia, Saunders, 2005; modified with permission from FR Rosendaal: Venous thrombosis: A multicausal disease. Lancet 353:1167, 1999.)*

Similar consideration should be given in determining the need, if any, to test the patient and family members for thrombophilias.

LABORATORY EVALUATION

Careful history taking and clinical examination are essential components in the assessment of bleeding and thrombotic risk. The use of laboratory tests of coagulation complement, but cannot substitute for, clinical assessment. No test exists that provides a global assessment of hemostasis. The bleeding time has been used to assess bleeding risk; however, it does not predict bleeding risk with surgery and it is not recommended for this indication. The PFA-100, an instrument that measures platelet-dependent coagulation under flow conditions, is more sensitive and specific for VWD than the bleeding time; however, it is not sensitive enough to rule out mild bleeding disorders. PFA-100 closure times are prolonged in patients with some, but not all, inherited platelet disorders. Also, its utility in predicting bleeding risk has not been determined.

For routine preoperative and preprocedure testing, an abnormal prothrombin time (PT) may detect liver disease or vitamin K deficiency that had not been previously appreciated. Studies have not confirmed the usefulness of an aPTT in preoperative evaluations in patients with a negative bleeding history. The primary use of coagulation testing should be to confirm the presence and type of bleeding disorder in a patient with a suspicious clinical history.

Because of the nature of coagulation assays, proper sample acquisition and handling is critical to obtaining valid results. In patients with abnormal coagulation assays who have no bleeding history, repeat studies with attention to these factors frequently results in normal values. Most coagulation assays are performed in sodium citrate anticoagulated plasma that is recalcified for the assay. Because the anticoagulant is in liquid solution and needs to be added to blood in proportion to the plasma volume, incorrectly filled or inadequately mixed blood collection tubes will give erroneous results. Vacutainer tubes should be filled to >90% of the recommended fill, which is usually denoted by a line on the tube. An elevated hematocrit (>55%) can result in a false value due to a decreased plasma-to-anticoagulant ratio.

Screening Assays The most commonly used screening tests are the PT, aPTT, and platelet count. The PT assesses the factors I (fibrinogen), II (prothrombin), V, VII, and X (Fig. 78-6). The PT measures the time for clot formation of the citrated plasma after recalcification and addition of thromboplastin, a mixture of TF and phospholipids. The sensitivity of the assay varies by the source of thromboplastin. The relationship between defects in secondary hemostasis (fibrin formation) and coagulation test abnormalities is shown in Table 78-4. To adjust for this variability, the overall sensitivity of different thromboplastins to reduction of the vitamin K–dependent clotting factors II, VII, IX, and X in anticoagulation patients is now expressed as the International Sensitivity Index (ISI). An inverse relationship exists between ISI and thromboplastin sensitivity. The international normalized ratio (INR) is then determined based on the formula: $INR = (PT_{patient}/PT_{normal\ mean})^{ISI}$.

The INR was developed to assess stable anticoagulation due to reduction of vitamin K–dependent coagulation factors; it is commonly used in the evaluation of patients with liver disease. Although it does allow comparison between laboratories, reagent sensitivity as used to determine the ISI is not the same in liver disease as with warfarin anticoagulation. In addition, progressive liver failure is associated with variable changes in coagulation factors; the degree of prolongation of either the PT or the INR only roughly predicts the bleeding risk. Thrombin generation has been shown to be normal in many patients with mild to moderate liver dysfunction. Because the PT only measures one aspect of hemostasis affected by liver dysfunction, we likely overestimate the bleeding risk of a mildly elevated INR in this setting.

The aPTT assesses the intrinsic and common coagulation pathways; factors XI, IX, VIII, X, V, and II; fibrinogen; prekallikrein;

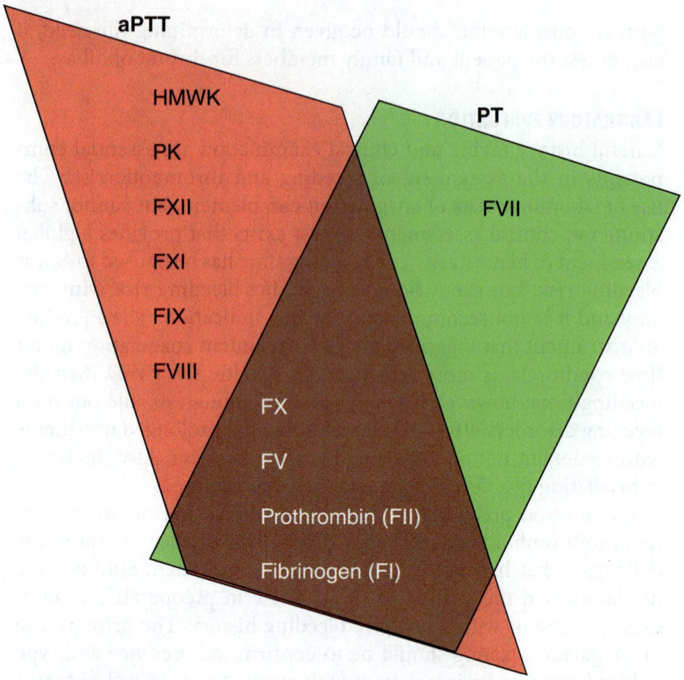

FIGURE 78–6 **Coagulation factor activity** tested in the activated partial thromboplastin time (aPTT) in red and prothrombin time (PT) in green, or both. F, factor; HMWK, high-molecular-weight kininogen; PK, prekallikrein.

TABLE 78-4 HEMOSTATIC DISORDERS AND COAGULATION TEST ABNORMALITIES

Prolonged Activated Partial Thromboplastin Time (aPTT)
No clinical bleeding—↓ factor XII, high-molecular-weight kininogen, prekallikrein
Variable, but usually mild, bleeding—↓ factor XI, mild ↓ factor VIII and factor IX
Frequent, severe bleeding—severe deficiencies of factors VIII and IX
Heparin and direct thrombin inhibitors
Prolonged Prothrombin Time (PT)
Factor VII deficiency
Vitamin K deficiency—early
Warfarin anticoagulation
Direct Xa inhibitors (rivaroxaban, apixaban)
Prolonged aPTT and PT
Factor II, V, X, or fibrinogen deficiency
Vitamin K deficiency—late
Direct thrombin inhibitors
Prolonged Thrombin Time
Heparin or heparin-like inhibitors
Direct thrombin inhibitors (e.g., dabigatran, argatroban, bivalirudin)
Mild or no bleeding—dysfibrinogenemia
Frequent, severe bleeding—afibrinogenemia
Prolonged PT and/or aPTT Not Corrected with Mixing with Normal Plasma
Bleeding—specific factor inhibitor
No symptoms, or clotting and/or pregnancy loss—lupus anticoagulant
Disseminated intravascular coagulation
Heparin or direct thrombin inhibitor
Abnormal Clot Solubility
Factor XIII deficiency
Inhibitors or defective cross-linking
Rapid Clot Lysis
Deficiency of α_2-antiplasmin or plasminogen activator inhibitor 1
Treatment with fibrinolytic therapy

high-molecular-weight kininogen; and factor XII (Fig. 78-6). The aPTT reagent contains phospholipids derived from either animal or vegetable sources that function as a platelet substitute in the coagulation pathways and includes an activator of the intrinsic coagulation system, such as nonparticulate ellagic acid or the particulate activators kaolin, celite, or micronized silica.

The phospholipid composition of aPTT reagents varies, which influences the sensitivity of individual reagents to clotting factor deficiencies and to inhibitors such as heparin and lupus anticoagulants. Thus, aPTT results will vary from one laboratory to another, and the normal range in the laboratory where the testing occurs should be used in the interpretation. Local laboratories can relate their aPTT values to the therapeutic heparin anticoagulation by correlating aPTT values with direct measurements of heparin activity (anti-Xa or protamine titration assays) in samples from heparinized patients, although correlation between these assays is often poor. The aPTT reagent will vary in sensitivity to individual factor deficiencies and usually becomes prolonged with individual factor deficiencies of 30–50%.

Mixing Studies Mixing studies are used to evaluate a prolonged aPTT or, less commonly PT, to distinguish between a factor deficiency and an inhibitor. In this assay, normal plasma and patient plasma are mixed in a 1:1 ratio, and the aPTT or PT is determined immediately and after incubation at 37°C for varying times, typically 30, 60, and/or 120 min. With isolated factor deficiencies, the aPTT will correct with mixing and stay corrected with incubation. With aPTT prolongation due to a lupus anticoagulant, the mixing and incubation will show no correction. In acquired neutralizing factor antibodies, notably an acquired factor VIII inhibitor, the initial assay may or may not correct immediately after mixing but will prolong or remain prolonged with incubation at 37°C. Failure to correct with mixing can also be due to the presence of other inhibitors or interfering substances such as heparin, fibrin split products, and paraproteins.

Specific Factor Assays Decisions to proceed with specific clotting factor assays will be influenced by the clinical situation and the results of coagulation screening tests. Precise diagnosis and effective management of inherited and acquired coagulation deficiencies necessitate quantitation of the relevant factors. When bleeding is severe, specific assays are urgently required to guide appropriate therapy. Individual factor assays are usually performed as modifications of the mixing study, where the patient's plasma is mixed with plasma deficient in the factor being studied. This will correct all factor deficiencies to >50%, thus making prolongation of clot formation due to a factor deficiency dependent on the factor missing from the added plasma.

Testing for Antiphospholipid Antibodies Antibodies to phospholipids (cardiolipin) or phospholipid-binding proteins (β_2-microglobulin and others) are detected by enzyme-linked immunosorbent assay (ELISA). When these antibodies interfere with phospholipid-dependent coagulation tests, they are termed *lupus anticoagulants*. The aPTT has variability sensitivity to lupus anticoagulants, depending in part on the aPTT reagents used. An assay using a sensitive reagent has been termed an *LA-PTT*. The dilute Russell viper venom test (dRVVT) and the tissue thromboplastin inhibition (TTI) test are modifications of standard tests with the phospholipid reagent decreased, thus increasing the sensitivity to antibodies that interfere with the phospholipid component. The tests, however, are not specific for lupus anticoagulants, because factor deficiencies or other inhibitors will also result in prolongation. Documentation of a lupus anticoagulant requires not only prolongation of a phospholipid-dependent coagulation test but also lack of correction when mixed with normal plasma and correction with the addition of activated platelet membranes or certain phospholipids (e.g., hexagonal phase).

Other Coagulation Tests The thrombin time and the reptilase time measure fibrinogen conversion to fibrin and are prolonged when the fibrinogen level is low (usually <80–100 mg/dL) or qualitatively abnormal, as seen in inherited or acquired dysfibrinogenemias, or when fibrin/fibrinogen degradation products interfere. The thrombin time, but not the reptilase time, is prolonged in the presence of heparin. The thrombin time is markedly prolonged in the presence of the direct thrombin inhibitor, dabigatran; a dilute thrombin time can be used to assess drug activity. Measurement of anti–factor Xa plasma inhibitory activity is a test frequently used to assess low-molecular-weight heparin (LMWH) levels, as a direct measurement of unfractionated heparin (UFH) activity, or to assess activity of the new direct Xa inhibitors rivaroxaban or apixaban. Drug in the patient sample inhibits the enzymatic conversion of an Xa-specific chromogenic substrate to colored product by factor Xa. Standard curves are created using multiple concentrations of drug and are used to calculate the concentration of anti-Xa activity in the patient plasma.

Laboratory Testing for Thrombophilia Laboratory assays to detect thrombophilic states include molecular diagnostics and immunologic and functional assays. These assays vary in their sensitivity and specificity for the condition being tested. Furthermore, acute thrombosis, acute illnesses, inflammatory conditions, pregnancy, and medications affect levels of many coagulation factors and their inhibitors. Antithrombin is decreased by heparin and in the setting of acute thrombosis. Protein C and S levels may be increased in the setting of acute thrombosis and are decreased by warfarin. Antiphospholipid antibodies are frequently transiently positive in acute illness. Testing for genetic thrombophilias should, in general, only be performed when there is a strong family history of thrombosis and results would affect clinical decision making.

Because thrombophilia evaluations are usually performed to assess the need to extend anticoagulation, testing should be performed in a steady state, remote from the acute event. In most instances, warfarin anticoagulation can be stopped after the initial 3–6 months of treatment, and testing can be performed at least 3 weeks later. As a sensitive marker of coagulation activation, the quantitative D-dimer assay, drawn 4 weeks after stopping anticoagulation, can be used to stratify risk of recurrent thrombosis in patients who have an idiopathic event.

Measures of Platelet Function The bleeding time has been used to assess bleeding risk; however, it has not been found to predict bleeding risk with surgery, and it is not recommended for use for this indication. The PFA-100 and similar instruments that measure platelet-dependent coagulation under flow conditions are generally more sensitive and specific for platelet disorders and VWD than the bleeding time; however, data are insufficient to support their use to predict bleeding risk or monitor response to therapy, and they will be normal in some patients with platelet disorders or mild VWD. When they are used in the evaluation of a patient with bleeding symptoms, abnormal results, as with the bleeding time, require specific testing, such as VWF assays and/or platelet aggregation studies. Because all of these "screening" assays may miss patients with mild bleeding disorders, further studies are needed to define their role in hemostasis testing.

For classic platelet aggregometry, various agonists are added to the patient's platelet-rich plasma and platelet aggregation is measured. Tests of platelet secretion in response to agonists can also be measured. These tests are affected by many factors, including numerous medications, and the association between minor defects in aggregation or secretion in these assays and bleeding risk is not clearly established.

ACKNOWLEDGMENT
Robert I. Handin, MD, contributed this chapter in the 16th edition, and some material from that chapter has been retained here.

79 Enlargement of Lymph Nodes and Spleen

Patrick H. Henry, Dan L. Longo

This chapter is intended to serve as a guide to the evaluation of patients who present with enlargement of the lymph nodes (*lymphadenopathy*) or the spleen (*splenomegaly*). Lymphadenopathy is a rather common clinical finding in primary care settings, whereas palpable splenomegaly is less so.

LYMPHADENOPATHY

Lymphadenopathy may be an incidental finding in patients being examined for various reasons, or it may be a presenting sign or symptom of the patient's illness. The physician must eventually decide whether the lymphadenopathy is a normal finding or one that requires further study, up to and including biopsy. Soft, flat, submandibular nodes (<1 cm) are often palpable in healthy children and young adults; healthy adults may have palpable inguinal nodes of up to 2 cm, which are considered normal. Further evaluation of these normal nodes is not warranted. In contrast, if the physician believes the node(s) to be abnormal, then pursuit of a more precise diagnosis is needed.

APPROACH TO THE PATIENT: Lymphadenopathy

Lymphadenopathy may be a primary or secondary manifestation of numerous disorders, as shown in Table 79-1. Many of these disorders are infrequent causes of lymphadenopathy. In primary care practice, more than two-thirds of patients with lymphadenopathy have nonspecific causes or upper respiratory illnesses (viral or bacterial), and <1% have a malignancy. In one study, 84% of patients referred for evaluation of lymphadenopathy had a "benign" diagnosis. The remaining 16% had a malignancy (lymphoma or metastatic adenocarcinoma). Of the patients with benign lymphadenopathy, 63% had a nonspecific or reactive etiology (no causative agent found), and the remainder had a specific cause demonstrated, most commonly infectious mononucleosis, toxoplasmosis, or tuberculosis. Thus, the vast majority of patients with lymphadenopathy will have a nonspecific etiology requiring few diagnostic tests.

CLINICAL ASSESSMENT

The physician will be aided in the pursuit of an explanation for the lymphadenopathy by a careful medical history, physical examination, selected laboratory tests, and perhaps an excisional lymph node biopsy.

The *medical history* should reveal the setting in which lymphadenopathy is occurring. Symptoms such as sore throat, cough, fever, night sweats, fatigue, weight loss, or pain in the nodes should be sought. The patient's age, sex, occupation, exposure to pets, sexual behavior, and use of drugs such as diphenylhydantoin are other important historic points. For example, children and young adults usually have benign (i.e., nonmalignant) disorders that account for the observed lymphadenopathy such as viral or bacterial upper respiratory infections; infectious mononucleosis; toxoplasmosis; and, in some countries, tuberculosis. In contrast, after age 50, the incidence of malignant disorders increases and that of benign disorders decreases.

The *physical examination* can provide useful clues such as the extent of lymphadenopathy (localized or generalized), size of nodes, texture, presence or absence of nodal tenderness, signs of inflammation over the node, skin lesions, and splenomegaly. A thorough ear, nose, and throat (ENT) examination is indicated in adult patients

TABLE 79-1 DISEASES ASSOCIATED WITH LYMPHADENOPATHY

1. Infectious diseases
   a. Viral—infectious mononucleosis syndromes (EBV, CMV), infectious hepatitis, herpes simplex, herpesvirus-6, varicella-zoster virus, rubella, measles, adenovirus, HIV, epidemic keratoconjunctivitis, vaccinia, herpesvirus-8
   b. Bacterial—streptococci, staphylococci, cat-scratch disease, brucellosis, tularemia, plague, chancroid, melioidosis, glanders, tuberculosis, atypical mycobacterial infection, primary and secondary syphilis, diphtheria, leprosy, *Bartonella*
   c. Fungal—histoplasmosis, coccidioidomycosis, paracoccidioidomycosis
   d. Chlamydial—lymphogranuloma venereum, trachoma
   e. Parasitic—toxoplasmosis, leishmaniasis, trypanosomiasis, filariasis
   f. Rickettsial—scrub typhus, rickettsialpox, Q fever
2. Immunologic diseases
   a. Rheumatoid arthritis
   b. Juvenile rheumatoid arthritis
   c. Mixed connective tissue disease
   d. Systemic lupus erythematosus
   e. Dermatomyositis
   f. Sjögren's syndrome
   g. Serum sickness
   h. Drug hypersensitivity—diphenylhydantoin, hydralazine, allopurinol, primidone, gold, carbamazepine, etc.
   i. Angioimmunoblastic lymphadenopathy
   j. Primary biliary cirrhosis
   k. Graft-versus-host disease
   l. Silicone-associated
   m. Autoimmune lymphoproliferative syndrome
   n. IgG4-related disease
   o. Immune reconstitution inflammatory syndrome (IRIS)
3. Malignant diseases
   a. Hematologic—Hodgkin's disease, non-Hodgkin's lymphomas, acute or chronic lymphocytic leukemia, hairy cell leukemia, malignant histiocytosis, amyloidosis
   b. Metastatic—from numerous primary sites
4. Lipid storage diseases—Gaucher's, Niemann-Pick, Fabry, Tangier
5. Endocrine diseases—hyperthyroidism
6. Other disorders
   a. Castleman's disease (giant lymph node hyperplasia)
   b. Sarcoidosis
   c. Dermatopathic lymphadenitis
   d. Lymphomatoid granulomatosis
   e. Histiocytic necrotizing lymphadenitis (Kikuchi's disease)
   f. Sinus histiocytosis with massive lymphadenopathy (Rosai-Dorfman disease)
   g. Mucocutaneous lymph node syndrome (Kawasaki's disease)
   h. Histiocytosis X
   i. Familial Mediterranean fever
   g. Severe hypertriglyceridemia
   k. Vascular transformation of sinuses
   l. Inflammatory pseudotumor of lymph node
   m. Congestive heart failure

Abbreviations: CMV, cytomegalovirus; EBV, Epstein-Barr virus.

with cervical adenopathy and a history of tobacco use. Localized or regional adenopathy implies involvement of a single anatomic area. Generalized adenopathy has been defined as involvement of three or more noncontiguous lymph node areas. Many of the causes of lymphadenopathy (Table 79-1) can produce localized *or* generalized adenopathy, so this distinction is of limited utility in the differential diagnosis. Nevertheless, generalized lymphadenopathy is frequently associated with nonmalignant disorders such as infectious mononucleosis (Epstein-Barr virus [EBV] or cytomegalovirus [CMV]), toxoplasmosis, AIDS, other viral infections, systemic lupus erythematosus (SLE), and mixed connective tissue disease. Acute and chronic lymphocytic leukemias and malignant lymphomas also produce generalized adenopathy in adults.

The site of localized or regional adenopathy may provide a useful clue about the cause. Occipital adenopathy often reflects an infection of the scalp, and preauricular adenopathy accompanies conjunctival infections and cat-scratch disease. The most frequent site of regional adenopathy is the neck, and most of the causes are benign—upper respiratory infections, oral and dental lesions, infectious mononucleosis, or other viral illnesses. The chief malignant causes include metastatic cancer from head and neck, breast, lung, and thyroid primaries. Enlargement of supraclavicular and scalene nodes is always abnormal. Because these nodes drain regions of the lung and retroperitoneal space, they can reflect lymphomas, other cancers, or infectious processes arising in these areas. Virchow's node is an enlarged left supraclavicular node infiltrated with metastatic cancer from a gastrointestinal primary. Metastases to supraclavicular nodes also occur from lung, breast, testis, or ovarian cancers. Tuberculosis, sarcoidosis, and toxoplasmosis are nonneoplastic causes of supraclavicular adenopathy. Axillary adenopathy is usually due to injuries or localized infections of the ipsilateral upper extremity. Malignant causes include melanoma or lymphoma and, in women, breast cancer. Inguinal lymphadenopathy is usually secondary to infections or trauma of the lower extremities and may accompany sexually transmitted diseases such as lymphogranuloma venereum, primary syphilis, genital herpes, or chancroid. These nodes may also be involved by lymphomas and metastatic cancer from primary lesions of the rectum, genitalia, or lower extremities (melanoma).

The size and texture of the lymph node(s) and the presence of pain are useful parameters in evaluating a patient with lymphadenopathy. Nodes <1.0 cm^2 in area (1.0 cm × 1.0 cm or less) are almost always secondary to benign, nonspecific reactive causes. In one retrospective analysis of younger patients (9–25 years) who had a lymph node biopsy, a maximum diameter of >2 cm served as one discriminant for predicting that the biopsy would reveal malignant or granulomatous disease. Another study showed that a lymph node size of 2.25 cm^2 (1.5 cm × 1.5 cm) was the best size limit for distinguishing malignant or granulomatous lymphadenopathy from other causes of lymphadenopathy. Patients with node(s) ≤ 1.0 cm^2 should be observed after excluding infectious mononucleosis and/or toxoplasmosis unless there are symptoms and signs of an underlying systemic illness.

The texture of lymph nodes may be described as soft, firm, rubbery, hard, discrete, matted, tender, movable, or fixed. Tenderness is found when the capsule is stretched during rapid enlargement, usually secondary to an inflammatory process. Some malignant diseases such as acute leukemia may produce rapid enlargement and pain in the nodes. Nodes involved by lymphoma tend to be large, discrete, symmetric, rubbery, firm, mobile, and nontender. Nodes containing metastatic cancer are often hard, nontender, and nonmovable because of fixation to surrounding tissues. The coexistence of splenomegaly in the patient with lymphadenopathy implies a systemic illness such as infectious mononucleosis, lymphoma, acute or chronic leukemia, SLE, sarcoidosis, toxoplasmosis, cat-scratch disease, or other less common hematologic disorders. The patient's story should provide helpful clues about the underlying systemic illness.

Nonsuperficial presentations (thoracic or abdominal) of adenopathy are usually detected as the result of a symptom-directed diagnostic workup. Thoracic adenopathy may be detected by routine chest radiography or during the workup for superficial adenopathy. It may also be found because the patient complains of a cough or wheezing from airway compression; hoarseness from recurrent laryngeal nerve involvement; dysphagia from esophageal compression; or swelling of the neck, face, or arms secondary to compression of the superior vena cava or subclavian vein. The differential diagnosis of mediastinal and hilar adenopathy includes primary lung disorders and systemic illnesses that characteristically involve mediastinal or hilar nodes. In the young, mediastinal adenopathy is associated with infectious mononucleosis and sarcoidosis. In endemic regions, histoplasmosis can cause unilateral paratracheal lymph node involvement that mimics lymphoma. Tuberculosis can also cause unilateral adenopathy. In older patients, the differential diagnosis includes primary lung cancer (especially among smokers), lymphomas, metastatic carcinoma (usually lung), tuberculosis, fungal infection, and sarcoidosis.

Enlarged intraabdominal or retroperitoneal nodes are usually malignant. Although tuberculosis may present as mesenteric lymphadenitis, these masses usually contain lymphomas or, in young men, germ cell tumors.

LABORATORY INVESTIGATION

The laboratory investigation of patients with lymphadenopathy must be tailored to elucidate the etiology suspected from the patient's history and physical findings. One study from a family practice clinic evaluated 249 younger patients with "enlarged lymph nodes, not infected" or "lymphadenitis." No laboratory studies were obtained in 51%. When studies were performed, the most common were a complete blood count (CBC) (33%), throat culture (16%), chest x-ray (12%), or monospot test (10%). Only eight patients (3%) had a node biopsy, and half of those were normal or reactive. The CBC can provide useful data for the diagnosis of acute or chronic leukemias, EBV or CMV mononucleosis, lymphoma with a leukemic component, pyogenic infections, or immune cytopenias in illnesses such as SLE. Serologic studies may demonstrate antibodies specific to components of EBV, CMV, HIV, and other viruses; *Toxoplasma gondii*; *Brucella*; and so on. If SLE is suspected, antinuclear and anti-DNA antibody studies are warranted.

The chest x-ray is usually negative, but the presence of a pulmonary infiltrate or mediastinal lymphadenopathy would suggest tuberculosis, histoplasmosis, sarcoidosis, lymphoma, primary lung cancer, or metastatic cancer and demands further investigation.

A variety of imaging techniques (computed tomography [CT], magnetic resonance imaging [MRI], ultrasound, color Doppler ultrasonography) have been used to differentiate benign from malignant lymph nodes, especially in patients with head and neck cancer. CT and MRI are comparably accurate (65–90%) in the diagnosis of metastases to cervical lymph nodes. Ultrasonography has been used to determine the long axis, short axis, and a ratio of long to short (L/S) axis in cervical nodes. An L/S ratio of <2.0 has a sensitivity and a specificity of 95% for distinguishing benign and malignant nodes in patients with head and neck cancer. This ratio has greater specificity and sensitivity than palpation or measurement of either the long or the short axis alone.

The indications for lymph node biopsy are imprecise, yet it is a valuable diagnostic tool. The decision to biopsy may be made early in a patient's evaluation or delayed for up to 2 weeks. Prompt biopsy should occur if the patient's history and physical findings suggest a malignancy; examples include a solitary, hard, nontender cervical node in an older patient who is a chronic user of tobacco; supraclavicular adenopathy; and solitary or generalized adenopathy that is firm, movable, and suggestive of lymphoma. If a primary head and neck cancer is suspected as the basis of a solitary, hard cervical node, then a careful ENT examination should be performed. Any mucosal lesion that is suspicious for a primary neoplastic process should be biopsied first. If no mucosal lesion is detected, an excisional biopsy of the largest node should be performed. Fine-needle aspiration should not be performed as the first diagnostic procedure. Most diagnoses require more tissue than such aspiration can provide, and it often delays a definitive diagnosis. Fine-needle aspiration should be reserved for thyroid nodules and for confirmation of relapse in patients whose primary diagnosis is known. If the primary physician is uncertain about whether to proceed to biopsy, consultation with a hematologist or medical oncologist should be helpful. In primary care practices, <5% of lymphadenopathy patients will require a biopsy. That percentage will be considerably larger in referral practices, i.e., hematology, oncology, or ENT.

Two groups have reported algorithms that they claim will identify more precisely those lymphadenopathy patients who should have a biopsy. Both reports were retrospective analyses in referral practices. The first study involved patients 9–25 years of age who had a node biopsy performed. Three variables were identified that predicted those young patients with peripheral lymphadenopathy who should undergo biopsy; lymph node size >2 cm in diameter and abnormal chest x-ray had positive predictive values, whereas recent ENT symptoms had negative predictive values. The second study evaluated 220 lymphadenopathy patients in a hematology unit and identified five variables (lymph node size, location [supraclavicular or nonsupraclavicular], age [>40 years or <40 years], texture [nonhard or hard], and tenderness) that were used in a mathematical model to identify patients requiring a biopsy. Positive predictive value was found for age >40 years, supraclavicular location, node size >2.25 cm^2, hard texture, and lack of pain or tenderness. Negative predictive value was evident for age <40 years, node size <1.0 cm^2, nonhard texture, and tender or painful nodes. Ninety-one percent of those who required biopsy were correctly classified by this model. Because both of these studies were retrospective analyses and one was limited to young patients, it is not known how useful these models would be if applied prospectively in a primary care setting.

Most lymphadenopathy patients do not require a biopsy, and at least half require no laboratory studies. If the patient's history and physical findings point to a benign cause for lymphadenopathy, careful follow-up at a 2- to 4-week interval can be used. The patient should be instructed to return for reevaluation if there is an increase in the size of the nodes. Antibiotics are not indicated for lymphadenopathy unless strong evidence of a bacterial infection is present. Glucocorticoids should not be used to treat lymphadenopathy because their lympholytic effect obscures some diagnoses (lymphoma, leukemia, Castleman's disease), and they contribute to delayed healing or activation of underlying infections. An exception to this statement is the life-threatening pharyngeal obstruction by enlarged lymphoid tissue in Waldeyer's ring that is occasionally seen in infectious mononucleosis.

SPLENOMEGALY

STRUCTURE AND FUNCTION OF THE SPLEEN

The spleen is a reticuloendothelial organ that has its embryologic origin in the dorsal mesogastrium at about 5 weeks of gestation. It arises in a series of hillocks, migrates to its normal adult location in the left upper quadrant (LUQ), and is attached to the stomach via the gastrolienal ligament and to the kidney via the lienorenal ligament. When the hillocks fail to unify into a single tissue mass, accessory spleens may develop in around 20% of persons. The function of the spleen has been elusive. Galen believed it was the source of "black bile" or melancholia, and the word *hypochondria* (literally, beneath the ribs) and the idiom "to vent one's spleen" attest to the beliefs that the spleen had an important influence on the psyche and emotions. In humans, its normal physiologic roles seem to be the following:

1. Maintenance of quality control over erythrocytes in the red pulp by removal of senescent and defective red blood cells. The spleen accomplishes this function through a unique organization of its parenchyma and vasculature (Fig. 79-1).
2. Synthesis of antibodies in the white pulp.
3. The removal of antibody-coated bacteria and antibody-coated blood cells from the circulation.

An increase in these normal functions may result in splenomegaly.

The spleen is composed of *red pulp* and *white pulp*, which are Malpighi's terms for the red blood–filled sinuses and reticuloendothelial

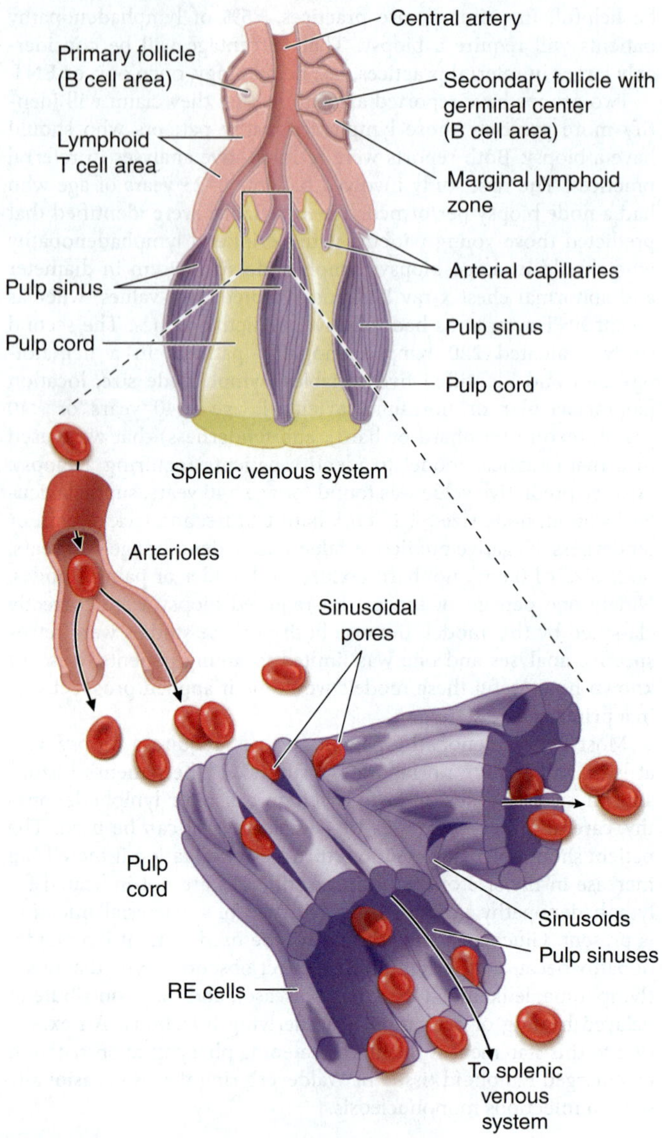

FIGURE 79-1 Schematic spleen structure. The spleen comprises many units of red and white pulp centered around small branches of the splenic artery, called *central arteries*. White pulp is lymphoid in nature and contains B cell follicles, a marginal zone around the follicles, and T cell–rich areas sheathing arterioles. The red pulp areas include pulp sinuses and pulp cords. The cords are dead ends. In order to regain access to the circulation, red blood cells must traverse tiny openings in the sinusoidal lining. Stiff, damaged, or old red cells cannot enter the sinuses. RE, reticuloendothelial. *(Bottom portion of figure from RS Hillman, KA Ault: Hematology in Clinical Practice, 4th ed. New York, McGraw-Hill, 2005.)*

cell–lined cords and the white lymphoid follicles arrayed within the red pulp matrix. The spleen is in the portal circulation. The reason for this is unknown but may relate to the fact that lower blood pressure allows less rapid flow and minimizes damage to normal erythrocytes. Blood flows into the spleen at a rate of about 150 mL/min through the splenic artery, which ultimately ramifies into central arterioles. Some blood goes from the arterioles to capillaries and then to splenic veins and out of the spleen, but the majority of blood from central arterioles flows into the macrophage-lined sinuses and cords. The blood entering the sinuses reenters the circulation through the splenic venules, but the blood entering the cords is subjected to an inspection of sorts. To return to the circulation, the blood cells in the cords must squeeze through slits in the cord lining to enter the sinuses that lead to the venules. Old and damaged erythrocytes are less deformable and are retained in the cords, where they are destroyed and their components recycled. Red cell–inclusion bodies such as parasites (Chaps. 248 and 250e), nuclear residua (Howell-Jolly bodies, see Fig. 77-6), or denatured hemoglobin (Heinz bodies) are pinched off in the process of passing through the slits, a process called *pitting*. The culling of dead and damaged cells and the pitting of cells with inclusions appear to occur without significant delay because the blood transit time through the spleen is only slightly slower than in other organs.

The spleen is also capable of assisting the host in adapting to its hostile environment. It has at least three adaptive functions: (1) clearance of bacteria and particulates from the blood, (2) the generation of immune responses to certain pathogens, and (3) the generation of cellular components of the blood under circumstances in which the marrow is unable to meet the needs (i.e., extramedullary hematopoiesis). The latter adaptation is a recapitulation of the blood-forming function the spleen plays during gestation. In some animals, the spleen also serves a role in the vascular adaptation to stress because it stores red blood cells (often hemoconcentrated to higher hematocrits than normal) under normal circumstances and contracts under the influence of β-adrenergic stimulation to provide the animal with an autotransfusion and improved oxygen-carrying capacity. However, the normal human spleen does not sequester or store red blood cells and does not contract in response to sympathetic stimuli. The normal human spleen contains approximately one-third of the total body platelets and a significant number of marginated neutrophils. These sequestered cells are available when needed to respond to bleeding or infection.

APPROACH TO THE PATIENT: Splenomegaly

CLINICAL ASSESSMENT

The most common *symptoms* produced by diseases involving the spleen are pain and a heavy sensation in the LUQ. Massive splenomegaly may cause early satiety. Pain may result from acute swelling of the spleen with stretching of the capsule, infarction, or inflammation of the capsule. For many years, it was believed that splenic infarction was clinically silent, which, at times, is true. However, Soma Weiss, in his classic 1942 report of the self-observations by a Harvard medical student on the clinical course of subacute bacterial endocarditis, documented that severe LUQ and pleuritic chest pain may accompany thromboembolic occlusion of splenic blood flow. Vascular occlusion, with infarction and pain, is commonly seen in children with sickle cell crises. Rupture of the spleen, from either trauma or infiltrative disease that breaks the capsule, may result in intraperitoneal bleeding, shock, and death. The rupture itself may be painless.

A palpable spleen is the major *physical sign* produced by diseases affecting the spleen and suggests enlargement of the organ. The normal spleen weighs <250 g, decreases in size with age, normally lies entirely within the rib cage, has a maximum cephalocaudad diameter of 13 cm by ultrasonography or maximum length of 12 cm and/or width of 7 cm by radionuclide scan, and is usually not palpable. However, a palpable spleen was found in 3% of 2200 asymptomatic, male, freshman college students. Follow-up at 3 years revealed that 30% of those students still had a palpable spleen without any increase in disease prevalence. Ten-year follow-up found no evidence for lymphoid malignancies. Furthermore, in some tropical countries (e.g., New Guinea), the incidence of splenomegaly may reach 60%. Thus, the presence of a palpable spleen does not always equate with presence of disease. Even when disease is present, splenomegaly may not reflect the primary disease but rather a reaction to it. For example, in patients with Hodgkin's disease, only two-thirds of the palpable spleens show involvement by the cancer.

Physical examination of the spleen uses primarily the techniques of palpation and percussion. Inspection may reveal fullness in the LUQ that descends on inspiration, a finding associated with a massively enlarged spleen. Auscultation may reveal a venous hum or friction rub.

Palpation can be accomplished by bimanual palpation, ballotment, and palpation from above (Middleton maneuver). For bimanual palpation, which is at least as reliable as the other techniques, the patient is supine with flexed knees. The examiner's left hand is placed on the lower rib cage and pulls the skin toward the costal margin, allowing the fingertips of the right hand to feel the tip of the spleen as it descends while the patient inspires slowly, smoothly, and deeply. Palpation is begun with the right hand in the left lower quadrant with gradual movement toward the left costal margin, thereby identifying the lower edge of a massively enlarged spleen. When the spleen tip is felt, the finding is recorded as centimeters below the left costal margin at some arbitrary point, i.e., 10–15 cm, from the midpoint of the umbilicus or the xiphisternal junction. This allows other examiners to compare findings or the initial examiner to determine changes in size over time. Bimanual palpation in the right lateral decubitus position adds nothing to the supine examination.

Percussion for splenic dullness is accomplished with any of three techniques described by Nixon, Castell, or Barkun:

1. *Nixon's method*: The patient is placed on the right side so that the spleen lies above the colon and stomach. Percussion begins at the lower level of pulmonary resonance in the posterior axillary line and proceeds diagonally along a perpendicular line toward the lower midanterior costal margin. The upper border of dullness is normally 6–8 cm above the costal margin. Dullness >8 cm in an adult is presumed to indicate splenic enlargement.
2. *Castell's method*: With the patient supine, percussion in the lowest intercostal space in the anterior axillary line (eighth or ninth) produces a resonant note if the spleen is normal in size. This is true during expiration or full inspiration. A dull percussion note on full inspiration suggests splenomegaly.
3. *Percussion of Traube's semilunar space*: The borders of Traube's space are the sixth rib superiorly, the left midaxillary line laterally, and the left costal margin inferiorly. The patient is supine with the left arm slightly abducted. During normal breathing, this space is percussed from medial to lateral margins, yielding a normal resonant sound. A dull percussion note suggests splenomegaly.

Studies comparing methods of percussion and palpation with a standard of ultrasonography or scintigraphy have revealed sensitivity of 56–71% for palpation and 59–82% for percussion. Reproducibility among examiners is better for palpation than percussion. Both techniques are less reliable in obese patients or patients who have just eaten. Thus, the physical examination techniques of palpation and percussion are imprecise at best. It has been suggested that the examiner perform percussion first and, if positive, proceed to palpation; if the spleen is palpable, then one can be reasonably confident that splenomegaly exists. However, not all LUQ masses are enlarged spleens; gastric or colon tumors and pancreatic or renal cysts or tumors can mimic splenomegaly.

The presence of an enlarged spleen can be more precisely determined, if necessary, by liver-spleen radionuclide scan, CT, MRI, or ultrasonography. The latter technique is the current procedure of choice for routine assessment of spleen size (normal = a maximum cephalocaudad diameter of 13 cm) because it has high sensitivity and specificity and is safe, noninvasive, quick, mobile, and less costly. Nuclear medicine scans are accurate, sensitive, and reliable but are costly, require greater time to generate data, and use immobile equipment. They have the advantage of demonstrating accessory splenic tissue. CT and MRI provide accurate determination of spleen size, but the equipment is immobile and the procedures are expensive. MRI appears to offer no advantage over CT. Changes in spleen structure such as mass lesions, infarcts, inhomogeneous infiltrates, and cysts are more readily assessed by CT, MRI, or ultrasonography. None of these techniques is very reliable in the detection of patchy infiltration (e.g., Hodgkin's disease).

DIFFERENTIAL DIAGNOSIS

Many of the diseases associated with splenomegaly are listed in Table 79-2. They are grouped according to the presumed basic mechanisms responsible for organ enlargement:

1. Hyperplasia or hypertrophy related to a particular splenic function such as reticuloendothelial hyperplasia (work hypertrophy) in diseases such as hereditary spherocytosis or thalassemia syndromes that require removal of large numbers of defective red blood cells; immune hyperplasia in response to systemic infection (infectious mononucleosis, subacute bacterial endocarditis) or to immunologic diseases (immune thrombocytopenia, SLE, Felty's syndrome).
2. Passive congestion due to decreased blood flow from the spleen in conditions that produce portal hypertension (cirrhosis, Budd-Chiari syndrome, congestive heart failure).
3. Infiltrative diseases of the spleen (lymphomas, metastatic cancer, amyloidosis, Gaucher's disease, myeloproliferative disorders with extramedullary hematopoiesis).

The differential diagnostic possibilities are much fewer when the spleen is "massively enlarged," palpable more than 8 cm below the left costal margin or has a drained weight of ≥1000 g (Table 79-3). The vast majority of such patients will have non-Hodgkin's lymphoma, chronic lymphocytic leukemia, hairy cell leukemia, chronic myeloid leukemia, myelofibrosis with myeloid metaplasia, or polycythemia vera.

LABORATORY ASSESSMENT

The major laboratory abnormalities accompanying splenomegaly are determined by the underlying systemic illness. Erythrocyte counts may be normal, decreased (thalassemia major syndromes, SLE, cirrhosis with portal hypertension), or increased (polycythemia vera). Granulocyte counts may be normal, decreased (Felty's syndrome, congestive splenomegaly, leukemias), or increased (infections or inflammatory disease, myeloproliferative disorders). Similarly, the platelet count may be normal, decreased when there is enhanced sequestration or destruction of platelets in an enlarged spleen (congestive splenomegaly, Gaucher's disease, immune thrombocytopenia), or increased in the myeloproliferative disorders such as polycythemia vera.

The CBC may reveal cytopenia of one or more blood cell types, which should suggest *hypersplenism*. This condition is characterized by splenomegaly, cytopenia(s), normal or hyperplastic bone marrow, and a response to splenectomy. The latter characteristic is less precise because reversal of cytopenia, particularly granulocytopenia, is sometimes not sustained after splenectomy. The cytopenias result from increased destruction of the cellular elements secondary to reduced flow of blood through enlarged and congested cords (congestive splenomegaly) or to immune-mediated mechanisms. In hypersplenism, various cell types usually have normal morphology on the peripheral blood smear, although the red cells may be spherocytic due to loss of surface area during their longer transit through the enlarged spleen. The increased marrow production of red cells should be reflected as an increased reticulocyte production index, although the value may be less than expected due to increased sequestration of reticulocytes in the spleen.

The need for additional laboratory studies is dictated by the differential diagnosis of the underlying illness of which splenomegaly is a manifestation.

SPLENECTOMY

Splenectomy is infrequently performed for diagnostic purposes, especially in the absence of clinical illness or other diagnostic tests that suggest underlying disease. More often, splenectomy is performed for symptom control in patients with massive splenomegaly, for disease control in patients with traumatic splenic rupture, or for correction of cytopenias in patients with hypersplenism or immune-mediated destruction of one or more cellular blood elements. Splenectomy is

TABLE 79-2 DISEASES ASSOCIATED WITH SPLENOMEGALY GROUPED BY PATHOGENIC MECHANISM

Enlargement Due to Increased Demand for Splenic Function	
Reticuloendothelial system hyperplasia (for removal of defective erythrocytes)	Leishmaniasis
Spherocytosis	Trypanosomiasis
Early sickle cell anemia	Ehrlichiosis
Ovalocytosis	Disordered immunoregulation
Thalassemia major	Rheumatoid arthritis (Felty's syndrome)
Hemoglobinopathies	Systemic lupus erythematosus
Paroxysmal nocturnal hemoglobinuria	Collagen vascular diseases
Pernicious anemia	Serum sickness
Immune hyperplasia	Immune hemolytic anemias
Response to infection (viral, bacterial, fungal, parasitic)	Immune thrombocytopenias
Infectious mononucleosis	Immune neutropenias
AIDS	Drug reactions
Viral hepatitis	Angioimmunoblastic lymphadenopathy
Cytomegalovirus	Sarcoidosis
Subacute bacterial endocarditis	Thyrotoxicosis (benign lymphoid hypertrophy)
Bacterial septicemia	Interleukin 2 therapy
Congenital syphilis	Extramedullary hematopoiesis
Splenic abscess	Myelofibrosis
Tuberculosis	Marrow damage by toxins, radiation, strontium
Histoplasmosis	Marrow infiltration by tumors, leukemias, Gaucher's disease
Malaria	
Enlargement Due to Abnormal Splenic or Portal Blood Flow	
Cirrhosis	Splenic artery aneurysm
Hepatic vein obstruction	Hepatic schistosomiasis
Portal vein obstruction, intrahepatic or extrahepatic	Congestive heart failure
Cavernous transformation of the portal vein	Hepatic echinococcosis
Splenic vein obstruction	Portal hypertension (any cause including the above): "Banti's disease"
Infiltration of the Spleen	
Intracellular or extracellular depositions	Hodgkin's disease
Amyloidosis	Myeloproliferative syndromes (e.g., polycythemia vera, essential thrombocytosis)
Gaucher's disease	
Niemann-Pick disease	Angiosarcomas
Tangier disease	Metastatic tumors (melanoma is most common)
Hurler's syndrome and other mucopolysaccharidoses	Eosinophilic granuloma
Hyperlipidemias	Histiocytosis X
Benign and malignant cellular infiltrations	Hamartomas
Leukemias (acute, chronic, lymphoid, myeloid, monocytic)	Hemangiomas, fibromas, lymphangiomas
Lymphomas	Splenic cysts
Unknown Etiology	
Idiopathic splenomegaly	Iron-deficiency anemia
Berylliosis	

necessary for staging of patients with Hodgkin's disease only in those with clinical stage I or II disease in whom radiation therapy alone is contemplated as the treatment. Noninvasive staging of the spleen in Hodgkin's disease is not a sufficiently reliable basis for treatment decisions because one-third of normal-sized spleens will be involved with Hodgkin's disease and one-third of enlarged spleens will be tumor-free. The widespread use of systemic therapy to test all stages of Hodgkin's disease has made staging laparotomy with splenectomy unnecessary. Although splenectomy in chronic myeloid leukemia (CML) does not affect the natural history of disease, removal of the massive spleen usually makes patients significantly more comfortable and simplifies their management by significantly reducing transfusion requirements. The improvements in therapy of CML have reduced the need for splenectomy for symptom control. Splenectomy is an effective secondary or tertiary treatment for two chronic B cell leukemias, hairy cell leukemia and prolymphocytic leukemia, and for the very rare splenic mantle cell or marginal zone lymphoma. Splenectomy in these diseases may be associated with significant tumor regression in bone marrow and other sites of disease. Similar regressions of systemic disease have been noted after splenic irradiation in some types of lymphoid tumors, especially chronic lymphocytic leukemia and prolymphocytic leukemia. This has been termed the *abscopal effect*. Such systemic tumor responses to local therapy directed at the spleen suggest that some hormone or growth factor produced by the spleen may affect tumor cell proliferation, but this conjecture is not yet substantiated.

TABLE 79-3 DISEASES ASSOCIATED WITH MASSIVE SPLENOMEGALY[a]

Chronic myeloid leukemia	Gaucher's disease
Lymphomas	Chronic lymphocytic leukemia
Hairy cell leukemia	Sarcoidosis
Myelofibrosis with myeloid metaplasia	Autoimmune hemolytic anemia
Polycythemia vera	Diffuse splenic hemangiomatosis

[a]The spleen extends >8 cm below the left costal margin and/or weighs >1000 g.

A common therapeutic indication for splenectomy is traumatic or iatrogenic splenic rupture. In a fraction of patients with splenic rupture, peritoneal seeding of splenic fragments can lead to *splenosis*—the presence of multiple rests of spleen tissue not connected to the portal circulation. This ectopic spleen tissue may cause pain or gastrointestinal obstruction, as in endometriosis. A large number of hematologic, immunologic, and congestive causes of splenomegaly can lead to destruction of one or more cellular blood elements. In the majority of such cases, splenectomy can correct the cytopenias, particularly anemia and thrombocytopenia. In a large series of patients seen in two tertiary care centers, the indication for splenectomy was diagnostic in 10% of patients, therapeutic in 44%, staging for Hodgkin's disease in 20%, and incidental to another procedure in 26%. Perhaps the only contraindication to splenectomy is the presence of marrow failure, in which the enlarged spleen is the only source of hematopoietic tissue.

The absence of the spleen has minimal long-term effects on the hematologic profile. In the immediate postsplenectomy period, leukocytosis (up to 25,000/μL) and thrombocytosis (up to 1×10^6/μL) may develop, but within 2–3 weeks, blood cell counts and survival of each cell lineage are usually normal. The chronic manifestations of splenectomy are marked variation in size and shape of erythrocytes (anisocytosis, poikilocytosis) and the presence of Howell-Jolly bodies (nuclear remnants), Heinz bodies (denatured hemoglobin), basophilic stippling, and an occasional nucleated erythrocyte in the peripheral blood. When such erythrocyte abnormalities appear in a patient whose spleen has not been removed, one should suspect splenic infiltration by tumor that has interfered with its normal culling and pitting function.

The most serious consequence of splenectomy is increased susceptibility to bacterial infections, particularly those with capsules such as *Streptococcus pneumoniae*, *Haemophilus influenzae*, and some gram-negative enteric organisms. Patients under age 20 years are particularly susceptible to overwhelming sepsis with *S. pneumoniae*, and the overall actuarial risk of sepsis in patients who have had their spleens removed is about 7% in 10 years. The case–fatality rate for pneumococcal sepsis in splenectomized patients is 50–80%. About 25% of patients without spleens will develop a serious infection at some time in their life. The frequency is highest within the first 3 years after splenectomy. About 15% of the infections are polymicrobial, and lung, skin, and blood are the most common sites. No increased risk of viral infection has been noted in patients who have no spleen. The susceptibility to bacterial infections relates to the inability to remove opsonized bacteria from the bloodstream and a defect in making antibodies to T cell–independent antigens such as the polysaccharide components of bacterial capsules. Pneumococcal vaccine should be administered to all patients 2 weeks before elective splenectomy. The Advisory Committee on Immunization Practices recommends that these patients receive repeat vaccination 5 years after splenectomy. Efficacy has not been proven for this group, and the recommendation discounts the possibility that administration of the vaccine may actually lower the titer of specific pneumococcal antibodies. A more effective pneumococcal conjugate vaccine that involves T cells in the response is now available (Prevenar, 7-valent). The vaccine to *Neisseria meningitidis* should also be given to patients in whom elective splenectomy is planned. Although efficacy data for *H. influenzae* type b vaccine are not available for older children or adults, it may be given to patients who have had a splenectomy.

Splenectomized patients should be educated to consider any unexplained fever as a medical emergency. Prompt medical attention with evaluation and treatment of suspected bacteremia may be life-saving. Routine chemoprophylaxis with oral penicillin can result in the emergence of drug-resistant strains and is not recommended.

In addition to an increased susceptibility to bacterial infections, splenectomized patients are also more susceptible to the parasitic disease babesiosis. The splenectomized patient should avoid areas where the parasite *Babesia* is endemic (e.g., Cape Cod, MA).

Surgical removal of the spleen is an obvious cause of hyposplenism. Patients with sickle cell disease often suffer from autosplenectomy as a result of splenic destruction by the numerous infarcts associated with sickle cell crises during childhood. Indeed, the presence of a palpable spleen in a patient with sickle cell disease after age 5 suggests a coexisting hemoglobinopathy, e.g., thalassemia or hemoglobin C. In addition, patients who receive splenic irradiation for a neoplastic or autoimmune disease are also functionally hyposplenic. The term *hyposplenism* is preferred to *asplenism* in referring to the physiologic consequences of splenectomy because asplenia is a rare, specific, and fatal congenital abnormality in which there is a failure of the left side of the coelomic cavity (which includes the splenic anlagen) to develop normally. Infants with asplenia have no spleens, but that is the least of their problems. The right side of the developing embryo is duplicated on the left so there is liver where the spleen should be, there are two right lungs, and the heart comprises two right atria and two right ventricles.

80 Disorders of Granulocytes and Monocytes

Steven M. Holland, John I. Gallin

Leukocytes, the major cells comprising inflammatory and immune responses, include neutrophils, T and B lymphocytes, natural killer (NK) cells, monocytes, eosinophils, and basophils. These cells have specific functions, such as antibody production by B lymphocytes or destruction of bacteria by neutrophils, but in no single infectious disease is the exact role of the cell types completely established. Thus, whereas neutrophils are classically thought to be critical to host defense against bacteria, they may also play important roles in defense against viral infections.

The blood delivers leukocytes to the various tissues from the bone marrow, where they are produced. Normal blood leukocyte counts are $4.3–10.8 \times 10^9$/L, with neutrophils representing 45–74% of the cells, bands 0–4%, lymphocytes 16–45%, monocytes 4–10%, eosinophils 0–7%, and basophils 0–2%. Variation among individuals and among different ethnic groups can be substantial, with lower leukocyte numbers for certain African-American ethnic groups. The various leukocytes are derived from a common stem cell in the bone marrow. Three-fourths of the nucleated cells of bone marrow are committed to the production of leukocytes. Leukocyte maturation in the marrow is under the regulatory control of a number of different factors, known as colony-stimulating factors (CSFs) and interleukins (ILs). Because an alteration in the number and type of leukocytes is often associated with disease processes, total white blood cell (WBC) count (cells per μL) and differential counts are informative. This chapter focuses on neutrophils, monocytes, and eosinophils. Lymphocytes and basophils are discussed in Chaps. 372e and 376, respectively.

NEUTROPHILS

MATURATION

Important events in neutrophil life are summarized in Fig. 80-1. In normal humans, neutrophils are produced only in the bone marrow. The minimum number of stem cells necessary to support hematopoiesis is estimated to be 400–500 at any one time. Human blood monocytes, tissue macrophages, and stromal cells produce CSFs, hormones required for the growth of monocytes and neutrophils in the bone marrow. The hematopoietic system not only produces enough neutrophils (~1.3×10^{11} cells per 80-kg person per day) to carry out physiologic functions but also has a large reserve stored in the marrow, which can be mobilized in response to inflammation or infection. An increase in the number of blood neutrophils is called *neutrophilia*, and the presence of immature cells is termed a *shift to the left*. A decrease in the number of blood neutrophils is called *neutropenia*.

Neutrophils and monocytes evolve from pluripotent stem cells under the influence of cytokines and CSFs (Fig. 80-2). The proliferation phase through the metamyelocyte takes about 1 week, while the maturation phase from metamyelocyte to mature neutrophil takes

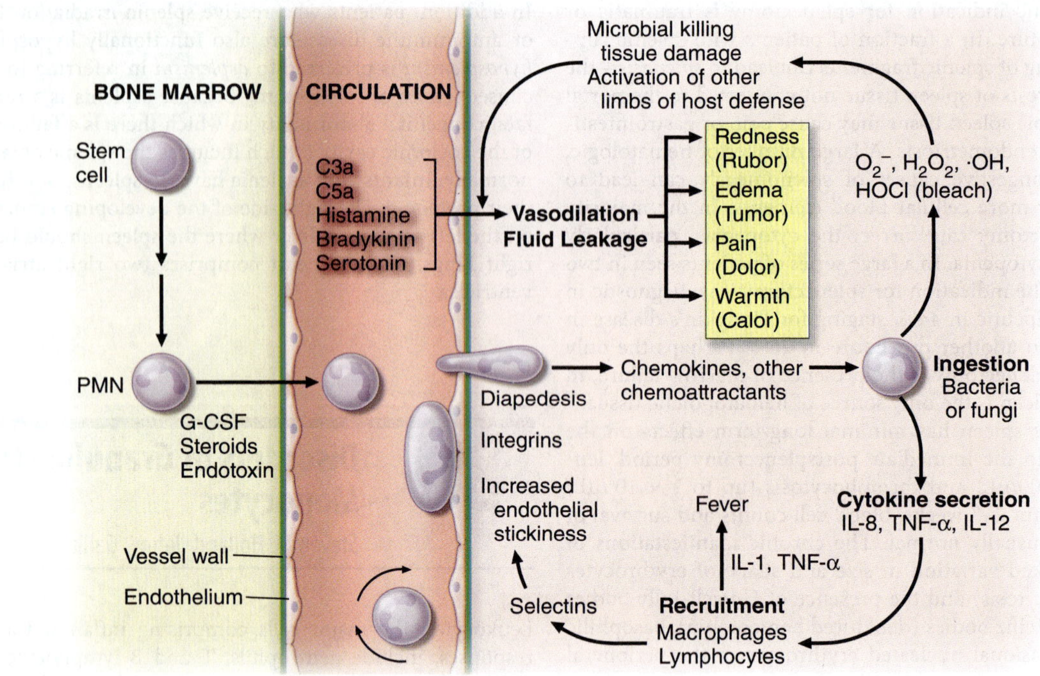

FIGURE 80-1 Schematic events in neutrophil production, recruitment, and inflammation. The four cardinal signs of inflammation (rubor, tumor, calor, dolor) are indicated, as are the interactions of neutrophils with other cells and cytokines. G-CSF, granulocyte colony-stimulating factor; IL, interleukin; PMN, polymorphonuclear leukocyte; TNF-α, tumor necrosis factor α.

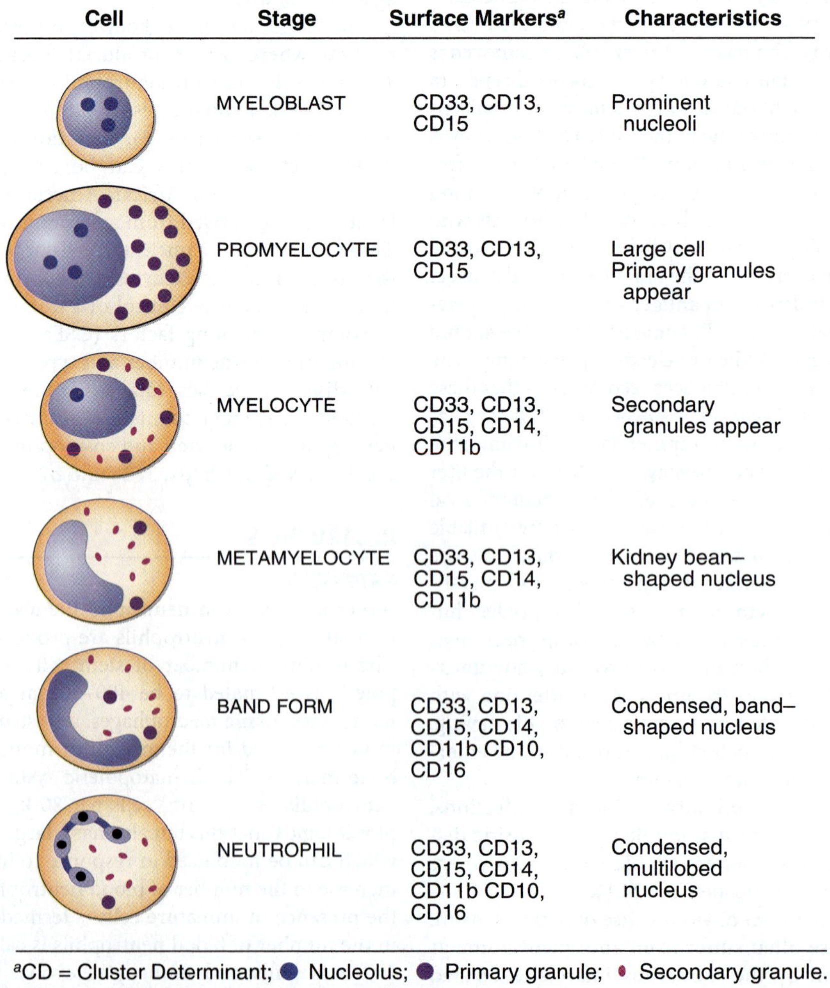

FIGURE 80-2 Stages of neutrophil development shown schematically. Granulocyte colony-stimulating factor (G-CSF) and granulocyte-macrophage colony-stimulating factor (GM-CSF) are critical to this process. Identifying cellular characteristics and specific cell-surface markers are listed for each maturational stage.

another week. The myeloblast is the first recognizable precursor cell and is followed by the *promyelocyte*. The promyelocyte evolves when the classic lysosomal granules, called the *primary*, or *azurophil, granules* are produced. The primary granules contain hydrolases, elastase, myeloperoxidase, cathepsin G, cationic proteins, and bactericidal/permeability-increasing protein, which is important for killing gram-negative bacteria. Azurophil granules also contain *defensins*, a family of cysteine-rich polypeptides with broad antimicrobial activity against bacteria, fungi, and certain enveloped viruses. The promyelocyte divides to produce the *myelocyte*, a cell responsible for the synthesis of the *specific*, or *secondary, granules*, which contain unique (specific) constituents such as lactoferrin, vitamin B_{12}–binding protein, membrane components of the reduced nicotinamide-adenine dinucleotide phosphate (NADPH) oxidase required for hydrogen peroxide production, histaminase, and receptors for certain chemoattractants and adherence-promoting factors (CR3) as well as receptors for the basement membrane component, laminin. The secondary granules do not contain acid hydrolases and therefore are not classic lysosomes. Packaging of secondary granule contents during myelopoiesis is controlled by CCAAT/enhancer binding protein-ε. Secondary granule contents are readily released extracellularly, and their mobilization is important in modulating inflammation. During the final stages of maturation, no cell division occurs, and the cell passes through the metamyelocyte stage and then to the band neutrophil with a sausage-shaped nucleus (Fig. 80-3). As the band cell matures, the nucleus assumes a lobulated configuration. The nucleus of neutrophils normally contains up to four segments (Fig. 80-4). Excessive segmentation (more than five nuclear lobes) may be a manifestation of folate or vitamin B_{12} deficiency or the congenital neutropenia syndrome of warts, hypogammaglobulinemia, infections, and myelokathexis (WHIM) described below. The Pelger-Hüet anomaly (Fig. 80-5), an infrequent dominant benign inherited trait, results in neutrophils with distinctive bilobed nuclei that must be distinguished from band forms. Acquired bilobed nuclei, pseudo Pelger-Hüet anomaly, can occur with acute infections or in myelodysplastic syndromes. The physiologic role of the normal multilobed nucleus of neutrophils is unknown, but it may allow great deformation of neutrophils during migration into tissues at sites of inflammation.

In severe acute bacterial infection, prominent neutrophil cytoplasmic granules, called *toxic granulations*, are occasionally seen. Toxic granulations are immature or abnormally staining azurophil granules. Cytoplasmic inclusions, also called *Döhle bodies* (Fig. 80-3), can be seen during infection and are fragments of ribosome-rich endoplasmic reticulum. Large neutrophil vacuoles are often present in acute

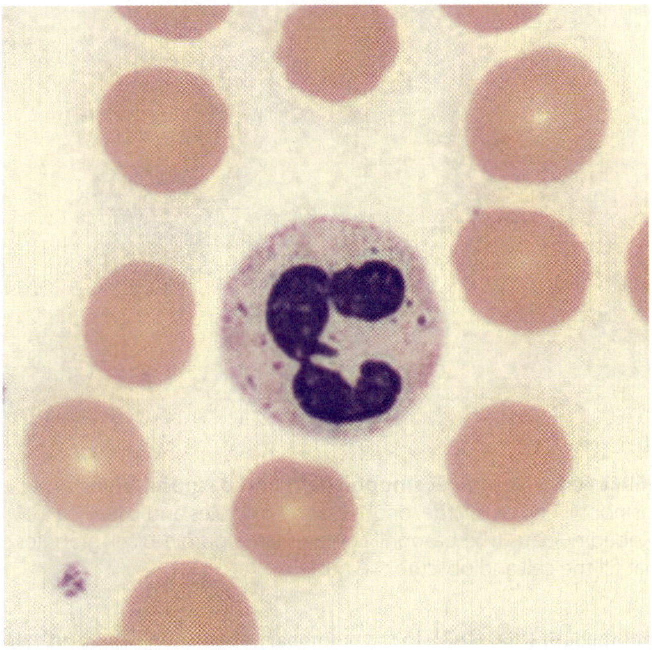

FIGURE 80-4 Normal granulocyte. The normal granulocyte has a segmented nucleus with heavy, clumped chromatin; fine neutrophilic granules are dispersed throughout the cytoplasm.

bacterial infection and probably represent pinocytosed (internalized) membrane.

Neutrophils are heterogeneous in function. Monoclonal antibodies have been developed that recognize only a subset of mature neutrophils. The meaning of neutrophil heterogeneity is not known.

The morphology of eosinophils and basophils is shown in Fig. 80-6.

MARROW RELEASE AND CIRCULATING COMPARTMENTS

Specific signals, including IL-1, tumor necrosis factor α (TNF-α), the CSFs, complement fragments, and chemokines, mobilize leukocytes from the bone marrow and deliver them to the blood in an unstimulated state. Under normal conditions, ~90% of the neutrophil pool is in the bone marrow, 2–3% in the circulation, and the remainder in the tissues (Fig. 80-7).

The circulating pool exists in two dynamic compartments: one freely flowing and one marginated. The freely flowing pool is about one-half the neutrophils in the basal state and is composed of those cells that are in the blood and not in contact with the endothelium. Marginated leukocytes are those that are in close physical contact with the

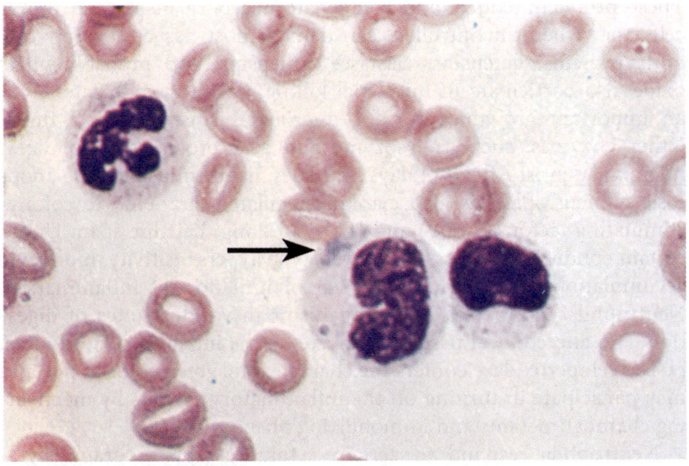

FIGURE 80-3 Neutrophil band with Döhle body. The neutrophil with a sausage-shaped nucleus in the center of the field is a band form. Döhle bodies are discrete, blue-staining, nongranular areas found in the periphery of the cytoplasm of the neutrophil in infections and other toxic states. They represent aggregates of rough endoplasmic reticulum.

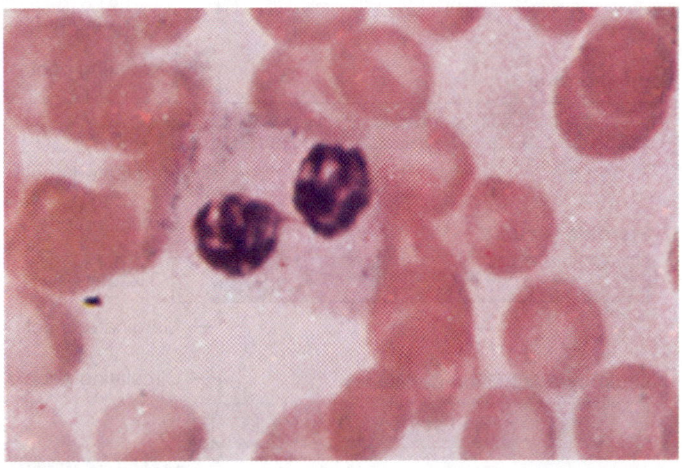

FIGURE 80-5 Pelger-Hüet anomaly. In this benign disorder, the majority of granulocytes are bilobed. The nucleus frequently has a spectacle-like, or "pince-nez," configuration.

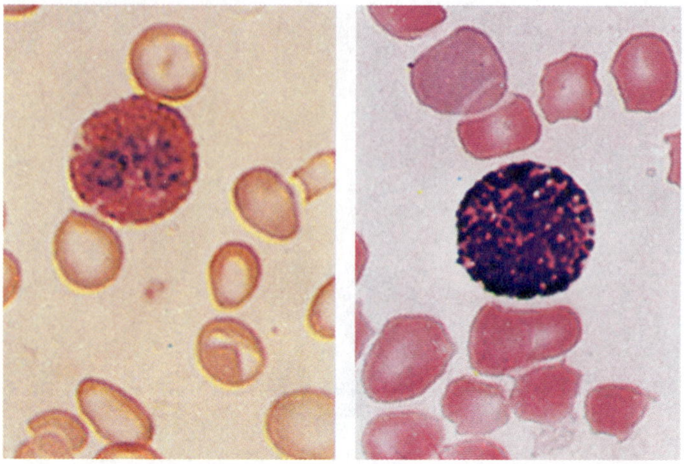

FIGURE 80-6 Normal eosinophil (*left*) and basophil (*right*). The eosinophil contains large, bright orange granules and usually a bilobed nucleus. The basophil contains large purple-black granules that fill the cell and obscure the nucleus.

endothelium (Fig. 80-8). In the pulmonary circulation, where an extensive capillary bed (~1000 capillaries per alveolus) exists, margination occurs because the capillaries are about the same size as a mature neutrophil. Therefore, neutrophil fluidity and deformability are necessary to make the transit through the pulmonary bed. Increased neutrophil rigidity and decreased deformability lead to augmented neutrophil trapping and margination in the lung. In contrast, in the systemic postcapillary venules, margination is mediated by the interaction of specific cell-surface molecules called *selectins*. Selectins are glycoproteins expressed on neutrophils and endothelial cells, among others, that cause a low-affinity interaction, resulting in "rolling" of the neutrophil along the endothelial surface. On neutrophils, the molecule L-selectin (cluster determinant [CD] 62L) binds to glycosylated proteins on endothelial cells (e.g., glycosylation-dependent cell adhesion molecule [GlyCAM1] and CD34). Glycoproteins on neutrophils, most importantly sialyl-Lewis^x (SLe^x, CD15s), are targets for binding of selectins expressed on endothelial cells (E-selectin [CD62E] and P-selectin [CD62P]) and other leukocytes. In response to chemotactic stimuli from injured tissues (e.g., complement product C5a, leukotriene B_4, IL-8) or bacterial products (e.g., *N*-formylmethionylleucylphenylalanine [f-met-leu-phe]), neutrophil adhesiveness increases through mobilization of intracellular adhesion proteins stored in specific granules to the cell surface, and the cells "stick" to the endothelium through *integrins*. The integrins are leukocyte glycoproteins that exist as complexes of a common CD18 β chain with CD11a (LFA-1), CD11b (called Mac-1, CR3, or the C3bi receptor), and CD11c (called p150,95 or CR4). CD11a/CD18 and CD11b/CD18 bind to specific endothelial receptors (intercellular adhesion molecules [ICAM] 1 and 2).

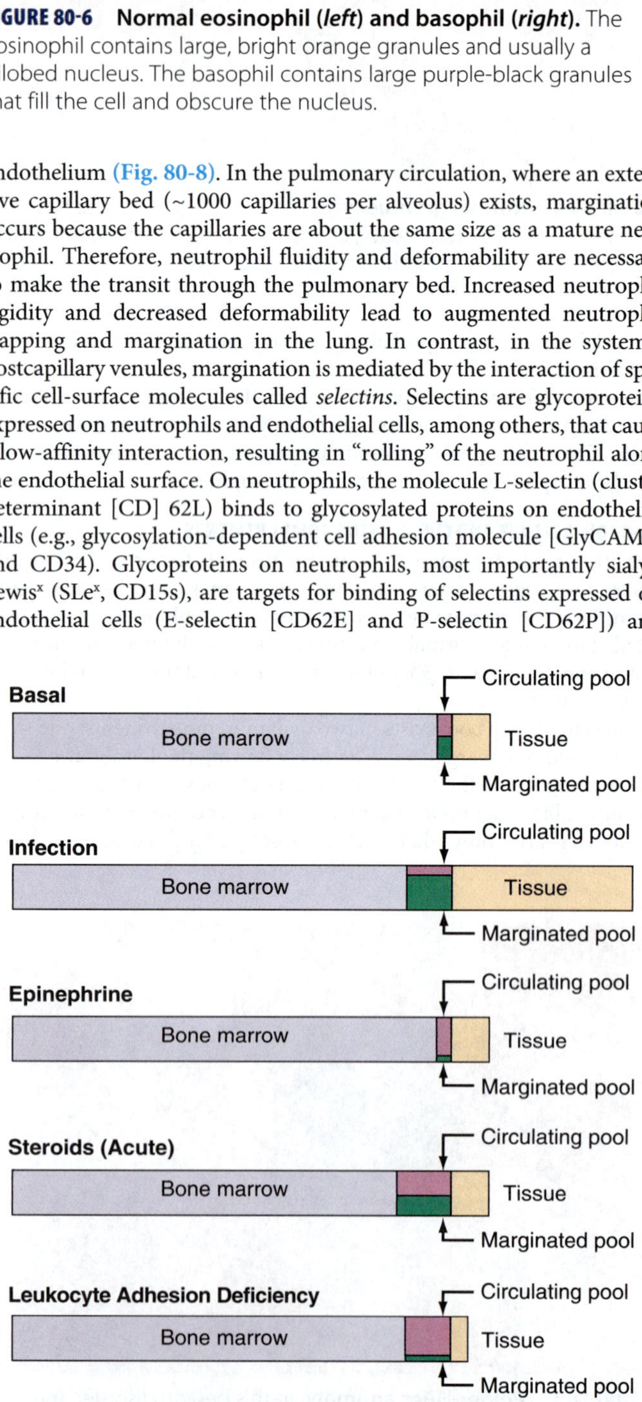

FIGURE 80-7 Schematic neutrophil distribution and kinetics between the different anatomic and functional pools.

On cell stimulation, L-selectin is shed from neutrophils, and E-selectin increases in the blood, presumably because it is shed from endothelial cells; receptors for chemoattractants and opsonins are mobilized; and the phagocytes orient toward the chemoattractant source in the extravascular space, increase their motile activity (chemokinesis), and migrate directionally (chemotaxis) into tissues. The process of migration into tissues is called *diapedesis* and involves the crawling of neutrophils between postcapillary endothelial cells that open junctions between adjacent cells to permit leukocyte passage. Diapedesis involves platelet/endothelial cell adhesion molecule (PECAM) 1 (CD31), which is expressed on both the emigrating leukocyte and the endothelial cells. The endothelial responses (increased blood flow from increased vasodilation and permeability) are mediated by anaphylatoxins (e.g., C3a and C5a) as well as vasodilators such as histamine, bradykinin, serotonin, nitric oxide, vascular endothelial growth factor (VEGF), and prostaglandins E and I. Cytokines regulate some of these processes (e.g., TNF-α induction of VEGF, interferon [IFN] γ inhibition of prostaglandin E).

In the healthy adult, most neutrophils leave the body by migration through the mucous membrane of the gastrointestinal tract. Normally, neutrophils spend a short time in the circulation (half-life, 6–7 h). Senescent neutrophils are cleared from the circulation by macrophages in the lung and spleen. Once in the tissues, neutrophils release enzymes, such as collagenase and elastase, which may help establish abscess cavities. Neutrophils ingest pathogenic materials that have been opsonized by IgG and C3b. Fibronectin and the tetrapeptide tuftsin also facilitate phagocytosis.

With phagocytosis comes a burst of oxygen consumption and activation of the hexose-monophosphate shunt. A membrane-associated NADPH oxidase, consisting of membrane and cytosolic components, is assembled and catalyzes the univalent reduction of oxygen to superoxide anion, which is then converted by superoxide dismutase to hydrogen peroxide and other toxic oxygen products (e.g., hydroxyl radical). Hydrogen peroxide + chloride + neutrophil myeloperoxidase generate hypochlorous acid (bleach), hypochlorite, and chlorine. These products oxidize and halogenate microorganisms and tumor cells and, when uncontrolled, can damage host tissue. Strongly cationic proteins, defensins, elastase, cathepsins, and probably nitric oxide also participate in microbial killing. Lactoferrin chelates iron, an important growth factor for microorganisms, especially fungi. Other enzymes, such as lysozyme and acid proteases, help digest microbial debris. After 1–4 days in tissues, neutrophils die. The apoptosis of neutrophils is also cytokine-regulated; granulocyte colony-stimulating factor (G-CSF) and IFN-γ prolong their life span. Under certain conditions, such as in delayed-type hypersensitivity, monocyte accumulation occurs within 6–12 h of initiation of inflammation. Neutrophils, monocytes, microorganisms in various states of digestion, and altered local tissue cells make up the inflammatory exudate, pus. Myeloperoxidase confers the characteristic green color to pus and may participate in turning off the inflammatory process by inactivating chemoattractants and immobilizing phagocytic cells.

Neutrophils respond to certain cytokines (IFN-γ, granulocyte-macrophage colony-stimulating factor [GM-CSF], IL-8) and produce cytokines and chemotactic signals (TNF-α, IL-8, macrophage inflammatory protein [MIP] 1) that modulate the inflammatory response. In the presence of fibrinogen, f-met-leu-phe or leukotriene B_4 induces IL-8 production by neutrophils, providing autocrine amplification of inflammation. *Chemokines* (*chemo*attractant cyto*kines*) are small proteins

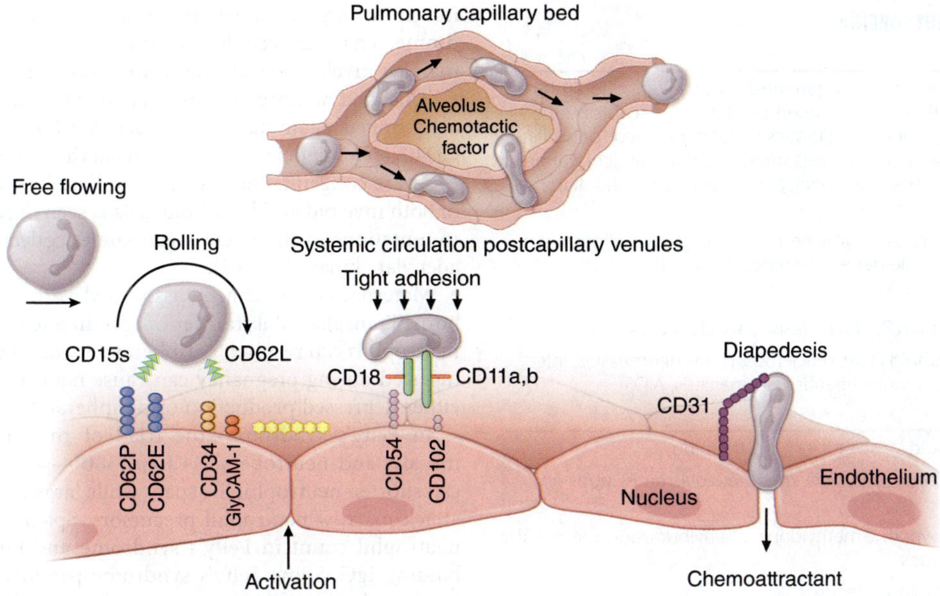

FIGURE 80-8 Neutrophil travel through the pulmonary capillaries is dependent on neutrophil deformability. Neutrophil rigidity (e.g., caused by C5a) enhances pulmonary trapping and response to pulmonary pathogens in a way that is not so dependent on cell-surface receptors. Intraalveolar chemotactic factors, such as those caused by certain bacteria (e.g., *Streptococcus pneumoniae*), lead to diapedesis of neutrophils from the pulmonary capillaries into the alveolar space. Neutrophil interaction with the endothelium of the systemic postcapillary venules is dependent on molecules of attachment. The neutrophil "rolls" along the endothelium using selectins: neutrophil CD15s (sialyl-Lewis^x) binds to CD62E (E-selectin) and CD62P (P-selectin) on endothelial cells; CD62L (L-selectin) on neutrophils binds to CD34 and other molecules (e.g., GlyCAM-1) expressed on endothelium. Chemokines or other activation factors stimulate integrin-mediated "tight adhesion": CD11a/CD18 (LFA-1) and CD11b/CD18 (Mac-1, CR3) bind to CD54 (ICAM-1) and CD102 (ICAM-2) on the endothelium. Diapedesis occurs between endothelial cells: CD31 (PECAM-1) expressed by the emigrating neutrophil interacts with CD31 expressed at the endothelial cell-cell junction. CD, cluster determinant; GlyCAM, glycosylation-dependent cell adhesion molecule; ICAM, intercellular adhesion molecule; PECAM, platelet/endothelial cell adhesion molecule.

produced by many different cell types, including endothelial cells, fibroblasts, epithelial cells, neutrophils, and monocytes, that regulate neutrophil, monocyte, eosinophil, and lymphocyte recruitment and activation. Chemokines transduce their signals through heterotrimeric G protein–linked receptors that have seven cell membrane–spanning domains, the same type of cell-surface receptor that mediates the response to the classic chemoattractants f-met-leu-phe and C5a. Four major groups of chemokines are recognized based on the cysteine structure near the N terminus: C, CC, CXC, and CXXXC. The CXC cytokines such as IL-8 mainly attract neutrophils; CC chemokines such as MIP-1 attract lymphocytes, monocytes, eosinophils, and basophils; the C chemokine lymphotactin is T cell tropic; the CXXXC chemokine fractalkine attracts neutrophils, monocytes, and T cells. These molecules and their receptors not only regulate the trafficking and activation of inflammatory cells, but specific chemokine receptors also serve as co-receptors for HIV infection (Chap. 226) and have a role in other viral infections such as West Nile infection and atherogenesis.

NEUTROPHIL ABNORMALITIES

Defects in the neutrophil life cycle can lead to dysfunction and compromised host defenses. Inflammation is often depressed, and the clinical result is often recurrent, severe bacterial and fungal infections. Aphthous ulcers of mucous membranes (gray ulcers without pus) and gingivitis and periodontal disease suggest a phagocytic cell disorder. Patients with congenital phagocyte defects can have infections within the first few days of life. Skin, ear, upper and lower respiratory tract, and bone infections are common. Sepsis and meningitis are rare. In some disorders, the frequency of infection is variable, and patients can go for months or even years without major infection. Aggressive management of these congenital diseases has extended the life span of patients well beyond 30 years.

Neutropenia The consequences of absent neutrophils are dramatic. Susceptibility to infectious diseases increases sharply when neutrophil counts fall below 1000 cells/μL. When the absolute neutrophil count (ANC; band forms and mature neutrophils combined) falls to <500 cells/μL, control of endogenous microbial flora (e.g., mouth, gut) is impaired; when the ANC is <200/μL, the local inflammatory process is absent. Neutropenia can be due to depressed production, increased peripheral destruction, or excessive peripheral pooling. A falling neutrophil count or a significant decrease in the number of neutrophils below steady-state levels, together with a failure to increase neutrophil counts in the setting of infection or other challenge, requires investigation. Acute neutropenia, such as that caused by cancer chemotherapy, is more likely to be associated with increased risk of infection than neutropenia of long duration (months to years) that reverses in response to infection or carefully controlled administration of endotoxin (see "Laboratory Diagnosis and Management," below).

Some causes of inherited and acquired neutropenia are listed in Table 80-1. The most common neutropenias are iatrogenic, resulting from the use of cytotoxic or immunosuppressive therapies for malignancy or control of autoimmune disorders. These drugs cause neutropenia because they result in decreased production of rapidly growing progenitor (stem) cells of the marrow. Certain antibiotics such as chloramphenicol, trimethoprim-sulfamethoxazole, flucytosine, vidarabine, and the antiretroviral drug zidovudine may cause neutropenia by inhibiting proliferation of myeloid precursors. Azathioprine and 6-mercaptopurine are metabolized by the enzyme thiopurine methyltransferase (TMPT), hypofunctional polymorphisms in which are found in 11% of whites and can lead to accumulation of 6-thioguanine and profound marrow toxicity. The marrow suppression is generally dose-related and dependent on continued administration of the drug. Cessation of the offending agent and recombinant human G-CSF usually reverse these forms of neutropenia.

Another important mechanism for iatrogenic neutropenia is the effect of drugs that serve as immune haptens and sensitize neutrophils or neutrophil precursors to immune-mediated peripheral destruction. This form of drug-induced neutropenia can be seen within 7 days of exposure to the drug; with previous drug exposure, resulting in preexisting antibodies, neutropenia may occur a few hours after

TABLE 80-1 CAUSES OF NEUTROPENIA

Decreased Production
Drug-induced—alkylating agents (nitrogen mustard, busulfan, chlorambucil, cyclophosphamide); antimetabolites (methotrexate, 6-mercaptopurine, 5-flucytosine); noncytotoxic agents (antibiotics [chloramphenicol, penicillins, sulfonamides], phenothiazines, tranquilizers [meprobamate], anticonvulsants [carbamazepine], antipsychotics [clozapine], certain diuretics, anti-inflammatory agents, antithyroid drugs, many others)
Hematologic diseases—idiopathic, cyclic neutropenia, Chédiak-Higashi syndrome, aplastic anemia, infantile genetic disorders (see text)
Tumor invasion, myelofibrosis
Nutritional deficiency—vitamin B_{12}, folate (especially alcoholics)
Infection—tuberculosis, typhoid fever, brucellosis, tularemia, measles, infectious mononucleosis, malaria, viral hepatitis, leishmaniasis, AIDS
Peripheral Destruction
Antineutrophil antibodies and/or splenic or lung trapping
Autoimmune disorders—Felty's syndrome, rheumatoid arthritis, lupus erythematosus
Drugs as haptens—aminopyrine, α-methyldopa, phenylbutazone, mercurial diuretics, some phenothiazines
Granulomatosis with polyangiitis (Wegener's)
Peripheral Pooling (Transient Neutropenia)
Overwhelming bacterial infection (acute endotoxemia)
Hemodialysis
Cardiopulmonary bypass

administration of the drug. Although any drug can cause this form of neutropenia, the most frequent causes are commonly used antibiotics, such as sulfa-containing compounds, penicillins, and cephalosporins. Fever and eosinophilia may also be associated with drug reactions, but often these signs are not present. Drug-induced neutropenia can be severe, but discontinuation of the sensitizing drug is sufficient for recovery, which is usually seen within 5–7 days and is complete by 10 days. Readministration of the sensitizing drug should be avoided, because abrupt neutropenia will often result. For this reason, diagnostic challenge should be avoided.

Autoimmune neutropenias caused by circulating antineutrophil antibodies are another form of acquired neutropenia that results in increased destruction of neutrophils. Acquired neutropenia may also be seen with viral infections, including infection with HIV. Acquired neutropenia may be cyclic in nature, occurring at intervals of several weeks. Acquired cyclic or stable neutropenia may be associated with an expansion of large granular lymphocytes (LGLs), which may be T cells, NK cells, or NK-like cells. Patients with large granular lymphocytosis may have moderate blood and bone marrow lymphocytosis, neutropenia, polyclonal hypergammaglobulinemia, splenomegaly, rheumatoid arthritis, and absence of lymphadenopathy. Such patients may have a chronic and relatively stable course. Recurrent bacterial infections are frequent. Benign and malignant forms of this syndrome occur. In some patients, a spontaneous regression has occurred even after 11 years, suggesting an immunoregulatory defect as the basis for at least one form of the disorder. Glucocorticoids, cyclosporine, and methotrexate are commonly used to manage these cytopenias.

Hereditary Neutropenias Hereditary neutropenias are rare and may manifest in early childhood as a profound constant neutropenia or agranulocytosis. Congenital forms of neutropenia include Kostmann's syndrome (neutrophil count <100/μL), which is often fatal and due to mutations in the antiapoptosis gene *HAX-1*; severe chronic neutropenia (neutrophil count of 300–1500/μL) due to mutations in neutrophil elastase (*ELANE*); hereditary cyclic neutropenia, or, more appropriately, cyclic hematopoiesis, also due to mutations in neutrophil elastase (*ELANE*); the cartilage-hair hypoplasia syndrome due to mutations in the mitochondrial RNA-processing endoribonuclease *RMRP*; Shwachman-Diamond syndrome associated with pancreatic insufficiency due to mutations in the Shwachman-Bodian-Diamond syndrome gene *SBDS*; the WHIM (*w*arts, *h*ypogammaglobulinemia, *i*nfections, *m*yelokathexis [retention of WBCs in the marrow]) syndrome, characterized by neutrophil hypersegmentation and bone marrow myeloid arrest due to mutations in the chemokine receptor *CXCR4*; and neutropenias associated with other immune defects, such as X-linked agammaglobulinemia, Wiskott-Aldrich syndrome, and CD40 ligand deficiency. Mutations in the G-CSF receptor can develop in severe congenital neutropenia and are linked to leukemia. Absence of both myeloid and lymphoid cells is seen in reticular dysgenesis, due to mutations in the nuclear genome-encoded mitochondrial enzyme adenylate kinase-2 (*AK2*).

Maternal factors can be associated with neutropenia in the newborn. Transplacental transfer of IgG directed against antigens on fetal neutrophils can result in peripheral destruction. Drugs (e.g., thiazides) ingested during pregnancy can cause neutropenia in the newborn by either depressed production or peripheral destruction.

In Felty's syndrome—the triad of rheumatoid arthritis, splenomegaly, and neutropenia (Chap. 380)—spleen-produced antibodies can shorten neutrophil life span, while large granular lymphocytes can attack marrow neutrophil precursors. Splenectomy may increase the neutrophil count in Felty's syndrome and lower serum neutrophil-binding IgG. Some Felty's syndrome patients also have neutropenia associated with an increased number of LGLs. Splenomegaly with peripheral trapping and destruction of neutrophils is also seen in lysosomal storage diseases and in portal hypertension.

Neutrophilia Neutrophilia results from increased neutrophil production, increased marrow release, or defective margination (Table 80-2). The most important acute cause of neutrophilia is infection. Neutrophilia from acute infection represents both increased production and increased marrow release. Increased production is also associated with chronic inflammation and certain myeloproliferative diseases. Increased marrow release and mobilization of the marginated leukocyte pool are induced by glucocorticoids. Release of epinephrine, as with vigorous exercise, excitement, or stress, will demarginate neutrophils in the spleen and lungs and double the neutrophil count in minutes. Cigarette smoking can elevate neutrophil counts above the normal range. Leukocytosis with cell counts of 10,000–25,000/μL occurs in response to infection and other forms of acute inflammation and results from both release of the marginated pool and mobilization of marrow reserves. Persistent neutrophilia with cell counts of ≥30,000–50,000/μL is called a *leukemoid reaction*, a term

TABLE 80-2 CAUSES OF NEUTROPHILIA

Increased Production
Idiopathic
Drug-induced—glucocorticoids, G-CSF
Infection—bacterial, fungal, sometimes viral
Inflammation—thermal injury, tissue necrosis, myocardial and pulmonary infarction, hypersensitivity states, collagen vascular diseases
Myeloproliferative diseases—myelocytic leukemia, myeloid metaplasia, polycythemia vera
Increased Marrow Release
Glucocorticoids
Acute infection (endotoxin)
Inflammation—thermal injury
Decreased or Defective Margination
Drugs—epinephrine, glucocorticoids, nonsteroidal anti-inflammatory agents
Stress, excitement, vigorous exercise
Leukocyte adhesion deficiency type 1 (CD18); leukocyte adhesion deficiency type 2 (selectin ligand, CD15s); leukocyte adhesion deficiency type 3 (FERMT3)
Miscellaneous
Metabolic disorders—ketoacidosis, acute renal failure, eclampsia, acute poisoning
Drugs—lithium
Other—metastatic carcinoma, acute hemorrhage or hemolysis

Abbreviation: G-CSF, granulocyte colony-stimulating factor.

TABLE 80-3 TYPES OF GRANULOCYTE AND MONOCYTE DISORDERS

	Cause of Indicated Dysfunction		
Function	**Drug-Induced**	**Acquired**	**Inherited**
Adherence-aggregation	Aspirin, colchicine, alcohol, glucocorticoids, ibuprofen, piroxicam	Neonatal state, hemodialysis	Leukocyte adhesion deficiency types 1, 2, and 3
Deformability		Leukemia, neonatal state, diabetes mellitus, immature neutrophils	
Chemokinesis-chemotaxis	Glucocorticoids (high dose), auranofin, colchicine (weak effect), phenylbutazone, naproxen, indomethacin, interleukin 2	Thermal injury, malignancy, malnutrition, periodontal disease, neonatal state, systemic lupus erythematosus, rheumatoid arthritis, diabetes mellitus, sepsis, influenza virus infection, herpes simplex virus infection, acrodermatitis enteropathica, AIDS	Chédiak-Higashi syndrome, neutrophil-specific granule deficiency, hyper IgE–recurrent infection (Job's) syndrome (in some patients), Down's syndrome, α-mannosidase deficiency, leukocyte adhesion deficiencies, Wiskott-Aldrich syndrome
Microbicidal activity	Colchicine, cyclophosphamide, glucocorticoids (high dose), TNF-α-blocking antibodies	Leukemia, aplastic anemia, certain neutropenias, tuftsin deficiency, thermal injury, sepsis, neonatal state, diabetes mellitus, malnutrition, AIDS	Chédiak-Higashi syndrome, neutrophil-specific granule deficiency, chronic granulomatous disease, defects in IFNγ/IL-12 axis

Abbreviations: IFNγ, interferon γ; IL, interleukin; TNF-α, tumor necrosis factor alpha.

often used to distinguish this degree of neutrophilia from leukemia. In a leukemoid reaction, the circulating neutrophils are usually mature and not clonally derived.

Abnormal Neutrophil Function Inherited and acquired abnormalities of phagocyte function are listed in Table 80-3. The resulting diseases are best considered in terms of the functional defects of adherence, chemotaxis, and microbicidal activity. The distinguishing features of the important inherited disorders of phagocyte function are shown in Table 80-4.

DISORDERS OF ADHESION Three main types of leukocyte adhesion deficiency (LAD) have been described. All are autosomal recessive and result in the inability of neutrophils to exit the circulation to sites of infection, leading to leukocytosis and increased susceptibility to infection (Fig. 80-8). Patients with LAD 1 have mutations in *CD18*, the common component of the integrins LFA-1, Mac-1, and p150,95, leading to a defect in tight adhesion between neutrophils and the endothelium. The heterodimer formed by CD18/CD11b (Mac-1) is also the receptor for the complement-derived opsonin C3bi (CR3). The *CD18* gene is located on distal chromosome 21q. The severity of the defect determines the severity of clinical disease. Complete lack of expression of the leukocyte integrins results in a severe phenotype in which inflammatory stimuli do not increase the expression of leukocyte integrins on neutrophils or activated T and B cells. Neutrophils (and monocytes) from patients with LAD 1 adhere poorly to endothelial cells and protein-coated surfaces and exhibit defective spreading, aggregation, and chemotaxis. Patients with LAD 1 have recurrent bacterial infections involving the skin, oral and genital mucosa, and respiratory and intestinal tracts; persistent leukocytosis (resting neutrophil counts of 15,000–20,000/μL) because cells do not marginate; and, in severe cases, a history of delayed separation of the umbilical stump. Infections, especially of the skin, may become necrotic with progressively enlarging borders, slow healing, and development of dysplastic scars. The most common bacteria are *Staphylococcus aureus* and enteric gram-negative bacteria. LAD 2 is caused by an abnormality of fucosylation of SLe^x (CD15s), the ligand on neutrophils that interacts with selectins on endothelial cells and is responsible for neutrophil rolling along the endothelium. Infection susceptibility in LAD 2 appears to be less severe than in LAD 1. LAD 2 is also known as *congenital disorder of glycosylation IIc* (CDGIIc) due to mutation in a GDP-fucose transporter (*SLC35C1*). LAD 3 is characterized by infection susceptibility, leukocytosis, and petechial hemorrhage due to impaired integrin activation caused by mutations in the gene *FERMT3*.

DISORDERS OF NEUTROPHIL GRANULES The most common neutrophil defect is myeloperoxidase deficiency, a primary granule defect inherited as an autosomal recessive trait; the incidence is ~1 in 2000 persons. Isolated myeloperoxidase deficiency is not associated with clinically compromised defenses, presumably because other defense systems such as hydrogen peroxide generation are amplified. Microbicidal activity of neutrophils is delayed but not absent. Myeloperoxidase deficiency may make other acquired host defense defects more serious, and patients with myeloperoxidase deficiency and diabetes are more susceptible to *Candida* infections. An acquired form of myeloperoxidase deficiency occurs in myelomonocytic leukemia and acute myeloid leukemia.

Chédiak-Higashi syndrome (CHS) is a rare disease with autosomal recessive inheritance due to defects in the lysosomal transport protein LYST, encoded by the gene *CHS1* at 1q42. This protein is required for normal packaging and disbursement of granules. Neutrophils (and all cells containing lysosomes) from patients with CHS characteristically have large granules (Fig. 80-9), making it a systemic disease. Patients with CHS have nystagmus, partial oculocutaneous albinism, and an increased number of infections resulting from many bacterial agents. Some CHS patients develop an "accelerated phase" in childhood with a hemophagocytic syndrome and an aggressive lymphoma requiring bone marrow transplantation. CHS neutrophils and monocytes have impaired chemotaxis and abnormal rates of microbial killing due to slow rates of fusion of the lysosomal granules with phagosomes. NK cell function is also impaired. CHS patients may develop a severe disabling peripheral neuropathy in adulthood that can lead to bed confinement.

Specific granule deficiency is a rare autosomal recessive disease in which the production of secondary granules and their contents, as well as the primary granule component defensins, is defective. The defect in killing leads to severe bacterial infections. One type of specific granule deficiency is due to a mutation in the CCAAT/enhancer binding protein-ε, a regulator of expression of granule components. A dominant mutation in *C/EBP-ε* has also been described.

CHRONIC GRANULOMATOUS DISEASE Chronic granulomatous disease (CGD) is a group of disorders of granulocyte and monocyte oxidative metabolism. Although CGD is rare, with an incidence of ~1 in 200,000 individuals, it is an important model of defective neutrophil oxidative metabolism. In about two-thirds of patients, CGD is inherited as an X-linked recessive trait; 30% of patients inherit the disease in an autosomal recessive pattern. Mutations in the genes for the five proteins that assemble at the plasma membrane account for all patients with CGD. Two proteins (a 91-kDa protein, abnormal in X-linked CGD, and a 22-kDa protein, absent in one form of autosomal recessive CGD) form the heterodimer cytochrome b-558 in the plasma membrane. Three other proteins (40, 47, and 67 kDa, abnormal in the other autosomal recessive forms of CGD) are cytoplasmic in origin and interact with the cytochrome after cell activation to form NADPH oxidase, required for hydrogen peroxide production. Leukocytes from patients with CGD have severely diminished hydrogen peroxide production. The genes involved in each of the defects have been cloned and sequenced and the chromosome locations identified. Patients with CGD characteristically have increased numbers of infections

TABLE 80-4 INHERITED DISORDERS OF PHAGOCYTE FUNCTION: DIFFERENTIAL FEATURES

Clinical Manifestations	Cellular or Molecular Defects	Diagnosis
Chronic Granulomatous Diseases (70% X-Linked, 30% Autosomal Recessive)		
Severe infections of skin, ears, lungs, liver, and bone with catalase-positive microorganisms such as *Staphylococcus aureus, Burkholderia cepacia* complex, *Aspergillus* spp., *Chromobacterium violaceum*; often hard to culture organism; excessive inflammation with granulomas, frequent lymph node suppuration; granulomas can obstruct GI or GU tracts; gingivitis, aphthous ulcers, seborrheic dermatitis	No respiratory burst due to the lack of one of five NADPH oxidase subunits in neutrophils, monocytes, and eosinophils	DHR or NBT test; no superoxide and H_2O_2 production by neutrophils; immunoblot for NADPH oxidase components; genetic detection
Chédiak-Higashi Syndrome (Autosomal Recessive)		
Recurrent pyogenic infections, especially with *S. aureus*; many patients get lymphoma-like illness during adolescence; periodontal disease; partial oculocutaneous albinism, nystagmus, progressive peripheral neuropathy, mental retardation in some patients	Reduced chemotaxis and phagolysosome fusion, increased respiratory burst activity, defective egress from marrow, abnormal skin window; defect in *CHS1*	Giant primary granules in neutrophils and other granule-bearing cells (Wright's stain); genetic detection
Specific Granule Deficiency (Autosomal Recessive and Dominant)		
Recurrent infections of skin, ears, and sinopulmonary tract; delayed wound healing; decreased inflammation; bleeding diathesis	Abnormal chemotaxis, impaired respiratory burst and bacterial killing, failure to upregulate chemotactic and adhesion receptors with stimulation, defect in transcription of granule proteins; defect in *CEBPE*	Lack of secondary (specific) granules in neutrophils (Wright's stain), no neutrophil-specific granule contents (i.e., lactoferrin), no defensins, platelet α granule abnormality; genetic detection
Myeloperoxidase Deficiency (Autosomal Recessive)		
Clinically normal except in patients with underlying disease such as diabetes mellitus; then candidiasis or other fungal infections	No myeloperoxidase due to pre- and posttranslational defects in myeloperoxidase deficiency	No peroxidase in neutrophils; genetic detection
Leukocyte Adhesion Deficiency		
Type 1: Delayed separation of umbilical cord, sustained neutrophilia, recurrent infections of skin and mucosa, gingivitis, periodontal disease	Impaired phagocyte adherence, aggregation, spreading, chemotaxis, phagocytosis of C3bi-coated particles; defective production of CD18 subunit common to leukocyte integrins	Reduced phagocyte surface expression of the CD18-containing integrins with monoclonal antibodies against LFA-1 (CD18/CD11a), Mac-1 or CR3 (CD18/CD11b), p150,95 (CD18/CD11c); genetic detection
Type 2: Mental retardation, short stature, Bombay (hh) blood phenotype, recurrent infections, neutrophilia	Impaired phagocyte rolling along endothelium; due to defects in fucose transporter	Reduced phagocyte surface expression of Sialyl-Lewis^x, with monoclonal antibodies against CD15s; genetic detection
Type 3: Petechial hemorrhage, recurrent infections	Impaired signaling for integrin activation resulting in impaired adhesion due to mutation in *FERMT3*	Reduced signaling for adhesion through integrins; genetic detection
Phagocyte Activation Defects (X-Linked and Autosomal Recessive)		
NEMO deficiency: mild hypohidrotic ectodermal dysplasia; broad-based immune defect: pyogenic and encapsulated bacteria, viruses, *Pneumocystis*, mycobacteria; X-linked	Impaired phagocyte activation by IL-1, IL-18, TLR, CD40L, TNF-α leading to problems with inflammation and antibody production	Poor in vitro response to endotoxin; impaired NF-κB activation; genetic detection
IRAK4 and MyD88 deficiency: susceptibility to pyogenic bacteria such as staphylococci, streptococci, clostridia; resistant to *Candida*; autosomal recessive	Impaired phagocyte activation by endotoxin through TLR and other pathways; TNF-α signaling preserved	Poor in vitro response to endotoxin; lack of NF-κB activation by endotoxin; genetic detection
Hyper IgE–Recurrent Infection Syndrome (Autosomal Dominant) (Job's Syndrome)		
Eczematoid or pruritic dermatitis, "cold" skin abscesses, recurrent pneumonias with *S. aureus* with bronchopleural fistulae and cyst formation, mild eosinophilia, mucocutaneous candidiasis, characteristic facies, restrictive lung disease, scoliosis, delayed primary dental deciduation	Reduced chemotaxis in some patients, reduced memory T and B cells; mutation in *STAT3*	Somatic and immune features involving lungs, skeleton, and immune system; serum IgE >2000 IU/mL; genetic testing
DOCK8 deficiency (autosomal recessive), severe eczema, atopic dermatitis, cutaneous abscesses, HSV, HPV, and molluscum infections, severe allergies, cancer	Impaired T cell proliferation to mitogens; mutation in *DOCK8*	Severe allergies, viral infections, high IgE, eosinophilia, low IgM, progressive lymphopenia, genetic detection
Mycobacteria Susceptibility (Autosomal Dominant and Recessive Forms)		
Severe extrapulmonary or disseminated infections with bacille Calmette-Guérin (BCG), nontuberculous mycobacteria, salmonella, histoplasmosis, coccidioidomycosis, poor granuloma formation	Inability to kill intracellular organisms due to low IFN-γ production or response; mutations in IFN-γ receptors, IL-12 receptors, IL-12 p40, *STAT1*, *NEMO*, *ISG15*, *GATA2*	Abnormally low or very high levels of IFN-γ receptor 1; functional assays of cytokine production and response; genetic detection
GATA2 Deficiency (Autosomal Dominant)		
Persistent or disseminated warts, disseminated mycobacterial disease, low monocytes, NK cells, B cells; hypoplastic myelodysplasia, leukemia, cytogenetic abnormalities, pulmonary alveolar proteinosis	Impaired macrophage activity, cytopenias; mutations in *GATA2*	Profound circulating monocytopenia, NK and B cell cytopenias; genetic detection

Abbreviations: C/EBPε, CCAAT/enhancer binding protein-ε; DHR, dihydrorhodamine (oxidation test); DOCK8, dedicator of cytokinesis 8; GI, gastrointestinal; GU, genitourinary; HPV, human papilloma virus; HSV, herpes simplex virus; IFN, interferon; IL, interleukin; IRAK4, IL-1 receptor–associated kinase 4; LFA-1, leukocyte function–associated antigen 1; MyD88, myeloid differentiation primary response gene 88; NADPH, nicotinamide–adenine dinucleotide phosphate; NBT, nitroblue tetrazolium (dye test); NEMO, NF-κB essential modulator; NF-κB, nuclear factor-κB; NK, natural killer; STAT1–3, signal transducer and activator of transcription 1–3; TLR, Toll-like receptor; TNF, tumor necrosis factor.

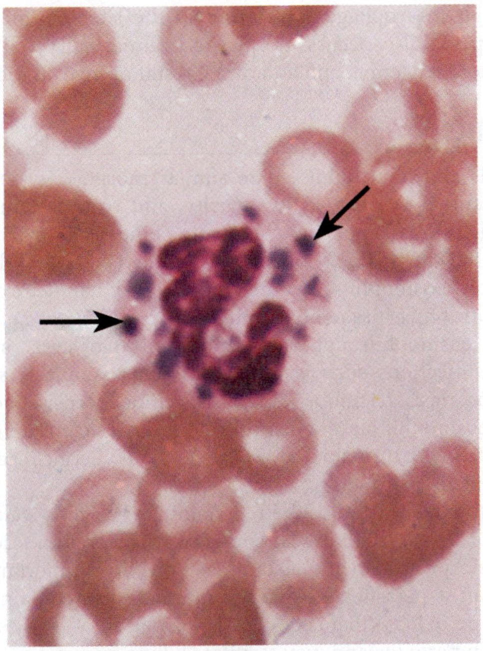

FIGURE 80-9 Chédiak-Higashi syndrome. The granulocytes contain huge cytoplasmic granules formed from aggregation and fusion of azurophilic and specific granules. Large abnormal granules are found in other granule-containing cells throughout the body.

due to catalase-positive microorganisms (organisms that destroy their own hydrogen peroxide) such as *S. aureus*, *Burkholderia cepacia*, and *Aspergillus* species. When patients with CGD become infected, they often have extensive inflammatory reactions, and lymph node suppuration is common despite the administration of appropriate antibiotics. Aphthous ulcers and chronic inflammation of the nares are often present. Granulomas are frequent and can obstruct the gastrointestinal or genitourinary tracts. The excessive inflammation is due to failure to downregulate inflammation, reflecting failure to inhibit the synthesis of, degradation of, or response to chemoattractants or residual antigens, leading to persistent neutrophil accumulation. Impaired killing of intracellular microorganisms by macrophages may lead to persistent cell-mediated immune activation and granuloma formation. Autoimmune complications such as immune thrombocytopenic purpura and juvenile rheumatoid arthritis are also increased in CGD. In addition, for unexplained reasons, discoid lupus is more common in X-linked carriers. Late complications, including nodular regenerative hyperplasia and portal hypertension, are increasingly recognized in long-term survivors of severe CGD.

DISORDERS OF PHAGOCYTE ACTIVATION Phagocytes depend on cell-surface stimulation to induce signals that evoke multiple levels of the inflammatory response, including cytokine synthesis, chemotaxis, and antigen presentation. Mutations affecting the major pathway that signals through NF-κB have been noted in patients with a variety of infection susceptibility syndromes. If the defects are at a very late stage of signal transduction, in the protein critical for NF-κB activation known as the NF-κB essential modulator (NEMO), then affected males develop ectodermal dysplasia and severe immune deficiency with susceptibility to bacteria, fungi, mycobacteria, and viruses. If the defects in NF-κB activation are closer to the cell-surface receptors, in the proteins transducing Toll-like receptor signals, IL-1 receptor–associated kinase 4 (IRAK4), and myeloid differentiation primary response gene 88 (MyD88), then children have a marked susceptibility to pyogenic infections early in life but develop resistance to infection later.

MONONUCLEAR PHAGOCYTES

The mononuclear phagocyte system is composed of monoblasts, promonocytes, and monocytes, in addition to the structurally diverse tissue macrophages that make up what was previously referred to as the reticuloendothelial system. Macrophages are long-lived phagocytic cells capable of many of the functions of neutrophils. They are also secretory cells that participate in many immunologic and inflammatory processes distinct from neutrophils. Monocytes leave the circulation by diapedesis more slowly than neutrophils and have a half-life in the blood of 12–24 h.

After blood monocytes arrive in the tissues, they differentiate into macrophages ("big eaters") with specialized functions suited for specific anatomic locations. Macrophages are particularly abundant in capillary walls of the lung, spleen, liver, and bone marrow, where they function to remove microorganisms and other noxious elements from the blood. Alveolar macrophages, liver Kupffer cells, splenic macrophages, peritoneal macrophages, bone marrow macrophages, lymphatic macrophages, brain microglial cells, and dendritic macrophages all have specialized functions. Macrophage-secreted products include lysozyme, neutral proteases, acid hydrolases, arginase, complement components, enzyme inhibitors (plasmin, α_2-macroglobulin), binding proteins (transferrin, fibronectin, transcobalamin II), nucleosides, and cytokines (TNF-α; IL-1, -8, -12, -18). IL-1 (Chaps. 23 and 372e) has many functions, including initiating fever in the hypothalamus, mobilizing leukocytes from the bone marrow, and activating lymphocytes and neutrophils. TNF-α is a pyrogen that duplicates many of the actions of IL-1 and plays an important role in the pathogenesis of gram-negative shock (Chap. 325). TNF-α stimulates production of hydrogen peroxide and related toxic oxygen species by macrophages and neutrophils. In addition, TNF-α induces catabolic changes that contribute to the profound wasting (cachexia) associated with many chronic diseases.

Other macrophage-secreted products include reactive oxygen and nitrogen metabolites, bioactive lipids (arachidonic acid metabolites and platelet-activating factors), chemokines, CSFs, and factors stimulating fibroblast and vessel proliferation. Macrophages help regulate the replication of lymphocytes and participate in the killing of tumors, viruses, and certain bacteria (*Mycobacterium tuberculosis* and *Listeria monocytogenes*). Macrophages are key effector cells in the elimination of intracellular microorganisms. Their ability to fuse to form giant cells that coalesce into granulomas in response to some inflammatory stimuli is important in the elimination of intracellular microbes and is under the control of IFN-γ. Nitric oxide induced by IFN-γ is an important effector against intracellular parasites, including tuberculosis and *Leishmania*.

Macrophages play an important role in the immune response (Chap. 372e). They process and present antigen to lymphocytes and secrete cytokines that modulate and direct lymphocyte development and function. Macrophages participate in autoimmune phenomena by removing immune complexes and other substances from the circulation. Polymorphisms in macrophage receptors for immunoglobulin (FcγRII) determine susceptibility to some infections and autoimmune diseases. In wound healing, they dispose of senescent cells, and they contribute to atheroma development. Macrophage elastase mediates development of emphysema from cigarette smoking.

DISORDERS OF THE MONONUCLEAR PHAGOCYTE SYSTEM

Many disorders of neutrophils extend to mononuclear phagocytes. Monocytosis is associated with tuberculosis, brucellosis, subacute bacterial endocarditis, Rocky Mountain spotted fever, malaria, and visceral leishmaniasis (kala azar). Monocytosis also occurs with malignancies, leukemias, myeloproliferative syndromes, hemolytic anemias, chronic idiopathic neutropenias, and granulomatous diseases such as sarcoidosis, regional enteritis, and some collagen vascular diseases. Patients with LAD, hyperimmunoglobulin E–recurrent infection (Job's) syndrome, CHS, and CGD all have defects in the mononuclear phagocyte system.

Monocyte cytokine production or response is impaired in some patients with disseminated nontuberculous mycobacterial infection who are not infected with HIV. Genetic defects in the pathways regulated by IFN-γ and IL-12 lead to impaired killing of intracellular bacteria, mycobacteria, salmonellae, and certain viruses (Fig. 80-10).

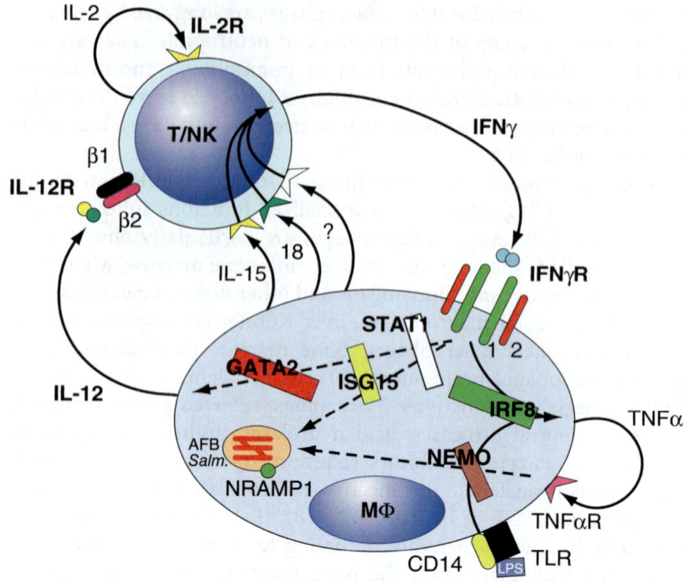

FIGURE 80-10 Lymphocyte-macrophage interactions underlying resistance to mycobacteria and other intracellular pathogens such as *Salmonella, Histoplasma,* and *Coccidioides*. Mycobacteria (and others) infect macrophages, leading to the production of IL-12, which activates T or NK cells through its receptor, leading to production of IL-2 and IFN-γ. IFN-γ acts through its receptor on macrophages to upregulate TNF-γ and IL-12 and kill intracellular pathogens. Other critical interacting molecules include signal transducer and activator of transcription 1 (STAT1), interferon regulatory factor 8 (IRF8), GATA2, and ISG15. Mutant forms of the cytokines and receptors shown in *bold type* have been found in severe cases of nontuberculous mycobacterial infection, salmonellosis and other intracellular pathogens. AFB, acid-fast bacilli; IFN, interferon; IL, interleukin; NEMO, nuclear factor-κB essential modulator; NK, natural killer; TLR, Toll-like receptor; TNF, tumor necrosis factor.

Certain viral infections impair mononuclear phagocyte function. For example, influenza virus infection causes abnormal monocyte chemotaxis. Mononuclear phagocytes can be infected by HIV using CCR5, the chemokine receptor that acts as a co-receptor with CD4 for HIV. T lymphocytes produce IFN-γ, which induces FcR expression and phagocytosis and stimulates hydrogen peroxide production by mononuclear phagocytes and neutrophils. In certain diseases, such as AIDS, IFN-γ production may be deficient, whereas in other diseases, such as T cell lymphomas, excessive release of IFN-γ may be associated with erythrophagocytosis by splenic macrophages.

Autoinflammatory diseases are characterized by abnormal cytokine regulation, leading to excess inflammation in the absence of infection. These diseases can mimic infectious or immunodeficient syndromes. Gain-of-function mutations in the TNF-α receptor cause TNF-α receptor–associated periodic syndrome (TRAPS), which is characterized by recurrent fever in the absence of infection, due to persistent stimulation of the TNF-α receptor (Chap. 392). Diseases with abnormal IL-1 regulation leading to fever include familial Mediterranean fever due to mutations in *PYRIN*. Mutations in *cold-induced autoinflammatory syndrome 1* (*CIAS1*) lead to neonatal-onset multisystem autoinflammatory disease, familial cold urticaria, and Muckle-Wells syndrome. The syndrome of *p*yoderma gangrenosum, *a*cne, and sterile *p*yogenic *a*rthritis (PAPA syndrome) is caused by mutations in *PSTPIP1*. In contrast to these syndromes of overexpression of proinflammatory cytokines, blockade of TNF-α by the antagonists infliximab, adalimumab, certolizumab, golimumab, or etanercept has been associated with severe infections due to tuberculosis, nontuberculous mycobacteria, and fungi (Chap. 392).

Monocytopenia occurs with acute infections, with stress, and after treatment with glucocorticoids. Drugs that suppress neutrophil production in the bone marrow can cause monocytopenia. Persistent severe circulating monocytopenia is seen in GATA2 deficiency, even though macrophages are found at the sites of inflammation. Monocytopenia also occurs in aplastic anemia, hairy cell leukemia, acute myeloid leukemia, and as a direct result of myelotoxic drugs.

EOSINOPHILS

Eosinophils and neutrophils share similar morphology, many lysosomal constituents, phagocytic capacity, and oxidative metabolism. Eosinophils express a specific chemoattractant receptor and respond to a specific chemokine, eotaxin, but little is known about their required role. Eosinophils are much longer lived than neutrophils, and unlike neutrophils, tissue eosinophils can recirculate. During most infections, eosinophils appear unimportant. However, in invasive helminthic infections, such as hookworm, schistosomiasis, strongyloidiasis, toxocariasis, trichinosis, filariasis, echinococcosis, and cysticercosis, the eosinophil plays a central role in host defense. Eosinophils are associated with bronchial asthma, cutaneous allergic reactions, and other hypersensitivity states.

The distinctive feature of the red-staining (Wright's stain) eosinophil granule is its crystalline core consisting of an arginine-rich protein (major basic protein) with histaminase activity, important in host defense against parasites. Eosinophil granules also contain a unique eosinophil peroxidase that catalyzes the oxidation of many substances by hydrogen peroxide and may facilitate killing of microorganisms.

Eosinophil peroxidase, in the presence of hydrogen peroxide and halide, initiates mast cell secretion in vitro and thereby promotes inflammation. Eosinophils contain cationic proteins, some of which bind to heparin and reduce its anticoagulant activity. Eosinophil-derived neurotoxin and eosinophil cationic protein are ribonucleases that can kill respiratory syncytial virus. Eosinophil cytoplasm contains Charcot-Leyden crystal protein, a hexagonal bipyramidal crystal first observed in a patient with leukemia and then in sputum of patients with asthma; this protein is lysophospholipase and may function to detoxify certain lysophospholipids.

Several factors enhance the eosinophil's function in host defense. T cell–derived factors enhance the ability of eosinophils to kill parasites. Mast cell–derived eosinophil chemotactic factor of anaphylaxis (ECFa) increases the number of eosinophil complement receptors and enhances eosinophil killing of parasites. Eosinophil CSFs (e.g., IL-5) produced by macrophages increase eosinophil production in the bone marrow and activate eosinophils to kill parasites.

EOSINOPHILIA

Eosinophilia is the presence of >500 eosinophils per μL of blood and is common in many settings besides parasite infection. Significant tissue eosinophilia can occur without an elevated blood count. A common cause of eosinophilia is allergic reaction to drugs (iodides, aspirin, sulfonamides, nitrofurantoin, penicillins, and cephalosporins). Allergies such as hay fever, asthma, eczema, serum sickness, allergic vasculitis, and pemphigus are associated with eosinophilia. Eosinophilia also occurs in collagen vascular diseases (e.g., rheumatoid arthritis, eosinophilic fasciitis, allergic angiitis, and periarteritis nodosa) and malignancies (e.g., Hodgkin's disease; mycosis fungoides; chronic myeloid leukemia; and cancer of the lung, stomach, pancreas, ovary, or uterus), as well as in Job's syndrome, DOCK8 deficiency (see below), and CGD. Eosinophilia is commonly present in helminthic infections. IL-5 is the dominant eosinophil growth factor. Therapeutic administration of the cytokines IL-2 or GM-CSF frequently leads to transient eosinophilia. The most dramatic hypereosinophilic syndromes are Loeffler's syndrome, tropical pulmonary eosinophilia, Loeffler's endocarditis, eosinophilic leukemia, and idiopathic hypereosinophilic syndrome (50,000–100,000/μL). IL-5 is the dominant eosinophil growth factor and can be specifically inhibited with the monoclonal antibody mepolizumab.

The idiopathic hypereosinophilic syndrome represents a heterogeneous group of disorders with the common feature of prolonged eosinophilia of unknown cause and organ system dysfunction, including the heart, central nervous system, kidneys, lungs, gastrointestinal tract, and skin. The bone marrow is involved in all affected individuals, but the most severe complications involve the heart and central nervous system. Clinical manifestations and organ dysfunction are highly variable. Eosinophils are found in the involved tissues and likely cause tissue damage by local deposition of toxic eosinophil proteins such as eosinophil cationic protein and major basic protein. In the heart, the pathologic changes lead to thrombosis, endocardial fibrosis, and restrictive endomyocardiopathy. The damage to tissues in other organ systems is similar. Some cases are due to mutations involving the platelet-derived growth factor receptor, and these are extremely sensitive to the tyrosine kinase inhibitor imatinib. Glucocorticoids, hydroxyurea, and IFN-α each have been used successfully, as have therapeutic antibodies against IL-5. Cardiovascular complications are managed aggressively.

The *eosinophilia-myalgia syndrome* is a multisystem disease, with prominent cutaneous, hematologic, and visceral manifestations, that frequently evolves into a chronic course and can occasionally be fatal. The syndrome is characterized by eosinophilia (eosinophil count >1000/μL) and generalized disabling myalgias without other recognized causes. Eosinophilic fasciitis, pneumonitis, and myocarditis; neuropathy culminating in respiratory failure; and encephalopathy may occur. The disease is caused by ingesting contaminants in L-tryptophan–containing products. Eosinophils, lymphocytes, macrophages, and fibroblasts accumulate in the affected tissues, but their role in pathogenesis is unclear. Activation of eosinophils and fibroblasts and the deposition of eosinophil-derived toxic proteins in affected tissues may contribute. IL-5 and transforming growth factor β have been implicated as potential mediators. Treatment is withdrawal of products containing L-tryptophan and the administration of glucocorticoids. Most patients recover fully, remain stable, or show slow recovery, but the disease can be fatal in up to 5% of patients.

Eosinophilic neoplasms are discussed in Chapter 135e.

EOSINOPENIA

Eosinopenia occurs with stress, such as acute bacterial infection, and after treatment with glucocorticoids. The mechanism of eosinopenia of acute bacterial infection is unknown but is independent of endogenous glucocorticoids, because it occurs in animals after total adrenalectomy. There is no known adverse effect of eosinopenia.

HYPERIMMUNOGLOBULIN E–RECURRENT INFECTION SYNDROME

The hyperimmunoglobulin E–recurrent infection syndrome, or Job's syndrome, is a rare multisystem disease in which the immune and somatic systems are affected, including neutrophils, monocytes, T cells, B cells, and osteoclasts. Autosomal *dominant* mutations in signal transducer and activator of transcription 3 (STAT3) lead to inhibition of normal STAT signaling with broad and profound effects. Patients have characteristic facies with broad nose, kyphoscoliosis, and eczema. The primary teeth erupt normally but do not deciduate, often requiring extraction. Patients develop recurrent sinopulmonary and cutaneous infections that tend to be much less inflamed than appropriate for the degree of infection and have been referred to as "cold abscesses." Characteristically, pneumonias cavitate, leading to pneumatoceles. Coronary artery aneurysms are common, as are cerebral demyelinated plaques that accumulate with age. Importantly, IL-17–producing T cells, which are thought responsible for protection against extracellular and mucosal infections, are profoundly reduced in Job's syndrome. Despite very high IgE levels, these patients do not have elevated levels of allergy. An important syndrome with clinical overlap with STAT3 deficiency is due to autosomal recessive defects in dedicator of cytokinesis 8 (DOCK8). In DOCK8 deficiency, IgE elevation is joined to severe allergy, viral susceptibility, and increased rates of cancer.

LABORATORY DIAGNOSIS AND MANAGEMENT

Initial studies of WBC and differential and often a bone marrow examination may be followed by assessment of bone marrow reserves (steroid challenge test), marginated circulating pool of cells (epinephrine challenge test), and marginating ability (endotoxin challenge test) (Fig. 80-7). In vivo assessment of inflammation is possible with a Rebuck skin window test or an in vivo skin blister assay, which measures the ability of leukocytes and inflammatory mediators to accumulate locally in the skin. In vitro tests of phagocyte aggregation, adherence, chemotaxis, phagocytosis, degranulation, and microbicidal activity (for *S. aureus*) may help pinpoint cellular or humoral lesions. Deficiencies of oxidative metabolism are detected with either the nitroblue tetrazolium (NBT) dye test or the dihydrorhodamine (DHR) oxidation test. These tests are based on the ability of products of oxidative metabolism to alter the oxidation states of reporter molecules so that they can be detected microscopically (NBT) or by flow cytometry (DHR). Qualitative studies of superoxide and hydrogen peroxide production may further define neutrophil oxidative function.

Patients with leukopenias or leukocyte dysfunction often have delayed inflammatory responses. Therefore, clinical manifestations may be minimal despite overwhelming infection, and unusual infections must always be suspected. Early signs of infection demand prompt, aggressive culturing for microorganisms, use of antibiotics, and surgical drainage of abscesses. Prolonged courses of antibiotics are often required. In patients with CGD, prophylactic antibiotics (trimethoprim-sulfamethoxazole) and antifungals (itraconazole) markedly diminish the frequency of life-threatening infections. Glucocorticoids may relieve gastrointestinal or genitourinary tract obstruction by granulomas in patients with CGD. Although TNF-α-blocking agents may markedly relieve inflammatory bowel symptoms, extreme caution must be exercised in their use in CGD inflammatory bowel disease, because it profoundly increases these patients' already heightened susceptibility to infection. Recombinant human IFN-γ, which nonspecifically stimulates phagocytic cell function, reduces the frequency of infections in patients with CGD by 70% and reduces the severity of infection. This effect of IFN-γ in CGD is additive to the effect of prophylactic antibiotics. The recommended dose is 50 $\mu g/m^2$ subcutaneously three times weekly. IFN-γ has also been used successfully in the treatment of leprosy, nontuberculous mycobacteria, and visceral leishmaniasis.

Rigorous oral hygiene reduces but does not eliminate the discomfort of gingivitis, periodontal disease, and aphthous ulcers; chlorhexidine mouthwash and tooth brushing with a hydrogen peroxide–sodium bicarbonate paste help many patients. Oral antifungal agents (fluconazole, itraconazole, voriconazole, posaconazole) have reduced mucocutaneous candidiasis in patients with Job's syndrome. Androgens, glucocorticoids, lithium, and immunosuppressive therapy have been used to restore myelopoiesis in patients with neutropenia due to impaired production. Recombinant G-CSF is useful in the management of certain forms of neutropenia due to depressed neutrophil production, including those related to cancer chemotherapy. Patients with chronic neutropenia with evidence of a good bone marrow reserve need not receive prophylactic antibiotics. Patients with chronic or cyclic neutrophil counts <500/μL may benefit from prophylactic antibiotics and G-CSF during periods of neutropenia. Oral trimethoprim-sulfamethoxazole (160/800 mg) twice daily can prevent infection. Increased numbers of fungal infections are not seen in patients with CGD on this regimen. Oral quinolones such as levofloxacin and ciprofloxacin are alternatives.

In the setting of cytotoxic chemotherapy with severe, persistent lymphocyte dysfunction, trimethoprim-sulfamethoxazole prevents *Pneumocystis jiroveci* pneumonia. These patients, and patients with phagocytic cell dysfunction, should avoid heavy exposure to airborne soil, dust, or decaying matter (mulch, manure), which are often rich in *Nocardia* and the spores of *Aspergillus* and other fungi. Restriction of activities or social contact has no proven role in reducing risk of infection for phagocyte defects.

Although aggressive medical care for many patients with phagocytic disorders can allow them to go for years without a life-threatening infection, there may still be delayed effects of prolonged antimicrobials and other inflammatory complications. Cure of most congenital phagocyte defects is possible by bone marrow transplantation, and rates of success are improving (Chap. 139e). The identification of specific gene defects in patients with LAD 1, CGD, and other immunodeficiencies has led to gene therapy trials in a number of genetic white cell disorders.

81e Atlas of Hematology and Analysis of Peripheral Blood Smears

Dan L. Longo

This is a digital-only chapter. It is available on the DVD that accompanies this book, as well as on Access Medicine/Harrison's Online, and the eBook and "app" editions of HPIM 19e.

Some of the relevant findings in peripheral blood, enlarged lymph nodes, and bone marrow are illustrated in this chapter. Systematic histologic examination of the bone marrow and lymph nodes is beyond the scope of a general medicine textbook. However, every internist should know how to examine a peripheral blood smear.

The examination of a peripheral blood smear is one of the most informative exercises a physician can perform. Although advances in automated technology have made the examination of a peripheral blood smear by a physician seem less important, the technology is not a completely satisfactory replacement for a blood smear interpretation by a trained medical professional who also knows the patient's clinical history, family history, social history, and physical findings. It is useful to ask the laboratory to generate a Wright's-stained peripheral blood smear and examine it.

Part 3: Genes, the Environment, and Disease

82 Principles of Human Genetics

J. Larry Jameson, Peter Kopp

IMPACT OF GENETICS AND GENOMICS ON MEDICAL PRACTICE

The prevalence of genetic diseases, combined with their potential severity and chronic nature, imposes great human, social, and financial burdens on society. Human genetics refers to the study of individual genes, their role and function in disease, and their mode of inheritance. Genomics refers to an organism's entire genetic information, the *genome*, and the function and interaction of DNA within the genome, as well as with environmental or nongenetic factors, such as a person's lifestyle. With the characterization of the human genome, genomics complements traditional genetics in our efforts to elucidate the etiology and pathogenesis of disease and to improve therapeutic interventions and outcomes. Following impressive advances in genetics, genomics, and health care information technology, the consequences of this wealth of knowledge for the practice of medicine are profound and play an increasingly prominent role in the diagnosis, prevention, and treatment of disease (Chap. 84).

Personalized medicine, the customization of medical decisions to an individual patient, relies heavily on genetic information. For example, a patient's genetic characteristics (genotype) can be used to optimize drug therapy and predict efficacy, adverse events, and drug dosing of selected medications (*pharmacogenetics*) (Chap. 5). The mutational profile of a malignancy allows the selection of therapies that target mutated or overexpressed signaling molecules. Although still investigational, genomic risk prediction models for common diseases are beginning to emerge.

Genetics has traditionally been viewed through the window of relatively rare single-gene diseases. These disorders account for ~10% of pediatric admissions and childhood mortality. Historically, genetics has focused predominantly on chromosomal and metabolic disorders, reflecting the long-standing availability of techniques to diagnose these conditions. For example, conditions such as trisomy 21 (Down's syndrome) or monosomy X (Turner's syndrome) can be diagnosed using cytogenetics (Chap. 83e). Likewise, many metabolic disorders (e.g., phenylketonuria, familial hypercholesterolemia) are diagnosed using biochemical analyses. The advances in DNA diagnostics have extended the field of genetics to include virtually all medical specialties and have led to the elucidation of the pathogenesis of numerous monogenic disorders. In addition, it is apparent that virtually every medical condition has a genetic component. As is often evident from a patient's family history, many common disorders such as hypertension, heart disease, asthma, diabetes mellitus, and mental illnesses are significantly influenced by the genetic background. These polygenic or multifactorial (complex) disorders involve the contributions of many different genes, as well as environmental factors that can modify disease risk (Chap. 84). Genome-wide association studies (GWAS) have elucidated numerous disease-associated loci and are providing novel insights into the allelic architecture of complex traits. These studies have been facilitated by the availability of comprehensive catalogues of human single-nucleotide polymorphism (SNP) haplotypes generated through the HapMap Project. The sequencing of whole genomes or exomes (the exons within the genome) is increasingly used in the clinical realm in order to characterize individuals with complex undiagnosed conditions or to characterize the mutational profile of advanced malignancies in order to select better targeted therapies.

Cancer has a genetic basis because it results from acquired somatic mutations in genes controlling growth, apoptosis, and cellular differentiation (Chap. 101e). In addition, the development of many cancers is associated with a hereditary predisposition. Characterization of the genome (and epigenome) in various malignancies has led to fundamental new insights into cancer biology and reveals that the genomic profile of mutations is in many cases more important in determining the appropriate chemotherapy than the organ in which the tumor originates. Hence, comprehensive mutational profiling of malignancies has increasing impact on cancer taxonomy, the choice of targeted therapies, and improved outcomes.

Genetic and genomic approaches have proven invaluable for the detection of infectious pathogens and are used clinically to identify agents that are difficult to culture such as mycobacteria, viruses, and parasites, or to track infectious agents locally or globally. In many cases, molecular genetics has improved the feasibility and accuracy of diagnostic testing and is beginning to open new avenues for therapy, including gene and cellular therapy (Chaps. 90e and 91e). Molecular genetics has also provided the opportunity to characterize the *microbiome*, a new field that characterizes the population dynamics of bacteria, viruses, and parasites that coexist with humans and other animals (Chap. 86e). Emerging data indicate that the microbiome has significant effects on normal physiology as well as various disease states.

Molecular biology has significantly changed the treatment of human disease. Peptide hormones, growth factors, cytokines, and vaccines can now be produced in large amounts using recombinant DNA technology. Targeted modifications of these peptides provide the practitioner with improved therapeutic tools, as illustrated by genetically modified insulin analogues with more favorable kinetics. Lastly, there is reason to believe that a better understanding of the genetic basis of human disease will also have an increasing impact on disease prevention.

The astounding rate at which new genetic information is being generated creates a major challenge for physicians, health care providers, and basic investigators. Although many functional aspects of the genome remain unknown, there are many clinical situations where sufficient evidence exits for the use of genetic and genomic information to optimize patient care and treatment. Much genetic information resides in databases or is being published in basic science journals. Databases provide easy access to the expanding information about the human genome, genetic disease, and genetic testing (Table 82-1). For example, several thousand monogenic disorders are summarized in a large, continuously evolving compendium, referred to as the *Online Mendelian Inheritance in Man* (OMIM) catalogue (Table 82-1). The ongoing refinement of bioinformatics is simplifying the analysis and access to this daunting amount of new information.

THE HUMAN GENOME

Structure of the Human Genome • ***HUMAN GENOME PROJECT*** The Human Genome Project was initiated in the mid-1980s as an ambitious effort to characterize the entire human genome. Although the prospect of determining the complete sequence of the human genome seemed daunting several years ago, technical advances in DNA sequencing and bioinformatics led to the completion of a draft human sequence in 2000 and the completion of the DNA sequence for the last of the human chromosomes in May 2006. Currently, facilitated by rapidly decreasing costs for comprehensive sequence analyses and improvement of bioinformatics pipelines for data analysis, the sequencing of whole genomes and exomes is used with increasing frequency in the clinical setting. The scope of a whole genome sequence analysis can be illustrated by the following analogy. Human DNA consists of ~3 billion base pairs (bp) of DNA per haploid genome, which is nearly 1000-fold greater than that of the *Escherichia coli* genome. If the human DNA sequence were printed out, it would correspond to about 120 volumes of *Harrison's Principles of Internal Medicine*.

In addition to the human genome, the genomes of numerous organisms have been sequenced completely (~4000) or partially (~10,000) (Genomes Online Database [GOLD]; Table 82-1). They include, among others, eukaryotes such as the mouse (*Mus musculus*),

TABLE 82-1 SELECTED DATABASES RELEVANT FOR GENOMICS AND GENETIC DISORDERS

Site	URL	Comment
National Center for Biotechnology Information (NCBI)	*http://www.ncbi.nlm.nih.gov/*	Broad access to biomedical and genomic information, literature (PubMed), sequence databases, software for analyses of nucleotides and proteins Extensive links to other databases, genome resources, and tutorials
National Human Genome Research Institute	*http://www.genome.gov/*	An institute of the National Institutes of Health focused on genomic and genetic research; links providing information about the human genome sequence, genomes of other organisms, and genomic research
Catalog of Published Genome-Wide Association Studies	*http://www.genome.gov/GWAStudies/*	Published high-resolution genome-wide association studies (GWAS)
Ensembl Genome browser	*http://www.ensembl.org*	Maps and sequence information of eukaryotic genomes
Online Mendelian Inheritance in Man	*http://www.ncbi.nlm.nih.gov/omim*	Online compendium of Mendelian disorders and human genes causing genetic disorders
Office of Biotechnology Activities, National Institutes of Health	*http://oba.od.nih.gov/oba*	Information about recombinant DNA and gene transfer; medical, ethical, legal, and social issues raised by genetic testing; medical, ethical, legal, and social issues raised by xenotransplantation
American College of Medical Genetics and Genomics	*http://www.acmg.net/*	Extensive links to other databases relevant for the diagnosis, treatment, and prevention of genetic disease
American Society of Human Genetics	*http://www.ashg.org*	Information about advances in genetic research, professional and public education, social and scientific policies
Cancer Genome Anatomy Project (CGAP)	*http://cgap.nci.nih.gov/*	Information about gene expression profiles of normal, precancer, and cancer cells
GeneTests	*http://www.genetests.org/*	International directory of genetic testing laboratories and prenatal diagnosis clinics; reviews and educational materials
Genomes Online Database (GOLD)	*http://www.genomesonline.org/*	Information on published and unpublished genomes
HUGO Gene Nomenclature	*http://www.genenames.org/*	Gene names and symbols
MITOMAP, a human mitochondrial genome database	*http://www.mitomap.org/*	A compendium of polymorphisms and mutations of the human mitochondrial DNA
International HapMap Project	*http://www.hapmap.org/*	Catalogue of haplotypes in different ethnic groups relevant for association studies and pharmacogenomics
ENCODE	*http://www.genome.gov/10005107*	*Encyclopedia* of *DNA Elements*; catalogue of all functional elements in the human genome
Dolan DNA Learning Center, Cold Spring Harbor Laboratories	*http://www.dnalc.org/*	Educational material about selected genetic disorders, DNA, eugenics, and genetic origin
The Online Metabolic and Molecular Bases of Inherited Disease (OMMBID)	*http://www.ommbid.com/*	Online version of the comprehensive text on the metabolic and molecular bases of inherited disease
Online Mendelian Inheritance in Animals (OMIA)	*http://omia.angis.org.au/*	Online compendium of Mendelian disorders in animals
The Jackson Laboratory	*http://www.jax.org/*	Information about murine models and the mouse genome
	http://www.informatics.jax.org	Mouse genome informatics

Note: Databases are evolving constantly. Pertinent information may be found by using links listed in the few selected databases.

Saccharomyces cerevisiae, *Caenorhabditis elegans*, and *Drosophila melanogaster*; bacteria (e.g., *E. coli*); and Archaea, viruses, organelles (mitochondria, chloroplasts), and plants (e.g., *Arabidopsis thaliana*). Genomic information of infectious agents has significant impact for the characterization of infectious outbreaks and epidemics. Other ramifications arising from the availability of genomic data include, among others, (1) the comparison of entire genomes (*comparative genomics*), (2) the study of large-scale expression of RNAs (*functional genomics*) and proteins (*proteomics*) to detect differences between various tissues in health and disease, (3) the characterization of the variation among individuals by establishing catalogues of sequence variations and SNPs (HapMap Project), and (4) the identification of genes that play critical roles in the development of polygenic and multifactorial disorders.

CHROMOSOMES The human genome is divided into 23 different chromosomes, including 22 autosomes (numbered 1–22) and the X and Y sex chromosomes (Fig. 82-1). Adult cells are *diploid*, meaning they contain two homologous sets of 22 autosomes and a pair of sex chromosomes. Females have two X chromosomes (XX), whereas males have one X and one Y chromosome (XY). As a consequence of meiosis, germ cells (sperm or oocytes) are haploid and contain one set of 22 autosomes and one of the sex chromosomes. At the time of fertilization, the diploid genome is reconstituted by pairing of the homologous chromosomes from the mother and father. With each cell division (mitosis), chromosomes are replicated, paired, segregated, and divided into two daughter cells.

STRUCTURE OF DNA DNA is a double-stranded helix composed of four different bases: adenine (A), thymidine (T), guanine (G), and cytosine (C). Adenine is paired to thymidine, and guanine is paired to cytosine, by hydrogen bond interactions that span the double helix (Fig. 82-1). DNA has several remarkable features that make it ideal for the transmission of genetic information. It is relatively stable, and the double-stranded nature of DNA and its feature of strict base-pair complementarity permit faithful replication during cell division. Complementarity also allows the transmission of genetic information from DNA → RNA → protein (Fig. 82-2). mRNA is encoded by the so-called sense or coding strand of the DNA double helix and is translated into proteins by ribosomes.

The presence of four different bases provides surprising genetic diversity. In the protein-coding regions of genes, the DNA bases are arranged into codons, a triplet of bases that specifies a particular amino acid. It is possible to arrange the four bases into 64 different triplet codons (4^3). Each codon specifies 1 of the 20 different amino acids, or a regulatory signal such as initiation and stop of translation. Because there are more codons than amino acids, the genetic code is degenerate; that is, most amino acids can be specified by several different codons. By arranging the codons in different combinations and in

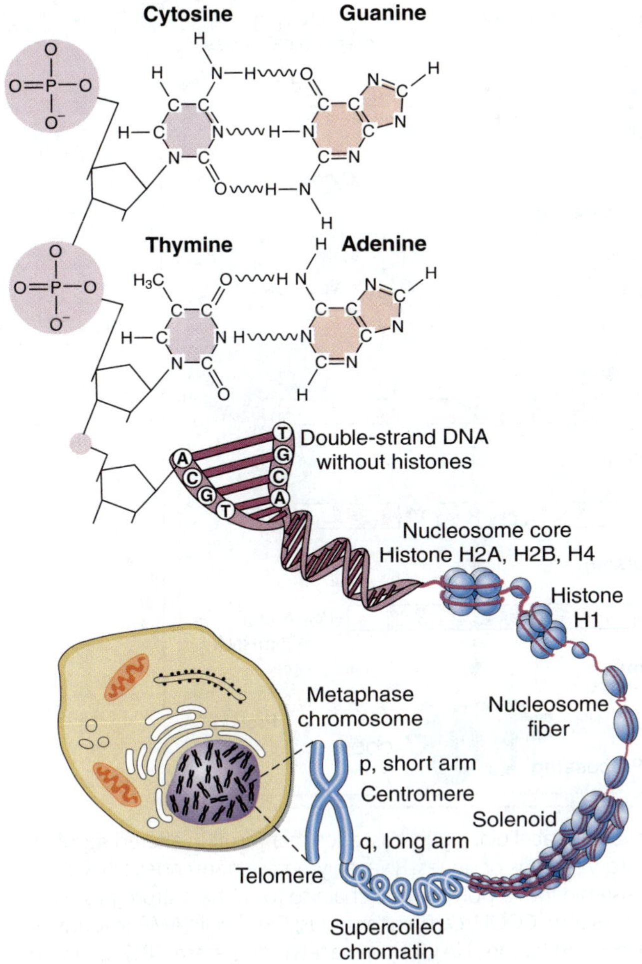

FIGURE 82-1 Structure of chromatin and chromosomes. Chromatin is composed of double-strand DNA that is wrapped around histone and nonhistone proteins forming nucleosomes. The nucleosomes are further organized into solenoid structures. Chromosomes assume their characteristic structure, with short (p) and long (q) arms at the metaphase stage of the cell cycle.

various lengths, it is possible to generate the tremendous diversity of primary protein structure.

DNA length is normally measured in units of 1000 bp (kilobases, kb) or 1,000,000 bp (megabases, Mb). Not all DNA encodes genes. In fact, genes account for only ~10–15% of DNA. Much of the remaining DNA consists of sequences, often of highly repetitive nature, the function of which is poorly understood. These repetitive DNA regions, along with nonrepetitive sequences that do not encode genes, serve, in part, a structural role in the packaging of DNA into chromatin (i.e., DNA bound to histone proteins, and chromosomes) and exert regulatory functions (Fig. 82-1).

GENES A *gene* is a functional unit that is regulated by transcription (see below) and encodes an RNA product, which is most commonly, but not always, translated into a protein that exerts activity within or outside the cell (Fig. 82-3). Historically, genes were identified because they conferred specific traits that are transmitted from one generation to the next. Increasingly, they are characterized based on expression in various tissues (*transcriptome*). The size of genes is quite broad; some genes are only a few hundred base pairs, whereas others are extraordinarily large (2 Mb). The number of genes greatly underestimates the complexity of genetic expression, because single genes can generate multiple spliced messenger RNA (mRNA) products (*isoforms*), which are translated into proteins that are subject to complex posttranslational modification such as phosphorylation. *Exons* refer to the portion of genes that are eventually spliced together to form mRNA. *Introns* refer to the spacing regions between the exons that are spliced out of precursor RNAs during RNA processing. The gene locus also includes regions that are necessary to control its expression (Fig. 82-2). Current estimates predict 20,687 protein-coding genes in the human genome with an average of about four different coding transcripts per gene. Remarkably, the exome only constitutes 1.14% of the genome. In addition, thousands of noncoding transcripts (RNAs of various length such as microRNAs and long noncoding RNAs), which function, at least in part, as transcriptional and posttranscriptional regulators of gene expression, have been identified. Aberrant expression of microRNAs has been found to play a pathogenic role in numerous diseases.

SINGLE-NUCLEOTIDE POLYMORPHISMS An SNP is a variation of a single base pair in the DNA. The identification of the ~10 million SNPs estimated to occur in the human genome has generated a catalogue of common genetic variants that occur in human beings from distinct ethnic backgrounds (Fig. 82-3). SNPs are the most common type of sequence variation and account for ~90% of all sequence variation. They occur on average every 100 to 300 bases and are the major source of genetic heterogeneity. Remarkably, however, the primary DNA sequence of humans has ~99.9% similarity compared to that of any other human. SNPs that are in close proximity are inherited together (e.g., they are linked) and are referred to as *haplotypes* (Fig. 82-4). The HapMap describes the nature and location of these SNP haplotypes and how they are distributed among individuals within and among populations. The haplotype map information, referred to as HapMap, is greatly facilitating GWAS designed to elucidate the complex interactions among multiple genes and lifestyle factors in multifactorial disorders (see below). Moreover, haplotype analyses are useful to assess variations in responses to medications (*pharmacogenomics*) and environmental factors, as well as the prediction of disease predisposition.

COPY NUMBER VARIATIONS Copy number variations (CNVs) are relatively large genomic regions (1 kb to several Mb) that have been duplicated or deleted on certain chromosomes (Fig. 82-5). It has been estimated that as many as 1500 CNVs, scattered throughout the genome, are present in an individual. When comparing the genomes of two individuals, approximately 0.4–0.8% of their genomes differ in terms of CNVs. Of note, de novo CNVs have been observed between monozygotic twins, who otherwise have identical genomes. Some CNVs have been associated with susceptibility or resistance to disease, and CNVs can be elevated in cancer cells.

Replication of DNA and Mitosis Genetic information in DNA is transmitted to daughter cells under two different circumstances: (1) somatic cells divide by *mitosis*, allowing the diploid ($2n$) genome to replicate itself completely in conjunction with cell division; and (2) germ cells (sperm and ova) undergo *meiosis*, a process that enables the reduction of the diploid ($2n$) set of chromosomes to the haploid state ($1n$).

Prior to mitosis, cells exit the resting, or G_0 state, and enter the cell cycle (Chap. 101e). After traversing a critical checkpoint in G_1, cells undergo DNA synthesis (S phase), during which the DNA in each chromosome is replicated, yielding two pairs of sister chromatids ($2n \rightarrow 4n$). The process of DNA synthesis requires stringent fidelity in order to avoid transmitting errors to subsequent generations of cells. Genetic abnormalities of DNA mismatch/repair include xeroderma pigmentosum, Bloom's syndrome, ataxia telangiectasia, and hereditary nonpolyposis colon cancer (HNPCC), among others. Many of these disorders strongly predispose to neoplasia because of the rapid acquisition of additional mutations (Chap. 101e). After completion of DNA synthesis, cells enter G_2 and progress through a second checkpoint before entering mitosis. At this stage, the chromosomes condense and are aligned along the equatorial plate at metaphase. The two identical sister chromatids, held together at the centromere, divide and migrate to opposite poles of the cell. After formation of a nuclear membrane around the two separated sets of chromatids, the cell divides and two daughter cells are formed, thus restoring the diploid ($2n$) state.

Assortment and Segregation of Genes During Meiosis Meiosis occurs only in germ cells of the gonads. It shares certain features with mitosis but involves two distinct steps of cell division that reduce the chromosome number to the haploid state. In addition, there is active recombination that generates genetic diversity. During the first cell division, two

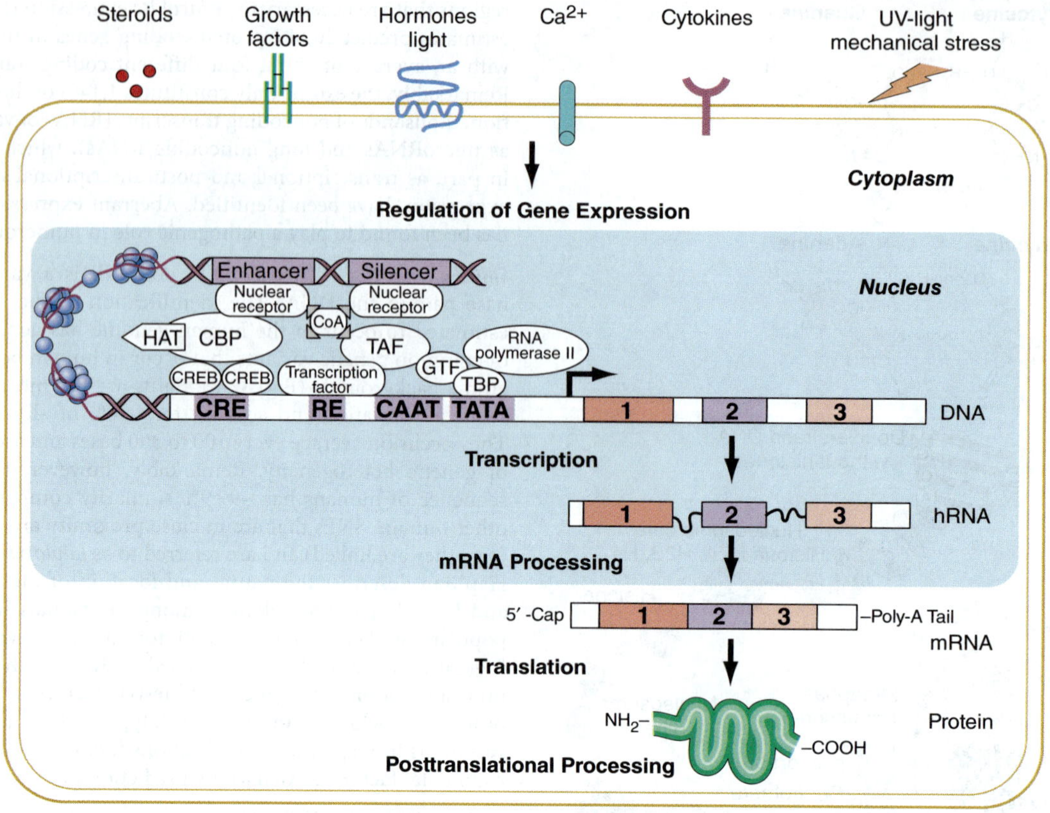

FIGURE 82-2 Flow of genetic information. Multiple extracellular signals activate intracellular signal cascades that result in altered regulation of gene expression through the interaction of transcription factors with regulatory regions of genes. RNA polymerase transcribes DNA into RNA that is processed to mRNA by excision of intronic sequences. The mRNA is translated into a polypeptide chain to form the mature protein after undergoing posttranslational processing. CBP, CREB-binding protein; CoA, co-activator; COOH, carboxyterminus; CRE, cyclic AMP responsive element; CREB, cyclic AMP response element–binding protein; GTF, general transcription factors; HAT, histone acetyl transferase; NH2, aminoterminus; RE, response element; TAF, TBP-associated factors; TATA, TATA box; TBP, TATA-binding protein.

sister chromatids ($2n \rightarrow 4n$) are formed for each chromosome pair and there is an exchange of DNA between homologous paternal and maternal chromosomes. This process involves the formation of *chiasmata*, structures that correspond to the DNA segments that cross over between the maternal and paternal homologues (Fig. 82-6). Usually there is at least one crossover on each chromosomal arm; recombination occurs more frequently in female meiosis than in male meiosis. Subsequently, the chromosomes segregate randomly. Because there are 23 chromosomes, there exist 2^{23} (>8 million) possible combinations of chromosomes. Together with the genetic exchanges that occur during recombination, chromosomal segregation generates tremendous diversity, and each gamete is genetically unique. The process of recombination and the independent segregation of chromosomes provide the foundation for performing linkage analyses, whereby one attempts to correlate the inheritance of certain chromosomal regions (or linked genes) with the presence of a disease or genetic trait (see below).

After the first meiotic division, which results in two daughter cells ($2n$), the two chromatids of each chromosome separate during a second meiotic division to yield four gametes with a haploid state ($1n$). When the egg is fertilized by sperm, the two haploid sets are combined, thereby restoring the diploid state ($2n$) in the zygote.

REGULATION OF GENE EXPRESSION

Regulation by Transcription Factors The expression of genes is regulated by DNA-binding proteins that activate or repress transcription. The number of DNA sequences and transcription factors that regulate transcription is much greater than originally anticipated. Most genes contain at least 15–20 discrete regulatory elements within 300 bp of the transcription start site. This densely packed promoter region often contains binding sites for ubiquitous transcription factors such as CAAT box/enhancer binding protein (C/EBP), cyclic AMP response element–binding (CREB) protein, selective promoter factor 1 (Sp-1), or activator protein 1 (AP-1). However, factors involved in cell-specific expression may also bind to these sequences. Key regulatory elements may also reside at a large distance from the proximal promoter. The globin and the immunoglobulin genes, for example, contain *locus control regions* that are several kilobases away from the structural sequences of the gene. Specific groups of transcription factors that bind to these promoter and enhancer sequences provide a combinatorial code for regulating transcription. In this manner, relatively ubiquitous factors interact with more restricted factors to allow each gene to be expressed and regulated in a unique manner that is dependent on developmental state, cell type, and numerous extracellular stimuli. Regulatory factors also bind within the gene itself, particularly in the intronic regions. The transcription factors that bind to DNA actually represent only the first level of regulatory control. Other proteins—*co-activators* and *co-repressors*—interact with the DNA-binding transcription factors to generate large regulatory complexes. These complexes are subject to control by numerous cell-signaling pathways and enzymes, leading to phosphorylation, acetylation, sumoylation, and ubiquitination. Ultimately, the recruited transcription factors interact with, and stabilize, components of the basal transcription complex that assembles at the site of the TATA box and initiator region. This basal transcription factor complex consists of >30 different proteins. Gene transcription occurs when RNA polymerase begins to synthesize RNA from the DNA template. A large number of identified genetic diseases involve transcription factors (Table 82-2).

The field of *functional genomics* is based on the concept that understanding alterations of gene expression under various physiologic and pathologic conditions provides insight into the underlying functional role of the gene. By revealing specific gene expression profiles, this knowledge may be of diagnostic and therapeutic relevance. The large-scale study of expression profiles, which takes advantage of microarray and bead array technologies, is also referred to as *transcriptomics*

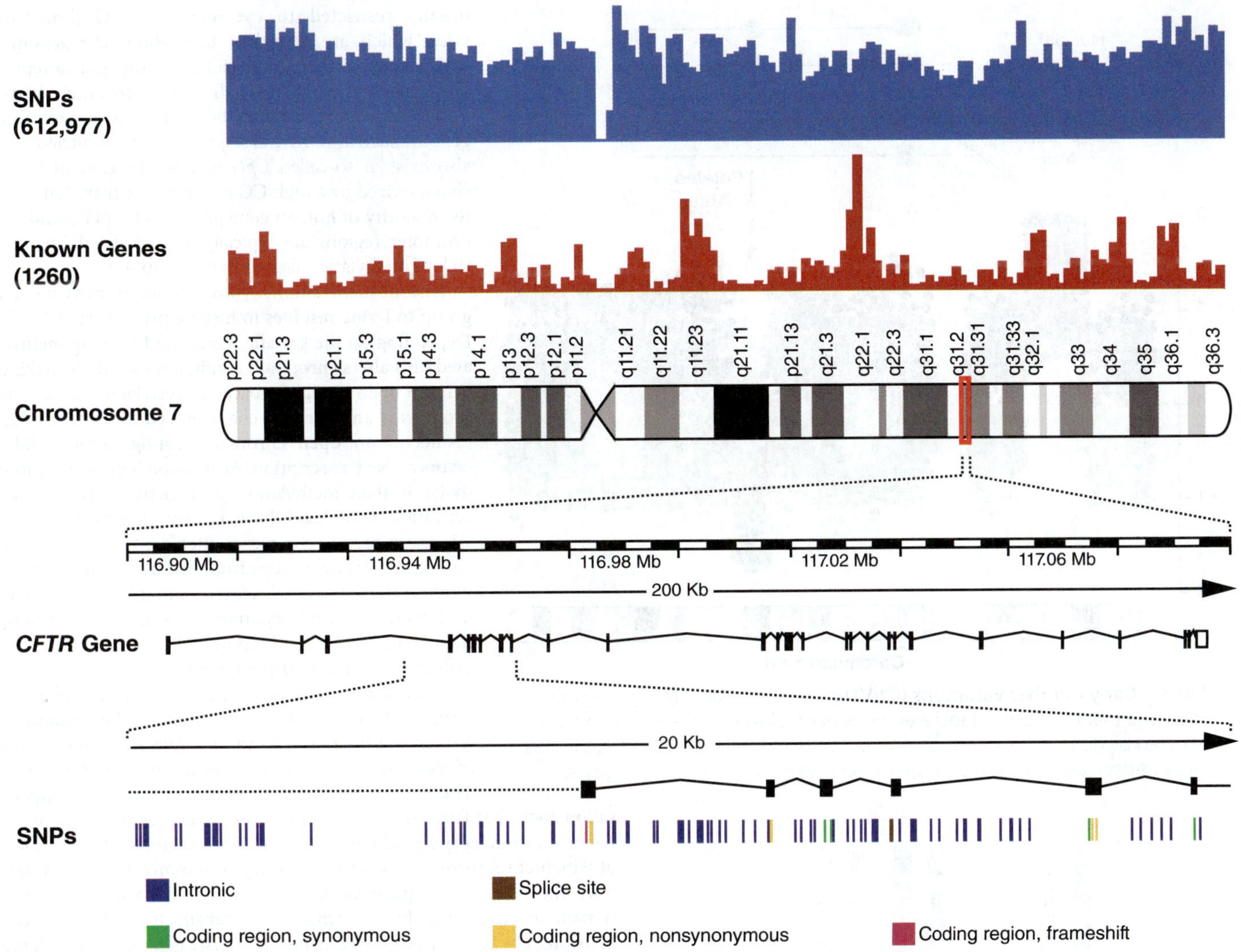

FIGURE 82-3 Chromosome 7 is shown with the density of single-nucleotide polymorphisms (SNPs) and genes above. A 200-kb region in 7q31.2 containing the *CFTR* gene is shown below. The *CFTR* gene contains 27 exons. More than 1900 mutations in this gene have been found in patients with cystic fibrosis. A 20-kb region encompassing exons 4–9 is shown further amplified to illustrate the SNPs in this region.

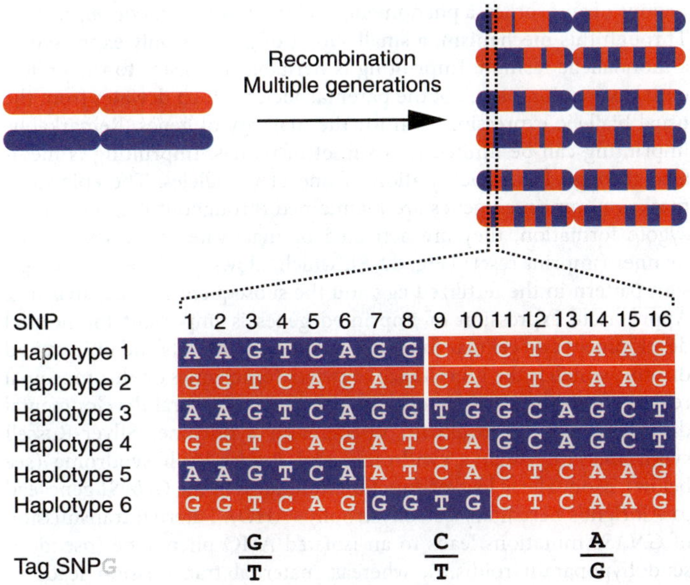

FIGURE 82-4 The origin of haplotypes is due to repeated recombination events occurring in multiple generations. Over time, this leads to distinct haplotypes. These haplotype blocks can often be characterized by genotyping selected Tag single-nucleotide polymorphisms (SNPs), an approach that facilitates performing genome-wide association studies (GWAS).

because the complement of mRNAs transcribed by the cellular genome is called the *transcriptome*.

Most studies of gene expression have focused on the regulatory DNA elements of genes that control transcription. However, it should be emphasized that gene expression requires a series of steps, including mRNA processing, protein translation, and posttranslational modifications, all of which are actively regulated (Fig. 82-2).

Epigenetic Regulation of Gene Expression *Epigenetics* describes mechanisms and phenotypic changes that are not a result of variation in the primary DNA nucleotide sequence, but are caused by secondary modifications of DNA or histones. These modifications include heritable changes such as X-inactivation and imprinting, but they can also result from dynamic posttranslational protein modifications in response to environmental influences such as diet, age, or drugs. The epigenetic modifications result in altered expression of individual genes or chromosomal loci encompassing multiple genes. The term *epigenome* describes the constellation of covalent modifications of DNA and histones that impact chromatin structure, as well as noncoding transcripts that modulate the transcriptional activity of DNA. Although the primary DNA sequence is usually identical in all cells of an organism, tissue-specific changes in the epigenome contribute to determining the transcriptional signature of a cell (transcriptome) and hence the protein expression profile (proteome).

Mechanistically, DNA and histone modifications can result in the activation or silencing of gene expression (Fig. 82-7). DNA methylation involves the addition of a methyl group to cytosine residues. This is

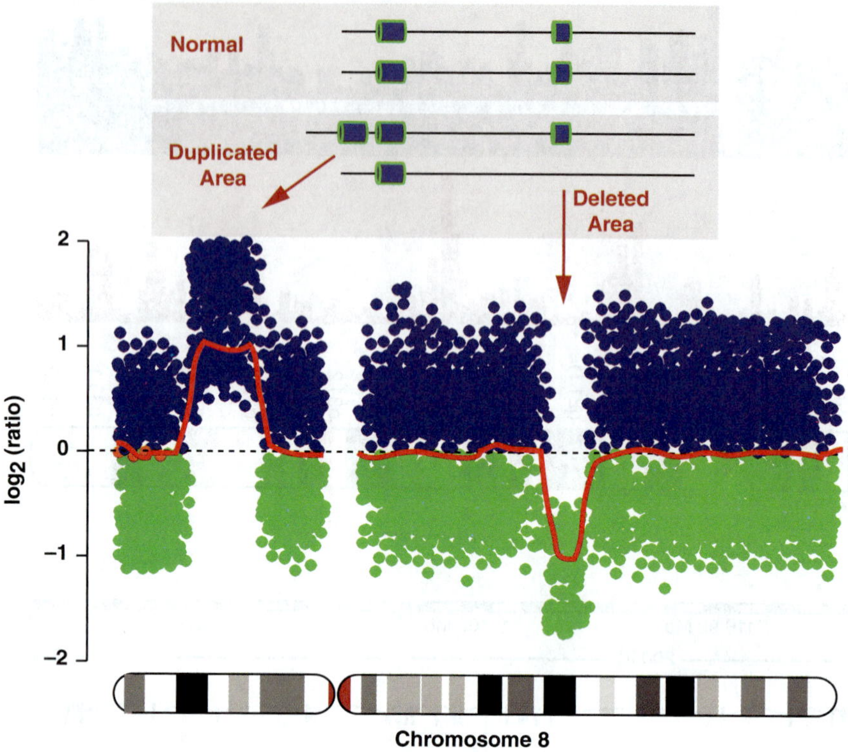

FIGURE 82-5 Copy number variations (CNV) encompass relatively large regions of the genome that have been duplicated or deleted. Chromosome 8 is shown with CNV detected by genomic hybridization. An increase in the signal strength indicates a duplication, a decrease reflects a deletion of the covered chromosomal regions.

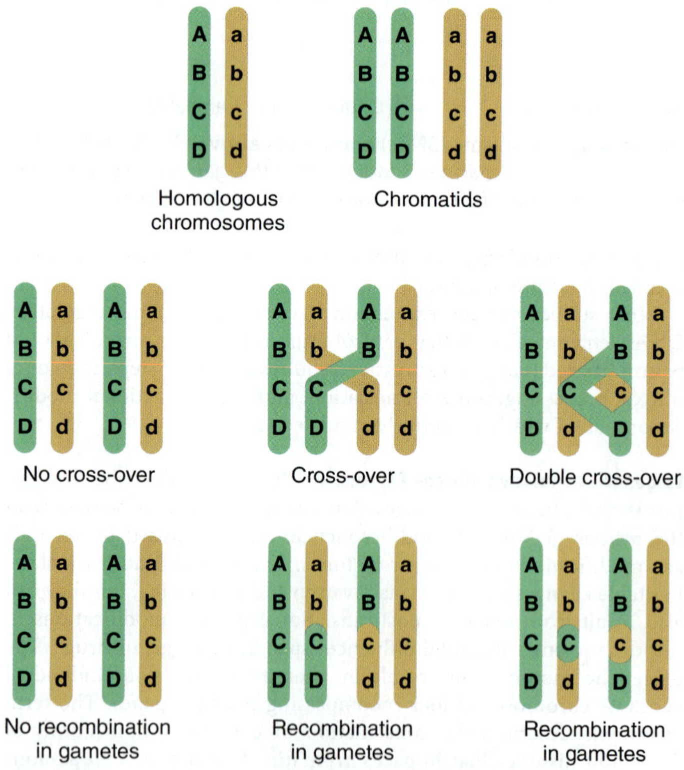

FIGURE 82-6 Crossing-over and genetic recombination. During chiasma formation, either of the two sister chromatids on one chromosome pairs with one of the chromatids of the homologous chromosome. Genetic recombination occurs through crossing-over and results in recombinant and nonrecombinant chromosome segments in the gametes. Together with the random segregation of the maternal and paternal chromosomes, recombination contributes to genetic diversity and forms the basis of the concept of linkage.

usually restricted to cytosines of CpG dinucleotides, which are abundant throughout the genome. Methylation of these dinucleotides is thought to represent a defense mechanism that minimizes the expression of sequences that have been incorporated into the genome such as retroviral sequences. CpG dinucleotides also exist in so-called *CpG islands*, stretches of DNA characterized by a high CG content, which are found in the majority of human gene promoters. CpG islands in promoter regions are typically unmethylated, and the lack of methylation facilitates transcription.

Histone methylation involves the addition of a methyl group to lysine residues in histone proteins (Fig. 82-7). Depending on the specific lysine residue being methylated, this alters chromatin configuration, either making it more open or tightly packed. Acetylation of histone proteins is another well-characterized mechanism that results in an open chromatin configuration, which favors active transcription. Acetylation is generally more dynamic than methylation, and many transcriptional activation complexes have histone acetylase activity, whereas repressor complexes often contain deacetylases and remove acetyl groups from histones. Other histone modifications, whose effects are incompletely characterized, include phosphorylation and sumoylation. Lastly, noncoding RNAs that bind to DNA can have a significant impact on transcriptional activity.

Physiologically, epigenetic mechanisms play an important role in several instances. For example, X-inactivation refers to the relative silencing of one of the two X chromosome copies present in females. The inactivation process is a form of dosage compensation such that females (XX) do not generally express twice as many X-chromosomal gene products as males (XY). In a given cell, the choice of which chromosome is inactivated occurs randomly in humans. But once the maternal or paternal X chromosome is inactivated, it will remain inactive, and this information is transmitted with each cell division. The *X-inactive specific transcript* (*Xist*) gene encodes a large noncoding RNA that mediates the silencing of the X chromosome from which it is transcribed by coating it with Xist RNA. The inactive X chromosome is highly methylated and has low levels of histone acetylation.

Epigenetic gene inactivation also occurs on selected chromosomal regions of autosomes, a phenomenon referred to as *genomic imprinting*. Through this mechanism, a small subset of genes is only expressed in a monoallelic fashion. Imprinting is heritable and leads to the preferential expression of one of the parental alleles, which deviates from the usual biallelic expression seen for the majority of genes. Remarkably, imprinting can be limited to a subset of tissues. Imprinting is mediated through DNA methylation of one of the alleles. The epigenetic marks on imprinted genes are maintained throughout life, but during zygote formation, they are activated or inactivated in a sex-specific manner (imprint reset) (Fig. 82-8), which allows a differential expression pattern in the fertilized egg and the subsequent mitotic divisions. Appropriate expression of imprinted genes is important for normal development and cellular functions. Imprinting defects and uniparental disomy, which is the inheritance of two chromosomes or chromosomal regions from the same parent, are the cause of several developmental disorders such as Beckwith-Wiedemann syndrome, Silver-Russell syndrome, Angelman's syndrome, and Prader-Willi syndrome (see below). Monoallelic loss-of-function mutations in the *GNAS1* gene lead to Albright's hereditary osteodystrophy (AHO). Paternal transmission of *GNAS1* mutations leads to an isolated AHO phenotype (pseudopseudohypoparathyroidism), whereas maternal transmission leads to AHO in combination with hormone resistance to parathyroid hormone, thyrotropin, and gonadotropins (pseudohypoparathyroidism type IA). These phenotypic differences are explained by tissue-specific imprinting of the *GNAS1* gene, which is expressed primarily from the maternal allele in the thyroid, gonadotropes, and the proximal renal tubule. In most other tissues, the *GNAS1* gene is expressed biallelically.

TABLE 82-2 SELECTED EXAMPLES OF DISEASES CAUSED BY MUTATIONS AND REARRANGEMENTS IN TRANSCRIPTION FACTOR CLASSES

Transcription Factor Class	Example	Associated Disorder
Nuclear receptors	Androgen receptor	Complete or partial androgen insensitivity (recessive missense mutations)
		Spinobulbar muscular atrophy (CAG repeat expansion)
Zinc finger proteins	WT1	WAGR syndrome: *W*ilms' tumor, *a*niridia, *g*enitourinary malformations, mental *r*etardation
Basic helix-loop-helix	MITF	Waardenburg's syndrome type 2A
Homeobox	IPF1	Maturity onset of diabetes mellitus type 4 (heterozygous mutation/haploinsufficiency)
		Pancreatic agenesis (homozygous mutation)
Leucine zipper	Retina leucine zipper (NRL)	Autosomal dominant retinitis pigmentosa
High mobility group (HMG) proteins	SRY	Sex reversal
Forkhead	HNF4α, HNF1α, HNF1β	Maturity onset of diabetes mellitus types 1, 3, 5
Paired box	PAX3	Waardenburg's syndrome types 1 and 3
T-box	TBX5	Holt-Oram syndrome (thumb anomalies, atrial or ventricular septum defects, phocomelia)
Cell cycle control proteins	P53	Li-Fraumeni syndrome, other cancers
Co-activators	CREB binding protein (CBP)	Rubinstein-Taybi syndrome
General transcription factors	TATA-binding protein (TBP)	Spinocerebellar ataxia 17 (CAG expansion)
Transcription elongation factor	VHL	von Hippel–Lindau syndrome (renal cell carcinoma, pheochromocytoma, pancreatic tumors, hemangioblastomas)
		Autosomal dominant inheritance, somatic inactivation of second allele (Knudson two-hit model)
Runt	CBFA2	Familial thrombocytopenia with propensity to acute myelogenous leukemia
Chimeric proteins due to translocations	PML-RAR	Acute promyelocytic leukemia t(15;17)(q22;q11.2-q12) translocation

Abbreviations: CREB, cAMP responsive element–binding protein; HNF, hepatocyte nuclear factor; PML, promyelocytic leukemia; RAR, retinoic acid receptor; SRY, sex-determining region Y; VHL, von Hippel–Lindau.

In patients with isolated renal resistance to parathyroid hormone (pseudohypoparathyroidism type IB), defective imprinting of the *GNAS1* gene results in decreased Gsα expression in the proximal renal tubules. Rett's syndrome is an X-linked dominant disorder resulting in developmental regression and stereotypic hand movements in affected girls. It is caused by mutations in the *MECP2* gene, which encodes a methyl-binding protein. The ensuing aberrant methylation results in abnormal gene expression in neurons, which are otherwise normally developed.

Remarkably, epigenetic differences also occur among monozygotic twins. Although twins are epigenetically indistinguishable during the early years of life, older monozygotic twins exhibit differences in the overall content and genomic distribution of DNA methylation and histone acetylation, which would be expected to alter gene expression in various tissues.

In cancer, the epigenome is characterized by simultaneous losses and gains of DNA methylation in different genomic regions, as well as repressive histone modifications. Hyper- and hypomethylation are associated with mutations in genes that control DNA methylation. Hypomethylation is thought to remove normal control mechanisms that prevent expression of repressed DNA regions. It is also associated with genomic instability. Hypermethylation, in contrast, results in the silencing of CpG islands in promoter regions of genes, including tumor-suppressor genes. Epigenetic alterations are considered to be more easily reversible compared to genetic changes, and modification of the epigenome with demethylating agents and histone deacetylases is being explored in clinical trials.

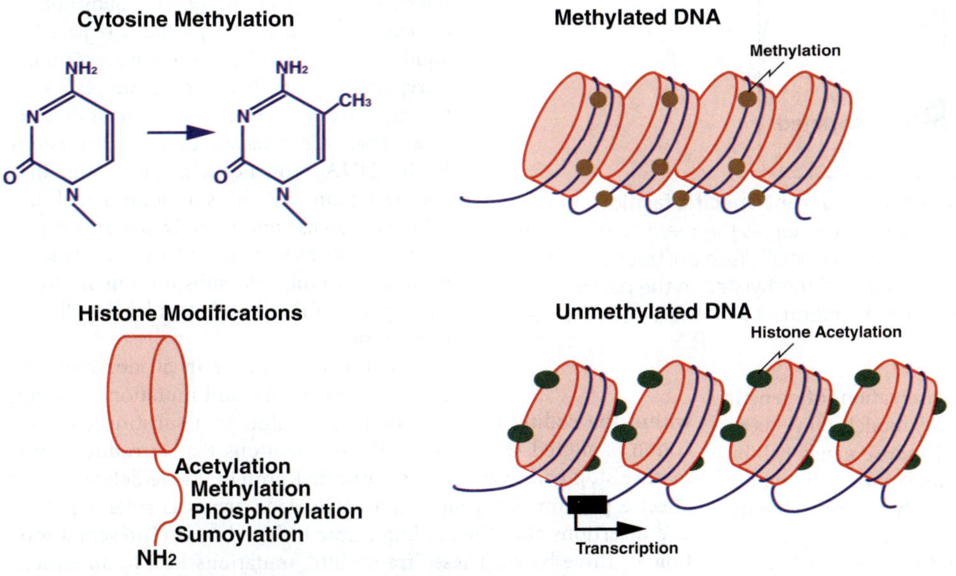

FIGURE 82-7 Epigenetic modifications of DNA and histones. Methylation of cytosine residues is associated with gene silencing. Methylation of certain genomic regions is inherited (imprinting), and it is involved in the silencing of one of the two X chromosomes in females (X-inactivation). Alterations in methylation can also be acquired, e.g., in cancer cells. Covalent posttranslational modifications of histones play an important role in altering DNA accessibility and chromatin structure and hence in regulating transcription. Histones can be reversibly modified in their amino-terminal tails, which protrude from the nucleosome core particle, by acetylation of lysine, phosphorylation of serine, methylation of lysine and arginine residues, and sumoylation. Acetylation of histones by histone acetylases (HATs), e.g., leads to unwinding of chromatin and accessibility to transcription factors. Conversely, deacetylation by histone deacetylases (HDACs) results in a compact chromatin structure and silencing of transcription.

MODELS OF GENETIC DISEASE

Several organisms have been studied extensively as genetic models, including *M. musculus* (mouse), *D. melanogaster* (fruit fly), *C. elegans* (nematode), *S. cerevisiae* (baker's yeast), and *E. coli* (colonic bacterium). The ability to use these evolutionarily distant organisms as genetic models that are relevant

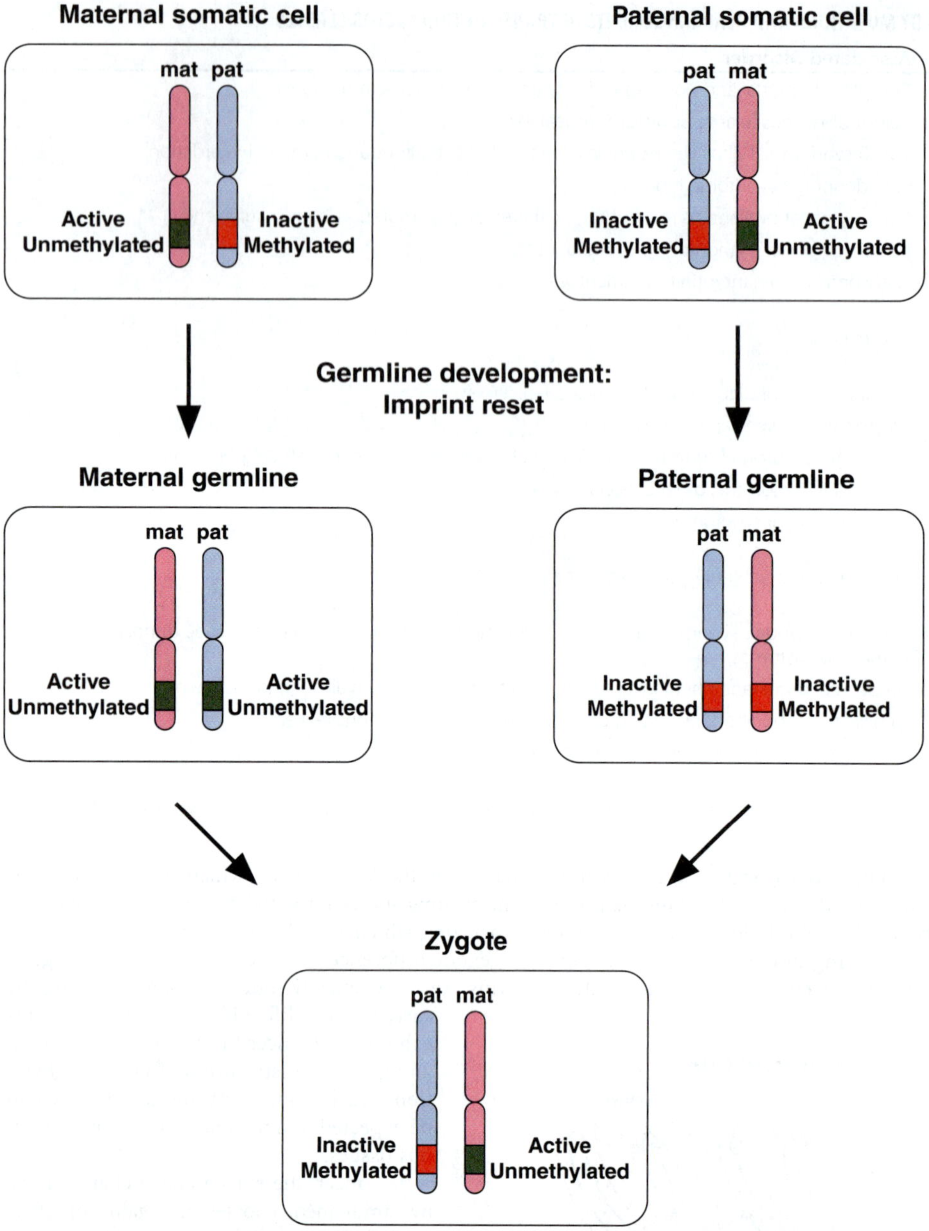

FIGURE 82-8 A few genomic regions are imprinted in a parent-specific fashion. The unmethylated chromosomal regions are actively expressed, whereas the methylated regions are silenced. In the germline, the imprint is reset in a parent-specific fashion: both chromosomes are unmethylated in the maternal (mat) germline and methylated in the paternal (pat) germline. In the zygote, the resulting imprinting pattern is identical with the pattern in the somatic cells of the parents.

to human physiology reflects a surprising conservation of genetic pathways and gene function. Transgenic mouse models have been particularly valuable, because many human and mouse genes exhibit similar structure and function and because manipulation of the mouse genome is relatively straightforward compared to that of other mammalian species. Transgenic strategies in mice can be divided into two main approaches: (1) expression of a gene by random insertion into the genome, and (2) deletion or targeted mutagenesis of a gene by homologous recombination with the native endogenous gene (knock-out, knock-in). Previous versions of this chapter provide more detail about the technical principles underlying the development of genetically modified animals. Several databases provide comprehensive information about natural and transgenic animal models, the associated phenotypes, and integrated genetic, genomic, and biologic data (Table 82-1).

TRANSMISSION OF GENETIC DISEASE

Origins and Types of Mutations A *mutation* can be defined as any change in the primary nucleotide sequence of DNA regardless of its functional consequences. Some mutations may be lethal, others are less deleterious, and some may confer an evolutionary advantage. Mutations can occur in the germline (sperm or oocytes); these can be transmitted to progeny. Alternatively, mutations can occur during embryogenesis or in somatic tissues. Mutations that occur during development lead to *mosaicism*, a situation in which tissues are composed of cells with different genetic constitutions. If the germline is mosaic, a mutation can be transmitted to some progeny but not others, which sometimes leads to confusion in assessing the pattern of inheritance. Somatic mutations that do not affect cell survival can sometimes be detected because of variable phenotypic effects in tissues (e.g., pigmented lesions in McCune-Albright syndrome). Other somatic mutations are associated with neoplasia because they confer a growth advantage to cells. Epigenetic events may also influence gene expression or facilitate genetic damage. With the exception of triplet nucleotide repeats, which can expand (see below), mutations are usually stable.

Mutations are structurally diverse—they can involve the entire genome, as in triploidy (one extra set of chromosomes), or gross numerical or structural alterations in chromosomes or individual genes (Chap. 83e). Large deletions may affect a portion of a gene or an entire gene, or, if several genes are involved, they may lead to a *contiguous gene syndrome*. Unequal crossing-over between homologous genes can result in fusion gene mutations, as illustrated by color blindness. Mutations involving single nucleotides are referred to as *point mutations*. Substitutions are called *transitions* if a purine is replaced by another purine base (A ↔ G) or if a pyrimidine is replaced by another pyrimidine (C ↔ T). Changes from a purine to a pyrimidine, or vice versa, are referred to as *transversions*. If the DNA sequence change occurs in a coding region and alters an amino acid, it is called a *missense mutation*. Depending on the functional consequences of such a missense mutation, amino acid substitutions in different regions of the protein can lead to distinct phenotypes.

Mutations can occur in all domains of a gene (Fig. 82-9). A point mutation occurring within the coding region leads to an amino acid substitution if the codon is altered (Fig. 82-10). Point mutations that introduce a premature stop codon result in a truncated protein. Large deletions may affect a portion of a gene or an entire gene, whereas small deletions and insertions alter the reading frame if they do not represent a multiple of three bases. These "frameshift" mutations lead to an entirely altered carboxy terminus. Mutations in intronic sequences or in exon junctions may destroy or create splice donor or splice acceptor sites. Mutations may also be found in the regulatory sequences of genes, resulting in reduced or enhanced gene transcription.

Certain DNA sequences are particularly susceptible to mutagenesis. Successive pyrimidine residues (e.g., T-T or C-C) are subject to the formation of ultraviolet light–induced photoadducts. If these pyrimidine dimers are not repaired by the nucleotide excision repair pathway, mutations will be introduced after DNA synthesis. The dinucleotide C-G, or CpG, is also a hot spot for a specific type of mutation. In this case, methylation of the cytosine is associated with

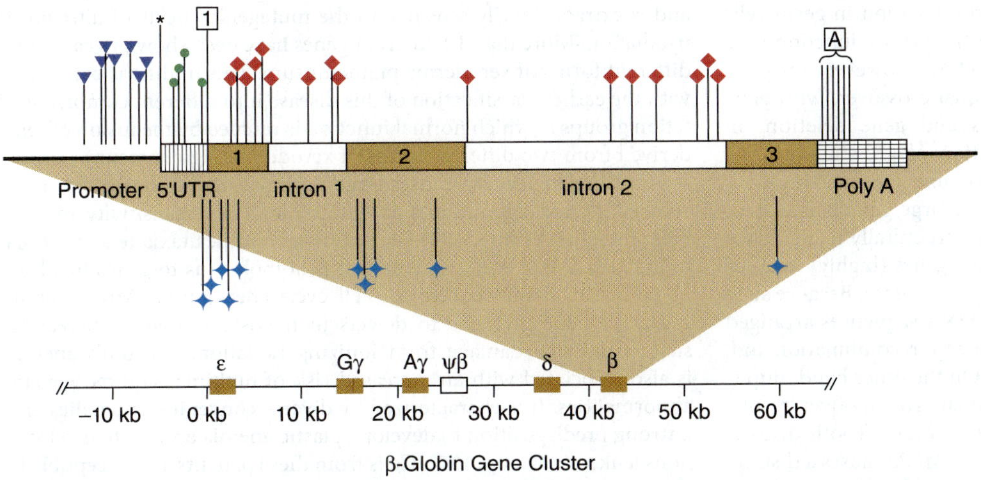

FIGURE 82-9 Point mutations causing β thalassemia as example of allelic heterogeneity. The β-globin gene is located in the globin gene cluster. Point mutations can be located in the promoter, the CAP site, the 5′-untranslated region, the initiation codon, each of the three exons, the introns, or the polyadenylation signal. Many mutations introduce missense or nonsense mutations, whereas others cause defective RNA splicing. Not shown here are deletion mutations of the β-globin gene or larger deletions of the globin locus that can also result in thalassemia. ▼, promoter mutations; *, CAP site; •, 5′UTR; 1, initiation codon; ♦, defective RNA processing; ✦, missense and nonsense mutations; A, Poly A signal.

an enhanced rate of deamination to uracil, which is then replaced with thymine. This C → T transition (or G → A on the opposite strand) accounts for at least one-third of point mutations associated with polymorphisms and mutations. In addition to the fact that certain types of mutations (C → T or G → A) are relatively common, the nature of the genetic code also results in overrepresentation of certain amino acid substitutions.

Polymorphisms are sequence variations that have a frequency of at least 1%. Usually, they do not result in a perceptible phenotype. Often they consist of single base-pair substitutions that do not alter the protein coding sequence because of the degenerate nature of the genetic code (synonymous polymorphism), although it is possible that some might alter mRNA stability, translation, or the amino acid sequence (nonsynonymous polymorphism) (Fig. 82-10). The detection of sequence variants poses a practical problem because it is often unclear whether it creates a mutation with functional consequences or a benign polymorphism. In this situation, the sequence alteration is described as *variant of unknown significance (VUS)*.

MUTATION RATES Mutations represent an important cause of genetic diversity as well as disease. Mutation rates are difficult to determine in humans because many mutations are silent and because testing is often not adequate to detect the phenotypic consequences. Mutation rates vary in different genes but are estimated to occur at a rate of ~10^{-10}/bp per cell division. Germline mutation rates (as opposed to somatic mutations) are relevant in the transmission of genetic disease. Because the population of oocytes is established very early in development, only ~20 cell divisions are required for completed oogenesis, whereas spermatogenesis involves ~30 divisions by the time of puberty and 20 cell divisions each year thereafter. Consequently, the probability of acquiring new point mutations is much greater in the male germline than the female germline, in which rates of aneuploidy are increased (Chap. 83e). Thus, the incidence of new point mutations in spermatogonia increases with paternal age (e.g., achondrodysplasia, Marfan's syndrome, neurofibromatosis). It is estimated that about 1 in 10 sperm carries a new deleterious mutation. The rates for new mutations are calculated most readily for autosomal dominant and X-linked disorders and are ~10^{-5}–10^{-6}/locus per generation. Because most monogenic diseases are relatively rare, new mutations account for a significant fraction of cases. This is important in the context of genetic counseling, because a new mutation can be transmitted to the affected individual but does not necessarily imply that the parents are at risk to transmit the disease to other children. An exception to this is when the new mutation occurs early in germline development, leading to *gonadal mosaicism*.

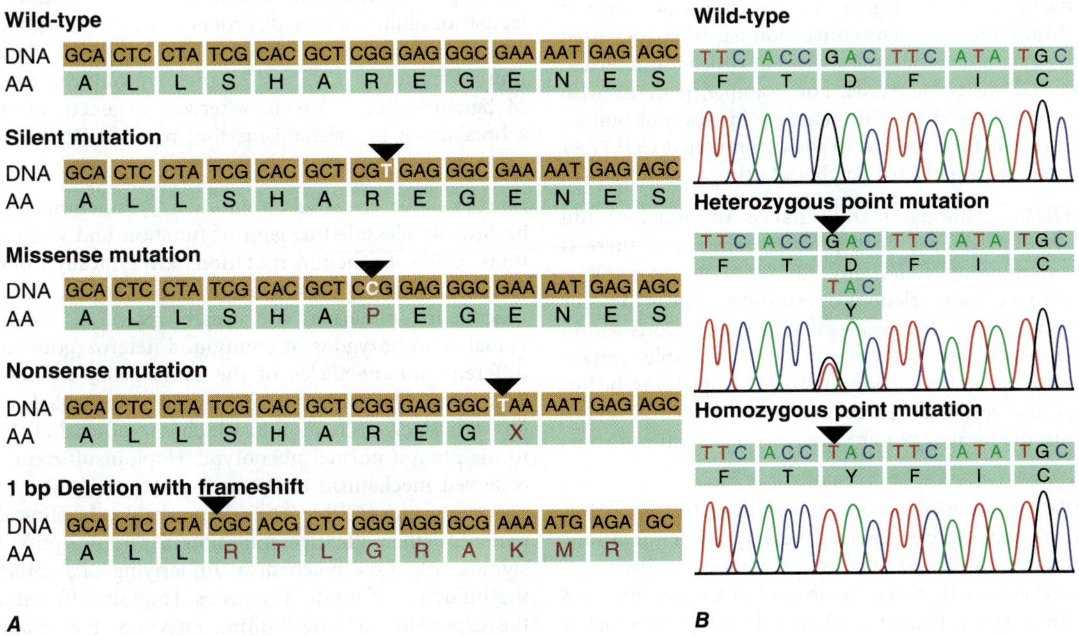

FIGURE 82-10 ***A.*** Examples of mutations. The coding strand is shown with the encoded amino acid sequence. ***B.*** Chromatograms of sequence analyses after amplification of genomic DNA by polymerase chain reaction.

UNEQUAL CROSSING-OVER Normally, DNA recombination in germ cells occurs with remarkable fidelity to maintain the precise junction sites for the exchanged DNA sequences (Fig. 82-6). However, mispairing of homologous sequences leads to unequal crossover, with gene duplication on one of the chromosomes and gene deletion on the other chromosome. A significant fraction of growth hormone (*GH*) gene deletions, for example, involve unequal crossing-over (Chap. 402). The *GH* gene is a member of a large gene cluster that includes a GH variant gene as well as several structurally related chorionic somatomammotropin genes and pseudogenes (highly homologous but functionally inactive relatives of a normal gene). Because such gene clusters contain multiple homologous DNA sequences arranged in tandem, they are particularly prone to undergo recombination and, consequently, gene duplication or deletion. On the other hand, duplication of the *PMP22* gene because of unequal crossing-over results in increased gene dosage and type IA Charcot-Marie-Tooth disease. Unequal crossing-over resulting in deletion of *PMP22* causes a distinct neuropathy called *hereditary liability to pressure palsy* (Chap. 459).

Glucocorticoid-remediable aldosteronism (GRA) is caused by a gene fusion or rearrangement involving the genes that encode aldosterone synthase (*CYP11B2*) and steroid 11β-hydroxylase (*CYP11B1*), normally arranged in tandem on chromosome 8q. These two genes are 95% identical, predisposing to gene duplication and deletion by unequal crossing-over. The rearranged gene product contains the regulatory regions of 11β-hydroxylase fused to the coding sequence of aldosterone synthetase. Consequently, the latter enzyme is expressed in the adrenocorticotropic hormone (ACTH)–dependent zona fasciculata of the adrenal gland, resulting in overproduction of mineralocorticoids and hypertension (Chap. 406).

Gene conversion refers to a nonreciprocal exchange of homologous genetic information. It has been used to explain how an internal portion of a gene is replaced by a homologous segment copied from another allele or locus; these genetic alterations may range from a few nucleotides to a few thousand nucleotides. As a result of gene conversion, it is possible for short DNA segments of two chromosomes to be identical, even though these sequences are distinct in the parents. A practical consequence of this phenomenon is that nucleotide substitutions can occur during gene conversion between related genes, often altering the function of the gene. In disease states, gene conversion often involves intergenic exchange of DNA between a gene and a related pseudogene. For example, the 21-hydroxylase gene (*CYP21A2*) is adjacent to a nonfunctional pseudogene (*CYP21A1P*). Many of the nucleotide substitutions that are found in the *CYP21A2* gene in patients with congenital adrenal hyperplasia correspond to sequences that are present in the *CYP21A1P* pseudogene, suggesting gene conversion as one cause of mutagenesis. In addition, mitotic gene conversion has been suggested as a mechanism to explain revertant mosaicism in which an inherited mutation is "corrected" in certain cells. For example, patients with autosomal recessive generalized atrophic benign epidermolysis bullosa have acquired reverse mutations in one of the two mutated *COL17A1* alleles, leading to clinically unaffected patches of skin.

INSERTIONS AND DELETIONS Although many instances of insertions and deletions occur as a consequence of unequal crossing-over, there is also evidence for internal duplication, inversion, or deletion of DNA sequences. The fact that certain deletions or insertions appear to occur repeatedly as independent events indicates that specific regions within the DNA sequence predispose to these errors. For example, certain regions of the *DMD* gene, which encodes dystrophin, appear to be hot spots for deletions and result in muscular dystrophy (Chap. 462e). Some regions within the human genome are rearrangement hot spots and lead to CNVs.

ERRORS IN DNA REPAIR Because mutations caused by defects in DNA repair accumulate as somatic cells divide, these types of mutations are particularly important in the context of neoplastic disorders (Chap. 102e). Several genetic disorders involving DNA repair enzymes underscore their importance. Patients with xeroderma pigmentosum have defects in DNA damage recognition or in the nucleotide excision and repair pathway (Chap. 105). Exposed skin is dry and pigmented and is extraordinarily sensitive to the mutagenic effects of ultraviolet irradiation. More than 10 different genes have been shown to cause the different forms of xeroderma pigmentosum. This finding is consistent with the earlier classification of this disease into different complementation groups in which normal function is rescued by the fusion of cells derived from two different forms of xeroderma pigmentosum.

Ataxia telangiectasia causes large telangiectatic lesions of the face, cerebellar ataxia, immunologic defects, and hypersensitivity to ionizing radiation (Chap. 450). The discovery of the ataxia telangiectasia mutated (*ATM*) gene reveals that it is homologous to genes involved in DNA repair and control of cell cycle checkpoints. Mutations in the *ATM* gene give rise to defects in meiosis as well as increasing susceptibility to damage from ionizing radiation. Fanconi's anemia is also associated with an increased risk of multiple acquired genetic abnormalities. It is characterized by diverse congenital anomalies and a strong predisposition to develop aplastic anemia and acute myelogenous leukemia (Chap. 132). Cells from these patients are susceptible to chromosomal breaks caused by a defect in genetic recombination. At least 13 different complementation groups have been identified, and the loci and genes associated with Fanconi's anemia have been cloned. HNPCC (Lynch's syndrome) is characterized by autosomal dominant transmission of colon cancer, young age (<50 years) of presentation, predisposition to lesions in the proximal large bowel, and associated malignancies such as uterine cancer and ovarian cancer. HNPCC is predominantly caused by mutations in one of several different mismatch repair (MMR) genes including MutS homologue 2 (*MSH2*), MutL homologue 1 and 6 (*MLH1, MLH6*), *MSH6*, *PMS1*, and *PMS2* (Chap. 110). These proteins are involved in the detection of nucleotide mismatches and in the recognition of slipped-strand trinucleotide repeats. Germline mutations in these genes lead to microsatellite instability and a high mutation rate in colon cancer. Genetic screening tests for this disorder are now being used for families considered to be at risk (Chap. 84). Recognition of HNPCC allows early screening with colonoscopy and the implementation of prevention strategies using nonsteroidal anti-inflammatory drugs.

UNSTABLE DNA SEQUENCES *Trinucleotide repeats* may be unstable and expand beyond a critical number. Mechanistically, the expansion is thought to be caused by unequal recombination and slipped mispairing. A premutation represents a small increase in trinucleotide copy number. In subsequent generations, the expanded repeat may increase further in length and result in an increasingly severe phenotype, a process called *dynamic mutation* (see below for discussion of anticipation). Trinucleotide expansion was first recognized as a cause of the fragile X syndrome, one of the most common causes of intellectual disability. Other disorders arising from a similar mechanism include Huntington's disease (Chap. 448), X-linked spinobulbar muscular atrophy (Chap. 452), and myotonic dystrophy (Chap. 462e). Malignant cells are also characterized by genetic instability, indicating a breakdown in mechanisms that regulate DNA repair and the cell cycle.

Functional Consequences of Mutations Functionally, mutations can be broadly classified as gain-of-function and loss-of-function mutations. Gain-of-function mutations are typically dominant (e.g., they result in phenotypic alterations when a single allele is affected). Inactivating mutations are usually recessive, and an affected individual is homozygous or compound heterozygous (e.g., carrying two different mutant alleles of the same gene) for the disease-causing mutations. Alternatively, mutation in a single allele can result in *haploinsufficiency*, a situation in which one normal allele is not sufficient to maintain a normal phenotype. Haploinsufficiency is a commonly observed mechanism in diseases associated with mutations in transcription factors (Table 82-2). Remarkably, the clinical features among patients with an identical mutation in a transcription factor often vary significantly. One mechanism underlying this variability consists in the influence of modifying genes. Haploinsufficiency can also affect the expression of rate-limiting enzymes. For example, haploinsufficiency in enzymes involved in heme synthesis can cause porphyrias (Chap. 430).

An increase in dosage of a gene product may also result in disease, as illustrated by the duplication of the *DAX1* gene in dosage-sensitive sex reversal (Chap. 410). Mutation in a single allele can also result in loss of function due to a dominant-negative effect. In this case, the mutated allele interferes with the function of the normal gene product by one of several different mechanisms: (1) a mutant protein may interfere with the function of a multimeric protein complex, as illustrated by mutations in type 1 collagen (*COL1A1*, *COL1A2*) genes in osteogenesis imperfecta (Chap. 427); (2) a mutant protein may occupy binding sites on proteins or promoter response elements, as illustrated by thyroid hormone resistance, a disorder in which inactivated thyroid hormone receptor β binds to target genes and functions as an antagonist of normal receptors (Chap. 405); or (3) a mutant protein can be cytotoxic as in α_1 antitrypsin deficiency (Chap. 314) or autosomal dominant neurohypophyseal diabetes insipidus (Chap. 404), in which the abnormally folded proteins are trapped within the endoplasmic reticulum and ultimately cause cellular damage.

Genotype and Phnotype • ***ALLELES, GENOTYPES, AND HAPLOTYPES*** An observed trait is referred to as a *phenotype*; the genetic information defining the phenotype is called the *genotype*. Alternative forms of a gene or a genetic marker are referred to as *alleles*. Alleles may be polymorphic variants of nucleic acids that have no apparent effect on gene expression or function. In other instances, these variants may have subtle effects on gene expression, thereby conferring adaptive advantages associated with genetic diversity. On the other hand, allelic variants may reflect mutations that clearly alter the function of a gene product. The common Glu6Val (E6V) sickle cell mutation in the *β-globin* gene and the ΔF508 deletion of phenylalanine (F) in the *CFTR* gene are examples of allelic variants of these genes that result in disease. Because each individual has two copies of each chromosome (one inherited from the mother and one inherited from the father), he or she can have only two alleles at a given locus. However, there can be many different alleles in the population. The normal or common allele is usually referred to as *wild type*. When alleles at a given locus are identical, the individual is *homozygous*. Inheriting identical copies of a mutant allele occurs in many autosomal recessive disorders, particularly in circumstances of consanguinity or isolated populations. If the alleles are different on the maternal and the paternal copy of the gene, the individual is *heterozygous* at this locus (Fig. 82-10). If two different mutant alleles are inherited at a given locus, the individual is said to be a *compound heterozygote*. *Hemizygous* is used to describe males with a mutation in an X chromosomal gene or a female with a loss of one X chromosomal locus.

Genotypes describe the specific alleles at a particular locus. For example, there are three common alleles (E2, E3, E4) of the apolipoprotein E (*APOE*) gene. The genotype of an individual can therefore be described as *APOE3/4* or *APOE4/4* or any other variant. These designations indicate which alleles are present on the two chromosomes in the *APOE* gene at locus 19q13.2. In other cases, the genotype might be assigned arbitrary numbers (e.g., 1/2) or letters (e.g., B/b) to distinguish different alleles.

A *haplotype* refers to a group of alleles that are closely linked together at a genomic locus (Fig. 82-4). Haplotypes are useful for tracking the transmission of genomic segments within families and for detecting evidence of genetic recombination, if the crossover event occurs between the alleles (Fig. 82-6). As an example, various alleles at the histocompatibility locus antigen (HLA) on chromosome 6p are used to establish haplotypes associated with certain disease states. For example, 21-hydroxylase deficiency, complement deficiency, and hemochromatosis are each associated with specific HLA haplotypes. It is now recognized that these genes lie in close proximity to the HLA locus, which explains why HLA associations were identified even before the disease genes were cloned and localized. In other cases, specific HLA associations with diseases such as ankylosing spondylitis (HLA-B27) or type 1 diabetes mellitus (HLA-DR4) reflect the role of specific HLA allelic variants in susceptibility to these autoimmune diseases. The characterization of common SNP haplotypes in numerous populations from different parts of the world through the HapMap Project is providing a novel tool for association studies designed to detect genes involved in the pathogenesis of complex disorders (Table 82-1). The presence or absence of certain haplotypes may also become relevant for the customized choice of medical therapies (pharmacogenomics) or for preventive strategies.

Genotype-phenotype correlation describes the association of a specific mutation and the resulting phenotype. The phenotype may differ depending on the location or type of the mutation in some genes. For example, in von Hippel–Lindau disease, an autosomal dominant multisystem disease that can include renal cell carcinoma, hemangioblastomas, and pheochromocytomas, among others, the phenotype varies greatly and the identification of the specific mutation can be clinically useful in order to predict the phenotypic spectrum.

ALLELIC HETEROGENEITY *Allelic heterogeneity* refers to the fact that different mutations in the same genetic locus can cause an identical or similar phenotype. For example, many different mutations of the β-globin locus can cause β thalassemia (Table 82-3) (Fig. 82-9). In essence, allelic heterogeneity reflects the fact that many different mutations are capable of altering protein structure and function. For this reason, maps of inactivating mutations in genes usually show a near-random distribution. Exceptions include (1) a founder effect, in which a particular mutation that does not affect reproductive capacity can be traced to a single individual; (2) "hot spots" for mutations, in which the nature of the DNA sequence predisposes to a recurring mutation; and (3) localization of mutations to certain domains that are particularly critical for protein function. Allelic heterogeneity creates a practical problem for genetic testing because one must often examine the entire genetic locus for mutations, because these can differ in each patient. For example, there are currently 1963 reported mutations in the *CFTR* gene (Fig. 82-3). Mutational analysis may initially focus on a panel of mutations that are particularly frequent (often taking the ethnic background of the patient into account), but a negative result does not exclude the presence of a mutation elsewhere in the gene. One should also be aware that mutational analyses generally focus on the coding region of a gene without considering regulatory and intronic regions. Because disease-causing mutations may be located outside the coding regions, negative results need to be interpreted with caution. The advent of more comprehensive sequencing technologies greatly facilitates concomitant mutational analyses of several genes after targeted enrichment, or even mutational analysis of the whole exome or genome. However, comprehensive sequencing can result in significant diagnostic challenges because the detection of a sequence alteration alone is not always sufficient to establish that it has a causal role.

PHENOTYPIC HETEROGENEITY *Phenotypic heterogeneity* occurs when more than one phenotype is caused by allelic mutations (e.g., different mutations in the same gene) (Table 82-3). For example, laminopathies are monogenic multisystem disorders that result from mutations in the *LMNA* gene, which encodes the nuclear lamins A and C. Twelve autosomal dominant and four autosomal recessive disorders are caused by mutations in the *LMNA* gene. They include several forms of lipodystrophies, Emery-Dreifuss muscular dystrophy, progeria syndromes, a form of neuronal Charcot-Marie-Tooth disease (type 2B1), and a group of overlapping syndromes. Remarkably, hierarchical cluster analysis has revealed that the phenotypes vary depending on the position of the mutation (*genotype-phenotype correlation*). Similarly, identical mutations in the *FGFR2* gene can result in very distinct phenotypes: Crouzon's syndrome (craniofacial synostosis) or Pfeiffer's syndrome (acrocephalopolysyndactyly).

LOCUS OR NONALLELIC HETEROGENEITY AND PHENOCOPIES *Nonallelic or locus heterogeneity* refers to the situation in which a similar disease phenotype results from mutations at different genetic loci (Table 82-3). This often occurs when more than one gene product produces different subunits of an interacting complex or when different genes are involved in the same genetic cascade or physiologic pathway. For example, osteogenesis imperfecta can arise from mutations in two different procollagen genes (*COL1A1* or *COL1A2*) that are located on different chromosomes, and at least eight other genes (Chap. 427). The effects of inactivating mutations in these two genes are similar because the protein products comprise different subunits

TABLE 82-3 SELECTED EXAMPLES OF LOCUS HETEROGENEITY AND PHENOTYPIC HETEROGENEITY

Phenotypic Heterogeneity

Gene, Protein	Phenotype	Inheritance	OMIM
LMNA, Lamin A/C	Emery-Dreifuss muscular dystrophy (AD)	AD	181350
	Familial partial lipodystrophy Dunnigan	AD	151660
	Hutchinson-Gilford progeria	AD	176670
	Atypical Werner's syndrome	AD	150330
	Dilated cardiomyopathy	AD	115200
	Early-onset atrial fibrillation	AD	607554
	Emery-Dreifuss muscular dystrophy (AR)	AR	604929
	Limb-girdle muscular dystrophy type 1B	AR	159001
	Charcot-Marie-Tooth type 2B1	AR	605588
KRAS	Noonan's syndrome	AD	163950
	Cardio-facio-cutaneous syndrome	AD	115150

Locus Heterogeneity

Phenotype	Gene	Chromosomal Location	Protein
Familial hypertrophic cardiomyopathy	*MYH7*	14q12	Myosin heavy chain beta
Genes encoding sarcomeric proteins	*TNNT2*	1q2	Troponin-T2
	TPM1	15q22.1	Tropomyosin alpha
	MYBPC3	11p11q	Myosin-binding protein C
	TNNI3	19q13.4	Troponin 1
	MYL2	12q23-24.3	Myosin light chain 2
	MYL3	3p	Myosin light chain 3
	TTN	2q24.3	Cardiac titin
	ACTC	15q11	Cardiac alpha actin
	MYH6	14q1	Myosin heavy chain alpha
	MYLK2	20q13.3	Myosin light-peptide kinase
	CAV3	3p25	Caveolin 3
Genes encoding nonsarcomeric proteins	*MTT1*	Mitochondrial	tRNA isoleucine
	MTTG	Mitochondrial	tRNA glycine
	PRKAG2	7q35-q36	AMP-activated protein kinase γ2 subunit
	DMPK	19q13.2-13.3	Myotonin protein kinase (myotonic dystrophy)
	FRDA	9q13	Frataxin (Friedreich's ataxia)
Polycystic kidney disease	*PKD1*	16p13.3-13.12	Polycystin 1 (AD)
	PKD2	4q21.-23	Polycystin 2 (AD)
	PKHD1	6p21.1-p12	Fibrocystin (AR)
Noonan's syndrome	*PTPN11*	12q24.1	Protein-tyrosine phosphatase 2c
	KRAS	12p12.1	KRAS

of the helical collagen fiber. Similarly, muscular dystrophy syndromes can be caused by mutations in various genes, consistent with the fact that it can be transmitted in an X-linked (Duchenne or Becker), autosomal dominant (limb-girdle muscular dystrophy type 1), or autosomal recessive (limb-girdle muscular dystrophy type 2) manner (Chap. 462e). Mutations in the X-linked *DMD* gene, which encodes dystrophin, are the most common cause of muscular dystrophy. This feature reflects the large size of the gene as well as the fact that the phenotype is expressed in hemizygous males because they have only a single copy of the X chromosome. Dystrophin is associated with a large protein complex linked to the membrane-associated cytoskeleton in muscle. Mutations in several different components of this protein complex can also cause muscular dystrophy syndromes. Although the phenotypic features of some of these disorders are distinct, the phenotypic spectrum caused by mutations in different genes overlaps, thereby leading to nonallelic heterogeneity. It should be noted that mutations in dystrophin also cause allelic heterogeneity. For example, mutations in the *DMD* gene can cause either Duchenne's or the less severe Becker's muscular dystrophy, depending on the severity of the protein defect.

Recognition of nonallelic heterogeneity is important for several reasons: (1) the ability to identify disease loci in linkage studies is reduced by including patients with similar phenotypes but different genetic disorders; (2) genetic testing is more complex because several different genes need to be considered along with the possibility of different mutations in each of the candidate genes; and (3) novel information is gained about how genes or proteins interact, providing unique insights into molecular physiology.

Phenocopies refer to circumstances in which nongenetic conditions mimic a genetic disorder. For example, features of toxin- or drug-induced neurologic syndromes can resemble those seen in Huntington's disease, and vascular causes of dementia share phenotypic features with familial forms of Alzheimer's dementia (Chap. 448). As in nonallelic heterogeneity, the presence of phenocopies has the potential to confound linkage studies and genetic testing. Patient history and subtle differences in phenotype can often provide clues that distinguish these disorders from related genetic conditions.

VARIABLE EXPRESSIVITY AND INCOMPLETE PENETRANCE The same genetic mutation may be associated with a phenotypic spectrum in different affected individuals, thereby illustrating the phenomenon of *variable expressivity*. This may include different manifestations of a disorder variably involving different organs (e.g., multiple endocrine neoplasia [MEN]), the severity of the disorder (e.g., cystic fibrosis), or the age of disease onset (e.g., Alzheimer's dementia). MEN 1 illustrates several of these features. In this autosomal dominant tumor syndrome, affected individuals carry an inactivating germline mutation that is inherited in an autosomal dominant fashion. After somatic inactivation of the alternate allele, they can develop tumors of the parathyroid gland, endocrine pancreas, and the pituitary gland (Chap. 408). However, the pattern of tumors in the different glands, the age at which tumors develop, and the types of hormones produced vary among affected individuals, even within a given family. In this example, the phenotypic variability arises, in part, because of the requirement for a second somatic mutation in the normal copy of the *MEN1* gene, as well as the large array of different cell types that are susceptible to the effects of *MEN1* gene mutations. In part, variable expression reflects the influence of modifier genes, or genetic background, on the effects of a particular mutation. Even in identical twins, in whom the genetic constitution is essentially the same, one can occasionally see variable expression of a genetic disease.

Interactions with the environment can also influence the course of a disease. For example, the manifestations and severity of hemochromatosis can be influenced by iron intake (Chap. 428), and the course of phenylketonuria is affected by exposure to phenylalanine in the diet (Chap. 434e). Other metabolic disorders, such as hyperlipidemias and porphyria, also fall into this category. Many mechanisms, including genetic effects and environmental influences, can therefore lead to variable expressivity. In genetic counseling, it is particularly important to recognize this variability, because one cannot always predict the course of disease, even when the mutation is known.

Penetrance refers to the proportion of individuals with a mutant genotype that express the phenotype. If all carriers of a mutant express the phenotype, penetrance is complete, whereas it is said to be *incomplete* or *reduced* if some individuals do not exhibit features of the phenotype. Dominant conditions with incomplete penetrance are characterized by skipping of generations with unaffected carriers transmitting the mutant gene. For example, hypertrophic obstructive cardiomyopathy (HCM) caused by mutations in the *myosin-binding protein C* gene is a dominant disorder with clinical features in only a subset of patients who carry the mutation (Chap. 283). Patients who have the mutation but no evidence of the disease can still transmit the disorder to subsequent generations. In many conditions with postnatal onset, the proportion of gene carriers who are affected varies with age. Thus, when describing penetrance, one has to specify age. For example, for disorders such as Huntington's disease or familial amyotrophic lateral sclerosis, which present later in life, the rate of penetrance is influenced by the age at which the clinical assessment is performed. *Imprinting* can also modify the penetrance of a disease. For example, in patients with Albright's hereditary osteodystrophy, mutations in the Gsα subunit (*GNAS1* gene) are expressed clinically only in individuals who inherit the mutation from their mother (Chap. 424).

SEX-INFLUENCED PHENOTYPES Certain mutations affect males and females quite differently. In some instances, this is because the gene resides on the X or Y sex chromosomes (X-linked disorders and Y-linked disorders). As a result, the phenotype of mutated X-linked genes will be expressed fully in males but variably in heterozygous females, depending on the degree of X-inactivation and the function of the gene. For example, most heterozygous female carriers of factor VIII deficiency (hemophilia A) are asymptomatic because sufficient factor VIII is produced to prevent a defect in coagulation (Chap. 141). On the other hand, some females heterozygous for the X-linked lipid storage defect caused by α-galactosidase A deficiency (Fabry's disease) experience mild manifestations of painful neuropathy, as well as other features of the disease (Chap. 432e). Because only males have a Y chromosome, mutations in genes such as *SRY*, which causes male-to-female sex reversal, or *DAZ* (deleted in azoospermia), which causes abnormalities of spermatogenesis, are unique to males (Chap. 410).

Other diseases are expressed in a sex-limited manner because of the differential function of the gene product in males and females. Activating mutations in the luteinizing hormone receptor cause dominant male-limited precocious puberty in boys (Chap. 411). The phenotype is unique to males because activation of the receptor induces testosterone production in the testis, whereas it is functionally silent in the immature ovary. Biallelic inactivating mutations of the follicle-stimulating hormone (FSH) receptor cause primary ovarian failure in females because the follicles do not develop in the absence of FSH action. In contrast, affected males have a more subtle phenotype, because testosterone production is preserved (allowing sexual maturation) and spermatogenesis is only partially impaired (Chap. 411). In congenital adrenal hyperplasia, most commonly caused by 21-hydroxylase deficiency, cortisol production is impaired and ACTH stimulation of the adrenal gland leads to increased production of androgenic precursors (Chap. 406). In females, the increased androgen level causes ambiguous genitalia, which can be recognized at the time of birth. In males, the diagnosis may be made on the basis of adrenal insufficiency at birth, because the increased adrenal androgen level does not alter sexual differentiation, or later in childhood, because of the development of precocious puberty. Hemochromatosis is more common in males than in females, presumably because of differences in dietary iron intake and losses associated with menstruation and pregnancy in females (Chap. 428).

Chromosomal Disorders Chromosomal or cytogenetic disorders are caused by numerical or structural aberrations in chromosomes. For a detailed discussion of disorders of chromosome number and structure, see Chap. 83e. Deviations in chromosome number are common causes of abortions, developmental disorders, and malformations. *Contiguous gene syndromes* (e.g., large deletions affecting several genes) have been useful for identifying the location of new disease-causing genes. Because of the variable size of gene deletions in different patients, a systematic comparison of phenotypes and locations of deletion breakpoints allows positions of particular genes to be mapped within the critical genomic region.

Monogenic Mendelian Disorders Monogenic human diseases are frequently referred to as *Mendelian disorders* because they obey the principles of genetic transmission originally set forth in Gregor Mendel's classic work. The continuously updated OMIM catalogue lists several thousand of these disorders and provides information about the clinical phenotype, molecular basis, allelic variants, and pertinent animal models (Table 82-1). The mode of inheritance for a given phenotypic trait or disease is determined by pedigree analysis. All affected and unaffected individuals in the family are recorded in a pedigree using standard symbols (Fig. 82-11). The principles of allelic segregation, and the transmission of alleles from parents to children, are illustrated in Fig. 82-12. One dominant (A) allele and one recessive (a) allele can display three Mendelian modes of inheritance: autosomal dominant, autosomal recessive, and X-linked. About 65% of human monogenic disorders are autosomal dominant, 25% are autosomal recessive, and 5% are X-linked. Genetic testing is now available for many of these disorders and plays an increasingly important role in clinical medicine (Chap. 84).

AUTOSOMAL DOMINANT DISORDERS These disorders assume particular relevance because mutations in a single allele are sufficient to cause the disease. In contrast to recessive disorders, in which disease pathogenesis is relatively straightforward because there is loss of gene function, dominant disorders can be caused by various disease mechanisms, many of which are unique to the function of the genetic pathway involved.

In autosomal dominant disorders, individuals are affected in successive generations; the disease does not occur in the offspring of unaffected individuals. Males and females are affected with equal frequency because the defective gene resides on one of the 22 autosomes (Fig. 82-13*A*). Autosomal dominant mutations alter one of the two alleles at a given locus. Because the alleles segregate randomly at meiosis, the probability that an offspring will be affected is 50%. Unless there is a new germline mutation, an affected individual has an affected parent. Children with a normal genotype do not transmit the disorder. Due to differences in penetrance or expressivity (see above), the

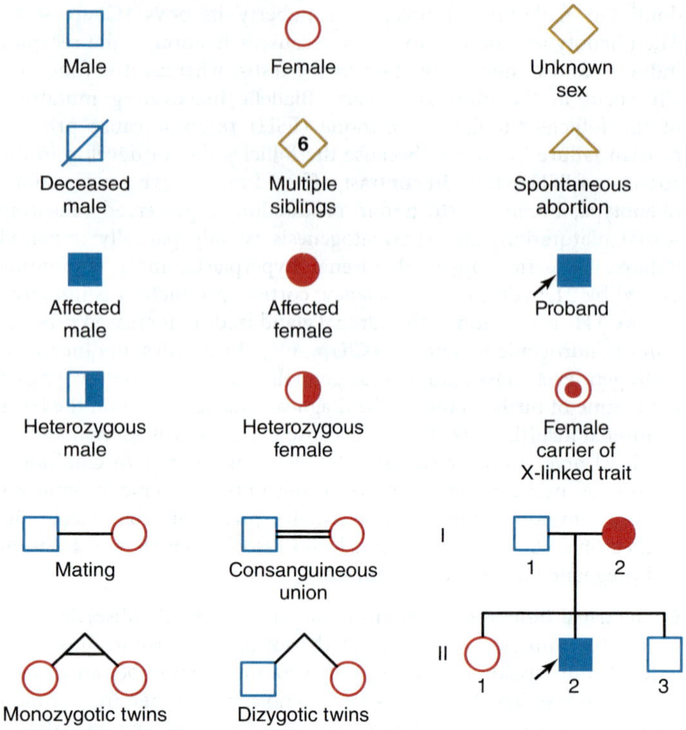

FIGURE 82-11 Standard pedigree symbols.

clinical manifestations of autosomal dominant disorders may be variable. Because of these variations, it is sometimes challenging to determine the pattern of inheritance.

It should be recognized, however, that some individuals acquire a mutated gene from an unaffected parent. De novo germline mutations occur more frequently during later cell divisions in gametogenesis, which explains why siblings are rarely affected. As noted before, new germline mutations occur more frequently in fathers of advanced age. For example, the average age of fathers with new germline mutations that cause Marfan's syndrome is ~37 years, whereas fathers who transmit the disease by inheritance have an average age of ~30 years.

AUTOSOMAL RECESSIVE DISORDERS In recessive disorders, the mutated alleles result in a complete or partial loss of function. They frequently involve enzymes in metabolic pathways, receptors, or proteins in signaling cascades. In an autosomal recessive disease, the affected individual, who can be of either sex, is a homozygote or compound heterozygote for a single-gene defect. With a few important exceptions, autosomal recessive diseases are rare and often occur in the context of parental consanguinity. The relatively high frequency of certain recessive disorders such as sickle cell anemia, cystic fibrosis, and thalassemia, is partially explained by a selective biologic advantage for the heterozygous state (see below). Although heterozygous carriers of a defective allele are usually clinically normal, they may display subtle differences in phenotype that only become apparent with more precise testing or in the context of certain environmental influences. In sickle

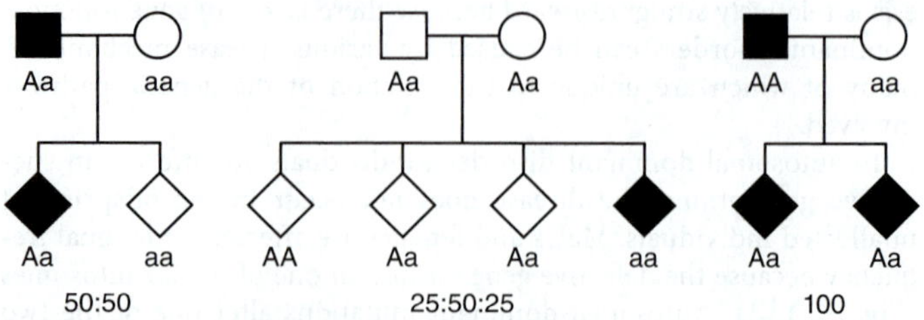

FIGURE 82-12 Segregation of alleles. Segregation of genotypes in the offspring of parents with one dominant (A) and one recessive (a) allele. The distribution of the parental alleles to their offspring depends on the combination present in the parents. Filled symbols = affected individuals.

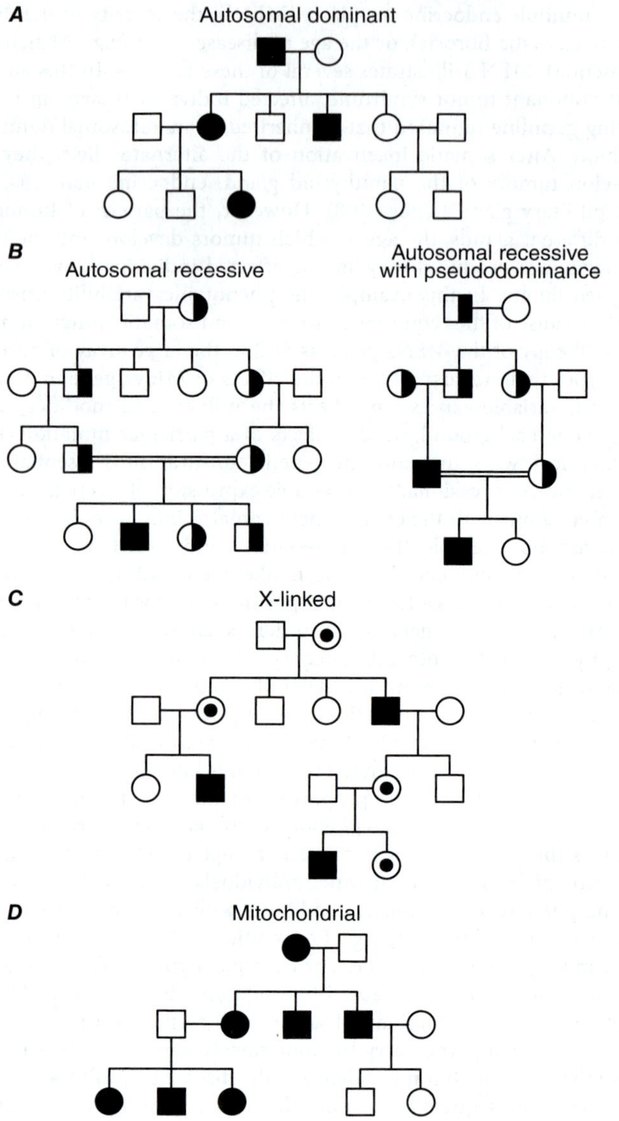

FIGURE 82-13 (*A*) Dominant, (*B*) recessive, (*C*) X-linked, and (*D*) mitochondrial (matrilinear) inheritance.

cell anemia, for example, heterozygotes are normally asymptomatic. However, in situations of dehydration or diminished oxygen pressure, sickle cell crises can also occur in heterozygotes (Chap. 127).

In most instances, an affected individual is the offspring of heterozygous parents. In this situation, there is a 25% chance that the offspring will have a normal genotype, a 50% probability of a heterozygous state, and a 25% risk of homozygosity for the recessive alleles (Figs. 82-10, 82-13B). In the case of one unaffected heterozygous and one affected homozygous parent, the probability of disease increases to 50% for each child. In this instance, the pedigree analysis mimics an autosomal dominant mode of inheritance (*pseudodominance*). In contrast to autosomal dominant disorders, new mutations in recessive alleles are rarely manifest because they usually result in an asymptomatic carrier state.

X-LINKED DISORDERS Males have only one X chromosome; consequently, a daughter always inherits her father's X chromosome in addition to one of her mother's two X chromosomes. A son inherits the Y chromosome from his father and one maternal X chromosome. Thus, the characteristic features of X-linked inheritance are (1) the absence of father-to-son transmission, and (2) the fact that all daughters of an affected male are obligate carriers of the mutant allele (Fig. 82-13C). The risk of developing disease due to a mutant X-chromosomal gene differs in the two sexes. Because males have only one X chromosome, they are hemizygous for the mutant allele; thus, they are more likely to develop the mutant phenotype, regardless of whether the mutation is dominant or recessive. A female may be either heterozygous or homozygous for the mutant allele, which may be dominant or recessive. The terms *X-linked dominant* or *X-linked recessive* are therefore only applicable to expression of the mutant phenotype in women. In addition, the expression of X-chromosomal genes is influenced by X chromosome inactivation.

Y-LINKED DISORDERS The Y chromosome has a relatively small number of genes. One such gene, the sex-region determining Y factor (*SRY*), which encodes the testis-determining factor (*TDF*), is crucial for normal male development. Normally there is infrequent exchange of sequences on the Y chromosome with the X chromosome. The *SRY* region is adjacent to the pseudoautosomal region, a chromosomal segment on the X and Y chromosomes with a high degree of homology. A crossing-over event occasionally involves the *SRY* region with the distal tip of the X chromosome during meiosis in the male. Translocations can result in XY females with the Y chromosome lacking the *SRY* gene or XX males harboring the *SRY* gene on one of the X chromosomes (Chap. 410). Point mutations in the *SRY* gene may also result in individuals with an XY genotype and an incomplete female phenotype. Most of these mutations occur de novo. Men with oligospermia/azoospermia frequently have microdeletions on the long arm of the Y chromosome that involve one or more of the azoospermia factor (*AZF*) genes.

Exceptions to Simple Mendelian Inheritance Patterns • ***MITOCHONDRIAL DISORDERS*** Mendelian inheritance refers to the transmission of genes encoded by DNA contained in the nuclear chromosomes. In addition, each mitochondrion contains several copies of a small circular chromosome (Chap. 85e). The mitochondrial DNA (mtDNA) is ~16.5 kb and encodes transfer and ribosomal RNAs and 13 core proteins that are components of the respiratory chain involved in oxidative phosphorylation and ATP generation. The mitochondrial genome does not recombine and is inherited through the maternal line because sperm does not contribute significant cytoplasmic components to the zygote. A noncoding region of the mitochondrial chromosome, referred to as D-loop, is highly polymorphic. This property, together with the absence of mtDNA recombination, makes it a valuable tool for studies tracing human migration and evolution, and it is also used for specific forensic applications.

Inherited mitochondrial disorders are transmitted in a matrilineal fashion; all children from an affected mother will inherit the disease, but it will not be transmitted from an affected father to his children (Fig. 82-13*D*). Alterations in the mtDNA that involves enzymes required for oxidative phosphorylation lead to reduction of ATP supply, generation of free radicals, and induction of apoptosis. Several syndromic disorders arising from mutations in the mitochondrial genome are known in humans and they affect both protein-coding and tRNA genes (Chap. 85e). The broad clinical spectrum often involves (cardio) myopathies and encephalopathies because of the high dependence of these tissues on oxidative phosphorylation. The age of onset and the clinical course are highly variable because of the unusual mechanisms of mtDNA transmission, which replicates independently from nuclear DNA. During cell replication, the proportion of wild-type and mutant mitochondria can drift among different cells and tissues. The resulting heterogeneity in the proportion of mitochondria with and without a mutation is referred to as *heteroplasmia* and underlies the phenotypic variability that is characteristic of mitochondrial diseases.

Acquired somatic mutations in mitochondria are thought to be involved in several age-dependent degenerative disorders affecting predominantly muscle and the peripheral and central nervous system (e.g., Alzheimer's and Parkinson's diseases). Establishing that an mtDNA alteration is causal for a clinical phenotype is challenging because of the high degree of polymorphism in mtDNA and the phenotypic variability characteristic of these disorders. Certain pharmacologic treatments may have an impact on mitochondria and/or their function. For example, treatment with the antiretroviral compound azidothymidine (AZT) causes an acquired mitochondrial myopathy through depletion of muscular mtDNA.

MOSAICISM Mosaicism refers to the presence of two or more genetically distinct cell lines in the tissues of an individual. It results from a mutation that occurs during embryonic, fetal, or extrauterine development. The developmental stage at which the mutation arises will determine whether germ cells and/or somatic cells are involved. Chromosomal mosaicism results from nondisjunction at an early embryonic mitotic division, leading to the persistence of more than one cell line, as exemplified by some patients with Turner's syndrome (Chap. 410). Somatic mosaicism is characterized by a patchy distribution of genetically altered somatic cells. The McCune-Albright syndrome, for example, is caused by activating mutations in the stimulatory G protein α (Gsα) that occur early in development (Chap. 424). The clinical phenotype varies depending on the tissue distribution of the mutation; manifestations include ovarian cysts that secrete sex steroids and cause precocious puberty, polyostotic fibrous dysplasia, café-au-lait skin pigmentation, growth hormone–secreting pituitary adenomas, and hypersecreting autonomous thyroid nodules (Chap. 412).

X-INACTIVATION, IMPRINTING, AND UNIPARENTAL DISOMY According to traditional Mendelian principles, the parental origin of a mutant gene is irrelevant for the expression of the phenotype. There are, however, important exceptions to this rule. *X-inactivation* prevents the expression of most genes on one of the two X chromosomes in every cell of a female. Gene inactivation through genomic imprinting occurs on selected chromosomal regions of autosomes and leads to inheritable preferential expression of one of the parental alleles. It is of pathophysiologic importance in disorders where the transmission of disease is dependent on the sex of the transmitting parent and, thus, plays an important role in the expression of certain genetic disorders. Two classic examples are the Prader-Willi syndrome and Angelman's syndrome (Chap. 83e). Prader-Willi syndrome is characterized by diminished fetal activity, obesity, hypotonia, mental retardation, short stature, and hypogonadotropic hypogonadism. Deletions of the paternal copy of the Prader-Willi locus located on the short arm of chromosome 15 result in a contiguous gene syndrome involving missing paternal copies of the *necdin* and *SNRPN* genes, among others. In contrast, patients with Angelman's syndrome, characterized by mental retardation, seizures, ataxia, and hypotonia, have deletions involving the maternal copy of this region on chromosome 15. These two syndromes may also result from *uniparental disomy*. In this case, the syndromes are not caused by deletions on chromosome 15 but by the inheritance of either two maternal chromosomes (Prader-Willi syndrome) or two paternal chromosomes (Angelman's syndrome). Lastly, the two distinct phenotypes can also be caused by an imprinting defect that impairs the resetting of the imprint during zygote development (defect in the father leads to Prader-Willi syndrome; defect in the mother leads to Angelman's syndrome).

Imprinting and the related phenomenon of allelic exclusion may be more common than currently documented, because it is difficult to examine levels of mRNA expression from the maternal and paternal alleles in specific tissues or in individual cells. Genomic imprinting, or uniparental disomy, is involved in the pathogenesis of several other disorders and malignancies (Chap. 83e). For example, hydatidiform moles contain a normal number of diploid chromosomes, but they are all of paternal origin. The opposite situation occurs in ovarian teratomata, with 46 chromosomes of maternal origin. Expression of the imprinted gene for insulin-like growth factor II (IGF-II) is involved in the pathogenesis of the cancer-predisposing Beckwith-Wiedemann syndrome (BWS) (Chap. 101e). These children show somatic overgrowth with organomegalies and hemihypertrophy, and they have an increased risk of embryonal malignancies such as Wilms' tumor. Normally, only the paternally derived copy of the *IGF-II* gene is active and the maternal copy is inactive. Imprinting of the *IGF-II* gene is regulated by *H19*, which encodes an RNA transcript that is not translated into protein. Disruption or lack of *H19* methylation leads to a relaxation of *IGF-II* imprinting and expression of both alleles. Alterations of the epigenome through gain and loss of DNA methylation, as well as altered histone modifications, play an important role in the pathogenesis of malignancies.

SOMATIC MUTATIONS Cancer can be considered a genetic disease at the cellular level (Chap. 101e). Cancers are monoclonal in origin, indicating that they have arisen from a single precursor cell with one or several mutations in genes controlling growth (proliferation or apoptosis) and/or differentiation. These acquired somatic mutations are restricted to the tumor and its metastases and are not found in the surrounding normal tissue. The molecular alterations include dominant gain-of-function mutations in oncogenes, recessive loss-of-function mutations in tumor-suppressor genes and DNA repair genes, gene amplification, and chromosome rearrangements. Rarely, a single mutation in certain genes may be sufficient to transform a normal cell into a malignant cell. In most cancers, however, the development of a malignant phenotype requires several genetic alterations for the gradual progression from a normal cell to a cancerous cell, a phenomenon termed *multistep carcinogenesis* (Chaps. 101e and 102e). Genome-wide analyses of cancers using deep sequencing often reveal somatic rearrangements resulting in fusion genes and mutations in multiple genes. Comprehensive sequence analyses provide further insight into genetic heterogeneity within malignancies; these include intratumoral heterogeneity among the cells of the primary tumor, intermetastatic and intrametastatic heterogeneity, and interpatient differences. These analyses further support the notion of cancer as an ongoing process of clonal evolution, in which successive rounds of clonal selection within the primary tumor and metastatic lesions result in diverse genetic and epigenetic alterations that require targeted (personalized) therapies. The heterogeneity of mutations within a tumor can also lead to resistance to target therapies because cells with mutations that are resistant to the therapy, even if they are a minor part of the tumor population, will be selected as the more sensitive cells are killed. Most human tumors express telomerase, an enzyme formed of a protein and an RNA component, which adds telomere repeats at the ends of chromosomes during replication. This mechanism impedes shortening of the telomeres, which is associated with senescence in normal cells and is associated with enhanced replicative capacity in cancer cells. Telomerase inhibitors provide a novel strategy for treating advanced human cancers.

In many cancer syndromes, there is an inherited *predisposition* to tumor formation. In these instances, a germline mutation is inherited in an autosomal dominant fashion inactivating one allele of an autosomal tumor-suppressor gene. If the second allele is inactivated by a somatic mutation or by epigenetic silencing in a given cell, this will lead to neoplastic growth (Knudson two-hit model). Thus, the defective allele in the germline is transmitted in a dominant mode, although tumorigenesis results from a biallelic loss of the tumor-suppressor gene in an affected tissue. The classic example to illustrate this phenomenon is retinoblastoma, which can occur as a sporadic or hereditary tumor. In sporadic retinoblastoma, both copies of the retinoblastoma (*RB*) gene are inactivated through two somatic events. In hereditary retinoblastoma, one mutated or deleted *RB* allele is inherited in an autosomal dominant manner and the second allele is inactivated by a subsequent somatic mutation. This two-hit model applies to other inherited cancer syndromes such as MEN 1 (Chap. 408) and neurofibromatosis type 2 (Chap. 118).

NUCLEOTIDE REPEAT EXPANSION DISORDERS Several diseases are associated with an increase in the number of nucleotide repeats above a certain threshold (Table 82-4). The repeats are sometimes located within the coding region of the genes, as in Huntington's disease or the X-linked form of spinal and bulbar muscular atrophy (SBMA; Kennedy's syndrome). In other instances, the repeats probably alter gene regulatory sequences. If an expansion is present, the DNA fragment is unstable and tends to expand further during cell division. The length of the nucleotide repeat often correlates with the severity of the disease. When repeat length increases from one generation to the next, disease manifestations may worsen or be observed at an earlier age; this phenomenon is referred to as *anticipation*. In Huntington's disease, for example, there is a correlation between age of onset and length of the triplet codon expansion (Chap. 444e). Anticipation has also been documented in other diseases caused by dynamic mutations in trinucleotide repeats (Table 82-4). The repeat number may also vary in a tissue-specific manner. In myotonic dystrophy, the CTG repeat may be tenfold greater in muscle tissue than in lymphocytes (Chap. 462e).

Complex Genetic Disorders The expression of many common diseases such as cardiovascular disease, hypertension, diabetes, asthma, psychiatric disorders, and certain cancers is determined by a combination of genetic background, environmental factors, and lifestyle. A trait is called *polygenic* if multiple genes contribute to the phenotype or *multifactorial* if multiple genes are assumed to interact with environmental factors. Genetic models for these complex traits need to account for genetic heterogeneity and interactions with other genes and the environment. Complex genetic traits may be influenced by modifier genes that are not linked to the main gene involved in the pathogenesis of the trait. This type of gene-gene interaction, or *epistasis*, plays an important role in polygenic traits that require the simultaneous presence of variations in multiple genes to result in a pathologic phenotype.

Type 2 diabetes mellitus provides a paradigm for considering a multifactorial disorder, because genetic, nutritional, and lifestyle factors are intimately interrelated in disease pathogenesis (Table 82-5) (Chap. 417).

TABLE 82-4 SELECTED TRINUCLEOTIDE REPEAT DISORDERS

Disease	Locus	Repeat	Triplet Length (Normal/Disease)	Inheritance	Gene Product
X-chromosomal spinobulbar muscular atrophy (SBMA)	Xq11-q12	CAG	11–34/40–62	XR	Androgen receptor
Fragile X syndrome (FRAXA)	Xq27.3	CGG	6–50/200–300	XR	FMR-1 protein
Fragile X syndrome (FRAXE)	Xq28	GCC	6–25/>200	XR	FMR-2 protein
Dystrophia myotonica (DM)	19q13.2-q13.3	CTG	5–30/200–1000	AD, variable penetrance	Myotonin protein kinase
Huntington's disease (HD)	4p16.3	CAG	6–34/37–180	AD	Huntingtin
Spinocerebellar ataxia type 1 (SCA1)	6p21.3-21.2	CAG	6–39/40–88	AD	Ataxin 1
Spinocerebellar ataxia type 2 (SCA2)	12q24.1	CAG	15–31/34–400	AD	Ataxin 2
Spinocerebellar ataxia type 3 (SCA3); Machado-Joseph disease (MD)	14q21	CAG	13–36/55–86	AD	Ataxin 3
Spinocerebellar ataxia type 6 (SCA6, CACNAIA)	19p13.1-13.2	CAG	4–16/20–33	AD	Alpha 1A voltage-dependent L-type calcium channel
Spinocerebellar ataxia type 7 (SCA7)	3p21.1-p12	CAG	4–19/37 to >300	AD	Ataxin 7
Spinocerebellar ataxia type 12 (SCA12)	5q31	CAG	6–26/66–78	AD	Protein phosphatase 2A
Dentatorubral pallidoluysian atrophy (DRPLA)	12p	CAG	7–23/49–75	AD	Atrophin 1
Friedreich's ataxia (FRDA1)	9q13-21	GAA	7–22/200–900	AR	Frataxin

Abbreviations: AD, autosomal dominant; AR, autosomal recessive; XR, X-linked recessive.

TABLE 82-5 GENES AND LOCI INVOLVED IN MONO- AND POLYGENIC FORMS OF DIABETES

Disorder	Genes or Susceptibility Locus	Chromosomal Location	Other Factors
Monogenic permanent neonatal diabetes mellitus	*KCNJ11* (inwardly rectifying potassium channel Kir6.2)	11p15.1	AD
	GCK (glucokinase)	7p15-p13	AR
	INS (insulin)	11p15.5	AR, hyperproinsulinemia
	ABCC8 (ATP-binding cassette, subfamily c, member 8; sulfonylurea receptor)	11p15.1	AD or AR
	GLIS3 (GLIS family zinc finger protein 3)	9p24.2	AR, diabetes, congenital hypothyroidism
Maturity-onset diabetes of the young (MODY): Monogenic forms of diabetes mellitus			
MODY 1	*HNF4α* (hepatocyte nuclear factor 4α)	20q12-q13.1	AD inheritance
MODY 2	*GCK* (glucokinase)	7p15-p13	
MODY 3	*HNF1α* (hepatocyte nuclear factor 1α)	12q24.2	
MODY 4	*IPF1* (insulin receptor substrate)	13q12.1	
MODY 5 (renal cysts, diabetes)	*HNF1β* (hepatocyte nuclear factor 1β)	17cen-q21.3	
MODY 6	*NeuroD1* (neurogenic differentiation factor 1)	2q32	
MODY 7	*KLF1* (Kruppel-like factor 1)	19p13.13-p13.12	
MODY 8	*CEL* (carboxyl ester lipase)	9q34.3	
MODY 9	*PAX4* (paired box transcription factor 4)	7q32	
MODY 10	*INS* (insulin)	11p15.5	
MODY 11	*BLK* (B-lymphocyte-specific tyrosine kinase)	8p23-p22	
Diabetes mellitus type 2; loci and genes linked and/or associated with susceptibility for diabetes mellitus type 2	Genes and loci identified by linkage/association studies		Heavily influenced by diet, energy expenditure, obesity
	PPARG, KCNJ11/ABCC8, TCF7L2, IGF2BP2, CDKAL1, SLC30A8, CDKN2A/B, HHEX, FTO, HNF1B, NOTCH2, THADA, ADAMSTS9, JAZF1, CDC122/CAMK1D, KCNQ1, TSPAN8/LGR5, IRS1, DUSP9, PROX1, BCK11A, G6PC2, GCKR, ADCY5, SLC2A2, WFS1, ZBED3, DGKB/TMEM195, GCK, KLF14, TP53INP1, GLIS3, TLE4, ADRA2A, CENTD2, CRY2, FADS1, MADD, MTNR1B, HMGA1, HNF1A, IGF1A, IGF1, C2CD4B, PRC1, VPS13C, ZFAND6, GIPR		

Abbreviations: AD, autosomal dominant; AR, autosomal recessive; MODY, maturity onset diabetes of the young.

The identification of genetic variations and environmental factors that either predispose to or protect against disease is essential for predicting disease risk, designing preventive strategies, and developing novel therapeutic approaches. The study of rare monogenic diseases may provide insight into some of the genetic and molecular mechanisms important in the pathogenesis of complex diseases. For example, the identification of the genes causing monogenic forms of permanent neonatal diabetes mellitus or maturity-onset diabetes defined them as *candidate genes* in the pathogenesis of diabetes mellitus type 2 (Tables 82-2 and 82-5). Genome scans have identified numerous genes and loci that may be associated with susceptibility to development of diabetes mellitus in certain populations. Efforts to identify susceptibility genes require very large sample sizes, and positive results may depend on ethnicity, ascertainment criteria, and statistical analysis. Association studies analyzing the potential influence of (biologically functional) SNPs and SNP haplotypes on a particular phenotype are providing new insights into the genes involved in the pathogenesis of these common disorders. Large variants ([micro]deletions, duplications, and inversions) present in the human population also contribute to the pathogenesis of complex disorders, but their contributions remain poorly understood.

Linkage and Association Studies There are two primary strategies for mapping genes that cause or increase susceptibility to human disease: (1) classic linkage can be performed based on a known genetic model or, when the model is unknown, by studying pairs of affected relatives; or (2) disease genes can be mapped using allelic association studies (Table 82-6).

GENETIC LINKAGE *Genetic linkage* refers to the fact that genes are physically connected, or linked, to one another along the chromosomes. Two fundamental principles are essential for understanding the concept of linkage: (1) when two genes are close together on a chromosome, they are usually transmitted together, unless a recombination event separates them (Figs. 82-6); and (2) the odds of a crossover, or recombination event, between two linked genes is proportional to the distance that separates them. Thus, genes that are farther apart are more likely to undergo a recombination event than genes that are very close together. The detection of chromosomal loci that segregate with a disease by linkage can be used to identify the gene responsible for the disease (*positional cloning*) and to predict the odds of disease gene transmission in genetic counseling.

Polymorphisms are essential for linkage studies because they provide a means to distinguish the maternal and paternal chromosomes in an individual. On average, 1 out of every 1000 bp varies from one person to the next. Although this degree of variation seems low (99.9% identical), it means that >3 million sequence differences exist between any two unrelated individuals and the probability that the sequence at such loci will differ on the two homologous chromosomes is high (often >70–90%). These sequence variations include variable number of tandem repeats (VNTRs), short tandem repeats (STRs), and SNPs. Most STRs, also called *polymorphic microsatellite markers*, consist of di-, tri-, or tetranucleotide repeats that can be characterized readily using the polymerase chain reaction (PCR). Characterization of SNPs, using DNA chips or beads, permits comprehensive analyses of genetic variation, linkage, and association studies. Although these sequence variations often have no apparent functional consequences, they provide much of the basis for variation in genetic traits.

In order to identify a chromosomal locus that segregates with a disease, it is necessary to characterize polymorphic DNA markers from affected and unaffected individuals of one or several pedigrees. One can

TABLE 82-6 GENETIC APPROACHES FOR IDENTIFYING DISEASE GENES

Method	Indications and Advantages	Limitations
Linkage Studies		
Classical linkage analysis (parametric methods)	Analysis of monogenic traits	Difficult to collect large informative pedigrees
	Suitable for genome scan	Difficult to obtain sufficient statistical power for complex traits
	Control population not required	
	Useful for multifactorial disorders in isolated populations	
Allele-sharing methods (nonparametric methods)	Suitable for identification of susceptibility genes in polygenic and multifactorial disorders	Difficult to collect sufficient number of subjects
Affected sib and relative pair analyses	Suitable for genome scan	Difficult to obtain sufficient statistical power for complex traits
Sib pair analysis	Control population not required if allele frequencies are known	Reduced power compared to classical linkage, but not sensitive to specification of genetic mode
	Statistical power can be increased by including parents and relatives	
Association Studies		
Case-control studies	Suitable for identification of susceptibility genes in polygenic and multifactorial disorders	Requires large sample size and matched control population
Linkage disequilibrium	Suitable for testing specific allelic variants of known candidate loci	False-positive results in the absence of suitable control population
Transmission disequilibrium test (TDT)	Facilitated by HapMap data, making GWAS more feasible	Candidate gene approach does not permit detection of novel genes and pathways
Whole-genome association studies	Does not necessarily need relatives	Susceptibility genes can vary among different populations

Abbreviation: GWAS, genome-wide association study.

then assess whether certain marker alleles cosegregate with the disease. Markers that are closest to the disease gene are less likely to undergo recombination events and therefore receive a higher linkage score. Linkage is expressed as a lod (logarithm of odds) score—the ratio of the probability that the disease and marker loci are linked rather than unlinked. Lod scores of +3 (1000:1) are generally accepted as supporting linkage, whereas a score of –2 is consistent with the absence of linkage.

ALLELIC ASSOCIATION, LINKAGE DISEQUILIBRIUM, AND HAPLOTYPES *Allelic association* refers to a situation in which the frequency of an allele is significantly increased or decreased in individuals affected by a particular disease in comparison to controls. Linkage and association differ in several aspects. Genetic linkage is demonstrable in families or sibships. Association studies, on the other hand, compare a population of affected individuals with a control population. Association studies can be performed as case-control studies that include unrelated affected individuals and matched controls or as family-based studies that compare the frequencies of alleles transmitted or not transmitted to affected children.

Allelic association studies are particularly useful for identifying susceptibility genes in complex diseases. When alleles at two loci occur more frequently *in combination* than would be predicted (based on known allele frequencies and recombination fractions), they are said to be in *linkage disequilibrium*. Evidence for linkage disequilibrium can be helpful in mapping disease genes because it suggests that the two loci are tightly linked.

Detecting the genetic factors contributing to the pathogenesis of common complex disorders remains a great challenge. In many instances, these are low-penetrance alleles (e.g., variations that individually have a subtle effect on disease development, and they can only be identified by unbiased GWAS) (Catalog of Published Genome-Wide Association Studies; Table 82-1) (Fig. 82-14). Most variants occur in noncoding or regulatory sequences but do not alter protein structure. The analysis of complex disorders is further complicated by ethnic differences in disease prevalence, differences in allele frequencies in known susceptibility genes among different populations, locus and allelic heterogeneity, gene-gene and gene-environment interactions, and the possibility of phenocopies. The data generated by the HapMap Project are greatly facilitating GWAS for the characterization of complex disorders. Adjacent SNPs are inherited together as blocks, and these blocks can be identified by genotyping selected marker SNPs, so-called *Tag SNPs*, thereby reducing cost and workload (Fig. 82-4). The availability of this information permits the characterization of a limited number of SNPs to identify the set of haplotypes present in an individual (e.g., in cases and controls). This, in turn, permits performing GWAS by searching for associations of certain haplotypes with a disease phenotype of interest, an essential step for unraveling the genetic factors contributing to complex disorders.

POPULATION GENETICS In population genetics, the focus changes from alterations in an individual's genome to the distribution pattern of different genotypes in the population. In a case where there are only two alleles, A and a, the frequency of the genotypes will be $p^2 + 2pq + q^2 = 1$, with p^2 corresponding to the frequency of AA, $2pq$ to the frequency of Aa, and q^2 to aa. When the frequency of an allele is known, the frequency of the genotype can be calculated. Alternatively, one can determine an allele frequency if the genotype frequency has been determined.

Allele frequencies vary among ethnic groups and geographic regions. For example, heterozygous mutations in the *CFTR* gene are relatively common in populations of European origin but are rare in the African population. Allele frequencies may vary because certain allelic variants confer a selective advantage. For example, heterozygotes for the sickle cell mutation, which is particularly common in West Africa, are more resistant to malarial infection because the erythrocytes of heterozygotes provide a less favorable environment for *Plasmodium* parasites. Although homozygosity for the sickle cell mutation is associated with severe anemia and sickle crises (Chap. 127), heterozygotes have a higher probability of survival because of the reduced morbidity and mortality from malaria; this phenomenon has led to an increased frequency of the mutant allele. Recessive conditions are more prevalent in geographically isolated populations because of the more restricted gene pool.

APPROACH TO THE PATIENT: **Inherited Disorders**

For the practicing clinician, the family history remains an essential step in recognizing the possibility of a hereditary predisposition to disease. When taking the history, it is useful to draw a detailed

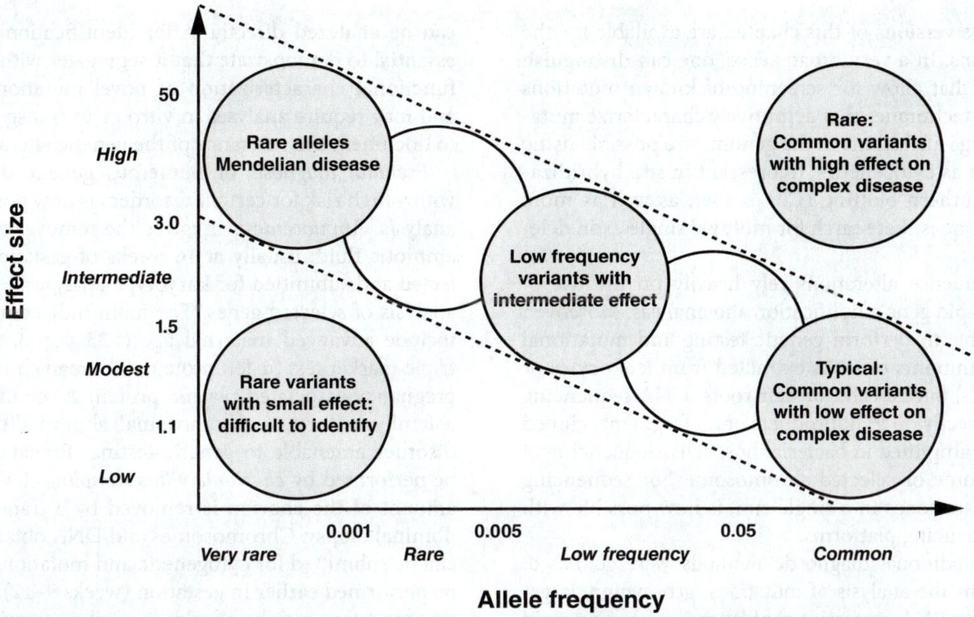

FIGURE 82-14 Relationship between allele frequency and effect size in monogenic and polygenic disorders. In classic Mendelian disorders, the allele frequency is typically low but has a high impact (single gene disorder). This contrasts with polygenic disorders that require the combination of multiple low impact alleles that are frequently quite common in the general population.

pedigree of the first-degree relatives (e.g., parents, siblings, and children), because they share 50% of genes with the patient. Standard symbols for pedigrees are depicted in Fig. 82-11. The family history should include information about ethnic background, age, health status, and deaths, including infants. Next, the physician should explore whether there is a family history of the same or related illnesses to the current problem. An inquiry focused on commonly occurring disorders such as cancers, heart disease, and diabetes mellitus should follow. Because of the possibility of age-dependent expressivity and penetrance, the family history will need intermittent updating. If the findings suggest a genetic disorder, the clinician should assess whether some of the patient's relatives may be at risk of carrying or transmitting the disease. In this circumstance, it is useful to confirm and extend the pedigree based on input from several family members. This information may form the basis for genetic counseling, carrier detection, early intervention, and disease prevention in relatives of the index patient (Chap. 84).

In instances where a diagnosis at the molecular level may be relevant, it is important to identify an appropriate laboratory that can perform the appropriate test. Genetic testing is available for a rapidly growing number of monogenic disorders through commercial laboratories. For uncommon disorders, the test may only be performed in a specialized research laboratory. Approved laboratories offering testing for inherited disorders can be identified in continuously updated online resources (e.g., GeneTests; Table 82-1). If genetic testing is considered, the patient and the family should be counseled about the potential implications of positive results, including psychological distress and the possibility of discrimination. The patient or caretakers should be informed about the meaning of a negative result, technical limitations, and the possibility of false-negative and inconclusive results. For these reasons, genetic testing should only be performed after obtaining *informed consent*. Published ethical guidelines address the specific aspects that should be considered when testing children and adolescents. Genetic testing should usually be limited to situations in which the results may have an impact on medical management.

IDENTIFYING THE DISEASE-CAUSING GENE

Genomic medicine aims to enhance the quality of medical care through the use of genotypic analysis (DNA testing) to identify genetic predisposition to disease, to select more specific pharmacotherapy, and to design individualized medical care based on genotype. Genotype can be deduced by analysis of protein (e.g., hemoglobin, apoprotein E), mRNA, or DNA. However, technologic advances have made DNA analysis particularly useful because it can be readily applied.

DNA testing is performed by mutational analysis or linkage studies in individuals at risk for a genetic disorder known to be present in a family. Mass screening programs require tests of high sensitivity and specificity to be cost-effective. Prerequisites for the success of genetic screening programs include the following: that the disorder is potentially serious; that it can be influenced at a presymptomatic stage by changes in behavior, diet, and/or pharmaceutical manipulations; and that the screening does not result in any harm or discrimination. Screening in Jewish populations for the autosomal recessive neurodegenerative storage disease Tay-Sachs has reduced the number of affected individuals. In contrast, screening for sickle cell trait/disease in African Americans has led to unanticipated problems of discrimination by health insurers and employers. Mass screening programs harbor additional potential problems. For example, screening for the most common genetic alteration in cystic fibrosis, the ΔF508 mutation with a frequency of ~70% in northern Europe, is feasible and seems to be effective. One has to keep in mind, however, that there is pronounced allelic heterogeneity and that the disease can be caused by about 2000 other mutations. The search for these less common mutations would substantially increase costs but not the effectiveness of the screening program as a whole. Next-generation genome sequencing permits comprehensive and cost-effective mutational analyses after selective enrichment of candidate genes. For example, tests that sequence all the common genes causing hereditary deafness are already commercially available. Occupational screening programs aim to detect individuals with increased risk for certain professional activities (e.g., α_1 antitrypsin deficiency and smoke or dust exposure). Integrating genomic data into electronic medical records is evolving and may provide significant decision support at the point of care, for example, by providing the clinician with genomic data and decision algorithms for the prescription of drugs that are subject to pharmacogenetic influences.

Mutational Analyses DNA sequence analysis is now widely used as a diagnostic tool and has significantly enhanced diagnostic accuracy. It is used for determining carrier status and for prenatal testing in monogenic disorders (Chap. 84). Numerous techniques, discussed in previous versions of this chapter, are available for the detection of mutations. In a very broad sense, one can distinguish between techniques that allow for screening of known mutations (screening mode) or techniques that definitively characterize mutations. Analyses of large alterations in the genome are possible using classic methods such as cytogenetics, fluorescent in situ hybridization (FISH), and Southern blotting (Chap. 83e), as well as more sensitive novel techniques that search for multiple single exon deletions or duplications.

More discrete sequence alterations rely heavily on the use of PCR, which allows rapid gene amplification and analysis. Moreover, PCR makes it possible to perform genetic testing and mutational analysis with small amounts of DNA extracted from leukocytes or even from single cells, buccal cells, or hair roots. DNA sequencing can be performed directly on PCR products or on fragments cloned into plasmid vectors amplified in bacterial host cells. Sequencing of all exons of the genome or selected chromosomes, or sequencing of numerous candidate genes in a single run, is now possible with next-generation sequencing platforms.

The majority of traditional diagnostic methods were gel-based. Novel technologies for the analysis of mutations, genotyping, large-scale sequencing, and mRNA expression profiles are undergoing rapid evolution. DNA chip technologies allow hybridization of DNA or RNA to hundreds of thousands of probes simultaneously. Microarrays are being used clinically for mutational analysis of several human disease genes, as well as for the identification of viral or bacterial sequence variations. With advances in high-throughput DNA sequencing technology, complete sequencing of the genome or an exome has entered the clinical realm. Although comprehensive sequencing of large genomic regions or multiple genes is already a reality, the subsequent bioinformatics analysis, assembly of sequence fragments, and comparative alignments remains a significant and commonly underestimated challenge. The discovery of incidental (or secondary) findings that are unrelated to the indication for the sequencing analysis but indicators of other disorders of potential relevance for patient care can pose a difficult ethical dilemma. It can lead to the detection of undiagnosed medically actionable genetic conditions, but can also reveal deleterious mutations that cannot be influenced, as numerous sequence variants are of unknown significance.

A general algorithm for the approach to mutational analysis is outlined in Fig. 82-15. The importance of a detailed clinical phenotype cannot be overemphasized. This is the step where one should also consider the possibility of genetic heterogeneity and phenocopies. If obvious candidate genes are suggested by the phenotype, they can be analyzed directly. After identification of a mutation, it is essential to demonstrate that it segregates with the phenotype. The functional characterization of novel mutations is labor intensive and may require analyses in vitro or in transgenic models in order to document the relevance of the genetic alteration.

Prenatal diagnosis of numerous genetic diseases in instances with a high risk for certain disorders is now possible by direct DNA analysis. *Amniocentesis* involves the removal of a small amount of amniotic fluid, usually at 16 weeks of gestation. Cells can be collected and submitted for karyotype analyses, FISH, and mutational analysis of selected genes. The main indications for amniocentesis include advanced maternal age (>35 years), an abnormal serum triple marker test (α-fetoprotein, β human chorionic gonadotropin, pregnancy-associated plasma protein A, or unconjugated estriol), a family history of chromosomal abnormalities, or a Mendelian disorder amenable to genetic testing. Prenatal diagnosis can also be performed by *chorionic villus sampling* (CVS), in which a small amount of the chorion is removed by a transcervical or transabdominal biopsy. Chromosomes and DNA obtained from these cells can be submitted for cytogenetic and mutational analyses. CVS can be performed earlier in gestation (weeks 9–12) than amniocentesis, an aspect that may be of relevance when termination of pregnancy is a consideration. Later in pregnancy, beginning at about 18 weeks of gestation, percutaneous umbilical blood sampling (PUBS) permits collection of fetal blood for lymphocyte culture and analysis. Recently, the entire fetal genome has been determined prenatally from cells taken from the mother's plasma through deep sequencing and the counting of parental haplotypes, or by inferring it from DNA sequences obtained from blood samples from the mother, father, and umbilical cord. These approaches enable screening for clinically relevant and deleterious alleles inherited from the parents, as well as for de novo germline mutations, and they may have the potential to change the diagnosis of genetic disorders in the prenatal setting.

In combination with in vitro fertilization (IVF) techniques, it is even possible to perform genetic diagnoses in a single cell removed from the four- to eight-cell embryo or to analyze the first polar body from an oocyte. Preconceptual diagnosis thereby avoids therapeutic abortions but is costly and labor intensive. It should be emphasized that excluding a specific disorder by any of these approaches is never equivalent to the assurance of having a normal child.

Mutations in certain cancer susceptibility genes such as *BRCA1* and *BRCA2* may identify individuals with an increased risk for the development of malignancies and result in risk-reducing interventions. The detection of mutations is an important diagnostic and

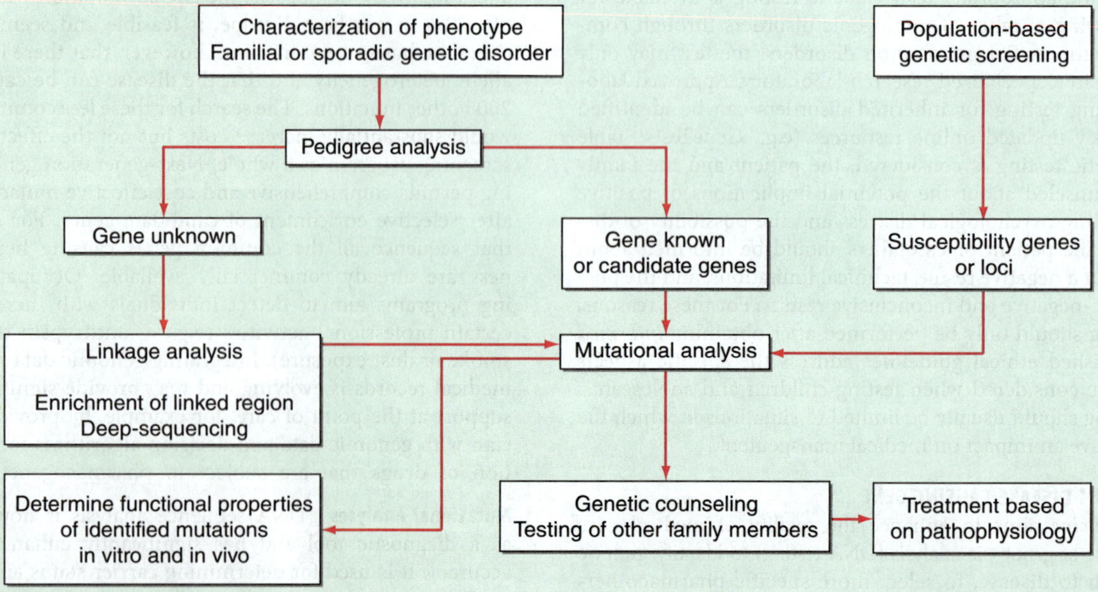

FIGURE 82-15 Approach to genetic disease.

prognostic tool in leukemias and lymphomas. The demonstration of the presence or absence of mutations and polymorphisms is also relevant for the rapidly evolving field of pharmacogenomics, including the identification of differences in drug treatment response or metabolism as a function of genetic background. For example, the thiopurine drugs 6-mercaptopurine and azathioprine are commonly used cytotoxic and immunosuppressive agents. They are metabolized by thiopurine methyltransferase (TPMT), an enzyme with variable activity associated with genetic polymorphisms in 10% of whites and complete deficiency in about 1 in 300 individuals. Patients with intermediate or deficient TPMT activity are at risk for excessive toxicity, including fatal myelosuppression. Characterization of these polymorphisms allows mercaptopurine doses to be modified based on TPMT genotype. Pharmacogenomics may increasingly permit individualized drug therapy, improve drug effectiveness, reduce adverse side effects, and provide cost-effective pharmaceutical care (Chap. 5).

ETHICAL ISSUES

Determination of the association of genetic defects with disease, comprehensive data of an individual's genome, and studies of genetic variation raise many ethical and legal issues. Genetic information is generally regarded as sensitive information that should not be readily accessible without explicit consent (*genetic privacy*). The disclosure of genetic information may risk possible discrimination by insurers or employers. The scientific components of the Human Genome Project have been paralleled by efforts to examine ethical, social, and legal implications. An important milestone emerging from these endeavors consists in the Genetic Information Nondiscrimination Act (GINA), signed into law in 2008, which aims to protect asymptomatic individuals against the misuse of genetic information for health insurance and employment. It does not, however, protect the symptomatic individual. Provisions of the U.S. Patient Protection and Affordable Care Act, effective in 2014, will fill this gap and prohibit exclusion from, or termination of, health insurance based on personal health status. Potential threats to the maintenance of genetic privacy consist in the emerging integration of genomic data into electronic medical records, compelled disclosures of health records, and direct-to-consumer genetic testing.

It is widely accepted that identifying disease-causing genes can lead to improvements in diagnosis, treatment, and prevention. However, the information gleaned from genotypic results can have quite different impacts, depending on the availability of strategies to modify the course of disease (Chap. 84). For example, the identification of mutations that cause MEN 2 or hemochromatosis allows specific interventions for affected family members. On the other hand, at present, the identification of an Alzheimer's or Huntington's disease gene does not currently alter therapy and outcomes. Most genetic disorders are likely to fall into an intermediate category where the opportunity for prevention or treatment is significant but limited (Chap. 84). However, the progress in this area is unpredictable, as underscored by the finding that angiotensin II receptor blockers may slow disease progression in Marfan's syndrome. Genetic test results can generate anxiety in affected individuals and family members. Comprehensive sequence analyses are particularly challenging because most individuals can be expected to harbor several serious recessive gene mutations.

The impact of genetic testing on health care costs is currently unclear. It is likely to vary among disorders and depend on the availability of effective therapeutic modalities. A significant problem arises from the marketing of genetic testing directly to consumers by commercial companies. The validity of these tests has not been defined, and there are numerous concerns about the lack of appropriate regulatory oversight, the accuracy and confidentiality of genetic information, the availability of counseling, and the handling of these results.

Many issues raised by the genome project are familiar, in principle, to medical practitioners. For example, an asymptomatic patient with increased low-density lipoprotein (LDL) cholesterol, high blood pressure, or a strong family history of early myocardial infarction is known to be at increased risk of coronary heart disease. In such cases, it is clear that the identification of risk factors and an appropriate intervention are beneficial. Likewise, patients with phenylketonuria, cystic fibrosis, or sickle cell anemia are often identified as having a genetic disease early in life. These precedents can be helpful for adapting policies that relate to genetic information. We can anticipate similar efforts, whether based on genotypes or other markers of genetic predisposition, to be applied to many disorders. One confounding aspect of the rapid expansion of information is that our ability to make clinical decisions often lags behind initial insights into genetic mechanisms of disease. For example, when genes that predispose to breast cancer such as *BRCA1* are described, they generate tremendous public interest in the potential to predict disease, but many years of clinical research are still required to rigorously establish genotype and phenotype correlations.

Genomics may contribute to improvements in global health by providing a better understanding of pathogens and diagnostics, and through contributions to drug development. There is, however, concern about the development of a "genomics divide" because of the costs associated with these developments and uncertainty as to whether these advances will be accessible to the populations of developing countries. The World Health Organization has summarized the current issues and inequities surrounding genomic medicine in a detailed report titled "Genomics and World Health."

Whether related to informed consent, participation in research, or the management of a genetic disorder that affects an individual or his or her family, there is a great need for more information about fundamental principles of genetics. The pervasive nature of the role of genetics in medicine makes it important for physicians and other health care professionals to become more informed about genetics and to provide advice and counseling in conjunction with trained genetic counselors (Chap. 84). The application of screening and prevention strategies will therefore require intensive patient and physician education, changes in health care financing, and legislation to protect patient's rights.

83e Chromosome Disorders

Nancy B. Spinner, Laura K. Conlin

This is a digital-only chapter. It is available on the DVD that accompanies this book, as well as on Access Medicine/Harrison's Online, and the eBook and "app" editions of HPIM 19e.

CHROMOSOME DISORDERS

Alterations of the chromosomes (numerical and structural) occur in about 1% of the general population, in 8% of stillbirths, and in close to 50% of spontaneously aborted fetuses. The 3×10^9 base pairs that encode the human genome are packaged into 23 pairs of chromosomes, which consist of discrete portions of DNA, bound to several classes of regulatory proteins. Technical advances that led to the ability to analyze human chromosomes immediately translated into the revelation that human disorders can be caused by an abnormality of chromosome number. In 1959, the clinically recognizable disorder, Down syndrome, was demonstrated to result from having three copies of chromosome 21 (trisomy 21). Very soon thereafter, in 1960, a small, structurally abnormal chromosome was recognized in the cells of some patients with chronic myelogenous leukemia (CML), and this abnormal chromosome is now known as the Philadelphia chromosome.

84 The Practice of Genetics in Clinical Medicine

Susan M. Domchek, J. Larry Jameson, Susan Miesfeldt

APPLICATIONS OF MOLECULAR GENETICS IN CLINICAL MEDICINE

Genetic testing for inherited abnormalities associated with disease risk is increasingly used in the practice of clinical medicine. Germline alterations include chromosomal abnormalities (Chap. 83e), specific gene mutations with autosomal dominant or recessive patterns of transmission (Chap. 82), and single nucleotide polymorphisms with small relative risks associated with disease. Germline alterations are responsible for disorders beyond classic Mendelian conditions with genetic susceptibility to common adult-onset diseases such as asthma, hypertension, diabetes mellitus, macular degeneration, and many forms of cancer. For many of these diseases, there is a complex interplay of genes (often multiple) and environmental factors that affect lifetime risk, age of onset, disease severity, and treatment options.

The expansion of knowledge related to genetics is changing our understanding of pathophysiology and influencing our classification of diseases. Awareness of genetic etiology can have an impact on clinical management, including prevention and screening for or treatment of a range of diseases. Primary care physicians are relied upon to help patients navigate testing and treatment options. Consequently, they must understand the genetic basis for a large number of genetically influenced diseases, incorporate personal and family history to determine the risk for a specific mutation, and be positioned to provide counseling. Even if patients are seen by genetic specialists who assess genetic risk and coordinate testing, primary care providers should provide information to their patients regarding the indications, limitations, risks, and benefits of genetic counseling and testing. They must also be prepared to offer risk-based management following genetic risk assessment. Given the pace of genetics, this is an increasingly difficult task. The field of clinical genetics is rapidly moving from single gene testing to multigene panel testing, with techniques such as whole-exome and -genome sequencing on the horizon, increasing the complexity of test selection and interpretation, as well as patient education and medical decision making.

COMMON ADULT-ONSET GENETIC DISORDERS

INHERITANCE PATTERNS

Adult-onset hereditary diseases follow multiple patterns of inheritance. Some are autosomal dominant conditions. These include many common cancer susceptibility syndromes such as hereditary breast and ovarian cancer (due to germline *BRCA1* and *BRCA2* mutations) and Lynch syndrome (caused by germline mutations in the mismatch repair genes *MLH1*, *MSH2*, *MSH6*, and *PMS2*). In both of these examples, inherited mutations are associated with a high penetrance (lifetime risk) of cancer, although risk is not 100%. In other conditions, although there is autosomal dominant transmission, there is lower penetrance, thereby making the disorders more difficult to recognize. For example, germline mutations in *CHEK2* increase the risk of breast cancer, but with a moderate lifetime risk in the range of 20–40%, as opposed to 50–70% for mutations in *BRCA1* or *BRCA2*. Other adult-onset hereditary diseases are transmitted in an autosomal recessive fashion where two mutant alleles are necessary to cause disease. Examples include hemochromatosis and *MYH*-associated colon cancer. There are more pediatric-onset autosomal recessive disorders, such as lysosomal storage diseases and cystic fibrosis.

The genetic risk for many adult-onset disorders is multifactorial. Risk can be conferred by genetic factors at a number of loci, which individually have very small effects (usually with relative risks of <1.5). These risk loci (generally single nucleotide polymorphisms [SNPs]) combine with other genes and environmental factors in ways that are not well understood. SNP panels are available to assess risk of disease, but the optimal way of using this information in the clinical setting remains uncertain.

Many diseases have multiple patterns of inheritance, adding to the complexity of evaluating patients and families for these conditions. For example, colon cancer can be associated with a single germline mutation in a mismatch repair gene (Lynch syndrome, autosomal dominant), biallelic mutations in *MYH* (autosomal recessive), or multiple SNPs (polygenic). Many more individuals will have SNP risk alleles than germline mutations in high-penetrance genes, but cumulative lifetime risk of colon cancer related to the former is modest, whereas the risk related to the latter is significant. Personal and family histories provide important insights into the possible mode of inheritance.

FAMILY HISTORY

When two or more first-degree relatives are affected with asthma, cardiovascular disease, type 2 diabetes, breast cancer, colon cancer, or melanoma, the relative risk for disease among close relatives ranges from two- to fivefold, underscoring the importance of family history for these prevalent disorders. In most situations, the key to assessing the inherited risk for common adult-onset diseases is the collection and interpretation of a detailed personal and family medical history in conjunction with a directed physical examination.

Family history should be recorded in the form of a pedigree. Pedigrees should convey health-related data on first- and second-degree relatives. When such pedigrees suggest inherited disease, they should be expanded to include additional family members. The determination of risk for an asymptomatic individual will vary depending on the size of the pedigree, the number of unaffected relatives, the types of diagnoses, and the ages of disease onset. For example, a woman with two first-degree relatives with breast cancer is at greater risk for a specific Mendelian disorder if she has a total of 3 female first-degree relatives (with only 1 unaffected) than if she has a total of 10 female first-degree relatives (with 7 unaffected). Factors such as adoption and limited family structure (few women in a family) should to be taken into consideration in the interpretation of a pedigree. Additional considerations include young age of disease onset (e.g., a 30-year nonsmoking woman with a myocardial infarction), unusual diseases (e.g., male breast cancer or medullary thyroid cancer), and the finding of multiple potentially related diseases in an individual (e.g., a woman with a history of both colon and endometrial cancer). Some adult-onset diseases are more prevalent in certain ethnic groups. For instance, 2.5% of individuals of Ashkenazi Jewish ancestry carry one of three founder mutation in *BRCA1* and *BRCA2*. Factor V Leiden mutations are much more common in Caucasians than in Africans or Asians.

Additional variables that should be documented are nonhereditary risk factors among those with disease (such as cigarette smoking and myocardial infarction; asbestos exposure and lung disease; and mantle radiation and breast cancer). Significant associated environmental exposures or lifestyle factors decrease the likelihood of a specific genetic disorder. In contrast, the absence of nonhereditary risk factors typically associated with a disease raises concern about a genetic association. A personal or family history of deep vein thrombosis in the absence of known environmental or medical risk factors suggests a hereditary thrombotic disorder. The physical examination may also provide important clues about the risk for a specific inherited disorder. A patient presenting with xanthomas at a young age should prompt consideration of familial hypercholesterolemia. The presence of trichilemmomas in a woman with breast cancer raises concern for Cowden syndrome, associated with *PTEN* mutations.

Recall of family history is often inaccurate. This is especially so when the history is remote and families lose contact or separate geographically. It can be helpful to ask patients to fill out family history forms before or after their visits, because this provides them with an opportunity to contact relatives. Ideally, this information should be embedded in electronic health records and updated intermittently. Attempts should be made to confirm the illnesses reported in the family history before making important and, in certain circumstances, irreversible management decisions. This process is often labor

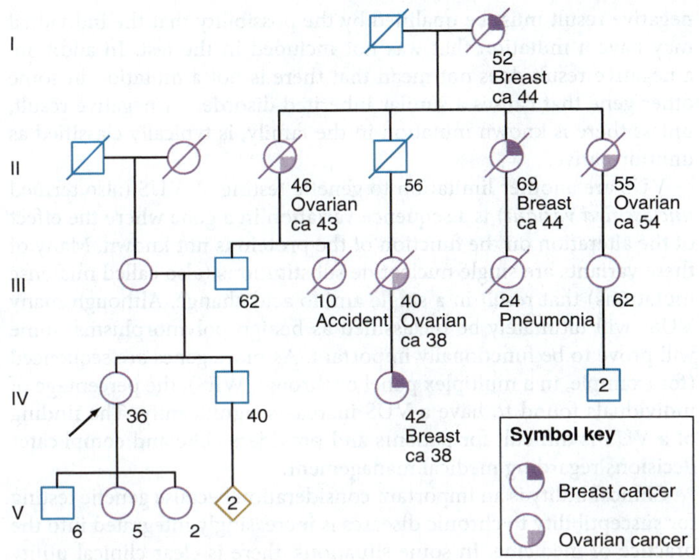

FIGURE 84-1 A 36-year-old woman (*arrow*) seeks consultation because of her family history of cancer. The patient expresses concern that the multiple cancers in her relatives imply an inherited predisposition to develop cancer. The family history is recorded, and records of the patient's relatives confirm the reported diagnoses.

intensive and ideally involves interviews of additional family members or reviewing medical records, autopsy reports, and death certificates.

Although many inherited disorders will be suggested by the clustering of relatives with the same or related conditions, it is important to note that disease penetrance is incomplete for most genetic disorders. As a result, the pedigree obtained in such families may not exhibit a clear Mendelian inheritance pattern, because not all family members carrying the disease-associated alleles will manifest clinical evidence of the condition. Furthermore, genes associated with some of these disorders often exhibit variable disease expression. For example, the breast cancer–associated gene *BRCA2* can predispose to several different malignancies in the same family, including cancers of the breast, ovary, pancreas, skin, and prostate. For common diseases such as breast cancer, some family members without the susceptibility allele (or genotype) may develop breast cancer (or phenotype) sporadically. Such phenocopies represent another confounding variable in the pedigree analysis.

Some of the aforementioned features of the family history are illustrated in Fig. 84-1. In this example, the proband, a 36-year-old woman (IV-1), has a strong history of breast and ovarian cancer on the paternal side of her family. The early age of onset and the co-occurrence of breast and ovarian cancer in this family suggest the possibility of an inherited mutation in *BRCA1* or *BRCA2*. It is unclear however, without genetic testing, whether her father harbors such a mutation and transmitted it to her. After appropriate genetic counseling of the proband and her family, the most informative and cost-effective approach to DNA analysis in this family is to test the cancer-affected 42-year-old living cousin for the presence of a *BRCA1* or *BRCA2* mutation. If a mutation is found, then it is possible to test for this particular alteration in other family members, if they so desire. In the example shown, if the proband's father has a *BRCA1* mutation, there is a 50:50 probability that the mutation was transmitted to her, and genetic testing can be used to establish the absence or presence of this alteration. In this same example, if a mutation is not detected in the cancer-affected cousin, testing would not be indicated for cancer-unaffected relatives.

GENETIC TESTING FOR ADULT-ONSET DISORDERS

A critical first step before initiating genetic testing is to ensure that the correct clinical diagnosis has been made, whether it is based on family history, characteristic physical findings, pathology, or biochemical testing. Such careful clinical assessment can define the phenotype. In the traditional model of genetic testing, testing is directed initially toward the most probable genes (determined by the phenotype), which prevents unnecessary testing. Many disorders exhibit the feature of locus heterogeneity, which refers to the fact that mutations in different genes can cause phenotypically similar disorders. For example, osteogenesis imperfecta (Chap. 427), long QT syndrome (Chap. 277), muscular dystrophy (Chap. 462e), and hereditary predisposition to breast (Chap. 108) or colon (Chap. 110) cancer can each be caused by mutations in a number of distinct genes. The patterns of disease transmission, disease risk, clinical course, and treatment may differ significantly depending on the specific gene affected. Historically, the choice of which gene to test has been determined by unique clinical and family history features and the relative prevalence of candidate genetic disorders. However, rapid changes in genetic testing techniques, as discussed below, may impact this paradigm. It is now technically and financially feasible to sequence many genes (or even the whole exome) at one time. The incorporation of multiplex testing for germline mutations is rapidly evolving.

METHODOLOGIC APPROACHES TO GENETIC TESTING

Genetic testing is regulated and performed in much the same way as other specialized laboratory tests. In the United States, genetic testing laboratories are Clinical Laboratory Improvement Amendments (CLIA) approved to ensure that they meet quality and proficiency standards. A useful information source for various genetic tests is *www.genetests.org*. It should be noted that many tests need to be ordered through specialized laboratories.

Genetic testing is performed largely by DNA sequence analysis for mutations, although genotype can also be deduced through the study of RNA or protein (e.g., apolipoprotein E, hemoglobin S, and immunohistochemistry). For example, universal screening for Lynch syndrome via immunohistochemical analysis of colorectal cancers for absence of expression of mismatch repair proteins is under way at multiple hospitals throughout the United States. The determination of DNA sequence alterations relies heavily on the use of polymerase chain reaction (PCR), which allows rapid amplification and analysis of the gene of interest. In addition, PCR enables genetic testing on minimal amounts of DNA extracted from a wide range of tissue sources including leukocytes, mucosal epithelial cells (obtained via saliva or buccal swabs), and archival tissues. Amplified DNA can be analyzed directly by DNA sequencing, or it can be hybridized to DNA chips or blots to detect the presence of normal and altered DNA sequences. Direct DNA sequencing is frequently used for determination of hereditary disease susceptibility and prenatal diagnosis. Analyses of large alterations of the genome are possible using cytogenetics, fluorescent in situ hybridization (FISH), Southern blotting, or multiplex ligation-dependent probe amplification (MLPA) (Chap. 83e).

Massively parallel sequencing (also called *next-generation sequencing*) is significantly altering the approach to genetic testing for adult-onset hereditary susceptibility disorder. This technology encompasses several high-throughput approaches to DNA sequencing, all of which can reliably sequence many genes at one time. Technically, this involves the use of amplified DNA templates in a flow cell, a very different process than traditional Sanger sequencing which is time-consuming and expensive.

Multiplex panels for inherited susceptibility are commercially available and include testing of a number of genes that have been associated with the condition of interest. For example, panels are available for Brugada syndrome, hypertrophic cardiomyopathy, and Charcot-Marie-Tooth neuropathy. For many syndromes, this type of panel testing may make sense. However, in other situations, the utility of panel testing is less certain. Currently available breast cancer susceptibility panels contain six genes or more. Many of the genes included in the larger panels are associated with only a modest risk of breast cancer, and the clinical application is uncertain. An additional problem of sequencing many genes (rather than the genes for which there is most suspicion) is the identification of one or more variants of uncertain significance (VUS), discussed below.

Whole-exome sequencing (WES) is also now commercially available, although largely used in individuals with syndromes unexplained by traditional genetic testing. As cost declines, WES may be more widely used. Whole-genome sequencing is also commercially available. Although it may be quite feasible to sequence the entire genome, there are many issues in doing so, including the daunting task of analyzing the vast amount of data generated. Other issues include: (1) the optimal way in which to obtain informed consent, (2) interpretation of frequent sequence variation of uncertain significance, (3) interpretation of alterations in genes with unclear relevance to specific human pathology, and (4) management of unexpected but clinically significant genetic findings.

Testing strategies are evolving as a result of these new genetic testing platforms. As the cost of multiple gene panels and WES continue to fall, and as interpretation of such test results improve, there may be a shift from sequential single-gene (or a few genes) testing to multigene testing. For example, presently, a 30-year-old woman with breast cancer but no family history of cancer and no syndromic features would undergo *BRCA1/2* testing. If negative, she would subsequently be offered *TP53* testing. Notably, a reasonable number of individuals offered *TP53* testing for Li-Fraumeni syndrome decline because mutations are associated with extremely high cancer risks (including childhood cancers) in multiple organs and there are no proven interventions to mitigate risk. Without features consistent with Cowden syndrome, the woman would not be routinely offered *PTEN* testing or testing for *CHEK2*, *ATM*, *BRIP*, *BARD*, *NBN*, and *PALB2*. However, it is now possible to synchronously analyze all of the aforementioned genes, for a nominally higher cost than *BRCA1/2* testing alone. Concerns about such panels include appropriate consent strategies related to unexpected findings, VUS, and unclear clinical utility of testing moderate-penetrance genes. Thus, changes from the traditional model of single-gene genetic testing should be done with caution (Fig. 84-2).

Limitations to the accuracy and interpretation of genetic testing exist. In addition to technical errors, genetics tests are sometimes designed to detect only the most common mutations. In addition, genetic testing has evolved over time. For example, it was not possible to obtain commercially available comprehensive large genomic rearrangement testing for *BRCA1* and *BRCA2* until 2006. Therefore, a negative result must be qualified by the possibility that the individual may have a mutation that was not included in the test. In addition, a negative result does not mean that there is not a mutation in some other gene that causes a similar inherited disorder. A negative result, unless there is known mutation in the family, is typically classified as uninformative.

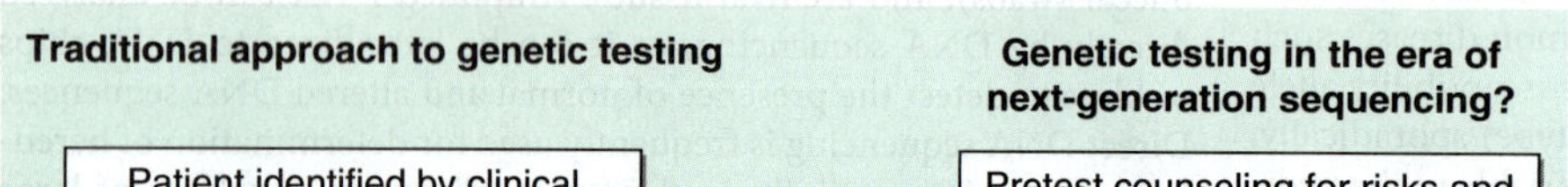

FIGURE 84-2 Approach to genetic testing.

VUS are another limitation to genetic testing. A VUS (also termed *unclassified variant*) is a sequence variation in a gene where the effect of the alteration on the function of the protein is not known. Many of these variants are single nucleotide substitutions (also called missense mutations) that result in a single amino acid change. Although many VUSs will ultimately be reclassified as benign polymorphisms, some will prove to be functionally important. As more genes are sequenced (for example, in a multiplex panel or through WES), the percentage of individuals found to have a VUS increases significantly. The finding of a VUS is difficult for patients and providers alike and complicates decisions regarding medical management.

Clinical utility is an important consideration because genetic testing for susceptibility to chronic diseases is increasingly integrated into the practice of medicine. In some situations, there is clear clinical utility to genetic testing with significant evidence-based changes in medical management decisions based on results. However, in many cases, the discovery of disease-associated genes has outpaced studies that assess how such information should be used in the clinical management of the patient and family. This is particularly true for moderate- and low-penetrance gene mutations. Therefore, predictive genetic testing should be approached with caution and only offered to patients who have been adequately counseled and have provided informed consent.

Predictive genetic testing falls into two distinct categories. Presymptomatic testing applies to diseases where a specific genetic alteration is associated with a near 100% likelihood of developing disease. In contrast, predisposition testing predicts a risk for disease that is less than 100%. For example, presymptomatic testing is available for those at risk for Huntington's disease; whereas, predisposition testing is considered for those at risk for hereditary colon cancer. It is important to note that for the majority of adult-onset disorders, testing is only predictive. Test results cannot reveal with confidence whether, when, or how the disease will manifest itself. For example, not everyone with the apolipoprotein E4 allele will develop Alzheimer's disease, and individuals without this genetic marker can still develop the disorder.

The optimal testing strategy for a family is to initiate testing in an affected family member first. Identification of a mutation can direct the testing of other at-risk family members (whether symptomatic or not). In the absence of additional familial or environmental risk factors, individuals who test negative for the mutation found in the affected family member can be informed that they are at general population risk for that particular disease. Furthermore, they can be reassured that they are not at risk for passing the mutation on to their children. On the other hand, asymptomatic family members who test positive for the known mutation must be informed that they are at increased risk for disease development and for transmitting the alteration to their children.

Pretest counseling and education are important, as is an assessment of the patient's ability to understand and cope with test results. Genetic testing has implications for entire families, and thus individuals interested in pursuing genetic testing must consider how test results might impact their relationships with relatives, partners, spouses, and children. In families with a known genetic mutation, those who test positive must consider the impact of their carrier status on their present and future lifestyles; those who test negative may manifest survivor guilt. Parents who are found to have a disease-associated mutation often express considerable anxiety and despair as they address the issue of risk to their children. In addition, some individuals consider options such as preimplantation genetic diagnosis in their reproductive decision making.

When a condition does not manifest until adulthood, clinicians and parents are faced with the question of whether at-risk children should be offered genetic testing and, if so, at what age. Although the matter is debated, several professional organizations have cautioned that genetic testing for adult-onset disorders should not be offered to children. Many of these conditions have no known interventions in childhood to prevent disease; consequently, such information can pose significant psychosocial risk to the child. In addition, there is concern that testing during childhood violates a child's right to make an informed decision regarding testing upon reaching adulthood. On the other hand, testing should be offered in childhood for disorders that may manifest early in life, especially when management options are available. For example, children with multiple endocrine neoplasia 2 (MEN 2) may develop medullary thyroid cancer early in life and should be considered for prophylactic thyroidectomy (Chap. 408). Similarly, children with familial adenomatous polyposis (FAP) due to a mutation in *APC* may develop polyps in their teens with progression to invasive cancer in the twenties, and therefore, colonoscopy screening is started between the ages of 10 and 15 years (Chap. 110).

INFORMED CONSENT

Informed consent for genetic testing begins with education and counseling. The patient should understand the risks, benefits, and limitations of genetic testing, as well as the potential implications of test results. Informed consent should include a written document, drafted clearly and concisely in a language and format that is understandable to the patient. Because molecular genetic testing of an asymptomatic individual often allows prediction of future risk, the patient should understand all potential long-term medical, psychological, and social implications of testing. There have long been concerns about the potential for genetic discrimination. The Genetic Information Nondiscrimination Act (GINA) was passed in 2008 and provides some protections related to job and health insurance discrimination. It is important to explore with patients the potential impact of genetic test results on future health as well as disability and life insurance coverage. Patients should understand that alternatives remain available if they decide not to pursue genetic testing, including the option of delaying testing to a later date. The option of DNA banking should be presented so that samples are readily available for future use by family members, if needed.

FOLLOW-UP CARE AFTER TESTING

Depending on the nature of the genetic disorder, posttest interventions may include: (1) cautious surveillance and awareness; (2) specific medical interventions such as enhanced screening, chemoprevention, or risk-reducing surgery; (3) risk avoidance; and (4) referral to support services. For example, patients with known deleterious mutations in *BRCA1* or *BRCA2* are strongly encouraged to undergo risk-reducing salpingo-oophorectomy and are offered intensive breast cancer screening as well as the option of risk-reducing mastectomy. In addition, such women may wish to take chemoprevention with tamoxifen, raloxifene, or exemestane. Those with more limited medical management and prevention options, such as patients with Huntington's disease, should be offered continued follow-up and supportive services, including physical and occupational therapy and social services or support groups as indicated. Specific interventions will change as research continues to enhance our understanding of the medical management of these genetic conditions and more is learned about the functions of the gene products involved.

Individuals who test negative for a mutation in a disease-associated gene identified in an affected family member must be reminded that they may still be at risk for the disease. This is of particular importance for common diseases such as diabetes mellitus, cancer, and coronary artery disease. For example, a woman who finds that she does not carry the disease-associated mutation in *BRCA2* previously discovered in the family should be reminded that she still requires the same breast cancer screening recommended for the general population.

GENETIC COUNSELING AND EDUCATION

Genetic counseling should be distinguished from genetic testing and screening, although genetic counselors are often involved in issues related to testing. Genetic counseling refers to a communication process that deals with human problems associated with the occurrence of risk of a genetic disorder in a family. Genetic risk assessment is complex and often involves elements of uncertainty. Counseling, therefore, includes genetic education as well as psychosocial counseling. Genetic counseling can be useful in a wide range of situations (Table 84-1). The role of the genetic counselor includes the following:

1. Gather and document a detailed family history.
2. Educate patients about general genetic principles related to disease risk, both for themselves and for others in the family.
3. Assess and enhance the patient's ability to cope with the genetic information offered.
4. Discuss how nongenetic factors may relate to the ultimate expression of disease.
5. Address medical management issues.
6. Assist in determining the role of genetic testing for the individual and the family.
7. Ensure the patient is aware of the indications, process, risks, benefits, and limitations of the various genetic testing options.
8. Assist the patient, family, and referring physician in the interpretation of the test results.
9. Refer the patient and other at-risk family members for additional medical and support services, if necessary.

Genetic counseling is generally offered in a nondirective manner, wherein patients learn to understand how their values factor into a particular medical decision. Nondirective counseling is particularly appropriate when there are no data demonstrating a clear benefit associated with a particular intervention or when an intervention is considered experimental. For example, nondirective genetic counseling is used when a person is deciding whether to undergo genetic testing for Huntington's disease. At this time, there is no clear benefit (in terms of medical outcome) to an at-risk individual undergoing genetic testing for this disease because its course cannot be altered by therapeutic interventions. However, testing can have an important impact on the individual's perception of advanced care planning and his or her interpersonal relationships and plans for childbearing. Therefore, the decision to pursue testing rests on the individual's belief system and values. On the other hand, a more directive approach is appropriate when a condition can be treated. In a family with FAP, colon cancer screening and prophylactic colectomy should be recommended for known *APC* mutation carriers. The counselor and clinician following this family must ensure that the at-risk family members have access to the resources necessary to adhere to these recommendations.

Genetic education is central to an individual's ability to make an informed decision regarding testing options and treatment. An adequate knowledge of patterns of inheritance will allow patients to understand the probability of disease risk for themselves and other family members. It is also important to impart the concepts of disease penetrance and expression. For most complex adult-onset genetic

TABLE 84-1 INDICATIONS FOR GENETIC COUNSELING
Advanced maternal age (>35 years)
Consanguinity
Previous history of a child with birth defects or a genetic disorder
Personal or family history suggestive of a genetic disorder
High-risk ethnic groups
Documented genetic alteration in a family member
Ultrasound or prenatal testing suggesting a genetic disorder

disorders, asymptomatic patients should be advised that a positive test result does not always translate into future disease development. In addition, the role of nongenetic factors, such as environmental exposures and lifestyle, must be discussed in the context of multifactorial disease risk and disease prevention. Finally, patients should understand the natural history of the disease as well as the potential options for intervention, including screening, prevention, and in certain circumstances, pharmacologic treatment or prophylactic surgery.

THERAPEUTIC INTERVENTIONS BASED ON GENETIC RISK FOR DISEASE

Specific treatments are available for a number of genetic disorders. Strategies for the development of therapeutic interventions have a long history in childhood metabolic diseases; however, these principles have been applied in the diagnosis and management of adult-onset diseases as well (Table 84-2). Hereditary hemochromatosis is usually caused by mutations in *HFE* (although other genes have been less commonly associated) and manifests as a syndrome of iron overload, which can lead to liver disease, skin pigmentation, diabetes mellitus, arthropathy, impotence in males, and cardiac issues (Chap. 428). When identified early, the disorder can be managed effectively with therapeutic phlebotomy. Therefore, when the diagnosis of hemochromatosis has been made in a proband, it is important to counsel and offer testing to other family members in order to minimize the impact of the disorder.

Preventative measures and therapeutic interventions are not restricted to metabolic disorders. Identification of familial forms of long QT syndrome, associated with ventricular arrhythmias, allows early electrocardiographic testing and the use of prophylactic antiarrhythmic therapy, overdrive pacemakers, or defibrillators. Individuals with familial hypertrophic cardiomyopathy can be screened by ultrasound, treated with beta blockers or other drugs, and counseled about the importance of avoiding strenuous exercise and dehydration. Those with Marfan's syndrome can be treated with beta blockers or

TABLE 84-2 EXAMPLE OF GENETIC TESTING AND POSSIBLE INTERVENTIONS

Genetic Disorder	Inheritance	Genes	Interventions
Oncologic			
Lynch syndrome (HNPCC)	AD	*MLH1, MSH2, MSH6, PMS2*	Early endoscopic screening; risk-reducing surgery
Familial adenomatous polyposis	AD	*APC*	Early and frequent endoscopy; prophylactic colectomy
Hereditary breast and ovarian cancer	AD	*BRCA1, BRCA2*	Risk reducing salpingo-oophorectomy; intensified breast surveillance including breast MRI; risk-reducing mastectomy
Hereditary diffuse gastric cancer	AD	*CDH1*	Prophylactic gastrectomy; enhanced breast cancer surveillance
Hematologic			
Factor V Leiden	AD	*F5*	Avoidance of thrombogenic risk factors
Hemophilia A	XL	*F8*	Factor VIII replacement
Hemophilia B	XL	*F9*	Factor IX replacement
Glucose 6-phosphate dehydrogenase deficiency	XL	*G6PD*	Avoidance of oxidant drugs and certain foods
Cardiovascular			
Hypertrophic cardiomyopathy	AD	>10 genes including *MYBPC3, MYH7, TNNT2, TPM1*	Echocardiographic screening; pharmacologic intervention; myomectomy
Long QT syndrome	AD, AR	>10 genes including *KCNQ1, SCN5A, KCNE1, KCNE2*	Electrocardiographic screening; pharmacologic intervention; implantable cardiac defibrillator devices
Marfan's syndrome	AD	*FBN1*	Echocardiographic screening; prophylactic beta blockers; aortic valve replacement as indicated
Gastrointestinal			
Familial Mediterranean fever	AR	*MEFV*	Colchicine
Hemochromatosis	AR	*HFE*	Phlebotomy
Pulmonary			
α_1 Antitrypsin deficiency	AR	*SERPINA1*	Avoidance of smoking and occupational and environmental toxins
Cystic fibrosis	AR	*CFTR*	Chest physiotherapy; agents to promote airway secretion clearance; *CFTR* modulators (G551D mutations); lung transplantation
Endocrine			
Neurohypophyseal diabetes insipidus	AD	*AVP*	Replace vasopressin
Familial hypocalciuric hypercalcemia	AD	*CASR*	Avoidance of parathyroidectomy
Multiple endocrine neoplasia type 2	AD	*RET*	Prophylactic thyroidectomy; screening for pheochromocytoma and hyperparathyroidism
Renal			
Polycystic kidney disease	AD, AR	*PKD1, PKD2, PKHD1*	Prevention of hypertension; prevention of urinary tract infections; kidney transplantation
Nephrogenic diabetes insipidus	XL, AR	*AVPR2, AQP2*	Fluid replacement; thiazides with or without amiloride
Neurologic			
Malignant hyperthermia	AD	*RYR1, CACNA1S*	Avoidance of precipitating anesthetics
Hyperkalemic periodic paralysis	AD	*SCN4A*	Diet rich in calcium and low in potassium; thiazides or acetazolamide
Duchenne's and Becker's muscular dystrophy	XL	*DMD*	Corticosteroids; physical therapy
Wilson's disease	AR	*ATP7B*	Zinc, trientene

Abbreviations: AD, autosomal dominant; AR, autosomal recessive; HNPCC, hereditary nonpolyposis colorectal cancer; MRI, magnetic resonance imaging; XL, X-linked.

angiotensin II receptor blockers and monitored for the development of aortic aneurysms.

The field of pharmacogenetics identifies genes that alter drug metabolism or confer susceptibility to toxic drug reactions. Pharmacogenetics seeks to individualize drug therapy in an attempt to improve treatment outcomes and reduce toxicity. Examples include thiopurine methyltransferase (TPMT) deficiency, dihydropyrimidine dehydrogenase deficiency, malignant hyperthermia, and glucose-6-phosphate deficiency. Despite successes in this area, it is not always clear how to incorporate pharmacogenetics into clinical care. For example, although there is an association with *CYP2C6* and *VKORC1* genotypes and warfarin dosing, there is no evidence that incorporating genotyping into clinical practice improves patient outcomes.

The identification of germline abnormalities that increase the risk of specific types of cancer is rapidly changing clinical management. Identifying family members with mutations that predispose to FAP or Lynch syndrome leads to recommendations of early cancer screening and prophylactic surgery, as well as consideration of chemoprevention and attention to healthy lifestyle habits. Similar principles apply to familial forms of melanoma as well as cancers of the breast, ovary, and thyroid. In addition to increased screening and prophylactic surgery, the identification of germline mutations associated with cancer may also lead to the development of targeted therapeutics, for example, the ongoing development of PARP inhibitors in those with *BRCA*-associated cancers.

Although the role of genetic testing in the clinical setting continues to evolve, such testing holds the promise of allowing early and more targeted interventions that can reduce morbidity and mortality. Rapid technologic advances are changing the ways in which genetic testing is performed. As genetic testing becomes less expensive and technically easier to perform, it is anticipated that there will be an expansion of its use. This will present challenges, but also opportunities. It is critical that physicians and other health care professionals keep current with advances in genetic medicine in order to facilitate appropriate referral for genetic counseling and judicious use of genetic testing, as well as to provide state-of-the-art, evidence-based care for affected or at-risk patients and their relatives.

85e Mitochondrial DNA and Heritable Traits and Diseases

Karl Skorecki, Doron Behar

This is a digital-only chapter. It is available on the DVD that accompanies this book, as well as on Access Medicine/Harrison's Online, and the eBook and "app" editions of HPIM 19e.

Mitochondria are cytoplasmic organelles whose major function is to generate ATP by the process of oxidative phosphorylation under aerobic conditions. This process is mediated by the respiratory electron transport chain (ETC) multiprotein enzyme complexes I–V and the two electron carriers, coenzyme Q (CoQ) and cytochrome c. Other cellular processes to which mitochondria make a major contribution include apoptosis (programmed cell death) and additional cell type–specific functions. The efficiency of the mitochondrial ETC in ATP production is a major determinant of overall body energy balance and thermogenesis. In addition, mitochondria are the predominant source of reactive oxygen species (ROS), whose rate of production also relates to the coupling of ATP production to oxygen consumption. Given the centrality of oxidative phosphorylation to the normal activities of almost all cells, it is not surprising that mitochondrial dysfunction can affect almost any organ system. Thus, physicians in many disciplines might encounter patients with mitochondrial diseases and should be aware of their existence and characteristics.

86e The Human Microbiome

Jeffrey I. Gordon, Rob Knight

This is a digital-only chapter. It is available on the DVD that accompanies this book, as well as on Access Medicine/Harrison's Online, and the eBook and "app" editions of HPIM 19e.

The technologies that allowed us to decipher the human genome have revolutionized our ability to delineate the composition and functions of the microbial communities that colonize our bodies and make up our *microbiota*. Each body habitat, including the skin, nose, mouth, airways, gastrointestinal tract, and vagina, harbors a distinctive community of microbes. Efforts to understand our microbiota and its collection of microbial genes (our *microbiome*) are changing our views of "self" and deepening our understanding of many normal physiologic, metabolic, and immunologic features and their interpersonal and intrapersonal variations. In addition, this area of research is beginning to provide new insights into diseases not previously known to have microbial "contributors" and is suggesting new strategies for treatment and prevention.

87e Network Medicine: Systems Biology in Health and Disease

Joseph Loscalzo

This is a digital-only chapter. It is available on the DVD that accompanies this book, as well as on Access Medicine/Harrison's Online, and the eBook and "app" editions of HPIM 19e.

The field of human biology has progressed over the last three centuries largely as a result of the reductionist approach to the scientific problems that challenge the discipline. Biologists study the experimental response of a variable of interest in a cell or organism while holding all other variables constant. In this way, it is possible to dissect the individual components of a biologic system and assume that a thorough understanding of a specific component (e.g., an enzyme or a transcription factor) will provide sufficient insight to explain the global behavior of that system (e.g., a metabolic pathway or a gene network, respectively). Biologic systems are, however, much more complex than this approach assumes and manifest behaviors that frequently (if not invariably) cannot be predicted from knowledge of their component parts characterized in isolation. Growing recognition of this shortcoming of conventional biologic research has led to the development of a new discipline, systems biology, *which is defined as the holistic study of living organisms or their cellular or molecular network components to predict their response to perturbations.* Concepts of systems biology can be applied readily to human disease and therapy and define the field of *systems pathobiology,* in which genetic or environmental perturbations produce disease and drug perturbations restore normal system behavior.

88 Stem Cell Biology

Minoru S. H. Ko

Stem cell biology is a rapidly expanding field that explores the characteristics and possible clinical applications of a variety of stem cells that serve as the progenitors of more differentiated cell types. In addition to potential therapeutic applications (Chap. 90e), patient-derived stem cells can also be used as disease models and as a means of testing drug efficacy. Stem cells and their niche are a major focus of medical research because they play central roles in tissue and organ homeostasis and repair, which are important aspects of aging and disease.

IDENTIFICATION, ISOLATION, AND DERIVATION OF STEM CELLS

Resident Stem Cells The definition of stem cells remains elusive. Stem cells were originally postulated as *unspecified* or *undifferentiated* cells that provide a source of renewal of skin, intestine, and blood cells throughout life. These *resident stem cells* have been identified in a variety of organs (e.g., epithelia of the skin and digestive system, bone marrow, blood vessels, brain, skeletal muscle, liver, testis, and pancreas) based on their specific locations, morphology, and biochemical markers.

Isolated Stem Cells Unequivocal identification of stem cells requires their separation and purification, usually based on a combination of specific cell-surface markers. These *isolated stem cells* (e.g., hematopoietic stem [HS] cells) can be studied in detail and used in clinical applications, such as bone marrow transplantation (Chap. 89e). However, the lack of specific cell-surface markers for other types of stem cells has made it difficult to isolate them in large quantities. This challenge has been partially addressed in animal models by genetically marking different cell types with green-fluorescent protein driven by cell-specific promoters. Alternatively, putative stem cells have been isolated from a variety of tissues as side population (SP) cells using fluorescence-activated cell sorting after staining with the Hoechst 33342 dye.

Cultured Stem Cells It is desirable to culture and expand stem cells in vitro to obtain a sufficient quantity for analysis and potential therapeutic use. Although the derivation of stem cells in vitro has been a major obstacle in stem cell biology, the number and types of *cultured stem cells* have increased progressively (Table 88-1). Cultured stem cells derived from resident stem cells are often called *adult stem cells* or *somatic stem cells* to distinguish them from *embryonic stem* (ES) and *embryonic germ* (EG) *cells*. However, considering the existence of embryo-derived, tissue-specific stem cells (e.g., trophoblast stem [TS] cells) and the possible derivation of similar cells from an embryo/fetus (e.g., neural stem [NS] cells), it is more appropriate to use the term, *tissue stem cells*.

Successful derivation of cultured stem cells (both embryonic and tissue stem cells) often requires the identification of necessary growth factors and culture conditions, mimicking the microenvironment or *niche* of the resident stem cells. Recently, long-term maintenance of tissue stem cells in vitro is increasingly possible by growing them as three-dimensional (3D) organoids, which contain both stem cells and niche cells (Chap. 92e). For example, intestinal stem cells can now be cultured as "epithelial mini-guts" in the presence of R-spondin, epidermal growth factor (EGF), and noggin on Matrigel. Similarly, lung stem cells can be cultured as self-renewing "alveolospheres." A growing list of cultured stem cells, although not comprehensive, is shown in Table 88-1. Please note that the establishment of cultured stem cells is often under dispute due to the difficulties in assessing the characteristics of these cells.

SELF-RENEWAL AND PROLIFERATION OF STEM CELLS

Symmetric and Asymmetric Cell Division The most widely accepted stem cell definition is a cell with a unique capacity to produce unaltered daughter cells (*self-renewal*) and to generate specialized cell types (*potency*). Self-renewal can be achieved in two ways. *Asymmetric cell division* produces one daughter cell that is identical to the parental cell and one daughter cell that is different from the parental cell and is a progenitor or differentiated cell. Asymmetric cell division does not increase the number of stem cells. *Symmetric cell division* produces two

TABLE 88-1 EXAMPLES OF CULTURED STEM CELLS

Name	Source
Embryonic stem cells (ES, ESC)	Blastocysts or immunosurgically isolated inner cell mass (ICM) from blastocysts
Embryonic germ cells (EG, EGC)	Primordial germ cells (PGCs) from embryos at E8.5–E12.5 (m); gonadal tissues from 5–11 week postfertilization embryo/fetus (h)
Trophoblast stem cells (TS, TSC)	Trophectoderm of E3.5 blastocysts, extraembryonic ectoderm of E6.5 embryos, and chorionic ectoderm of E7.5 embryos (m)
Extraembryonic endoderm cells (XEN)	ICM from blastocysts (m)
Embryonal carcinoma cells (EC)	Teratocarcinoma—a type of cancer that develops in the testes and ovaries (m, h)
Mesenchymal stem cells (MS, MSC)	Bone marrow, muscle, adipose tissue, peripheral blood, and umbilical cord blood (m, h)
Multipotent adult stem cells (MAPC)	Bone marrow mononuclear cells (m, h); postnatal muscle and brain (m)
Spermatogonial stem cells (SS, SSC)	Newborn testis (m)
Germline stem cells (GS, GSC)	Neonatal testis (m)
Multipotent adult germline stem cells (maGSC)	Adult testis (m)
Neural stem cells (NS, NSC)	Fetal and adult brain (subventricular zone, ventricular zone, and hippocampus) (m, h)
Unrestricted somatic stem cells (USSC)	Mononuclear fraction of cord blood (h)
Epistem cells (EpiSC)	Early postimplantation epiblast (m)
Induced pluripotent stem cells (iPS, iPSC)	Variety of terminally differentiated cells and tissue stem cells (m, h)
Multilineage-differentiating stress-enduring (MUSE) cells	Adult human bone marrow stromal cells and dermal fibroblasts
Urine-derived stem cells (USC)	Urine (h)
Lung stem cells	Lung (m, h)
Amniotic fluid-derived stem (AFS) cells	Amniotic fluid (m, h)
Umbilical cord blood stem cells	Umbilical cord (h)
Adipose stem cells (AST)	Fat (m, h)
Cardiac stem cells	Heart (m, h)
Renal stem cells	Renal papilla (m, h)
Crypt stem cells	Intestine (m, h)
Colon stem cells (CoSC)	Colon (m, h)
Hepatic stem cells	Liver (m, h)
Dental pulp stem cells (DPSC)	Dental pulp (m, h)
Hair follicle stem cells	Hair (m, h)

Abbreviations: h, human; m, mouse.

identical daughter cells. For stem cells to proliferate in vitro, they must divide symmetrically.

Unlimited Expansion In Vitro Resident stem cells are often quiescent and divide infrequently. However, once the stem cells are successfully cultured in vitro, they often acquire the capacity to divide continuously and the ability to proliferate beyond the normal passage limit typical of primary cultured cells (sometimes called *immortality*). These features are primarily seen in ES cells but have also been demonstrated for tissue stem cells, such as NS cells and mesenchymal stem (MS) cells, thereby enhancing the potential of these cells for therapeutic use (Table 88-1).

Stability of Genotype and Phenotype The capacity to actively proliferate is often associated with the accumulation of chromosomal abnormalities and mutations. Mouse ES cells appear to be an exception to this rule and tend to maintain their euploid karyotype and genome integrity. By contrast, human ES cells appear to be more susceptible to mutations after long-term culture. However, it is also important to note that even euploid mouse ES cells can form teratomas when injected into immunosuppressed animals, raising concerns about the possible formation of tumors after transplanting actively dividing stem cells.

POTENCY AND DIFFERENTIATION OF STEM CELLS

Developmental Potency The term *potency* is used to indicate a cell's ability to differentiate into multiple specialized cell types. The current lack of knowledge about the molecular nature of potency requires the experimental manipulation of stem cells to demonstrate their potency. For example, in vivo testing can be done by injecting stem cells into mouse blastocysts or immunosuppressed adult mice and determining how many different cell types are formed from the injected cells. However, these in vivo assays are not applicable to human stem cells. In vitro testing can be performed by differentiating cells in various culture conditions to determine how many different cell types are formed from the cells. The formal test of self-renewal and potency is performed by demonstrating that a single cell possesses such abilities in vitro (*clonality*). Cultured stem cells are tentatively grouped according to their potency (Fig. 88-1). Only some examples are shown, because many cultured stem cells, especially human cells, lack definitive information about their developmental potency.

From Totipotency to Unipotency *Totipotent cells* can form an entire organism autonomously. Only a fertilized egg (zygote) possesses this feature. *Pluripotent cells* (e.g., ES cells) can form almost all of the body's cell lineages (endoderm, mesoderm, and ectoderm), including germ cells. *Multipotent cells* (e.g., HS cells) can form multiple cell lineages but cannot form all of the body's cell lineages. *Oligopotent cells* (e.g., NS cells) can form more than one cell lineage but are more restricted than multipotent cells. Oligopotent cells are sometimes called *progenitor cells* or *precursor cells*; however, these terms are often more strictly used to define partially differentiated or lineage-committed cells (e.g., myeloid progenitor cells) that can divide into different cell types but lack self-renewing capacity. *Unipotent cells* or *monopotent cells* (e.g., spermatogonial stem [SS] cells) can form a single differentiated cell lineage.

Potency \ Source	Preimplantation	Embryonic, fetal	Postnatal	Adult
Totipotent	Zygote^{m,h}			
Pluripotent	ES^{m,h}	EG^{m,h} EpiSC^{m}	GS^{m} iPS^{m,h} USSC^{h}	EC^{m,h} iPS^{m,h} maGSC^{m}
Multipotent				MS^{m,h}
Oligopotent	TS^{m}			NS^{m,h}
Unipotent	XEN^{m}			SSC^{m}
Terminally differentiated cells				

FIGURE 88-1 Potency and source developmental stage of cultured stem cells. For abbreviations of stem cells, see Table 88-1. Note that stem cells are often abbreviated with or without "cells," e.g., ES cells or ESCs for embryonic stem cells. h, human; m, mouse.

Nuclear Reprogramming Development naturally progresses from totipotent fertilized eggs to pluripotent epiblast cells to multipotent cells and, finally, to terminally differentiated cells. According to Waddington's epigenetic landscape, this is analogous to a ball moving down a slope. The reversal of the terminally differentiated cells to totipotent or pluripotent cells (called *nuclear reprogramming*) can thus be seen as an uphill gradient. Nuclear reprogramming has been achieved using *nuclear transplantation*, or *nuclear transfer* (NT), procedures (often called "cloning"), where the nucleus of a differentiated cell is transferred into an enucleated oocyte. Although this is an error-prone procedure with a very low success rate, live animals have been produced using adult somatic cells as donors in sheep, mice, and other mammals. In mice, it has been demonstrated that ES cells derived from blastocysts made by somatic cell NT are indistinguishable from normal ES cells. NT can potentially be used to produce *patient-specific ES cells* carrying a genome identical to that of the patient, although such strategies have not been pursued due to ethical issues and technical challenges. Recent success in generating human ES cells by NT has rekindled an interest in this area; however, the limited supply of human oocytes will still be a major problem for clinical applications of NT.

An alternative approach that has become a method of choice is the direct conversion of terminally differentiated cells into ES-like cells (called induced pluripotent stem [iPS] cells) by overexpressing a combination of key transcription factors (TFs). The original method was to infect mouse embryonic fibroblast cells with retrovirus vectors carrying four TFs [*Pou5f1* (*Oct4*), *Sox2*, *Klf4*, and *Myc*] and to identify rare ES-like cells in culture. This approach was soon adapted to human cells, followed by a more refined procedure (e.g., the use of fewer TFs, different cell types, and different gene-delivery methods). Because a clinical trial using iPS cells is imminent, the safety of iPS-based therapy is a major concern and a variety of measures are being taken to ensure the safety. For example, it has now become a standard to use footprint-free methods such as an episomal vector, Sendai virus vector, and synthetic mRNAs to deliver reprogramming factors into cells, resulting in the production of patient-specific iPS cells with minimal alteration of their genetic makeup. In addition to cell replacement therapy, disease-specific iPS cells are expected to play a role in modeling human disease in vitro and in screening drugs for personalized medicine.

It has also become possible to convert one type of terminally differentiated cell (e.g., fibroblast cell) into another type of terminally differentiated cell (e.g., cardiac muscle, neuron, or hepatocyte) by overexpressing specific sets of TFs (called direct reprogramming). Direct reprogramming can bypass the step of making iPS cells, possibly providing the safer route to desired cell types for therapy; however, the technology is currently limited by its low efficiency.

Stem Cell Plasticity, Transdifferentiation, and Facultative Stem Cells The prevailing paradigm in developmental biology is that once cells are differentiated, their phenotypes are stable. However, more recent studies show that tissue stem cells, which have traditionally been thought to be lineage-committed multipotent cells, possess the capacity to differentiate into cell types outside their lineage restrictions (called *transdifferentiation*). For example, HS cells may be converted into neurons as well as germ cells. This feature may provide a means to use tissue stem cells derived directly from a patient for therapeutic purposes, thereby eliminating the need to use embryonic stem cells or elaborate procedures such as nuclear reprogramming of a patient's somatic cells. However, more strict criteria and rigorous validation are required to establish tissue stem cell plasticity. For example, observations of transdifferentiation may reflect cell fusion, contamination with progenitor cells from other cell lineages, or persistence of pluripotent embryonic cells in adult organs. Therefore, the assignment of potency to each cultured stem cell in Fig. 88-1 should be considered with caution. Whether transdifferentiation exists and can be used for therapeutic purposes remains to be determined conclusively. A similar, but distinct, concept is the facultative stem cell, which is defined as a unipotent cell or a terminally differentiated cell that can function as a stem cell upon tissue injury. The presence of such cells has been proposed for some organs such as liver, intestine, pancreas, and testis, but is still debated.

Directed Differentiation of Stem Cells Pluripotent stem cells (e.g., ES and iPS cells) can differentiate into multiple cell types, but in culture, they normally differentiate into heterogeneous cell populations in a stochastic manner. However, for therapeutic uses, it is desirable to direct stem cells into specific cell types (e.g., insulin-secreting beta cells). This is an active area of stem cell research, and protocols are being developed to achieve this goal. In any of these directed cell differentiation systems, the cell phenotype must be evaluated critically. Alternatively, the heterogeneity of the cell population derived from pluripotent stem cells can be actively exploited, as different types of cells interact with each other in culture and further enhance their own differentiation. In some instances, e.g., optic cup, self-organizing tissue morphogenesis has been demonstrated in 3D culture.

MOLECULAR CHARACTERIZATION OF STEM CELLS

Genomics and Proteomics In addition to standard molecular biological approaches, high-throughput genomics and proteomics have been extensively applied to the analysis of stem cells. For example, DNA microarray analyses have revealed the expression levels of essentially all genes and identified specific markers for some stem cells. Chromatin immunoprecipitation coupled with next-generation sequencing technologies, capable of producing billions of sequence reads in a single run, has revealed chromatin modifications ("epigenetic marks") relevant to stem cell properties. Similarly, the protein profiles of stem cells have been assessed by using mass spectrometry. These methods are beginning to provide a novel means to characterize and classify various stem cells and the molecular mechanisms that give them their unique characteristics.

ES Cell Regulation It is important to identify genes involved in the regulation of stem cell function and to examine the effects of altered gene expression on ES and other stem cells. For example, core networks of TFs such as *Pou5f1* (*Oct4*), *Nanog*, and *Sox2*, govern key gene regulatory pathways/networks for the maintenance of self-renewal and pluripotency of mouse and human ES cells. These TF networks are modulated by specific external factors through signal transduction pathways, such as leukemia inhibitory factor (*Lif*)/*Stat3*, mitogen-activated protein kinase 1/3 (*Mapk1/3*), the transforming growth factor β (TGFβ) superfamily, and *Wnt*/glycogen synthase kinase 3 beta (*Gsk3b*). Inhibitors of *Mapk1/3* and *Gsk3b* signaling enhance the derivation of ES cells and help maintain ES cells in full pluripotency ("ground" or "naive state"). Recent data also indicate that 20–25 nucleotide RNAs, called microRNAs (miRNAs), play an important role in regulating stem cell function by repressing the translation of their target genes. For example, it has been shown that miR-21 regulates cell cycle progression in ES cells and miR-128 prevents the differentiation of hematopoietic progenitor cells. These types of analyses should provide molecular clues about the function of stem cells and lead to a more effective means to manipulate stem cells for future therapeutic use.

89e Hematopoietic Stem Cells

David T. Scadden, Dan L. Longo

This is a digital-only chapter. It is available on the DVD that accompanies this book, as well as on Access Medicine/Harrison's Online, and the eBook and "app" editions of HPIM 19e.

All of the cell types in the peripheral blood and some cells in every tissue of the body are derived from hematopoietic (*hemo*: blood; *poiesis*: creation) stem cells. If the hematopoietic stem cell is damaged and can no longer function (e.g., due to a nuclear accident), a person would survive 2–4 weeks in the absence of extraordinary support measures. With the clinical use of hematopoietic stem cells, tens of thousands of lives are saved each year (Chap. 139e). Stem cells produce hundreds of billions of blood cells daily from a stem cell pool that is estimated to be only in the tens of thousands. How stem cells do this, how they persist for many decades despite the production demands, and how they may be better used in clinical care are important issues in medicine.

The study of blood cell production has become a paradigm for how other tissues may be organized and regulated. Basic research in hematopoiesis includes defining stepwise molecular changes accompanying functional changes in maturing cells, aggregating cells into functional subgroups, and demonstrating hematopoietic stem cell regulation by a specialized microenvironment; these concepts are worked out in hematology, but they offer models for other tissues. Moreover, these concepts may not be restricted to normal tissue function but extend to malignancy. Stem cells are rare cells among a heterogeneous population of cell types, and their behavior is assessed mainly in experimental animal models involving reconstitution of hematopoiesis. Thus, much of what we know about stem cells is imprecise and based on inferences from genetically manipulated animals.

90e Applications of Stem Cell Biology in Clinical Medicine

John A. Kessler

This is a digital-only chapter. It is available on the DVD that accompanies this book, as well as on Access Medicine/Harrison's Online, and the eBook and "app" editions of HPIM 19e.

Damage to an organ initiates a series of events that lead to the reconstruction of the damaged tissue, including proliferation, differentiation, and migration of various cell types; release of cytokines and chemokines; and remodeling of the extracellular matrix. Endogenous stem and progenitor cells are among the cell populations that are involved in these injury responses. In normal steady-state conditions, an equilibrium is maintained in which endogenous stem cells intrinsic to the tissue replenish dying cells. After tissue injury, stem cells in organs such as the liver and skin have a remarkable ability to regenerate the organ, whereas other stem cell populations, such as those in the heart and brain, have a much more limited capability for self-repair. In rare circumstances, circulating stem cells may contribute to regenerative responses by migrating into a tissue and differentiating into organ-specific cell types. The goal of stem cell therapies is to promote cell replacement in organs that are damaged beyond their ability to self-repair.

91e Gene Therapy in Clinical Medicine

Katherine A. High

This is a digital-only chapter. It is available on the DVD that accompanies this book, as well as on Access Medicine/Harrison's Online, and the eBook and "app" editions of HPIM 19e.

Gene transfer is a novel area of therapeutics in which the active agent is a nucleic acid sequence rather than a protein or small molecule. Because delivery of naked DNA or RNA to a cell is an inefficient process, most gene transfer is carried out using a vector, or gene delivery vehicle. These vehicles have generally been engineered from viruses by deleting some or all of the viral genome and replacing it with the therapeutic gene of interest under the control of a suitable promoter. Gene transfer strategies can thus be described in terms of three essential elements: (1) a vector, (2) a gene to be delivered, sometimes called the transgene, and (3) a physiologically relevant target cell to which the DNA or RNA is delivered. The series of steps in which the vector and donated DNA enter the target cell and express the transgene is referred to as *transduction*. Gene delivery can take place in vivo, in which the vector is directly injected into the patient, or, in the case of hematopoietic and some other target cells, ex vivo, with removal of the target cells from the patient, followed by return of the gene-modified autologous cells to the patient after manipulation in the laboratory. The latter approach effectively combines gene transfer techniques with cellular therapies (Chap. 90e).

92e Tissue Engineering

Anthony Atala

This is a digital-only chapter. It is available on the DVD that accompanies this book, as well as on Access Medicine/Harrison's Online, and the eBook and "app" editions of HPIM 19e.

Tissue engineering is a field that applies principles of regenerative medicine to restore the function of various organs by combining cells with biomaterials. It is multidisciplinary, often combining the skills of physicians, cell biologists, bioengineers, and material scientists, to recapitulate the native three-dimensional architecture of an organ, the appropriate cell types, and the supportive nutrients and growth factors that allow normal cell growth, differentiation, and function. Tissue engineering is a relatively new field, originating in the late 1970s. Early studies focused on efforts to create skin substitutes using biomaterials and epithelial skin cells with a goal of providing barrier protection for patients with burns. The early strategies employed a tissue biopsy, followed by ex vivo expansion of cells seeded on scaffolds. The cell–scaffold composite was later implanted back into the same patient, where the new tissue would mature. However, there were many hurdles to overcome. The three major challenges in the field of tissue engineering involved: (1) the ability to grow and expand normal primary human cells in large quantities; (2) the identification of appropriate biomaterials; and (3) the requirement for adequate vascularization and innervation of the engineered constructs.

Part 5: Aging

93e World Demography of Aging

Richard M. Suzman, John G. Haaga

This is a digital-only chapter. It is available on the DVD that accompanies this book, as well as on Access Medicine/Harrison's Online, and the eBook and "app" editions of HPIM 19e.

Population aging is transforming the world in dramatic and fundamental ways. The age distributions of populations have changed and will continue to change radically, due to long-term declines in fertility rates and improvements in mortality rates. This transformation, known as the Demographic Transition, is also accompanied by an epidemiologic transition, in which noncommunicable chronic diseases are becoming the major causes of death and contributors to the burden of disease and disability. A concomitant of population aging is the change in key ratios expressing "dependency" of one form or another—the ratio of adults in the workforce to those typically out of the workforce, such as infants, children, retired "young old" (those still active but in ways other than paid work), and the oldest old. Global aging will affect economic growth, migration, patterns of work and retirement, family structures, pension and health systems, and even trade and the relative standing of nations. Both absolute numbers (the size of an age group) and ratios (the ratio of those in working ages to dependents such as the young or retired, or the ratio of children to older people) are important. The size of age groups might affect the number of hospital beds needed, whereas the ratio of children to older people could affect the relative demand for pediatricians and geriatricians.

94e The Biology of Aging

Rafael de Cabo, David G. Le Couteur

This is a digital-only chapter. It is available on the DVD that accompanies this book, as well as on Access Medicine/Harrison's Online, and the eBook and "app" editions of HPIM 19e.

THE IMPACT OF AGING ON MEDICINE

Aging and old age are among the most significant challenges facing medicine this century. The aging process is the major risk factor underlying disease and disability in developed nations, and older people respond differently to therapies developed for younger adults (usually with less effectiveness and more adverse reactions). Modern medicine and healthier lifestyles have increased the likelihood that younger adults will now achieve old age. However, this has led to rapidly increasing numbers of older people, often encumbered with age-related disorders that are predicted to overwhelm health care systems. Improved health in old age and further extension of the human healthspan are now likely to result primarily from increased understanding of the biology of aging, age-related susceptibility to disease, and modifiable factors that influence the aging process.

PART 6: Nutrition and Weight Loss

95e Nutrient Requirements and Dietary Assessment

Johanna Dwyer

This is a digital-only chapter. It is available on the DVD that accompanies this book, as well as on Access Medicine/Harrison's Online, and the eBook and "app" editions of HPIM 19e.

Nutrients are substances that are not synthesized in sufficient amounts in the body and therefore must be supplied by the diet. Nutrient requirements for groups of healthy persons have been determined experimentally. The absence of essential nutrients leads to growth impairment, organ dysfunction, and failure to maintain nitrogen balance or adequate status of other nutrients. For good health, we require energy-providing nutrients (protein, fat, and carbohydrate), vitamins, minerals, and water. Requirements for organic nutrients include 9 essential amino acids, several fatty acids, glucose, 4 fat-soluble vitamins, 10 water-soluble vitamins, dietary fiber, and choline. Several inorganic substances, including 4 minerals, 7 trace minerals, 3 electrolytes, and the ultratrace elements, must also be supplied by diet.

96e Vitamin and Trace Mineral Deficiency and Excess

Robert M. Russell, Paolo M. Suter

This is a digital-only chapter. It is available on the DVD that accompanies this book, as well as on Access Medicine/Harrison's Online, and the eBook and "app" editions of HPIM 19e.

Vitamins are required constituents of the human diet since they are synthesized inadequately or not at all in the human body. Only small amounts of these substances are needed to carry out essential biochemical reactions (e.g., by acting as coenzymes or prosthetic groups). Overt vitamin or trace mineral deficiencies are rare in Western countries because of a plentiful, varied, and inexpensive food supply; food fortification; and use of supplements. However, multiple nutrient deficiencies may appear together in persons who are chronically ill or alcoholic. After gastric bypass surgery, patients are at high risk for multiple nutrient deficiencies. Moreover, subclinical vitamin and trace mineral deficiencies, as diagnosed by laboratory testing, are quite common in the normal population, especially in the geriatric age group. Conversely, because of the widespread use of nutrient supplements, nutrient toxicities are gaining pathophysiologic and clinical importance.

97 Malnutrition and Nutritional Assessment

Douglas C. Heimburger

Malnutrition can arise from primary or secondary causes, resulting in the former case from inadequate or poor-quality food intake and in the latter case from diseases that alter food intake or nutrient requirements, metabolism, or absorption. *Primary* malnutrition occurs mainly in developing countries and under conditions of political unrest, war, or famine. *Secondary* malnutrition, the main form encountered in industrialized countries, was largely unrecognized until the early 1970s, when it was appreciated that persons with adequate food supplies can become malnourished as a result of acute or chronic diseases that alter nutrient intake or metabolism, particularly diseases that cause acute or chronic inflammation. Various studies have shown that protein-energy malnutrition (PEM) affects one-third to one-half of patients on general medical and surgical wards in teaching hospitals. The consistent finding that nutritional status influences patient prognosis underscores the importance of preventing, detecting, and treating malnutrition.

Definitions for forms of PEM are in flux. Traditionally, the two major types of PEM have been *marasmus* and *kwashiorkor*. These conditions are compared in Table 97-1. Marasmus is the end result of a long-term deficit of dietary energy, whereas kwashiorkor has been understood to result from a protein-poor diet. Although the former concept remains essentially correct, evidence is accumulating that PEM syndromes are distinguished by two main features: insufficient dietary intake and underlying inflammatory processes. Energy-poor diets with minimal inflammation cause gradual erosion of body mass, resulting in classic marasmus. By contrast, inflammation from acute illnesses such as injury or sepsis or from chronic illnesses such as cancer, lung or heart disease, or HIV infection can erode lean body mass even in the presence of relatively sufficient dietary intake, leading to a kwashiorkor-like state. Quite often, inflammatory illnesses impair appetite and dietary intake, producing combinations of the two conditions.

Consensus committees have proposed the following revised definitions. *Starvation-related malnutrition* is suggested for instances of chronic starvation without inflammation, *chronic disease–related malnutrition* when inflammation is chronic and of mild to moderate degree, and *acute disease– or injury-related malnutrition* when inflammation is acute and of a severe degree. However, because distinguishing diagnostic criteria for these conditions have not been universally adopted, this chapter integrates the older and newer terms.

MARASMUS (STARVATION–RELATED MALNUTRITION) AND CACHEXIA (CHRONIC DISEASE–RELATED MALNUTRITION)

Marasmus (starvation–related malnutrition) is a state in which virtually all available body fat stores have been exhausted due to starvation without systemic inflammation. *Cachexia* (chronic disease–related malnutrition) is a state that involves substantial loss of lean body mass in the presence of chronic systemic inflammation. Conditions that produce cachexia tend to be chronic and indolent, such as cancer and chronic pulmonary disease, whereas, in high-income countries, the classic setting for marasmus is in patients with anorexia nervosa. These conditions are relatively easy to detect because of the patient's starved

TABLE 97-1 COMPARISON OF MARASMUS/CACHEXIA AND KWASHIORKOR/ACUTE MALNUTRITION

Feature	Marasmus (Starvation–Related Malnutrition) and Cachexia (Chronic Disease–Related Malnutrition)	Kwashiorkor (Acute Disease– or Injury–Related Malnutrition)[a]
Clinical setting	Prolonged ↓ energy and protein intake with or without systemic inflammation	Acute ↓ energy and protein intake with substantial systemic inflammation
Time course to develop	Months or years	Weeks
Clinical features	Starved appearance (body mass index <18.5)	Normal body mass index (although loss of body mass may be masked by edema)
	Reduced triceps skinfold	Easy hair pluckability[b]
	Reduced midarm muscle circumference	Edema
Laboratory findings	Serum albumin normal (marasmus, no inflammation) or decreased (cachexia, with inflammation)	Serum albumin <2.8 g/dL
		Total iron-binding capacity <200 μg/dL
		Lymphocytes <1500/μL
		Anergy
Clinical course	Reasonably preserved responsiveness to short-term stress	Infections
		Poor wound healing, decubitus ulcers, skin breakdown
Mortality risk	Low unless related to underlying disease	High
Diagnostic criteria	Triceps skinfold <3 mm	Serum albumin <2.8 g/dL
	Midarm muscle circumference <15 cm	At least one of the following:
		Poor wound healing, decubitus ulcers, or skin breakdown
		Easy hair pluckability[b]
		Edema

[a]The findings used to diagnose kwashiorkor/acute malnutrition must be unexplained by other causes. [b]Tested by *firmly* pulling a lock of hair from the top (not the sides or back), grasping with the thumb and forefinger. An average of three or more hairs removed easily and painlessly is considered abnormal hair pluckability.

appearance. The diagnosis is based on fat and muscle wastage resulting from prolonged calorie deficiency and/or inflammation. Diminished skinfold thickness reflects the loss of fat reserves; reduced arm muscle circumference with temporal and interosseous muscle wasting reflects the catabolism of protein throughout the body, including in vital organs such as the heart, liver, and kidneys.

Routine laboratory findings in cachexia/marasmus are relatively unremarkable. The creatinine-height index (24-h urinary creatinine excretion compared with normal values based on height) is low, reflecting the loss of muscle mass. Occasionally, the serum albumin level is reduced, but it remains above 2.8 g/dL when systemic inflammation is absent. Despite a morbid appearance, immunocompetence, wound healing, and the ability to handle short-term stress are reasonably well preserved in most patients.

Pure starvation–related malnutrition is a chronic, fairly well adapted form of starvation rather than an acute illness; it should be treated cautiously in an attempt to reverse the downward trend gradually. Although nutritional support is necessary, overly aggressive repletion can result in severe, even life-threatening metabolic imbalances such as hypophosphatemia and cardiorespiratory failure (*refeeding syndrome*). When possible, oral or enteral nutritional support is preferred; treatment started slowly allows readaptation of metabolic and intestinal functions (Chap. 98e).

KWASHIORKOR (ACUTE DISEASE– OR INJURY–RELATED MALNUTRITION)

By contrast, *kwashiorkor* (acute disease– or injury–related malnutrition) in developed countries occurs mainly in connection with acute, life-threatening conditions such as trauma and sepsis. The physiologic stress produced by these illnesses increases protein and energy requirements at a time when intake is often limited. A classic scenario is an acutely stressed patient who receives only 5% dextrose solutions for periods as brief as 2 weeks. Although the etiologic mechanisms are not fully known, the protein-sparing response normally seen in starvation is blocked by the stressed state and by carbohydrate infusion.

In its early stages, the physical findings of kwashiorkor/acute malnutrition are few and subtle. Initially unaffected fat reserves and muscle mass give the deceptive appearance of adequate nutrition. Signs that support the diagnosis include easy hair pluckability, edema, skin breakdown, and poor wound healing. The major sine qua non is severe reduction of levels of serum proteins such as albumin (<2.8 g/dL) and transferrin (<150 mg/dL) or of iron-binding capacity (<200 μg/dL). Cellular immune function is depressed, as reflected by lymphopenia (<1500 lymphocytes/μL in adults and older children) and lack of response to skin test antigens (*anergy*).

The prognosis of adult patients with full-blown kwashiorkor/acute malnutrition is not good even with aggressive nutritional support. Surgical wounds often dehisce (fail to heal), pressure sores develop, gastroparesis and diarrhea can occur with enteral feeding, the risk of gastrointestinal bleeding from stress ulcers is increased, host defenses are compromised, and death from overwhelming infection may occur despite antibiotic therapy. Unlike treatment of marasmus, therapy for kwashiorkor entails aggressive nutritional support to restore better metabolic balance rapidly (Chap. 98e).

PHYSIOLOGIC CHARACTERISTICS OF HYPOMETABOLIC AND HYPERMETABOLIC STATES

The metabolic characteristics and nutritional needs of hypermetabolic patients who are stressed from injury, infection, or chronic inflammatory illness differ from those of hypometabolic patients who are unstressed but chronically starved. In both cases, nutritional support is important, but misjudgments in selecting the appropriate approach may have serious adverse consequences.

The *hypometabolic* patient is typified by the relatively less stressed but mildly catabolic and chronically starved individual who, with time, will develop cachexia/marasmus. The *hypermetabolic* patient stressed from injury or infection is catabolic (experiencing rapid breakdown of body mass) and is at high risk for developing acute malnutrition/kwashiorkor if nutritional needs are not met and/or the illness does not resolve quickly. As summarized in Table 97-2, the two states are distinguished by differing perturbations of metabolic rate, rates of protein breakdown (*proteolysis*), and rates of gluconeogenesis. These differences are mediated by proinflammatory cytokines and counterregulatory hormones—tumor necrosis factor, interleukins 1 and 6, C-reactive protein, catecholamines (epinephrine and norepinephrine), glucagon, and cortisol—whose levels are relatively reduced in hypometabolic patients and increased in hypermetabolic patients. Although insulin levels are also elevated in stressed patients, insulin resistance in the target tissues blocks insulin-mediated anabolic effects. Physiologic

TABLE 97-2 PHYSIOLOGIC CHARACTERISTICS OF HYPOMETABOLIC AND HYPERMETABOLIC STATES

Physiologic Characteristics	Hypometabolic, Nonstressed Patient (Risk for Starvation/Marasmus)	Hypermetabolic, Stressed Patient (Risk for Kwashiorkor/Acute Malnutrition)
Cytokines, catecholamines, glucagon, cortisol, insulin	↓	↑
Metabolic rate, O_2 consumption	↓	↑
Proteolysis, gluconeogenesis	↓	↑
Ureagenesis, urea excretion	↓	↑
Fat catabolism, fatty acid utilization	Relative ↑	Absolute ↑
Adaptation to starvation	Normal	Abnormal

characteristics of patients at risk for chronic disease–related malnutrition are less predictable and likely represent a mixture of the two extremes depicted in Table 97-2.

Metabolic Rate In starvation and semistarvation, the resting metabolic rate falls between 10% and 30% as an adaptive response to energy restriction, slowing the rate of weight loss. By contrast, the resting metabolic rate rises in the presence of physiologic stress in proportion to the degree of the insult. The rate may increase by ~10% after elective surgery, 20–30% after bone fractures, 30–60% with severe infections such as peritonitis or gram-negative septicemia, and as much as 110% after major burns.

If the metabolic rate (energy requirement) is not matched by energy intake, weight loss results—slowly in hypometabolism and quickly in hypermetabolism. Losses of up to 10% of body mass are unlikely to be detrimental; however, greater losses in acutely ill hypermetabolic patients may be associated with rapid deterioration in body functions.

Protein Catabolism The rate of endogenous protein breakdown (*catabolism*) to supply energy needs normally falls during uncomplicated energy deprivation. After ~10 days of total starvation, an unstressed individual loses about 12–18 g of protein per day (equivalent to ~60 g of muscle tissue or ~2–3 g of nitrogen). In contrast, in injury and sepsis, protein breakdown accelerates in proportion to the degree of stress, reaching 30–60 g/d after elective surgery, 60–90 g/d with infection, 100–130 g/d with severe sepsis or skeletal trauma, and >175 g/d with major burns or head injuries. These losses are reflected by proportional increases in the excretion of urea nitrogen, the major by-product of protein breakdown.

Gluconeogenesis The major aim of protein catabolism during a state of starvation is to provide the glucogenic amino acids (especially alanine and glutamine) that serve as substrates for endogenous glucose production (*gluconeogenesis*) in the liver. In the hypometabolic/starved state, protein breakdown for gluconeogenesis is minimized, especially as ketones derived from fatty acids become the substrate preferred by certain tissues. In the hypermetabolic/stress state, gluconeogenesis increases dramatically and in proportion to the degree of the insult to increase the supply of glucose (the major fuel of reparation). Glucose is the only fuel that can be utilized by hypoxemic tissues (*anaerobic glycolysis*), white blood cells, and newly generated fibroblasts. Infusions of glucose partially offset a negative energy balance but do not significantly suppress the high rates of gluconeogenesis in catabolic patients. Hence, adequate supplies of protein are needed to replace the amino acids used for this metabolic response.

In summary, a hypometabolic patient is adapted to starvation and conserves body mass through reduction of the metabolic rate and use of fat as the primary fuel (rather than glucose and its precursor amino acids). A hypermetabolic patient also uses fat as a fuel but rapidly breaks down body protein to produce glucose, with consequent loss of muscle and organ tissue and danger to vital body functions.

MICRONUTRIENT MALNUTRITION

The same illnesses and reductions in nutrient intake that lead to PEM often produce deficiencies of vitamins and minerals as well (Chap. 96e). Deficiencies of nutrients that are stored in small amounts (such as the water-soluble vitamins) occur because of loss through external secretions, such as zinc in diarrhea fluid or burn exudate, and are probably more common than is generally recognized.

Deficiencies of vitamin C, folic acid, and zinc are relatively common in sick patients. Signs of scurvy, such as corkscrew hairs on the lower extremities, are found frequently in chronically ill and/or alcoholic patients. The diagnosis can be confirmed by determination of plasma vitamin C levels. Folic acid intakes and blood levels are often less than optimal, even among healthy persons; with illness, alcoholism, poverty, or poor dentition, these deficiencies are common. Low blood zinc levels are prevalent in patients with malabsorption syndromes such as inflammatory bowel disease. Patients with zinc deficiency often exhibit poor wound healing, pressure ulcer formation, and impaired immunity. Thiamine deficiency is a common complication of alcoholism but may be prevented by therapeutic doses of thiamine in patients treated for alcohol abuse.

Patients with low plasma vitamin C levels usually respond to the doses in multivitamin preparations, but patients with deficiencies should be supplemented with 250–500 mg/d. Folic acid is absent from some oral multivitamin preparations; patients with deficiencies should be supplemented with ~1 mg/d. Patients with zinc deficiencies resulting from large external losses sometimes require oral supplementation with 220 mg of zinc sulfate one to three times daily. For these reasons, laboratory assessments of the micronutrient status of patients at high risk are desirable.

Hypophosphatemia develops in hospitalized patients with remarkable frequency and generally results from rapid intracellular shifts of phosphate in underweight or alcoholic patients receiving intravenous glucose (Chap. 63). The adverse clinical sequelae are numerous; some, such as acute cardiopulmonary failure, are collectively called *refeeding syndrome* and can be life-threatening.

GLOBAL CONSIDERATIONS

Many developing countries are still faced with high prevalences of the classic forms of PEM: marasmus and kwashiorkor. *Food insecurity*, which characterizes many poor countries, prevents consistent dietary sufficiency and/or quality and leads to endemic or cyclic malnutrition. Factors threatening food security include marked seasonal variations in agricultural productivity (rainy season–dry season cycles), periodic droughts, political unrest or injustice, and disease epidemics (especially of HIV/AIDS). The coexistence of malnutrition and disease epidemics exacerbates the latter and increases complications and mortality rates, creating vicious cycles of malnutrition and disease.

As economic prosperity improves, developing countries have been observed to undergo an epidemiologic transition, a component of which has been termed the *nutrition transition*. As improved economic resources make greater dietary diversity possible, middle-income populations (e.g., in southern Asia, China, and Latin America) typically begin to adopt lifestyle habits of industrialized nations, with increased consumption of energy and fat and decreased levels of physical activity. These changes lead to rising levels of obesity, metabolic syndrome, diabetes, cardiovascular disease, and cancer, sometimes coexisting in populations with persistent undernutrition.

Micronutrient deficiencies also remain prevalent in many countries of the world, impairing functional status and productivity and increasing mortality rates. Vitamin A deficiency impairs vision and increases morbidity and mortality rates from infections such as measles. Mild to moderate iron deficiency may be prevalent in up to 50% of the world, resulting from poor dietary diversity coupled with periodic blood loss and pregnancies. Iodine deficiency remains prevalent, causing goiter, hypothyroidism, and cretinism. Zinc deficiency is endemic in many populations, producing growth retardation, hypogonadism, and dermatoses and impairing wound healing. Fortunately, public health supplementation programs have substantially improved vitamin A and zinc status in developing countries during the past two decades, reducing mortality rates from measles, diarrheal diseases, and other manifestations. However, with the advancing nutrition transition and a shift toward nutritionally related chronic noncommunicable conditions, it is estimated that nutrition remains one of the three greatest contributors of risk for morbidity and mortality worldwide.

NUTRITIONAL ASSESSMENT

Because interactions between illness and nutrition are complex, many physical and laboratory findings reflect both underlying disease and nutritional status. Therefore, the nutritional evaluation of a patient requires an integration of history, physical examination, anthropometrics, and laboratory studies. This approach helps both to detect nutritional problems and to prevent the conclusion that isolated findings indicate nutritional problems when they do not. For example, hypoalbuminemia caused by an inflammatory illness does not necessarily indicate malnutrition.

TABLE 97-3 NUTRITIONAL DEFICIENCY: THE HIGH-RISK PATIENT

Underweight (body mass index <18.5) and/or recent loss of ≥10% of usual body mass
Poor intake: anorexia, food avoidance (e.g., psychiatric condition), or NPO[a] status for more than ~5 days
Protracted nutrient losses: malabsorption, enteric fistulas, draining abscesses or wounds, renal dialysis
Hypermetabolic states: sepsis, protracted fever, extensive trauma or burns
Alcohol abuse or use of drugs with antinutrient or catabolic properties: glucocorticoids, antimetabolites (e.g., methotrexate), immunosuppressants, antitumor agents
Impoverishment, isolation, advanced age

[a]Nil per os (nothing by mouth).

Nutritional History Elicitation of a nutritional history is directed toward the identification of underlying mechanisms that put patients at risk for nutritional depletion or excess. These mechanisms include inadequate intake, impaired absorption, decreased utilization, increased losses, and increased requirements for nutrients.

Individuals with the characteristics listed in Table 97-3 are at particular risk for nutritional deficiencies.

Physical Examination Physical findings that suggest vitamin, mineral, and protein-energy deficiencies and excesses are outlined in Table 97-4. Most of the physical findings are not specific for individual nutrient deficiencies and must be integrated with historic, anthropometric, and laboratory findings. For example, follicular hyperkeratosis on the back of the arms is a fairly common, normal finding. However, if it is widespread in a person who consumes few fruits and vegetables and smokes regularly (increasing ascorbic acid requirements), vitamin C deficiency is likely. Similarly, easily pluckable hair may be a consequence of chemotherapy but suggests acute malnutrition/kwashiorkor in a hospitalized patient who has poorly healing surgical wounds and hypoalbuminemia.

Anthropometric Measurements Anthropometric measurements provide information on body muscle mass and fat reserves. The most practical and commonly used measurements are body weight, height, triceps skinfold (TSF), and midarm muscle circumference (MAMC). Body weight is one of the most useful nutritional parameters to follow in patients who are acutely or chronically ill. Unintentional weight loss during illness often reflects loss of lean body mass (muscle and organ tissue), especially if it is rapid and is not caused by diuresis. Such weight loss can be an ominous sign since it indicates use of vital body protein stores for metabolic fuel. The reference standard for normal body weight, body mass index (BMI: weight in kilograms divided by height, in meters, squared), is discussed in Chap. 416. BMI values <18.5 are considered underweight; <17, significantly underweight; and <16, severely wasted. Values of 18.5–24.9 are normal; 25–29.9, overweight; and ≥30, obese.

Measurement of skinfold thickness is useful for estimating body fat stores, because ~50% of body fat is normally located in the subcutaneous region. This measurement can also permit discrimination of fat mass from muscle mass. The triceps is a convenient site that is generally representative of the body's overall fat level. A thickness <3 mm suggests virtually complete exhaustion of fat stores. The MAMC can be used to estimate skeletal muscle mass, calculated as follows:

$$\text{MAMC (cm)} = \text{upper arm circumference (cm)} - [0.314 \times \text{TSF (mm)}]$$

Laboratory Studies A number of laboratory tests used routinely in clinical medicine can yield valuable information about a patient's nutritional status if a slightly different approach to their interpretation is used. For example, abnormally low serum albumin levels, low total iron-binding capacity, and anergy may have a distinct explanation, but collectively they may represent kwashiorkor. In the clinical setting of a hypermetabolic, acutely ill patient who is edematous and has easily pluckable hair and inadequate protein intake, the diagnosis of acute malnutrition/kwashiorkor is clear-cut. Commonly used laboratory tests for assessing nutritional status are outlined in Table 97-5. The table also provides tips to avoid the assignment of nutritional significance to tests that may be abnormal for nonnutritional reasons.

ASSESSMENT OF CIRCULATING (VISCERAL) PROTEINS The serum proteins most commonly used to assess nutritional status include albumin, total iron-binding capacity (or transferrin), thyroxine-binding prealbumin (or transthyretin), and retinol-binding protein. Because they have different synthesis rates and half-lives (the half-life of serum albumin is ~21 days, whereas those of prealbumin and retinol-binding protein are ~2 days and ~12 h, respectively), some of these proteins reflect changes in nutritional status more quickly than do others. However, rapid fluctuations can also make shorter-half-life proteins less reliable.

Levels of circulating proteins are influenced by their rates of synthesis and catabolism, "third spacing" (loss into interstitial spaces), and, in some cases, external loss. Although an adequate intake of calories and protein is necessary for optimal circulating protein levels, serum protein levels generally do not reflect protein intake. For example, a drop in the serum level of albumin or transferrin often accompanies significant physiologic stress (e.g., from infection or injury) and is not necessarily an indication of malnutrition or poor intake. A low serum albumin level in a burned patient with both hypermetabolism and increased dermal losses of protein may not indicate malnutrition. However, adequate nutritional support of the patient's calorie and protein needs is critical for returning circulating proteins to normal levels as stress resolves. Thus low values by themselves do not define malnutrition, but they often point to increased risk of malnutrition because of the hypermetabolic stress state. As long as significant physiologic stress persists, serum protein levels remain low, even with aggressive nutritional support. However, if the levels do not rise after the underlying illness improves, the patient's protein and calorie needs should be reassessed to ensure that intake is sufficient.

ASSESSMENT OF VITAMIN AND MINERAL STATUS The use of laboratory tests to confirm suspected micronutrient deficiencies is desirable because the physical findings for those deficiencies are often equivocal or nonspecific. Low blood micronutrient levels can predate more serious clinical manifestations and also may indicate drug-nutrient interactions.

ESTIMATING PROTEIN AND ENERGY REQUIREMENTS

A patient's basal energy expenditure (BEE, measured in kilocalories per day) can be estimated from height, weight, age, and sex with the Harris-Benedict equations:

$$\text{Men: BEE} = 66.47 + 13.75W + 5.00H - 6.76A$$
$$\text{Women: BEE} = 655.10 + 9.56W + 1.85H - 4.68A$$

In these equations, W is weight in kilograms, H is height in centimeters, and A is age in years. After these equations are solved, total energy requirements are estimated by multiplying BEE by a factor that accounts for the stress of illness. Multiplying by 1.1–1.4 yields a range 10–40% above basal that estimates the 24-h energy expenditure of the majority of patients. The lower value (1.1) is used for patients without evidence of significant physiologic stress; the higher value (1.4) is appropriate for patients with marked stress such as sepsis or trauma. The result is used as a 24-h energy goal for feeding.

When it is important to have a more accurate assessment, energy expenditure can be measured at the bedside by indirect calorimetry. This technique is useful in patients who are thought to be hypermetabolic from sepsis or trauma and whose body weight cannot be ascertained accurately. Indirect calorimetry can also be useful in patients who have difficulty weaning from a ventilator and whose energy needs therefore should not be exceeded to avoid excessive CO_2 production. Patients at the extremes of weight (e.g., obese persons) and/or age are good candidates as well, because the Harris-Benedict equations were developed from measurements in adults with roughly normal body weights.

Because urea is a major by-product of protein catabolism, the amount of urea nitrogen excreted each day can be used to estimate the rate of protein catabolism and determine whether protein intake is adequate to

TABLE 97-4 PHYSICAL FINDINGS OF NUTRITIONAL DEFICIENCIES

Clinical Findings	Possible Deficiency or Form of Malnutrition	Possible Excess
Hair, nails		
Corkscrew hairs and unemerged coiled hairs	Vitamin C	
Easily pluckable hair	Acute malnutrition	
Flag sign (transverse depigmentation of hair)	Acute malnutrition	
Sparse hair	Biotin, zinc; acute malnutrition	Vitamin A
Transverse ridging of nails	Acute malnutrition	
Skin		
Cellophane appearance	Acute malnutrition	
Cracking ("flaky-paint" or "crazy-pavement" dermatosis)	Acute malnutrition	
Follicular hyperkeratosis	Vitamins A, C	
Petechiae (especially perifollicular)	Vitamin C	
Purpura	Vitamins C, K	
Pigmentation, scaling of sun-exposed areas	Niacin	
Poor wound healing, decubitus ulcers	Vitamin C, zinc; acute malnutrition	
Scaling	Vitamin A, essential fatty acids, biotin	Vitamin A
	Zinc (hyperpigmented)	
Yellow pigmentation sparing sclerae (benign)		Carotene
Eyes		
Night blindness	Vitamin A	
Papilledema		Vitamin A
Perioral		
Angular stomatitis	Riboflavin, pyridoxine, niacin	
Cheilosis (dry, cracking, ulcerated lips)	Riboflavin, pyridoxine, niacin	
Oral		
Atrophic lingual papillae (slick tongue)	Riboflavin, niacin, folate, vitamin B_{12}, iron; acute malnutrition	
Glossitis (scarlet, raw tongue)	Riboflavin, niacin, pyridoxine, folate, vitamin B_{12}	
Hypogeusesthesia, hyposmia	Zinc	
Swollen, retracted, bleeding gums (if teeth present)	Vitamin C	
Bones, joints		
Beading of ribs, epiphyseal swelling, bowlegs	Vitamin D	
Tenderness, subperiosteal hemorrhage in children	Vitamin C	
Neurologic		
Confabulation, disorientation	Thiamine (Korsakoff's psychosis)	
Drowsiness, lethargy, vomiting		Vitamin A
Dementia	Niacin, vitamin B_{12}, folate	
Headache		Vitamin A
Ophthalmoplegia	Thiamine, phosphorus	
Peripheral neuropathy (e.g., weakness, paresthesias, ataxia, footdrop, and decreased tendon reflexes, fine tactile sense, vibratory sense, and position sense)	Thiamine, pyridoxine, vitamin B_{12}	Pyridoxine
Tetany	Calcium, magnesium	
Other		
Edema	Thiamine; acute malnutrition	
Heart failure	Thiamine ("wet" beriberi), phosphorus	
Hepatomegaly	Acute malnutrition	Vitamin A
Parotid enlargement	Acute malnutrition (consider also bulimia)	
Sudden heart failure, death	Vitamin C	

offset it. Total protein loss and protein balance can be calculated from urinary urea nitrogen (UUN) as follows:

$$\text{Protein catabolic rate (g/d)} = [\text{24-h UUN (g)} + 4] \times 6.25 \text{ (g protein/g nitrogen)}$$

The value of 4 g added to the UUN represents a liberal estimate of the unmeasured nitrogen lost in the urine (e.g., creatinine and uric acid), sweat, hair, skin, and feces. When protein intake is low (e.g., less than ~20 g/d), the equation indicates both the patient's protein requirement and the severity of the catabolic state (Table 97-5). More substantial protein intakes can raise the UUN because some of the ingested (or intravenously infused) protein is catabolized and converted to UUN. Thus, at lower protein intakes, the equation is useful for estimating *requirements*, and at higher protein intakes it is useful for assessing protein *balance*.

$$\text{Protein balance (g/d)} = \text{protein intake} - \text{protein catabolic rate}$$

TABLE 97-5 LABORATORY TESTS FOR NUTRITIONAL ASSESSMENT

Test (Normal Values)	Nutritional Use	Causes of Normal Value Despite Malnutrition	Other Causes of Abnormal Value
Serum albumin (3.5–5.5 g/dL)	2.8–3.5 g/dL: Protein depletion or systemic inflammation <2.8 g/dL: Possible acute malnutrition or severe inflammation Increasing value reflects positive protein balance	Dehydration Infusion of albumin, fresh-frozen plasma, or whole blood	**Low** *Common:* Infection and other stress, especially with poor protein intake Burns, trauma Congestive heart failure Fluid overload Severe liver disease *Uncommon:* Nephrotic syndrome Zinc deficiency Bacterial stasis/overgrowth of small intestine
Serum prealbumin, also called transthyretin (20–40 mg/dL; lower in prepubertal children)	10–15 mg/dL: Mild protein depletion or inflammation 5–10 mg/dL: Moderate protein depletion or inflammation <5 mg/dL: Severe protein depletion or inflammation Increasing value reflects positive protein balance	Chronic renal failure	Similar to serum albumin
Serum total iron-binding capacity (240–450 μg/dL)	<200 μg/dL: Protein depletion or inflammatory state; possible acute malnutrition Increasing value reflects positive protein balance More labile than albumin	Iron deficiency	**Low** Similar to serum albumin **High** Iron deficiency
Prothrombin time (2.0–15.5 s)	Prolongation: vitamin K deficiency		**Prolonged** Anticoagulant therapy (warfarin) Severe liver disease
Serum creatinine (0.6–1.6 mg/dL)	<0.6 mg/dL: Muscle wasting due to prolonged energy deficit Reflects muscle mass		**High** Despite muscle wasting: Renal failure Severe dehydration
24-h urinary creatinine (500–1200 mg/d, standardized for height and sex)	Low value: muscle wasting due to prolonged energy deficit	>24-h collection Decreasing serum creatinine	**Low** Incomplete urine collection Increasing serum creatinine Neuromuscular wasting
24-h urinary urea nitrogen (UUN; <5 g/d; depends on level of protein intake)	*Determine level of catabolism* (as long as protein intake is ≥10 g below calculated protein loss or <20 g total, and as long as carbohydrate intake has been at least 100 g) 5–10 g/d: Mild catabolism or normal fed state 10–15 g/d: Moderate catabolism >15 g/d: Severe catabolism *Estimate protein balance* Protein balance = protein intake − protein loss where protein loss (protein catabolic rate) = [24-h UUN (g) + 4] × 6.25. Adjustments required in burn patients and others with large nonurinary nitrogen losses and in patients with fluctuating levels of blood urea nitrogen (e.g., in renal failure)		
Blood urea nitrogen (8–23 mg/dL)	<8 mg/dL: Possibly inadequate protein intake 12–23 mg/dL: Possibly adequate protein intake >23 mg/dL: Possibly excessive protein intake If serum creatinine is normal, use BUN. If serum creatinine is elevated, use BUN/creatinine ratio. (Normal range is essentially the same as for BUN.)		**Low** Severe liver disease Anabolic state Syndrome of inappropriate antidiuretic hormone **High** Despite poor protein intake: Renal failure (Use BUN/creatinine ratio.) Congestive heart failure Gastrointestinal hemorrhage

98e Enteral and Parenteral Nutrition Therapy

Bruce R. Bistrian, L. John Hoffer, David F. Driscoll

This is a digital-only chapter. It is available on the DVD that accompanies this book, as well as on Access Medicine/Harrison's Online, and the eBook and "app" editions of HPIM 19e.

When correctly implemented, specialized nutritional support (SNS) plays a major and often life-saving role in medicine. SNS is used for two main purposes: (1) to provide an appropriate nutritional substrate in order to maintain or replenish the nutritional status of patients unable to voluntarily ingest or absorb sufficient amounts of food, and (2) to maintain the nutritional and metabolic status of adequately nourished patients who are experiencing systemic hypercatabolic effects of severe inflammation, injury, or infection in the course of persistent critical illness. Patients with permanent major loss of intestinal length or function often require lifelong SNS. Many patients who require treatment in chronic-care facilities receive enteral SNS, most often because their voluntary food intake is deemed insufficient or because impaired chewing and swallowing create a high risk of aspiration pneumonia.

INDEX

Page numbers in **bold** indicate the start of the main discussion of the topic. Page numbers followed by "f" or "t" refer to the page location of figures and tables, respectively, and a "v" indicates a video on the DVD. Numbers containing "e-" followed by a number (e.g., 91e-3) refer to pages in the e-chapters on the DVD.

INDEX

INDEX

INDEX

INDEX

INDEX

INDEX

INDEX

INDEX

INDEX

INDEX

INDEX

INDEX

INDEX

INDEX

INDEX

INDEX

INDEX

INDEX

INDEX

INDEX

INDEX

INDEX

INDEX

G

INDEX

INDEX

INDEX

INDEX

INDEX

INDEX

INDEX

INDEX

INDEX

INDEX

INDEX

INDEX

INDEX

INDEX

INDEX

INDEX

INDEX

INDEX

INDEX

INDEX

INDEX

INDEX

INDEX

INDEX

INDEX

INDEX

INDEX

INDEX

INDEX

INDEX

INDEX

INDEX

INDEX

INDEX

INDEX

X

INDEX

INDEX